Encyclopedia of

Nursing Research, Second Edition

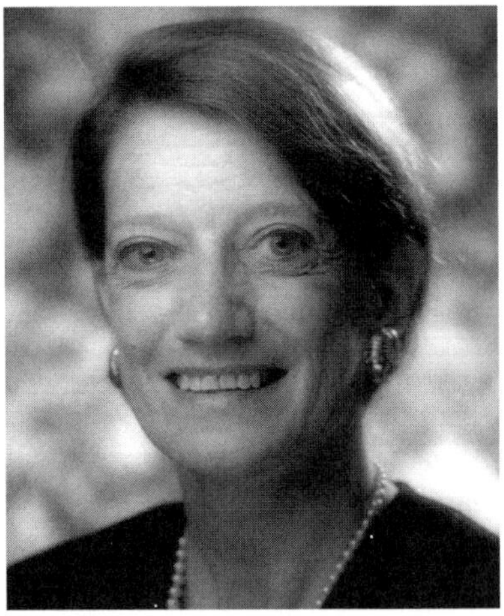

Joyce J. Fitzpatrick, PhD, MBA, RN, FAAN, is the Elizabeth Brooks Ford Professor of Nursing, Frances Payne Bolton School of Nursing, Case Western Reserve University in Cleveland Ohio where she was Dean from 1982 through 1997. She has received numerous honors and awards including the *American Journal of Nursing* Book of the Year Award 18 times. Dr. Fitzpatrick is widely published in nursing and health care literature. She is senior editor of the *Annual Review of Nursing Research* series, now in its 23rd volume. In 1998 Dr. Fitzpatrick was senior editor of the first volume of the classic *Encyclopedia of Nursing Research* as well as a series of Research Digests, including *Nursing Research Digest, Maternal Child Health Nursing Research Digest, Geriatric Nursing Research Digest,* and *Psychiatric Mental Health Nursing Research Digest.* She has coedited four books focused on nurses and the internet: *Internet Resources for Nurses* (2000) and *Nurses Guide to Consumer Health Web Sites* (2001), *Essentials of Internet Use for Nurses* (2002) and *Internet for Nursing Research* (2004). Dr. Fitzpatrick has provided consultation on nursing education and research throughout the world, including universities and health ministries in Africa, Asia, Australia, Europe, Latin America, and the Middle East.

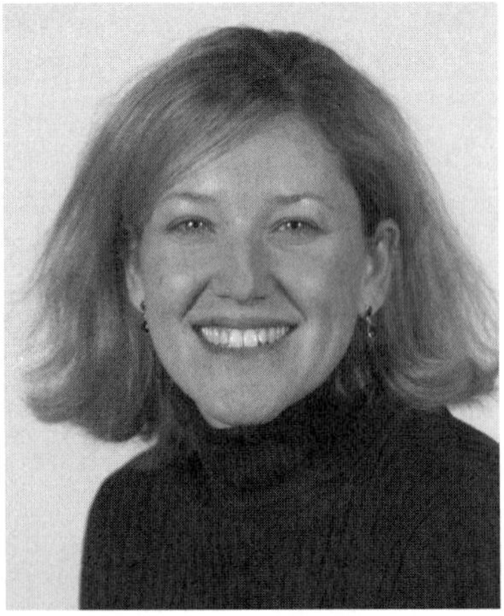

Meredith Wallace, PhD, APRN-BC, has been a nurse since she completed her BSN degree Magna Cum Laude at Boston University in 1988. Following this, she earned an MSN in medical-surgical nursing with a specialty in geriatrics from Yale University and a PhD in nursing research and theory development at New York University. During her time at NYU she was awarded a predoctoral fellowship at the Hartford Institute for Geriatric Nursing. In this capacity she became the original author and editor of *Try This: Best Practices in Geriatric Nursing* series. In 2001, she won the Springer Publishing Company Award for Applied Nursing Research. She was the Managing Editor of the *Journal of Applied Nursing Research* and is currently the research brief editor for the journal. She is the author of numerous journal articles and book chapters. Dr Wallace published *Prostate Cancer: Nursing Assessment Management and Care,* in April 2002, which won the *American Journal of Nursing* Book of the Year Award. Preceding this, she was the Associate Editor of *The Geriatric Nursing Research Digest*, which also won the *American Journal of Nursing* Book of the Year Award in 2002. She is the recent recipient of the Eastern Nursing Research Society/John A. Hartford Foundation junior investigator award. Dr. Wallace is currently an Associate Professor and the Elizabeth DeCamp McInerney Chair in Health Sciences at Fairfield University School of Nursing, in Fairfield, CT.

Encyclopedia of Nursing Research, Second Edition

Joyce J. Fitzpatrick, PhD, RN, FAAN
Editor-in-Chief

Meredith Wallace, PhD, APRN-BC
Associate Editor

SPRINGER PUBLISHING COMPANY

Springer Publishing Company, Inc.
11 West 42nd Street
New York, NY 10036

Acquisitions Editor: Ruth Chasek
Production Editor: Sara Yoo
Cover design by Joanne Honigman
Typeset by International Graphic Services, Inc., Newtown, PA

07 08 09 / 5 4 3 2

Library of Congress Cataloging-in-Publication Data

Encyclopedia of nursing research / Joyce J. Fitzpatrick and Meredith Wallace [editors]. — 2nd ed.
p. ; cm.
Includes bibliographical references and index.
ISBN 0-8261-9812-0 978-0-8261-9812-9
1. Nursing—Research—Encyclopedias. 2. Evidence-based nursing—Encyclopedias. I. Fitzpatrick, Joyce J., 1944- . II. Wallace, Meredith, PhD, RN.
[DNLM: 1. Nursing Research—Encyclopedias—English. 2. Evidence-Based Medicine—methods. WY 13 E5632 2006]
RT81.5.E53 2006
610.73'072—dc22 2005017674

Printed in the United States of America by Maple-Vail Book Manufacturing Group.

Contents

ADVISORY BOARD

PREFACE

This second edition of the *Encyclopedia of Nursing Research* (ENR), like the first, is a comprehensive, yet concise and authoritative guide to existing nursing research literature. It charts the course of nursing research since 1983 when the first edition of the *Annual Review of Nursing Research* (ARNR) was published.

The original edition of ENR, published in 1998, grew from a long-standing commitment of the publisher, Dr. Ursula Springer, to the field of nursing, and my commitment to nurse scholars around the globe. The original encyclopedia followed 15 years of publication of the ARNR series. This second edition of ENR follows publication of 22 volumes of ARNR and incorporates the research topics included in the ARNR series. Through these formative years of nursing science, I have had the privilege of serving as editor of the ARNR series and witnessing the rapid growth of knowledge and expertise in nursing research. Having served as editor for the first edition of ENR, I am joined in this edition by Meredith Wallace, the Associate Editor.

Nurse researchers and graduate students in nursing will be the primary audience for this edition of ENR. Yet, as with the first edition, nurses in all phases of education, from basic to doctoral, from formal university and college-based programs to continuing education offerings, within all health systems, will find this an important introduction to current nursing research topics. The alphabetical list of entries is provided to assist the reader in quickly finding the relevant term. While every effort was made to include the most comprehensive list of entries, based on both a literature review of key terms in journals and the ARNR series and the expert advice of the Advisory Board members, we are cognizant of the fact that some terms may have been overlooked. Thus, we encourage readers to advise us of new terms that should be added to the already extensive list.

This project has been one of the most rewarding endeavors of my professional career. It has been met with a great deal of professional interest and, most importantly, an extra measure of enthusiasm by students at all levels. The References section lists the most critical references on each topic. It is this attention to key references that may be of most use to graduate students who wish to pursue a topic in more depth.

This publication would not have been possible without the experts in nursing research who authored the hundreds of entries. Each author, some of whom have contributed multiple entries, deserves thanks for the written entries, for the willingness to respond to strict guidelines and page and reference limitations, and, of course, for adhering to a very demanding time line for publication. Distilling one's life work into a few hundred words is often the most difficult accomplishment.

We also are indebted to the colleagues who served as members of the Advisory Board for both the first and second editions of ENR. I thank each of you for your input into the terms to be included here, the suggestions of potential contributors, and your willingness to plunge into yet another publishing project with me.

As with any large continuing project such as this, a true team effort is necessary for a quality project. First, my thanks to Dr. Ursula Springer for conceiving the project and asking me to undertake the editing at a time when my commitments were at a peak. I am glad that I did not hesitate. To the Springer staff who facilitated the production at the many levels, I owe a huge thank you, most especially to Ruth Chasek, Senior Nursing Editor, who saw the project through its many stages. I also acknowledge the endless energy, dedication, and expertise of Meredith Wallace, Associate Editor for this edition. There was never too daunting a task for Meredith as we worked tirelessly over the past 2 years to complete the project. A number of students assisted Meredith and me in our activities for this edition of ENR. I would like to thank Ali Salman and Yi-Hui Lee, PhD candidates at Case Western Reserve University, Frances Payne Bolton School of Nursing, and Kara Diffley, Lindsey Neptune, and Christine McGurk, undergraduate students at Fairfield University School of Nursing. I am certain that there are numerous other graduate students who assisted the authors in completing their entries. We hope that this edition of ENR will continue to be rewarding to them in their future academic and professional careers.

Joyce J. Fitzpatrick
Editor-in-Chief

CONTRIBUTORS

Lauren S. Aaronson, PhD, RN, FAAN
Professor
University of Kansas
School of Nursing
Kansas City, KS
Data Analysis; Fatigue; Grantsmanship; Sampling

Faye G. Abdellah, EdD, ScD, RN, FAAN
Dean & Professor Emeritus
Uniformed Services University of the Health Sciences
Graduate School of Nursing
Bethesda, MD
History of Nursing Research

Ivo L. Abraham, PhD, RN, FAAN
Visiting Professor
University of Pennsylvania
School of Nursing
Philadelphia, PA
Applied Research; Experimental Research; Quasi-Experimental Research

Raeda Fawzi AbuAlRub, PhD, RN
Assistant Professor
Jordan University of Science and Technology
College of Nursing
Irbid, Jordan
Social Support

Donna L. Algase, PhD, RN, FAAN
Josephine M. Sana Collegiate Professor of Nursing
University of Michigan
School of Nursing
Ann Arbor, MI
Activities of Daily Living

Elaine J. Amella, PhD, APRN, BC
Associate Professor and Associate Dean for Research
Medical University of South Carolina
College of Nursing
Charleston, SC
Dysphagia

Gene Cranston Anderson, PhD, RN, FAAN
Edward J. & Louise Mellen Professor of Nursing
Case Western Reserve University
Frances Payne Bolton School of Nursing
Cleveland, OH
Kangaroo Care

Ida Androwich, PhD, RNC, FAAN
Professor
School of Nursing
Loyola University Medical Center
Maywood, IL
Nursing Informatics; Nursing Information Systems

Karen J. Aroian, PhD, RN, FAAN
Katharine Faville Professor of Nursing Research
Wayne State University
College of Nursing
Detroit, MI
Immigrant Women

Carol A. Ashton, PhD, RN
Director of Nursing Research
LDS, Cottonwood, and Alta View Hospitals
Salt Lake City, UT
Research Utilization

Joan K. Austin, DNS, RN, FAAN
Distinguished professor
Indiana University
School of Nursing
Indianapolis, IN
Attitudes; Chronic Conditions in Childhood; Epilepsy

Kay C. Avant, PhD, RN, FAAN
Associate Professor
University of Texas
School of Nursing
Austin, TX
Concept Analysis; Nursing Diagnosis

Cynthia Guerrero Ayres, PhD, RN
Director
Health Systems and Collaborations—New Jersey
American Cancer Society—Eastern Division
North Brunswick, NJ
Clinical Preventive Services Delivery

Terry A. Badger, PhD, APRN, BC
Professor
University of Arizona
College of Nursing
Tucson, AZ
Depression in Families

Judith A. Baigis, PhD, RN, FAAN
Associate Dean for Research and Scholarship
Georgetown University
School of Nursing and Health Studies
Washington, DC
Health Conceptualization

Tamilyn Bakas, DNS, RN
Associate Professor, Department of Adult Health
Indiana University
School of Nursing
Indianapolis, IN
Stroke

Suzanne Bakken, DNSc, RN, FAAN
Alumni Professor of Nursing & Professor of Biomedical Informatics
Columbia University
School of Nursing
New York, NY
Formal Nursing Languages; SNOMED International; Unified Language Systems

Jane Barnsteiner, PhD, RN, FAAN
Professor and Director
University of Pennsylvania
School of Nursing
Philadelphia, PA
Online Journal of Knowledge Synthesis for Nursing

Mara M. Baun, DNSc, FAAN
Lee & Joseph D. Jamail Distinguished Professor
University of Texas Health Sciences Center at Houston
School of Nursing
Houston, TX
Pet Therapy

Cheryl Tatano Beck, DNSc, CNM, FAAN
Professor
University of Connecticut
School of Nursing
Storrs, CT
Meta-Analysis; Phenomenology; Replication Studies

Sandra C. Garmon Bibb, DNSc, RN
Assistant Professor
Uniformed Services University of the Health Sciences
Graduate School of Nursing
Bethesda, MD
Leininger's Theory of Culture Care Diversity and Universality; Population Health

Carol E. Blixen, PhD, RN
Senior Nurse Researcher
Cleveland Clinic Foundation
Department of Nursing Education and Research
Cleveland, OH
Osteoarthritis

Ella Blot, MA, RN, GNP
New York University
Division of Nursing
New York, NY
Urinary Incontinence

Rebecca J. Bonugli, MSN, RN
Clinical Instructor
University of Texas Health Science Center
School of Nursing
San Antonio, TX
Serious Mental Illness

Joan L. Bottorff, PhD, RN
Professor and UBC Distinguished University Scholar
University of British Columbia
School of Nursing
Vancouver, British Colombia
Canada
Nurse-Patient Interaction; Nurse-Patient Relationship

Meg Bourbonniere, PhD, RN
Assistant Professor
Yale University
School of Nursing
New Haven, CT
Physical Restraints

Diane K. Boyle, PhD, RN
Associate Professor
University of Kansas
School of Nursing
Kansas City, KS
Job Satisfaction

Barbara Braden, PhD, RN, FAAN
Professor and Dean, Graduate College
Creighton University Medical Center
School of Nursing
Omaha, NE
Computerized Decision Support Systems

Geraldine Britton, PhD, FNP
Assistant Research Professor
Decker School of Nursing
Binghamton University
Binghamton, NY
Osteoporosis

Dorothy Brooten, PhD, FAAN
Professor
Florida International University
School of Nursing
Miami, FL
Clinical Trials; Transitional Care

Emma J. Brown, PhD, RN
Associate Professor and Chatlos Endowed Chair
University of Central Florida
School of Nursing
Orlando, FL
Urban Health Research: Nursing Research in Urban Neighborhoods

Helen Kogan Budzynski, PhD, FAAN
Faculty Emeritus
University of Washington
School of Nursing
Seattle, WA
Biofeedback

Vern L. Bullough, PhD, RN, FAAN
Distinguished Professor Emeritus
State University of New York
Stony Brook, NY
Gender Research; Sex and Gender

Andrea Calaluce, BSN, RN
Yale New Haven Hospital
New Haven CT
Adult Pulmonary Medicine
Milford, CT
Parkinson's Disease

Sara L. Campbell, DNS, RN, CNAA, BC
Associate Professor and Associate Dean
Illinois State University
Mennonite College of Nursing
Bloomington, IL
Feminist Research Methodology

Suzanne Hetzel Campbell, PhD, APRN, IBCLC
Assistant Professor
Fairfield University
School of Nursing
Fairfield, CT
Breast-feeding

Victoria Champion, DNS, RN, FAAN
Associate Dean of Research
Indiana University
School of Nursing
Indianapolis, IN
Breast Cancer Screening

Jeeyae Choi, RN, MS
Doctoral Student
Columbia University
School of Nursing
New York, NY
Formal Nursing Languages

Norma J. Christman, PhD, RN, FAAN
Associate Professor Emeritus
University of Kentucky
College of Nursing
Lexington, KY
Preoperative Psychological Preparation for Surgery

Deborah A. Chyun, PhD, RN
Associate Professor
Yale University
School of Nursing
New Haven, CT
Angina; Cardiovascular Disease

Amy Coenen, PhD, RN, FAAN
Associate Professor
University of Wisconsin
College of Nursing
Milwaukee, WI
International Classification for Nursing Practice (ICNP®)

Marlene Zichi Cohen, PhD, RN, FAAN
John S. Dunn, Sr., Distinguished Professor in Oncology Nursing
University of Texas Health Science Center at Houston
School of Nursing
Houston, TX
Descriptive Research; Nursing Assessment

Kathleen Byrne Colling, PhD, RN
Assistant Research Scientist
University of Michigan
School of Nursing
Ann Arbor, MI
Middle-Range Theories of Dementia Care

Karen Corcoran, BSN, RN
Staff Nurse
Greenwich Hospital
Greenwich, CT
Family Satisfaction With End-of-Life Care

Inge B. Corless, PhD, RN, FAAN
Professor
Massachusetts General Hospital
Institute of Health Professions
Boston, MA
Hospice; Terminal Illness

Cynthia L. Corritore, PhD
Associate Professor
Creighton University
College of Business Administration
Omaha, NE
Computerized Decision Support Systems

Colleen Corte, PhD, RN
Postdoctoral Research Fellow
University of Michigan
School of Medicine
Ann Arbor, MI
Self-Concept Disturbances and Eating Disorders

Jessica Shank Coviello, MSN, RN
Lecturer
Yale University
School of Nursing
New Haven, CT
Angina; Cardiovascular Disease

Barbara J. Daly, PhD, RN, FAAN
Associate Professor
Case Western Reserve University
Frances Payne Bolton School of Nursing
Cleveland, OH
Critical Care Nursing

Jennifer P. D'Auria, PhD, RN, CPNP
Associate Professor
University of North Carolina Chapel Hill
School of Nursing
Chapel Hill, NC
Bibliometrics

Sabina De Geest, PhD, RN
Director
University of Basel
Institute of Nursing Science
Basel, Switzerland
Applied Research; Medications in Older Persons

Alice S. Demi, PhD, RN, FAAN
Professor
Georgia State University
Byrdine F. Lewis School of Nursing
Atlanta, GA
Delphi Technique; Grief; Suicide

Karen E. Dennis, PhD, RN, FAAN
Professor
University of Central Florida
School of Nursing
Orlando, FL
Obesity as Cardiovascular Risk Factor

Danielle Deveau, BS, MPS
Research Analyst
California State University, Fresno
Central California Center for Health & Human Services
Fresno, CA
HIV Symptom Management and Quality of Life

Mary Jo Devereaux
Hospital Librarian
Community Medical Center
Scranton, PA
Orem's Self-Care Deficit Nursing Theory

Elizabeth C. Devine, PhD, RN, FAAN
Professor
University of Wisconsin-Milwaukee
College of Nursing
Milwaukee, WI
Patient Education

Nancy Diekelmann, PhD, RN, FAAN
Helen Denne Schulte Professor
University of Wisconsin-Madison
School of Nursing
Madison, WI
Hermeneutics

Rose Ann DiMaria-Ghalili, PhD, RN
Assistant Professor
West Virginia University
Robert C. Byrd Health Science Center
School of Nursing
Charleston, WV
Nutrition in the Elderly

Fabienne Dobbels, MSc
Katholieke Universiteit Leuven
Center for Health Services and Nursing Research
Leuven, Belgium
Medications in Older Persons

Joanne McCloskey Dochterman, PhD, RN, FAAN
Professor
University of Iowa
College of Nursing
Iowa City, IA
Nursing Interventions Classification (NIC); Taxonomy

Moreen Donahue, DNP, RN
Sr. Vice President Patient Care Services
Greenwich Hospital
Greenwich, CT
Clinical Judgment

Sue K. Donaldson, PhD, RN, FAAN
Dean and Professor
Johns Hopkins University
School of Nursing
Baltimore, MD
Basic Research

Dianna Hutto Douglas, DNS, RN, CNS
Associate Professor
Louisiana State University
School of Nursing
New Orleans, LA
Empathy

Annemarie Dowling-Castronovo, MA, APRN, BC
Assistant Clinical Professor
New York University
Division of Nursing
New York, NY
Gerontological Advanced Practice Nursing

Jacqueline Dunbar-Jacob, PhD, RN, FAAN
Dean and Professor
University of Pittsburgh
School of Nursing
Pittsburgh, PA
Adherence/Compliance; Behavioral Research

Patricia C. Dykes, DNSc, RN
Senior Nurse Informatician
Partners HealthCare
Wellesley, MA
Clinical Judgment

Karen L. Elberson, PhD, RN
Associate Professor and Associate Dean
Uniformed Services University of the Health Sciences
Graduate School of Nursing
Bethesda, MD
Capitation; Health Indicators

Jennifer Harrison Elder, PhD, RN, FAAN
Associate Professor
University of Florida
College of Nursing
Gainesville, FL
Child Abuse and Neglect

Marsha L. Ellett, DNS, RN, CGRN
Associate Professor
Indiana University
School of Nursing
Indianapolis, IN
Enteral Tube Placement

Veronica F. Engle, PhD, GNP, APRN, BC, FAAN
Professor
University of Tennessee
School of Nursing
Memphis, TN
Newman's Theory of Health

Janet Enslein, MA, RN
Assistant Professor of Nursing
St. Ambrose University
School of Nursing
Davenport, IA
Ethnography

Carol Diane Epstein, PhD, RN, FCCM
Associate Professor
Fairfield University
School of Nursing
Fairfield, CT
Critical Care Nursing

W. Scott Erdley, DNS, RN
Clinical Assistant Professor
University at Buffalo
School of Nursing
Buffalo, NY
Electronic Network

Lois K. Evans, DNSc, RN, FAAN
Viola MacInnes/Independence Professor in Nursing
University of Pennsylvania
School of Nursing
Philadelphia, PA
Physical Restraints

Melissa Spezia Faulkner, DSN, RN
Associate Professor
Department of Maternal-Child Nursing
University of Illinois at Chicago
Chicago, IL
Diabetes

Jacqueline Fawcett, PhD, RN
Professor, College of Nursing & Health Sciences
University of Massachusetts-Boston
College of Nursing & Health Sciences
Boston MA
(Dorothy) Johnson's Behavioral System Model

Suzanne L. Feetham, PhD, RN, FAAN
Professor Emeritus
University of Illinois at Chicago
College of Nursing
Chicago, IL
Director of Division of Clinical Quality
Bureau of Primary Health Care
Health Resources and Services Administration
Bethesda, MD
Family Care; Family Health

Donna Fick, PhD, RN
Associate Professor of Nursing, College of Health and Human Development
Associate Professor of Medicine, Department of Psychiatry
The Pennsylvania State University
University Park, PA
Ageism

Joseph M. Filakovsky, MSN, APRN, CCNS, CS, FAHA
Doctoral Student
Case Western Reserve University
Frances Payne Bolton School of Nursing
Cleveland, OH
Computer-Aided Instruction

Mary L. Fisher, PhD, RN, CNAA, BC
Associate Professor
Indiana University
School of Nursing
Indianapolis, IN
Cost Analysis of Nursing Care; Health Services Administration

Ellen Flaherty, PhD, APRN, BC
Director of Quality Improvement
Village Care of New York
New York, NY
Geriatric Interdisciplinary Teams

Robin Fleschler, PhD, RNC, CNS, NP
Assistant Professor
University of Texas Medical Branch
School of Nursing Medical Branch
Galveston, TX
Evidence-Based Practice

Beverly C. Flynn, PhD, RN, FAAN
Professor
Indiana University
School of Nursing
Indianapolis, IN
Community Health

Marquis D. Foreman, PhD, RN, FAAN
Professor
University of Illinois at Chicago
College of Nursing
Chicago, IL
Delirium

Frances Foster, MS, RN, CS
Adult Health Nurse Practitioner
Massachusetts General Hospital
Boston, MA
Functional Health Patterns

Jeanne C. Fox, PhD, RN
Professor Emeritus
School of Nursing
University of Virginia
School of Nursing
Charlottesville, VA
Mental Health Services Research

Emily Fox-Hill, PhD, RN
Associate Professor
University of Tennessee
College of Nursing
Memphis, TN
Newman's Theory of Health

Maureen A. Frey, PhD, RN
Director of Research and Advanced Practice
Children's Hospital of Michigan
Detroit, MI
(Imogene) King's Conceptual System and Theory of Goal Attainment

Sara T. Fry, PhD, RN, FAAN
Henry R. Luce Professor of Nursing Ethics
Boston College
School of Nursing
Chestnut Hill, MA
Research in Nursing Ethics; Rights of Human Subjects

Terry Fulmer, PhD, RN, FAAN
The Erline Perkins McGriff Professor and Division Head
New York University
Division of Nursing
New York, NY
Acute Care of the Elderly; Elder Mistreatment

Carol D. Gaskamp, PhD, RN
Assistant Professor
University of Texas Austin
School of Nursing
Austin, TX
Quality of Life

Rauda Gelazis, PhD, RN, CS
Associate Professor
Ursuline College
Breen School of Nursing
Pepper Pike, OH
Individual Nursing Therapy

Deborah L. Gentile, MSN, RN
Doctoral Student
University of Wisconsin-Milwaukee
College of Nursing
Milwaukee, WI
Patient Education

Phyllis B. Giovannetti, ScD, RN
Professor
University of Alberta
Faculty of Nursing
Edmonton, Alberta
Canada
Nursing Workload Measurement Systems; Patient Classification

Barbara Given, PhD, RN
Professor
Michigan State University
College of Nursing
East Lansing, MI
Family Care

Barbara A. Goldrick, MPH, PhD, RN, CIC
Nurse Consultant
Chatham, MA
Nosocomial Infections

Marion Good, PhD, RN, FAAN
Professor
Case Western Reserve University
Frances Payne Bolton School of Nursing
Cleveland, OH
Music Therapy; Pain; Pain Management: A Mid-Range Theory

Patricia A. Grady, PhD, RN, FAAN
Director
National Institutes of Health
National Institute of Nursing Research
Bethesda, MD
National Institutes of Health; National Institute of Nursing Research

Judith R. Graves, PhD, RN, FAAN
Professor, College of Nursing
Adjunct Associate Professor
Department of Medical Informatics
School of Medicine
University of Utah
Salt Lake City, UT
Bibliographic Retrieval Systems; Representation of Knowledge for Computational Modeling in Nursing: The Arcs© Program; Secondary Data Analysis; Sigma Theta Tau International Nursing Research Classification System; Virginia Henderson International Nursing Library

Bobbe Ann Gray, PhD, RNC
Assistant Professor
Wright State University
College of Nursing and Health
Dayton, OH
Childbirth Education

Hurdis M. Griffith, PhD, RN, FAAN
Professor and Dean Emeritus
Rutgers University
College of Nursing
Newark, NJ
Clinical Preventive Services Delivery; Current Procedural Terminology-Coded Services

Deborah Gross, DNSc, RN, FAAN
Professor
Rush University
College of Nursing
Chicago, IL
Mother-Infant/Toddler Relationships

Sheila Grossman, PhD, APRN
Professor
Fairfield University
School of Nursing
Fairfield, CT
Genetics; Mentoring

Sarah Hall Gueldner, DSN, RN, FAAN
Dean and Professor
Binghamton University
Decker School of Nursing
Binghamton, NY
Osteoporosis

Linda C. Haber, DNS, RN, CS
Clinical Specialist
Veterans Affairs
Northern Indiana Health Care System
Fort Wayne, IN
Family Theory and Research

Barbara K. Haight, DrPH, RNC, FAAN
Professor Emeritus
Medical University of South Carolina
College of Nursing
Charleston, SC
Reminiscence and Life Review

Edward J. Halloran, PhD, RN, FAAN
Associate Professor
University of North Carolina Chapel Hill
School of Nursing
Chapel Hill, NC
Henderson's Model; Nurse Staffing; Nursing Studies Index

Charlene M. Hanson, EdD, RN, CS, FAAN
Professor
Georgia Southern University
Center for Rural Health and Research
Statesboro, GA
Advanced Practice Nurses

Gail A. Harkness, DrPH, RN, FAAN
Professor Emeritus
University of Connecticut
School of Nursing
Storrs, CT
Infection Control

Gretchen Harwood, MS, RN
Doctoral Student
The Ohio State University
Columbus, OH
Smoking Cessation

Emily J. Hauenstein, PhD, LCP, APRN, BC
Associate Professor
University of Virginia
School of Nursing
Charlottesville, VA
Depression in Women; Mental Health in Public Sector Primary Care

Laura Hayman, PhD, RN, FAAN
Professor
New York University
Division of Nursing
New York, NY
Cardiovascular Risk Factors: Cholesterol; Nutrition in Infancy and Childhood

Marion Hemstrom-Krainess, DNSc, RN, CS
Assistant Professor
Case Western Reserve University
Frances Payne Bolton School of Nursing
Cleveland, OH
Wellness

Eileen M. Hermann, RN, BSN, MHS
Critical Care Nurse Educator, Cardiovascular Services
Hartford Hospital
Hartford, CT
Bowel Elimination Among Older Adults

Patricia A. Higgins, PhD, RN
Assistant Professor
Case Western Reserve University
Frances Payne Bolton School of Nursing
Cleveland, OH
Failure to Thrive (Adult)

Martha N. Hill, PhD, RN, FAAN
Professor and Dean
John Hopkins University
School of Nursing
Baltimore, MD
Hypertension

Mary Angelique Hill, MSN, RN, CPN
Associate Professor of Nursing
Lake City Community College
Lake City, FL
Boykin & Schoenhofer: The Theory of Nursing as Caring

Marilyn Hockenberry, PhD, RN-CS, PNP, FAAN
Professor of Pediatrics
Baylor College of Medicine
Nurse Scientist, Director
Center for Nursing Research
Texas Children's Hospital
Houston, TX
Cancer in Children

Diane Holditch-Davis, PhD, RN, FAAN
Professor
University of North Carolina at Chapel Hill
School of Nursing
Chapel Hill, NC
Parenting

Barbara J. Holtzclaw, PhD, RN, FAAN
Professor Emeritus
University of Texas Health Science Center
School of Nursing
San Antonio, TX
Fever/Febrile Response; Shivering; Thermal Balance

William L. Holzemer, PhD, RN, FAAN
Professor and Associate Dean
University of California San Francisco
School of Nursing
San Francisco, CA
Nursing Education; Substruction

June Andrews Horowitz, RN, PhD, FAAN
Professor
Boston College
William F. Connell School of Nursing
Chestnut Hill, MA
Postpartum Depression

Carol Noll Hoskins, PhD, RN, FAAN
Professor
New York University
Division of Nursing
New York, NY
Breast Cancer: Psychosocial Adjustment to Illness

Susan Houston, PhD, RN, CNAA, FAAN
Professor
University of Texas at Austin
School of Nursing
Austin, TX
Managed Care

Heddy Bishop Hubbard, MPH, RN, FAAN
Staff Member
Agency for Healthcare Quality and Research
Rockville, MD
Health Services Research

Ronda G. Hughes, PhD, MHS, RN
Senior Health Scientist Administrator
Agency for Healthcare Research and Quality
Rockville, MD
Patient Safety

Ann Hurley, DNSc, RN, FAAN
Executive Director
Center for Excellence in Nursing Practice
Brigham and Women's Hospital
Brookline, MA
Mental Status Measurement: The Mini-Mental State Examination

Sally A. Hutchinson, PhD, RN, FAAN
Professor
University of Florida
College of Nursing
Jacksonville, FL
Grounded Theory; Research Interviews (Qualitative)

Kathleen Huttlinger, PhD, RN
Professor
Kent State University
College of Nursing
Kent, OH
Content Analysis; Exploratory Studies; Participant Observation

Gail L. Ingersoll, EdD, RN, FAAN
Professor & Director of Clinical Nursing Research
University of Rochester
School of Nursing
Rochester, NY
Evaluation; Health Systems Delivery; Organizational Redesign

Pamela Magnussen Ironside, PhD, RN
Assistant Professor
University of Wisconsin-Madison
School of Nursing
Madison, WI
Hermeneutics

Michele Freeman Irwin, BSN, RN
New York University
Division of Nursing
New York, NY
Neuroleptic Use in Nursing Homes

Sharol F. Jacobson, PhD, RN, FAAN
Associate Dean for Research and Practice and Professor
University of Alabama
School of Nursing
Tucsaloosa, AL
Cultural/Transcultural Focus

Ada Jacox, PhD, RN, FAAN
Director, Clinical Practice Guidelines Program
University of Virginia
Charlottesville, VA
Pain

Loretta Sweet Jemmott, PhD, RN, FAAN
van Ameringen Professor in Psychiatric Mental Health Nursing, and Co-Director of the Center for Health Disparities Research
University of Pennsylvania
School of Nursing
Philadelphia, PA
Urban Health Research: Nursing Research in Urban Neighborhoods

Carole P. Jennings, PhD, RN, FAAN
Associate Professor and Deputy Director
Center for Health Policy, Research and Ethics
College of Nursing and Health Science
George Mason University
Fairfax, VA
Health Policy

Jean E. Johnson, PhD, RN, FAAN
Professor Emeritus
University of Rochester
School of Nursing
Rochester, NY
Surgery

Marion Johnson, PhD, RN
Professor Emeritus
University of Iowa
College of Nursing
Iowa City, IA
Benchmarking in Health Care; Nursing Outcomes Classification

Dorothy A. Jones, EdD, RNc, FAAN
Professor
Boston College
William F. Connell School of Nursing
Chestnut Hill, MA
Functional Health Patterns; Nursing Practice Models

Josette Jones, PhD, RN, BC
Assistant Professor
Indiana University
School of Nursing and School of Informatics
Indianapolis, IN
Telehealth

Evanne Juratovac, RN, MSN, CS
Lecturer and Project Coordinator
Prentiss Care Networks
University Center on Aging and Health
Case Western Reserve University
Frances Payne Bolton School of Nursing
Cleveland, OH
Disparities in Minority Mental Health

Maureen Keckeisen, RN, MN, CCRN
Clinical Nurse Specialist
Transplant/Surgical Specialties ICU
UCLA Medical Center
Department of Nursing
Los Angeles, CA
Hemodynamic Monitoring

Gwen Brumbaugh Keeney, PhD, RN, CNM
Clinical Assistant Professor
University of Illinois at Chicago
College of Nursing
Chicago, IL
Primary Health Care

Lisa Skemp Kelley
University of Iowa
College of Nursing
Iowa City, IA
Qualitative Research

Susan J. Kelley, PhD, RN, FAAN
Dean and Professor
College of Health and Human Sciences
Georgia State University
Atlanta, GA
Grandparents Raising Grandchildren

Alice R. Kempe, PhD, CS
Associate Professor
Ursuline College
Breen School of Nursing
Pepper Pike, OH
Family Caregiving and the Seriously Mentally Ill; Homelessness and Related Mood Disorders

Mary E. Kerr, PhD, RN, FAAN
Professor and
UPMC Health System Chair of Nursing Science
University of Pittsburgh
School of Nursing
Pittsburgh, PA
Cerebral Ischemia; Nursing Diagnosis

Shaké Ketefian, EdD, RN
Professor
University of Michigan
School of Nursing
Ann Arbor, MI
Research in Nursing Ethics

HaeSook Kim, RN, BSN
Graduate Student
University of Michigan
School of Nursing
Ann Arbor, MI
Activities of Daily Living

Hesook Suzie Kim, PhD, RN
Professor Emerita
University of Rhode Island
Kingston, RI
Professor
Buskerud University College
Kongsberg, Norway
Action Science; Discourse Analysis; Narrative Analysis

Karin T. Kirchhoff, PhD, RN, FAAN
Professor
University of Utah
College of Nursing
Salt Lake City, UT
Nurse Researcher in the Clinical Setting

Kenn M. Kirksey, PhD, RN, APRN, BC
Associate Professor of Nursing
California State University, Fresno
Department of Nursing
Fresno, CA
HIV Symptom Management and Quality of Life

Mia Kobayashi, MSN, RN, CNM
Doctoral Candidate
New York University
Division of Nursing
New York, NY
End-of-Life Planning and Choices; Unlicensed Assistive Personnel

Katharine Kolcaba, PhD, RN, C
Associate Professor
University of Akron
College of Nursing
Akron, OH
Comfort

Heidi V. Krowchuk, PhD, RN, FAAN
Associate Professor
University of North Carolina at Greensboro
School of Nursing
Greensboro, NC
Child Lead Exposure Effects; Failure to Thrive (Child)

Helen Lach, PhD, RN
Assistant Professor
St. Louis University
School of Nursing
St. Louis, MO
Dizziness in the Elderly

Cheryl A. Larson, MS, RN
Doctoral Candidate
University of Arizona
College of Nursing
Tucson, AZ
Spirituality

Marjorie Thomas Lawson, PhD, APRN, BC, FNP
Associate Professor
University of Southern Maine
College of Nursing and Health Professions
Portland, ME
Interpersonal Communication: Nurse-Patient

Regina Placzek Lederman, RN, FAAN
Professor
University of Texas Medical Branch
School of Nursing
Galveston, TX
Maternal Anxiety and Adaptation During Pregnancy

Yi-Hui Lee, MSN, RN
PhD Candidate
Case Western Reserve University
Frances Payne Bolton School of Nursing
Cleveland, OH
HIV Risk Behavior

Elizabeth R. Lenz, PhD, RN, FAAN
Dean and Professor
Ohio State University
College of Nursing
Columbus, OH
Doctoral Education

Eugene Levine, PhD
Professor Emeritus
Uniformed Services University of the Health Sciences
Graduate School of Nursing
Bethesda, MD
Quantitative Research

Wendy Lewandowski, PhD, RN, CS
Assistant Professor
Kent State University
College of Nursing
Kent, OH
Community Mental Health

Irene Daniels Lewis, DNS, APN, FAAN
College of Applied Sciences and Arts
San Jose State University
School of Nursing
San Jose, CA
Ethnogeriatrics

Judith A. Lewis, PhD, RNC, FAAN
Professor
Virginia Commonwealth University
School of Nursing
Richmond VA
Genetics

Patricia Liehr, PhD, RN
Professor and Director of Doctoral Program
Florida Atlantic University
College of Nursing
West Palm Beach, FL
Middle-Range Theories

Deborah F. Lindell, ND, APRN, BC
Assistant Professor of Nursing
Case Western Reserve University
Frances Payne Bolton School of Nursing
Cleveland, OH
Grounded Theory

Ada M. Lindsey, PhD, RN, FAAN
Dean and Professor Emeritus
University of Nebraska Medical Center
College of Nursing
Omaha, NE
Research Careers

Adrianne D. Linton, PhD, RN
Associate Professor
University of Texas Health Science Center at San Antonio
School of Nursing
San Antonio, TX
Wandering

Terri H. Lipman, PhD, CRNP, FAAN
Associate Professor
University of Pennsylvania
School of Nursing
Pediatric Nurse Practitioner
Division of Endocrinology
Children's Hospital of Philadelphia
Philadelphia, PA
Clinical Decision Making

Doris Troth Lippman, PhD, APRN
Professor
Fairfield University
School of Nursing
Fairfield, CT
Psychosocial Interventions (PSI)

Jane Lipscomb, PhD, RN, FAAN
Associate Professor
University of Maryland
School of Nursing
Baltimore, MD
Workplace Violence

Juliene G. Lipson, PhD, RN, FAAN
Professor
University of California San Francisco
School of Nursing
San Francisco, CA
Immigrant Women

Marilyn J. Lotas, PhD, RN
Associate Dean for Student Services and Director BSN Program
Associate Professor
Case Western Reserve University
Frances Payne Bolton School of Nursing
Cleveland, OH
Prevention of Preterm and Low-Birthweight Births

Courtney H. Lyder, ND
University of Virginia Medical Center
Professor of Nursing
Professor of Internal Medicine and Geriatrics
University of Virginia
School of Nursing
Charlottesville, VA
Pressure Ulcers

Brenda L. Lyon, DNS, RN
Professor
Indiana University
School of Nursing
Indianapolis, IN
Job Stress; Stress; Stress Management

Meridean Maas, PhD, RN, FAAN
Emeritus Professor and Director of the John A. Hartford Center of Geriatric Nursing Excellence
University of Iowa
College of Nursing
Iowa City, IA
Nursing Outcomes Classification

Linda Manfrin-Ledet, DNS, APRN
Assistant Professor of Nursing
Nicholls State University
Department of Nursing
Thibodaux, LA
Violence

Kiran Mangrola, MSN, RN, CS-GNP
New York University
Division of Nursing
New York, NY
Acute Care of the Elderly

Anne Manton, PhD, APRN, FAAN
Psychiatric Mental Health Nurse Practitioner
Cape Cod Hospital
Emergency Nursing

Lucy N. Marion, PhD, RN, FAAN
Professor and Dean
Medical College of Georgia
School of Nursing
Augusta, GA
Primary Care

Patricia A. Martin, PhD, RN
Dean and Professor
Wright State University
College of Nursing and Health
Dayton, OH
Nurse Researcher in the Clinical Setting; Organizational Culture; Research Dissemination

Linda J. Mayberry, PhD, RN, FAAN
Associate Professor
Director, Muriel and Virginia Pless Center for Nursing Research
New York University
Division of Nursing
New York, NY
Postpartum Depression

Angela Barron McBride, PhD, RN, FAAN
Distinguished Professor and University Dean Emerita
Indiana University
School of Nursing
Indianapolis, IN
Feminist Research Methodology; Women's Health

Melen R. McBride, PhD, RN
Stanford University
Stanford Geriatric Education Center
School of Medicine
Palo Alto, CA
Ethnogeriatrics

Maureen P. McCausland, DNSc, RN, FAAN
Senior Vice President, Chief Nursing Officer and Patient Care Services
University of Wisconsin-Madison Hospital and Clinic
Madison, WI
Primary Nursing

Sandee Graham McClowry, PhD, RN, FAAN
Professor
New York University
Division of Nursing
New York, NY
Mental Disorders Prevention

Ruth McCorkle, PhD, FAAN
Florence S. Wald Professor of Nursing
Yale University
School of Nursing
New Haven, CT
Chronic Illness

Susan H. McCrone, PhD, RN
Associate Professor
West Virginia University
Robert C. Byrd Health Science Center
School of Nursing
Morgantown, WV
Coronary Artery Bypass Graft (CABG) Surgery

Deborah Dillon McDonald, PhD, RN
Associate Professor
University of Connecticut
School of Nursing
Storrs, CT
Health Care Communication

Graham J. McDougall, Jr., PhD, RN, FAAN
Professor
University of Texas at Austin
School of Nursing
Austin, TX
Cognitive Interventions; Self-Efficacy

Beverly J. McElmurry, EdD, RN, FAAN
Professor and Associate Dean
University of Illinois at Chicago
College of Nursing
Chicago, IL
Primary Health Care

Elizabeth McGann, DNSc, RN, CS
Chairperson
Quinnipiac University
Department of Nursing
School of Health Sciences
Hamden, CT
Pulmonary Changes in Elders

Mary L. McHugh, PhD, RN, BC
Associate Professor and
Director, Professional Development and Extended Studies
University of Colorado Health Sciences Center
School of Nursing
Denver, CO
Artificial Intelligence; Nursing Intensity

Mary J. McNamee, PhD, RN
Associate Professor and Director
Office of Student Equity and Multicultural Affairs
University of Nebraska Medical Center
Omaha, NE
Homeless Health; Research Careers

Barbara Medoff-Cooper, PhD, RN, FAAN
Helen M. Shearer Professor in Nutrition
University of Pennsylvania
School of Nursing
Philadelphia, PA
Neurobehavioral Development and Nutritive Sucking

Paula M. Meek, PhD, RN
Assistant Professor
University of Arizona
College of Nursing
Tucson, AZ
Instrumentation; Reliability; Validity

Sue E. Meiner, EdD, APRN, BC, GNP
Assistant Professor
University of Nevada, Las Vegas
School of Nursing
Las Vegas, NV
Gastroesophageal Reflux Disease

Janet C. Meininger, PhD, RN, FAAN
Professor
University of Texas Health Sciences Center at Houston
School of Nursing
Houston, TX
Observational Research Design

Afaf Ibrahim Meleis, PhD, FAAN
Dean of Nursing
University of Pennsylvania
School of Nursing
Philadelphia, PA
Immigrant Women; International Nursing Research; Transitions and Health

Victoria Menzies, PhD, RN
Center for the Study of Complementary and Alternative Therapies
University of Virginia
School of Nursing
Charlottesville, VA
Complementary and Alternative Practices and Products (CAPPs)

Bonnie L. Metzger, PhD, RN, FAAN
Professor
University of Michigan
School of Nursing
Ann Arbor, MI
Time Series Analysis

Margaret Shandor Miles, PhD, RN, FAAN
Professor
University of North Carolina at Chapel Hill
School of Nursing
Chapel Hill, NC
Parental Response to the Birth and Hospitalization of a High-Risk Infant; Parenting

Koen Milisen, PhD, RN
Center for Health Services and Nursing Research
Katholieke Universiteit Leuven
Leuven, Belgium
Medications in Older Persons

Nancy Houston Miller, BSN, RN
Associate Director
Stanford Cardiac Rehabilitation Program
Stanford University Medical Center
Palo Alto, CA
Smoking/Tobacco as a Cardiovascular Risk Factor

Peggy A. Miller, MS, RN
Research Coordinator
University of Kansas
School of Nursing
Kansas City, KS
Job Satisfaction

Susan M. Miovech, PhD, RNC
Assistant Professor
Holy Family University
School of Nursing & Allied Health Professions
Philadelphia, PA
Fetal Monitoring

Merle H. Mishel, PhD, RN, FAAN
Kenan Professor of Nursing
University of North Carolina, Chapel Hill
School of Nursing
Chapel Hill, NC
Uncertainty in Illness

Ethel L. Mitty, EdD, RN
Adjunct Clinical Professor of Nursing
New York University
Division of Nursing
New York, NY
End-of-Life Planning and Choices; Unlicensed Assistive Personnel

Wanda K. Mohr, PhD, RN, FAAN
Associate Professor
University of Medicine and Dentistry of New Jersey
School of Nursing
Newark, NJ
Children Exposed to Intimate Partner Violence; Intimate Partner Violence

Mary Moller, MSN, RN
Doctoral Student
Case Western Reserve University
Frances Payne Bolton School of Nursing
Cleveland, OH
Schizophrenia

Rita Monsen, DSN, MPH, RN
Interim Executive Director
Genetic Nursing Credentialing Commission, Inc.
Keuka Park, NY
Genetics

Kristen S. Montgomery, PhD, RN
Assistant Professor
University of South Carolina
College of Nursing
Columbia, SC
Fitzpatrick's Rhythm Model; Pregnancy; Watson's Theory of Human Caring

Shirley M. Moore, PhD, RN, FAAN
Professor and Associate Dean for Research
Case Western Reserve University
Frances Payne Bolton School of Nursing
Cleveland, OH
Pain Management: A Mid-Range Theory; Theoretical Framework

Susan K. Moore, LMSW-ACP
Independent Consultant
San Antonio, TX
Minority Women Offenders

Sue Moorhead, PhD, RN
Associate Professor
University of Iowa
College of Nursing
Iowa City, IA
Nursing Outcomes Classification; Quality of Care

Patricia Moritz, PhD, RN, FAAN
Professor and Dean
University of Colorado Health Sciences Center
School of Nursing
Denver, CO
Funding

Diana Lynn Morris, PhD, RN, FAAN
Associate Professor
Case Western Reserve University
Frances Payne Bolton School of Nursing
Cleveland, OH
Parse's Theory of Nursing: Human Becoming Theory; Watson's Theory of Human Caring

Barbara Munro, PhD, RN, FAAN
Dean and Professor
Boston College
School of Nursing
Chestnut Hill, MA
Data Management; Quantitative Research Methodology; Statistical Techniques

Shirley A. Murphy, PhD, RN, FAAN
Professor Emeritus
University of Washington
School of Nursing
Seattle, WA
Disaster Nursing

Carol M. Musil, PhD, RN
Associate Professor
Case Western Reserve University
Frances Payne Bolton School of Nursing
Cleveland, OH
Cohort Design; Family Caregiving to Frail Elders; Pilot Study

Madeline A. Naegle, PhD, APRN-BC, FAAN
Professor
New York University
Division of Nursing
New York, NY
Substance Abuse and Addiction Among Registered Nurses

Yolanda Narvaez-Edwards, RN, BSN
Graduate Student
University of Texas Health Science Center
School of Nursing
San Antonio, TX
Minority Women Offenders

Alvita Nathaniel, DSN, APRN, BC
Assistant Professor
West Virginia University
School of Nursing
Morgantown, WV
Moral Distress; Moral Reckoning

Mary Duffin Naylor, PhD, RN, FAAN
Professor
University of Pennsylvania
School of Nursing
Philadelphia, PA
Transitional Care

Kathleen M. Nokes, PhD, RN, FAAN
Professor
Hunter College, CUNY
Hunter-Bellevue School of Nursing
New York, NY
HIV/AIDS Care and Treatment

Jeanne M. Novotny, PhD, RN, FAAN
Dean and Professor
Fairfield University
School of Nursing
Fairfield, CT
Nursing Education

Cassandra Okechukwu, RN, MSN, MPH
Research Coordinator/Clinical Instructor
University of Maryland
School of Nursing
Baltimore, MD
Workplace Violence

Lisa Onega, PhD, RN, FNP, GNP, CS
Associate Professor, Hartford Foundation Gerontology Fellow
Radford University
School of Nursing
Radford, VA
Ethnography

Ann L. O'Sullivan, PhD, CRNP, FAAN
Professor
University of Pennsylvania
School of Nursing
Philadelphia, PA
Adolescence; Adolescent Pregnancy and Parenting; Infant Injury

Joanne O'Sullivan, PhD, APRN, BC, FNP
Assistant Professor
Graduate Program of Nursing
Massachusetts Institute of Health Professions
Boston, MA
Homelessness

Mary H. Palmer, PhD, RNC, FAAN
Umphlet Distinguished Professor in Aging
University of North Carolina at Chapel Hill
School of Nursing
Chapel Hill, NC
Prostate Cancer

Jin-Hwa Park, MA, RN, GNP
New York University
Division of Nursing
New York, NY
Chronic Gastrointestinal Symptoms

John R. Phillips, PhD, RN
Professor Emeritus
New York University
School of Education
New York, NY
(Martha E.) Rogers Science of Unitary Persons

Linda R. Phillips, PhD, RN, FAAN
Professor
University of Arizona
College of Nursing
Tucson, AZ
Clinical Nursing Research

Sally Phillips, PhD, RN
Director of Bioterrorism Preparedness Research Program
Agency for Health Care Research and Quality
Rockville, MD
Caring; Nursing Process

Joanne M. Pohl, PhD, APRN, BC, FAAN
Associate Professor, Associate Dean for Community Partnerships
University of Michigan
School of Nursing
Ann Arbor, MI
Nursing Centers

Denise F. Polit, PhD
President
Humanalysis, Inc.
Saratoga Springs, NY
Data Collection Methods

Sue A. Popkess-Vawter, PhD, RN, ARNP
Professor
University of Kansas
School of Nursing
Kansas City, KS
Weight Management

Demetrius J. Porche, DNS, RN
Associate Dean of Research & Evaluation and Professor
Louisiana State University Health Sciences Center
School of Nursing
New Orleans, LA
Violence

Eileen J. Porter, PhD, RN
Associate Professor
University of Missouri
School of Nursing
Columbia, MO
Widows and Widowers

Lorrie L. Powel, PhD, RN
Associate Professor
School of Nursing
College of Health and Public Affairs
University of Central Florida
Orlando, FL
Cancer Survivorship; Prostate Cancer

Diane Shea Pravikoff, PhD, RN
Director of Research/ Professional Liaison
CINAHL Information Systems
Glendale, CA
Cumulative Index to Nursing and Allied Health Literature

Jana L. Pressler, PhD, RN
Assistant Dean for Research, Professor, College of Nursing
University of Oklahoma
College of Nursing
Oklahoma City, OK
Fitzpatrick's Rhythm Model

Mary T. Quinn Griffin, PhD, RN
Assistant Professor
Case Western Reserve University
Frances Payne Bolton School of Nursing
Cleveland, OH
Health Conceptualization; Parse's Theory of Nursing: Human Becoming Theory; Roy Adaptation Model

Joanne W. Rains, DNS, RN
Dean and Associate Professor
Indiana University East
Division of Nursing
Richmond, IN
Collaborative Research

Barbara Rakel, MA, RN
Advanced Practice Nurse Supervisor
University of Iowa Hospitals and Clinics
Iowa City, IA
Ethnography

Pamela G. Reed, PhD, RN, FAAN
Professor
University of Arizona
College of Nursing
Tucson, AZ
Peplau's Theoretical Model; Spirituality

Barbara Resnick, PhD, CRNP, FAAN, FAANP
Associate Professor
University of Maryland
School of Nursing
Baltimore, MD
Continuing Care Retirement Communities

Virginia Richardson, DNS, RN, CPNP
Assistant Dean for Student Affairs
Associate Professor
Indiana University
School of Nursing
Indianapolis, IN
Pediatric Primary Care

Susan K. Riesch, DNSc, RN, FAAN
Professor, School of Nursing
University of Wisconsin-Madison
School of Nursing
Madison, WI
Nursing Centers

Mary Anne Rizzolo, EdD, RN, FAAN
Director for Professional Development
National League for Nursing
New York, NY
Research on Interactive Video

Beverly L. Roberts, RN, PhD, FAAN, FGSA
Arline H. and Curtis F. Garvin Professor of Nursing
Frances Payne Bolton School of Nursing
Case Western Reserve University
Cleveland, OH
Falls; Functional Health

Karen R. Robinson, PhD
Non Clinical Lecturer in Gastroenterology
Institute of Infection, Immunity and Inflammation
University Hospital
Queens Medical Center
Nottingham, United Kingdom
Current Procedural Terminology-Coded Services; Denial in Coronary Heart Disease

Bonnie Rogers, PhD, COHN-S, LNCC, FAAN
Associate Professor and Director, Occupational Safety and Health
Education and Research Center
University of North Carolina at Chapel Hill
School of Public Health
Chapel Hill, NC
Nursing Occupational Injury and Stress

Norma Martinez Rogers, PhD, RN
Assistant Professor
University of Texas Health Science Center
School of Nursing
San Antonio, TX
Minority Women Offenders

Carol A. Romano, MS, RN, FAAN
Director, Nursing Information Systems and Quality Assurance
Warren Grant Magnuson Clinical Center
National Institutes of Health
Bethesda, MD
Data Stewardship

Eileen Virginia Romeo, MSN, RN
Doctoral Student
Case Western Reserve University
Frances Payne Bolton School of Nursing
Cleveland, OH
Orem's Self-Care Deficit Nursing Theory

Marlene M. Rosenkoetter, PhD, RN, FAAN
Professor
Medical College of Georgia
School of Nursing
Atlanta, GA
Retirement

Virginia K. Saba, EdD, RN, FAAN, FACMI
Distinguished Scholar, Adjunct
Georgetown University
School of Nursing and Health Studies
Washington, DC
Home Health Care Classification System; Home Health Systems; Nursing Informatics; Nursing Information Systems

Ali Salman, MD, RN
PhD Candidate
Case Western Reserve University
Frances Payne Bolton School of Nursing
Cleveland, OH
Depression and Cardiovascular Diseases; Hypertension

Helen A. Schaag, RN, MSN, MA
Project Director, CPAP Research Study
University of Kansas
School of Nursing
Kansas City, KS
Caregiver; Home Care Technologies

Karen L. Schumacher, PhD, RN
Assistant Professor
University of Pennsylvania
School of Nursing
Philadelphia, PA
Transitions and Health

Elizabeth A. Schlenk, PhD, RN
Assistant Professor
University of Pittsburgh
School of Nursing
Pittsburgh, PA
Patient Contracting

Donald F. Schwarz, MD, MPH, MBA
Deputy Physician-in-Chief
Chief, Craig-Dalsimer Division of Adolescent Medicine
University of Pennsylvania
Schools of Medicine and Nursing
Philadelphia, PA
Adolescence; Adolescent Pregnancy and Parenting; Infant Injury

Judith Kennedy Schwarz, PhD, RN
Consultant, Ethics and End-of-Life Care
New York, NY
Advance Directives

Joan L. Shaver, PhD, RN, FAAN
Professor and Dean
University of Illinois at Chicago
College of Nursing
Chicago, IL
Sleep

Nelma B. Shearer, PhD, RN
Assistant Professor
College of Nursing
Arizona State University
Tempe, AZ
Peplau's Theoretical Model

Caryn A. Sheehan, MSN, RN
Assistant Professor
St. Anselm College
Department of Nursing
Manchester, NH
Pender's Health Promotion Model

Mary Shelkey, PhD, RN, ARNP
Assistant Professor
Seattle University
College of Nursing
Seattle, WA
Alzheimer's Disease

Deborah Shelton, PhD, RN, CNA, BC
Associate Professor of Nursing
University of Connecticut
School of Nursing
Storrs, CT
Child Delinquents

Shyang-Yun Pamela K. Shiao, PhD, RN, FAAN
Associate Professor
University of Texas
Health Sciences Center School of Nursing
Houston, TX
Endotracheal Suctioning in Newborns: NICU Preterm Infant Care

Elaine K. Shimono, MA, RN
Clinical Director
Psychiatry Care Center
Mount Sinai Medical Center
New York, NY
(Martha E.) Rogers Science of Unitary Persons

Mary Cipriano Silva, PhD, RN, FAAN
Professor Emeritus
George Mason University
College of Nursing and Health Science
Fairfax, VA
Clinical Professor
School of Public Health and Health Sciences
University of Massachussetts
Amherst, MA
Ethics of Research; Philosophy of Nursing

Carol E. Smith, PhD, RN
Professor
University of Kansas
School of Nursing
Kansas City, KS
Caregiver; Home Care Technologies; Quality of Life

Marlaine C. Smith, PhD, RN, AHN-C, FAAN
Professor and Associate Dean for Academic Affairs
University of Colorado Health Sciences Center
School of Nursing
Denver, CO
Caring

Mary Jane Smith, PhD, RN
Professor and Associate Dean for Graduate Academic Affairs
West Virginia University
Robert C. Byrd Health Science Center
School of Nursing
Morgantown, WV
Drinking and Driving Among Adolescents; Middle-Range Theories

Bernard Sorofman, PhD
Professor
University of Iowa
College of Pharmacy
Iowa City, IA
Ethnography

Susan M. Sparks, PhD, RN, FAAN
Project Officer
National Library of Medicine
Bethesda, MD
Electronic Network

Ann M. Stalter, MS, RN
Clinical Instructor
Wright State University
College of Nursing and Health
Dayton, OH
Vulnerable Populations

Theresa Standing, PhD, RN
Assistant Professor
Case Western Reserve University
Frances Payne Bolton School of Nursing
Cleveland, OH
Triangulation

Els Steeman, MSN
Center for Health Services and Nursing Research
Katholieke Universiteit Leuven
Leuven, Belgium
Medications in Older Persons

Karen Farchaus Stein, PhD, RN, FAAN
Associate Professor of Nursing
University of Michigan
School of Nursing
Ann Arbor, MI
Self-Concept Disturbances and Eating Disorders

Joanne Sabol Stevenson, PhD, RN, FAAN
Professor Emeritus
Ohio State University College of Nursing
Columbus, OH
and
Rutgers College of Nursing
Newark, NJ
Adult Health; Alcohol Dependence; Drug Abuse; Geriatrics

Kathleen Stone, PhD, RN, FAAN
Professor Emeritus
Ohio State University
College of Nursing
Columbus, OH
Endotracheal Suctioning

Patricia W. Stone, PhD, MPH, RN
Assistant Professor
Columbia University
School of Nursing
New York, NY
Patient Safety

Ora L. Strickland, PhD, RN, FAAN
Professor
Emory University
Nell Hodgson School of Nursing
Atlanta, GA
Measurement and Scales

Neville E. Strumpf, PhD, RN, FAAN
Edith Clemmer Steinbright Professor in Gerontology
Director of the Center for Gerontologic Nursing Science
University of Pennsylvania
School of Nursing
Philadelphia, PA
Physical Restraints

Sheri Stucke, PhD, FNP
Kresge Center Research Assistant
Decker School of Nursing
Binghamton University
Binghamton, NY
Osteoporosis

Hussein A. Tahan, DNSc, RN, CNA
Director of Nursing, Cardiovascular Services
Columbia University Medical Center
New York-Presbyterian Hospital
New York, NY
Case Management

Hsin-Yi (Jean) Tang, PhD, RN
Teaching Associate
University of Washington
School of Nursing
Seattle, WA
Biofeedback

Siew Tzuh Tang, DNSc
Assistant Professor
College of Nursing
National Yang-Ming University
Taipei, Taiwan
Chronic Illness

Susan Dale Tannenbaum, RN, BSN
Staff Nurse—Cardiac Unit
Johns Hopkins University
School of Nursing
Baltimore, MD
Hypertension

Anita J. Tarzian, MS, RN
Research Associate
University of Maryland
School of Nursing
Baltimore, MD
Descriptive Research

Roma Lee Taunton, PhD, RN, FAAN
Senior Scientist
University of Kansas Medical Center
School of Nursing
Kansas City, KS
Job Satisfaction; Outcome Measures

Ann Gill Taylor, EdD, RN, FAAN
Betty Norman Norris Professor of Nursing and
Director, Center for the Study of Complementary and Alternative Therapies
University of Virginia School of Nursing
Charlottesville, VA
Complementary and Alternative Practices and Products (CAPPs)

Diana L. Taylor, PhD, RN, FAAN
Professor Emeritus, Department of Family Health Care Nursing
Adjunct Professor, Center for Reproductive Health Policy & Research
University of California, San Francisco
San Francisco, CA
Menstrual Cycle; Premenstrual Syndrome

Debera Jane Thomas, DNS, RN, CS
Associate Professor
Florida Atlantic University
Boca Raton, FL
Case Study as a Method of Research

Mary E. Tiedeman, PhD, RN
Associate Professor, College of Nursing
Brigham Young University
College of Nursing
Provo, UT
Roy Adaptation Model

Sara Torres, PhD, RN, FAAN
Dean and Professor
University of Medicine and Dentistry of New Jersey
School of Nursing
Newark, NJ
Children Exposed to Intimate Partner Violence; Intimate Partner Violence

Toni Tripp-Reimer, PhD, RN, FAAN
Professor and Associate Dean
University of Iowa
College of Nursing
Iowa City, IA
Ethnography; Qualitative Research

Barbara S. Turner, DNSc, RN, FAAN
Professor and Associate Dean
Duke University
School of Nursing
Durham, NC
Informed Consent

Doris C. Vahey, PhD
Special Projects Consultant
Mount Sinai Hospital
New York, NY
Patient Satisfaction

Barbara Valanis, PhD, FAAN
Director of Nursing Research
Kaiser-Permanente Center for Health Research
Portland, OR
Consortial Research

Connie Vance, RN, EdD, FAAN
Professor, School of Nursing
The College of New Rochelle
School of Nursing
New Rochelle, NY
Mentoring

Patricia E. H. Vermeersch, PhD, RN
Assistant Professor
Wright State University
School of Nursing and Health
Dayton, OH
Delirium

Joyce A. Verran, PhD, RN, FAAN
Professor
University of Arizona
College of Nursing
Tucson, AZ
Instrumentation; Reliability; Validity

Antonia M. Villarruel, PhD, RN, FAAN
Professor
Director, Center for Health Promotion
University of Michigan
Ann Arbor, MI
Health Disparities

Ladislov Volicer, PhD, MD
Boston University
School of Medicine
Boston, MA
Geriatric Research Education and Clinical Center
Edith Nourse Rogers Memorial Veterans Hospital
Bedford, MA
Mental Status Measurement: The Mini-Mental State Examination

Madeline Musante Wake, PhD, RN
Provost, Marquette University
Marquette University
Milwaukee, WI
International Classification for Nursing Practice (ICNP®)

Patricia Hinton Walker, PhD, RN, FAAN
Dean and Professor
Uniformed Services University of the Health Sciences
Graduate School of Nursing
Bethesda, MD
Capitation; Case Management; Neuman Systems Model

Lynn I. Wasserbauer, PhD, RN
Assistant Professor
University of Akron
College of Nursing
Akron, OH
Experimental Research; Quasi-Experimental Research

Clarann Weinert, SC, PhD, RN, FAAN
Professor & Director
Center for Research on Chronic Health Conditions in Rural Dwellers
College of Nursing
Montana State University-Bozeman
Bozeman, MT
Longitudinal Survey; Rural Health

Joan Stehle Werner, DNSc, RN
Professor
University of Wisconsin-Eau Claire
College of Nursing and Health Sciences
Eau Claire, WI
Coping

Mary Ellen Wewers, PhD, MPH, RN, FAAN
Professor
Ohio State University
College of Nursing
Columbus, OH
Smoking Cessation

Ann Whall, PhD, RN, FAAN, FGSA
Professor and
Associate Director, University of Michigan Geriatrics Center
University of Michigan
School of Nursing
Ann Arbor, MI
Middle-Range Theories of Dementia Care

Margaret A. Wheatley, RN, MSN
Instructor
Case Western Reserve University
Frances Payne Bolton School of Nursing
Cleveland, OH
Disparities in Minority Mental Health

Sharon A. Wilkerson, PhD, RN
Associate Professor of Nursing
Purdue University
School of Nursing
West Lafayette, IN
(Dorothy) Johnson's Behavioral System Model

Carolyn A. Williams, PhD, RN, FAAN
Dean and Professor
University of Kentucky
School of Nursing
Lexington, KY
Populations and Aggregates

Danny G. Willis, RN, MN
Doctoral Candidate
Louisiana State University
School of Nursing
New Orleans, LA
Violence

Celia E. Wills, PhD, RN
Associate Professor
Michigan State University
College of Nursing
East Lansing, MI
Mental Health in Public Sector Primary Care; Mental Health Services Research

Holly Skodol Wilson, PhD, RN, FAAN
Professor Emeritus
University of California San Francisco
School of Nursing
San Francisco, CA

Grounded Theory; Research Interviews (Qualitative)

Sarah A. Wilson, PhD, RN
Associate Professor
Marquette University
College of Nursing
Milwaukee, WI

Death and Dying

Chris Winkelman, PhD, RN
Assistant Professor
Case Western Reserve University
Frances Payne Bolton School of Nursing
Cleveland, OH

Physiological Monitoring

May L. Wykle, PhD, RN, FAAN, FGSA
Dean and Florence Cellar Professor of Gerontological Nursing
Director, University Center on Aging & Health
Case Western Reserve University
Frances Payne Bolton School of Nursing
Cleveland, OH

Depression in Older Adults

JoAnne M. Youngblut, PhD, RN, FAAN
Professor
Florida International University
School of Nursing
Miami, FL

Causal Modeling; Structural Equation Modeling

Renzo Zanotti, PhD
Professor
University of Padova
Padova, Italy

Scientific Development

Jaclene A. Zauszniewski, PhD, RNC, FAAN
Kate Hanna Harvey Professor of Community Health Nursing
Case Western Reserve University
Frances Payne Bolton School of Nursing
Cleveland, OH

Depression in Older Adults; Factor Analysis; Resourcefulness

Cora D. Zembrzuski, PhD, APRN
Lecturer and Clinical Coordinator
Community Health Nursing
Yale University
New Haven, CT

Bowel Elimination Among Older Adults; Hydration and Dehydration in Older Adults

Tamara L. Zurakowski, PhD, CRNP
Lecturer
University of Pennsylvania
School of Nursing
Philadelphia, PA

(Florence) Nightingale

List of Entries

A

Action Science

Action science is an approach to generating knowledge for practice by engaging practitioners in that process through reflection on their own behavioral worlds of practice (Argyris, Putnam, & Smith, 1985; Schön, 1983). Schön contrasts action science as advanced by these authors with the traditional, positivistic science, which he calls technical rationality. Technical rationality for professional practice is concerned with "knowing that," whereas action science is oriented to "knowing how" in practice. Although knowing how in practice contributes to the creation of knowledge that is not available from traditional research, what practitioners actually design in their practice may be limiting, routinized, and self-sealing. Hence, action science addresses generation of knowledge through reflection that fulfills the functions of discovery and change. Action science is primarily oriented to studying individual practitioners in their practice and generation of knowledge from individuals' practice; however, it can be applied to organizational behaviors and organizational intervention.

R. Putnam (1992) suggests that action science is based on three philosophical premises: (a) human practice involves meaning making, intentionality in action, and normativity from the perspective of human agency; (b) human practice goes on in an interdependent milieu of behavioral norms and institutional politics; and (c) the epistemology of practice calls for the engagement of practitioners in generating knowledge. Action science thus is a method and philosophy for improving practice and generating knowledge. Argyris (1987) suggests further that action science is an interventionist approach in which three prerequisites must be established for the research to ensue: (a) a creation of normative models of rare universes that are free of defensive routines, (b) a theory of intervention that can move practitioners and organizations from the present to a new desirable universe, and (c) a theory of instruction that can be used to teach new skills and create new culture.

Action science holds that actions in professional practice are based on practitioners' theories of action. Theories of action are learned and organized as repertoires of concepts, schemata, and propositions and are the basis on which practitioners' behavioral worlds are created in specific situations of practice. Argyris, Putnam, and Smith (1985) identified espoused theories and theories-in-use as two types of theories of action. Espoused theories of action are the rationale expressed by practitioners as guiding their actions in a situation of practice, whereas theories-in-use refers to theories that are actually used in practice. Theories-in-use are only inferable from the actions themselves, and practitioners usually are not aware of or not able to articulate their theories-in-use except through careful reflection and self-dialogue.

Argyris and Schön (1974) and Argyris, Putnam, and Smith (1985) identified Model I theories-in-use as a type that seals practitioners from learning and produces routinization and ineffectiveness in practice. Model II theories-in-use are proposed within action science as an intervention for Model I theories-in-use. Model II theories-in-use encompass principles of valid information, free and informed choice in action, and internal commitment. Reflection and learning are the two key processes necessary for the transformation from Model I theories-in-use to Model II theories-in-use. Action science, then, aims to engage both practitioners and researchers in this process of transformation through the creation of a normative model of rare universe and application of theories of intervention and instruction.

Knowledge of practitioners' theories-in use and espoused theories provides a descriptive understanding about the patterns of inconsistencies between theories-in-use and espoused theories recalled in actual practice. Through action science, practitioners engaged in Model II theories-in-use produce practice knowledge that informs their approach to practice without routinization or the self-sealing mode. In addition, action science generates knowledge regarding the process involved in self-awareness and the learning of new theories-in-use through reflective practice and practice design.

Research process in action science calls for the cooperative participation of practitioner and researcher through the phases of description, discovery of theories-in-use, and intervention. Transcriptions of actual practice by the researcher or narratives of actual practice by the practitioner are analyzed together in order to describe and inform reflectively the nature of practice and theories-in-use. R. Putnam (1996) suggests the use of the ladder of inference as a tool to discover practitioners' modes of thinking and action as revealed in transcripts or narratives. The research process is not oriented to the analysis of action transcripts or narratives by a researcher independent of the practitioner. It involves a post-practice face-to-face discussion (interview) between the researcher and the practitioner. Such session, are used to get at the reconstructed reasoning of practitioners regarding critical moments of the practice and to provide opportunities for reflection on the thinking and doing that were involved in the practice. Through such sessions, the researcher also acts as an interventionist by engaging the practitioner to move toward new learning.

Nursing practice is a human-to-human service that occurs in the context of health care. Nurses practice within on-line conditions that are complex not only with respect to clients problems but also in terms of organizational elements of the health care environment. Nursing practice is not based simply on linear translations of relevant theoretical knowledge that governs the situation of practice but has to be derived and designed from the nurse's knowledge of and responses to the competing and complex demands of the situation (Kim, 1994). In addition, as the action scientists suggest, nursing practice in general, as well as particular nursing actions, may be entrenched with routinization or frozen within Model I theories-in-use.

On the other hand, a great deal of nursing as practiced may be exemplary and creatively designed and enacted. The general aim of action science for nursing is then to improve nursing practice by freeing nurses from self-sealing practices and engaging them in the process of learning and participatory research.

HESOOK SUZIE KIM

Activities of Daily Living

Ability to care for oneself and meet basic needs is fundamental to maintaining health and independence. The term "activities of daily living" (ADL) is used to refer to the set of skills that constitute these essential abilities. ADL are evaluated for many purposes, such as to assess current capabilities, to determine care requirements, to gauge progress or response to intervention, and to evaluate outcomes. Thus, ADL are useful to many health disciplines and professions across a wide range of health care settings and populations for addressing both clinical and research goals.

ADL are generally viewed hierarchically from the most basic of human skills (e.g., ability to feed oneself) to somewhat higher ones (e.g., ability to bathe and dress oneself). Higher still are those more complex skills necessary to maintain independence in the community, such as using the telephone, doing household chores, and managing one's finances. This higher level skill set is usually distinguished from the more basic ones by use of the term "instrumental activities of daily living" or IADL. ADL and IADL are also part of the broader concept of functional assessment, which generally encompasses more domains, such as cognitive and social functioning.

Many scales have been developed to measure ADL and IADL. Among the most widely used are the Katz Index of Activities of Daily Living, the Barthel Index, and the Functional Independence Measure, each of which addresses basic ADL. These and similar scales encompassing IADL can be used alone, together, or in combination with other measures of function, depending upon the purpose and breadth of the assessor's goals.

ADL scales vary, not only in the range and complexity of skills they include, but also in the way skills are rated. Generally, each scale measures along one dimension, such as difficulty in performing a skill (e.g., performs with ease) or type of support (e.g., physical, cognitive) or level of assistance (e.g., single person assist) needed to perform a skill. Dichotomous and ordinal scaling approaches are most common. The scaling model is especially important in determining not only the dimension of ADL to be assessed, but also in determining the scale's sensitivity to change. Although ADL and IADL assessments have been used for many years, the prevalence of dichotomous and broad ordinal scaling models has led to only a limited understanding of the pattern of ADL and IADL change over time for various patient populations.

ADL scales can be used to elicit information from various informants including the individual being assessed, a family member or informal caregiver, a health professional, or research staff. To obtain accurate ADL ratings it is essential to consider the informant's knowledge of the individual's abilities and any motivations of the informant that may color responses. Further, it is also important to distinguish between what the informant says the individual can do, what the individual actually can do, and what the individual is expected to do, all of which may or may not actually correspond with one another (Smith & Clark, 1995). Even when obtaining ratings of actual rather than reported performance, accuracy can be a problem. An evaluator should take care to note, or control when possible, both environmental factors (e.g., familiarity, glare, and noise), and personal factors (e.g., fatigue or depression), when conducting and interpreting assessments of ADL performance.

The application of ADL and IADL measures to particular clinical populations is a new approach that is beginning to gain notice, much as quality of life measures have been specified to various clinical populations. Such specific ADL measures may be applied best when the most commonly affected ADL and related performance limitations are known for a given population. In these situations, the assessment can be targeted toward the most relevant ADL and scaled more meaningfully to the nature of the difficulty encountered. For example, knowing that a person with dementia is unable to dress themselves independently is useful; but knowing that the person needs help with sequencing the steps involved in selecting and donning appropriate clothing is substantially more useful in supporting a higher level of independence for the individual. This approach to the assessment of ADL may be most beneficial in a clinical context where prescriptions for the kinds and levels of ADL assistance are made. One disadvantage of specifying ADL assessments to particular populations is that the narrowed view may result in a failure to identify uncommon areas of difficulty.

In sum, ADL and IADL are widely used concepts in nursing and health care practice and research because they are valuable in understanding the impact of illness or injury on a person's everyday life and in determining their needs for assistance in support of continued independence. Particular approaches to assessing ADL and IADL should be selected based on the purpose of the assessment and the quality of information available from informants. Careful consideration should be given to factors that may affect ADL and IADL ratings so that the most accurate assessment can be made. Tailored approaches for specific patient populations are emerging as the next advancement in ADL measurement.

DONNA L. ALGASE
HAESOOK KIM

Acute Care of the Elderly

Older people have a greater prevalence of chronic diseases and disorders that lead to hospitalization. On average, people over 65 are hospitalized more than three times as often as younger individuals, and the length of their stay is estimated to be 50% longer than that of younger individuals. Nursing research that defines the evidence for practice interventions is needed for patients of all ages, and especially for the elderly (Fulmer & Mezey, 2002). Nursing research that provides the basis for best practice for hospitalized elders is often embedded in interdisciplinary studies. For example, in one study, 244 patients aged 70 years and older were enrolled in a geriatric care program which used a geriatric resource-nurse intervention to improve the quality of care received by the hospitalized elderly. The intervention decreased patients' length of stay and improved quality indicators (Inouye et al., 1993a, 1993b). In another study, Palmer and colleagues were able to demonstrate improved care through the use of an ACE (Acute Care of the Elderly) unit, in which protocols for skin care, urinary-incontinence management, and pressure-ulcer prevention were used (Palmer, Landefeld, Kresevic, & Kowal, 1994).

ACE units have shown improved outcomes among older patients who have been hospitalized. A widely cited study conducted by Landefeld, Palmer, and Kresevic (1995) demonstrated that patients admitted to an ACE unit were more likely to improve in activities of daily living (ADL) and were less likely to be institutionalized. Asplund, Gustafson, and Jacobsson (2000) also demonstrated that ACE units reduce the institutionalization rate of hospitalized elders. Siegler, Glick, and Lee (2002) found that the commonality of the ACE unit was their interdisciplinary care and focus on functional improvement, patient and staff satisfaction, and reduction of length of stay. In a prospective study of 804 patients 80 years of age or older, 42% of the elderly patients with no baseline dependencies at admission had developed one or more limitations within 2 months (Hart, 2002). Individuals older than 65 years of age are more likely to be admitted to acute care from the emergency department than other age groups. The hospitalized elderly are at an increased risk for poor outcomes such as increased length of stay, readmissions, functional decline, and iatrogenic complications, as compared with other age groups. There is a 33% rate of readmission within 3 months and complications such as acute confusion and nosocomial infections, which are common among the elderly, resulting in increased morbidity and mortality. Fifty-eight percent of patients who are hospitalized will experience at least one iatrogenic complication (Hart).

Data for acute care are also found in research that looks at "nurse sensitive" indicators for patient outcomes. For example, hospital staff has been shown to make a difference in patient outcomes (Aiken, Sloane, Lake, Sochalski, & Weber, 1999; Kovner & Gergen, 1998). Nurse accountability and models of patient and nursing administration also have been examined (Mark, Salyer, Geddes, & Smith, 1998; Scherb, Rapp, Johnson, & Maas, 1998). These studies provide some information regarding outcomes for the elderly, but intensive effort needs to be focused on understanding the differences between outcomes for younger individuals versus older individuals in the case of hospital care. For example, do older adults have different cardiac output after coronary artery bypass surgery than younger individuals when other variables are held constant, such as premorbid conditions? Such parameters are needed for the improvement of care for the elderly. A study conducted by Kleinpell and Ferrans (1998) explored functional status and quality of life outcomes for elderly patients after ICU hospitalization; survival rates 4 to 6 months after discharge were examined in patients aged 45 and older. In this study, the severity of the illness was a predictor of ICU outcome; age was not.

Historically, elders were not considered to be "suitable candidates" for surgeries and treatments that today are considered routine. In the early 1970s, individuals over the age of 65 were excluded from surgical intensive care units, as it was felt that the cost-benefit was not going to be in favor of the older patient. Today individuals in their 80s and 90s undergo open-heart surgery and require appropriate postoperative care that only a surgical intensive care unit can provide.

Ethical issues abound regarding elders during a hospitalization. For example, if there is an insufficient number of beds in an intensive care unit, should older individuals be sent out to the floor before younger individuals? Are scarce resources allocated to younger individuals before they are used to care for the elderly? Further, elder abuse, a serious and potentially fatal syndrome, is frequently overlooked when elders come into the hospital with severe symptoms, such as bilateral bruising, histories incompatible with injuries, and overt fear of caregivers. These issues are a part of acute care of the elderly and need to be addressed with rigorous research studies. Studies involving younger individuals need to be replicated among older adults to discern differences between the age cohorts.

TERRY FULMER
KIRAN MANGROLA

Adherence/Compliance

Adherence is defined as the degree to which behavior corresponds to a recommended therapeutic regimen (Haynes, Taylor, & Sackett, 1979). Numerous terms have been used to describe this behavior, including compliance, therapeutic alliance, and patient cooperation. Although the literature is filled with discussion of the acceptability of these terms and the differences between them, most investigators view the terms as synonymous and independent of the decision to engage in a particular therapeutic regimen. The most complete literature can be obtained from structured databases with the term *compliance.*

Adherence to health care regimens has been discussed in the literature since the days of Plato. However, little systematic attention was given to this phenomenon until the 1970s, when there was a proliferation of research. One of the first reviews of the literature was published in *Nursing Research* (Marston, 1970). Since that time there has been a profusion of research from a variety of disciplines. The majority of the research has been focused on patient adherence, although there is a smaller body of literature on the adherence of research staff to clinical protocols and a growing body of literature on provider adherence to treatment guidelines.

One of the issues that continues to arise in discussions of patient adherence is patient autonomy. Is nonadherence a patient right or is adherence a patient responsibility? This argument presumes that the patient is aware of his or her own behavior and has consciously decided not to follow a treatment regimen. The literature suggests that fewer than 20% of patients with medication regimens consciously decide not to engage in a treatment program. Those patients who have decided to follow the regimen but do not carry it out are unaware of episodic lapses in behavior or have difficulty in integration of the health care regimen into their lives. The most common reasons given by patients for lapses in adherence are forgetting and being too busy. This group comprises on average 40% to 50% or more of patients in a treatment regimen.

The problem of nonadherence is costly in terms of dollars and lives. The national pharmacy council estimates that nonadherence to pharmacological therapies costs approximately $100 billion annually (Grahl, 1994).

Although the cost of nonadherence to nonpharmacological therapies has not been estimated, the contribution to morbidity and mortality is high. Failures to quit smoking, to lose and maintain weight, to exercise regularly, to engage in safe sex practices, to avoid excess alcohol, and to use seat belts contribute significantly to declines in functional ability as well as to early mortality. Further data suggest that nonadherence to pharmacological as well as nonpharmacological therapies contributes to excess hospitalization and complication rates (Dunbar-Jacob & Schlenk, 1996).

Poor adherence then is a significant problem of direct relevance to nursing. Nurse practitioners may prescribe or recommend therapies. Home health and community nurses provide education and assistance in carrying out health care advice. Hospital, clinic, and office nurses provide education regarding treatment plans. There is a need for intervention studies that will guide practice as nurses prepare and support patients in the conduct of treatment regimens.

Research on adherence has been focused heavily on the determination of the extent of the problem and on predictors or contributing factors. Recent reports by the Cochrane Collaboration suggested that just 36 randomized controlled studies have evaluated interventions to improve medication adherence and examine both adherence and clinical indicators as outcomes. Fewer still have examined adherence to lifestyle behaviors. Most of these used general educational or behavioral counseling interventions. Just 1/3 of the interventions were found to have an effect on both adherence and outcome. Strategies that showed effectiveness were those that included components of self-management and/or enhanced attention by health professionals.

One problem in evaluating interventions and identifying relevant predictors is that of measurement. Most clinical studies have relied on self-report of adherence. There is a growing body of evidence indicating that individuals do not report accurately and those reports are biased toward an overestimate of performance. Thus, alternative strategies are being used to obtain better information, such as electronic monitors, PDAs and other technologies.

Future research on adherence should address strategies by which nurses can improve adherence to treatment regimens with attention directed toward various age groups, clinical populations, and regimen behaviors. The research would benefit from theoretical approaches to the problem of patient adherence and the design of intervention strategies. Effective strategies delivered by nurses have considerable promise of a favorable impact on health outcomes and costs (Dunbar-Jacob & Schlenk, 1996).

JACQUELINE DUNBAR-JACOB

Adolescence

Adolescence is a developmental stage distinct from childhood and adulthood. At what age the label *adolescence* is appropriate depends on the data source. The *Guide to Clinical Preventive Services* (U.S. Preventive Services, 1996a) uses ages 11 to 24 years. The most meaningful approach to this stage is to separate adolescence into three periods: (a) early adolescence, ages 10 to 14; (b) middle adolescence, ages 15 to 19; and (c) late adolescence, ages 20 to 24. During this transitional period adolescents reach physical and sexual maturity, develop more sophisticated reasoning ability, and make important educational and occupational decisions that will shape their adult careers.

The actual number of adolescents and their proportion in the U.S. population is increasing. This group represented 14% of the population in 1990, 13.9% in 1993, and 14.2% in 2002. Of the adolescent population, those between ages 10 and 14 years represent 53% compared to 47% between ages 15 and 19 years (U.S. Bureau of the Census, 2003). As a result, the cohort of adolescents will likely continue to increase in size. According to Day (1996) reasons for this increase include the fact that "baby boomers" are having children later in life, non-White populations are experiencing high fertility rates, and a large number of immigrants are in their 20s. Also, the percentage of adolescents within the White population (12.8%) is lower than that within the Hispanic (17.5%) or Black populations (17.1%). In 2001, the adolescent population between the ages of 10 and 19 consisted of 63.2% Whites not of Hispanic origin, 14.7% Blacks, 15.6% Hispanics, 3.6% Asian/Pacific Islanders, and 1% American Indians, Eskimos, and Aleuts; therefore, it is crucial for nurses to be culturally competent in order to care for adolescents (Health Research Service Administration, 2001; American Medical Association, 1999).

Common concerns by adolescents and their parents have been documented (Neinstein, Radzik, & Sherer, 2002). Adolescents' concerns include parental conflicts, peer interpersonal concerns, identity, school, social situations, depression, medical problems, psychosomatic issues, safety, and prospects for the future. Parents' concerns include acting-out behaviors, risk-taking, emotional lability, drug and alcohol use, academic problems, sexual activity, eating disorders, safety issues, peer influences, psychosomatic problems, and "wasting time." The authors concluded that any adolescent concern should lead to assessment. When problems involve high-risk violent or self-injurious behavior or a severe or chronic disorder, referral is required. Other issues can generally be handled by discussion and reassurance with family, health care providers, or other community resources.

Most adolescent mortality and morbidity results from behavior and lifestyle and therefore is preventable. Many behavior patterns developed during adolescence continue into adulthood, and most of the leading health problems of adults are those associated with behaviors initiated early in life (e.g., smoking). In the past 10 years, major advances have been made in understanding the health beliefs of adults and how these beliefs influence health-related behaviors. As our focus has turned to the early origins of health beliefs and behaviors, adolescence has increasingly become a focus of investigations. Researchers are making some progress in understanding how parental health attitudes and behaviors, social norms, peer pressures, and mass media affect teenagers; health-related beliefs and lifestyles. There is still much to learn regarding cognitive aspects (attitude, beliefs, perceptions), emotional aspects (feelings, concerns, moods, personality), social effects (norms, culture, environment, socioeconomic status), and biobehavioral (neurohormonal, psychoneuroimmunological) influences on the health practices of adolescents.

Before working with adolescents, nurses must understand how the egocentrism of this period influences behavior. Elkind (1984) described the "imaginary audience" as one consequence of adolescent egocentrism, that is, the assumption that everyone around them is watching them and is concerned about their appearance and behavior. Hence, they are very self-conscious and often go to extreme lengths to avoid what they are convinced will be mortifying experiences. Another consequence of the adolescent egocentrism and self-centeredness is the "personal fable," which is a set of beliefs in the uniqueness of one's feelings and one's immortality. Others often describe this belief as "It won't happen to me"—the story we tell ourselves, whether having sex without protection, driving fast, smoking, or drinking, that other people may experience the negative consequences but we will not.

Romer (2003) offered an excellent overview of research on risk reduction to promote the health of adolescents. Two important concepts related to adolescent lifestyles are (a) how adolescents organize their lives and pattern their behavior in ways that put them at lower or higher risk for serious health problems; and (b) how these patterns develop, persist, or cease at different times during the life span. Research topics included decision making, problem solving, peer and parental influence, personality, and specific risks: suicide, alcohol and other substance use, sexual activity, and gambling behaviors.

Most of the health problems of adolescents have their origins in environmental or behavioral factors. Reducing adolescent morbidity and mortality requires strategies that involve multiple approaches delivered through multiple settings, including schools, the mass media, communities, families, and health care settings. In addition, legislation that prevents adolescents' access to cigarettes, alcohol, and guns can promote health. Regardless of the approach, it is essential that all nurses understand how to provide culturally competent health care for adolescents.

ANN L. O'SULLIVAN
DONALD F. SCHWARZ

Adolescent Pregnancy and Parenting

The incidence of adolescent pregnancy has declined steadily in the U.S. since 1990 when rates peaked at 116.3 pregnancies per 1,000 teenage women (Ventura, Abma, Mosher, & Henshaw, 2003). The rate in 1999 was 86.7/1,000 (a decline of 25.4%). Similarly, the rate of births to adolescents has decreased. The 2002 rate of 42.9 births per 1,000 young women was 31% lower than the 1991 rate of 61.8 births/1,000. Adolescent birth rates have declined for all racial and ethnic groups and for all age subgroups: those under 15, those 15–17 years and those 18–19 years. Since 1990 the rate of decline in births has been slower for Hispanics than for non-Hispanic Whites or Blacks. In 1991, the Black teen birth rate at 118/1,000 young women was higher than that for Hispanics (105/1,000). By 2001 the Hispanic rate was 86/1,000 compared with the non-Hispanic Black rate of 74 births/1,000 or the non-Hispanic White rate of 30/1,000 adolescent women (Child Trends, 2003). Some of the declines in rates across all groups have been attributed to revisions in Census population estimates in 2000. This effect is greatest for Hispanic, Asian/Pacific Islander, and Native American adolescent girls (Arias, MacDorman, Strobino, & Gwyer, 2003).

Much research has been focused on understanding the impact of adolescent pregnancy and birth and on the development of programs to prevent pregnancy. Controversy remains about whether a single birth to an adolescent has negative effects on the life of that young woman or her infant (Geronimus, 2003). Also controversial is whether adolescent parenting prevention programs work (DiCenso, Guyatt, Willan, & Griffith, 2002; Kirby, 2002; Elfenbein & Felice, 2003). These programs have tended to focus broadly on issues ranging from abstinence, hormonal contraceptive and condom use, public policy change for welfare support for young mothers, and male-focused efforts.

In contrast, growing evidence suggests that parenting interventions may make a difference in outcomes for teens' infants (Coren, Barlow, & Stewart-Brown, 2003). Successful programs have included both group and individual interventions, programs that are home-based and those that require participation at a center or institution, and programs that involve both majority and minority teens. Early Head Start programs funded by the National Institute on Child Health and Human Development have recently begun to show promising outcomes with respect to maternal school attendance as well as child development (Love et al., 2002). Programs have not yet begun to look at the processes within the programs that have correlated with success by the infants.

ANN L. O'SULLIVAN
DONALD F. SCHWARZ

Adult Health

Human adulthood refers to the stages or phases of the life cycle after childhood and adolescence. It is the longest period of the life course. Physical, intellectual, educational, occupational, social, economic, spiritual, and health-related changes characterize the multiple stages of adulthood. The changes that take place in adulthood are of importance to nursing for two reasons. First is that adults, especially older adults, comprise the largest population served by nurses. Second is that adults are the parents or guardians of infants, children, and adolescents and the informal caregivers of elders. Adults make up the "family" that is the basic unit of nursing care; thus, they are the direct or indirect clients for essentially all of nursing care.

Ideally, nursing care and client education about self-care would be designed to produce the maximum positive benefit for clients. However, rarely are nursing actions designed to fit within the specific life stage, developmental stage, or personal contextual reality of adult clients.

The study of adult development is a 20th century phenomenon, ostensibly because people did not live long enough to merit inquiry in previous centuries. One notable exception was a treatise by Queletet published in 1842, entitled *A Treatise on Man and the Development of His Faculties*. G. Stanley Hall and E. L. Thorndike were two early 20th century scholars of the adult years. In mid-20th century, Erik Erikson (1959) published a set of life stages that expressed the middle-class norms of the 1940s and 1950s. Fortunately, he lived long enough to revise them and add additional stages as people lived ever longer. From 1960 through 1980, Neugarten (1968) and other investigators at the University of Chicago generated much of the work that serves as the foundation of extant theory on adult development.

The life-span perspective of adult development and aging is oriented to the scientific study of adult life stages and critical situations that most closely fits within the nursing goal to maximize quality of life for as much of the life span as possible. The life-span perspective focuses on change, continuity, and discontinuity over the life course. Each stage of adulthood has normative patterns, and as one stage folds into the next, personal changes occur and integration of these changes is necessitated. This process may produce anxiety, anger, frustration, and physiological stress responses during the transition while the conflicts between the old and the new self are resolved and the changes are integrated into the self-system. These stress responses frequently present to health care providers in the form of accidents, chemical abuse, violence, or acute or chronic illness. The conditions are rarely perceived or treated within the developmental context. Rather adults are decontextualized by health care professionals, who treat the immediate symptoms or condition while ignoring the adult context in which it occurs (Stevenson, 1993). Furthermore, health researchers, including nurse investigators, do not study health or care phenomena within the context of the adult life course.

One conception of the health of adults that has wide appeal in the medical community is attributable to Dubos (1965), who defined health as a state of equilibrium, adaptation, and harmony. Dunn (1980) went beyond mere equilibrium and devised the new concept of higher-level wellness. Dunn's concept of higher-level wellness embodied the idea of actualizing and maximizing human potential through the pursuit of three sub-goals: making progress toward a higher level of functioning, having an open-ended expanding goal to seek a fuller potential, and progressing toward a more integrated and mature human existence through the entire life course. Pender (1996; 2002) attempted to incorporate both Dunn's actualizing focus and Dubos's concept of health as maintaining stability through adaptation to the environment. According to Pender's thesis, health is the optimization of inherent and acquired human potential through goal-directed behavior, informed self-care, and satisfying relationships with others. Adjustments are made as needed to maintain structural integrity and harmony within the context of the environment. WHO representatives redefined health as a "resource" for everyday life, not an outcome or end product to be obtained at some definable point in time. According to the highly influential WHO Ottawa Charter (Kaplan, 1992), good health is viewed as a resource that goes hand in hand with social, economic, and personal development, and it is a critically important resource for attaining and maintaining a high-level quality of life for the entire life course. The goal is to "live long and die short;" this implies avoiding chronic diseases and disabilities and dying of old age at the natural end of the human life span.

The prevailing theories about physical normality and the adult stages have changed since the 1960s. The prolongation of physical well-being has become a norm as humans are living ever longer, even in third world countries. Although the stages of adulthood differ by theorist, the middle stages have been expanded to accommodate the acceleration of longevity. Young adulthood lasts from about 18 to about 29; the core or traditional middle years encompass the years from 30 to 50 (50 was the average life span in 1900); the new middle years cover the years from about 51 to either 65 or 70, depending on the theorist. Young old age covers the period from either 65 or 70 to 75; middle old age extends to 85, and old-old age, or the frail age, is 85 and beyond. The latter three ages are relatively new designations and are evolving. It is quite likely that during the first 3 decades of the 21st century, as the baby boomers move into the higher age brackets, the old-old age designation will move upward and begin at age 90 or higher.

Different aspects of development are dominant in different stages of adulthood. The biological self reaches its peak in the middle 20s, and then a very gradual decline in physiological efficiency in organ systems occurs during the next 7 or 8 decades. The rate of change is mediated by genetics, lifestyle, and environment, but everyone experiences the decline. There is a rise in cognitive abilities in young adulthood that does not peak for most until middle age, and these abilities then decline at an even slower rate than the physical parameters. Emotional and spiritual development is postulated to continue well into old age and to peak near death for the cognitively and emotionally healthy. Any of these norms may be altered for individuals by genetics, mental or physical illness, catastrophic emotional events, or other significant situations. In the ideal world, health professionals would be cognizant of the developmental stage of each adult client and formulate care to match the needs and context of that stage (Stevenson, 1993). This ideal assumes that the necessary knowledge base exists, but it does not.

Although much has been learned, there is great difficulty in trying to separate the impact of lifestyle from what is ultimately possible for adult health under ideal conditions. This is true not only for the biological possibilities but also for the socioemotional realm and for the development of intellect, creativity, and wisdom. Much of the extant research is plagued by the inability of researchers to disentangle the overlay of familial and cultural expectations, cohort-specific life experiences, the environment, and idiosyncratic tendencies. What is generally considered normal for men or women during the major stages of adult life is open to criticism as being tied to specific historical periods (e.g., studies done in the 1950s or the 1980s), to expectations within an age cohort (e.g., those whose childhood occurred during the early years of television versus the internet age), to gender differences that were influenced by prevailing values and expectations (e.g., prewomen's liberation or sexual liberation), or to physical adult health status in light of varying mores about smoking, fat or carbohydrate intake, and exercise.

Cultural, cohort, and gender-expectation biases can be overcome to some extent with cross-cultural or cross-sequential designs. Nurse researchers were challenged to do more of their adult health research contextually tied to the specific adult ages and stages of their subjects (Stevenson, 1993). Even now, most nursing research either erroneously lumps three or more distinct adult stages into one group (e.g., 25 to 60) or makes up anti-developmental age categories (e.g., 25 to 45, 45 to 65, and 65 and above). Developmental and situational confounders abound in data categorized and analyzed in this anti-theoretical manner. Findings would be more valid and reliable, even about purely physiological phenomena, if scientifically based adult life stages were used as the grouping categories in research on adult health.

JOANNE SABOL STEVENSON

Advance Directives

Since the early 1970s, Americans have been encouraged to complete advance directives to ensure that physicians and family members will know their end-of-life treatment wishes in the event that they become unable to participate in decision making. Many Americans fear becoming trapped in a dehumanizing medical system that ignores their personal goals and wishes, robs them of privacy and dignity, and prolongs their dying with painful and ineffective technological interventions. Health care providers, educators, and those involved in health care policy maintain that, in order to avoid unwanted end-of-life situations, decisionally capable adults can extend their current autonomy into the future by participating in advance care planning and completing advance directives (ADs).

There are two general forms that these legal documents take. The *instructive directive* (i.e., living will) aims to direct future medical interventions by stipulating in writing a preferred course of action such as the refusal of particular therapies, or less commonly, requesting that all life-extending measures be used, in the event that the patient loses the ability to directly participate in health care decisions. Although each state stipulates and defines the conditions under which ADs become operational, honoring the instructions in living wills is invariably contingent upon a clinician's determination that the patient has lost decisional capacity and that he or she has a "terminal" or "incurable" condition. Both of these qualifying conditions require a medical judgment to be made.

The *proxy directive* (i.e., durable power of attorney for health care) designates a person to function as a surrogate decision maker and make all medical decisions in the event that the patient loses decision-making capacity. Treatment decisions made by the surrogate are expected to be consistent with those that would have been made by the now incompetent patient, a standard of decision making known as "substituted judgment." Some state statutes combine written and appointment directions in one document. A decision not to attempt cardiopulmonary resuscitation is another form of ADs and is usually made by a surrogate following a physician recommendation, when the physician determines that a resuscitation attempt would either be medically futile or extraordinarily burdensome in light of the patient's current condition.

Since 1976, when the first so-called "right-to-die" case involving Karen Ann Quinlan was decided, members of the public, religious groups, and health care professionals have engaged in a vigorous debate about the acceptability of stopping life-prolonging treatment and allowing death to occur. The individuals at the center of these early "right-to-die" cases were almost always young adults who had lost decisional capacity, often as a result of a traumatic injury, and left no written documentation or clear verbal instructions about their end-of-life treatment wishes. Their family members had to petition the courts in order to stop unwanted life-prolonging treatments. In 1990, the United States Supreme Court upheld Missouri's evidentiary standard that required "clear and convincing evidence" of the then vegetative Nancy Cruzan's wishes before permitting her family to discontinue the tube feedings that were sustaining her life.

In order to better inform the public about the expected benefits of advance directives and encourage their use, Congress passed the Patient Self-Determination Act of 1990. This Federal legislation requires all health care institutions to inform newly admitted patients about ADs and offer them assistance in completing a directive. Individual state legislatures have provided additional support for ADs; all 50 states have completed some form of statutory recognition of these documents. Despite a great deal of effort and subsequent publicity that included syndicated newspaper columns by Ann Landers and "Dear Abby" among other attempts to educate and motivate the public about these documents, completion rates for advance directives continue to range from 4% to 25% (Perkins, 2000). Even when patients have completed an AD, clinicians observe that they are often unavailable, or not applicable in many situations involving critically ill adults (Tonelli, 1996).

Researchers are now examining how ADs actually function in various clinical settings, and are exploring whether the presence of an AD ensures compliance with patients' end-of-life treatment wishes. Others are questioning the very relevance of ADs to advance care planning (Perkins, 2000; Drought & Koenig, 2002). Nonetheless, surveys of patients and health care professionals have consistently demonstrated widespread support for the *idea* of ADs as an effective means to ensure that end-of-life interventions conform with patients' wishes. Studies have found that while ADs are reassuring to patients who complete them, they do not ensure that a patient's end-of-life wishes will be followed. In a study by Tierney et al. (2001), investigators found that discussions about ADs improved the care satisfaction of elderly patients with chronic illnesses, but a second study found that having an 'instructional' AD did not increase the likelihood that family decision makers would make treatment choices that accurately reflected the patient's end-of-life wishes as stipulated in the AD (Ditto et al., 2001). Ditto and colleagues also found that family members' predictions of what the patient would want were correct less than 70% of the time, and families were two to three times as likely to make errors of over-treatment as under-treatment—e.g., approving life-sustaining treatments the patient would not have wanted under the circumstances.

In a study by geriatric nurse researchers that aimed to explore advance care planning (ACP) and end-of-life care for nursing home residents who were hospitalized during the last 6 weeks of life, Happ and colleagues (2002) found that the primary focus of ACP in the nursing home was on cardiopulmonary resuscitation preferences. By so limiting ACP discussions, end-of-life treatment choices were inappropriately constrained and oversimplified, with the result that the benefits of palliative or hospice end-of-life interventions were underutilized. In another study, researchers aimed to evaluate the effect of an ACP intervention on the completion of ADs and patient satisfaction among persons with HIV/AIDS. Although the rate of completion for ADs went from 16.4% to 40.7% following three face-to face counseling sessions about ADs, it was subsequently noted that 23% of the completed ADs were deemed legally invalid (Ho, Thiel, Rubin, & Singer, 2000).

Another group of researchers compared the accuracy of substituted judgments made by primary care physicians, hospital-based physicians, and family surrogates on behalf of elderly outpatients, and explored the effectiveness of ADs in improving the accuracy of those judgments. Coppola, Ditto, Danks, and Smucker (2001) found that familiarity with the patient's AD did not improve the accuracy of substituted judgments for primary care physicians or family surrogates; it did increase the accuracy of the judgments made by hospital-based physicians.

Drought and Koenig (2002), nurse ethicists, conducted an ethnographic, longitudinal study of terminally ill patients with solid tumor cancer or AIDS that explored the difficult medical decisions each patient faced in the course of their illness and treatment. These researchers concluded that shared decision making is illusory, terminal patients frequently resist advance care planning, and hold values other than autonomy as important. They cited substantial support for their observations that no studies to date have shown that ADs significantly facilitated end-of-life decision making, truly direct care, or saved resources at the end of life.

Many commentators noted the following difficulties associated with use of instructive directives: incomplete information, the inability to anticipate future medical conditions, and uncertainty regarding the meaning and intent of written instructions. These problems of interpretation require clinicians to seek information from others in the attempt to determine what the patient "really meant" (Tonelli, 1996). Tonelli and others concluded that, because of the limitations associated with the use of instructive directives, proxy directives are the preferred form of AD (Dexter, Wolinsky, Gramelspachar, Eckert, & Tierney, 2003; Perkins, 2000; Tonelli). Clearly, there is a need for further research to explore whether ADs facilitate good end-of-life care, and nurses are ideally situated to direct and participate in furthering understanding of these documents.

JUDITH KENNEDY SCHWARZ

Advanced Practice Nurses

Advanced practice nursing is described as the application of an expanded range of practical, theoretical, and research-based therapeutics to phenomena experienced by patients within a specialized clinical area of the larger discipline of nursing (Hamric, Spross, & Hanson, 1996). The history and evolution of advanced practice nursing is a tapestry of patient care provided by expert nurses who have expanded the boundaries and scope of the practice of nursing.

Advanced practice nurses (APNs) need basic core competencies to fulfill the advanced practice nursing role. These competencies include skills in expert clinical practice, consultation, teaching and coaching, research, leadership, collaboration, change agency, and ethical decision making. APNs offer high levels of autonomous decision making in the assessment, diagnosis, and management of patients. Conceptually, the practice is nursing-based, with emphasis on health promotion, disease prevention, and education of patients and families. Advanced practice nurses must have a graduate degree in nursing in a chosen specialty and are differentiated by the ability to carry out direct, expert clinical practice. Although advanced practice nursing is an evolving field, currently the role of the APN is limited to nurse practitioners, clinical nurse specialists, certified nurse midwives, and certified registered nurse anesthetists, who provide direct clinical care for patients.

One of the hallmarks of advanced practice nursing is the commitment to collaboration with other disciplines. Advanced practice nurses work within the designated scope of practice and collaborate with or refer to other professional colleagues those patients and problems that fall beyond the expertise of APNs.

Advanced practice nursing and the practice roles, issues, and evaluation of the four groups of APNs (nurse practitioners, certified nurse midwives, certified registered nurse anesthetists, and clinical nurse specialists) serve as a rich and comprehensive base for nursing research. Patient-centered outcomes research that explores outcomes of patients served by APNs is central to the health care system that is unfolding in the United States. The overused Office of Technology Assessment study of 1986, which evidenced the safety and satisfaction of using APNs to improve access to health care, can no longer be cited as the only research support for the education and practice of APNs. Health policy–based nursing research that explores workforce demographics, cost, reimbursement, and privileging, as well as the credentialing and regulation of APNs, is an undisputed data need. Nursing research focused in the realm of managed care and interdisciplinary, collaborative approaches to care is a highly sought after commodity. Research into the education and evaluation of APNs is critical to health policy forecasting and workforce planning.

Advanced practice nurse researchers who engage in clinical practice are the key to most of the research topics outlined above. Clinically based research networks that allow for data generation on patient outcomes are the single most important research agenda for the decade. Advanced nursing practice research, as a part of nursing as a whole, offers researchers the ability to explore new and expanding areas that support the use of expert nurses as competent, sought-after providers of primary and specialty care for the American people.

CHARLENE M. HANSON

Ageism

Ageism is defined as a negative attitude or bias toward older people that can lead to a belief that older people cannot or should not participate in certain activities or be given the same opportunities as younger persons (Holohan-Bell & Brummel-Smith, 1999). Ageism, according to geriatrician Robert Butler in his book *Why Survive*, suggests that there is a deep and profound prejudice against older people (Butler, 1975).

By 2030, it is projected that over 20% of the population will be 65 and older. Almost all health care personnel will find themselves at one time or another caring for the elderly. In fact, the majority of nurses will spend most of their career caring for older adults in a variety of settings. As these challenges are met, it is necessary to continually examine the development of attitudes and roles in the prevention of ageism. Older persons may be discriminated against because of the way they look, speak, or function in a society that values productivity, economic wealth, speed, youth, and beauty.

How to define aging and the aging process is a controversial topic. Prejudice and stereotyping may lead to policies for rationing health care: withholding treatment based on age alone, a lack of qualified personnel to care for older adults, the underrepresentation of older adults in clinical trials, and the underrecognition of geriatric problems and syndromes (Haight, Christ, & Dias, 1994; Bogardus, Yneh, & Shekelle, 2003; Alliance for Aging Research, 2003). Ageism may also be seen on a personal level when a nurse or other health care worker has low expectations of an older person's ability to perform a task. Ageism may lead staff to perceive that an older adult does not "know what is going on" and individuals may be excluded from decision making during hospitalization and care. Ageism may exist on a population level when older adults are excluded from disease screening or primary prevention programs.

Nursing research in ageism has centered on several main areas including education, student and practicing nurse's attitudes, socio-political issues, clinical care, and biological issues such as the differentiation of normal aging and disease processes. Several early nursing studies highlighted the problem of student attitudes toward aging and care of the older adult, the lack of trained professionals in gerontology, and the need for more research in gerontology.

The older population that is at the greatest risk of prejudice and stereotyping, however, are persons with mental illness, dementia, and mental retardation. The diagnosis of dementia often stigmatizes both the patient and the family. Research by Beck and others has helped explain aggressive behaviors in persons with dementia by illustrating the need for individualized care and behavioral systems theory to understand aggression in Alzheimer's disease patient. This has promoted autonomy and personal control in the care of persons with dementia, and has highlighted the need for greater resources to care for older adults with mental illness (Rice, Beck, & Stevenson, 1997; Buckwalter, Maas, & Reed, 1997; Beck et al., 1997; Sherrell, Anderson, & Buckwalter, 1998). Other research on dementia has advanced the understanding of persons with dementia and has exposed myths often held about this population (Strumpf & Evans, 1988; Evans, Strumpf, Allen-Taylor, et al., 1997; Sherrel & Buckwalter, 1997; Frengley & Mion, 1998; Minnick, Mion, Leipzig, Lamb, & Palmer, 1998; Mezey & Fulmer, 1998; Brod, Stewart, & Sands, 1999; Volicer, Hurley, & Camberg, 1999; Fick & Foreman, 2000; Fick, Agostini, & Inouye, 2002). This research is important as it forces the reexamination of stereotypes held about older persons with dementia, and influences both care and treatment of older persons.

Ageism will continue to be important in almost every area of geriatric nursing research. Ageism will influence both the type of research that is done and the public dissemination of research. Researchers must describe the relationship of ageism with qualitative and quantitative research in the areas of ethics, workplace studies, decision making and informed consent research, genetics, health promotion and preventive screening, cancer, presentations of disease, symptom research, biomarkers of aging, quality of life, barriers to treatment, nursing home care and organizational studies, resource utilization in health care, dementia care, mental health, and the care of the disabled older adult.

Researchers have agreed that past experiences with the elderly and faculty role models affect attitudes (Wilhite & Johnson, 1976;

Chaisson, 1980; Penner, Ludenia, & Mead, 1984; Fox & Wold, 1996). Several government and privately funded programs are promoting positive attitudes toward older adults by showcasing geriatric nursing as a challenging and attractive specialty for practicing nurses, bringing national attention to nursing care of the elderly, reaching out to hospital, home care, and nursing home nurses, and illustrating the need for more advanced practice nurses and basic gerontology content in baccalaureate nursing programs (Abraham et al., 1999; Fulmer & Abraham, 1998; Titler & Mentes, 1999).

Nursing has had a vital role in combating ageism and continues to be in a key position to minimize ageist attitudes in the future. Nurses must be involved in future studies to investigate these important and relevant areas of research. In addition, nurses must be prominent in other relevant arenas (intergenerational linkages, global attitudes on aging) that challenge stereotypes of aging and promote appropriate views and care of older adults. Perhaps the most lasting and powerful way to combat ageism is through the mentoring of other practicing nurses, nurses in training, and young adults, and through active dialogue with older persons.

Donna Fick

Alcohol Dependence

The DSM-IV (American Psychiatric Association, 1994) diagnostic term for alcoholism is alcohol dependence. Although many people still use the older term "alcoholism." Alcohol dependence is a chronic relapsing disease involving craving for, loss of control over, physical dependence on, and higher than normal tolerance for alcohol. The excessive intake of alcohol over time leads to social, emotional, and physical damage to health, interpersonal/familial relationships, and occupational status. It is a primary disease with genetic, psychological, lifestyle, and environmental causal influences that have not been adequately differentiated to date.

Alcohol is a solvent that permeates all body cells, including the blood-brain barrier, and has lipid-dissolving qualities. It is this latter quality that leads to findings that moderate drinking decreases fatty plaques in blood vessels and thus decreases the risk for heart attacks. Alcohol is a depressant drug and continued abuse leads to negative psychological and physical detriments including hypertension, cardiac arrhythmias, cardiomyopathy, hemorrhagic stroke, liver damage, distortions and errors in conceptual thought processes, memory decrements, depression, increased risk for all types of accidents, and risk for suicide.

Measuring alcohol intake presents research challenges. The amount of alcohol in a standard drink differs across countries and is made more complex by the fact that beer, wine, and other drinks may contain differing percentages of pure alcohol. Generally in the U.S. a standard drink is 12 ounces (oz.) of beer or wine cooler, 5 oz. of wine, or 1.5 oz. of 80 proof distilled spirits; that is, approximately 12 grams of pure alcohol per drink. Collecting data about alcohol intake is complex; in addition to the basic measure of a standard drink, it is crucial to determine the number of drinks consumed in a week or a month, the duration of the current and any prior patterns of alcohol intake, the number of drinks consumed in one drinking episode (binge drinking is defined as five or more drinks for a man and four or more for a woman during one episode), and the number of binge episodes during the past month/year.

Although many survey instruments and biomarkers exist to measure the amounts and effects of alcohol intake, no single approach is valid and reliable for men and women; across age groups; or for differentiating among binge drinking, alcohol abuse, and alcohol dependence. Blood alcohol level only reveals intake within recent hours, but does not inform about recurring or chronic intake. Carbohydrate deficient transferrin informs about longer term heavy drinking, but has acceptable sensitivity and specificity primarily for young adult and middle-aged men; it is much less valid for older men and for women of all ages. Most other biomarkers are not specific to alcohol effects, but simply report abnormalities in liver enzymes or hematological contents. There is also a measurement issue related to abstinence in comparison groups; it is essential to separate out "sick quitters" from lifelong abstainers or very low quantity users. Otherwise the results of studies are contaminated by the presence of subjects with alcohol-related sequelae (i.e. sick quitters) in the abstainer group.

Young adults, especially men, have the highest rate of drinking, binge drinking, and heavy drinking. Women at all ages drink less, but are at higher risk for negative effects of alcohol. The reasons have not been clearly explicated, but lower body water to lipid content and less muscle mass are generally accepted facts. More controversial is the hypothesis that women produce much less alcohol dehydrogenase, thus increasing the time necessary for first pass metabolism and prolonging the half-life of pure alcohol in body systems. Whatever the cause, women experience higher levels of cardiac, liver, and other system dysfunctions and psychological distress (depression and suicide attempts) earlier in their drinking histories and at much lower quantities compared to men. These findings led to the NIAAA (1995) guideline for moderate drinking of two standard drinks per day for young and middle adult men and one standard drink per day for non-pregnant women of all ages and elderly men.

Fetal alcohol syndrome (FAS) and alcohol-related birth defects (ARBD) are manifestations of neuro-developmental insults that result from alcohol ingestion by the mother during pregnancy. The negative effects are especially marked during periods of fetal brain growth spurts and continue during the postnatal period for breast-fed infants of drinking mothers. Consequences of FAS, and the milder form ARBD, include impaired attention, intelligence, memory, motor coordination, complex problem solving, and abstract thinking. There are also physical stigmata that attend FAS including abnormal facial features and other anatomical alterations (Connor & Streissguth, 1996).

Alcohol consumption differs among the three main ethnic groups in the U.S. (Caetano, Clark, & Tan, 1998). In general frequent heavy drinking and binge drinking has decreased among White men (from 20% in 1984 to 12% in 1995), but has remained stable among Black and Hispanic men (15% and 18% respectively in both years). Frequent heavy drinking is much less prevalent among all groups of women (2–5%). Within-group differences exist for ethnic minorities depending on where they were born. Asians, Pacific Islanders, and Hispanics who were born in the U.S. have higher rates of heavy drinking than those who immigrated to the U.S. Unfortunately, Blacks and Hispanics who have alcohol problems are much less likely to seek treatment compared to Whites.

Alcohol dependence is treatable with medication regimens (especially for detoxification), individual and family counseling, support groups, and self-help groups—primarily Alcoholics Anonymous and the 12 Step Program. Relapses are common, but the key is to get the drinker back into treatment and after-care following each relapse and eventually sobriety can be attained and maintained. Family solidarity is required to stop all cover-ups on behalf of the drinker. It is important that the drinker experience the full consequences of the drinking without being rescued so that continued denial of the effects of the drinking becomes impossible.

The research opportunities in this field are myriad. At the fundamental science level research is needed on the root causes of alcohol dependence including the role of genetics. The reasons for the excess risk among women merit considerably more research attention. Social, behavioral, and cultural studies are in order to address the many unanswered questions about adolescent drinking, college binge drinking, late onset alcohol dependence among elders, and differential risk for alcohol problems among ethnic minorities. Theory-based interventions should be developed and tested to enhance the case finding, referral, and successful treatment for adolescents, women, minorities, elderly persons, and white men. In the area of measurement, the current paper and pencil survey instruments are biased toward white men and toward the young and middle aged. New biomarkers must be developed that are sensitive and specific for women and for older adults. These are but a few of the many areas available for future inquiry.

JOANNE SABOL STEVENSON

Alzheimer's Disease

Alzheimer's disease (AD) is a progressively degenerative neurological disorder (syndrome) that results in impaired cognition, mood, behavior, and function. Dr. Alois Alzheimer (1906) first described the disorder in a published case report on a 52-year-old patient who suffered from psychosis, memory loss, agnosia (impaired sensory perception), apraxia (impairments in carrying out tasks), and aphasia (impaired communication). After the patient's death, Dr. Alzheimer performed an autopsy and discovered clumps—senile plaques—and knots—neurofibrillary tangles—in the patient's brain (Dharmarajan & Ugalino, 2003).

One hundred years later, despite decades of research, there remains no known etiology or cure for the disease. The diagnosis relies on a thorough clinical history and physical examination, including mental status testing, both to establish a diagnosis and to rule out other causes of dementia, such as brain tumors, metabolic disorders, or infection. Many genetic and nongenetic factors, such as estrogen, nonsteroidal anti-inflammatory medication, and apolipoprotein (apoE) alleles, have been speculatively associated with AD; researchers continue to discover definitive links between these factors and the illness.

Due to the lack of a diagnostic marker and the associated difficulties in diagnosing early-stage AD, precise prevalence rates are difficult to determine. Although a rare familial form of AD (afflicting people between 30 and 60 years of age) exists the disease is more prevalent as people age. Dementia, notably AD, affects only 1% of those between 60 and 64 years of age, with the number of cases doubling every 5 years in people over 65 (Beers & Berkow, 2000). In 2000, 40% (1.8 million) of people over 85 years of age were estimated to be afflicted with the disease. As a result of the rapidly aging U.S. population, the next 50 years is expected to show a threefold increase in the number of people with AD (Hebert, Scherr, Bienias, Bennett, & Evans, 2003).

Alzheimer's disease has a protracted downward trajectory. The average length of the disease is 8 years, but it can span up to 20 years (National Institute of Aging, 1995). As a result of its progressively degenerative course, symptom progression is typically divided into three stages: mild, moderate, and severe. Mild symptoms consist of personality changes, memory loss, and impaired word finding. As the disease progresses, the initial symptoms worsen, with AD sufferers often developing increased behavioral problems such as wandering, physical and verbal aggression, and resistance to personal care (grooming and hygiene). In the severe stage, the AD sufferer is profoundly cognitively and functionally disabled, typically requiring 24-hour care. Death usually results from an infectious process such as pneumonia.

Care is provided primarily by family members, and an estimated 75% of older adults with dementia are cared for at home (Dunkin & Anderson-Hanley, 1998). This care is primarily uncompensated and includes emotional, physical, and financial assistance. As the disease progresses, families are increasingly burdened in trying to provide care, often suffering adverse personal physical and psychosocial consequences (Ory, Hoffman, Yee, Tennstedt, & Schultz, 1999). AD causes severe cognitive impairments, and families are often forced to make decisions for the AD sufferer (e.g., whether to resuscitate or whether to institutionalize), without the guidance of advance directives.

Treatments for AD are multiple and vary by illness stage. Pharmacologic treatments include medications to improve cognition, treat depression, or treat behavioral symptoms (e.g., physical aggression or agitation). Because each person with AD experiences a unique confluence of symptoms, treatment strategies require careful tailoring to meet the respective needs of each person.

Researchers have discovered decreased levels of acetylcholine in the brains of AD sufferers; thus, acetylcholinesterase inhibitors are indicated in the mild to moderate stages of AD to slow the progressive cognitive decline. Some families have reported that these drugs resulted in some amelioration of behavioral symptoms. Certain behavioral symptoms, such as physical aggression or agitation, may require antipsychotic medications. However, these drugs often are associated with increased confusion, resulting in decreased function, and therefore require a careful risk-benefit analysis and ongoing evaluation of their effectiveness. Benzodiazepines are generally not useful for the control of behavioral symptoms and have been associated with increased falls in older adults (Frenchman, Capo, & Hass, 2000). Depression is a common comorbid condition with AD, requiring early recognition and treatment—both pharmacologic and non-pharmacologic—aimed at maximizing function and minimizing additional disability.

Certain behavioral symptoms (e.g., wandering, verbal aggressiveness, or resistance to personal grooming) do not respond favorably to pharmacologic therapy. These symptoms require environmental modifications and behavioral strategies. AD sufferer's agnosia, combined with other cognitive deficits (e.g., memory loss or lack of insight/judgment), often results in unsafe behaviors. For instance, AD sufferers may turn on stoves and then forget to turn them off. They may inadvertently drink toxic substances or step into a bathtub of scalding water. Driving becomes increasingly unsafe. Each AD sufferer needs to be evaluated for possible sources of injury, and strategies must be initiated to safeguard living environments. In institutional settings, similar types of environmental modifications are needed to ensure the person's safety. Many assisted living and skilled nursing facilities have dedicated units designed to address the specific needs of this population.

Behavioral strategies are extremely varied, typically successful, and do not have the unfavorable side-effect profiles of many of the medications used to treat behavioral symptoms. Diversion and redirection to a preferred activity remain highly successful strategies to deal with problems related to the AD sufferer's short- and long-term memory loss. Reality orientation is often unsuccessful, so validation therapy (Feil, 2002) is the preferred form of communication. Validation therapy techniques include carefully attending to a confused older adult's expressions of impaired cognition (e.g., thinking past events are occurring in the present) and responding with acceptance and empathy. In communicating with confused older adults, careful attention also needs to be taken to provide implements such as hearing aides or glasses, to compensate for sensory losses.

Physical restraints typically increase agitation and are not associated with a decrease in falls (Strumpf, Robinson, Wagner, & Evans, 1998). Individual and family therapy should be encouraged, to assist families in planning and preparing for the sufferer's future needs. Support groups, in particular the Alzheimer's support groups, are also an excellent source of information and assistance. In the latter stage of AD, hospice is another source of family support.

AD research is overwhelmingly biomedical, attempting to uncover a cause, better treatment, or a cure for the illness. Many behavioral strategies have been researched and reported to be clinically successful in treating AD, including music therapy, reminiscence therapy, strategies to prevent wandering, and therapy animals. Although positive results have been reported in utilizing behavioral strategies, the methodological limitations of the studies (small sample sizes, sampling bias, short evaluation periods, and lack of consideration of confounding variables) affect the scientific rigor of these findings (Beavis, Simpson, & Graham, 2002).

The rapidly aging U.S. society and subsequent increase in the number of people with

AD afford unique nursing opportunities and challenges. Most AD sufferers live in the community and are cared for by their families. Families interface with the health care delivery system at various points in time along the trajectory. It is then that nurses, in collaboration with people in other disciplines, can provide needed assistance to families struggling to manage in the face of this devastating illness.

MARY SHELKEY

Angina

Angina pectoris, a major manifestation of myocardial ischemia, is found in 13.7% of women and 21% of men aged 65–69 (Mittlemark et al., 1993). In women aged 70–84 the prevalence is 19% and in those 85 and older it is 24.7%. In men aged 70 and older the prevalence of angina is 27.3%. Although angina usually indicates the presence of underlying coronary heart disease (CHD), myocardial ischemia can result from a variety of conditions that lead to an imbalance between oxygen supply and demand, for example, left ventricular hypertrophy and aortic valve stenosis. Myocardial ischemia, however, frequently occurs in the absence of angina or its equivalents (jaw pain, numbness, dyspnea, fatigue, or nonspecific symptoms related to transient left ventricular dysfunction). Angina, therefore, is neither a reliable nor sensitive marker of myocardial ischemia. Many elderly have atypical findings or have totally asymptomatic CHD. Nursing research, therefore, must be directed at these different CHD presentations.

Atypical angina manifested by nontypical chest, shoulder, or back pain, dyspnea, pulmonary edema, and cardiac arrhythmias (Gibbons, Bachulis, & Allen, 1999), along with atypical presentation of myocardial infarction (MI) are common the prevalence increasing with increasing age (Tresch & Alla, 2001). The presence of chest pain with MI may occur in fewer than 20% of the elderly presenting with MI. Atypical symptoms or absence of symptoms may not only lead to underdiagnosis of CHD, but in the setting of MI, to delay in seeking treatment and in diagnosis (Tresch & Alla). This may contribute to a higher morbidity and mortality (Tresch & Alla). Differentiation of atypical symptoms from other chronic conditions is difficult, and MI may not even be suspected. Individuals may often present with dyspnea, gastrointestinal (GI) symptoms, syncope, stroke, confusion, faintness, giddiness, weakness, or restlessness. The individual who has suffered an unrecognized MI days to weeks earlier may in fact present to the hospital in heart failure (HF) or with recurrent angina. MI may also be the result of another primary process causing an increase in demand or a decrease in flow, such as intercurrent illness, GI bleed, or HF. Since prompt recognition and treatment of MI is crucial to limiting infarct size and preserving myocardial function, it is vital that nursing research address issues central to atypical presentation (Reilly, Dracup, Dattolo, & King, 1994; Dracup & Moser, 1991; Funk, Naum, Milner, & Chyun, 2001) such as: identification of anginal equivalents, factors that delay decision to seek treatment (perception of symptoms and expectations), caregiver reactions to symptoms, health care provider recognition, assessment strategies, and educational interventions aimed at reducing delay in seeking treatment.

Despite the limitation of using angina as a sole marker of CHD, the presence of angina supports the diagnosis of CHD and is useful in assessing disease progression and efficacy of medical management. However, implementation of primary and secondary CHD prevention has been shown to be lacking and health care provider noncompliance with established guidelines is high (Feder, Griffiths, Eldridge, & Spence, 1999; Rolka, Fagot, Campagna, & Narayan, 2001). Nursing has an important role in studying dissemination and adoption of guidelines for secondary prevention established by the American College of Cardiology (ACC)/American Heart Association (AHA) to the elderly and their health care providers (Smith et al., 2001; Pearson et al., 2002; Williams et al., 2002; Gibbons, Chatterjee, et al., 1999), with careful attention to use of aspirin, encouragement of physical activity, and control of lipids, HTN, obesity, and smoking, along with side effects associated with these interventions (Abete et al., 2001). In addition, nursing research focused on provider and patient-related factors contributing to inadequate CHD risk factor control is urgently needed, along with strategies to improve compliance with guidelines.

The importance and feasibility of optimizing self-management of CHD risk factors, including from a nursing perspective, have been demonstrated. Additional studies are needed in the elderly population, who are often excluded from intervention trials, and who are often confronted with comorbidites and a lack of social and financial resources. In addition, consideration of psychosocial factors specific to the elderly that influence CHD management is also warranted. Psychosocial (social support and interactions and relationships between persons managing the condition), personal (self-efficacy, denial, lack of motivation, educational, lifestyle, beliefs and past experience with management), environmental, and cultural influences which may contribute to CHD management and quality of life which may be affected by control of CHD, have not been widely studied in the elderly population. Anxiety and depression, may not only adversely affect CHD-risk-reduction behaviors, but have a role in the development of CHD and adverse CHD outcomes (Hegleson & Heidi, 1999; Sullivan, LaCroix, Spertus, & Hecht, 2000; van Elderen, Maes, & Dusseldore, 1999). The importance of depression and social support has been well documented especially in individuals with CHD (Stuart-Shor, Buselli, Carroll, & Forman, 2003); however, few interventional studies have extended these findings. Psychosocial and educational factors have been linked to how individuals perceive their own health status and manage chronic illness; these require further study, along with the influence of other comorbid conditions.

While assessment and management of typical and atypical angina are important problems, myocardial ischemia and infarction can also exist in the total absence of signs and symptoms, and unrecognized MI is common (Tresch & Alla, 2001). Individuals with asymptomatic ischemia tend to have a higher incidence of asymptomatic MI, underscoring the importance of detecting ischemia early in its course. Silent episodes outnumber symptomatic episodes in patients with chronic stable angina, unstable angina, and in asymptomatic patients following MI. Silent ischemia, present in 50,000 to 100,000 persons following MI and in 3 million persons with angina, along with symptomatic ischemia during daily activities, extent of CHD, the degree of left ventricular dysfunction, unstable angina, is associated with an adverse prognosis. Asymptomatic ischemia may also occur in the absence of known CHD and is frequently found in individuals with lower extremity arterial disease and diabetes. Recently, it has been shown that in older adults with type 2 diabetes (T2DM) without known CHD, 22% have CHD in the absence of symptoms (Wackers et al., 2004). Widespread screening of the elderly for asymptomatic CHD, however, has not been accomplished, so the true prevalence in the elderly population is not known.

The asymptomatic nature of CHD, particularly in individuals with diabetes mellitus (DM), presents a unique challenge in primary and secondary prevention as the large areas of potentially jeopardized myocardium are commonly found in these individuals. Not only are these individuals at risk for adverse CHD outcomes, but without cues such as angina, the individual may not be motivated to engage in control of CHD risk factors (Rockwell & Riegel, 2001) or know how to modify their activities. Although it has been shown that intensive lifestyle interventions and medical management in individuals with known CAD who also have asymptomatic myocardial ischemia may improve outcomes, little is known about the behavioral (Chyun & Minicucci, 2002; Chyun & Melkus, 2002) and psychological factors (Chyun, Melkus, et al.) that may contribute to control of CHD risk factors in this population. Additionally, in individuals with known CHD undergoing revascularization, quality of life (QOL) has been shown to predict long-term outcomes, disease progression, and response to therapy; however, little is known regarding QOL in individuals with asymptomatic myocardial ischemia (Chyun, Khuwatsamrit et al., 2003). Much needs to be determined regarding the individual and health care system factors that contribute to self-management of T2DM and CHD risk factors, as well as interventions that will successfully reduce their burden of risk.

Nursing also has an important role in identifying individuals with asymptomatic ischemia. Early studies suggested that a defect in pain perception may account for lack of anginal awareness (Droste & Roskamm, 1983). Recently, the presence of asymptomatic myocardial ischemia has been strongly linked to the presence of cardiac autonomic neuropathy (Chyun, Young, et al., 2003), yet standardized autonomic testing is infrequently used in clinical practice. Nursing also should share the responsibility for expanding the knowledge base of timing and circadian variation of episodes of asymptomatic myocardial ischemia and the psychosocial, environmental, cultural, and pathologic factors influencing the individual's response to pain. Although research is limited in the area, certain personality traits—those who score lower on levels of nervousness, dominance, and excitability, and higher on the masculinity scale—have been associated with silent ischemia (Droste & Roskamm; Stuart-Shor et al., 2003). Further research utilizing personality characteristics, not only to identify asymptomatic individuals but as a basis for patient education, is warranted. Identifying ischemia triggers, such as daily activities and mental stress, and assisting the person to recognize other vague symptoms associated with ischemia may allow more aggressive management of the condition.

Although ST-segment monitoring has been shown to be a reliable measure of myocardial ischemia following thrombolytic therapy or coronary angioplasty, it has not been widely used in monitoring the elderly for asymptomatic myocardial ischemia, even in the acute care setting. Most contemporary monitoring systems provide the capability to monitor ST-segment changes, without extra costs to the individual and with minimal time commitment by nursing staff (Drew & Krucoff, 1999). Nursing, therefore, has several unique opportunities to participate in assessing elderly individuals with or at high risk of asymptomatic myocardial ischemia, as well as to correlate the presence of asymptomatic episodes with precipitating factors, psychosocial factors, response to medications, and adverse outcomes. As current studies progress, asymptomatic myocardial ischemia, is likely to receive increasing attention. Nursing must be prepared to implement educational interventions and document their efficacy, as well as play an active role in assisting the individual in the recognition and management of asymptomatic disease.

Deborah A. Chyun
Jessica Shank Coviello

Applied Research

In an attempt to differentiate between various types of research, the scientific community uses a myriad of terms, which, however, tend to fall into a discrete classification. On the one end, terms such as *basic*, *fundamental*, and *theoretical* research are used to refer to research focused on discovering fundamental principles and processes governing physical and life phenomena. On the other end, we find such terms as *applied*, *clinical*, *practical*, and *product research*. These refer to the application of the findings of basic/fundamental/theoretical research to generate research aimed at answering focused and problem-specific questions. Though it is the subject of ongoing debate, it is assumed that there are fundamental principles and processes that are core to the nursing discipline and its central tenets of health, patient, nurse, and environment. In addition, it is assumed that nursing draws on fundamental principles and processes discovered in other disciplines to generate new knowledge about nursing and patient care.

Under these assumptions, applied research in nursing can be defined. The etymology of *applied* goes back to the Latin *ad-plicare*, meaning to put something (a law, a test, etc.) into practical operation. Applied research in nursing, then, refers to research aimed at concrete and practical issues and questions of concern to the delivery of nursing care. The most evident type of applied research is intervention research—from exploratory investigations to rigorous clinical trials. This type of applied research is aimed at providing answers to questions about the effectiveness and efficacy of nursing interventions.

Yet nonintervention (or descriptive) research may be categorized as applied research as well if it meets the general criterion of being focused on concrete and practical issues and questions about nursing care. For instance, understanding the dynamics of clinical and subclinical noncompliance in transplant patients and their relationship to the occurrence of adverse posttransplant events helps nurses and other health professionals in developing interventions to enhance adherence to prescribed drug regimens (De Geest, Borgermans, et al., 1995). Developing risk profiles for institutionalization among various cohorts of community-dwelling elderly furthers the knowledge base for designing preventive strategies and models of care for patients, caregivers, and families (Abraham, Currie, Neese, Yi, Thompson-Heisterman, 1994; Steeman, Abraham, & Godderis, 1997).

In addition to effectiveness and efficacy, applied research in nursing also refers to cost calculations of nursing interventions. Managing the costs of care is a major issue in health care, and health care workers need evidence about the cost-effectiveness of the interventions used. For instance, implementation of a modified isolation protocol incorporating only those elements with supported effectiveness in the care of heart transplant recipients can be a source of considerable cost savings (De Geest, Kesteloot, Degryse, & Vanhaecke, 1995). Clinical and cost comparisons of preoperative skin preparation procedures in coronary artery bypass graft (CABG) patients provides additional data to support the necessary process of altering routine nursing practice to evidence-based nursing (De Geest et al., 1996).

IVO L. ABRAHAM
SABINA DE GEEST

Artificial Intelligence

The term *artificial intelligence* (AI) was first used in 1956 at a computer conference at Dartmouth College. Artificial intelligence has been variously defined as: the design and operation of computer systems capable of improved performance based on (a) experience (i.e., learning), (b) the computerization of activities that people believe involve thinking (such as problem solving and decision making), and (c) the development of computer systems that exhibit what people describe as intelligence, or the ability to reason and learn from experience. All three defined areas—machine learning, decision making, and reasoning—have produced distinct lines of research.

Typical areas of AI research include cognitive models of human learning, machine learning models, case-based learning models, and neural network research. The Navy Center for Applied Research in Artificial Intelligence conducts advanced research in several of these fields, especially those of machine learning, sensor-based control of autonomous activity, integration of a variety of reasoning to support complex decision making, and neural networks. Other major centers of AI development are located at Massachusetts Institute of Technology, the University of Georgia, and SRI International (produces commercial AI products).

Four capabilities have been identified for a computer to be able to produce an artificially intelligent product. First, it must be programmed with natural language processing to enable successful communication in a human language. Second, it must have a strategy for knowledge representation so that it can store its own knowledge base as well as the information input by the user. Third, it must have programming that provides it with one or more information-processing and problem-solving strategies. Fourth, it must have machine learning strategies programmed. The research areas in AI that hold the most promise for nursing applications are machine learning, expert systems, and knowledge engineering and representation. The fourth requirement needs further definition because how a machine learns mimics a human process that may not be known to all readers.

Much work has been done on machine learning and reasoning in Defense Department laboratories. Machine learning requires the machine to evaluate its own performance and to change its decision-making strategies when performance success drops below predetermined acceptability levels. In general, this area of research focuses on pattern recognition and pattern reconstruction. Pattern recognition is a major source of human understanding, and making changes in mental protein-solving patterns is one definition of learning. Learning has been defined as adaptation to new circumstances by extrapolating the parameters of the problem and the deficiencies of the old problem-solving pattern to newly constructed patterns. The new patterns are tested until a more successful pattern is found. Thus, pattern recognition and elaboration is defined as the nature of learning.

When machines are programmed to recognize ineffectiveness of existing patterns and to construct and test changes in those patterns until a new pattern proves more successful, they are considered to exhibit machine learning. This area of research has produced significant new knowledge and applications in the defense industry. Of greater interest to nursing, it also led to new understandings about human reasoning and ways to improve human thinking, problem solving, and decision making. Woolery, Grzymala-Busse, Summers, & Budjhardjo (1991) examined the use of machine learning for development of expert systems in nursing.

The term *AI* has been used to deter to both expert systems and true artificially intelligent systems. The confusion stems from differences among users in the meaning of the term *intelligence*. The AI literature discusses two capacities of human intelligence: reasoning and learning from experience. All expert systems reason; that is, they apply one or more problem-solving strategies to specific information provided by a user and produce expert advice (or a decision) as a product. When humans perform this process, they are using reason. Some AI researchers add the requirement for machine learning to the definition of AI. Computer systems that are sophisticated enough to analyze their own performance and change their processing strategies in response to "experience" are said to learn. The capacity to learn is what differentiates AI from expert decision-support systems that do not achieve the level of true intelligence. It is typical to find the terms *AI* and *expert system* used interchangeably. However, the term *AI* should be restricted to systems that both reason and learn from experience.

In nursing the majority of publications that list AI as a search keyword address computerized nursing expert systems, which are usually clinical decision-support tools. The terms *expert systems* and *decision-support systems* are used interchangeably. Primarily, these are systems that help support decisions about nursing assessment or care planning. Much work also has been done on nurse staffing and scheduling systems, such as the MEDICUS or GRASP systems. These are management decision support systems that could also be considered expert systems for management. Decision-support systems may serve as an online reference without much reasoning ability. Poison control centers use such systems to determine the lethality and antidotes (if any) to a variety of substances considered to be poisonous to human beings.

Other types of expert systems accept data input from the user and provide a recommended course of action based on a preprogrammed problem-solving strategy. Still others guide the user in the selection of one or more problem-solving algorithms. The latter system may not offer action recommendations but merely serve to support a logical, systematic approach to the user's own problem-solving abilities.

Another line of nursing scholarship in the field of AI involves knowledge engineering in nursing (Chase, 1988). Knowledge engineering is a subfield of AI that seeks to understand the ways in which nursing experts conceptualize and define nursing problems and how they think about developing problem-solving strategies. Knowledge representation studies focus on a component of knowledge engineering. This field seeks methods of representing (programming and storing) information and human thinking processes in the computer. Knowledge is ultimately extracted from study of the ways that highly successful experts mentally depict external reality (knowledge representation) and from study of experts' problem-solving techniques, strategies, and approaches.

Just as a hammer is a tool that expands the power of the human hand, the computer is a tool that can expand the power of the human mind. Artificial intelligence can greatly enhance the power of human cognition. The knowledge base of health science has increased exponentially over the past 20 years. The amount and complexity of information available for clinical situations can easily exceed the ability of an unaided nurse to use that information clinically. The human mind evolved to function under relatively simple survival conditions, not to integrate multiple, highly complex, technical sources of information nor to calculate interaction effects and probable outcomes of many variables. Unassisted, people cannot do that kind of work with an acceptable degree of consistency. Yet that level of information processing is exactly what modern science (and the U.S. legal system) demands of nurses. When the requirements of a task exceed human performance parameters, people must have tools that expand their capabilities. Artificial intelligence is one type of tool that can be developed to support and expand nurses' cognitive abilities so that they can function in the sophisticated health care environment.

MARY L. MCHUGH

Attitudes

An attitude can be defined as the person's summary evaluation (like or dislike) associated with an object. An attitude object can be anything that is discriminated by the person. Attitudes are dispositions to evaluate objects and to respond. These responses are typically divided into three types: cognitive, affective, and behavioral (Eagly, 1992). Cognitive responses are beliefs or thoughts associated with the attitude object. Affective responses consist of emotions such as positive or negative feelings associated with the object. Behavioral responses are actions toward the attitude object that reflect favorable or unfavorable evaluations (Stroebe & Stroebe, 1995). Attitudes are thought to be acquired both directly through personal experience with an attitude object and indirectly through social learning (e.g., classical conditioning and modeling) from other persons (Baron & Byrne, 1994).

The primary reason attitudes are relevant for nursing practice is their relationship to health behavior. Although attitudes had long been assumed to influence behavior, early research failed to support a strong causal relationship between them. It was the inability to predict behavior from attitudes that led to new approaches to understanding attitudes. Social psychology has two different schools of thought about how attitudes affect behaviors, reflected in two models: expectancy-value and automatic attitude activation (Ajzen, 2001).

The rationale behind the expectancy-value model is that the process linking attitudes to behaviors is a reasoned one. According to this model (Fishbein & Ajzen, 1975), attitudes influence behavior through behavioral intentions or the intention to engage in the behavior. The direct antecedents of these behavioral intentions are (a) the attitude toward the behavior and (b) the subjective norm, which is the person's perception of the extent to which important others think that he or she should engage in the behavior. Ajzen (1988) revised this model by including additional concepts. The most popular revision is the theory of planned behavior; it proposes an additional predictor of behavioral intention, perceived behavioral control, which is the person's perception of how easy or difficult it will be to perform the behavior. Proponents of expectancy-value models point out that the degree of correspondence between the specificity of the attitude and the specificity of the behavior is important. If the correspondence between level of specificity of the attitude and the behavior are similar, attitudes are stronger predictors of behavior. For example, an attitude toward a specific object (taking hypertension medication) would be a better predictor of the behavior of taking hypertension medication than would a more global attitude toward maintaining a healthy lifestyle. The major criticism of these models is that they do not account for other causes of behavior. Current research focuses on these other causes such as past behavior, habit, personality traits, and self-identity (Ajzen, 2001).

The attitude-accessibility model, which was developed by Fazio and Williams (1986), proposed that attitudes are not carefully reasoned as proposed in the expectancy-value model. In contrast, this model proposes that attitudes are automatically accessed in memory without conscious awareness and influence behavior directly (Baron & Byrne, 1994). An important component of this model is attitude accessibility, or the ease with which attitudes can be brought from memory. The more accessible the attitude, the greater the strength of the association in memory between the attitude object and its evaluation, the more readily the attitude is activated, and the stronger the attitude's in fluence on behavior. Therefore, anything that would lead to an attitude becoming more accessible would lead to behaviors that are consistent with the attitude. For example, when the attitude is derived from direct experience with the attitude object, attitude accessibility is more rapid, and the relationship between attitudes and behavior is stronger (Eagly, 1992).

Attitude toward having a chronic condition has been found to be associated with adjustment. For example, in children with chronic epilepsy, attitudes toward epilepsy have been associated with depression symptoms (Dunn, Austin, & Huster, 1999). The attitude-behavior relationship is also relevant for nursing practice because nurses commonly intervene to assist persons in changing health behaviors. The expectancy-value model of attitude has been used much more extensively as a framework to guide health behavior than has the automatic attitude activation model (Stroebe & Stroebe, 1995). For example, Blue, Wilbur, and Marston-Scott (2001) used the theory of planned behavior to study exercise behavior in blue-collar workers. The expectancy-value model and its extension, the theory of planned behavior, provide frameworks on which to build nursing interventions by providing an understanding about the beliefs and perceptions that shape attitudes and subjective norms. With further development the automatic attitude activation model will have implications for nursing practice through improving the understanding of circumstances when intentions to stop negative health behaviors (e.g., overeating) are not predictive of the behavior (Stroebe & Stroebe, 1995). Also relevant to nursing practice are strategies for changing attitudes, such as social influence and message-based persuasion (Wood, 2000).

JOAN K. AUSTIN

B

Basic Research

Basic research includes all forms of scholarly inquiry for the purpose of demonstrating the existence or elucidation of phenomena. Basic research is conducted without intent to address specific problems or real-world application of knowledge. The discipline of nursing is primarily applied rather than basic, although basic research is a part of the discipline (Donaldson, S. K., & Crowley, 1978). As a discipline and a science, nursing is informed by knowledge from basic and applied research, and nursing disciplinary knowledge is integrated into the broader context of the whole of human knowledge.

The origins of nursing research trace back to Florence Nightingale (Woodham-Smith, 1951). Over time, the majority of the scholarly work is best categorized as applied rather than basic research in that nursing research has been conducted for the primary purpose of solving problems related to human health. Nursing seeks knowledge from the perspective of the human experience of health. Human perceptions and experiences of health are studied with the intent to generate knowledge to solve problems through nursing care and practice.

There is a cadre of nurses who were doctorally prepared in the basic sciences, both social and biological, as part of the U.S. Public Health Service Nurse Scientist Training Program from 1962 until the late 1970s. Nurses with doctoral degrees in basic sciences were prepared to contribute as basic researchers, and then they adapted their knowledge and skills to conduct nursing research. Despite the growing number and popularity of doctoral programs in nursing, small numbers of nurses continue to pursue degrees in the basic sciences in the United States. This educational path is used more often in countries where doctoral programs in nursing are not available. Another link between the basic sciences and nursing has evolved as a result of doctoral students in nursing pursuing a graduate minor in a basic science or a postdoctoral fellowship in a basic science. These basic research programs for nurses with doctoral degrees in nursing are facilitated by nurses with doctoral degrees in basic research disciplines. Nurse researchers often engage in basic research to generate knowledge that may lead to new perspectives for applied research in nursing.

All clinical research in nursing is by definition applied research. Studies using animal subjects are often applied rather than basic research in nursing. Animal research is categorized as applied research if the work is designed to answer a clinical question, such as how does mammalian (e.g., rat) skeletal muscle adapt to non-weight-bearing conditions equivalent to bed rest (Kasper, Maxwell, & White, 1996)? In contrast, research involving human subjects or human cells and tissue might be basic research, particularly if the intent of the study is to elucidate an inherent mechanism.

Sue K. Donaldson

Behavioral Research

An examination of behavioral research is best begun by examining what it is and differentiating it from related areas of research. Behavioral research within nursing generally refers to the study of health-related behaviors of persons. Studies may include the following areas: (a) health-promoting behaviors such as exercise, diet, immunization, and smoking cessation; (b) screening behaviors such as mammography, breast self-examination, and prostate examinations; and (c) therapeutic behaviors such as adherence to treatment regimen, blood glucose monitoring, participation in cardiac rehabilitation programs, and treatment-related appointment keeping. The research spans medical and psychiatric populations. It is directed toward an understanding of the nature of behavior and health relationships and to the modification of behaviors that affect health. It has been estimated that over half of premature deaths could be prevented if health behaviors were altered.

Behavioral research has its roots in learning theories that arose in the early part of the 20th century. Classical or respondent conditioning was followed by instrumental or operant conditioning and evolved into the cognitive-behavioral theories that dominate the field today. In classical conditioning an unconditioned stimulus is paired with a conditioned stimulus, resulting in the development of a conditioned response. Much of the research emphasizes conditioned physiological responses. An example is found in the study of anticipatory nausea and vomiting during chemotherapy. In this case, chemotherapy (unconditioned stimulus) may induce nausea and vomiting. After several exposures to chemotherapy in a particular setting (conditioned stimulus), the setting itself may induce nausea and vomiting (conditioned response) prior to and independent of the actual administration of the chemotherapy (unconditioned stimulus). Another example is reciprocal inhibition or desensitization in which anxiety is viewed similarly as a conditioned response to stimuli. An incompatible response (relaxation) is paired with progressively stronger levels of the conditioned stimulus in order to inhibit anxiety responses.

With instrumental or operant conditioning, behavior is seen as arising from environmental stimuli or random exploratory actions, which are then sustained by the occurrence of positive reinforcement following the behavior. Laws have been established that address the identification of reinforcers, the schedules of administration of reinforcers for initiation and maintenance of behavior, and strategies for the extinction of behavior. In this model, motivation is seen as a state of deprivation or satiation with regard to reinforcers. Numerous strategies have evolved from this work, including but not limited to contracting and tailoring, which have been used in studies of patient adherence; token economies, which have been used in studies on unit management with the mentally ill or developmentally delayed; and contingency management, which has been used in the promotion of treatment behaviors such as exercise.

As the operant model has expanded over time, self-management has evolved as a special case of contingency management. With self-management the individual is responsible for establishing intermediate goals, monitoring progress toward those goals, and administering self-reinforcement for success. Self-management has been studied particularly for chronic, long-term regimens such as those for diabetes, asthma, and cardiovascular disease.

In both of these models there is an emphasis on behavior rather than motivation or personality or relationships, beyond that of the reinforcing behaviors of significant others. The history of the behavior is of less interest than the factors that currently sustain the behavior. An empirical model is used with an assessment of the frequency or intensity of the behavior over time, the stimulus conditions that precede the behavior, and the consequent or reinforcing events that follow the behavior. Intervention is then directed to the specific areas targeted by the initial assessment. Detailed assessment continues through the course of intervention and often through a period following intervention to assess maintenance or generalization.

Each of the cognitive-behavioral models identifies a cognitive feature as a major motivational determinant of behavior. Self-efficacy theory postulates the role of perceived capability to engage in a behavior under various conditions. The theory of reasoned action postulates that intention to engage in a behavior is significant and is influenced by beliefs regarding behavioral outcomes and attitudes toward the behavior. The health belief model postulates that one's perceptions about the illness in terms of its threat (severity and susceptibility), as well as the perception of the benefits and barriers to engaging in the behavior, influence intentions and subsequently behavior. However, the common sense model of illness proposes that the individual's own model of the illness influences his or her illness or treatment-related behaviors.

Behavioral research can be distinguished from psychosocial research, which tends to emphasize adjustment and coping as well as predictor and moderator variables arising from the psychological state or the social environment of the person. Behavioral research, including cognitive-behavioral studies, emphasizes behavior. In the classical and instrumental models, observable behavior is stressed. In the cognitive-behavioral model, both observable and covert behaviors are stressed. Within nursing much of the behavioral research has addressed participation in treatment, exercise, sexual behaviors, health promotion, breast self-examination and mammography utilization, childbirth and maternal behaviors, behavioral symptoms of dementia, self-management in chronic conditions, management of alcohol or drug dependency, and the role of biofeedback in such behaviors as pelvic floor muscle exercise in incontinence and heart rate variability. Unlike psychosocial studies, factors such as personality, coping strategies, and socioeconomic status are not primary interests; however, they may be of interest in determining reinforcers and stimulus conditions.

There is an additional body of behavioral research that tends to be interdisciplinary in nature and is of relevance to nursing. There are studies in the community to modify health behaviors within populations and studies within multicenter clinical trials that attempt to influence the health behavior or protocol-related behaviors of research participants. Also there is a broad set of studies to identify the relationship between behavior and disease etiology, such as studies of the role of exercise on the maintenance of function in the older adult, mechanisms of addiction in smoking behavior, and the effect of neurotransmitters on eating behaviors.

Given the prevalence of lifestyle behaviors that adversely affect health and the management of illness, research to understand and modify those behaviors would benefit the individual as well as the population. There is a need for nursing research to expand into the interdisciplinary arenas, particularly in the examination of health behavior change in the community, studies within multicenter clinical trials, and the etiological relationship between behavior and health and illness. Further, many of the studies in nursing have been descriptive in nature or have focused on the development of assessment instruments. Although few of the studies have examined how to intervene with behaviors that contribute to the development or progression of illness, this research would be useful to better direct interventions with patients.

This paper was supported in part by a National Institute of Nursing Research grant (5 P30 NR03924) and a National Heart, Lung, and Blood Institute grant (1 UO1HL48992).

JACQUELINE DUNBAR-JACOB

Benchmarking in Health Care

Benchmarking is a structured process used to discover, compare, and incorporate the best practices of high-performing organizations for the purpose of improving the benchmarking organization's performance. It was first used in the late 1970s by the Xerox Corporation and soon became popular in other industries. The introduction of benchmarking in industry was aligned with total quality management (TQM) and continuous quality improvement (CQI). When used correctly, benchmarking offers the opportunity for exponential improvement rather than the incremental changes most frequent with traditional quality improvement methods. As health care became more industrialized, with enormous pressure to increase efficiency, quality, and customer satisfaction, health care organizations began to adopt benchmarking. As in other industries, benchmarking is often used in conjunction with TQM, CQI, other quality assurance programs, or competitive analysis in health care organizations. It has been used to improve business processes, management processes, and clinical processes in health care organizations.

Benchmarking is most effectively introduced in an organization with a preexisting culture of process orientation and analysis. It is a continuous, ongoing process that requires planning, analysis, and adoption of new processes. Processes to be benchmarked are identified during the planning phase, and because benchmarking costs can be significant, it is important that the organization identify key processes for improving performance. Performance data to be used as benchmarks must be identified and available for analysis and comparison with selected high performers. Selection of organizations to benchmark against is another major decision during the planning phase. The organization may choose internal benchmarking to compare performance of similar operations or divisions within the organization, within one operation or division over time, or with findings from research literature.

However, to reap the full benefit of benchmarking the organization must move to external benchmarking and comparisons with other organizations. External benchmarking may be conducted with like organizations in a geographical region, with similar organizations in a collaborative project, with recognized high performers in health care, or with high-performance industries outside health care. Identification and comparison with high performers is costly and time consuming and may be more efficiently handled by a consulting group or benchmarking clearinghouse that does benchmarking for health care organizations and has access to data from similar organizations recognized as high performers.

Analysis requires two discrete sets of data: (1) the benchmarks, or performance measures, to be used in comparing the benchmarking organization's performance against the selected high performers; and (2) a thorough description of the operational process being benchmarked in the organization using benchmarking and the comparison organizations. This operational description is often referred to as process mapping and is essential to identifying practices in the comparison organizations that enable them to be high performers. Identification of these "best" practices is a necessary prerequisite to the analysis, identification, and adoption of practices that can improve the benchmarking organization's performance. Implementation of operational processes identified through benchmarking, followed by reevaluation of the selected performance measures, is a cyclical process that is repeated until performance goals have been reached and maintained over time.

Although benchmarking has the potential to assist health care organizations to make quantum improvements in operational and delivery systems, it also has the potential to increase stress and cost and to be counterproductive if used inappropriately or improperly. Because benchmarking is in its infancy in health care, a number of pitfalls must be avoided. A common problem is comparing the benchmarks (performance measures) and not looking at the process to find out how the high-performing organization achieves performance and how it differs from the benchmarking organization's performance. Truly effective benchmarking requires in-depth, personal examination of the reasons for the high performer's success. It also requires that performance and productivity measures be consistent with the philosophy and objectives of the organization (Smeltzer, Leighty, & Williams-Brinkley, 1997). Problems also may arise from an inadequate study design, inadequate data analysis, and inadequate preparation of the organization for benchmarking.

Benchmarking studies have only recently been published in health care literature. Many of these studies are reported as case studies that provide information about the process being used, the organizational changes made, and the outcomes achieved through the benchmarking process. Examples of business and management processes studied include workers' compensation process, admissions process, scheduling systems, and operating room use. Studies of benchmarking with clinical processes (Bankert, Daughtridge, Meehan, & Colburn, 1996; Czarnecki, 1996) and patient populations (Clare, Sargent, Moxley, & Forthman, 1995; Lauver, 1996) are reported in the literature and often contain cost information as well as patient outcomes. Although consulting organizations have accumulated comparative data from the organizations they service, this information may surface in the literature slowly, if at all. To determine the usefulness of benchmarking for achieving improvements in health care organizations, more evaluative studies are needed to assess the effectiveness of benchmarking for improving the cost and quality of services provided by health care organizations.

MARION JOHNSON

Bibliographic Retrieval Systems

Classifying knowledge in books and other documents is in the domain of library and information sciences. Books and other documents are considered "physical objects" that can be classified in a number of ways; however, subject classification is considered the most significant characteristic. Whereas scientists in a field identify the knowledge of the field, bibliographic classifiers organize the knowledge produced by the scientists (Landgridge, 1992). The classification system is used to index the literature and thus serves a purpose of location and retrieval of the indexed documents. When the classification system is accompanied by an alphabetical list of terms with cross-references, it is called a thesaurus (Landgridge, 1992).

The major bibliographic classification schemes dealing with the nursing literature are implemented in computerized bibliographic database retrieval systems for nursing and medicine. Computerized bibliographic databases based on specialty-subject thesauri are available for many other reference disciplines of psychology, education, sociology, and so forth.

Access to bibliographic databases is either through a search service offered by the primary developer of the classification system or is licensed for use by bibliographic retrieval services that provide access to multiple bibliographic databases. Fees for such services vary considerably.

A bibliographic retrieval system is a special type of information retrieval system. The information that is stored (and retrieved) provides citations of documents represented in the system. Citations commonly include the article author, title, and the exact location of the article (the title of the journal in which it is published, journal volume and issue number, and pages). Other document types (books, videos, etc.), if incorporated in the system, have descriptors appropriate for that document type. Other data that help to locate a specific document—for example, accession number and author address—will be added to the database by the producer of the system. Abstracts are usually included.

Computerized bibliographic retrieval systems have three components: (a) the classification system for the field of knowledge (subject headings, thesaurus, controlled vocabulary); (b) a database of documents indexed with the controlled vocabulary of the classification system; and (c) the retrieval system search engine (software). The quality of retrieval is a function of all three elements. The controlled vocabulary must adequately represent the literature in the field. Terms from the controlled vocabulary must be accurately assigned to the documents in the field. The search software logic with which searches are done facilitates certain types of searches and hinders others, thereby affecting the quality of the retrieval.

Nursing has long been dissatisfied with bibliographic databases that index the nursing literature. In part, this is because the vocabulary used by major systems has not satisfactorily reflected nursing terminology. Systems oriented toward nursing literature overcome some of this difficulty by classifying things of importance in nursing but not in medicine, such as nursing theoretical frameworks.

Another long-standing disappointment in the profession has been the inability to locate nursing research by variables studied. This is because variable names are sometimes so far out on the classification tree that they are usually not suitable for subject headings. This makes sense because variables usually represent the new nomenclature in a field. These new terms are frequently renamed or incorporated into another term or they may disappear altogether. Vocabularies need more stability than is characteristic of research variable names. Because variable names are not always included in bibliographic classifications, articles are not indexed by the names of variables studied in the research.

The results section of research articles, where the variable names reside, is rarely used for assigning index terms (Horowitz, R. S., & Fuller, 1982). The identification of variable names as keywords by researchers is of little use. Currently, there is no way to tell whether an author-identified term or a classifier-assigned subject heading is a research variable name or just another topic the article is "about." It is fair to say that "aboutness" indexing has a serious impact on retrievals of interest to researchers (Weinberg, B. H., 1987).

Research document representation in nursing-related databases is a problem for several reasons. First, if a controlled vocabulary is inadequate for any reason, indexers cannot assign terms to adequately represent documents. Second, research by nurses that is published outside the field may be in journals that are not indexed by the database developers in the domain. Third, bibliographic databases are limited to the published research literature. Frequently, the published literature fails to reflect adequately the knowledge being generated in a field. Cost of publishing and availability of reviewers limit the number of articles that can be published. Publication bias against small studies with nonsignificant findings and perhaps of parochial interest works against publication of clinical research in nursing. With more focus on statistical meta-analysis strategies, these studies might be combined and thus yield valuable new knowledge. The consequence of large amounts of fugitive research lies not just in the invisibility of knowledge to the discipline but results in a significant waste of resources to duplicate work that has already been done or to identify work that needs to be done.

The strategy or "logic" that software uses to search databases determines how documents can be retrieved and how accurately the document set of interest can be retrieved. Although other search strategies are becoming available, the primary search strategy used by bibliographic retrieval systems in nursing and related fields is based on Boolean logic. The searcher must fully understand the logic used by the search system and how it is implemented in the database of interest.

Boolean logic is based in set theory, which is a way of combining sets of things—in this case, search terms in documents. The *operators*, called Boolean operators, dictate how the documents containing the terms will be combined. The operator *and* causes all the documents containing one term, *x*, and all documents containing another search term, *y*, to be combined into the set of documents that contain both *x* and *y*. This set of documents is called the search result.

The operator *or* results in a set of documents that have either the term *x* or *y*. It includes the set of documents that have both *x* and *y*. Other common operators are *not, adjacent, includes, excludes, begins with*. Generally, the more Boolean operators a system makes available, the more accurate the search that can be performed.

Accuracy is a generic term that refers to the concepts of sensitivity and specificity of the search result. In Boolean search systems of bibliographic databases, sensitivity and specificity are inversely related: the search either results in many documents that are not relevant but includes most that are relevant or it results in a few of the most relevant documents being found but fails to turn up others of relevance.

In addition to Boolean operators, common bibliographic database retrieval systems will have tags that identify other salient features of documents in the field; for example, the language the article is written in, document type, and whether the article is about humans or other animals. These characteristics can be used to further delimit a search.

Researchers are interested in scientific findings, not documents (Doyle, 1986; Weinberg, B. H., 1987). All that can be obtained from a bibliographic database search is a list of citations of documents or perhaps the full text of some documents that may or may not contain research findings. The accuracy of these searches can be extremely low, depending on the complexity of the search.

The scientific knowledge is the research result or findings; however, bibliographic classification is done to organize the scientific knowledge produced after it has been embodied in documents (Landgridge, 1992). When viewed this way, perhaps the results of research should not be part of a literature classification system because the results are the knowledge, not the document with the knowledge. Or perhaps this was and is the only legitimate method available to library and information scientists when approaching the literature of all disciplines.

Nonetheless, research knowledge can be indexed by its variables (Graves, 1997; Weiner, Stowe, Shirley, & Gilman, 1981) and linked to its source (the researchers); if published, the dissemination history of the study (bibliographic citations) can be provided. The Virginia Henderson International Nursing Library makes the nursing research that is in the *Registry of Nursing Research* accessible by directly indexing the studies by variable names as well as by researcher and by subject headings (see "The Virginia Henderson International Nursing Library").

JUDITH R. GRAVES

Bibliometrics

Bibliometrics is broadly defined as the application of mathematical and statistical methods to published scientific literature in a disciplinary field (Pritchard, 1969). Bibliometric research methods are based on a literary model of science. Using bibliometrics, information scientists assume that published research documents reflect new knowledge in a scientific field and that references in these reports represent relationships among scientists and their work.

Bibliometrics is a useful research methodology for describing and visually representing the communication structure of a scientific field. It has been used successfully to evaluate such things as emergence, change, and communication networks in specialty areas. Bibliometric methods have been helpful in identifying the foundational fields (i.e., other scientific fields) that have driven the genesis of a new scientific field. They also can be used to identify prominent scientists or documents that have influenced the intellectual development of a scientific field. Thus, bibliometric studies may provide insights into the historical and sociological evolution of nursing science as well as the design of information retrieval systems in nursing.

Research questions addressed by bibliometric studies generally fall into one of four categories: (a) characterization of a scholarly community, (b) evolution of a scholarly community, (c) evaluation of scholarly contributions, and (d) diffusion of ideas from within and across disciplines (Borgman, 1990). Citation data are often used in bibliometric studies and are generally collected from bibliographies, abstracting and indexing services, citation indexes, and primary journals. Typically, the references of research journal articles are analyzed in bibliometric studies. Bibliographic attributes such as authors, citations, and textual content are used as variables in bibliometric research.

Citation analysis is the best-known bibliometric strategy. It is a set of strategies for studying relationships among cited and citing literature in a scientific field. Bibliographic coupling and co-citation analysis use citation analysis to demonstrate linkage of citation data. In bibliographic coupling, the focus is on the citing literature; that is, the number of references two articles have in common reflects the similarity of their subject matter. In co-citation analysis the focus is on the cited literature, that is, the number of times two documents are cited together in the reference lists of later publications. Sets of co-cited document pairs may be grouped together and mapped, using graphical display techniques such as cluster analysis and multidimensional scaling. The unit of analysis for co-citation analysis studies can also be journals (journal co-citation analysis) or authors (author co-citation analysis). Co-word analysis is another bibliometric strategy based on the analysis of co-occurrence of keywords used to index documents or articles. This method is useful for mapping content in a research field or for tracing the evolution of networks of problems in a disciplinary field.

Bibliometric strategies are practical and may be applied to citation data that are readily accessible on citation indexes and online electronic databases. No subjective judgments are made by the researcher about what literature best defines a scientific field or specialty area. It is the scholars themselves who publish in the scientific literature that determine the intellectual base of the specialty area. However, citation data can portray only what the scientific community in a field of study has recognized by way of publication. In addition, bibliometrics does not have a theory that integrates the methods and techniques used in the analysis of citations. Therefore, it is important that the investigator clearly delimit the specialty area to be investigated, be familiar with the field of interest, and interpret citation data in conjunction with other sources of information relevant to the area of interest.

Review of Research

There have been at least five bibliometric investigations of the nursing literature. Garfield (1985), an information scientist, conducted a journal citation study on core nursing journals indexed in the 1983 *Social Sciences Citation Index*, using citation data from 1981 to 1983. Four bibliometric studies have been conducted by nurse researchers. Messler (1974) conducted a citation analysis investigating the growth of maternity nursing knowledge as reflected in published nursing practice literature from 1909 to 1972. Wilford (1989) used citation analysis techniques to study citation patterns depicted in the references of a random sample of 310 nursing dissertations from 1947 to mid-1987. Johnson (1990) conducted a bibliometric analysis using the technique of keyword analysis to describe the evolution of the holistic paradigm in the field of nursing. D'Auria (1994) used citation analysis techniques, including author co-citation analysis, to demonstrate the feasibility of using author co-citation analysis for identifying emerging networks of researchers in the subfield of maternal and child health nursing from 1976 to 1990. Further bibliometric analyses of the research literature from the general field or subfields of nursing will provide a baseline for describing and interpreting citation data in the field of nursing.

At this point in the development of nursing science, it is critical that nurse scholars create ways to increase the visibility and retrieval of scientific information being generated in the field. Bibliometric methods can provide a way to track disciplinary influences and the identities of nurse scientists and scientists from other disciplines whose interests are shaping the generation of scientific information in nursing. The findings of bibliometric studies will provide nurse scholars with a guide for scholarship for doctoral students and researchers in the field of nursing that may differ from information that has been passed down as traditional wisdom. Thus, the findings of bibliometric studies will open up new avenues for debate and hypotheses generation in regard to the evolution of nursing science.

As the nursing research literature continues to grow, rigorous and systematic bibliometric research of citation data may contribute working models of the development of nursing science that could be used to evaluate scientific progress. By discovering trends in disciplinary and interdisciplinary linkages, nurse scholars can identify underdeveloped or neglected areas of research in nursing science. Evaluating the degree of scientific activity in research areas would help nurse scholars determine if research resources are allocated correctly as well as assist them in determining the need for new journals and books in the field of nursing. It will also provide an avenue by which nurse scholars may access scientific information and prevent the loss of information generated in the field of nursing.

JENNIFER P. D'AURIA

Biofeedback

While in the past, biofeedback for chronic symptom patterns has been thought to be simply training muscles and body functioning through operant conditioning, now it is more common to consider the brain and central nervous system as the central focus of treatment. It is, after all, the electrical-biochemical systems through which all bodily activity is finally determined. To focus on the brain/neural pathway acknowledges the mind-body interface and the centrality of the brain in the disease process.

The use of biofeedback and its accompanying belief in helping persons master self-regulation of body function and optimum states has been greatly impacted by the cellular research in the recent years. While on the one hand, groups of neuroscientists have explored the progress of using stem cells as a way of repairing organs, another movement in research has realized exciting possibilities in tracing evidence of the capability of the body to perform neurogenesis and neuroplasticity (Kempermann, Kuhn, & Gage, 1997; Eriksson et al., 1998; Kempermann & Gage, 1999; Bjorklund & Lindvall, 2000; Magavi, Leavigtt, & Macklis, 2000). Early evidence of the possibility of generating growth or regrowth in neural tissue was reported by Marion Diamond (1988). In these early studies, Diamond stimulated brain growth in older rats by enriching the environment. From this study were derived the studies by Budzynski (1996), Budzynski and Budzynski (1997) to improve cognitive functioning of elderly humans by enhancing the brain with neurofeedback and light/sound stimulation.

Results of studies on cellular restoration of nerve tissue together with reports of improvement of body functioning through neurofeedback suggested that changes in bodily functioning can be reached through the brain. By managing appropriate change in the EEG or the brain's electrical activity, the body not only can rid itself of chronic symptoms but can also heal itself. These new directions for intervention are reaching consumers of health care.

There are over 100 nurse professionals in the Biofeedback Certification of America (BCIA), the certifying body for biofeedback/neurofeedback. There are untold other nurses practicing without current certification. Many of these practitioners are performing exciting biofeedback/neurofeedback work with target chronic problems, such as attention deficit disorder, epilepsy, stroke, mild head injury, migraines, and other symptom patterns. But they practice outside the mainstream of nursing's institutions of care. They practice privately alongside multiple other health disciplines. Other schisms are that these practitioners are not inclined to undertake research, and those who are doing research (often in universities) have little access to practice settings. The nursing biofeedback field could advance markedly if these activities and professionals could merge, as has medicine, to develop research based programs for specific target clinical problems.

Nursing biofeedback research has shown effective changes in patient symptoms through application of complementary techniques. A review of biofeedback/self-management training research by nurses prior to 1997 indicated favorable patient outcomes when performing management of stress symptoms, progressive relaxation, reduction of tension with EMG training, hand warming, training during childbirth, respiratory training, and heart rate variability training. These publications predominantly indicated individual efforts to inform the field of their respective specialized treatments. Over the years since then, there is very little shift to indicate that *programs of care* by nurses have proliferated. Also, fewer biofeedback studies have been generated in nursing publications. But there is evidence that research methods and physiologic measurement has markedly improved—many articles using feedback are competitive in nonnursing journals.

It is informative to point out the following: Chronic symptom patterns such as advanced heart failure, sudden cardiac arrest, incontinence following surgery, and elderly cognitive decline as listed above have not previously been treated with feedback training. Physiologic indicators with a psychological self-care orientation are used to demonstrate change. These above studies are few in number, but recently the kinds and quality of noninvasive instrumentation on the market are allowing researchers to trace change in bodily and psychological processes—EEG, heart rate variability, blood sugar levels, blood flow, CO2, and respiratory activity, to name a few. The stage is set for offering feedback to any number of chronic problems which have heretofore been neglected. Lynda Kirk, the new President of the Association for Applied Psychophysiology and Biofeedback, a nurse, recognized the dominance of the brain in feedback by quoting William James on the latest cover of *AAPB Biofeedback*: "The greatest thing, then, is to make the nervous system our ally instead of our enemy."

HELEN KOGAN BUDZYNSKI
HSIN-YI (JEAN) TANG

Bowel Elimination Among Older Adults

Bowel elimination is the end process of digestion resulting from interactions of the central and autonomic nervous systems, and endocrine, gastrointestinal and musculoskeletal systems. Three major bowel elimination problems have been studied and consistently have been shown to affect the older population: constipation, incontinence, and colorectal cancer (American Cancer Society, 2003a; Hogstel, 2001; Memorial Sloan-Kettering Cancer Center, 2003; Vogelzang, 1999).

Constipation, defined as the accumulation of feces in the lower intestines with difficulty evacuating this waste, is the most common complaint among older adults (Abrams, Beers, Berkow, & Fletcher, 1995). According to Annells and Koch (2002), laxatives have become the most commonly sought treatment for constipation. More than one third of older adults use weekly laxatives to reduce strain and enhance fecal elimination (Reiss & Evans, 2002). Research findings demonstrate that increasing fiber and fluid in the diet significantly decreases the need for laxative use and stool softeners (Howard, West, & Ossip-Klein, 2000; Robinson & Rosher, 2002).

Vogelzang (1999) cited seven reasons for constipation in the elderly. Multiple medications (polypharmacy) had been identified as a primary reason for constipation, especially in nursing home residents. Six or more medications have been shown to adversely effect motility of the digestive tract (Vogelzang). Older adults living at home may be at an even higher risk for overdose related to self-medication with over-the-counter drugs (Vogelzang). In addition, limited income influences the quality of food purchased and the degree of fiber-rich foods incorporated into the older adult's diet. Annual income is less than $6,000 in 40% of older Americans, leaving them limited funds for groceries. Most do not take advantage of funded food programs. Selection of the same foods is common, leading to a poorly balanced diet (Vogelzang). Non-healthy snacking throughout the day also counteracts appetite as well as bowel regularity. Lack of social interaction, physical inactivity, nausea caused by contaminated food due to unclean food preparation, and inadequate cooking skills also have been identified as contributing factors to risk for constipation (Vogelzang). Constipation can be controlled by a well-balanced diet high in fiber, adequate hydration (at least 6–8 eight-ounce glasses of water/day), along with increased activity (Hinrichs, Huseboe, Tang, & Titler, 2001).

Fecal incontinence has been shown to contribute to decreased social activity (Giebel, Lefering, Troidl, & Blochl, 1998). Older adults are embarrassed that incontinence may occur in public, so they tend to limit outside activity with friends and family. There exists a strong correlation between urinary and fecal incontinence (Chassagne et al., 1999). In a survey conducted by Giebel and colleagues, 500 randomly selected older adults in Germany responded to a questionnaire about bowel habits. It was found that 4.8% were unable to control solid stool, whereas 19.6% experienced at least one type of incontinence. Women had more of a problem with pasty or liquid stools. They also experienced an urgent sensation to quickly reach the toilet. Men described soiling their underwear as most problematic. Controlling flatus was also described as a concern. Findings suggest that the lack of control associated with bowel habits plus the reduction in activities necessitate interventions aimed at education about intestinal health and dietary change. Another study done on fecal incontinence enrolling 1,186 older adults 60 years of age and older in a long-term care setting identified five risk factors associated with fecal incontinence: (1) history of urinary incontinence, (2) neurological disease, (3) poor mobility, (4) severe cognitive decline, and (5) age greater than 70 (Chassagne et al.). Fecal incontinence associated with impaction and diarrhea occurred in 234 (20%) of the sample. The study showed an association between permanent fecal incontinence and overall poor health in older adults.

Approximately 90% of individuals with colorectal cancer are over 50 years of age (American Cancer Society, 2003a). The United States Preventive Task Force recommends individuals beginning at age 50 be screened for colorectal cancer as follows: (a) yearly fecal occult blood test, (b) flexible sigmoidoscopy every 5 years, (c) colonoscopy every 5–10 years (American Cancer Society; Donovan & Syngal, 1998). Screening can reduce risk by up to 75% (Donovan, & Syngal). Those with a family history of colon cancer and/or polyps should be screened at a younger age and more frequently.

Borum (1998) evaluated the relationship of age with screening for colorectal cancer. A retrospective chart review of 200 patients over 50 years old in an ambulatory clinic showed that more rectal exams were done on 50–60 year olds than on 60–70 year olds. These results indicate that less screening is done in the older elderly than the younger elderly. As aggressive screening diminishes, risk for colorectal cancer increases (Borum).

Diet plays an important role in the prevention of colorectal cancer. Negri, Franceschi, Parpinel, and La Vecchia (1998) researched fiber intake and the risk of colorectal cancer. Dietary habits of patients (1,225 with colon cancers, 728 with rectal cancers, and 4,154 with no history of cancer) were studied. The data indicated that dietary fiber has a protective effect against colorectal cancer. High fiber diets may protect against colorectal cancer by allowing brief mucosal exposure to carcinogens. The longer stool remains in the intestine, the more likely the chance of cancer.

Caygill, Charlett, and Hill (1998) investigated the relationship between intake of high fiber and risk of breast and bowel cancer. The study showed cereal and vegetables protect against both colorectal and breast cancer. Fruit had no protective effect on colorectal or breast cancer. However, fruit was shown to be more protective against cancers of the upper digestive tract (Caygill, Charlett, & Hill).

In summary, older adults are at risk for developing bowel elimination complications, which may be associated with the physiological changes occurring with advancing age and lack of screening. Screening for cancer needs to be done on all elderly, regardless of advanced age. Diets high in fiber, adequate hydration, increased activity, and education programs encourage prevention of complications.

CORA D. ZEMBRZUSKI
EILEEN M. HERMANN

Boykin & Schoenhofer: The Theory of Nursing as Caring

The theory Nursing as Caring (Boykin & Schoenhofer, 1993, 2001) provides a conceptual framework for the nature of nursing as a caring discipline and profession. Embodying the aesthetic and personal realms of knowing in nursing (Carper, 1978; Chinn & Kramer, 2004; Boykin, Parker, & Schoenhofer, 1994), the theory incorporates the artistic and empathic aspects of nursing situations as personal caring connections between the nurse and the nursed as they occur in the moment. The theory of Nursing as Caring is essential to the core essence of nursing, providing a structure for practice, administration, education, and research.

Major assumptions/fundamental beliefs underlying the transformational model of the theory of Nursing as Caring include:

- persons are caring by virtue of their humanness
- persons are caring, moment to moment
- persons are whole and complete in the moment
- personhood is a process of living grounded in caring
- personhood is enhanced through participating in nurturing relationships with caring others
- nursing is both a discipline and a profession

(Boykin & Schoenhofer, 2001a, p. 11).

The focus of Nursing as Caring is that nursing, both as a discipline and as a profession, "involves the nurturing of persons living and growing in caring" (Boykin & Schoenhofer, 2001a, p. 12). Central concepts include *caring*, characterized by altruistic actions and the recognition of value and connectedness between the nurse and the nursed, the *nursing situation*, "a shared lived experience in which the caring between nurse and nursed enhances personhood" (Boykin & Schoenhofer, p. 13), and the *caring between*, a personal connection encounter between the nurse and the nursed "within which personhood is nurtured" (Boykin & Schoenhofer, p. 14).

An integral component of Nursing as Caring, the *Dance of Caring Persons*, represents the circular nature of caring grounded in the valuing of one another (the nurse and the nursed) as unique caring individuals (Boykin & Schoenhofer, 2001a; Boykin, Schoenhofer, Smith, St. Jean, & Aleman, 2003). This element of the theory acknowledges the need for a paradigm shift from the traditional top-down hierarchical structures present in health care organizations to circular structures of mutuality and respect found within nurse-client collaborative partnerships.

Research approaches developed within the context of the theory of Nursing as Caring include focusing on the discovery of the meaning of lived caring, and the understanding of value experienced in nursing situations (Boykin & Schoenhofer, 2001a). A qualitative group phenomenology approach was utilized to provide insight into the meaning of lived caring. Research participants generated data in focus group settings and also developed the synthesis of meaning (Schoenhofer, Bingham, & Hutchins, 1998). Qualitative research methodologies grounded in dialogue and description and interpreted as themes characterize research into the value experienced in nursing situations (Boykin & Schoenhofer, 2001b; Boykin et al., 2003).

Nursing as Caring guides research by providing a broad conceptual framework for the development of middle-range theories that address more specific phenomena of nursing as caring in areas of nursing practice, administration, and education. Examples of developments of such mid-range theoretical models based on the theory of Nursing as Caring include the *theory of technological competence as caring in critical care nursing* (Locsin, 1998); Dunphy's (1998) *"circle of caring" model for advanced practice nursing* which focuses on caring processes; and the *caring-based nursing model* that grounded an acute care unit in the perspective of nursing as caring (Boykin et al., 2003). Future directions include the development of new methods of nursing inquiry appropriate to the study of Nursing as Caring allowing for research of the meaning of nursing within the lived experience of the nursing situation (Boykin & Schoenhofer, 2001a).

MARY ANGELIQUE HILL

Breast Cancer: Psychosocial Adjustment to Illness

Classified as a chronic disease, the demands of breast cancer extend over time, with some phases characterized by more demands and stress than others. Acceptance of the diagnosis, treatment decisions, emotional distress related to physical change and loss, alterations in lifestyle, uncertainty, and need for information and support are ongoing issues (Loveys & Klaich, 1991; Walker, Nail, Larsen, Magill, & Schwartz, 1996). Although the diagnostic and immediate postoperative phases are particularly stressful (Northouse, 1990), emotional distress (Hoskins et al., 1996b), distress from side effects (Walker et al., 1996), and limitations in role performance and sense of control may last longer.

Although adjustment has been commonly conceptualized as quality of life, the breadth of the broad conceptualization inhibits definitive studies of its dimensions and predictors. Adjustment has, however, been conceptualized in many ways, including role performance (Derogatis, 1983), sexual function (Lasry, 1991), emotional symptoms (Hoskins et al., 1996b; Pasacreta, 1997), cognitive function (Cimprich, 1995), self-esteem, and body image. To address the issue of multiple interpretations and dimensions, Dow, Ferrell, Haberman, and Eaton (1999) conducted a qualitative study of 687 survivors of various kinds of cancer and identified themes of struggle among independence-dependence, wholeness, life purpose, reclaiming life, multiple losses, control, and surviving cancer from a family perspective. Narrowing the focus of quality of life to breast cancer survivors, Ferrell, Grant, Funk, Otis-Green, and Garcia (1998) concluded that adjustment involves demands across the physical, psychological, social, and spiritual domains.

Similarly, Aaronson (1990) recognized the multidimensionality of quality of life and proposed the four major dimensions of functional status, symptoms related to the disease and treatment, psychological functioning, and social functioning. In general, it is agreed that the broad domains of adjustment to breast cancer may be conceptualized as psychological (Walker, Nail, & Croyle, 1999), physical (Given & Given, 1992; Cohen, Kahn, & Steeves, 1998; Wyatt & Friedman, 1998), and social (Tulman & Fawcett, 1990; Northouse, Dorris, & Charron-Moore, 1995).

The adjustment process has a strong effect on the family as a system (Cooley & Moriarty, 1997; Germino, 1998). Usual roles are altered with resultant interpersonal tension in both patients and partners (Lewis & Hammond, 1996). The factor of time is reflected in longitudinal studies of emotional and physical adjustment in both patients and partners. In their seminal study of 50 newly diagnosed breast cancer patients and spouses, Northouse and Swain (1987) noted that the emotional distress and mood disturbance among the spouses at 3-days post-surgery differed significantly from population norms. The distress and disturbance continued to 18 months. Higher emotional distress and lower adjustment among spouses (Given & Given, 1992), as compared to patients, may continue for as long as 3 years. As the person most intimately involved in the events related to the patient's illness and treatment, the partner struggles with fear of the cancer, demands placed on personal life (Samms, 1999), and feelings of being ineffectual. As demands escalate, increased depression among partners affects marital adjustment (Zahlis & Shands, 1993). Studies in which the partner, identified by the patient as the person most intimately involved in the breast cancer experience are rare and require furthur resources.

Finally, the wide variety of predictors of adjustment include life stress, age (Lehto & Cimprich, 1999), stage of disease (Zabalegui, 1999), time since diagnosis (Irvine, Brown, Crooks, Roberts, & Browne, 1991), initial emotional status (Iscoe, Williams, & Osoba, 1991), previous diagnosis of cancer (Northouse, Laten, & Reddy, 1995), perceived support (Northouse, Dorris, & Charron-Moore, 1995; Hoskins et al., 1996a, 1996b), social integration (Loveys & Klaich, 1991), side effects and associated distress (Wilson & Morse, 1991; Budin, 1998), and uncertainty (Christman, 1990).

CAROL NOLL HOSKINS

Breast Cancer Screening

Breast cancer is a disease for which there is no foreseeable cure, and indications are that the incidence will remain high. The American Cancer Society estimates that more than 211,300 women were diagnosed with breast cancer in 2003, and almost 39,800 will die. Although breast cancer remains a significant form of cancer mortality for women, in 1996 an overall decrease in mortality was reported. Because treatment is extremely effective with Stage I tumors, increases in mammography screening have influenced breast cancer mortality. When discovered early, breast cancer victims may anticipate a 97% chance for complete cure. Prospective mortality-based studies have demonstrated the effectiveness of mammography screening, particularly in women 50–70 years of age, and therefore most organizations recommend periodic screening beginning at age 50.

Recently, mammography recommendations have been expanded to include women 40 to 49. Consequently, both the American Cancer Society and the National Cancer Institute now recommend screening beginning at age 40. Obviously, breast cancer screening by mammography does not magically become effective at age 40 or 50 or 60, and one mistake that fueled controversy was comparing one decade to another. Comparing women aged 40 to 49 with women 50 and over creates artificial boundaries that cause much confusion. Now that the American Cancer Society and National Cancer Institute are in agreement, energy may be focused on other issues.

The effectiveness of clinical breast examination is not as clear as that of mammography, although it is currently recommended. Some studies demonstrating a mortality decrease for mammography have included clinical breast examination, but the independent effect of the latter has not been studied. In addition, the efficacy of breast self-examination (BSE) has been documented although not in randomized, prospective mortality-based trials. To date, retrospective studies have found that BSE may detect an earlier stage of disease or smaller tumor size.

Despite its apparent effectiveness, breast cancer screening is not used to its fullest advantage. While screening rates may approach 70% to 74%, rates are lower for minorities and women over 65. The rates for consistent mammography screening at recommended intervals are not good. Rates for mammography in 2000 ranged from 57%–72%. Rates for clinical breast examination and mammography were higher, ranging between 37.3% and 69%. Recent data indicate that women may report BSE practice as frequently as seven to eight times a year but have low proficiency scores.

It is obvious that breast cancer screening has the potential to reduce mortality and morbidity from this dreaded disease. Breast cancer screening rates, although increasing, are not optimal. Most problematic is the fact that women do not follow current recommendations for screening. Minority rates for follow-up are dismal, and access to care is a real issue. This health-promoting detection activity is of primary importance to nurses in all areas of practice. Nurses are in an optimal position to increase all three screening methods (mammography, clinical breast examination, and BSE). Interventions to promote mammography and teach BSE can be carried out during general health promotion or while women are being seen for other reasons. Clinical breast examination is a skill that should be learned by all nurse practitioners and conducted yearly on all women aged 20 and over.

Several important theoretical variables have been tested for relationships to breast cancer screening—in particular, mammography and BSE. The theory that has generated the most research is the *health belief model.* The health belief model was initially conceptualized in the early 1950s to predict preventive behaviors such as influenza inoculations (Rosenstock, 1966). As originally formulated, the health belief model included the variable of perceived threat to health, which included the concepts of risk of contracting the disease (perceived susceptibility) and personal cost should the disease be contracted (perceived seriousness). In addition, benefits and barriers to taking a preventive action were predicted to influence the health behavior. In 1988, the concept of self-efficacy, or perceived confidence in carrying out a preventive behavior, was added to the health belief model.

Other theories that have been used to predict breast cancer screening have included Fishbein and Ajzen's (1975) theory of reasoned action, which postulates that two major concepts are related to breast cancer screening: (a) beliefs and evaluations of these beliefs and (b) social influence. Social influence is also composed of two components: beliefs of significant others and the influence of significant others on the individual. Most recently, the transtheoretical model has been tested with mammography use and found to predict behavior (Prochaska et al., 1994). This model defines the outcome in terms of stages of preparedness to engage in a health-promoting activity. In addition to the factors involved in these models, descriptive research suggests that breast cancer screening is influenced by knowledge, previous health habits, particular demographic characteristics, and health care systems.

A number of studies spanning over a decade have used various models to predict mammography screening. In general, attitudinal variables such as perceived susceptibility, perceived benefits to screening, and perceived barriers to screening have been predictive of mammography. Rakowski and coworkers (1992) found that perceived pros (benefits) and cons (barriers) varied across stages of mammography. The most consistent predictors of mammography use have been physician recommendation and barriers. The latter have included perceived lack of need, fear of results, fear of radiation, cost, pain, time, and inconvenience. Recently, the transtheoretical model has been used for predicting mammography by postulating that women move through a series of stages from precontemplation, or not thinking about mammography, to maintenance of mammography over time.

Descriptive studies to predict BSE have spanned the past 2 decades. Again, the variables of perceived susceptibility, benefits, and barriers have been significantly related to BSE. A less significant prediction of BSE compliance has been physician recommendation. Instead, women who were taught personally and returned a demonstration have been found to comply at higher rates. A major problem with BSE research has been the measurement of outcomes. In many earlier studies women were asked how many times they examined their breasts, and this was used as the operational measure of compliance. Later, self-report proficiency scales were widely used. Research has shown that there is often little correlation between reported frequency and proficiency, indicating that even if women practice BSE, they may not be doing it proficiently enough to detect lumps.

Actual measurement of BSE proficiency also has been problematic. The best studies have used trained observers to watch women either complete BSE or identify silicon lumps embedded in models. Subjective norms, as identified in the theory of reasoned action, have been predictive in some studies. Most research has identified low to moderate correlations between attitudinal variables and BSE. Perceived confidence for completing self-examination has been one of the strongest predictors.

Intervention research for both mammography and BSE has systematically built on the descriptive studies of earlier decades. Interventions have ranged from multistrategy community interventions to individual patient-oriented interventions. Many of the individually focused interventions targeted perceptions of risk, benefits, and barriers. Multistrategy interventions often targeted physician recommendation, which had been found to be an important predictor of mammography screening. Various ways of delivering messages have been tried, including the media, telephone delivery, tailored letters or postcards, and in-person counseling. Access has been identified as a problem, as shown by the fact that persons in health maintenance organizations (HMOs) consistently have higher rates of mammography screening than do patients in private medical practice. Access-enhancing interventions have included the use of mobile vans, which provide easier access for women with transportation problems. Costs of mammography for indigent women continue to be a problem, although agencies such as the American Cancer Society and Little Red Door have helped to defray these costs. Social network interventions have been effective with minority groups. Peer leaders can sometimes be important links for low-income, African American, or Hispanic women. Most interventions, especially those based on sound theory, have been successful in increasing mammography.

Interventions addressing BSE often focus on teaching women the correct skills for practice. Many of the interventions use educational strategies, with or without counseling, related to the theoretical constructs of perceived susceptibility, benefits, and barriers. Many studies have used reminder systems or self-prompts to increase practice. Interventions have ranged from handing out pamphlets to one-to-one teaching sessions with return demonstrations. Studies using models to identify lumps have been the most vigorous. Studies that include personal demonstrations, guided feedback, and both cognitive and personal instruction evidence the greatest increase in proficiency.

Descriptive and intervention studies based on similar theories of breast cancer screening have extended over the past 2 decades. The major difference in relation to promoting mammography is the addition of physician recommendation. Physician recommendation is important both because medical advice is related to mammography and because an order may be necessary to obtain a mammogram. For BSE, personal teaching has been found to be a most important predictor. We now know enough about breast cancer screening to make certain recommendations for nursing practice. For both BSE and mammography, clinicians must take into account the individual's perceptions about her susceptibility to breast cancer. If this perceived susceptibility is unrealistically low, efforts must be made to paint a more accurate picture. Perceived benefits and barriers to both mammography and BSE also should be addressed and individualized strategies developed. For BSE teaching, the set of skills needed to complete this exam and observation of proficiency will be important. A major future direction related to mammography will be to increase interval compliance.

Breast cancer screening research has broad implications for increasing other health behaviors, such as colorectal or prostate screening. Preventive behaviors such as the use of skin protection and adherence to low-fat diets can also be targeted for intervention trials. Finally, nurses must actively encourage public policy decisions that increase screening access for all people.

Victoria Champion

Breast-Feeding

Breast-feeding continues to be the gold standard for feeding infants, as it provides nutritional, immunological, cognitive, and psychological benefits for young children. Recently, a burgeoning body of research in the immunological and biochemical sciences has continued to identify the unique properties and unreplicable living tissue transferred to infants and children through breast-feeding. These studies have made the connection between breast-feeding and a decreased risk of illness and health problems in infants and children, supporting its importance and necessity to the health of humans (Heinig, 2001). Once seen as a personal lifestyle choice, documentation of the superiority of breast-feeding to the health and well-being of infants, children, and women, has led to the recognition that breast-feeding is a health care behavior. There continues to be a large discrepancy in the United States between breast-feeding rates, especially according to income, education, race, and ethnicity (Ahluwalia, Morrow, Hsia, & Grummer-Strawn, 2003). When breast-feeding is examined as a health care behavior, nurses have an opportunity for health promotion and disease prevention among mother-child dyads which can affect all of society. The Healthy People 2010 (2000) national health objectives target, 75% initiation of breast-feeding, 50% breast-feeding at 6 months, and 25% breast-feeding children until 1 year of age.

Breast-feeding has an international and interdisciplinary focus. Many professionals from various arenas of health care and the sciences are interested in lactation and the field continues to grow; however, experts, especially lactation consultants, are still underutilized. Nurses have intimate contact with women at key times to make a difference in their breast-feeding experiences. The majority of nursing breast-feeding research relates to promotion, protection, and support of breast-feeding.

Breast-feeding researchers in nursing examined the policies and practices that impact breast-feeding initiation. Nurse scientists continue to develop instruments to assess breast-feeding (Dennis, 2002; Riordan, Bibb, Miller, & Rawlins, 2001). More research is needed into nurses' influence on the decision to breast-feed and their roles in promoting and reinforcing women's decision. Investigators have demonstrated the importance of health care professionals' recommendations to mothers (Ahluwalia et al., 2003). Nurses need updated education based on research to provide this support at critical times, and to identify women at risk for complications early on, so that interventions can be initiated and referrals made in a timely fashion to preserve the breast-feeding relationship. They need to be aware of new research on breast-feeding in areas such as: breast reduction/augmentation surgery, HIV status, medical conditions, and drugs. Careful assessment of the benefits and risks of *not* breast-feeding should be in the forefront in nursing research.

The advent of the Breastfeeding-Friendly Hospital Initiative in 1997 in the United States by United Nations Children's Fund (UNICEF) encouraged the identification of practices that impact breast-feeding duration. Studies have demonstrated the negative effect on breast-feeding initiation and duration of: labor medications, vigorous suctioning, forcing baby to breast, ineffective positioning, early introduction of pacifiers, delayed feedings, routine separation of mother and baby, failure of nurses to frequently assess breast-feeding encounters, use of supplements, and provision of gift packs with promotional materials for artificial infant milk (Auerbach, 2000). In contrast, a meta-analysis of over 35 studies demonstrated that breast-feeding educational programs had the greatest single effect on initiation and short-term duration of breast-feeding, although support programs did increase both short and long-term duration (Guise et al., 2003).

In a thorough review of the literature from 1990-2000, Dennis (2002) examined breast-feeding initiation and duration and concluded that mothers who weaned prior to 6 months postpartum experienced perceived difficulties with breast-feeding. These studies identified those *least* likely to breast-feed as: young, low income, ethnic minority, unsupported, full-time employed women with a negative attitude toward breast-feeding and low confidence in their ability to breast-feed.

Partners and nonprofessionals were most supportive, hospital routines were often detrimental to breast-feeding, and health care professionals who lacked knowledge related to breast-feeding were seen as negative sources of support providing inaccurate and inconsistent advice (Dennis). These results provide a target population for intervention and indicate that even as knowledge has grown, the shift from knowledge to practice is painful and takes time (Hong, Callister, & Schwartz, 2003).

A major population needing attention focused on breast-feeding are low-income women, especially women of color within this group. African-American women have among the lowest rates of breast-feeding in the United States (Ahluwalia et al., 2003), 45% report ever breast-feeding (compared to 66% and 68% of Hispanic and white women) (Bentley, Dee, & Jensen, 2003). Reasons given by women for not breast-feeding include: embarrassment, a lack of social acceptability of breast-feeding (both public and private), work or school, the difficulty keeping the infant close, and lack of support.

Nurse scientists are using different methodologies to study breast-feeding, including: ethnographies, phenomenological studies, historical-cultural approaches, and ecological perspectives. Theoretical frameworks used to explore the health behavior of breast-feeding include the theory of planned behavior, the health belief model, social cognitive theory using the concept of self-efficacy, and the social ecological framework. Nurses are exhibiting a stronger role in publishing studies examining breast-feeding education, support, and prenatal and postnatal interventions to support the mother and infant. Researchers have demonstrated the importance of peer and social support, the effect of hospital interventions, the need for comprehensive breast-feeding education and support, communication-related barriers, socioeconomic issues, the effect of values and practice, and most importantly the culturally relevant issues that influence breast-feeding choices.

Clinical issues being explored by nurse scientists include: biological benefits of breast-feeding to the mother, breast-feeding and circumcision, HIV and breast-feeding, lactation mastitis, and positioning and attachment. The influence of the health care delivery system, community, and society/culture cannot be ignored.

Challenges related to the study of breast-feeding include three major areas: the lack of consistency in the definition of breast-feeding (e.g., exclusivity), making comparison of studies tedious if not impossible; the difficulty measuring cross-cultural effects (lack of reliability and validity studies of major breast-feeding instruments with various cultures); and the development of prospective designs and randomized controlled trials.

Although breast-feeding is now recognized as a right of mothers, a health care behavior contributing to the reduction of infant and maternal morbidity and mortality rates, less expensive than artificial milk supplementation and more environmentally friendly, the national breast-feeding goals are far from being met. Federal funding for breast-feeding research in the United States demonstrates an incongruity with the national priorities for breast-feeding. Only 13.7% ($5.6 million out of $40.4 million available) of federal research funds from 1994 to 1996 were awarded to projects having an impact on the Healthy People 2000 goals for increasing the incidence and duration of breast-feeding. In contrast, 27 projects (7.5% or $4.1 million) involved the use of human milk composition and technologies to improve artificial milks (Brown, Bair, & Meier, 2003). Nurses need to be at the forefront in protecting, promoting, and supporting breast-feeding for the health of society. This will require exploring the ways that cultural norms and structures at all levels support or interfere with breast-feeding for all women and ways in which nursing can make a difference.

SUZANNE HETZEL CAMPBELL

C

Cancer in Children

Pediatric oncology represents only a small fraction of the discipline of oncology. However, the numerous advances in the diagnosis and treatment of childhood cancer have resulted in significant improvements in survival. Approximately 75% of all children diagnosed with malignant neoplasms will survive more than 5 years (Smith & Gloeckler Reis, 2002).

The annual incidence of childhood cancer is 15.6 per 100,000 children ages birth to 19 years (U.S. Cancer Statistics Working Group, 2003). There is a slightly higher incidence in males (16.5 per 100,000) compared to females (14.6 per 100,000). There are approximately 12,400 children and adolescents less than 20 years of age diagnosed each year with cancer (Smith & Gloeckler Ries, 2002). Childhood cancer is the third leading cause of death in children ages 1 to 19 years (Arias, McDorman, Strobino, & Guyer, 2003). For children of all ages, leukemia is the most frequent type of cancer, followed by brain tumors and lymphomas. Tumors of the kidney and soft tissue are more common in African Americans, whereas tumors of the bone are more common in Caucasians.

The cause of childhood cancer is not known. Some childhood cancers, in particular retinoblastoma, Wilms tumor, and neuroblastoma demonstrate patterns of inheritance that suggest a genetic basis for the disorder. Chromosome abnormalities have been found in acute leukemia and lymphoma as well as in other pediatric solid tumors. Wilms tumor is associated with an increased incidence of congenital anomalies. Children with syndromes caused by abnormal numbers of chromosomes (e.g., Down syndrome) have an increased incidence of cancer (Gurney & Bondy, 2002). Children with immune deficiencies are at greater risk for developing cancer. Despite the lack of knowledge about the origin of cancer, there is some information on risk factors that increase the likelihood of children developing cancer. Environmental agents such as exposure to ionizing radiation have been found to cause cancer in children (Gurney & Bondy).

Major areas of pediatric oncology nursing research include psychosocial care needs, physical impact of cancer, nursing care procedures, nursing professional issues, and management of health care resources. A review by Hinds, Hockenberry, and Schum (2002) found that the majority of published studies (70%) are related to psychosocial care needs of the child and family. Only 5.5% of the published studies were on nursing care procedures, and less than 5% were on nursing professional issues. Most studies (78.2%) were published in nursing journals and of those, 67% were published in cancer nursing journals. While increased attention on nursing research has occurred over the past 10 years, many areas of pediatric oncology nursing have yet to be explored.

The emphasis on psychosocial care needs of children with cancer and families has changed over the past 20 years, due to the improvement in childhood cancer survival. Nursing research in the 1980s focused on grief and loss experienced by the parents and siblings of children who died of cancer. Researchers studied how care was provided in the home care environment, the needs of parents facing the loss of a child, and terminal care costs. As survival improved, chronic illness and its impact on the child and family living with a cancer took center stage. In recent years researchers have evaluated perceptions of clinical trials and understanding of the consent process, while continuing to evaluate stress and coping in the child and family. Adolescent risk-taking behaviors is a new research area as survival rates continue to improve and childhood cancer survivors move toward adulthood.

In order to evaluate the status of the current research on symptom management in individuals with cancer, the National Institutes of Health recently held a State of the Science Conference on Symptom Management in Cancer: Pain, Depression, and Fatigue (NIH, 2002). The review of existing research revealed that efforts to manage symptoms of cancer and its treatments have not kept pace with new advances in the causes and cures for cancer. Three landmark studies have addressed distressing cancer events and symptoms from the specific perspective of the child and their families (Hedstrom, Haglund, Skolin, & von Essen, 2003; Woodgate & Degner, 2003; Collins et al., 2000). Hedstrom et al. discovered that the most common causes of distress in a group of 121 children with cancer were treatment-related pain, nausea, and fatigue. Collins et al. described the most common physical symptoms (prevalence > 35%) in a group of 160 children with cancer as lack of energy, pain, drowsiness, nausea, cough, and lack of appetite. Woodgate and Degner evaluated expectations and beliefs about childhood cancer symptoms in a group of 39 children and their family members and found that these individuals expected to experience suffering as part of the cancer treatment. The families felt unrelieved or uncontrolled symptoms were necessary for cure. Nurse researchers have evaluated pain management issues, complications of central venous access, blood product infusion methods, and chest tube care.

Also, a relatively new area of symptom management research focus is the evaluation of fatigue in children and adolescents with cancer. Fatigue has been found to be one of the most distressing symptoms experienced during childhood cancer treatment. The prevalence of this symptom confirms the need to explore the interrelationships between fatigue and other symptoms commonly experienced by children with cancer. This symptom has been evaluated from both qualitative and quantitative research perspectives. Fatigue measurement instruments have been developed and tested during the past 5 years. Multi-center trials have been implemented to evaluate this symptom in children with cancer.

As survival for childhood cancer continues to improve, nursing investigations are focusing on survivorship issues and quality of life following the diagnosis and treatment of cancer. Nursing studies have documented the adverse effects of central nervous system (CNS) treatment on cognitive, academic, and psychosocial functioning. Interventions designed to minimize the adverse effects of central nervous system therapy are now being conducted.

Docherty (2003) recently completed a review of the published literature on symptom experiences of children and adolescents with cancer. This review revealed no longitudinal symptom management study designs, limited use of conceptual models or theories, frequent adaptation of adult instruments as symptom measures, and no attention to the impact of these symptoms on the children's lives.

It is evident from the recent childhood cancer pain literature that there is still much to be gained from continued research. The importance of striving for symptom relief in children cannot be over emphasized. Recognition and acknowledgment of the beliefs and expectations of children and their parents regarding cancer-related symptoms (Woodgate & Degner, 2003) should continue to be a major research focus. Limited research is found regarding assessment of pain in children with cancer. Longitudinal studies evaluating the trajectory of pain over time are not found. The effective use of pain management teams in hospital settings and their relationship with cancer center staff need further development and evaluation. Continued exploration of the most effective drug regimens and methods of delivery should be pursued for children experiencing all types of cancer pain. Finally, utilization of research findings in the clinical setting is lacking. More innovative, creative methods for dissemination of our knowledge of cancer pain and its management must be explored.

MARILYN HOCKENBERRY

Cancer Survivorship

As we move forward in the new millennium more people are living with cancer than dying from it (National Cancer Institute [NCI], 2003). Indeed barring death by other causes, 63% of adults treated for cancer are alive 5 years after diagnosis, accounting for 10 million cancer survivors (NCI). For most people this means that cancer has gone from a death sentence to a chronic disease. This success has resulted from continued advances made both in the laboratory and at the bedside.

The word *survivor* is derived from the Middle French *survivre,* to outlive, and from the Latin *supervivere*, to live more (Merriam-Webster Online, 2004). Thus, cancer survivorship is the period of time after the diagnosis and treatment of cancer through the remainder of life (NCI, 2003). It encompasses the physical, psychosocial, and economic sequelae of cancer diagnosis and its treatment and issues related to health care delivery, access, and follow-up care among both pediatric and adult survivors of cancer (NCI).

The current focus on cancer survivorship is in large part a result of the visionary efforts of the National Coalition for Cancer Survivorship (NCCS). Founded in 1986, it was established to refocus attention from people victimized by cancer to people living with and surviving cancer (NCCS, 2003). The NCCS evolved from a peer-support organization to what is now a formidable advocacy group setting public policy priorities on behalf of people with cancer. Moreover, as a result of the efforts of the NCCS as well as other grassroots organizations, in 1996 the NCI created the Office of Cancer Survivorship (OCS) in recognition of the large number of individuals now surviving cancer and their unique and unstudied needs. Since its inception the OCS has funded initiatives geared towards the stimulation of research on long-term cancer survivorship. Thus, although the concept of cancer survivorship is relatively young, these novel efforts have provided important structure for a small but rapidly increasing field of cancer survivorship research.

In his annual report to the nation, Dr. Andrew von Eschenbach of the National Cancer Institute identified areas of focus for survivorship research. They included long-term follow-up of childhood cancer survivors and issues faced by cancer survivors from underserved populations (NCI, 2003). These areas are uniquely relevant to nursing practice and therefore represent important areas for future research as the number of cancer survivors increases in the coming decades. Findings of studies related to these foci will be discussed.

Cancer survivorship research originated from studies conducted with adolescent and adult survivors of pediatric cancers culminating from 3 decades of successful treatment for pediatric cancers. Recent statistics indicate that 1 in 1,000 20-year-olds is a childhood cancer survivor (Meadows, Krejmas, & Belasco, 1980). Ironically, the same treatment that produced successful response rates can also cause long-term adverse effects (Smith, M., & Hare, 2004). For many pediatric cancer survivors, survivorship is marked by the occurrence of treatment-related late effects, i.e., side effects that do not resolve or that arise after completion of therapy, and may result in physical, social, and emotional consequences. Such effects include a plethora of physical, intellectual, pubertal, and reproductive manifestations, as well as the potential for secondary cancers (Swartz, 1999). These effects represent a lifelong risk that often negatively influence quality of life and may be linked to the practice of high-risk lifestyle behaviors, including smoking and consumption of alcohol, practices that are further complicated in this population because of their genetic predisposition and previous exposure to cytotoxic agents (Larcombe, Mott, & Hunt, 2002; Swartz).

An important vehicle for addressing some of these and other childhood cancer survivor concerns is the Childhood Cancer Survivor Study (CCCS). Funded by the National Cancer Institute, the CCCS is a collaborative, multi-institutional, longitudinal survey of over 14,500 5-year childhood cancer survivors initially diagnosed between 1970 and 1986. Survivors who participated in the study completed baseline and follow-up questionnaires including items related to organ system functioning, health habits, psychosocial health, fertility, and second malignancies. Highlights of four studies reporting initial findings were: (a) a statistically significant excess of secondary malignancies, the most common being breast cancer, thyroid cancer, meningioma, sarcoma, and bone cancer (Neglia et al., 2001); (b) reduced general physical and mental health, and activity and functional limitations when compared with siblings (Hudson et al., 2003); (c) increased use of special education services when compared with siblings (23% vs. 8%) (Mitby et al., 2003); and (d) increased reports of depressive and somatic distress when compared with siblings (Zebrack et al., 2002). These important findings provide insight into a variety of concerns relevant to childhood cancer survivors. As a result of this work, the CCCS has laid the groundwork for further examination into other issues that will provide additionally important contributions to childhood cancer survivors.

Cancer survivors from underserved populations may include the elderly, those with low income and educational levels, survivors from ethnic and cultural minorities, and those who live in remote areas (Rowland, Aziz, Tesauro, & Feuer, 2001). As increasing numbers of people from underserved populations are diagnosed and treated for cancer, significant differences have been reported with respect to patterns of cancer-specific survival and relative risks of cancer death (Surveillance Epidemiology and End Results [SEER], 2004), as well as other issues such as access to care (Shavers & Brown, 2002), cost of treatment (Brandeis, Pashos, Henning, & Litwin, 2001), access to educational and emotional support services (Wilson, Andersen, & Meischke, 2000), and meaning of cancer (Phillips, Cohen, & Moses, 1999). These differences have implications for the adaptation to and survival of cancer. Moreover, these factors may be complicated by poorer overall health status as a result of comorbidities or lifestyle.

In a review of the current state of knowledge of cancer survivorship among ethnic minorities and medically underserved groups, Aziz and Rowland (2002) found that research related to the impact of ethnic and minority groups on issues of survivorship is largely related to epidemiologic analysis of cancer risk and survival. Thus, research related to issues of the underserved and cancer survivorship is needed. Some of their findings included the following: (a) a majority of studies of late effects of treatment of secondary cancers were conducted on Caucasian survivors of cancer; (b) while there is a growing body of literature on sociocultural and behavioral determinants of cancer decision making, few studies explored interventions in underserved populations and; (c) culturally relevant measures that capture concerns of cancer survivors were largely absent.

The number of people with cancer is expected to reach 2.6 million by the year 2050. Thus, there is a growing emphasis on conducting research that improves the understanding of cancer survivors. Needed are intervention studies that develop or test strategies to promote optimal health status in survivors of cancer, information on survivors of cancer who have previously been understudied, and research on the impact of cancer on the family (Rowland et al., 2001). Nurse researchers have the potential to make a significant contribution to improving the lives of people who live with cancer.

LORRIE L. POWEL

Capitation

Capitation, a form of payment for health services, is usually associated with managed care. This form of payment is a change from fee-for-service payments as a method of compensation to capitation for services and to negotiation of reduced payments to health-care providers (Schramm, 1996). Kongsvedt (1995) defined capitation specifically as "prepayment for services on a per member per month (PMPM) basis" (p. 76). Capitation can also be defined as a fixed payment per health plan enrollee being paid to a provider for a defined set of services for a prescribed period of time (Knowlton, 1996). Under capitation, providers or provider organizations receive the same amount of dollars every month (PMPM rate) for each enrolled member regardless of how expensive the services are or whether the member actually received services. Capitation payments are usually calculated on the capitation equivalent of average fee-for-service revenues of the provider or provider organization (based on actual or existing data for the population of interest) and vary according to the age and gender of the enrolled members. In some cases, the capitation rate is also based on risk, or on expected high utilization of service based on risk, or on specific conditions such as use of illegal drugs, selected chronic illness, and so forth.

Although health care reform as a legislative agenda is no longer relevant, market-driven reform is rapidly changing the structure and terminology of health care delivery to managed care. Managed care has grown out of the need to control escalating health care costs and has become accepted as an inevitable way for health care to be delivered. Managed health care organizations are not new. They grew out of the private sector when prepaid plans were implemented in health maintenance organizations (HMOs). Implemented in the 1970s, HMO providers first shared the risk of financing health care for an enrolled population. Providers (primarily physicians) were offered the choice of collecting a fee for service from the patient or having the HMO pay the physician directly out of a prepaid per capita payment (capitation) for health services. Any excess revenue generated above expenses could be shared by providers, and enrollees (members) were also able to save health insurance premiums by reducing unnecessary hospital admissions and lengths of stays. Many forms of managed care organizations besides HMOs exist, but the challenge for all these provider organizations is to remove inefficiencies and reduce costs from the current fee-for-service systems and through capitation to improve the quality and coordination of care across the continuum.

In many cases, one capitated payment is in place that covers care across the continuum. In other situations, a blended capitation rate such as $*x* PMPM may exist for primary care services, with an additional capitated pool of #*xx* for referral services, and $*xxx* for inpatient or institutional care. Capitation affects nurses in all care settings across the continuum, from the staff nurse in acute care to the home health nurse to the primary care nurse practitioner. Awareness of the value of prevention, health promotion, and coordination of care in order to reduce unplanned visits and unexpected admissions is key to success in a capitated managed care system. New nursing roles of case management and primary care provider in community-based settings offer opportunities created by managed care and challenges to manage care within specific limited resources.

Research related to capitation in the context of managed care is health systems research, health services research, or evaluation research. Holzemer and Reilly (1994) used the term *variations research* as an important strategy designed to improve the quality of care while controlling costs. They proposed an outcomes model (based on the work of Donabedian) that allowed for measurement of variability related to client or population (age, gender, risk, etc.), variability of providers (such as advanced practice nurses vs. physicians), variability of interventions or process of care, and variability in outcomes of care (which may include quality indicators, costs, cost savings, and patient/provider satisfaction).

Research related to capitation may involve assessment of risk for population-based care and determining the appropriate capitation based on variability within different populations. Community health assessment performed by community health nurses may be used for these types of assessments. Research related to capitation may involve study of the different uses and types of providers or processes of care needed to achieve required outcomes at a particular price (capitation rate PMPM). Finally, the research may focus on the cost savings of a particular intervention, for example, transitional models of care between hospital and home or the use of case management models to reduce inappropriate utilization of care.

The unit of analysis in research related to capitation is of paramount importance. Nurse researchers may study the client and client characteristics, the provider or provider system, specific interventions, or outcomes. Outcomes research is of great interest to managed care companies that are implementing capitation models. These companies desire quality outcomes (functional and clinically relevant changes) in the client and client satisfaction with the care, and they want them in a cost-effective manner. Variations research is an attempt to control confounding variables such as risk, severity of illness, and client characteristics that influence outcomes of care. Risk adjustment of outcomes is complex but must be addressed in variations research. Use of information systems to obtain data related to costs and other outcomes from organizational databases must be addressed. The issue of decisions related to data substitution and use of proxies to handle missing data is a relevant issue for health systems researchers who study the impact or effectiveness of capitation in the context of managed care.

Finally, an important issue is educating practicing nurses, current nurse researchers, and future students in the risk, cost, and quality issues related to capitation in managed care. The rapid increase in managed care organizations and systems has introduced new terms and concepts into medical and nursing language.

More current literature suggests that providers are turning to fee-for-service charges to make up revenue lost under capitation (Dalzell, 2002). Nonetheless, even though health care on a fixed, per-capita budget has lost favor of late, many trends are cyclical just as this trend may be (Dalzell, 2002).

PATRICIA HINTON WALKER
UPDATED BY KAREN L. ELBERSON

Cardiovascular Disease

Cardiovascular diseases (CVD), which include stroke, hypertension (HTN), arrhythmias, coronary heart disease (CHD), and heart failure (HF) are major contributors to mortality and morbidity. Although the most prevalent form of CVD is HTN, the majority of CVD deaths are attributed to CHD. The prevalence and incidence of CHD increase dramatically with age and CHD is the leading cause of death in the elderly, with 84% of all CHD deaths in those 65 years of age or older (American Heart Association [AHA], 2001). Angina, sudden death and myocardial infarction (MI) are the major manifestations of CHD. Twenty-five percent of men and 38% of women will die within 1 year of their MI (AHA). Although HF may result from valvular dysfunction and other conditions, the majority of cases of HF are attributable to CHD with approximately 22% of men and 46% of women disabled by heart failure post-MI (AHA). Despite the importance of CHD, prevention and management of CHD are only beginning to be studied in the elderly population. The Second World Assembly on Aging in 2002 addressed the international issue of supporting patients in both primary and secondary prevention of CHD and HF that are so prevalent in the geriatric population. Although control of hypertension and dyslipidemia have been shown to reduce CVD mortality and morbidity in both middle-aged and elderly individuals, the efficacy of other measures such as lowering homocysteine and fibrinogen levels, quitting smoking, exercising or weight reduction are not yet established in the elderly. Nevertheless, such measures appear to be warranted (Kannel, 1997; Gladdish & Rajkumar, 2001). Much of our current knowledge, however, is still based on studies conducted with non-elderly individuals.

CHD and subsequent MI are potentially preventable conditions. The recent publication of the standards of care for both dyslipidemia (Adult Treatment Panel III [ATP III] Guidelines, 2001) and hypertension (Chobanian et al., 2003) do not make guidelines specific to different adult age groups. Older and younger adults are classified by their risk factors, with increasing age yielding a higher risk score in the Framingham Risk Profile. Research aimed at prevention must address the importance of established risk factors in the elderly, as well as identifying new risk factors specific to the elderly population. Age-related differences exist between younger and elderly individuals regarding cardiac risk factors, and the role of conventional cardiac risk factors remains controversial. In addition, diabetes mellitus is a prevalent problem, and is considered a CHD equivalent (ATP III). Diabetes is also associated with an increased risk of recurrent MI, HF, and death following MI. Knowledge of diabetes management in relation to the of development of CHD and MI, as well as to long-term outcomes, however, is limited.

Secondly, although information regarding patient management of cardiac risk factors is limited, recent trials of lipid-lowering agents have demonstrated a beneficial effect on morbidity and mortality (Mostaghel & Waters, 2003). Large multicenter hypertension trials have also begun to demonstrate the efficacy of aggressive hypertension treatment in reducing risk of CHD (Puddey, 2000). Identification and evaluation of the efficacy of other preventive interventions, therefore, need to be documented, as well as individual characteristics that contribute to better risk factor control. Nursing also has an important role in studying methods and adequacy of dissemination of guidelines for primary prevention of CHD established by the AHA, not only to the public, but to health care providers (Williams et al., 2002). Levels of physical activity and control of lipids, HTN, obesity, and smoking need to be determined, along with side effects of these interventions. Management of diet and exercise may pose special challenges; medications to treat hypertension and lipid abnormalities may not be well-tolerated and the potential for side effects and drug interactions is increased in the setting of polypharmacy. Finally, consideration of psychosocial factors is warranted. Psychosocial influences, which may contribute to control cardiac risk factors, and quality of life, which may be affected by control of cardiac risk factors, however, have not been widely studied in the elderly population.

Advanced age is known to be associated with an increased risk of in-hospital death following MI, and a beginning understanding of prognostic factors for short-term mortality is available (Normand et al., 1997; Chyun et al., 2002). Efficacy of monitoring for complications, and methods to prepare individuals and their caregivers for discharge, within a shortened hospital stay, however, need to be studied. Awareness of prognostic factors can assist in identifying patients at risk of short-term mortality so that interventional nursing care can be targeted, delivered to, and assessed in high-risk individuals. Many individuals who are eligible for aspirin or beta-blocker therapy following MI do not receive these medications upon discharge. Discrepancies between other medications known to have a survival benefit—ACE inhibitors, lipid lowering agents—may also exist and need to be documented, along with reasons for any discrepancy. Although coronary revascularization procedures—angioplasty or bypass surgery—are being used more frequently, nursing research is also needed to document post-discharge complications and long-term management of underlying CHD. Hospitalization for acute MI or revascularization may provide the only opportunity to maximize CHD management, as well as link the individual to a cardiac rehabilitation program following discharge.

Older age has consistently been associated with poorer long-term outcomes—death, recurrent MI, and CHF—following MI. Although acute MI-related prognostic factors are beginning to be identified (Chyun et al., 2002), information on post-discharge factors that may have contributed to these outcomes, as well as to use of health care services, has not been documented. It is unknown how patients manage their cardiac condition, control specific cardiac risk factors, or if they participate in cardiac rehabilitation. Nor is it known what factors contribute to or prevent successful CHD management in the elderly. Angina and psychosocial factors may contribute to long-term management of CHD and adverse outcomes, yet only limited information is available on these possible influences (Stuart-Shor et al., 2003). These data are crucial prior to much-needed interventional studies aimed at decreasing the substantial mortality and morbidity associated with CHD and MI. Potential psychosocial factors that may contribute to poorer long-term outcomes, therefore, need to be identified. Educational strategies directed specifically to the needs of the elderly and their caregivers also need to be identified and tested. In addition, factors, such as the impact of functional status, which has been linked to mortality require further study in the elderly population with CHD.

Functional status has been shown to be an important prognostic factor after MI, even after adjustment for other prognostic factors, yet it has not been widely studied, despite higher levels of functional disability in the elderly. Functional loss appears to be proceeded by a decline in physical performance, and early functional limitations or mild impairments that are not evident clinically have been shown to predict subsequent functional dependence (Gill, Williams, Mendes de Leon, & Tinettit, 1997). Subjects at risk of functional decline may be identified early, prior to loss of function, so that interventions may be targeted. Although physical performance and functional status may influence participation in a cardiac rehabilitation program, both can be greatly improved through exercise rehabilitation. Therefore, low levels at outset should not prohibit participation.

Cardiac rehabilitation, including exercise rehabilitation, has been shown to improve exercise tolerance and assist in control of cardiac risk factors; however, few studies are available that address these issues in the elderly (Lavie & Milani, 1995; Pasquali, Alexander, & Peterson, 2001). Although physical activity is central to management of CHD, and it is recommended that men and women should be strongly encouraged to participate in exercise-based cardiac rehabilitation and that special efforts be made to overcome obstacles to entry and participation, the elderly, particularly elderly women, are referred to and enroll less frequently than younger individuals (Lavie & Milani, 1995). Despite improvements in functional status, anxiety, depression, mobility, health care resource consumption, and mortality with exercise, the majority of older adults report having no regular exercise and most report not having walked a mile in the past year. The reasons that individuals do not enroll in cardiac rehabilitation have not been well defined, but probably result from a combination of physical, psychosocial, and economic factors. Barriers to participation, therefore, need to be explored and strategies for improving access and maintaining participation tested.

Prevalence of HF in the elderly MI population increases with increasing age, and following MI, older age has been shown to be related to the development of HF despite normal systolic function. Normal age-related changes in the elderly also appear to affect diastolic, rather than systolic function. HF is associated with decreased quality of life and a decrease in functional capacity. While multidisciplinary teams, focusing on coordination of inpatient, outpatient and home care have demonstrated positive outcomes in terms of functional capacity, length of stay, readmission rates, self-care knowledge, patient satisfaction, and quality of life (Rich et al., 1995; Venner & Solitro-Seelbinder, 1996; Naylor et al., 1994; Stanley & Prasun, 2002; Grady et al., 2000), and prognostic factors for readmission have been identified, HF remains the leading cause of hospitalization in the elderly. Additional interventional studies are needed on management of common problems in this population—monitoring for deterioration in clinical status, medication, dietary and fluid adjustment, social support, and noncompliance—as well as in innovative strategies, such as use of structured exercise programs, in HF management. In addition, with the recent publication of new guidelines for HF, a new staging system expands the continuum of care to encompass prevention and includes screening and treatment targets for people at high risk for developing heart failure (Hunt et al., 2001). As HF will continue to be an important problem in the elderly population, nursing research should focus on evaluating nursing interventions that reduce hospital admission and improve quality of life.

JESSICA SHANK COVIELLO
DEBORAH A. CHYUN

Cardiovascular Risk Factors: Cholesterol

Coronary heart disease (CHD) is a major cause of morbidity and premature mortality in men and women in the United States, the industrialized world, and many developing countries. Atherosclerotic-CHD processes begin early in life and are influenced over time by the interaction of genetic and potentially modifiable environmental factors including health-related lifestyle behaviors. Hypercholesterolemia, elevated serum total cholesterol (TC), is recognized as an independent risk factor for CHD. Low-density lipoprotein cholesterol (LDL-C), the major atherogenic lipoprotein, typically constitutes 60%–70% of serum TC and is the primary target of cholesterol-lowering therapy. In 1988, based on available epidemiological and clinical data, the National Cholesterol Education Program (NCEP) Adult Treatment Panel (ATP) issued the first guidelines for identifying and managing hypercholesterolemia in adults. Throughout the past 16 years, results of numerous randomized controlled trials confirmed that lowering LDL-C was important in primary and secondary prevention of CHD. The most recent revision of these guidelines (Executive Summary of the Third Report of the National Cholesterol Education Program, 2001), referred to as ATP III, continues to focus on LDL-C as the primary target of risk reduction therapy, considers other lipid and nonlipid risk factors, and emphasizes therapeutic lifestyle change (TLC) and pharmacological therapies for reducing individual risk and the public health burden of CHD. With continued emphasis on identification of individuals at risk and more attention to adherence-enhancing strategies, ATP III incorporates numerous roles for nurses and nursing across health care settings where lipid abnormalities are diagnosed and treated.

ATP III continues to define hypercholesterolemia as TC ≥ 240 mg/dl (6.21 mmol/L) for individuals 20 years of age and older; TC levels of 200–239 mg/dl are considered borderline high and < 200 mg/dl is considered desirable. LDL-C levels are categorized as follows: very high (≥ 190 mg/dl), high (160–189 mg/dl), borderline high (130–159 mg/dl), above optimal (100–129 mg/dl), and optimal (< 100 mg/dl). Results of very recent clinical trials suggested that LDL-C lowering beyond 100 mg/dl in secondary prevention (after an acute coronary event) was associated with improved cardiovascular outcomes and raised questions regarding the currently established cutpoints for LDL-C (Cannon et al., 2004; Nissen et al., 2004; Topol, 2004). The National Cholesterol Education Program (NCEP) has not revised the 1991 definitions and guidelines for management of hypercholesterolemia in children and adolescents in the United States; however, the American Heart Association's (AHA) recent guidelines for primary prevention are consistent with NCEP definitions: acceptable TC (< 170 mg/dl [4.4 mmol/L]), borderline TC (170–199 mg/dl), elevated TC (≥ 200 mg/dl) (Kavey et al., 2003). Similar to adults, both lipid and nonlipid risk factors are addressed, LDL-C levels are targeted as the basis for treatment decisions, and TLC is the cornerstone of treatment. LDL-C levels ≤ 110 mg/dl are considered acceptable for children and adolescents without comorbidities; LDL-C < 100 mg/dl is recommended for children and adolescents with diabetes. ATP III recommends a fasting lipoprotein profile (TC, LDL-C, high-density lipoprotein cholesterol [HDL-C], and triglyceride) should be obtained once every 5 years in adults aged 20 years or older. A basic principle of prevention is emphasized throughout ATP III: the intensity of risk-reduction therapy should be adjusted to an individual's absolute risk.

The Framingham projections of 10-year absolute CHD risk (i.e., the percent probability of having a CHD event in 10 years) are used to identify and risk-stratify individuals. In addition to LDL-C, risk determinants include: presence or absence of CHD and other clinical forms of atherosclerotic disease, cigarette smoking, hypertension (blood pressure ≥ 140/90 mm Hg or on antihypertensive medication), low HDL-C (< 40 mg/dl), family history of premature CHD, and age (men ≥ 45 years, women ≥ 55 years). The category of highest risk (10-year risk > 20%) includes CHD and CHD risk equivalents (other clinical forms of atherosclerotic disease, diabetes) has a goal of LDL-C defined as < 100 mg/dl. The intermediate risk category (10-year risk ≤ 20%) includes multiple (2+) risk factors and has goal LDL-C as 130 mg/dl; the lowest risk category (10-year risk < 10%) includes 0–1 risk factors with LCL-C goal of 160 mg/dl.

The cornerstone of treatment for hypercholesterolemia and other lipid abnormalities is therapeutic lifestyle change (TLC) with emphasis on dietary modification, increased physical activity and normalization of body weight. Important components of the TLC diet are saturated fat (less than 7% of total calories), polyunsaturated fat (up to 10% of total calories) and monounsaturated fat (up to 20% of total calories). Less than 200 mg/day of dietary cholesterol, 50–60% of total calories from carbohydrates and approximately 15% of total calories from protein are recommended. Other key components of the TLC diet include viscous fiber, plant stanols/sterols, and soy protein. Considerable variation in response to dietary modification has been observed in males and females across the life span. Variations in serum TC, for example (ranging from 3% to 14%) are attributed to individual differences in biological mechanisms, baseline TC levels, nutrient composition of baseline diets, and adherence over time to the prescribed dietary regimen.

The first priority of pharmacological therapy is to achieve the appropriate LDL-C goal (as defined by the individual's category of risk). ATP III recommends the use of HMG-CoA reductase inhibitors (statins) as first-line therapeutic agents. In a meta-analysis of clinical trials, the average reduction in TC in over 30,000, middle-aged men followed for over 5 years was 20%, the average reduction in LDL-C was 28%, and the decline in triglyceride averaged 13% (LaRosa, He, & Vupputuri, 1999). Results of a very recent secondary prevention trial suggested that early and continued lowering of LDL-C with an intensive lipid-lowering (statin) regimen provides greater protection against death or major cardiovascular events than a standard regimen (Cannon et al., 2004). Other pharmacological agents currently used in treatment of dyslipidemia in adults include bile-acid binding resins, niacin, and fibrates. Decisions to initiate LDL-C lowering drug therapy, the type and dosage of agent to be used, and the schedule for monitoring individual response to therapy are based on the individual's baseline risk status. Normally, the patient's response is evaluated about 6 weeks after starting drug therapy. Relatedly, TLC continues throughout (and beyond) the duration of pharmacotherapy.

Consistent with recommendations of the 33rd Bethesda Conference on preventive cardiology (Ockene, Hayman, Pasternak, Schron, & Dunbar-Jacob, 2002), ATP III identifies and targets adherence-enhancing interventions that consider the characteristics of the individual patient, the provider, and systems of health care delivery. Case management by nurses within the context of multidisciplinary team approaches is considered an integral component of increasing adherence to therapeutic regimens for hypercholesterolemia and other lipid abnormalities.

Assessment and management of hypercholesterolemia and other lipid abnormalities is an important component of both individual/ high risk and population-based approaches to CVD risk reduction. Current evidence-based guidelines, including ATP III and the AHA primary prevention guidelines for children and youth, consider both lipid and nonlipid risk factors, target LDL-C in algorithms for assessment and treatment considerations, and emphasize TLC as the cornerstone of treatment. Therapeutic regimens including pharmacotherapy and TLC are based on the individual's risk status; treatment outcomes are optimized with case management by nurses within the context of a multidisciplinary team approach. Directions for future research build on and extend current programs of nursing and multidisciplinary research focused on innovative models for primary and secondary prevention of CVD across the life span and with emphasis on both quality and cost as outcomes (Allen et al., 2002). In addition, current recommendations emphasize family-based approaches to CVD risk reduction; however, minimal data exist regarding strategies for effective implementation in clinical practice.

LAURA HAYMAN

Caregiver

The term *caregiver* is defined as an individual who assists ill person(s), helps with a patient's physical care, typically lives with the patient, and does not receive monetary compensation for the help. A more descriptive definition of a caregiver is a person who not only performs common caregiver responsibilities (i.e., providing physical, social, spiritual, financial management, and technical care) but also advocates for the ill person within health care systems and society as a whole. The caregiver role is often anticipated in relationship to elders, yet rarely is there preparation for caregiving to one's child or one's spouse.

Delineating the role of the caregiver reveals potential problems they experience. Direct patient care encompasses much more than physical care; it also necessitates learning an extensive amount of information about illness, symptoms, medications, technological treatments, and how to relate to health care professionals (Smith, 1995). Caregivers also must be prepared for emergencies and be capable to respond. Usually the caregiver must also maintain their personal responsibilities, whether as breadwinner, housekeeper, or both. The caregiver's relationship with the patient, the caregiver's age and life developmental stage, the patient's illness severity, and the suddenness and amount of the change in the patient's need for caregiving have been predictive of caregiver burnout in various illness populations such as cancer care with home chemotherapy, cardiac rehabilitation, muscle deterioration, and dementia victims (Biegel, Sales, & Schultz, 1991).

The indirect familial caregiver tasks include designating others to assist with patient care, exchanging information, and maintaining decision making among appropriate persons. Caregivers also have numerous expectations for themselves and from others around them to perform various psychosocial tasks such as coping with changes in role, grieving the loss of the health and personality of their loved one, releasing tension, resolving uncertainty or guilt, and providing positive regard for those with whom they interact.

Because the caregiver by definition is laden with tasks and expectations, it is no wonder that the major area of research has been caregiver burden and negative outcomes on caregivers' physical, mental, and financial health. The majority of burden studies have been descriptive and correlational and have resulted in identification of multiple factors recognized as being significant for burden: characteristics of the care needed by the patient that are often measured as illness demands. Numerous variables (e.g., demographic information, developmental stage, social support) that have been studied in relation to caregiver experience are influential yet not universally predictive of caregiver burden (Biegel et al., 1991). Research across disciplines identifies significant negative health outcomes of caregiving (reduced physical function, immune status, wound healing, greater fatigue, mortality, and cardiovascular disease) (Beach, Schultz, Yee, & Jackson, 2000; Federal Interagency Forum on Aging, 2000; Given & Given, 1998; Schultz & Beach, 1999; Silver & Wellman, 2002). The majority of caregivers experience depression, social isolation, financial strain, sleep deprivation with daytime sleepiness, and inefficient use of family resources (Fitzgerald, 2003; Smith, 1996). These caregiver problems directly influence patient outcomes, resulting in complications and high health service use (Smith, Pace, et al., 2002). Smith's (1994) research indicated caregivers' motives for helping consistently explain variance in their depression, coping, and quality of life (Smith, Kleinbeck, Boyle, Kochinda, & Parker, 2002).

Problem-solving ability is lauded as essential and caregivers' ability to solve problems can avert patient problems (National Family Caregivers Association, 2002; Schultz, 2000), yet only a handful of studies on problem solving in caregiving were found and not all had positive outcomes (Roberts et al., 1995). Unique research on the positive aspects of caregiving is being conducted by Smith under the concept of caregiving effectiveness. Effective caregiving is defined as family provision of technical, physical, and emotional care that results in optimal patient health and quality of life and minimal technological side effects (e.g., catheter infections) while maintaining the caregiver's health and quality of life. Nursing interventions have been found efficacious for caregiver problems of depression, sleep deprivation, social isolation, and lack of access to evidence-based information, caregiving and complex technology problem solving. These interventions include counseling, peer support, high-quality internet information, and contacts with experts. For example, there is a dearth of research on caregiving with lifelong technology dependence that begins unexpectedly in middle life (when teenagers and elder family members also need assistance) and continues on a trajectory of intermittent disease exacerbations and slow, progressive decline (Collins, Stommel, Wang, & Given, 1994; DiMartini et al., 1998; Howard & Malone, 1996).

The most widely recommended clinical yet unverified approach is to provide guidelines to manage specific caregiving problems (Schultz, Lustig, Handler, & Martire, 2002). A step-by-step approach is an essential caregiving skill. Step-by-step guidelines on computer algorithms can guide systematic thinking and develop skills for solving stressful problems (Smith et al., 2003; Wilkinson & Mynors-Wallis, 1994). The state of the science report on computer-based algorithms that aid patients to make step-by-step decisions about treatment options concluded that improved knowledge, attitudes, and lower health services used resulted from patients' use of algorithms (Agency for Health Care Policy and Research [AHCPR], 1998). The Cochrane review and randomized trial results concur, adding that patients with step-by-step decision aids had realistic treatment expectations, satisfaction with care, and lowered anxiety (O'Connor et al., 2002). The more successful problem-solving algorithms included logical, easily-remembered steps, multi-perspective (psychological and physical) information, long-term access, and booster repetition, all tailored to a specific group with common problems (Shaw, McTavish, Hawkins, Gustafson, & Pingree, 2000).

Research should continue on the culturally-related aspects of caregiving strategies used in various ethnic groups (Picot, 1995). Another contemporary focus in caregiving research should be the caregiving family, as research has clearly indicated that multiple members of families are involved in providing direct and indirect care, both to the patient and in support of the primary caregiver (Smith CE, 1996). In addition to the caregiving family, the caregiving neighborhood or parish should be a focus of study. In some countries giving care is a way of life that extends to friends, neighbors, and society. In the Netherlands the term *mantlezork* is used to define caregiving. This term is translated as the "care cloak," protecting not only the patient but also the caregiver. In the U.S., Share the Care, a program designed for the care of people with cancer, is an example of *mantlezork* (Lakey, Singh, Warnock, Elliott, & Rajotte, 1995).

Historically, research on the topic of caregivers has come from the literature on aging in which burden and supportive interventions have been studied. Interventions tested include teaching mastery of caregiving tasks, social interventions such as support groups or telephone contacts, and direct clinical services such as counseling and respite care. Outcomes of many of these intervention studies indicated that in the short term, the interventions may reduce caregiver stress in a limited way but the burden returns when the interventions cease. Research with midlife caregivers reveals the need for interventions on resource management (Smith, 1993b) and motivation to help (Smith, 1994a). Further research is needed to test more interventions and match the timing of the intervention with the developmental life stage of the caregiver.

CAROL E. SMITH
HELEN A. SCHAAG

Caring

Caring has been identified as a central concept in the discipline of nursing. In the past 25 years theory and research on caring have grown steadily, contributing to a substantive body of knowledge that can be referred to as caring science. While criticism has been levied against this body of literature for its lack of conceptual clarity, there seems to be a growing international consensus in nursing that knowledge about caring is key to understanding human health, healing, and quality of life. One analysis (Morse, Bottoroff, et al., 1991) elaborated five perspectives of caring in nursing literature as: (a) a human trait or condition of being human, (b) a moral imperative, (c) an affect, (d) an interpersonal interaction, and (e) a therapeutic intervention. In another analysis of caring theory, Boykin and Schoenhafer (1990) argue for a multidimensional approach that poses ontological (meaning of caring), anthropological (meaning of being a caring person), and ontical (function and ethic of caring) questions to fully understand the concept. Watson (2001) defined caring as an ontology, a way of being, or a quality of consciousness that potentiates healing. She also defined caring as an ethic or moral imperative for relating with the other in which the humanity of the person is preserved. Swanson (1991) defined caring as "a nurturing way of relating to a valued other toward whom one feels a personal sense of commitment and responsibility" (p. 165). She identified five processes by which caring is enacted: knowing, being with, doing for, enabling, and maintaining belief.

Three reviews of the research literature on caring have been published. Swanson (1999) summarized and categorized the research related to caring in nursing science and Sherwood (1997) reported a meta-synthesis of the qualitative research on caring. Smith (2004) reviewed the research related to Watson's theory of human caring. Many different designs and methods have been used to investigate caring including descriptive qualitative designs, surveys, phenomenology, and quasi-experimental designs using standardized scales and physiological measurement.

Swanson (1999) reviewed 130 databased articles, chapters, and books on caring published between 1980 and 1996. The studies were categorized into five levels: the capacity for caring (characteristics of caring persons);

concerns and commitments (beliefs or values that underlie nursing caring); conditions (what affects, enhances or inhibits the occurrence of caring); caring actions (what caring means to nurses and clients and what it looks like); and caring consequences (outcomes of caring). In her summary of 30 qualitative studies that described outcomes of caring and noncaring relationships Swanson found that outcomes of caring for the recipients of care were: emotional and spiritual well-being (dignity, self-control, personhood); enhanced healing; and enhanced relationships. Consequences of noncaring were humiliation, fear, and feeling out of control, desperate, helpless, alienated, and vulnerable. Nurses who care report a sense of personal and professional satisfaction and fulfillment while noncaring is related to outcomes of becoming hardened, oblivious, depressed, frightened, and worn down.

Sherwood's (1997) meta-synthesis of 16 qualitative studies revealed four patterns of nurse caring: interaction, knowledge, intentional response, and therapeutic outcomes. Caring was defined within content, context, process, and therapeutic or healing outcomes. Two types of caring knowledge and skills were identified as person-centered and technical-physical.

Smith (2004) reviewed 40 studies published between 1988 and 2003 that focused specifically on Watson's theory of transpersonal caring. Four major categories of research were identified: the nature of nurse caring, nurse caring behaviors as perceived by clients and nurses, human experiences and caring needs, and evaluating outcomes of caring in nursing practice and education. The highest number of studies were focused on nurse caring behaviors as perceived by clients or nurses. It is important to note that while patients rank behaviors such as knowledge and technological competence as the most important nurse caring behaviors, nurses rank behaviors such as presence, honoring dignity, and touch as most important. These differences suggest that nurses do not consider competence with medical and technical skills within the realm of nurse caring behaviors, but patients do. Patient vulnerability and the "taken for granted" nature of the instrumental activities by nurses might explain the differences. An expanding area of research is related to evaluating outcomes of caring. Research is indicating that caring-based activities impact mood following miscarriage, patient satisfaction, pain and symptom distress in patients with cancer, well-being, and even blood pressure.

Watson's (2002) compendium of instruments to assess and measure caring is an important contribution toward the advancement of research in the field. This text provides background on 21 instruments, citations of work in which they were used, and a copy of the tools. Some of these tools are: (a) the Caring Assessment Report Evaluation Q-sort (CARE-Q) to measure perceptions of nursing caring behavior, (b) the Caring Behavior Inventory (CBI) to measure that which is associated with the process of caring, (c) the Caring Behavior Assessment Tool (CBA) and the Caring Assessment Tool (CAT) to measure patient perceptions of nurse caring behaviors, (d) the Nyberg Caring Attribute Scale (CAS) to measure caring attributes of nurses, and (e) the Caring Efficacy Scale (CES) to measure the belief in one's ability to express a caring orientation and develop caring relationships.

The future of research in caring is promising. An international community of scholars is actively building knowledge in caring science. The International Association for Human Caring (IAHC) meets annually to disseminate the work of its members and the *International Journal in Human Caring* publishes research and scholarship that expands caring science. Scholars are examining the transtheoretical linkages between caring theories and other nursing conceptual systems (Watson & Smith, 2002). Important research questions center on the relationship between caring and healing outcomes, the qualities of a caring consciousness, the ontological competencies and types of nursing therapeutics that are caring-based, and the types of environments and communities that facilitate caring. Nursing is the discipline that is studying the relationship between caring relationships and healing. Research needs to move beyond examining caring in nurse-patient relationships to caring in relationships with family, friends, God, etc. and how these relationships affect health and healing outcomes. It will be important to study both caregiver and recipient outcomes of caring theory-based models of practice in different settings. Swanson (1999) offered several suggestions for future research related to caring: developing measures of caring capacity, examining the effects of nurturing and experience on caring capacity, identifying and measuring the competing variables that may confound the links between caring actions and their outcomes, moving from studying the individual as unit of analysis to studying aggregates, and developing clinical trials to test the effectiveness of caring-based therapeutics in promotion of health and well-being. Different designs and methods must be used to capture the emerging questions in the field. Multiple ways of knowing from empirics to aesthetics are required to explore all dimensions of caring phenomena. A model of research that integrates these multiple perspectives and ways of knowing may be the preferred epistemological model for studying caring (Quinn, Smith, Ritenbaugh, Swanson, & Watson, 2003).

SALLY PHILLIPS
UPDATED BY MARLAINE C. SMITH

Case Management

Case management (CM) is a growing patient care delivery structure that has been implemented in almost all care settings including acute, subacute, ambulatory (emergency departments and outpatient clinics), long-term, health insurance organizations, community-based centers, and palliative/hospice. Despite the fact that CM has been recognized as an effective and desirable approach to care delivery for the patient and the health care organization, there continues to be little consensus as to what CM is, which resulted in the absence of a standard or universal definition. The literature contains multiple definitions for CM, and each definition frequently depends on the setting and model that is used, the discipline that employs it, and the type of personnel used to accomplish the functions (Cohen & Cesta, 1997); that is, those who assume the role of the case manager.

There is no clear agreement in the literature about the definition and component activities/elements of CM practice. There also exists considerable confusion regarding what constitutes CM, who is best to assume the case manager's role, and which professional discipline owns or should own the accountability for the practice of CM. Some healthcare professionals view CM as a patient care delivery system; others see it as a process or an approach to better care delivery and outcomes. This difference in perception results in differences in the scope of CM practice. For example, when CM is viewed as a delivery system, its scope is wide and entails a continuum of care focus that transcends beyond one care setting or an episode of illness. However, as an approach to care or a process, it tends to be narrow, short-term, and focuses on one episode of illness/care, addresses the main issue(s) at that point in time, and takes place in a specific care setting.

There are multiple case management models in use today; however, all share similar aims: to improve health care delivery (access, continuity, and quality), eliminate fragmentation and duplication of services, and control or reduce costs. Models include private or independent case management, social case management, primary care case management, nursing case management, advanced practice case management, telephonic case management, disability case management (including rehabilitation and vocational counseling), chronic care, worker's compensation, and insurance case management (Cesta & Tahan, 2003). Regardless of the model, core functions identified are integration of care across the continuum, consumer advocacy, coordination of services among providers, and direct delivery of services to meet patient needs efficiently and effectively attending to cost and the use of resources (Cohen & Cesta, 1997; Cesta & Tahan).

When attempting to define CM, one must examine the views of two professionally credible and leading groups in the delineation of the knowledge base for CM. These are the American Nurses Association (ANA) and the Case Management Society of America (CMSA). The ANA defines CM as:

> . . . A dynamic and systematic collaborative approach to providing and coordinating health care services to a defined population. It is a participative process to identify and facilitate options and services for meeting individuals' health needs, while decreasing fragmentation and duplication of care and enhancing quality, cost-effective outcomes . . . (American Nurse Credentialing Center [ANCC], 1999, p. 3)

The CMSA defines CM as:

> . . . A collaborative process which assesses, plans, implements, coordinates, monitors, and evaluates options and services to meet an individual's health needs through communication and available resources to promote quality cost-effective outcomes . . . (CMSA, 2002)

Case management as a concept and role function is not new. It has been used by mental health providers, public health nurses, and social services for about a century. The use of CM in the U.S. goes back to the last quarter of the 19th century in the provision of care for the immigrants by the settlement houses (in 1860), and in coordinating public human services by the first Board of Charities in Massachusetts (in 1863) (Tahan, 1998). Around the turn of the 20th century, the use of CM became popular in the public health sector and in community-based social work services in the form of "case coordination." After World War II and in the 1950s, CM branched into the area of mental health especially to keep veterans out of the hospital (Tahan).

Major emphasis in the past was on the recipient of care and the coordination of services to meet the needs of the patient or client. However, more recently (especially since the mid-1980s), case management has become a dominant and desired approach to care and cost savings in the context of market-driven health care reform. The federal government enhanced the use of case management during the 1970s by way of funding certain community-based demonstration projects. However, the nurse case management model was first introduced in 1985 as a relatively new outgrowth of primary nursing and as a strategy to counteract the nursing shortage and meet the demands of the prospective payment system. This case management model emphasized early assessment and intervention, comprehensive care planning, and service system referrals to specialty providers (Cohen & Cesta, 1997). In the early 1990s and due to the proliferation of managed care, nursing case management models increasingly became interdisciplinary in structure; hence, the case management model of today focuses on interprofessional collaboration, with the case manager assuming the role of the gatekeeper of health care delivery and services.

Case management and managed care are two dominant concepts in discussion today in relation to the challenges of managing patients and resources in a cost-conscious and quality health care delivery system. Although managed care and case management are used to achieve effective management of care, it is important to differentiate between these two terms. Managed care can be described as a general system of care delivery that has replaced fee-for-service systems of care for improved management of resources, costs, quality, and effectiveness of health services. Case management, on the other hand, is a process of care that may be used as one strategy to control costs and inappropriate use of resources and services in a managed care system. Nursing case management provides outcomes-oriented care with attention to appropriate hospital length of stay and access to services, monitors use of patient care services based on type of client, integrates and coordinates clinical services, fosters continuity of care in the context of interdisciplinary and collaborative practice, and enhances patient and provider satisfaction (Cohen & Cesta, 1997; Cesta & Tahan, 2003).

The literature describing CM practice and its outcomes is focused on select areas associated with the design, structure, roles, processes, implementation, and evaluation of these CM models; however, the absence of theoretical underpinnings for these descriptions is dominant. Nurse scholars have pursued the conduct of CM evaluative research to validate its value, aims, and outcomes, i.e., cost-effectiveness and quality care. Although it is evident in the literature that research supports these goals and strengthens the benefits of implementing CM strategies for the provision of care, the ability to link these outcomes to the CM system has not been as strong because of the lack of clear or standardized definitions for either CM or CM interventions or outcome measures/indicators. In addition, there seems to be a lack of clear theoretical frameworks that define the relationships between the structure and processes of CM interventions and their effect on outcomes, or that integrate the different aspects of CM practice (Tahan, 2003).

The CM research literature shows that CM models are rarely appropriately evaluated, and in some instances the variables examined are loosely defined or measured. In most of the studies the research design, data collection, and sampling methods seem to be an "afterthought." The dominant approach to CM evaluation is the examination of cost and quality outcomes employing performance improvement and outcomes-measurement study designs. The dominant research studies are basically retrospective attempts at validating the value of CM. Although in some cases structure, process, and outcome variables are examined, evaluating the interrelationships among the variables or how they affect each other remains lacking. The majority of the published studies are primarily descriptive in nature and tend to ignore examining the effects of confounding variables (e.g., denials and appeals management, interdependence among multiple professionals including the physicians) that may have influenced the results obtained. Therefore, the significance and utility of these studies are compromised (Tahan, 2003).

Issues of cost, quality, access to care, and scope of services should be examined when evaluating CM delivery models, especially because of the claim that they are implemented to improve access to care, enhance quality, and control costs. The examination of these variables is essential so that the implications of CM for health policy decisions can be heightened. Very rarely a combination of these four variables is examined. The combination of variables most commonly used is cost and quality or access and quality. This existing limitation may be attributed to the challenge of conducting a study that combines the four types of variables. Such studies are also known to be complex, costly, time consuming, and require the coordination of a professional with specialized knowledge base in CM practice and research methods. Other challenges are attributed to the confusion of identifying the classification of the variables studied, such as readmission rate, complication rate, and length of stay, which are defined as both cost and quality variables depending on the researcher conducting the evaluation. Such confusion results from the lack of theoretical underpinnings of CM practice, con model frameworks, or standard definitions of the variables examined (Tahan, 2003).

Designing a study that evaluates the interconnectedness and relationships of structure, process(es), and outcomes of CM models is not an easy task. Research related to CM can be approached by evaluation research, experimental or quasi-experimental designs, or qualitative methods. However, because of the challenge of matching, randomizing, or controlling for control and experimental groups, quasi-experimental research is frequently used. CM research may focus on the processes of care (describing and differentiating CM models of care delivery) or on the outcomes of care that frequently include outcomes indicators such as quality and cost measures. Examples may include decreased length of stay, reduced hospitalization or rehospitalization rates, nonroutine visits to providers and emergency departments, and consumer satisfaction. However, outcome studies must not dominate the research without attention to the specific structure (context of care delivery) and processes (tasks, activities, and behaviors) of care that may influence evaluation studies of CM practice.

Data collection may be facilitated through the use of patient questionnaires, self-report instruments completed by those providing CM services, or large data sets from health care provider agencies or payers. Issues and considerations related to CM roles and functions must be addressed. Two of the most significant issues related to the implementation of CM roles and research related to CM are educational preparation and ethical competence of the case manager. Because this practice arena continues to be changing rapidly, it has been difficult for educators to clearly define core competencies of the case manager and to be clear about the necessary level of educational preparation. Also, the various models of CM require attention to the structure of care, whom the case manager works for, and the primary purpose of the CM role. These issues impact the research designs and questions, depending on setting, type of case manager, and population managed by case managers.

Another critical issue related to CM that affects practice and research is that of ethics. Because many case managers face competing loyalties and priorities, the question of ensuring ethical competence becomes as important as clinical, intellectual, financial, and administrative competence. Cohen and Cesta (1997) identified six challenges to be addressed in practice and research as the role of case manager continues to evolve: (a) fidelity to the unique needs of individual patients, (b) competing loyalties, (c) resolving role conflicts, (d) owning responsibilities to underserved populations, (e) identifying personal biases, and (f) balancing care for others with appropriate self-care. Additional important ethical issues are consumer advocacy, balancing access to care and services with cost-effectiveness, and ensuring that consumers' rights and safety are protected.

Patricia Hinton Walker
Updated by Hussein A. Tahan

Case Study as a Method of Research

There are many references to case study in the literature, but there is little agreement about what a case study actually is. Case study is described by some as a research method (Yin, R., 1989), a data collection method, and a reporting method (Lincoln & Guba, 1985). Others argue that "case study is not a methodologic choice, but a choice of object to be studied . . . case study is defined by interest in individual cases, not by methods of inquiry" (Stake, 1994, p. 236).

Thirty years ago case study was a popular design for nursing research. Today it is used less frequently in nursing because of the development of more sophisticated methods of research. Disciplines such as nursing, medicine, psychology, sociology, anthropology, ethics, and history frequently use case study as a teaching method. Used as a research method, case study can be quantitative; but because of the narrative nature of the case study, it is often used as a qualitative method. Case studies can be as simple as a single, brief case or very complex, examining a large number of variables. It is also used for hypothesis testing and theory generation.

Generally, case study is defined as an intensive systematic study of an entity or entities with definable boundaries, conducted within the context of the situation and examining in-depth data about the background, environmental characteristics, culture, and interactions (Bromley, 1986). Used as a research method, case study can be exploratory, descriptive, interpretive, experimental, or explanatory. The level of analysis also varies from factual or interpretive to evaluative, with the unit of analysis a single person, family, community, or institution.

Case studies must be conducted within the context of the individual or group of individuals because beliefs and values are an integral element in defining and influencing the behavior and experience of people. To determine if the conclusions of a case study can be applied to other situations, the case-in-context must be delineated. Another characteristic of case studies is that they are present-oriented. Even though historical data about the entity being studied is included in the research, the study focus is on the present.

One purpose of case study is to expand the understanding of phenomena about which little is known. The data then can be used to formulate hypotheses and plan larger studies. Other purposes of case study include theory testing, description, and explanation. For example, the intensive analysis involved in case study is appropriate to answer questions of explanation, such as why subjects think or behave in certain ways. The case study approach also can be used when a problem has been identified and a solution needs to be found.

The research process for case study design is similar to techniques used in other designs. First, the purpose and the research questions are developed. Questions of what, how, and why are appropriate for case study designs. A theoretical framework may be used to guide the case study. This helps identify assumptions that the researcher may have about the phenomenon at the beginning of the study.

At the outset of the study the unit of analysis must be clearly delineated. The unit of analysis can be an individual, family, organization, or event. Clearly identifying the unit of analysis has implications for data collection and the study protocol. The protocol should list how subjects will be recruited, what constitutes data (documents, letters, interviews, field observation, etc.), what resources will be needed, and a tentative time line for data collection. The protocol may need to be modified as the study progresses and problems emerge. The protocol also identifies a plan for data analysis and reporting the data.

There are two basic designs in case study research. The first is the single-case design, which is used when a case represents a typical, extreme, critical, unique, or revelatory case. Multiple-case designs draw inferences and interpretations from a group of cases. When the purpose of the study is theory generation, multiple-case design is appropriate. Multiple-case designs also are useful to add depth to explanatory and descriptive studies.

Data for case study can be quantitative or qualitative and often include both in the same study. To improve the rigor of the study, three principles of data collection are employed: (a) multiple sources of data are used; (b) a case study base is developed using field notes, audio- or videotapes, logs, documents, and narratives; and (c) an audit trail is evident whereby the reader can follow the researcher's process from question to conclusion (Lincoln & Guba, 1985).

Data analysis in case study is not well developed. Methods for analyzing qualitative data include content analysis, analytic induction, constant comparison, and phenomenological analysis. "Unlike statistical analysis, there are few fixed formulas [for data analysis] . . . much depends on an investigator's own style or rigorous thinking . . . and careful consideration of alternative interpretations" (Yin, R., 1989, p. 105). Methods for analyzing quantitative data are similar to those in any quantitative study and would depend on the research questions.

Case study reports are presented in a variety of ways, from formal written narratives to creative montages of photographs, videotape, and arts and craft work. Most case study reports in nursing, however, are formal written narratives. The written product of case study is often artistic in its composition. There are no rules or standardized ways to write a report, but most case studies include an explanation of the problem or issue and a detailed description of the context and processes surrounding the phenomenon under investigation. A discussion of the results is also included in the report, which can contain inferences about how these results fit with the existing literature and practice implications.

The standard measures of reliability and validity apply to case studies that are quantitative. When a qualitative study meets the criteria for credibility, transferability, dependability, and confirmability, it is considered to be trustworthy. Credibility of the interpretations is supported by techniques such as triangulation of data collection methods, negative case analysis, and checking the interpretation with the participants themselves. Transferability (or fittingness) is an indication of whether the findings or conclusions of the study fit in other contexts and fit with the existing literature. When another person is able to follow the researcher's audit trail or the process and procedures of the inquiry, then the study is considered to be dependable. Confirmability is achieved when the results, conclusions, and recommendations are supported in the data and the audit trail is evident.

Conducting case studies requires a researcher who is flexible and comfortable with ambiguity. It is essential that the investigator be open to the idea that there is more than one "truth." It is necessary for the researcher to be aware of his or her own assumptions, preconceived ideas and values, and of how these impact data collection and analysis.

Case studies are essential to nursing because they are an excellent way to study phenomena within the context in which they occur. Because nurses believe in the uniqueness of human beings, case study is a method to capture this uniqueness and afford a way to gain knowledge about human interaction and behavior as it is situated within time and culture.

DEBERA JANE THOMAS

Causal Modeling

Causal modeling refers to a class of theoretical and methodological techniques for examining cause-and-effect relationships, generally with nonexperimental data. Path analysis, structural equation modeling, covariance structure modeling, and LISREL modeling have slightly different meanings but often are used interchangeably with the term causal modeling. Path analysis usually refers to a model that contains observed variables rather than latent (unobserved) variables and is analyzed with multiple regression procedures. The other three terms generally refer to models with latent variables with multiple empirical indicators that are analyzed with iterative programs such as LISREL or EQS. A common misconception is that these models can be used to establish causality with nonexperimental data; however, statistical techniques cannot overcome restrictions imposed by the study's design. Nonexperimental data provide weak evidence of causality regardless of the analysis techniques applied.

A causal model is composed of latent concepts and the hypothesized relationships among those concepts. The researcher constructs this model a priori based on theoretical or research evidence for the direction and sign of the proposed effects. Although the model can be based on the observed correlations in the sample, this practice is not recommended. Empirically derived models capitalize on sample variations and often contain paths that are not theoretically defensible; findings from empirically constructed models should not be interpreted without replication in another sample.

Most causal models contain two or more stages; they have independent variables, one or more mediating variables, and the final outcome variables. Because the mediating variables act as both independent and dependent variables, the terms *exogenous* and *endogenous* are used to describe the latent variables. Exogenous variables are those whose causes are not represented in the model; the causes of the endogenous variables are represented in the model.

Causal models contain two different structures. The measurement model includes the latent variables, their empirical indicators (observed variables), and associated error variances. The measurement model is based on the factor analysis model. A respondent's position on the latent variables is considered to cause the observed responses on the empirical indicators, so arrows point from the latent variable to the empirical indicator. The part of the indicator that cannot be explained by the latent variable is the error variance generally due to measurement.

The structural model specifies the relationships among the latent concepts and is based on the regression model. Each of the endogenous variables has an associated explained variance, similar to R^2 in multiple regression. The paths between latent variables represent hypotheses about the relationship between the variables. The multistage nature of causal models allows the researcher to divide the total effects of one latent variable on another into direct and indirect effects. Direct effects represent one latent variable's influence on another that is not transmitted through a third latent variable. Indirect effects are the effects of one latent variable that are transmitted through one or more mediating latent variables. Each latent variable can have many indirect effects but only one direct effect on another latent variable.

Causal models can be either recursive or nonrecursive. Recursive models have arrows that point in the same direction; there are no feedback loops or reciprocal causation paths. Nonrecursive models contain one or more feedback loops or reciprocal causation paths. Feedback loops can exist between latent concepts or error terms.

An important issue for nonrecursive models is identification status. Identification status refers to the amount of information (variances and covariances) available, compared to the number of parameters that are to be estimated. If the amount of information equals the number of parameters to be estimated, the model is "just identified." If the amount of information exceeds the number of parameters to be estimated, the model is "overidentified." In both cases, a unique solution for the parameters can be found. With the use of standard conventions, recursive models are almost always overidentified. When the amount of information is less than the number of parameters to be estimated, the model is "underidentified" or "unidentified," and a unique solution is not possible. Nonrecursive models are underidentified unless instrumental latent variables (a latent variable for each path that has a direct effect on one of the two latent variables in the reciprocal causation relationship but only an indirect effect on the other latent variable) can be specified.

Causal models can be analyzed with standard multiple regression procedures or structural equation analysis programs, such as LISREL or EQS (see "Structural Equation Modeling"). Multiple regression is appropriate when each concept is measured with only one empirical indicator. Path coefficients (standardized regression coefficients, or βs) are estimated by regressing each endogenous variable on the variables that are hypothesized to have a direct effect on it. Fit of the model is calculated by comparing total possible explained variance for the just identified model with the total explained variance of the proposed overidentified model (Pedhazur, 1982). Data requirements for path analysis are the same as those for multiple regression: (a) interval or near-interval data for the dependent measure; (b) interval, near-interval, or dummy-, effect-, or orthogonally coded categorical data for the independent measures; and (c) 5 to 10 cases per independent variable. Assumptions of multiple regression must be met.

In summary, causal modeling techniques provide a way to more fully represent the complexities of the phenomenon, to test theoretical models specifying causal flow, and to separate the effects of one variable on another into direct and indirect effects. Although causal modeling cannot be used to establish causality, it provides information on the strength and direction of the hypothesized effects. Thus, causal modeling enables investigators to explore the process by which one variable might affect another and to identify possible points for intervention.

JoAnne M. Youngblut

Cerebral Ischemia

Cerebral ischemia is defined as inadequate blood flow to the brain to meet metabolic and nutritive needs of the brain tissue (Edvinsson, MacKenzie, & McCulloch, 1993). The severity of ischemia depends on the severity and duration of the reduction in cerebral blood flow (CBF) adversely affecting various functional and metabolic processes as CBF decreases (Heiss & Rosner, 1983). The brain stores no oxygen and little glucose, and is thus dependent on a constant supply of oxygen and glucose from the blood.

Cerebral ischemia may be focal or global, depending on whether a part of the brain or the entire brain is ischemic. Focal cerebral ischemia occurs when a major cerebral artery becomes occluded or constricted from arterial spasm, emboli, or thrombosis. Global ischemia occurs from an overall decrease in CBF, for example after cardiac arrest. Global oxygen deprivation of the brain may also occur as a result of asphyxia, anemia, hypoxia, or near drowning. Nurses are responsible for identifying individuals at risk for focal or global cerebral ischemia. Nursing assessment of early symptoms of cerebral ischemia can allow for intervention and minimize the probability of permanent damage.

Spielmeyer first described "ischemic cell change" in 1922, (Spielmeyer, 1922), and Brierley presented the time course for neuronal change during a low flow state and provided evidence of the threshold for cerebral anoxic ischemia (Brierley, Brown, & Meldrum, 1971; Chiang, Kowada, Ames, Wright, & Majno, 1968). He observed and described in further detail the process of ischemic cell change (Brierley, 1973). With the initial decrease in blood flow, oxygen, and/or glucose to the brain, the contour of cells, the nucleus, and nucleolus remain unchanged. There is disruption of mitochondria and an increase in the astrocyte processes surrounding the neurons. As the ischemic process continues, there is neuronal shrinkage, changes within organelles in the cytoplasm, and the cell is further surrounded by astrocytic processes. As the nucleus continues to shrink and the cytoplasm becomes more amorphous, incrustations begin to form. Finally, as the incrustations disappear and the cytoplasm becomes increasingly homogeneous, astrocytes proliferate and lipid phagocytes form in preparation for removal of the now "ghost cell." As the flow lowers and the mitochondria fail, energy sources change from an aerobic to an anaerobic pathway, with a corresponding increase in lactic acid production, metabolic derangement, and loss of ion and transmitter homeostasis. If this process continues unchecked, there will be inadequate energy to maintain the sodium potassium pump across the cell membrane (Jones et al., 1981). Researchers have increasingly detailed the process in an attempt to identify and improve the brain's tolerance to recover from an ischemic challenge.

Servetus, in the 16th century, first presented the idea that blood flowed through the lungs; he was burned at the stake for his efforts. William Harvey (1578–1657) supported Servetus' findings by describing the flow of blood through the body. Nearly 200 years later, oxygen was discovered by Priestley, and Steele and Lavoisier made the connection that oxygen contributed to the production of "heat" or energy. Adolf Fick, in 1870, defined blood flow as the quantity of a substance, such as oxygen, that is taken up by a specific organ over a unit of time (Fick, 1870; Obrist, 2001). The first "measures" of CBF involved direct and indirect observations of intracranial vessels (Roy & Sherrington, 1890). It was not until 1945, when Kety and Schmidt applied the Fick principle to diffusible gas, nitrous oxide, that one was able to estimate cerebral blood flow (Kety, 1950; Kety & Schmidt, 1948).

Kety was the first person to measure global CBF in humans using vascular transit time. The technique was modified by Lassen and Ingvar when Xe-133, a highly diffusible gas, was injected into the internal carotid artery (Lassen & Ingvar, 1972). Multiple extracranial detectors traced the transit time of the radiation from the Xe-133 as it flowed through the brain, providing focal CBF measures. Diffusible tracers are now combined with tomographic reconstruction such as computed tomography, PET, or magnetic resonance imaging (MRI), to calculate vascular transit time. For example, stable xenon-enhanced CT scanning measures CBF via conventional scanner interfaced with computer hardware and software and directs the delivery of xenon gas transit throughout brain regions. Serial CT scans are conducted during the inhalation of a gas mixture containing 30% xenon, 30% to 60% oxygen, and room air. The serial images are stored and regional flows are calculated.

CBF is also estimated from measurement of cerebral blood volume. One way to estimate cerebral blood volume is using a gradient-echo planar system on MR systems. The dynamic contrast-enhanced susceptibility-weighted perfusion imaging technique involves giving a bolus of paramagnetic contrast material (i.e., gadolinium). The contrast media is traced and the amount of signal attenuation is proportional to the cerebral blood volume. With a series of multi-slice measurements, one may generate a time-density curve, and the area under the curve provides an index of relative blood volume (Grandin, 2003). Similar techniques are adapted to CT scanners with the capability for rapid sequential scanning.

The threshold for irreversible brain damage from cerebral ischemia is generally defined as below 20 ml/100g of tissue/minute (Jones et al., 1981; Yonas, Sekhar, Johnson, & Gur, 1989). CBF below this level alters the functioning of the mitochondria to produce energy. Studies show that the threshold for irreversible brain damage are volume and time dependent. Global brain ischemia that is sustained for longer than 4 to 5 minutes will result in permanent brain damage (Brierley, Meldrum, & Brown, 1973). The majority of studies show that above 23 ml/100g/minute, little impairment occurs; however, below 20 ml/100g/minute symptoms of neurologic impairment develop (Branston, Symon, Crockard, & Pasztor, 1974). Below 18–20 ml/100g/minute evidence of diminished electrical activity by evoked potentials or electroencephalogram occurs (Sundt, Sharbrough, Anderson, & Michenfelder, 1974). Below 15 ml/100g/minute is considered to be a threshold for synaptic transmission (Astrup, Siesjo, & Symon, 1981). In addition, factors including temperature, drug administration, and individual variation contribute to the complexity of defining this threshold. Recent work focuses on methods that "noninvasively" detect, track changes in, or treat cerebral ischemia.

The determination and prediction of cerebral ischemia is only as good as the technique used to detect low flow states. Absolute CBF of the cerebral vessels combined with a marker of tissue response would provide the ultimate information in the evaluation of cerebral ischemia. However, the perfect technique is not yet available.

Future directions in cerebral ischemia include the development of noninvasive techniques to measure regional blood flow that have increased sensitivity and resolution. As techniques become increasingly more portable and useable, there will be a translation from the radiology department to application by nurses in the community or at the bedside to assess, predict, and identify patients at risk for cerebral ischemia.

MARY E. KERR

Child Abuse and Neglect

Child abuse and neglect, often referred to by the broader term "child maltreatment," are recognized as major social and mental health problems throughout the world (Bonner, Logue, Kaufman, & Niec, 2001). In the United States, child maltreatment has been identified as a national emergency and one of our nation's "most compelling problems" (U.S. Department of Health and Human Services, 1998). All forms of child maltreatment pose major threats to the integrity of families and society at large and are known to be associated with a variety of mental health concerns as well as criminal activity (Gelles & Cornell, 1990; Hobbs, Hanks, & Wynne, 1999).

Child maltreatment can be differentiated in terms of acts of commission (i.e., physical abuse, sexual abuse, and/or psychological maltreatment) and caregiver omission (i.e., abandonment, neglect) (Cowen, 1999). "Child abuse" is legally defined as "Any form of cruelty to a child's physical, moral or mental well-being" (Nolan & Nolan-Haley,

1990, p. 239). Examples of child abuse include overt physical abuse such as hitting, grabbing, burning, and shaking as well as emotional abuse that may be more subtle and difficult to detect. While reports of physical abuse still dominate the literature, there has been increasing interest in other acts of commission, particularly sexual abuse. However, to focus on sexual abuse alone, as is the recent trend, may be limiting as other important experiences commonly co-occur with sexual abuse that need identification and intervention (Dong, Anda, Dube, Giles, & Felitti, 2003).

Child emotional abuse and neglect are very common but have traditionally been, and continue to be, understudied, perhaps because professionals have difficulty recognizing and defining these terms. Generally speaking, child emotional abuse and neglect refer to a caregiver-child relationship that is characterized by patterns of harmful but nonphysical interactions with the child. Unlike other types of abuse that are performed in secret, this emotional maltreatment is often publicly demonstrated (Glaser, 2002). Children who frequently witness family violence and abuse are also described as psychologically maltreated (Dong et al., 2003). "Neglect" has been defined as the "chronic failure of a parent or caretaker to provide children under 18 with basic needs such as food, clothing, shelter, medical care, educational opportunity, protection, and supervision" (Bonner et al., 2001, p. 1016). Currently efforts are underway to further define the concepts of emotional abuse and neglect (Glaser, 2002) so that important research questions related to the prevalence, risk factors, and long-term effects of this type of maltreatment can be answered.

Different forms of child abuse and neglect frequently coexist. For example, Clauseen and Crittenden (1991) found that 90% of children who had been physically abused and neglected had also been psychologically maltreated. Another important factor worthy of further investigation is the finding that psychological maltreatment was more strongly predictive of impairment in child development than the severity of physical abuse (Glaser, 2002). Researchers are faced with the challenge of clearly defining each type of maltreatment so it can be studied separately, while also evaluating the potential influence of one type of maltreatment on another. For example, in longitudinal studies of physical abuse, mechanisms are needed to determine, if possible, sequelae of physical abuse versus coexisting emotional abuse and neglect. Other related questions include whether coexistence of two or more types of maltreatment more adversely affect child prognosis than a single type of maltreatment, and whether current treatment modalities should be modified to address maltreatment coexistence.

Male victims and perpetrators are also underrepresented in the literature, perhaps because females are traditionally more likely to volunteer for research studies or because male child abuse victims are less likely to report. Gender differences are found in many areas of psychology and child-related research. For example, literature suggests that females are more likely to be victims of child sexual abuse, whereas males are more likely to suffer more physical abuse (Behl, Conyngham, & May, 2003). The first step in addressing this concern and other gender issues is to obtain accurate gender-specific prevalence data. Then efforts can be directed toward determining if child and/or perpetrator gender constitute risk factors and how those findings might be incorporated into prevention programs and intervention development.

The relationship between the caregiver and child is "nested" within the family that is, in turn, significantly influenced by each family member's personal belief system and history as well as the social environment and culture. Yet, to date, the effect and interaction of these personal, social, and cultural influences have not been adequately studied. Ferrari (2002) provided a useful model for studying the predictive effect of cultural factors on parenting behaviors and definitions of maltreatment in three ethnic groups. Noting how the commonly used term "ethnicity" is complex and vague, the author defined three concepts associated with ethnicity (maschismo, familism, valuing children) and defined them for study. Measuring these components, the author also examined the possibility of intergenerational transmission of abuse among cultures. This is another area warranting continued research.

Child maltreatment is clearly a specific and challenging area of inquiry that is in need of further research to develop and empirically validate effective diagnostic, treatment, and prevention programs for all forms of child maltreatment. Since the publication of Kempe, Silverman, Steele Droegenmuller, and Silver's seminal article over 4 decades ago (1962), there have been promising trends in the development of relevant multidisciplinary theoretical models and increased focus for child maltreatment research. However, several important knowledge gaps remain. These include the need for (a) more specificity and differentiation regarding the type of maltreatment that is studied and reported, (b) more adequate conceptualization and research in the understudied areas of child emotional abuse and neglect, (c) examination of the coexistence and interaction of different forms of maltreatment, (d) more information regarding both male victims and perpetrators, and (e) examination of cultural influences upon child-rearing practices and definitions of maltreatment.

In addition to focusing on the previously discussed knowledge gaps, future research must also address important methodological issues. These include developing and using more standardized measures for identifying and differentiating forms of child maltreatment, measuring outcomes through recidivism data, conducting longitudinal studies to evaluate the children's health, academic performance, and psychological adjustment, and developing culturally sensitive diagnostic and evaluative measures to ensure accurate representation and assessment of ethnically diverse children and families. Nurses are educationally, clinically, and ethically well positioned to lead the way in advancing this important area of science.

JENNIFER ELDER

Child Delinquents

Child delinquents (juveniles between the ages of 7 and 12) constitute a population not usually recognized as needing services to prevent them from becoming tomorrow's serious, violent, and chronic juvenile offenders. The most violent behaviors demonstrated by delinquent youth are homicide and sex offenses. Although the number of cases involving offenses included in the FBI's Violent Crime Index (criminal homicide, forcible rape, robbery, and aggravated assault) decreased by 8% between 1997 and 1998 (FBI, 1999), for children under the age of 12, child arrests for violent crimes increased by 45%. Overall, child delinquents arrested in 1997 were more likely to be charged with a violent crime, a weapons offense, or a drug law violation than a property offense (Snyder, 2001). A larger proportion of these young child delinquents, as compared with later onset delinquents, become serious, violent, and chronic offenders (Loeber, Farrington, & Petechuk, 2003).

To treat youth who have committed some violent act, an understanding of violence in the lives of children is necessary. Violent behavior has specific risk factors and more common forms of violence that vary by gender, age and race/ethnicity. Risk factors for violence include 2 or more hours of media violence daily, history of physical fighting, harsh spanking as a form of discipline, carrying weapons, exposure to domestic violence, history of suicidal attempts, bullying, fear of attack at school, crime victimization, maltreatment, and sexual abuse (Brown & Bzostek, 2003).

For infants and young children, the primary locus of violence is in the home. Health consequences of abuse include permanent brain damage from shaken baby syndrome and homicide. The perpetrators are almost always a parent or other relative. The homicide rate for infants is higher than for any age group up to age 17 (Gells, 2002). Surviving toddlers exposed to domestic violence experience depression and psychological distress and are more likely than other children to be physically violent (Gells, 2003). Media violence and violence in the schools, which includes bullying and physical fighting, are more common sources of violence in middle childhood. Data indicate that chances of being bullied in school are higher for 6th graders than for any other group up to grade 12 (DeVoe et al., 2002). For teens, homicide and suicide increase rapidly and the risk of being a victim of sexual assault, aggravated assault, and robbery also increases (Minino, Arias, Kochanek, Murphy, & Smith, 2002).

Differences in violence experiences by race and ethnicity and by type of violence also exist. These factors reflect social factors related to family structure, income, education level, and neighborhood characteristics. Black infants are four times as likely to be murdered than Hispanic or white infants (Overpeck, Brenner, Trumble, Trifiletti, & Berendes, 1998). Black teens are twice as likely to be murdered as Hispanic teens and about 12 times as likely to be murdered as white teens (Anderson, 2002). Black youth are more likely to have been abused (U.S. Department of Health and Human Services, 2003a) and more likely to report being victims of aggravated assault and robbery than their Hispanic or white counterparts (Hawkins et al., 2000).

As might be expected, there are variations in the types of violence experienced by males and females. Females at any age are more likely to be victims of sexual abuse and rape (Finkelhor & Hashima, 2001). Males under the age of 8 are more likely to be victims of physical abuse in the home, a trend that changes to female teens between ages 12 to 17. Both male and female students are equally likely to report dating violence, but females are more likely to suffer significant injury from such violence (Hawkins et al., 2000).

A public health strategy used for public health risks should be applied to preventing serious and violent juvenile delinquency, with a focus on targeting early risk factors associated with persistent disruptive child behavior. Because it is not possible to accurately predict which children will progress from serious problem behaviors to delinquency (Loeber, Farrington, & Petechuk, 2003), it is better to address problem behaviors before they become more serious. Interventions delivered early are most effective to prevent child delinquency, whether these interventions focus on the individual child, the home and family, or the school and community.

The most promising prevention programs for child delinquency focus on several risk domains at a time (Herrenkohl, Hawkins, Chung, Hill, & Battin-Pearson, 2001) in an effort to shift the balance toward a greater number of protective domains. To achieve this effect, multisystemic programs designed to target the child, family, school, peers, and the community have proven most effective. These include parent training and family therapy in combination with classroom and behavior management programs.

The first step toward obtaining effective treatment is to provide families with access to mental health and other services. The delay between symptom onset and help seeking contributes to poor behavioral health outcomes. Awareness and use of culturally congruent approaches reduce the challenges to implementing interventions. Interventions must deal with the multiple problems stemming from generations of dysfunctional families. To be effective, these public health interventions must address both the social conditions and institutions that impact family functioning.

While the very early detection of emotional and behavior problems is a public health goal, results have been limited. Juvenile justice systems continue to be dumping grounds for children who are inadequately served by other institutions (Kupperstein, 1971; Office of Juvenile Justice and Delinquency Prevention, 1995).

DEBORAH SHELTON

Child Lead Exposure Effects

Childhood lead poisoning is recognized as the most important preventable pediatric environmental health problem in the United States. The adverse health effects of lead exposure in early childhood are well documented. Lead poisoning is defined as exposure to environmental lead that results in whole blood lead concentrations ≥ 10 μg/dL (micrograms/deciliter) (U.S. Centers for Disease Control and Prevention, 1992). Exposure to environmental lead begins in the prenatal period when physiologic stress mobilizes lead from its storage in maternal bone into the blood, where it easily crosses the placenta and is deposited in fetal tissue. Depending on the level of lead present in the environment, the exposure can continue as infants and children develop. Absorption of lead is dependent on age and nutritional status; young children and those who have diets high in fats are most susceptible. Lead is most commonly ingested through exposure to lead-contaminated paint and the resulting dust, soil, and paint chips. Once ingested, lead is distributed in the blood and eventually is deposited in bone and teeth.

Whole blood lead levels (BLL) greater than 10 μg/dL put children at risk for developing a variety of health problems. At high level exposures (BLL > 20 μg/dL), damage to the nervous, hematopoietic, endocrine, and renal systems can occur. At lower level exposures, these health problems include altered cognitive and neurobehavioral processes. Researchers have suggested that some of these effects may be seen in children with BLL as low as 5 μg/dL (Lamphear, Deitrich, Auinger, & Cox, 2000; Landrigan, 2000; Needleman & Landrigan, 2004).

Direct results of primary and secondary efforts at prevention of lead toxicity have significantly reduced BLL among young U.S. children within the last 30 years. The major sources of environmental lead exposure have been greatly decreased through the elimination of lead in gasoline, the banning of lead-based paint for residential use, and the elimination of lead solder from food and beverage cans. Despite the success of these efforts, lead poisoning continues to occur in about 5% of children 5 years of age and younger, and much higher levels of lead poisoning have consistently been documented among low-income, urban, and African-American children living in older housing in the Midwest and Northeast (Pirkle et al., 1994).

Childhood lead poisoning was first described in the late 1800s by Gibson and colleagues (Gibson, Love, Hendle, Bancroft, & Turner, 1892), who encountered a case of peripheral paralysis in a young child and described the similarities of the case to that of chronic lead poisoning in adults. Gibson speculated that the source of the lead poisoning was paint, and he described the long-lasting effects of the exposure. Unfortunately, most of Gibson's observations were ignored, as the prevailing view of the time was that once a child survived lead poisoning, there were no lasting effects. It was not until the early 1970s that cross-sectional and longitudinal studies of low-level lead exposure were conducted.

These early studies of lead exposure involved comparisons of a lead-exposed group and a comparison group on intelligence test measures. As knowledge accumulated and research strategies became more sophisticated, researchers began to assess the influence of covariates, such as parental intelligence, socioeconomic status, and parental education level (Gatsonis & Needleman, 1992). Though conflicting results were common, lead exposure and neurobehavioral deficits remained significantly associated.

Although few nurse researchers have investigated the effects of low-level lead exposure on the neurobehavioral development of children, low-level lead exposure certainly falls within the realm of the phenomena of concern to the discipline. Lead exposure is unquestionably of clinical significance; until all lead is removed from the environment, clinicians will be faced both with screening children for lead exposure and treating the effects of this preventable public health problem. The deleterious effects of lead exposure have been known for a hundred years; however, progress in prevention has been slow. Some of the reasons for this are related to society's indifference to problems of poor and vulnerable populations. Until recently, lead exposure was thought to be a problem only for poor inner-city minority populations, and parenting practices were thought to contribute to the problem. Also, many considered the elimination of lead in gasoline and paint sufficient to eradicate the problem of lead poisoning. The Centers for Disease Control (CDC), in 1992, issued comprehensive guidelines for preventing and treating the problem of childhood lead exposure. These guidelines were issued after the CDC accumulated large amounts of scientific evidence from animal and human studies that supported the hypothesis that the deleterious effects of lead exposure occurred at levels previously thought to be harmless.

The earliest studies of lead poisoning were conducted on children who had BLL ≥ 60 μg/dL and were symptomatic. During the 1970s, researchers focused on asymptomatic children who had BLL in the 40–50 μg/dL. Conclusions about the effects of lead exposure were difficult to make from these studies because of their methodological shortcomings. In 1979, researchers conducted a major investigation of large cohorts of asymptomatic children and used shed deciduous teeth rather than BLL to measure lead exposure (Needleman et al., 1979). These researchers controlled for major confounding variables and concluded that BLL was associated with lower IQ, decreased attention span, and poor speech and language skills in the children studied. Long-term follow-up of these children led the researchers to conclude that the effects of low-level lead exposure (equivalent to BLL ≤ 25 μg/dL) persisted throughout young adulthood; failure to complete high school, reading disabilities, and delinquency were behaviors exhibited by children who had elevated BLL at age 7 (Needleman, Riess, Tobin, Biesecker, & Greenhouse, 1996).

Scientists criticized the work done by Needleman and his colleagues (1979) because the study lacked baseline data about early cognitive abilities of the subjects. For instance, it was proposed that the affected children may have had neurological deficits at birth that would lead them to certain behaviors (increased mouthing) that predisposed them to be lead exposed. To address this issue, subsequent studies were designed to follow large numbers of subjects from birth through early school age and major outcomes (e.g., IQ level, motor development, cognitive development) were measured, while large numbers of covariates were controlled. Numerous investigators using comparable designs reported similar findings; thus a solid consensus among investigators began to emerge that lead was toxic at extremely low concentrations. Research with lead-exposed primates strengthened the consensus, and the toxic level of lead was redefined by the CDC as a BLL ≤ 10 μg/dL.

Researchers continue to study the effects of low-level lead exposure on the development of children. While these efforts are worthwhile, future efforts could focus on (a) identifying mediators of lead exposure effects, (b) investigating the effects of lowering blood lead levels (chelation) on the neurobehavioral outcomes of children, (c) investigating the synergistic effects of other environmental exposures on neurocognitive development, and (d) investigating the effects of providing educational materials about reducing environmental lead exposure to families of low-level exposed children. Any efforts that address the primary prevention of the problem would help to protect thousands of children against the long-lasting effects of lead exposure.

Heidi V. Krowchuk

Childbirth Education

Childbirth education focuses on the learning needs of expectant families and covers a broad range of topics from the physical care needs of expectant women to the psycho-socio-cultural needs of the new family. The goal of childbirth education is to assist families in acquiring the knowledge and skills necessary to achieve a healthy transition through the childbearing process and initial phases of parenthood. Classes range from courses designed for those considering pregnancy through courses dealing with infant care needs and early parenting issues.

Nurses are the professional practitioners who assume the primary responsibility for teaching childbirth education classes within the United States. Nurses are in a unique position to serve as childbirth educators because of their broad base of knowledge including both the behavioral and biological sciences. In addition, nursing's focus on caring and emphasis on client education enable nurses to guide families toward their childbirth goals with sensitivity using appropriate educational methods. Nurses are the health professionals within the hospital environment who provide the majority of hands-on care and labor support. Thus, nurses are in a strategic position to act as patient advocates and to provide anticipatory guidance regarding the decision making that is often required during a birth within an increasingly complex health care system.

Formal childbirth education in the United States began with the classes in hygiene, nutrition, and baby care provided by the American Red Cross. During the early part of the 20th century, classes on childbirth and family care became increasingly available to American women. However, the classes provided little information regarding coping with the stresses related to labor. With the shift from the female controlled, social model of childbirth to the medical illness model of childbirth that occurred during the first half of the 20th century, the scientific community paid increasing attention to the control of pain during labor. Thus, classes initially focused on management of pain related to childbirth (Ondeck, 2000).

Contemporary childbirth education dates back to the work of Dick-Read, Lamaze, and Bradley. The notion of pain during labor as secondary to fear and the use of psychological conditioning methods to reduce both the fear and the pain became the basis for "natural childbirth." While philosophical differences still exist among childbirth education methods, common aspects of all programs include education on: (a) the physical process of labor, (b) physical and psychological conditioning methods, and (c) supportive assistance during the birthing process.

A review of the Cumulative Index to Nursing and Allied Health Literature (CINAHL) for the years 1997–2003 reveals 173 published research-based articles listed under the keywords "childbirth education." A wide variety of topics are covered including: (a) postpartum skills such as parenting and breastfeeding; (b) classes for special populations such as grandparents, siblings, fathers, teens, disabled persons, and preparenthood couples; (c) effects of mother-friendly and baby-friendly hospital protocols; (d) self-care measures during pregnancy and labor such as nutrition, fitness, pain control, breathing, and relaxation techniques; (e) effects of medical interventions such as epidural anesthesia, analgesics, and cesarean deliveries; (f) caregiver effects focusing on the outcomes achieved by midwives and doulas; and (g) childbirth educator competencies and teaching methods.

Expectant fathers are currently the focus of many research efforts. Greenhalgh, Slade, and Spiby (2000) reported that fathers attending childbirth education classes who wished to avoid information perceived as threatening had significantly less fulfilling childbirth experiences than similar fathers who did not attend classes. This finding questions whether traditional mother-focused childbirth education classes meet the varying needs of fathers, some of whom are eager to participate in the childbirth experience and others who are reluctant to do so. Diemer's (1997) quasi-experimental study comparing traditional prenatal classes with classes using father-focused discussion groups found a decrease in psychological symptoms and greater improvement in spousal relationships for men attending father-focused groups. The need for attention to the special interests of fathers was also supported by the work of

McElligott (2001) and Smith (1999) who reported men's need for information about their unique contribution to the childbearing experience.

Prenatal education related to breast-feeding continues to be a major focus of research. Cox and Turnbull (1998) reported that attending a breast-feeding workshop significantly increased both women's confidence level and the length of time the women breastfed their infants. Britton's (1998) qualitative study of the sources used by women for breast-feeding information identified discord between women's expectations of breastfeeding and the reality of the experience. This study underscored the continuing need for prenatal breast-feeding education courses and development of peer-support and self-help groups.

A third area receiving continuing attention concerns childbirth education methods and content. The need for use of adult learning principles and identification of specific learner needs is continually reinforced. In addition, extension of the traditional childbirth education program to include gender-specific information on early parenting skills is supported (Callaghan, Jones, & Leonard, 2001; Schmied, Myors, Wills, & Cook, 2002).

Lamaze International (2002) presented a position paper for the 21st century which identifies the need to reshape the birth environment to be supportive of women's confidence, control, and comfort as well as maintaining rewarding family interactions through encouragement and support. With the advent of the mother-friendly and baby-friendly initiatives, additional research is needed to identify educational needs of both consumers and practitioners that will support cost-effective, collaborative policies and high levels of consumer satisfaction. In addition, continued examination of the traditional course content in light of the needs of fathers and special populations is required. Use of the internet as a media for childbirth education has not been reported in the literature. Online courses and support groups may provide a fruitful avenue for childbirth educators wishing to provide high-quality, yet convenient, classes for today's busy families.

BOBBE ANN GRAY

Children Exposed to Intimate Partner Violence

Given the magnitude of this problem, there is a growing awareness of the potential harm to children exposed to violence within families. Following a 2-year analysis of violence and children, the American Academy of Pediatrics issued a policy statement indicating that the U.S. is experiencing an epidemic of children exposed to violence. Despite recognition that domestic violence seriously threatens the health and emotional well-being of children, only recently have researchers focused on children affected by domestic violence. There has been intense advocacy and legislative action to combat violence against women; however serious concerns about their children did not appear in the research literature until recently (Mohr, Lutz, Fantuzzo, & Perry, 2000).

Children who live in homes where partner violence occurs are at risk for developing a range of emotional, physical, and behavioral symptoms. Research suggested that they are at serious risk of developing a host of aggressive, antisocial, or fearful and inhibited behaviors and deficits in social skills (Farrell & Bruce, 1997). They are reported to have impaired concentration and difficulties in school performance (Schwab-Stone et al., 1999; Delaney-Black et al., 2002) and higher levels of alcohol abuse as adults (Dube, Anda, Felitti, Edwards, & Croft, 2002). They perform overall at lower levels than nonexposed children on a variety of measures of cognitive and motor development (Jaycox et al., 2002). Children who witness domestic violence demonstrated higher levels of depression and anxiety than counterparts in nonviolent homes (Berman et al.; Hurt, Malmud, Brodsky, & Giannetta, 2001; Cuffe et al., 1998; Jaycox et al.). They see violence as an acceptable form of resolving interpersonal conflicts and they are at risk for potential deviance in future social relationships (Hurt et al.).

Children from families with domestic violence are at risk of suffering physical violence themselves. The link between marital conflict and child maltreatment has received much attention in the past 10 to 15 years. It has been observed that children of battered women are at an increased risk of being abused themselves, with estimates of an overlap between spousal abuse and child abuse ranging from 30% to 60% (Hartley, 2002; Dong et al., 2003).

In addition, child exposure to family violence can be deadly. Dube et al. (2001) examined the relationship between the risk of suicide attempts and adverse childhood experiences and the number of such experiences. The researchers conducted a retrospective cohort study of 17,337 adult health maintenance organization members who attended a primary care clinic in San Diego within a 3-year period (1995–1997). Subjects completed a survey about childhood abuse and household dysfunction, suicide attempts (including age at first attempt), and multiple other health-related issues. The researchers discovered a powerful relationship between adverse childhood experiences and risk of attempted suicide throughout the life span. Alcoholism, depressed affect, and illicit drug use, which are strongly associated with such experiences, appeared to partially mediate this relationship.

Finally, in a landmark intervention study, Stein and a multidisciplinary group of colleagues (2003) evaluated the effectiveness of a collaboratively designed school-based cognitive behavioral group therapy intervention. The 10-session intervention significantly decreased symptoms of posttraumatic stress disorder (PTSD) in students who were exposed to violence and experiencing distress.

There is a dearth of research conducted by nursing scholars on children exposed to violence. Some recent work has been published on the issue of children's reactions to exposure to family homicide, which may be considered within the context of family or intimate partner violence. Clements and Burgess (2002) conducted interviews with 13 children ages 9 to 11 years during the initial 1 to 3 months after a family homicide and provided insight into themes of bereavement. A major finding in the study was that the witnessing or hearing the news of a family member homicide was a powerful associative factor for childhood PTSD and for complicated bereavement.

In sum, nursing research concerned with victims' children is scant when compared to what is being studied by psychologists, physicians, and social workers. Findings in all cases comparing children exposed to domestic violence with children from nonviolent homes indicate that this exposure (a) has an adverse impact across a range of child functioning, (b) produces different adverse effects at different ages, (c) increases the risk of child abuse, and (d) is associated with other risk factors such as poverty and parental substance abuse. However, comprehensive reviews of this literature indicate no reliable information about the impact of particular types or frequencies of domestic violence on children or the impact of various degrees of exposure on children's functioning and across time. Close inspection of the child impact research indicates that it does not provide a substantial basis to inform strategic national policies and systemwide action due to many gaps and inadequacies. Some of these include retrospective analysis, no longitudinal studies unsubstantiated reports of child exposure or the violent episode itself, exclusive use of the CBCL as opposed to instruments that are more domain specific, and others (for more in-depth discussion on shortcomings of this literature, see Mohr, Lutz, Fantuzzo, & Perry, 2000). Yet, without accurate, reliable information about the prevalence and nature of children's exposure to domestic violence, prevention and intervention efforts cannot be designed for, and public and private resources cannot be appropriately targeted to the affected children.

Effective responses and effective interventions depend on responses to several questions. First, how many children are exposed to domestic violence, and what is the nature of these children's exposure? Second, how do these traumatic events uniquely affect the course of healthy development for child victims? Third, what factors increase risk for, or provide protection against, the potentially deleterious effects of child exposure to domestic violence? Fourth, what types of interventions can mitigate these specific negative effects? Responses to these critical questions require a scientifically rigorous research agenda, leading to the development of a trustworthy database.

Nurses are often the first care providers identifying and assessing not only adult victims but their children. Their presence in the area of adult victimology is laudable, but nurse scholars are relatively absent in the discussion surrounding the child victims—as invisible as the children themselves a scant 2 decades ago.

WANDA K. MOHR
SARA TORRES

Chronic Conditions in Childhood

There is no one accepted definition of a childhood chronic condition; however, a research consortium on chronic illness in childhood recommended that it be defined on two levels: duration of the condition and impact on the child's functioning (Perrin et al., 1993). In a definition based on duration, a chronic condition is one that has lasted or is expected to last more than 3 months (Perrin et al.). This definition would include recurring acute conditions (e.g., repeated ear infections) as well as those that are expected from the onset to be long-term (e.g., diabetes). In a definition based on impact on the child, a chronic condition would be one that limits the child's functioning or leads to the child's receiving additional medical attention beyond that expected for a child the same age. A recent trend is to address morbidities that are often associated with risk-taking behavior such as alcohol use, substance use, contraceptive use, and being overweight (Brown et al., 1999).

Prevalence estimates for childhood chronic conditions, or the number of children with chronic conditions at any given point in time, vary according to the definition used. Estimates of prevalence range from less than 5% to more than 30% (Newacheck & Taylor, 1992); they tend to be higher when the definition is based on duration and lower when the definition is based on impact on the child's functioning. In 2001, more than 4 out of 5 children (83%) were rated as having very good or excellent health by their parents; about 8% of school-age children were reported to have their activities limited because of a chronic condition (Federal Interagency Forum on Child and Family Statistics).

Risk factors for health problems have been identified. Boys have more limitations from chronic conditions than do girls. School-age children (ages 5–17 years) are twice as likely to have a chronic condition as preschoolers (under 5 years). Children living in lower-income families are less healthy than children living in families of higher income. There is also a trend for Black and Hispanic families to have poorer health than White, non-Hispanic children. In contrast, White adolescents have the highest rates of substance use such as smoking cigarettes, drinking alcohol, and using marijuana (Brown et al., 1999). There are also changes in the prevalence of health problems experienced by children. For example, pediatric AIDS cases are declining. In contrast, asthma is increasing among all children, with the highest increases in children who are under 4 years (National Center for Health Statistics).

A large amount of research has been carried out to investigate children with chronic conditions. There is an increasing emphasis on assessing the health-related quality of life of these children. This research has established that, compared to the general population peers, children with chronic conditions are at risk for a poorer quality of life related to physical, psychological, social, and academic functioning. Moreover, the families of these children are at increased risk for adjustment problems.

Two major approaches to sample selection are used in research on children with chronic conditions and their families: noncategorical and categorical. The major assumption behind the noncategorical approach is that there are many commonalities in the experience of families of children with chronic conditions. These researchers generally study samples in which many different chronic conditions are represented. In contrast, researchers using the categorical approach generally study samples that are homogeneous in regard to chronic condition. An example of nursing research using the categorical approach is the research on behavior problems in children with epilepsy (Austin, Dunn, & Huster, 2000). Even though there has been much discussion about which approach is better to use, the current thinking is that the purpose of the research should determine the approach used. In nursing, both approaches are needed to provide important information that will improve nursing care of children with chronic conditions and their families.

In the past decade there has been a strong trend to study chronic illness from the perspective of the person who is chronically ill. Many of these nurse researchers use qualitative methods to learn about the illness experience (Thorne & Patterson, 2000). This focus on the subjective experience is also reflected in a number of scales being developed to measure chronically ill children's perceptions of the quality of life. Another trend is the increasing focus on interventions to help children cope with a chronic condition. For example, common interventions for children with diabetes include educational programs, psychosocial interventions (e.g., coping skills training, psychotherapy, stress management, and social support groups), and family intervention (Grey, 2000).

Joan K. Austin

Chronic Gastrointestinal Symptoms

Chronic gastrointestinal (GI) symptoms—which include frequent bowel-related abdominal pain, reflux, dyspepsia, constipation, painless diarrhea, and fecal incontinence (Talley et al., 2001)—may be common among the public (Talley et al.), but for the health provider they are also among the most difficult conditions to read and treat. When a chronic gastrointestinal pathology cannot be identified, it is more generally diagnosed as Irritable Bowel Syndrome (IBS) or Functional Bowel Disorder (FBD) (Heitkemper, Jarrett, Caudell, & Bond, 1998).

IBS is a recurrent disorder characterized by chronic abdominal pain, bloating, and altered bowel patterns. It is the most common disorder treated by gastroentrologists (American Gastroenterological Association, 2002; Fass et al., 2001) and is more commonly found among women than men. IBS has also been found to contribute to lowering of economic and other quality-of-life factors. One study showed that 15.4 million people in the United States suffer from IBS regularly, with most missing three times as many work days as those without symptoms (13.4 days vs. 4.9 days), costing employers $1.6 billion in direct costs and another $19.2 billion in indirect costs (American Gastroenterological Association).

Although the etiology of IBS has not been clearly identified, it is thought to be related to such factors as the following: (a) abnormal GI motility, described as high-amplitude propagating contractions or delayed transit of gas; (b) visceral hypersensitivity; (c) enteric infection; (d) autonomic dysfunction; and (e) dysregulation of brain-bowel interactions. In addition, stress and psychological affliction are important psychosocial factors in IBS (American Gastroenterological Association, 2002; Fass et al., 2001); however, these are only partially correlated with symptoms and are not sufficient to explain reports of chronic, recurrent IBS. Although there are several pathophysiologies of IBS based on this etiology, further studies are needed to clarify such findings.

There are multiple potential causes for IBS, and the diagnosis of each case must be based relative to the symptoms (Rome criteria). Symptoms include at least 12 weeks of abdominal discomfort or pain in the preceding

12 months, accompanied by two or three of the following additional features: (a) the pain or discomfort is relieved with defecation, (b) the onset of the pain or discomfort is associated with a change in the frequency of the movement of stool, and/or (c) the onset of the pain or discomfort is associated with a change in the form of the stool. In addition, cumulatively supportive symptoms include: (a) abnormal stool frequency (for research purposes, "abnormal" may be defined as more than three times a day and less than three times a week), (b) abnormal stool form (lumpy/hard or loose/watery stool), (c) abnormal stool passage (straining, urgency, or feeling of incomplete evacuation), (d) passage of mucus, and (e) bloating or feeling of abdominal distention (Thompson et al., 2000).

Management of IBS is based on the dominant symptoms, their severity, and psychosocial factors. It is also imperative in the management of IBS that the patient take responsibility as an active participant in his or her treatment. Nurses can engage patients by encouraging them to write down their symptoms and times of occurrence in a diary, which can also be used to monitor the daily food intake, activities, and events of the patient in order to identify possible exacerbating factors. If, on examination of the diary, symptoms prove mild, prescription medication may not be needed, though in general the patient will benefit from normal daily activities that include dietary and lifestyle modification (Ringel, Sperber, & Drossman, 2001). Once the patient has monitored symptoms for 2 to 3 weeks by writing them in the symptom diary, certain foods and other agents that worsen symptoms can be identified and avoided. However, nurses should remind patients not to be overly restrictive in their diet to avoid the risk of malnutrition. Some studies recommend a high fiber diet to resolve symptoms, even though it may initially cause bloating and flatulence. However, although helpful in treating constipation, maintaining high levels of fiber intake is controversial when used to relieve diarrhea and abdominal pain (American Gastroenterological Association, 2002).

In cases in which individuals with IBS do not respond to physiological treatments, psychological factors should be considered. Several psychological procedures have been studied in IBS patient therapy trials, including cognitive-behavioral treatment, stress management, dynamic/interpersonal psychotherapy, hypnotherapy, and relaxation/arousal reduction training (Ringel, Sperber, & Drossman, 2001; Drossman, 1995). Due to methodological limitations, however, there are as yet no comparative data demonstrating that one psychological intervention is superior to any other for any given patient group or set of conditions (American Gastroenterological Association, 2002). Several recent findings in nursing research have focused on the relationship between gastrointestinal symptoms and women (Heitkemper et al., 1998), the effects of coping with stress among women with gastrointestinal disorders (Drossman et al., 2000), differences in patients' and physicians' perceptions about women with IBS (Heitkemper, Carter, Ameen, Olden, & Cheng, 2002), and the sense of coherence and quality of life in women with and without IBS (Motzer, Hertig, Jarrett, & Heitkemper, 2003). These studies supply information suggesting that GI symptoms in some women are linked to the following: (a) reproductive cycling (increased GI symptoms at menses), (b) negative health outcome due to maladaptive coping and decreased self-perceived ability concurrent with or in response to a history of abuse, (c) discordance between patients' and physicians' views about IBS, and (d) reduced sense of coherence and holistic quality of life.

The care of patients with chronic GI symptoms is particularly challenging because the diagnosis is never assured and symptomatic treatments are not always successful. Diagnosis and treatment tailored on the basis of individual need should be carefully performed. In addition, establishing an effective relationship between the patient and the health provider requires patience, education, and reassurance for vital therapeutic management. Future studies are needed to determine the degree to which the modification of management will improve symptom treatment, clinical outcomes, and the patient's overall quality of life. Finally, the treatments that are consistently effective for all symptoms should be further investigated.

JIN-HWA PARK

Chronic Illness

The practice of nursing has long been identified with the care and comfort of the chronically ill. It is apparent, however, that the health care delivery system, in general, has not adequately responded to the changing needs of the population, particularly in terms of the increasing numbers of chronically ill adults. Currently, in the United States, by age 70, a majority of the U.S. population copes with the effects of at least one chronic illness (Nesse, 2002). Blendon and colleagues (2001) reported that when asked what they thought were the most important health problems facing the nation, over 80% of respondents identified three chronic illnesses: cancer, human immunodeficiency virus (HIV)/acquired immunodeficiency syndrome (AIDS), and heart disease as the top three.

Chronic illness includes a broad spectrum of diseases that differ significantly from one another in their underlying causes, modes of treatment, symptoms, and effects on a person's life and activity. Chronic illness refers to diseases that are caused by nonreversible pathology; are characterized by a slow progressive decline in normal physiological function; are permanent with cure unlikely; and require long-term surveillance, leaving residual disability (Hwu, Coates, & Boore, 2001). Families are drained physically, emotionally, and financially. There is often upheaval of relations among the patient, family, and other members of society. Overall, chronic illnesses vary greatly in their developmental course. Some conditions improve over time, some stabilize, and others are progressively degenerating and debilitating.

From the societal perspective, living with a chronic illness is a major source of health care utilization. In the United States, chronic diseases account for three quarters of health care costs (Vlieland, 2003). Specifically, Druss and colleagues (2001) indicated that almost half of U.S. health care costs in 1996 were borne by persons with one or more of five chronic conditions: mood disorders, diabetes, heart disease, asthma, and hypertension. In addition, the nonmedical costs are substantial due to lack of productivity. Druss and colleagues (2002) reported that the most expensive chronic illness at a population level was ischemic heart disease; at the per capita level it was respiratory malignancies. The conditions with the greatest disability (including bed days, missed workdays, and rates of impairment in activities of daily living and instrumental activities of daily living) relative to expenditures were mood disorders, chronic obstructive pulmonary disease, and arthropathies.

The traditional approach to studying chronic illness has been limited, focusing on the medical model. A new health paradigm—a care-oriented model of illness—has emerged. The concept of health is more readily measured in terms of maximizing physical, psychological, social, and spiritual well-being. In this paradigm, a holistic health-focused model has become accepted with a resulting change towards care of the whole person as well as the family. In addition, in chronic disease management, all clinical decisions need to be individualized, because they usually involve choices between possible outcomes that may be viewed differently by different patients. Vlieland (2003) recognized that a constant tailoring of care to the actual needs of individual patients as well as the complexity and long duration of the disease are the distinguishing features of chronic disease management. Another related framework that has emerged is the self and family management in chronic illness (Grey, Knafl, Gilliss, & McCorkle, in press).

Pollock (1987) provided an initial review of nursing research related to adaptation to chronic illness. More recently, Fitzpatrick and Goeppinger (2000) edited ten chapters that reflected a variety of chronic illnesses and a full range of interventions to manage them. Valuable contributions to increase our understanding have come from first-person accounts of patients' experiences (Thorne & Patterson, 2000). Other noteworthy efforts have been expanded to families, including ethnically diverse families (Chesla & Rungreangkulkij, 2001). Other important contributions have focused particularly on nursing interventions. For example, Frich (2003) concluded that nursing interventions for patients with diabetes can improve psychosocial and health outcomes in terms of facilitating adherence to regimens or behavior changes (greater self-care skills), patient satisfaction, good clinical outcomes (reduction in plasma glucose, decreased blood pressure and cholesterol), and cost savings.

Research related to improving the quality of life for people with chronic illness should be a national priority given that people are living much longer and better with conditions that used to be fatal. The existing literature is limited in several critical ways. Much of the research in chronic illness addresses a particular illness or disability. Findings may be applied too narrowly or too inclusively to illnesses with markedly different demands. The landscape of chronic illness is diverse and complex, presenting a vast range of symptoms and trajectories, accomplished by a variety of demands over the natural history of the diseases. Research to date has focused on only specific phases of the trajectory of specific diseases, and not on the unfolding of illness related to developmental tasks over the entire course of an illness. The impact of chronic illness on the patient, well family members, and key caregivers differs and depends on when an illness strikes in the family and on each member's individual development. Many complex management interventions are eventually aimed at improving or maintaining the patient's independent participation in society. Outcome measures covering this dimension are rarely applied. In order to capture these complex relationships, designs that include mixed methods will be essential.

RUTH MCCORKLE
SIEW TZUH TANG

Clinical Decision Making

Clinical decision making is the process nurses use to gather patient information, evaluate the information, and make judgments that result in the provision of patient care (White, Nativio, Kobert, & Enberg, 1992). Clinical decision-making ability is defined as the ability by which a clinician identifies, prioritizes, establishes plans, and evaluates data. Decision making is central to professional nursing and has vital links to patient-care outcomes (Catolico, Navas, Sommer, & Collins, 1996).

Researchers have investigated the process, types, and quality of clinical decision making. Catolico and colleagues (1996) studied decision making of practicing staff nurses. It was demonstrated that nurses with better communication skills had a greater frequency of actual decision-making practices. Intuition was a critical component of clinical decision making in a qualitative study of 10 novice nurse practitioners (Kosowski & Roberts, 2003). Some researchers have looked at approaches such as informatics or algorithms to aid decision making. Akers (1991) showed that nurses who used algorithms to aid their decision making utilized more thorough patient assessment and a more informed nursing response, which resulted in better patient management. Another critical issue is the educational level and preparation of the nurses who are formulating decisions. Studies have explored the decision-making process of student nurses, staff nurses, and nurse practitioners. A group of nursing students were given didactic and interactive teaching sessions on clinical decision making. Students' decision making was in accordance with the decision making of experts significantly more often than that of the student nurses who did not receive the decision-making content (Shamian, 1991). A study in the United Kingdom demonstrated that nurses having a college education were significantly better at decision making than their colleagues educated in diploma programs (Girot, 2000). Advanced practice nurses in specialty practices tend to generate fewer hypotheses in their clinical decision making. Those nurses must be aware that formulating a diagnosis too early in the data-gathering phase precludes the possibility of considering all options (Lipman & Deatrick, 1997).

When investigating the decision-making process, researchers have utilized simulations, together with interviews regarding the thought processes individuals use to reach decisions. The quality of decision making is defined as having the ability to make frequently required decisions (Catolico et al., 1996). That aspect of decision making has been studied by using computer-assisted simulations requiring nurses to make decisions in controlled clinical situations. To investigate clinical decision making by nurse practitioners, the nurses care for patients via computer and interactive videos. To more objectively assess student clinical competencies, the clinical decision-making skills of nurse practitioner students were evaluated using a standardized simulated patient encounter (Stroud, Smith, Edlund, & Erkel, 1999).

Various factors have been shown to affect clinical decision making, such as the experience and the knowledge base of the nurse. Those with case-related experiences are more likely to choose appropriate interventions. A study of nurse practitioners by White and colleagues (1992) concluded that case content expertise is crucial for clinical decision making from the aspect of understanding the significance of the data acquired and in making the correct decision. Nurses' decision making is also affected by the sociodemographics of the patient. Age, sex, race, religion, and socioeconomic status can impact on decision making. Racial disparities in health care may be due to racial biases when formulating clinical decisions. Non-white patients presenting to the emergency department with chest pain are hospitalized less often than white patients (Pope et al., 2000). There was a significant difference in reports of suspected abuse after the evaluation of fractures between minority and non-minority children (Lane, Rubin, Monteith, & Christian, 2002). Competent clinical decision making by nurses requires being cognizant of potential biases.

Decision making is critical to nursing practice. Gathering, organizing, and prioritizing data are major components of the process. Continued research in this area can foster the development of decision-making skills in novice nurses and cultivate high clinical decision-making ability in expert nurses.

TERRI H. LIPMAN

Clinical Judgment

Clinical judgment has been defined as the process by which nurses come to understand problems, issues, or concerns of patients, attend to salient information, and respond in concerned and involved ways. Clinical judgment occurs within a framework of clinical, legal, ethical, and regulatory standards and is closely aligned with phenomena such as critical thinking, decision making, problem solving and the nursing process (Benner, Tanner, & Chelsa, 1996).

Expert clinical judgment is held in high regard by nurses as it is generally viewed as essential for provision of safe, effective nursing care and the promotion of desired outcomes. Nursing research has been conducted on the processes of clinical judgment with the intent of better understanding how nurses identify relevant information from the vast amounts of information available and then how information is used to make inferences about patient status and appropriate interventions. The complexity of the clinical judgment process has brought about collaboration of nurse researchers with multidisciplinary experts from a broad array of scientific backgrounds including cognitive psychology, informatics, phenomenology, and statistics.

The body of research on clinical judgment generated by interdisciplinary collaboration has been categorized into two disparate theoretical classifications: the "rationalistic" and the "phenomenological" perspectives. In this context, the term "rationalistic" describes scientific inquiry into the deliberate, conscious, and analytic aspects of clinical judgment (Benner et al., 1996). Examples include research on the role of information processing, diagnostic reasoning (Tanner, Padrick, Westfall, & Putzier, 1987) and decision analysis (Schwartz, Gorry, Kassirer, & Essig, 1973) in the clinical judgment process. The term "phenomenological" refers to research on the skill-acquisition component of clinical judgment as advanced by Benner et al. in the Novice to Expert Model (Benner & Tanner, 1987; Benner et al., 1996).

Information processing theory and diagnostic reasoning are based on the work of Newell and Simon (1972b) and Elstein (Elstein, Shulman, & Sprafka, 1978) and collectively describe problem-solving behavior and the effect of memory and the environment on problem solving. These theories hold that human information processing capacity is restricted by short-term memory and effective problem-solving ability is dependent on adoption of strategies to overcome human limitations. Information processing theory and diagnostic reasoning have been applied widely to the study of clinical judgment and the use of information in the clinical judgment process. Published research suggested that nurses and physicians use a similar process for clinical judgment which involves information gathering, early hypothesis generation and then additional information gathering to confirm or rule out a suspected diagnosis or clinical problem. According to the "rationalistic theories," early hypothesis generation "chunks" data and is an effective strategy for conserving short-term memory (Corcoran, 1986; Elstein et al., 1978; Tanner et al., 1987). While knowledge generated from work completed in the fields of information processing and diagnostic reasoning has been descriptive in nature, decision analysis is a prescriptive approach to decision making and involves the process of weighing cues and employing mathematical models (generally made possible through expert systems) to determine the course of action most likely to produce desired outcomes.

Corcoran (1986) used an information-processing approach and verbal-protocol technique to compare care-planning strategies used by hospice nurses. She found that unlike novice nurses, the overall approach of expert nurses differed by case complexity with a systematic approach employed for less complex cases and an exploratory approach for cases of greater complexity. In addition, expert nurses generated more alternative actions during the treatment planning process, were better able to evaluate alternative actions, and developed better care plans than did novices.

Tanner et al. (1987) used verbal responses to videotape vignettes to describe and compare the cognitive strategies of diagnostic reasoning used by nursing students and practicing nurses. They found that practicing nurses were more likely to employ a systematic approach and to be more accurate in diagnosis than the students. Henry (1991) examined the effect of patient acuity on clinical decision making of experienced and inexperienced critical care nurses using computerized simulations. Findings suggest that inexperienced nurses collected more data and had poorer patient outcomes than experienced nurses.

Salantera, Eriksson, Junnola, Salminen, and Lauri (2003) employed simulated case descriptions and the think-aloud method to compare and describe the process of information gathering and clinical judgment by nurses and physicians working with cancer patients. The authors found that while nurses and physicians identify similar problems, they employ divergent approaches to information gathering and clinical judgment.

Unlike the objective, detached approach to the study of clinical judgment characteristic of the rationalistic perspective, the phenomenological perspective holds that intuition is a legitimate and essential aspect of clinical judgment and is the feature that distinguishes expert human judgment from that of expert systems (Benner & Tanner, 1987). Benner's work is based on the skill acquisition model advanced by Dreyfus. According to this model, there are six key aspects of intuitive judgment: pattern recognition, similarity recognition, commonsense understanding, skilled know-how, sense of salience, and deliberative rationality (Benner & Tanner). Much of the research related to Benner's work and the Novice to Expert Model relates to the relationships that exist between nursing knowledge, clinical expertise and intuition.

The Novice to Expert Model is based on Benner's early work where a phenomenological approach was used to interview and observe nurses with varying degrees of clinical expertise. In the interview process, nurses were asked to describe outstanding clinical situations from their practice. Benner found that a holistic grasp of clinical situations is a necessary precursor to expert clinical judgment (Benner, 1984). Subsequent research has supported these findings and has teased out differences in clinical judgment between clinicians with varying levels of experience (Corcoran, 1986). In a six-year interpretive study of nursing practice, Benner et al. (1996) identified five interrelated aspects of clinical judgment: (1) disposition towards what is good and right; (2) extensive practical knowledge; (3) emotional responses to the context of a clinical situation; (4) intuition; and (5) the role of narrative in understanding a patient's story, meanings, intents and concerns. The authors suggested that these aspects play a significant role in clinical judgment and deserve equal consideration along with the aspects arising from the "rationalistic" perspective of clinical judgment

Research on clinical judgment identified two divergent but legitimate perspectives. The challenge for future research is to integrate these perspectives to study the impact of integrated models on clinical reasoning and patient outcomes. Synthesis holds promise for promoting evidence-base practice (EBP). Rationalistic models can be employed in the form of guideline-based tools to bring the best evidence to patient care. Phenomenological models hold potential for bringing effectiveness to EBP by providing a holistic evaluation of patient systems. A holistic perspective would serve as a guide to clinicians in the care of individuals through identification and application of evidence which is most relevant at the local level and for individual patients.

Patricia C. Dykes
Moreen Donahue

Clinical Nursing Research

Clinical nursing research is both broadly and narrowly defined. Broadly, it denotes any research of relevance to nursing practice that is focused on care recipients, their problems and needs. This broad definition stems from the 1960s, when a major change occurred in nursing science. Prior to the 1960s the research of nurses had focused on nurses and the profession of nursing including major questions of interest related to nursing education and the way in which nurses practiced within care delivery structures (i.e., hospitals). The reasons for these foci are many, but for the most part they stem from the dearth of nurses with advanced degrees at that time and the fact that nurses with advanced degrees were educated in other disciplines (e.g., education).

In the late 1950s and 1960s a major shift occurred, driven by three factors. First, leaders in nursing successfully lobbied for the institution of the nurse scientist program through the federal government, which provided financial support for nurses to be educated in the sciences (e.g., physiology, biology, anthropology, psychology). Second, nurse theorists such as Faye Abdellah, Virginia Henderson, Imogene King, Ida Orlando, Hildegard Peplau, and Martha Rogers began to formulate conceptual models to direct nursing practice, and attention was focused on designing research that more or less was guided by those models (or at least the substantive areas circumscribed by the models). Third, as more nurses attained advanced degrees, doctoral education with a major in nursing finally became a reality, and the focus of nursing research shifted more firmly away from nurses and nursing education to the practice of clinical nursing. The broad definition of clinical nursing research, then, was originally formulated to differentiate between the research conducted by nurses prior to the 1960s, which focused on nurses, to the major shift in focus on practice.

Strongly influenced by the establishment of the Center for Nursing Research (at present the National Institute of Nursing Research) in the National Institutes of Health (NIH), clinical nursing research has recently taken on a narrower definition, modeled after the definition of clinical trials (large-scale experiments designed to test the efficacy of treatment on human subjects) used at NIH. This narrow definition limits clinical nursing research to only those studies that focus on testing the effects of nursing interventions on clinical or "nurse sensitive" outcomes.

In addition to an evolution in definition, clinical nursing research also has changed in form and complexity over time. Early clinical nursing research was characterized by a focus on circumscribed areas of inquiry using experimental and quasi-experimental methodologies. Investigators were few and tended to work in isolation. Prompted by metatheorists such as Dickoff, James, and Wiedenbach (1968) and methodologists such as Abdellah and Levine (1965) and Mabel Wandelt (1970), nurse scientists were advised to derive questions directly from problems encountered in their clinical practice and to strive to develop and test interventions to solve these problems. Often an investigator conducted single studies on different problems rather than series of studies focused on different aspects of the same problem. As a result, study results tended to be context-bound and limited in generalizability to other settings, samples, or problems. The relationship between theory development and research was discussed abstractly but not explicitly operationalized, and a philosophy of knowledge building, rather than problem solving, had not yet developed.

The next stage in the evolution occurred with the realization that little was known about many of the phenomena of concern to nurses. This heralded a period during which emphasis shifted away from experimental methods to exploratory/descriptive methods, such as grounded theory. Guided by the metaparadigm of nursing (person, nursing, health, environment), nurse scientists began focusing on discovering and naming the concepts of relevance for study in nursing, delineating the structure of these concepts, and hypothesizing about the relationships of these concepts in theoretical systems.

More recently, clinical nursing research has become clearly defined as a cumulative, evolutionary process. Investigators are still advised to derive questions from clinical problems, but the focus is on knowledge generation, specifically the generation and testing of middle-range theory (a theory that explains a class of human responses), for example, self-help responses, symptom experience and management, and family responses to caregiving. Because knowledge is viewed as cumulative, investigators usually study various aspects of one particular concept or response; studies build on one another, and each study adds a new dimension of understanding about the concept of interest. This approach to clinical nursing research requires investigators to use multiple methodologies in their programs of research, including (a) inductive techniques to discover knowledge from data; (b) deductive techniques to test hypotheses that are either induced or deduced; and (c) instrumentation to increase the sensitivity, reliability, and validity of the measurement system designed for the concept.

The methodologies being used include qualitative methods such as ethnomethodology, grounded theory, and phenomenology and quantitative methods ranging from traditional experimental methods and designs to less traditional methods, such as path analysis and latent variable modeling. Because human responses change over time based on contextual factors or treatments (independent variables) applied by the nurse investigator and because understanding the nature of change often is at the crux of the theory building, skills in measuring change also may be required. This has resulted in the need for many investigators to incorporate techniques such as time series analysis and individual regression into their research.

Understanding the human responses of concern to nurses can also require an understanding of cellular mechanisms that are best studied in animal models and a coupling of biological techniques such as radioimmunoassay and electron microscopy, with psychosocial techniques such as neurocognitive assessment or self-report of psychological states. In addition, measurement of different units of analysis (e.g., individual, family, organization) may be required, along with strategies for understanding the effect of care contexts (e.g., social, physical, organizational environments) on the human response of concern. Needless to say, single investigators rarely have all the skills needed to advance the understanding of a particular concept. As a consequence, single investigators are becoming more and more a thing of the past as teams of scientists, including nurses and individuals from other disciplines, collaborate in the knowledge-building endeavor.

Nursing is concerned with human responses and is based on the assumption that humans are holistic and embedded in history and various environments. Clinical nursing research is about generating a body of knowledge on which nurses can base practice. It is about assuring the efficacy and safety of nursing actions, substantiating the effect of nursing actions on patient outcomes, and conserving resources (costs, time, and effort) while effecting the best possible results. It is about identifying strategies for improving the health of the population and promoting humanization within a health care environment that has a natural tendency to be mechanistic, compartmentalized, and focused on short-term rather than long-term gain. It is about client advocacy, client protection, and client empowerment. The challenge of clinical nursing research is to develop an understanding of human response through theory generation and testing while developing measurement systems and using research methods that capture the holism of the client and the holistic nature of the health care experience.

LINDA R. PHILLIPS

Clinical Preventive Services Delivery

Empirical support of preventive health care and health promotion has grown considerably over the past decade, demonstrating that the short-term investment in preventive care could avert health problems and medical costs over time (U.S. Preventive Services Task Force, 2000). Many serious disorders can be prevented or postponed by immunizations, chemoprophylaxis, and healthier lifestyles, or detected with screening and treated effectively (U.S. Public Health Service, 1994). However, many preventive care services are frequently not being delivered by clinicians in practice.

Despite the benefits of preventive care services, such as cancer screening and immunizations, utilization of specific preventive care services in New Jersey remain below state and national goals. Documented barriers to the implementation of these services included (a) clinician uncertainty about what services to offer, to whom, and how often; (b) lack of reimbursement and associated time constraints; (c) clinician attitudes and lack of knowledge about preventive services; (d) patient attitudes, confusion, and lack of understanding about clinical preventive services; and (e) lack of organized systems to facilitate the delivery of services (Griffith, Dickey, & Kamerow, 1995).

Clinicians are confronted with different recommendations regarding preventive care practices from the HPs they contract with. Multiple recommendations for preventive care sometimes conflict with each other, leaving clinicians confused about which services to provide. Literature shows that lack of a standardized approach to the delivery of clinical preventive services (CPS) is a barrier to implementation (Griffith et al., 1995).

HP medical directors seek recommendations from government agencies and professional organizations in selecting CPS their HP should recommend. Some medical directors work with a committee of practicing member clinicians, obtaining feedback regarding recommendations they should provide. However, some medical directors decide what should be recommended on their own, reviewing original empirical research to supplement the national guidelines, particularly for newer or more controversial services (Fox & Cuite, 2001). In either circumstance, HP medical directors work independently from other HPs.

Through a partnership between the New Jersey Association of Health Plans and Rutgers College of Nursing, nine NJ HP medical directors were brought together to form a coalition to identify a set of CPS guidelines that all plans could endorse as priorities for implementation. In meeting this objective, these HPs will be able to provide contracting clinicians with information on the value of preventive services to their patients, compensating for uneven knowledge and skill that many clinicians have in the area of prevention.

Sisk (1998) discussed that initiatives to improve consistency, both scientific evidence and clinical practice, are increasingly focusing on managed care plans and integrated delivery systems. HPs should be able to implement guidelines, particularly because plans are being held accountable for care provided. HPs have leverage, if not control, over clinicians utilizing patterns.

The New Jersey Association of Health Plans and Rutgers College of Nursing collaborated in this concerted effort with nine HPs in NJ, HPs covering 4.8 million New Jerseyans that represent 98% of the state's HMO market. Medical directors from competing HPs brought to the table expertise on CPS, discussed the current knowledge of evidence-based practice, and established a consistent set of guidelines to which all of the nine HPs agreed.

Agreed-upon guidelines of the coalition were based on the evidence-based U.S. Preventive Services Task Force (USPSTF) guidelines. The USPSTF, a body of preventive care experts convened by the U.S. Public Health Services, conducted comprehensive evaluation of the scientific evidence for CPS, including counseling interventions, screening tests, immunizations, and chemoprophylaxis (Fox & Cuite, 2001). Therefore, the coalition agreed on the value of these evidence-based guidelines as the standard for which preventive care should be delivered to the general population.

Seventy areas identified by the USPSTF for preventive care were reviewed by each medical director, individually through questionnaires and collectively through coalition meetings. Two rounds of questionnaires were sent to the medical directors to assess their HP's level of agreement and/or disagreement with the USPSTF guidelines. Positively stated recommendations that the medical directors disagreed on were addressed at subsequent coalition meetings to promote consensus. A third questionnaire was then sent to the medical directors, requesting them to rank order these guidelines according to priority for implementation.

Using consensus-building strategies including three Delphi rounds and four coalition meetings over the course of a year, medical directors were able to identify a subset of USPSTF guidelines that all HPs could endorse as priorities for implementation in clinician practice. Medical directors discussed that these guidelines serve as the minimum for which preventive care services should be delivered and do not replace the clinicians' judgment based on patient risk. However, implementation of these guidelines will ensure that all patients receive a consistent level of preventive care.

Decisions made at each level were based on scientific evidence and needs of their members at large. Their decision to include only those guidelines with good to fair evidence to support the recommendation that the condition be specifically considered in a periodic health examination, a level of strength "A" or "B" recommendation as determined by the USPSTF, illustrates their commitment to sound and safe practice for their members. They also identified diabetes mellitus (DM) as a growing problem that warrants attention. Although there is no evidence-based recommendation to screen for DM as a preventive measure, the medical directors identified methods to screen for complications of this disease. They unanimously agreed that clinicians should provide services to prevent morbidity and/or mortality in this population.

Conflicting and confusing guidelines are detrimental to the delivery of preventive care and create a major barrier to CPS delivery. This project used a systematic approach to reach consensus among medical directors from competing HPs regarding CPS. It provides a template for other HPs nationwide to come to consensus on guidelines that support clinicians in the delivery of CPS.

CYNTHIA GUERRERO AYRES
HURDIS M. GRIFFITH

Clinical Trials

A clinical trial is a prospective controlled experiment with patients. There are many types of clinical trials, ranging from studies to prevent, detect, diagnose, control, and treat health problems to studies of the psychological impact of a health problem and ways to improve people's health, comfort, functioning, and quality of life.

The universe of clinical trials is divided differently by different scientists. Clinical trials are often grouped into two major classifications, randomized and nonrandomized studies. A randomized trial is defined as an experiment in which therapies under investigation are allocated by a chance mechanism. Randomized clinical trials are comparative experiments that investigate two or more therapies. Nonrandomized clinical trials usually involve only one therapy, on which information is collected prospectively and the results compared to historical data. Comparing prospective data with historical control data introduces biases from many sources. These potential biases are usually of such magnitude that the results of nonrandomized studies are often ambiguous and not universally accepted unless the therapeutic effect is very large. These same biases are not present to the same degree in randomized trials. Recent development and use of mega-trials represents one variation.

The mega-trial is a large, simple, randomized trial analyzed on an "intent to treat" basis. In mega-trials randomization serves to achieve identical allocation groups (equal distribution of bias) where there is poor experimental control and large between-subject variation. Results of mega-trials cannot readily be generalized because their conclusions are observations, not causal hypotheses and therefore not testable. Mega-trials can be repeated but not replicated. Mega-trials dispense with the scientific aim of maximum experimental control to remove or minimize bias and instead use randomization to achieve equal distribution of bias between groups (Charlton, 1995).

In clinical drug trials, following approval by the Food and Drug Administration (FDA), three phases of clinical trials begin. Phase I studies generally establish whether a treatment is safe and at what dosages. Phase II studies assess the efficacy of treatments after their safety and feasibility has been established in Phase I. Phase III studies compare effectiveness of Phase II treatments against currently accepted treatments.

Some scientists divide clinical trials into three groups: (a) exploratory (initial trials investigating a novel idea), (b) confirmatory (designed to replicate results of exploratory trials), and (c) explanatory (designed to modify or better understand an established point). Other scientists divide the universe into two groups, such as pragmatic (practical benefits to the overall subject population treated) and explanatory (Viscoli, Bruzzi, & Glauser, 1995).

Issues surrounding clinical trials include biasing, expense of clinical trials, small sample sizes, and ethical issues. There are many biases that can compromise a clinical trial, such as observer bias, interviewer bias, use of nonvalidated instruments, uneven subject recruitment by physicians, and individual subject factors. Recent concerns have focused on bias in sample selection.

To date, the majority of clinical trials have included a limited segment of the U.S. population, that is, mainly middle-class, married, White males with little to no inclusion of women and minorities. This lack of diversity in trial samples has yielded results that are not always generalizable and effective. Research also has demonstrated bias due to subject factors. For example, subjects were more likely to participate in clinical trials on multiple sclerosis if they had a higher than median income and were disabled from work (Schwartz, C. E., & Fox, 1995). Suggested approaches to reduce selection bias include (a) using a broad recruitment base to reduce patient and physician biasing factors and (b) facilitating subject transportation to the study site.

Clinical trials are expensive and resource-intensive. As a result, subject numbers are generally limited to the minimum number needed to demonstrate a significant effect not caused by chance. However, small clinical trials may not provide convincing evidence of intervention effects. Small clinical trials are valuable in (a) challenging conventional but untested therapeutic wisdom, (b) providing data on number of events rather than number of patients and thus may be sufficient to identify the best therapy, and (c) serving as a basis for overview and meta-analysis (Sackett & Cook, 1993).

To deal with the issue of small sample sizes, meta-analysis is increasingly being used. Meta-analysis (quantitative overview) is a systematic review that employs statistical methods to combine and summarize the results of several trials. Well-conducted meta-analyses are the best method of summarizing all available unbiased evidence on the relative effects of treatment (Richards, S. M., 1995). In a meta-analysis the individual studies are weighted according to the inverse of the variance; that is, more weight is given to studies with more events. Arrangement of the trials according to event rate in the controls, effect sizes, and quality of the trials or according to covariables of interest supplies unique information. If carried out prospectively, the technique provides information on the need for another trial, the number of subjects necessary to determine the validity of past trends and the type of subjects who might be benefited.

Ethical issues in clinical trials include issues of informed consent, withholding of treatment, and careful monitoring of clinical trial results. Additional issues of informed consent include assuring that subjects thoroughly understand potential risks and benefits of participation and any effects on their care should they decide to withdraw at any point in the study. Issues of withholding treatment include increasing subject risk or subject benefit if there is reasonable evidence of positive effects of the intervention or treatment. Careful monitoring of the effects of interventions or treatment is necessary to stop the trial if there is associated morbidity or mortality and extending the intervention or treatment to the control group in the event of significantly positive treatment effects.

Clinical trials remain the principal way to collect scientific data on the value of interventions and treatment. However, in designing and evaluating clinical trials, rigor of method, including careful evaluation of potential biasing factors, is essential. Meta-analysis provides a summary of all available, unbiased evidence on the relative effects of treatment. However, rigor of methods used to conduct the meta-analysis also must be evaluated.

DOROTHY BROOTEN

Cognitive Interventions

Cognitive interventions have been defined as mechanisms designed to change cognitive function, such as attention, concentration, or memory (Baltes & Danish, 1980). An intervention may be defined as a programmatic attempt at altering the course of life-span developmental phenomena. Interventions may be classified as concrete technologies involving such parameters as the goal (enrichment, prevention, or alleviation), the target behavior (attention, cognition, memory, or perception), the setting (family, classroom, community, or hospital), and the mechanism (training, practice, or health delivery). Nurse scientists have broadened the scope of their research in health and illness by including multivariate models of affective, cognitive, and behavioral interventions. This review describes the research of nurse scientists in two areas: (1) the integrative reviews of nonpharmacological interventions, and (2) programs of research in chronic illness, medication adherence, and pain. These programs are examples, and are not presented as a comprehensive review of cognitive intervention research from nurse scientists.

Eller (1999) reviewed the research on guided imagery, visualization, cognitive-behavioral techniques for symptom management of stress, anxiety, depression, and for reducing blood pressure, pain, and the side effects of chemotherapy. McDougall (1999) reviewed cognitive-behavioral interventions designed to improve cognitive function in older adults without cognitive impairment. Snyder and Chlan (1999) reviewed the research on music therapy designed to manage pain, decrease anxiety and aggressive behaviors, and improve performance and well-being. Even though the three integrative reviews were framed within the paradigm of complementary and alternative therapies, they illuminated the vast differences between and among the interventions. Three major differences in the interventions emerged from these comprehensive reviews: (1) dose (number of sessions and length of exposure), (2) the target populations, and (3) the methodologies.

Chronic illness, such as cancer, HIV, and fibromyalgia, do not have cure as their primary goal for treatment. Therefore, palliation, symptom management, and health promotion become important day-to-day activities to maintain function and live with the illness. A number of intervention studies to ameliorate symptoms from chemotherapy treatment are published. Since chemotherapy often causes individuals to experience cognitive difficulties and physical fatigue, which last over time, the programs of two researchers are illustrated. Elderly cancer survivors reported difficulty with attention, concentration, and memory. Women undergoing treatment for breast cancer have difficulty with attention fatigue, and cancer survivors may suffer cognitive losses. McDougall (2001) tested the effectiveness of an efficacy-based intervention designed to improve memory performance, memory self-efficacy, and metamemory in older adult cancer survivors and those with other chronic conditions. A total of 78 older adults (58 Fs, 20 Ms) with an average age of 82 years participated in the eight-session program. Individuals were grouped by chronic condition: cancer = 11, arthritis = 16, heart disease = 32, and other = 19. The cancer group was older, $M = 84.82$, reported greater memory decline, and had lower self-reported instrumental activities of daily living scores. The cancer group made significant gains in short-term memory of immediate and delayed story recall, memory-efficacy ($M_1 = 48.22$, $M_2 = 58.00$), and metamemory (subjective memory evaluation) change ($M_1 = 2.18$, $M_2 = 2.50$). The responses of a group of elderly to training varied depending on their health status.

Cimprich and Ronis (2003) tested the efficacy of a natural environment intervention, delivered 120 minutes per week of exposure, in the home of the individual. Capacity to direct attention was assessed with objective measures at two time points: 2 weeks before surgery and 2 weeks after surgery. Compared with the control group, the intervention group showed greater ability to direct attention. These two studies are examples of programs of research in which aspects of cognitive function have been used as outcomes of health promotion interventions.

A unique program of research is the work of Stuifbergen, Becker, Blozis, Timmerman, & Kullberg (2003). Over more than 10 years of systematic inquiry, she has demonstrated that cognitive behavioral health-promotion interventions reduce the burden of illness and improve the health of women with multiple sclerosis (MS).

Older adults are particularly vulnerable to medication errors, whether intentional or unintentional. With older adults, age, cognitive function, and presence of depression are known to influence compliance and adherence behaviors. Two programs of research, emphasizing technology, are relevant to this review. Fulmer and her team (1999) tested two experimental interventions: video telephone and standard telephone against a control group receiving usual care. Compliance was determined as the percent of therapeutic coverage as recorded by Medication Event Monitoring System (MEMS) caps. The experimental groups, while not significantly different from each other, showed greater medication compliance than the control group, which worsened at 8 weeks.

Insel and Cole (2004) also incorporated the MEMS as a mechanism to enhance the availability of environmental cues to not only remember to take medications, but also to remember if the medications were taken as intended. The primary outcome measure, the percentage of days in which the correct number of doses was taken, significantly increased. The intervention focused on providing external memory cues to older adults responsible for self-management of medications. The cues assist in both remembering to perform the intended action (prospective memory) and remembering if the action was performed as intended (source monitoring). Therefore, the cues used both visual placement in salient places surrounding the time of day medicines need to be taken and also provided a way for older people to check if they have taken the medicines as desired. The interventions were tailored to the unique needs/lifestyle of the individual and embedded in the context of their living situation. These two studies provide examples in which the use of a commercially available technology produces significant health outcomes to assist older adults to maintain their independence.

Nurse researchers are making progress in developing cognitive interventions to manage pain. Two programs of research are described here. Wells-Federman and her team (Wells-Federman, Arnstein, & Caudill, 2002) provided a cognitive-behavioral treatment pain-management intervention to chronic pain patients. Physicians who determined that these individuals did not receive relief from pain and suffering after they had undergone multiple evaluations and treatments referred all individuals to the research project. The intervention was a group pain-management program that met once per week for 10 consecutive weeks. Topics explored during these weekly sessions were the role of lifestyle factors such as diet, activity, and physical and emotional tension. As a result of the intervention, pain intensity lowered by 18% and depression scores were reduced by 29%. In addition self-efficacy for pain management increased 36%. This intervention demonstrated that cognitive behavioral treatment reduced suffering and improved the well-being of persons with chronic pain.

Good, Anderson, Stanton-Hicks, Grass, and Makii (2002) evaluated the results of three nonpharmacological interventions delivered to 311 patients following gynecological surgery: jaw relaxation, music, combination of relaxation and music and a control group. Participants in the intervention groups practiced the technique for 2 minutes preoperatively and received coaching. The investigators evaluated sensation and distress of pain, opioid intake, or patient-controlled analgesia (PCA), and sleep. The intervention groups experienced less pain than the control group only receiving PCA. When combined with PCA, the three interventions had the same effects, that is a 9% to 29% reduction in pain. Those individuals who slept well had less pain on the following day.

With the greatly increasing older population, the cognitive function of older adults remains a great concern. Research focused on maintaining cognitive function and promoting improved cognitive function is actively being investigated. The future holds great promise for the ability of science to assist older adults in maintaining cognitive function necessary for quality of life.

GRAHAM J. MCDOUGALL, JR.

Cohort Design

A cohort design is a time-dimensional design to examine sequences, patterns of change or growth, or trends over time. A cohort is a group with common characteristics or experiences during a given time period. Cohorts generally refer to age groups or to groups of respondents who follow each other through formal institutions such as universities or hospitals or informal institutions such as a family. Populations also can be classified according to other time dimensions, such as time of diagnosis, time since exposure to a treatment, or time since initiating a behavior. A cohort might be graduates of nurse practitioner programs in the years 1995, 2000, 2005 or siblings in blended families. Cohort designs were originally used by epidemiologists and demographers but are increasingly used in studies conducted by nurses and other researchers in the behavioral and health sciences.

In the most restrictive sense a cohort design refers to a quasi-experimental design in which some cohorts are exposed to a treatment or event and others are not. The purpose of a cohort design is to determine whether two or more groups differ on a specific outcome measure. Cohort designs are useful for drawing causal inferences in quasi-experimental studies because cohort groups are expected to differ only minimally on background characteristics. Recall that a quasi-experimental design lacks random assignment of subjects to groups. Although the groups in a cohort design may not be as comparable as randomly assigned groups, archival records or data on relevant variables can be used to compare cohorts that received a treatment with those that did not. Because simple comparisons between cohorts may suffer from a number of design problems, such as biased sample selection, intervening historical events that may influence the outcome variable, maturation of subjects, and testing effects, a strong cohort design can account for many of these threats to the internal validity of a study.

There are two major types of cohort design: cohort design with treatment partitioning and the institutional cycles design. In a cohort design with treatment partitioning, respondents are partitioned by the extent of treatment (amount or length) received. In the institutional cycles design, one or more earlier cohorts are compared with the experimental cohort on the variable(s) of interest. The institutional cycles cohort design is strengthened if a nonequivalent nontreatment group is measured at the same time as the experimental group. A well-planned cohort design can control for the effects of age or experience when these might confound results in a pretest-posttest design or when no pretest measures of experimental subjects are available. Cohort designs might utilize a combination of cross-sectional and longitudinal data.

The term *cohort studies* broadly refers to studies of one or more cohort groups to examine the temporal sequencing of events over time. Cohort studies may eventually lead to hypotheses about causality between variables and to experimental designs. Most cohort designs are prospective (e.g., the Nurses' Health Study, in which 100,000 nurses were enrolled in 1976 and have been followed since) although some are retrospective.

There are a number of types of cohort studies. The panel design, in which one or more cohorts are followed over time, is especially useful for describing phenomena. Trend studies are prospective designs used to examine trends over time. In trend studies, different subsamples are drawn from a larger cohort at specified time points to look at patterns, rates, or trends over time (Polit & Hungler, 1995). Panel designs with multiple cohorts are used to study change in the variable(s) of interest over time, to examine differences between cohort groups in variables, and to identify different patterns between groups. In a panel study with multiple cohorts, the groups can enter the study at different points in time, and the effects of aging can be differentiated from the effect of being a member of a particular cohort group (Woods & Catanzaro, 1988). A prospective study is a variation of a panel design in which a cohort free of an outcome but with one or more risk factors is followed longitudinally to determine who develops the health outcome. The prospective design is used to test hypotheses about risk factors for disease or other health outcomes. Some authors limit the term *cohort study* to designs in which exposed and nonexposed subjects are studied prospectively or retrospectively from a specific point.

A major problem with prospective studies of all types is subject attrition from death, refusal, or other forms of loss. The loss of subjects in a prospective study may lead to biased estimates about the phenomena of interest.

Carol M. Musil

Collaborative Research

Collaborative research involves cooperation of individuals, agencies, and organizations in the planning, implementation, evaluation, and dissemination of research activities. Ideal collaboration brings the perspectives of nursing practice, research, and education to bear on complex issues of health and nursing. The research process, context, design, and needed resources for collaborative projects are not unique within the research arena. The unique feature involves the configuration of a research team whose members bring varying expertise, perspectives, and authority within an institution or agency.

Two prevailing trends support collaboration, namely, constrained resources and sociopolitical accountability. With diminishing resources to fund research and to deliver health care, partnerships can be an effective and efficient way to use human, fiscal, and material resources. Pooling resources of a variety of individuals, agencies, and disciplines can maximize the potential of all participants and contribute to a greater outcome.

Related to scarce resources is the call for increased accountability of research efforts. If finite resources are to be allocated, society and specific funding sources ask that the project demonstrate societal relevance and a connection to public concerns. Through partnerships with consumers, communities, or current practitioners, relevant and timely issues are more likely to emerge as inquiry topics.

Potential collaborators fall into several categories. Individuals can come to the project with expertise in the research process or in a substantive clinical area. Individuals can contribute the perspective of education, service, or research. Agencies or institutions can participate as collaborators, bringing specific human or material resources. Population groups can contribute the perspective and wisdom of a community. Nursing literature also advocates international collaborative efforts.

Collaborative research involves multiple advantages. One potential advantage is a strengthened process and improved outcome through the contribution from multiple individuals with varying expertise and perspectives. Investigator bias can be reduced with multiple inputs. Multisite partnerships give a potential of larger sample size over a shorter time frame and the benefits of built-in replication. Resources and potential funding sources can be increased through collaboration. The possibility of greater dissemination of findings increases with more participants. Collaboration with clinical agencies can help identify potential student clinical placement and supports a context for research that is compatible with the realities of nursing practice. Additionally, innovations in nursing practice or policy are more likely to be adopted if those involved in implementation participated in the inquiry process. Finally, collaborative interaction can enhance professional creativity, collegiality, and productivity.

Although benefits exist, collaborative research also presents distinct disadvantages. Most disadvantages are related to interpersonal issues and the complexities of pulling together different perspectives, priorities, and styles. Teamwork requires clear communication, trust, openness, administrative coordination, and distinct role delineation. Without those features, the integrity of the research and the professional productivity of the collaborators are at risk. Another disadvantage of collaboration is the possibility of multiple review boards and organizational protocols. Collaboration also may add to the time commitment.

Five major types of collaborative research described in the nursing literature are the traditional model, health care setting model, unification model, consortium model, and participatory action research. Each model has advantages and disadvantages.

In the traditional model, individual researchers from the same or different institutions work together. In this model, researchers learn from the expertise of each other. The usual equal distribution of experience and expertise means that the research tasks can be divided. The project ideas can be critiqued by two or more researchers with training in the research process or in a substantive area. Detrimental characteristics of the traditional model relate to the necessity of decreased teaching load for researchers with an educational appointment and the need for resources of funding and research assistance. Examples of the traditional model abound.

In the health care model, research occurs within a clinical institution under the leadership of an employed nurse researcher. Collaborators include the clinical staff and the nurse researcher. The strongest merit of this model is the development of practice-relevant research; and because clinicians are involved, there is ownership, accepted innovation, and practice based on scientific research. In this model, subjects are easily accessible, and interdisciplinary collaboration is easily arranged. Disadvantages involve the potential for poor generalizability, investigator bias, role conflict, and scarce research funding.

In the unification model, academic researchers from educational institutions and clinicians from health care agencies collaborate as equal partners. Benefits include combined resources from education and service, practice-relevant research, and enhanced collegiality. Disadvantages relate to the complexity of blending two institutions' perspectives and priorities, the challenges of meeting time and place, and the need to decrease teaching or work load for the researchers.

The consortium model involves individuals from multiple health care agencies in a geographic region. This model provides the benefits of cost sharing, large subject pool, decreased data collection time, and the momentum and inspiration of a shared project. Because of the geographic distance between sites, communication and decision making present major challenges. Multiple agencies also introduce multiple protocols or review boards. Researchers in this model often report an ambiguity regarding their role in the project.

The participatory action research (PAR) model combines community participation, research, and action to solve pressing social problems. This mode of inquiry involves the community as an equal partner at every step of the process. Benefits include empowerment of local communities, development of lay leadership, and resolution of real-life situations. Disadvantages involve a long time commitment and difficulty in obtaining funding.

Collaborative efforts can be enhanced by the explicit discussion and written communication of guidelines. Thiele (1989) mentioned three significant issues that require attention: "questions of authorship, contribution and recognition of effort" (p. 150). Written agreement among collaborators should clarify role responsibilities for each participant, decision-making processes, tentative time schedules, spin-off projects, and subsequent use of data. Engebretson and Wardell (1997) listed the requisite personal attributes as "trustworthiness, competence, and flexibility" (p. 43) and the requisite relationship attributes as "acceptance, validation, and commitment" (p. 44) and often synergy and fun.

JOANNE W. RAINS

Comfort

Comfort has been conceptualized as a holistic outcome of nursing care and defined as the experience of having needs for relief, ease, and transcendence addressed or met in four contexts of experience. The four contexts for experiencing comfort were derived from the literature on holism and were labeled physical, psychospiritual, environmental, and sociocultural (Kolcaba, 1991). Relief, ease, and transcendence, three types of comfort, were derived from a concept analysis of comfort (Kolcaba & Kolcaba, 1991).

Comfort care is nursing care that is intended to enhance a patient's comfort beyond its previous baseline. Comfort care consists of goal-directed, comforting activities (the process of comforting) through which enhanced comfort (the desired end product or outcome) is achieved. The process is initiated by the nurse after an assessment of the comfort needs of the patient/family. Because the specified product or goal is enhanced comfort, a successful process is evaluated by comparing comfort levels before and after interventions that are targeted towards comfort. The process is incomplete until the product of enhanced comfort is achieved (Dretske, 1988; Kolcaba, 2003).

Kolcaba (1994, 2003) provides a theoretical framework for practicing comfort care and for generating nursing research about comfort. Briefly, the theory states that interventions should be designed and implemented to address unmet comfort needs of patients and their families. Because comfort is a basic human need, patients and families often assist nursing efforts towards enhanced comfort. (In fact, some self-comforting measures can be negative, such as alcohol or drug abuse.) The effectiveness of comforting interventions is perceived in the context of existing intervening variables. Intervening variables are factors that recipients bring to the situation and upon which nurses have little influence, such as financial status, existing social support, previous experience with health care, and religious beliefs. Enhanced comfort strengthens patients and their families during stressful health care situations, thereby facilitating health-seeking behaviors (HSBs).

Schlotfeldt (1975) discussed HSBs in terms of those that are internal (fertility, healing), external (self-care, functional status), or leading to a peaceful death. Consistent with holism, conscious and subconscious experiences influence motivation for patients/families to engage in HSBs. Because HSBs are constructive, they are reciprocally and positively related to comfort. Comfort Theory states that patient/family comfort is the immediate goal of comforting interventions, and HSBs, specific to health-related goals, are subsequent outcomes.

Comfort Theory is focused on enhancing patient/family comfort for altruistic and pragmatic reasons. Patients/families want to be comforted by nurses in stressful health-care situations. Because comfort is related to subsequent desirable health and institutional outcomes, the outcome of enhanced comfort is elevated in stature among other more technical and narrow outcomes. It is a holistic and nursing-sensitive outcome that is congruent with recent mandates to measure nursing effectiveness in terms of positive and desirable patient/family goals (Magvary, 2002).

The Theory of Comfort directs research in several ways. First, it guides nurses to test relationships between particular holistic interventions and comfort. Second, it guides nurses to test relationships between comfort and setting-related HSBs. If the relationship is positive, nurses have a pragmatic rationale for enhancing patient comfort. Third, it guides nurses to test relationships between HSBs and institutional outcomes.

Qualitative studies have been conducted to determine the nature of comforting nursing actions and what comfort means to patients. Journal publications by these authors did not define or operationalize the outcome of comfort. Several empirical tests of Comfort Theory have been conducted by Kolcaba and associates (Kolcaba, 2003).These comfort studies demonstrated significant differences between treatment and comparison groups on comfort over time. The following interventions were tested: (a) types of immobilization for persons after coronary angiogram, (b) guided imagery for women going through radiation therapy for early breast cancer, (c) cognitive strategies for persons with urinary frequency and incontinence, (d) hand massage for persons near end of life, and (e) generalized comfort measures for women during first and second stages of labor. In each study, interventions were targeted to all attributes of comfort relevant to the research settings, comfort instruments were adapted from the General Comfort Questionnaire (Kolcaba, 2003), and there were at least two measurement points, usually three, to capture change in comfort over time.

To demonstrate that comfort is an important mission for nursing, additional tests of Comfort Theory should be conducted, including attention to increased functional status, faster progress during rehabilitation, faster healing, or peaceful death (when appropriate). Institutional outcomes could include decreased length of stay for hospitalized patients, decreased readmissions, and higher patient satisfaction.

KATHARINE KOLCABA

Community Health

Community health is influenced by environmental, biomedical, organizational, and behavioral factors and encompasses a broad definition of health. For example, good jobs, education, safe neighborhoods, access to health and social services, and recreation and leisure activities all promote community health. Community health is a process of health promotion and disease prevention in which community leaders identify community problems and assets, create consensus on goals, take action, and reach goals. Key aspects of this process are community development and multisectoral interventions, including health policy and community participation. Ongoing community-wide efforts assess and monitor progress in achieving explicitly stated community goals, for example, those adapted from *Healthy People 2010* (U.S. Department of Health and Human Services [USDHHS], 2000).

Because the health of people is affected by broad contextual factors, nurses, particularly community health nurses, must collaborate with other disciplines in developing a knowledge base for community health. Useful theories and models that can be applied to the study of community health include cultural change theories, social change theories, critical theories, community development, diffusion of innovation, ecological models, community participation, community power, and community decision making.

Community health research can be classified in different ways. For example, categorical programs include large-scale interdisciplinary studies such as the Minnesota Heart Health Program, the Pawtucket Heart Health Program, and the Stanford Five-City Project. Noncategorical programs include Healthy Cities and action research. Epidemiological research includes community needs, assets assessments, and risk factors for disease. Finally, there are evaluations of community health interventions. Increasingly, nurses are conducting community health research and involving other disciplines and the community in the process.

Opportunities for nursing research in community health are enormous. The growth of managed care is placing increased demands on state and local public health systems to assure the continuation of vital programs. Research in managed care and its impact on community health is needed to assure accountability of essential services. The extent to which underserved populations receive care within cost-containment strategies should be studied. The development of community coalitions for health throughout the country requires further study. Most major health programs—for example, Assessment Protocol for Excellence in Public Health (APEX/PH), Planned Approach to Community Health (PATCH), Healthy Cities and Communities, and HIV/AIDS Community Planning—involve the development of community coalitions as part of the community health process.

Research is needed to explain under what conditions coalitions succeed in promoting community health programs and policies. How effective are these programs and policies in changing key community health indicators of success? Nursing interventions, such as nurse-managed clinics or community nursing centers, need further research. What are the critical factors that sustain successful nurse-managed services at the local level? To what extent are these services being integrated into the networks of provider services? Dissemination of research findings is also important. For example, what are the characteristics of successful nurse-managed services that can be applied elsewhere and in what types of communities?

Likewise, the challenges are enormous. Nurses can take the lead in interdisciplinary research collaboration. The skills for community health research require the expertise of many disciplines in addition to nursing, including epidemiology, health economics, medicine, dentistry, health policy, statistics, and urban planning. The challenge is to share the expertise of each discipline as well as share the credit and rewards of collaboration. Although the time is ripe for funding such research efforts, such funding is highly competitive in the current health care arena.

The concept of community health incorporates a broad definition of health, one that recognizes the multiple community factors that support and impinge on health. Scientific inquiry that includes both qualitative and quantitative research approaches is needed to further build the body of knowledge relevant to the theory and practice of community health.

BEVERLY C. FLYNN

Community Mental Health

Over the past 50 years, the community mental health movement has had a tremendous impact on psychiatric nursing, taking psychiatric nurses into communities and freeing them from their almost exclusive practices in large state hospitals. Nursing research in the area of community mental health has steadily increased, the United Kingdom having contributed most to this body of literature, especially in recent years. Historic influences in the United States (U.S.) and United Kingdom (U.K.) created different climates from which nursing research in each of these countries emerged.

From the early 19th century until the 1960s, mental hospitals, or "asylums," constituted the major treatment resource for the mentally ill in both the U.S. and U.K. Advances in the use of psychotropic medications and government policy directives in each country spurred movement of mentally ill patients into the community. The historic report, *Action for Mental Health*, presented to the U.S. Congress in 1961, recommended a shift to community-based care. This was followed in 1963 by the enactment of the Community Mental Health Centers Act, which authorized $150 million in federal funds to develop comprehensive community mental health centers (Miller, 1981). The U.K. followed suit in 1962 when British politician Enoch Powell presented his *Hospital Plan for England* to Parliament; however, it was not until the publication of the 1975 White Paper, *Better Services for the Mentally Ill*, that any real increase in resources were initiated (Bonner, 2000).

The shift from hospital to community posed challenges for psychiatric nursing in both countries. Most psychiatric nurses in the U.S. were educated through hospital-based programs, making them ill equipped to take on the demands of an expanded community role. Although the findings of several early descriptive studies (Hess, 1969; Hicks, Deloughery, & Gebbie, 1971) show psychiatric nurses functioning in diverse roles, nursing leaders (Mereness, 1983) during this period expressed concern that too often nurses in community mental health adopt "residual roles," resulting from their lack of education in psychiatric theory and unequal status among fellow professionals.

In the U.K., social workers were the primary professionals delivering care to mentally ill patients in the community. Nursing was represented by the part-time activity of hospital-based psychiatric nurses who were seen merely as a technology through which psychiatrists could extend their authority beyond the confines of the hospital (Bonner, 2000). In both countries, the main role for community psychiatric nurses during these early years was the task of administering depot injections to patients with severe mental disorders.

The 1970s and 1980s were characterized by role differentiation and expansion for community psychiatric nurses in both countries. In the U.S., there was recognition of the need for advanced educational preparation of psychiatric nurses to meet the challenges of this evolving role (DeYoung & Tower, 1971). The findings of one descriptive study (Davis & Underwood, 1976) show that, although half of the nurses employed in four community mental health centers earned a bachelor's degree and provided some consultation and counseling, most of their time was spent performing traditional functions. With increased educational opportunities, funded largely by the National Institute of Mental Health (NIMH) in the 1980s, psychiatric nurses grew more sophisticated and diversified. They began to function as therapists for individuals, families, and groups and to serve as case managers and coordinators of community services. Psychiatric home care nursing also began to flourish during this period as reimbursement for these services became available (Fagin, 2001). Although nursing research related to community mental health was still scarce, an early intervention study (Slavinsky & Krauss, 1982), funded by the NIMH, characterized nurses' commitment to the care of psychiatric patients in the community and their skill in developing innovative programs for this population.

The drive for autonomy for community psychiatric nurses in the U.K. was away from psychiatry and "general nursing." Their "professionalization" and expansion was largely achieved through their successful incursion into primary health care and distancing from mental health teams. Government initially supported community psychiatric nurses' efforts in building new relationships with general practitioners, and even funded their training (Godin, 2000). Community psychiatric nurses expanded in number, and also in the range of therapeutic approaches used in their practices. As their self-image as professionals and their relationships with general practitioners grew, however, their caseloads became comprised of patients with less severe problems (Godin, 1996). The findings of one U.K. study (Barratt, 1989) show community psychiatric nurses' self-perceived roles becoming more differentiated, emphasizing prevention, counseling, and a variety of therapies for certain patient populations. Another study (Wetherill, Kelly, & Hore, 1987), investigating the effectiveness of a structured home intervention to improve patient compliance in alcohol treatment and recovery, demonstrates the growing ability of community psychiatric nurses in the U.K. to develop innovative interventions and expand their practices to include a varied clientele base.

In the U.S., psychiatric nurses continued to develop pivotal roles in a variety of community treatment modalities. In one national survey of assertive outreach programs, findings show that 88% had a psychiatric nurse as an integral member of the treatment team (Deci, Santos, Hiott, Schoenwald, & Dias, 1995). Over time, psychiatric clinical nurse specialists became recognized as independent practitioners, eligible for third-party reimbursement, and active in caring for seriously mentally ill patients (Iglesias, 1998; White, 2000); however, research addressing specific psychiatric nursing interventions for this population was still quite limited (Beebe, 2001; Rabbins et al., 2000). The "Decade of the Brain" in the 1990s brought the medicalization of psychiatric practice. In response to the challenge of integrating biologic knowledge into clinical practice, psychiatric nurses working in community mental health centers and in private practice in the U.S. sought prescriptive authority. Current nursing research reflects efforts to understand prescribing practices of advanced-practice psychiatric nurses (Talley & Richens, 2001) and identify barriers to prescriptive practice (Kaas, Dahl, Dehn, & Frank, 1998).

By the 1990s, community psychiatric nurses in the U.K. were numerically the most dominant occupational group within community mental health care; however, this also meant that they were perceived as responsible for many of its failures. Criticism was primarily directed toward their decision to shift focus away from the care of patients with severe mental illnesses in favor of work in primary health care. Many also questioned the effectiveness of their work in primary care, contending that counseling-based interventions were of unproven worth with people experiencing minor, self-limiting problems, and were not cost effective (Hannigan, 1997). Not only were community psychiatric nurses directed to reappraise the value they placed upon serving those with severe mental illness, they were also directed to develop and apply evidence-based interventions with this population.

One needs only to scan recent reviews of nursing research to gain an appreciation of the effort that has and is being put forth by psychiatric nurses in the U.K. to meet this mandate. The nursing literature is replete with studies investigating the clinical impact of specific interventions with severely mentally ill patients. Examples include nursing interventions for early detection of medication side effects (Jordan, Tunnicliffe, & Sykes, 2002), for identifying psychiatric illness in the elderly (Waterreus, Blanchard, & Mann, 1994), for providing sex education to mentally ill patients (Woolf & Jackson, 1996), for delivering a "psychosocial intervention" to families caring for a relative with schizophrenia (Brooker & Butterworth, 1991), and for using an "insight program" with patients diagnosed with schizophrenia (Pelton, 2001). While psychiatric nurses throughout the world can use the wealth of knowledge gained from these studies, it is equally important that research be directed toward testing nursing interventions within the context of specific communities and different cultures, and that nursing research in this area become more interdisciplinary in nature. It is also important that nurse researchers study the effects of disparity and stigma in access to community mental health care across the life span.

WENDY LEWANDOWSKI

Complementary and Alternative Practices and Products (CAPPS)

A large percentage of persons worldwide are using complementary and alternative practices and products (CAPPs), referred to also as "complementary and alternative medicine" (CAM), and, more recently, integrative medicine (NIH, 2003). However, the term CAM is not a true descriptor in that use of these practices and products is not limited to medicine. Integrative medicine is the newest term added to the range of definitions related to the concept of "complementary and alternative" medicine. The term "integrative" is increasingly used by clinicians and researchers, reflecting findings in the survey literature that suggested most people use CAPPs in conjunction with, rather than as an alternative to, conventional or mainstream medical services (NCCAM, 2003; Ni et al., 2002).

Despite any confusion in use of terms, surveys indicated that a significant percentage of the adult population in the United States (ranging from 30% to 45% at the beginning of the new millennium) is trying a variety of these ancient and modern CAPPs to treat a variety of symptoms and conditions (Eisenberg et al., 1993, 1998; Ni et al., 2002). A parallel trend is the increasing use of CAPPs among senior citizens, specifically in the aging U.S. population. A recent national sample study has shown that 30% of people aged 65 and older used at least one CAPP modality compared with 46% of those younger than age 65 ($p = < .001$) (Ai & Bolling, 2002). These surveys indicate, also, that the American public is spending billions of dollars for CAPPs, most of which is not reimbursed by third-party payers.

In response to the increasing interest of the American people in the healing potential of CAPPs, the Federal Government created in 1992 the Office of Alternative Medicine (OAM) (elevated in 1999 to the National Center for Complementary and Alternative Medicine [NCCAM]). The mission of the NCCAM is to assure users, through rigorous research studies, that the CAPPs widely used by the American people do what the practitioners of these modalities and the manufacturers of these products claim. It is acknowledged today that anecdotes about efficacy and effectiveness of practices for which there are not plausible explanations are insufficient, thereby giving importance to well-designed and well-executed research.

The term complementary medicine/therapies was introduced during the decade of the 1970s in the United Kingdom and refers to those practices and products that link the most appropriate therapies to meet the individual's physical, mental, emotional, and spiritual needs. In some cultures the term "alternative" refers to those practices and products that are provided in place of conventional health care, many of which are outside the realm of accepted health-care theory and practices in the United States. Still today, practices and products categorized as complementary and alternative reflect a broad spectrum of modalities and beliefs. Consequently, what is defined as such varies based upon professional or occupational perspective. Among the early initiatives of the NCCAM was identification of broad categories of CAPPs as a beginning to the classification of the more than 200 modalities that are reported to have more than 10,000 uses. These categories fall under the rubrics of alternative medical systems (e.g., homeopathy, naturopathy); mind-body interventions (e.g., mental imagery, music therapy); biologically based therapies (e.g., dietary supplements, herbal products); manipulative and body-based methods (e.g., massage, chiropractic); and energy therapies (e.g., qi gong, therapeutic touch, electromagnetic energy fields as in magnet therapy). The NCCAM fosters research to reduce barriers that keep promising therapies from emerging. To promote research in CAPPs, OAM initially established 10 research centers across the country, one of which is directed by a nurse. NCCAM has since enlarged this number to 13 research centers across the country and has reported plans to develop international research centers as well (NCCAM). Interested persons seeking state-of-the-science information on selected CAPPs may access a Public Information Clearinghouse Database, and the Evaluations Section of NCCAM may be accessed at the web site http://nccam.nih.gov/ (NCCAM, 2003; Taylor, 1998).

Selected complementary and alternative practices have been studied sufficiently to provide conclusive evidence of effectiveness. For example, there are data to support a number of behavioral and relaxation practices used to treat pain and insomnia. However, data currently available are insufficient to be definitive that one practice or procedure is more effective than another for a given condition. Yet, because of psychosocial differences among persons, as well as variations in personality traits among individuals, one procedure or product may be more suited than another for a given person (NIH Technology Assessment Panel, 1996; Owens, Taylor, & DeGood, 1999).

The challenge today for health care professionals is to become and stay informed regarding indications and contraindications for use of the myriad of procedures and products that patients are using, including the potential interactions of natural products with pharmaceuticals, foods, and lifestyles. Movement to offer some content about CAPPs within the curricula of schools of nursing, medicine, and pharmacy is evident. However, while faculty responsible for the integration of this content sometimes desire to include it, there appears to be less agreement among faculty on the practical aspects of its integration (Gaydos, 2001; Kligler, 1996). A more recent effort of the NCCAM focuses on introduction of CAPPs information into allopathic, osteopathic, nursing, dental, and pharmacy schools to capture the attention of young health professionals (Taylor, Menzies, & Boyden, 2001).

The main issue regarding research in CAPPs is not the adversarial position, e.g., "CAPPs vs mainstream," but the more scholarly position of asking whether an intervention is effective or not; is it safe or not? (NCCAM, 2001). Rigorous programs of research involving any of these practices and products may begin with basic questions:

What's going on with a particular therapy in the investigator's target population? How do individual differences, as assessed by a given measurement tool, influence what happens or does not happen in the use of a particular therapy for management of a specified symptom? From general questions such as these, coupled with extensive literature reviews and consultation with experts, more specific questions about the use of these therapies in patient care evolve to guide the investigator's research.

Because nursing takes the position that patients' perceptions, thoughts, and feelings are an important part of their reality, these influence the nature of inquiry and the choice of outcome measures. Focusing on individual differences among patients when assessing use, efficacy, and effectiveness of CAPPs permits the investigator to analyze disparate patient care findings and synthesize these into questions that will add to the body of knowledge about these therapies (Owens et al., 1999). Findings resulting from research studies testing the efficacy of CAPPs may lead to knowledge that can be useful in making reliable predictions and linking appropriate therapies to a person for promotion of health or symptom management (Taylor, 1998).

Definitions of complementary and alternative procedures and products (CAPPs) and estimates of consumer use will continue to change as researchers complete rigorous scientific studies in this area. While health consumers today are empowered to take control of their health care outcomes, a large number of nurses and other health care professionals still lack knowledge about CAPPs, thus creating a barrier to consumers achieving their goal. Rigorous clinical studies continue to be needed to provide evidence of treatment efficacy for many symptoms and conditions. Research monies are available for competitive research proposals through the NCCAM and other departments within the National Institutes of Health. Consumer demand and pressure will continue to drive integration of selected CAPPs into the conventional health care system as well as prompting the need for continued rigorous science in this field. These factors foster optimism and increase the potential for additional evidence-based holistic care, facilitating the safe integration of selected CAPPs into health care.

Ann Gill Taylor
Victoria Menzies

Computer-Aided Instruction

Computer-aided instruction is an educational method in which specially designed computer programs are delivered to learners as replacement or adjunct to standard classroom or practical experience. This form of instruction may be offered in a classroom setting by an instructor. Instruction may be offered in the form of clinical simulation, where the program reproduces a virtual scenario similar to what the learner would experience in a live, clinical situation; it may also be used in adaptive testing which tailors the testing in response to a learner's ability. Computer-aided instruction may also be offered in an interactive format for purposes of mastering theory in addition to clinical/psychomotor skills. Ayoub et al. (1998) proposed that use of an interactive computer classroom will help foster the development of critical thinking within groups at all levels of education. Utilization of this model of education becomes increasingly relevant in a basic or advanced practitioner role with the advent of the increasingly restricted clinical time allotments to students and faculty. Problem-solving skill development is impacted, and not uncommonly, places students with inadequate knowledge and insufficient clinical skills in situations which can ultimately prove harmful to patients (Weis & Guyton-Simmons, 1998).

One of the biggest impediments to broader use of the computer as an instructional device in the period from the late 1980s through the early 1990s was anxiety regarding computer use, commonly referred to as "technophobia" (Geibart, 2000). Age is also a factor, with older students exhibiting more anxiety than younger ones about computer technology. Initial attempts to integrate the computer into education were limited to using the device as an alternative to paper-and-pencil assignments and testing. Gibbons, Bachulis, and Allen (1999) compared a group of 45 students who were asked to design a computer program on a relevant clinical topic and compared this group to another group assigned a paper-and-pencil independent study. Students with the computer assignments expressed more satisfaction with their assignment. Ravert (2002) reviewed nine educational programs (five medical, four nursing) utilizing clinical simulation as a part of their instructional program and found that only one of the nine, at a medical school located outside the United States, did not score positively as favoring computer simulation as a part of its academic program. Simulation lends itself to a number of learning opportunities, particularly with complex patients and patients utilizing complex medical technologies normally seen in a critical care area. The study of pathophysiologic process also lends itself well to simulation (Hart, 2000).

Computer adaptive testing which adapts to the individual's ability forms the basis for many of the specialty practice and achievement examinations taken by practitioners. Probably the most familiar form of this type of testing is the National Council Licensing Examination (NCLEX) which was started in 1994. Forker and McDonald (1996) note that with the increased availability of microcomputers in schools, exclusive use of traditional paper-and-pencil testing is changing. It is safe to assume that this would be the case with computer simulation activities as well. It can also be assumed that with the almost daily advances in web-based technology, clinical education as well as education of a more theoretical nature, such as epidemiology or bioethics, will continue to lend itself to this mode of education.

The technology surrounding computer-aided instruction and testing will continue to expand greatly in the future. Distance learning will continue to become more widely used and embraced by educators throughout the world. Clinical simulation in the form of virtual reality will take the learner to new heights in very realistic learning adventures. As the use of computers in and out of the classroom continues to increase, research exploring the outcomes of this educational method will be forthcoming.

Joseph M. Filakovsky

Computerized Decision Support Systems

Although there is no clear agreement about how to define Computerized Decision Support Systems (DSSs), most would agree that a DSS can be defined in general as a computerized system used to aid decision making related to semi-structured problems. But some incorrectly include under the umbrella of DSS software that are not truly DSSs, such as expert systems. While differentiation is fuzzy, in general a true DSS is a collection of software programs, at the core of which are mathematical and statistical modeling components which act with real data to facilitate decision making. A defining characteristic of DSSs is that they are proactive. They provide rapid responses to real situations based on real data, models, and established guidelines. They are designed to be flexible, and allow ad hoc queries and easy changing of parameters in order to accommodate clinician intuition and judgment.

DDS systems vary in terms of complexity and scope, ranging from simple provision of integrated reports to use of inferencing methods to determine complex associations between pieces of data. While their goal is to facilitate effective decision making, they deal with problems that are relatively unstructured. For example, such a system might be used to predict how a new patient care treatment might affect the average duration of patient stay in an institutional setting.

The ultimate goal of any DSS is to help clinicians overcome their cognitive resource limitations for processing and storage as well as problem solving in an increasingly complex medical environment. DSSs do this by helping clinicians to manage information overload in order to properly assess all of the relevant information and generate systematic and reasonable therapy. This has the net effect of facilitating standardization of care, reducing errors, and improving quality of care.

Healthcare DSS systems use actual patient data to provide information that can help clinicians make decisions. Wyatt and Spiegelhalter (1990) add the requirement that a medical DSS generate case-specific advice. The use of DSSs in clinical decision support can be divided into two categories: diagnostic and therapeutic.

There are several types of diagnostic DSSs. First are systems generating differential diagnoses. Such systems provide lists of possible diagnoses based on given clinical data. However, such systems are often problematic as the potential benefit for the differential diagnosis-generating DSS to inform caregivers about additional relevant diagnoses can be outweighed by the "noise" that arises from the presentation of irrelevant or inappropriately ranked diagnostic choices (Weiner & Pifer, 2000). Another type of DSS is based on a rule in/out model. These are used by caregivers to rule in or out a small set of diagnoses based on a given set of objective clinical signs and symptoms. They function like a second opinion and have been successful in limited application (Weiner & Pifer). A third type of DSS is used for computer-aided review of clinical tests such as radiographs or pathology specimen evaluation (Alberdi et al., 2000; Peters, 1996). Such systems help caregivers to interpret results, and have again had success in limited application.

Therapeutic DSSs focus on decision making in point of care treatment. Some focus on medication dosing, with the goal of reducing errors and complications. Others manage complex processes such as ventilation and oxygenation (East et al., 1999). Most therapeutic DSSs focus on compliance of caregivers with established quality-of-care guidelines, such as embedding hypertension guidelines within the hypertensive patient record (McAlister, Covvy, Tong, Lee, & Wigle, 1986). Their goal is to generate, at the point-of-care, patient-specific evidence-based therapy instructions that can be carried out by different clinicians with little interclinician variability. Individualization of patient therapy is preserved by these explicit protocols since they are driven by individual patient data (Morris, 2001). A good example in nursing of such a DSS is the Braden System (Bergstrom, 1997). This is a DSS that guides the caregiver through risk assessment and then suggests risk-based care tailored to the specific patient risk-factors based on published guidelines. However, while the use of DSSs in therapeutics seems reasonable, research is need that demonstrate their benefits in terms of outcome measures (Weiner & Pifer, 2000).

Nursing research in the area of informatics has a history of perhaps 25 years, most of which has been heavily invested in the basic work necessary for the building of DSS systems. This basic work includes the development and identification of classification systems, taxonomies, vocabularies, best practices, essential data elements, and types of information used in nursing research and nursing decision making (McCormick & Jones, 1998; Werley, Devine, Zorn, Ryan, & Westra, 1991; Benner, 1984). While nurse informaticists have also developed circumscribed DDS systems using these building blocks, research related to the accuracy of the decisions and the efficacy of these systems in improving outcomes is fairly limited (Johnston, Langton, Haynes, & Mathieu, 1994). One study was located which tested the accuracy of a DSS system in using assessment data with a forward chaining inference engine to identify nursing diagnoses and interventions appropriate to the patient (Hendrickson & Paganelli, 1994). A few studies have moved beyond these basic issues to test the effectiveness of specific DSS systems in producing nursing decisions that result in better outcomes of care (Cuddigan, Logan, Evans, & Hoesing, 1988; Petrucci et al., 1992). Some have also moved to development of decision support systems based on established guidelines (Bowles, 2003). Future research will likely focus on how DSSs can help nurses help patients make decision in scenarios characterized by the need for careful deliberation about alternatives due to the risk or uncertainty of the outcomes or the value-laden nature of the decision (O'Connor et al., 1997).

In 1993, the National Institute of Nursing Research (NINR) constituted an expert panel on Nursing Informatics. They were charged with setting research priorities for nursing informatics as part of the National Nursing Research Agenda. In carrying out this mandate, the panel identified seven foci for research, and within each focus, these experts assessed the state of the science, then identified and prioritized more specific research needs (NINR, 1993). These foci were: (a) using data, information, and knowledge to deliver and manage patient care; (b) defining and describing data and information for patient care; (c) acquiring and delivering knowledge from and for patient care; (d) investigating new technologies to create tools for patient care; (e) applying patient-care ergonomics to the patient-nurse-machine interaction; (f) integrating systems for better patient care; and (g) evaluating the effects of nursing information systems. Similarly, in 2001 lawmakers provided the Agency for Health Research and Quality (AHRQ) with $50 million to undertake a major research initiative investigating the problem of medical errors. Among funded projects now under way are four different studies (two in adult and two in pediatric populations) assessing the impact of using handheld DSSs in ambulatory care settings (Ortiz & Clancy, 2003).

Health care delivery today is so complex that it is currently straining the resources of the country, and multifaceted clinical decisions are being made in an environment of rapidly escalating intensity. As DSS systems are developed to produce specific patient-care protocols that have been validated through using rigorous methodologies, these systems have the potential to decrease harmful variation in care, improve clinical decision making, reduce errors, optimize outcomes of care, and cut health care costs.

BARBARA BRADEN
CYNTHIA L. CORRITORE

Concept Analysis

Concept analysis is a strategy used for examining concepts for their semantic structure. Although there are several methods for conducting concept analysis, all of the methods have the purpose of determining the defining attributes or characteristics of the concept under study. Some uses of a concept analysis are refining and clarifying concepts in theory, practice, and research and arriving at precise theoretical and operational definitions for research or for instrument development. Concept analysis has been used in other disciplines, particularly philosophy and linguistics, for many years. However, the techniques have only recently been "discovered" by nurses interested in semantics and language development in the discipline.

Concept analysis is a useful tool for nurses conducting research. Because the outcome of a concept analysis is a set of defining characteristics that tell the researcher "what counts" as the concept, it allows the researcher to (a) formulate a clear, precise theoretical and/or operational definition to be used in the study; (b) choose measurement instruments that accurately reflect the defining characteristics of the concept to be measured; (c) determine if a new instrument is needed (if no extant measure adequately reflects the defining characteristics); and (d) accurately identify the concept when it arises in clinical practice or in qualitative research data.

Concept analyses were relatively rare in nursing research until the early 1980s but have increased dramatically in number over the past 2 decades. Concept analysis is particularly relevant to a young science such as nursing. The process, regardless of method, requires rigorous thinking about the language used to describe the phenomena of concern to the discipline. Doing a concept analysis causes the researcher to be much more aware of and sensitive to the use of language in research. A conscious awareness of the language chosen to represent phenomena is necessary if nursing scientists are to develop a comprehensible body of knowledge for the discipline.

It is also necessary for thoughtful practitioners to be aware of the language of the discipline. How nurses think about and describe the problems and solutions relevant to their practice is of paramount importance in helping the consumer of nursing care and the policymakers who influence the practice milieu to understand what nursing is and what nurses do. If nurses do not have a central core of well-defined concepts to describe their practice, then confusion and ambiguity will persist, and the development of nursing science will suffer.

Concept analysis has become a useful adjunct to nursing research. The outcome of a concept analysis significantly facilitates communication between researchers and practitioners alike. By specifying the defining characteristics of a concept, the researcher or practitioner makes it clear what counts as the concept so that anyone else reading about it or discussing it understands what is meant. Being clear about meaning allows better communication between scientists and practitioners about the usefulness and appropriateness of nursing language.

There is considerable discussion in the literature about which method of analysis is the most useful. Regardless of the method used, concept analyses can contribute significant insights into the phenomena of concern to nurses.

KAY C. AVANT

Consortial Research

Consortial research is a form of collaborative research that can be used to increase the quantity and quality of nursing research within clinical settings. It involves cooperative efforts among researchers at several institutions. The sites have formal, well-defined administrative and working relationships that spell out agreed-upon roles and responsibilities.

Consortial studies are done for a number of reasons: (a) to achieve the required sample size when studying a low-prevalence disease; (b) to increase the ethnic diversity or other characteristics of a sample, thus increasing generalizability of results; (c) to shorten the time line for conducting the study by simultaneously recruiting subjects at multiple sites; (d) to provide mentoring to more junior researchers and staff nurses; (e) to share resources, tasks, and costs when external funding is not available; and (f) to increase opportunities for replication and dissemination.

Consortial studies may be conceived by one or a few investigators, who draft the initial proposal then recruit colleagues at other sites to participate in the study. These other investigators may be involved in helping to refine the proposal before it is submitted for funding. When the purpose of the consortium is more focused on mentoring junior colleagues or is a way to share resources and costs, it is more likely that development of the proposal will be a group endeavor from the start. In the latter case, the choice of topic may be generated by an advisory or steering committee. Whichever approach is taken, the pool of ideas generated by expertise from several institutions creates synergy that leads to more creative and productive research.

To conduct these multisite studies, one site usually serves a coordinating function for the study. Most often in externally funded studies, the coordinating center is responsible for identifying or developing questionnaires or other data collection forms, for data collection and processing procedures, and for receiving and centrally analyzing the study data. The oversight role of the coordinating center includes development and implementation of a quality control plan to assure standardization of sample identification, recruitment, and data collection procedures. Scientific issues for the conduct of the study are usually managed by a steering committee, often composed of the principal investigator from each participating site and a few key individuals at the coordinating center. Standing or ad hoc subcommittees of the steering committee are often formed to propose standards and oversee the work on specific aspects of the study. For example, the subcommittees bring proposals for publications and presentations, participant safety and endpoints, or clinical aspects before the steering committee for approval. The degree to which the steering committee is involved in development of protocols, questionnaires, and so forth, as opposed to approving those developed by the coordinating center, varies by study and the reason the consortium was created.

In a consortium formed primarily for the purpose of sharing resources, mentoring junior researchers, replicating a previous study, or disseminating results, the steering committee may be composed of representatives appointed by each participating institution. In such cases the steering committee often serves the purpose of setting priorities for the activities of the consortium. Funding of studies conducted by a consortium may take several forms. When external funding is involved, the two most common types are (a) providing one large grant to a coordinating center, which then subcontracts with each clinical site, and (b) providing individual grants to each participating institution with a separate grant to the coordinating center. The first approach gives the coordinating center budgetary leverage when a site is not performing up to par. This is an advantage for involving a new site or increasing the number of subjects enrolled at existing sites by redistributing funds from the nonperforming site. The second approach requires that each site meet the commitments for the good of the overall study. A third model, used when external funding is not available, shares the cost of the research among participating institutions within the consortium.

In medical treatment research and public health prevention research, consortial arrangements have been a preferred structure for large randomized trials that must recruit substantial populations in a relatively short time, provide intervention, and have sufficient follow-up time to generate adequate statistical power to compare the effects of treatment on the study outcomes. Nursing has generally had less experience with this approach, although consortia of schools of nursing with several practice settings have been formed to facilitate the conduct of collaborative clinical nursing research (Rizzuto & Mitchell, 1988a, 1988b, 1990; Schutzenofer & Potter, 1989; Zalar, Welches, & Walker, 1985).

It may be expected that consortial research will increase as nursing researchers do more experimental research. Another factor that may promote consortial research in nursing is the changing health care system. As health care systems increase the number of contractual arrangements in attempts to provide cost-effective, integrated care across the continuum of patient needs, consortial research is likely to become more common.

BARBARA VALANIS

Content Analysis

Content analysis is a data analysis technique that is commonly used in qualitative research and focuses on structuring particular topics or domains of interest from unstructured data. It is a time-consuming process that involves organizing, identifying, coding, and making categories from patterns of data that are reflective of the topics (Patton, 1990). The topics or domains of interest are descriptive names chosen by the researcher and are sometimes also referred to as category labels (Morse, J. M., & Field, 1995). Historically, early content analysis focused on linguistic and observational data. However, in addition to information derived from interviews and casual or structured observations, researchers may analyze written text from special documents, archival records, field logs, and diaries or may develop schemes to analyze visual data from pictures or videotapes.

Content analysis begins with reading the text or written transcription of an interview, notes from an observation, or some other mode of data collection. The investigator reads the completed text and determines the main ideas or topics of the transcription or observation. The investigator then rereads the text and numbers and assigns a code to each segment or group of lines from the transcription. Sometimes this may also be called labeling. Segments may consist of a single word or line, multiple words or lines, one or more paragraphs, or a pictorial schema and may vary according to the chosen topic or topics. The codes developed by the investigator reflect some commonality, such as an action or behavior, an event, thought, concept, and so forth. Line segments or groups of lines are separated and are grouped into categories, and the categories are grouped according to the topics that were identified by the investigator.

Topics or domains of interest may be chosen prior to a study, as with a focused study, or after the first interview. A focused qualitative study centers on one particular area of interest or intent, such as metaphorical analysis or feminist research. Another kind of focused study might center on a particular phenomenon like leadership style, body adornment among adolescent girls, or a demonstration of how caring activities are performed, to name a few.

The researcher may also chose to develop topics after a first interview or observation. Sometimes the topics seem to arise naturally from the data, whereas at other times the researcher must decide on and develop the topics from the information given. Developing a topic may be similar to making an index for a book or file labels (Patton, 1990). The researcher reads through the transcript of the interview or observation and begins to sort and organize the interview data according to likenesses and similarities. The researcher usually gets a sense of the main topics that pervade the text soon after the transcribing process is complete and after the first reading. This organization of the data may be done by hand or by using one of the many computer software packages that are available to assist organization of qualitative data.

J. M. Morse and Field (1995) suggest using between 10 and 15 main topics per study. They caution against making topics too specialized as only very small amounts of data will be able to fit into each. On the other hand, too many topics can cause confusion, and the researcher may have difficulty in remembering what categories go into each topic as the study progresses and more data are collected. With each subsequent interview or observation, the topics may be combined or subdivided into multiple categories as the need arises. As repetitive patterns arise, relationships between the categories and then between topics may be seen. Often the relationships may occur at the same time or be concurrent with each other. For example, in a study of adolescent face care, the topics "blemish care" and "facial scrubbing" are related and occur at the same time. In the same study, the topic "facial preparation" occurs or is antecedent to the topics of "blemish care" and "facial scrubbing," whereas the topical area "making up the face" may occur as a consequence of one of the earlier categories that was formed (Morse & Field). Some researchers choose to quantify part of the analysis by counting frequency and sequencing of particular words, phrases, or topics.

The major reliability and validity issues of content analysis involve the subjective nature of the researcher-determined topics or category labels. What should be included within each topic should be clearly defined and should be clearly different from the others so that the results are mutually exclusive. The easiest way to determine reliability in a study that uses content analysis is to have two or more readers, other than the researcher, agree that the topics are appropriate for a particular study and that data can easily be organized under each. This is typically carried out by having the researcher randomly choosing a part of the study and having the readers look over the text and the topics independent of each other. A consensus of the readers would indicate the study's reliability.

Validity in content analysis can be achieved by determining the extent that the topics represent what they are intended to represent. If the topics are based on a conceptual framework or a particular focus, they must be justified, described, and explained in terms of being representative of that conceptual framework or focus. Therefore, topics that are developed to reflect a conceptual framework or focus must be consistent with the original definitions described by that framework. However, because content analysis is often used in exploratory and descriptive research, a conceptual orientation may not be used.

KATHLEEN HUTTLINGER

Continuing Care Retirement Communities

A continuing care retirement community (CCRC) is a type of facility that provides housing, meals, and other services, including nursing home care, for older adults in exchange for a one-time capital investment or entrance fee, and a monthly service fee. Most CCRCs are sponsored by religious or other nonprofit organizations, but for-profit organizations have entered into the retirement business as well. The CCRC is usually constructed as a village or community, and the individual remains within this community for the remainder of his or her life. All CCRCs have a written contract that residents must sign. The terms of the contract vary, and have been separated into three categories by the American Association of Homes for the Aged: (1) Type A homes are "all inclusive" as they offer guaranteed nursing care in the nursing facility at no increase in the residents' monthly fee; (2) Type B CCRCs do not guarantee unlimited nursing home care but have a contractual agreement to provide a specific number of days per year or lifetime of the resident in the nursing facility; and (3) Type C CCRCs are based on a typical fee-for-service approach. Financial stability, particularly of Type A and Type B CCRCs, depends on high occupancy rates in the independent living apartments and maintaining the residents' optimal health and function so as to need fewer health care services.

The number of CCRCs has increased dramatically (50%) during the 1980s and has continued to grow. CCRCs are located throughout the United States although five states (Pennsylvania, California, Florida, Illinois, and Ohio) are home to more than one-third of the nations' CCRCs. Despite the growth of CCRCs, proportionally they account for a smaller percentage of senior housing than previously. This is due to the dramatic increase in assisted living facilities.

Generally older adults who live in CCRCs are those who were never married, or married without children, are well educated, and health conscious (Krauskopf, Brown, Tokarz, & Bogutz, 1993; Petit, 1994; Resnick, 1989, 1998a). Initially CCRCs were for affluent older adults; however CCRCs are becoming more affordable and attracting those with more moderate incomes (Kitchen & Rouche, 1990). The decision to move into a CCRC requires a good deal of planning and adjustment for older adults, especially if they are relocating to another city or state, and/or moving from a large home to a smaller apartment.

The initial research in CCRCs focused on the adjustment to the community and the impact this had on the older adult. Resnick (1989), using a qualitative approach, described the challenges of adjustment to a CCRC and identified groups of individuals who were particularly at risk for relocation stress: (a) those who had experienced a recent loss, (b) those with a decline in mental status, and (c) the young-old (60 to 70 years) age group. Anticipating problems and letting residents know that they might have certain feelings helped residents in the adjustment process. The study also identified the need for frequent follow-up in the first 6 months to a year following the move-in as many residents did not begin to grieve over their losses until they fully completed the work of the move. Petit (1994) implemented the findings of this work as she developed the role of the wellness nurse in a CCRC.

The majority of the nursing research done in CCRCs has been on the health practices and health promotion of these individuals (Adams, 1996; Crowley, 1996; Resnick, 1998a; Resnick, Palmer, Jenkins, & Spellbring, 2000; Resnick, 2003). Generally these are descriptive surveys in which residents are asked about specific health behaviors such as getting vaccinations, monitoring cholesterol and dietary fat intake, exercise activity, alcohol and nicotine use, and participation in health screenings including mamograms, Pap tests, stools for occult blood, or prostate examinations. The majority of residents in the CCRCs studied did get yearly flu vaccines and a pneumonia vaccine, and approximately 61% had an up-to-date tetanus booster. A smaller percentage (approximately 30%) monitored their diets. About 50% of those living in CCRCs drink alcohol regularly, only a small percent use nicotine (11%), and under 50% exercise regularly. Approximately 40% to 50% of the residents get yearly mamograms, 31% to 37% get Pap tests, 65% to 80% get prostate examinations, approximately 60% have stools checked for blood yearly, and a little over 50% monitor their skin for abnormal growths regularly. Overall there is better participation in health promoting activities of older adults living in CCRCs when compared to older adults in the community (Blustein & Weiss, 1998; Smith et al., 1999). The findings, however, suggest that even in this population continued education is needed to encourage personal decision making related to health promotion activities. The findings can also be used to develop interventions to improve specific health behaviors.

In a series of analyses examining the relationships between health behaviors among residents of CCRCs, age was the only variable that was significantly related to health behaviors and accounted for 7% of the variance. With increased age the residents participated in fewer health-promoting or preventive behaviors. Age, gender, physical and mental health, self-efficacy expectations, outcome expectations, and stage of change related to exercise directly and/or indirectly influenced exercise behavior in the residents (Resnick, 1998a; Resnick et al., 2000; Resnick & Nigg, 2003). The influence of these variables on exercise behavior was supported in a qualitative study (Resnick & Spellbring, 2000) which focused on what helped older adults in a CCRC adhere to a regular walking program and what decreased their willingness to adhere. Crowley (1996) also considered the health behaviors of older adults in a CCRC and the outcomes of a wellness program which encouraged regular exercise. A total of 21% of the 225 residents exercised, and case reports identified positive outcomes such as weight loss and improved recovery following a fracture. Resnick (1999) explored the incidences and predictors of falls in a CCRC and found that the number of falls was the only variable associated with having an injurious fall. Resnick (1998b, 1999) also used a combined qualitative and quantitative approach to explore what increased or decreased residents' willingness to participate in and actual performance of activities of daily of living, such as bathing, dressing, and ambulating. Personality (i.e., determination), beliefs in their ability, the unpleasant sensations associated with the activity, goals, and fears, such as the fear of falling, were identified as common themes that influenced performance of functional activities. Based on quantitative findings, motivation (self-efficacy expectations, outcome expectations, and the personality component of motivation) as well as physical condition (standing balance and lower extremity contractures) were the most important predictors of functional performance in these individuals. Although not extensively studied, Russell (1996) considered the care-seeking behavior of older adults living in a CCRC. This was a qualitative study using ethnographic field research that incorporated semi-structured interviews, participant observation, and focus group interviews. The care-seeking process was described as sequential phases and stages that evolved over time. Resnick (2003) tested the impact of an individualized approach to health promotion in these sites, and Resnick and Andrews (2002) tested an educational intervention to help older adults make end-of-life treatment preferences. Some work has also been done to test exercise interventions in these settings (Resnick, Wagner & House, 2003; Vaitkevicius et al., 2002).

CCRCs continue to be a viable living environment for older adults. In order for these facilities to keep costs down and remain lucrative it is imperative that there be a focus on maintaining health and function. Continued research needs to build on the preliminary findings from exploratory studies and begin to develop and test interventions that will help older adults in CCRCs maintain their health and function. For example, many CCRCs have "wellness programs" which are nursing driven. The outcomes of these programs need to be considered both from a health perspective as well as a fiscal perspective. Other important areas of research within CCRCs that nursing should consider include care processes around relocation to different levels of care, end-of-life issues, injury prevention, health-care utilization patterns and the impact this has on nursing care services.

BARBARA RESNICK

Coping

Coping is one of the most prolific topics in all of nursing research. Thousands of studies have been conducted by nurse researchers on coping, mainly with chronic illness, acute conditions, and treatment stress; family responses related to illness/disease; child/adolescent illness and hospitalization; specific illness, disease, diagnosis, medical treatment, and hospitalization stressors; caregiving, and sequelae such as distress. Prominent are studies of individuals and families facing chronic illness. The most frequent disease/illness situations in nursing coping research are cancer and cardiac disease or events. Coping is an exceedingly important area of nursing research since coping has important observable and measurable effects on health outcomes.

With few exceptions, coping in nursing research is defined using the definition and theory of psychologists Lazarus and Folkman (1984). They define coping as "constantly changing cognitive and behavioral efforts to manage specific external and/or internal demands that are appraised as taxing or exceeding the resources of the person" (p. 141). This definition accentuates the fact that coping is a process requiring effort, free of positive or negative evaluation, focusing on "what the person actually thinks or does" (p. 142).

Nursing research portrays coping as part of a dynamic process consisting of a stressor, appraisal, resources, coping, and outcomes. Stress in this perspective is defined as a "relationship between the person and the environment that is appraised by the person as taxing or exceeding his or her resources and endangering his or her well-being" (Lazarus & Folkman, 1984, p. 19). Stress involves appraisal of the stressor for well-being (primary appraisal) and what can be done to manage the situation (secondary appraisal). Stressors in nursing research can be categorized as an "internal or external event, condition, situation, and/or cue" (Werner, Frost, & Orth, 2000, p. 10) that has the potential to bring about or actually activates significant physical, psychological, social, or spiritual reactions. They can be either normative or catastrophic.

Lazarus and Folkman (1984) also distinguish between problem-focused and emotion-focused coping. Problem-focused strategies are "directed at managing or altering the problem causing the distress" (p. 150). Emotion-focused coping is "coping that is directed at regulating emotional response to the problem" (p. 150).

Other coping theories tested in nursing research with individuals include Scott, Oberst, and Dropkin's Stress-Coping Model incorporating anxiety in the stress and coping process. The theory most often employed in nursing research on family coping is the Resiliency Model of Family Stress, Adjustment, and Adaptation (McCubbin & McCubbin, 1996).

Coping resources examined in nursing can be categorized as social, psychological, spiritual, and other, such as finances and education. The social resource most studied is social support (Underwood, 2000). Nursing research has shown that social support "works through main, mediating, and moderating (buffering) mechanisms" (Underwood, p. 372). These processes are active and dynamic, and there is evidence that specific functions of social support and other resources become important in certain situations and specific phases of illness, health crisis, or treatment. Generalizations indicate that context determines social support needs; social support can come from a variety of sources such as confidant or network; perceived support availability is often more strongly related to coping effectiveness than actual support received; social support has both positive and negative aspects; and there is a negative association between social support and deleterious outcomes such as depression and anxiety (Underwood). Instruments most frequently utilized for measuring social support with individuals are Norbeck's Social Support Questionnaire and Weinert's Personal Resource Questionnaire. Evidence is growing that support is an important family resource, particularly when families are faced with caregiving stress/burden. Family instruments include McCubbin and colleagues' Social Support Index, and Fink's Family Social Support Index (DeMarco, Ford-Gilboe, Friedemann, McCubbin, & McCubbin, 2000).

Hardiness is the psychological resource most studied in nursing coping research (Ford-Gilboe & Cohen, 2000). Hardiness, a personality phenomenon encompassing commitment, challenge, and control, especially health-related hardiness conceptualized by Pollock, has been shown to be related to positive health outcomes for adults. Emerging as important in family nursing research, there is support that hardiness mediates "the relationships between stressful life events and family adaptation" (Ford-Gilboe & Cohen, p. 427). It includes control, challenge, commitment, and confidence. Evidence is growing that hardiness enhances coping for both individuals and families.

Other coping resources gaining nursing research attention include hope, control, sense of coherence, and self-efficacy. Antonovsky defined sense of coherence as an enduring orientation rendering events and stimuli comprehensible, manageable, and meaningful. Family sense of coherence is conceptualized as an "explanation of how these resources may contribute to health" (Antonovsky, 1998, p. 8).

Coping can be differentiated as coping style or coping strategies (behaviors). Coping style suggests typical responses across situations. Coping strategies are what people actually do in the face of stress. Nurse researchers examine coping strategies much more frequently than coping styles. Choice of strategies has been found to differ based on illness phase, specific stressors, and/or resources. People in many health/illness situations use a mix of problem-focused and emotion-focused strategies. Theoretically, problem-focused strategies are specifically tailored to the situation, while more global emotion-focused strategies are used across situations (Lazarus & Folkman, 1984). Instruments used most often to assess coping strategies in nursing research are the Jaloweic Coping Scale, the Ways of Coping Questionnaire, and the Family APGAR.

Over the last decade, there has been remarkable growth in the nursing research on coping in several areas. One of these areas is family coping. Another area is coping in children/adolescents (Stewart, 2003), where Lazarus and Folkman's theory is most often applied. Most of these studies concentrate on serious illness, traumatic situations, and developmental transitions. While most investigations tap stressors specific to the situation, many also focus on behaviors based on Ryan-Wenger's taxonomy of children's coping strategies. Another newer area is spiritual coping (Baldacchino & Draper, 2001). Many researchers have found that spiritual coping strategies enhance positive health outcomes.

Specific findings of nursing coping investigations are numerous; several generalizations stem from the research. Problem-focused coping is consistently related to positive health outcomes and general well-being. Optimism is an important strategy for individuals, facilitating constructive action, choice among options, and retaining control. Positive social support for adults, children, and families is related to positive health outcomes, and may function through obtaining assistance, supporting self-esteem, receipt of advice or information, and/or presence of a confidant. Use of spiritual resources or coping strategies, such as prayer or religious attendance, is related to positive health outcomes. Exerting control is also associated with positive outcomes. Emotion-focused strategies, often associated with more negative outcomes, can be beneficial, especially in situations where there are few options. Coping strategies change over the course of illness stages. Less desirable coping strategies are associated with negative outcomes. Finally, coping strategies perceived by participants as most effective are often not those they engage in frequently.

Research designs most frequently used are descriptive/correlational and qualitative or interpretive. Longitudinal research is becoming more prevalent. Most studies employ self-report instruments, but interviews are gaining in popularity. Nurse researchers investigating coping are too numerous to mention, coming from all nursing specialty areas and many countries. Exemplary programs of research include those of Grey, Hagedoorn, Hinds, Hoskins, Jaloweic, J. Johnson, M. McCubbin, Nail, Northouse, and Ryan-Wenger.

JOAN STEHLE WERNER

Coronary Artery Bypass Graft (CABG) Surgery

Coronary artery bypass graft surgery, a common treatment for coronary artery disease (CAD), provides significant improvement in symptoms in 76%–90% of the patients (Rahimtola, 1982). An estimated 800,000 surgeries are performed worldwide each year (Borowicz et al., 2002) with 519,000 performed in the United States in 2000 (American Heart Association, 2001). Although CABG surgery succeeds in treating physiological problems, a significant number of patients report feelings of anxiety and depression pre- and/or postoperatively and depression has been linked to morbidity and mortality (Borowicz et al.).

Research findings support the relationship of depression, anxiety, or a combination of the two with risk for cardiovascular disease (CVD), independent of classic risk factors, in patients with established CAD and in previously healthy individuals. Prevalence rates for patients with CVD range from 16%–23%, for clinical depression, and 31.5% and 60% for depressive symptoms (Pignay-Demaria, Lesperance, Demaria, Frasure-Smith, & Perrault, 2003).

Evidence that depression and anxiety have prognostic importance in determining CABG surgery outcomes supports the development of pre- and postoperative nursing assessment strategies to identify patients at risk for adverse events. Nurses can play pivotal roles in identifying patients who need further evaluation, providing education about the effects of depression and anxiety on CABG surgery outcomes, and developing and evaluating interventions aimed at ameliorating the effects of these risk factors on postoperative morbidity and mortality.

Demand for CABG surgery exceeds resources in many developed countries, leading to waiting lists. The experience of waiting for surgery has been studied from quantitative as well as qualitative perspectives. Patients on waiting lists experienced anxiety, depression, and negative impacts on quality of life (Screeche-Powell & Owens, 2003; Fitzsimmons, Parahoo, & Stringer, 2000; Teo et al., 1998; Jonsdottir & Baldursdottir, 1998). Levels of anxiety and depression in patients awaiting CABG surgery were significantly reduced in a randomized controlled trial of a nurse-led shared care intervention (McHugh et al., 2001).

Longitudinal studies of the impact of psychological variables on outcomes of CABG surgery demonstrate that recovery is neither simple nor experienced consistently in all patients. Although some studies included the measurement of both anxiety and depression, most examined the impact of depression on recovery. Researchers have found that anxiety levels significantly decreased over time and remained linear. Relationships between anxiety and depression over time were relatively weak while those relationships, at the same points in time, were relatively strong (Duits, Boeke, Taams, Passchier, & Erdman,

1997; Duits et al., 1999). Postoperative anxiety was directly related to perception of pain with the strongest relationship on postoperative day two. In a study of 38 males, 80% scored in the moderate range of anxiety preoperatively with anxiety-prone reactivity persisting in 38.9% of the patients postoperatively. These patients exhibited significantly more sleep disturbances, energy deficits, tiredness, immobility, and a lower quality of life (Edell-Gustafsson & Hetta, 1999).

Recently-reported longitudinal studies evaluating depression pre- and postoperatively report prevalence ranging from 16–50% preoperatively and 19–61% postoperatively. Almost all studies used self-report questionnaires for measuring depression. Subjects' (n = 50 to 336) mean ages ranged from 54 to 65 years, represented a 3:1 male-to-female ratio, and ranged from 85%–100% Caucasian.

An issue in evaluating patients for depression is the timing of the evaluation. Poston, Haddock, Conard, Jones, and Spertus (2003) found depression 1 month after surgery to be a better predictor of depression at 6 months than the preoperative score. Pirraglia, Peterson, Williams-Russo, Gorkin, and Charlson (1999) identified other predictors of postoperative depression: poor social support, at least one stressful life event in the last year, low level of education, and moderate to severe dyspnea. Hypothermia during CABG has been associated with higher levels of postoperative emotional distress (Khatri et al., 2001), and early extubation has been associated with fewer patients with depressive symptoms on day three postoperatively (Silbert et al., 2001).

Depression has consistently been associated with adverse outcomes after CABG surgery. Investigators (Perski et al., 1998; Scheier et al., 1999; Saur et al., 2001) have found depressive symptoms, pre- or postoperatively to predict postoperative cardiac events (unstable angina, myocardial infarction (MI), repeat CABG, or angioplasty) and were positively correlated with the rate of readmission for cardiac events. Connerney, Shapiro, McLaughlin, Bagiella, and Sloan (2001) determined that patients meeting criteria for major depressive disorder at discharge were significantly more likely to experience a cardiac-related event than were those who failed to meet the criteria (including those with depressive symptoms). Furthermore, depression was a predictor independent of classic cardiovascular risk factors.

In a study investigating the impact of depression on mortality, Baker, Andrew, Schrader, and Knight (2001) found mortality rates to be six times higher among the patients with preoperative symptoms of depression. Blumenthal et al. (2003) also identified higher mortality rates for patients with moderate to severe depression at baseline and mild or moderate to severe depression that persisted from baseline to 6 months. Limitations of these reviewed studies include low enrollment of women, racial homogeneity, high rates of refusal to participate, high attrition, and use of self-report measures to evaluate anxiety and depression.

Several studies have addressed gender differences in recovery from CABG surgery. Vaccarino et al. (2003) found that women were older and more often had unstable angina, congestive heart failure, lower physical function, and more depressive symptoms in the month before surgery. Younger women were at a higher risk of in-hospital death than men, a difference decreasing with age (Vaccarino, Abramson, Veledar, & Weintraub, 2002). Postoperatively, for women but not men only, pain was correlated with depressive symptomatology and functional impairment (Con, Linden, Thompson, & Ignaszewski, 1999) and women had a more difficult recovery, unexplained by illness severity, presurgery health status, or other patient characteristics.

Postoperative neuropsychological deficits are a common complication of cardiac surgery, with incidence ranging from 25%–80% (Borowicz, Goldsborough, Selnes, & McKhann, 1996). Although investigators have found that changes in anxiety and depression did not influence changes in neuropsychological performance (Andrew, Baker, Kneebone, & Knight, 2000), multiple investigators have found that anxiety and depression impact perception of cognitive functioning (Vingerhoets, De Soete, & Jannes, 1995; Khatri et al., 1999). Factors predictive of post-CABG cognitive deficits were preexisting cognitive deficits, greater age, lower premorbid intelligence, and, at 3 months postsurgery, patients who received their first CABG surgery without cardiopulmonary bypass (Millar, Asbury, & Murray, 2001; Van Dijk et al., 2002).

Based upon several reviews of recent data, symptoms of depression and, to some extent, anxiety may be associated with cardiac events and mortality through multiple pathophysiological pathways. These include exerting a direct influence on health-related lifestyle behaviors (smoking, poor diet, low activity levels, poor adherence to treatment), effects on of hyperactivation of the hypothalamic-pituitary-adrenal and/or sympathomedullary axes, diminished heart rate variability, myocardial and ventricular instability in reaction to mental stress, alteration in platelet receptors and/or reactivity, and the inflammatory processes. To date, no one mechanism has been identified as the causal link between psychological states and cardiac events.

Although the benefits of short-term preoperative interventions have been examined in only one randomized controlled study of patients awaiting CABG surgery (McHugh et al., 2001), clinical experience suggests that routine screening and effective treatment preoperatively may decrease postoperative anxiety and depression and facilitate recovery. There is general agreement that early postoperative intervention should be offered to patients experiencing depression and/or anxiety. Some studies have shown that early psychological intervention may be associated with reduction in length of hospital stay, analgesic use, less subjective tension, and postsurgical morbidity (Mumford, Schlesinger, & Glass, 1982; Ashton et al., 1997; Perski et al., 1999; Karlsson, Berglin, & Larsson, 2000). A stress-management program, based upon relaxation techniques, offered 3 months after the MI or CABG surgery improved emotional well-being, daily activities, and several social parameters (Trzcieniecka-Green & Steptoe, 1996). Data is also accumulating about the efficacy of selective serotonin reuptake inhibitors on the treatment of depression (specifically sertraline and fluoxetine) in patients with cardiovascular disease (CVD). To date, no studies investigating the effect of antidepressants after CABG surgery have been published. Clearly, there is a need for large, randomized trials of both antidepressants and psychosocial interventions post CABG surgery to determine their efficacy, especially since depression has clearly been linked to increased morbidity and mortality.

Susan H. McCrone

Cost Analysis of Nursing Care

Cost analysis of nursing care reflects a body of administrative studies that focus on quantifying nursing costs needed to deliver care to individual clients or aggregates in a variety of settings, employing a variety of practice models and analysis tools. All cost analysis is based on assumptions that must be examined and made explicit when reporting findings (Friedman, De La Mare, Andrews, & McKenzie, 2002).

Much of the research on cost analysis of nursing care has focused on "costing out" nursing services for the purpose of measuring productivity, comparing costs of various nursing delivery models, charging individual patients for true nursing costs, and relating nursing costs to other cost models, most notably Diagnostic Related Group (DRG) categories. The need and motivation for these costing efforts have evolved with the economic underpinnings of the health care system, as have the methodologies and setting focuses. For example, most studies in the 1980s were performed in acute-care hospitals, whereas more studies now relate to other settings.

Today, cost analysis of nursing care focuses on justifying the cost effectiveness of professional practice models, evaluating redesign efforts, and monitoring and controlling nursing costs within an ever-tightening, cost-conscious health care environment. Within the context of rising capitation penetration, cost analysis is essential to accurate capitation bidding and financial viability of the parent organization. As "best practices" benchmarking pushes the envelope of competitive bidding, demonstrating cost-effective nursing practice becomes essential to securing managed care contracts.

Cost analysis research is a type of nursing administrative research that evaluates aspects of the delivery of nursing care. More recently, this type of research has been performed in a multidisciplinary fashion under the broader rubric of health services administration research.

Cost analysis studies always have been relevant to decision making by nursing administrators in selecting delivery models, treatment protocols, and justifying budgets; but such studies may become central to the survival of the entire profession for the future. As cross-trained, unlicensed assistive personnel (UAPs) proliferate, nurse administrators must struggle to support the cost-effectiveness of professional nursing practice. Larger questions of appropriate skill mix cannot be determined solely on a cost per hour of service, cost per case, or cost per DRG basis. New studies are needed that will combine traditional cost analysis with differential outcome analysis to secure a larger picture of the "true cost-benefit ratio" for specific nursing models.

The most notable characteristic of cost analysis studies is the variety of definitions, variables, and measurement tools used in the studies. Eckhart (1993) performed a comprehensive review of 73 studies published from the early 1980s through 1990, focusing on costing-out nursing. Because of the impact of DRGs, length of stay (LOS) was a consistent variable. Length of stay was found to correlate highly to nursing work performed, whether measured by acuity indexes, nursing care hours, nursing costs, patient charges, or percent of nursing costs to hospital costs. These studies focused on in-patient settings, so little is known about cost analysis of nursing in nonacute settings that are the emerging focus of health care. Not all DRG categories have been studied, and there has been little validity or reliability reported on the instruments used to measure related variables. Definitions critical to this area of study must be standardized. For example, which nursing staff or other care providers are included in direct care calculations? What support services are included in indirect care calculation? What role should overhead and depreciation costs of nursing-related resources play?

Another major area of dispute for costing studies is the lack of a standard acuity measure because of the proprietary nature of most acuity systems. One study (Phillips, Castorr, Prescott, & Soeken, 1992) compared GRASP and Medicus acuity systems to the Patient Intensity for Nursing Index (PINI). PINI significantly correlated with both systems ($p < .0001$), but the shared variability was only 44% and 49% respectively. Shared variability between GRASP and Medicus was only 34%, and it was concluded that the two acuity systems do not measure nursing resource use in the same way. Neither system was predictive of PINI items "knowledge deficit, emotional status, severity of illness, or potential for injury." Such PINI items as "hours of care, task/procedure complexity, and mobility" were significant predictors of both Medicus and GRASP scores (Phillips et al., 1992). These findings seem to indicate that task aspects of professional practice are measured by these systems but that interpersonal and observational aspects may not be fully appreciated. This work was confirmed by Cockerill, Pallas, Bolley, and Pink (1993) whose study compared case costs for patients across six acuity systems. Variances in estimated hours of care across workload measurement tools were statistically significant and varied by up to 30%. It is impossible to distinguish between true differences in case costs and measurement error across institutions in these circumstances. More study is needed to normalize acuity systems before cross-institutional data will be meaningful.

Cost and efficiency of nursing procedures or treatments continue to be studied. Capasso and Munro (2003) compared two wound treatments (saline vs. hydrogel). Although both were comparable for wound closure rate and cost of treatment supplies, one was significantly more expensive. The saline treatment required a higher number of home nursing visits, accounting for the difference in cost. Clearly, such analyses demonstrate the multifactorial nature of costing research and the need to look beyond the obvious in doing such analyses.

Another fertile area for cost analysis is to evaluate cost differences among professional practice models. However, most of these studies use proprietary practice models that are difficult to duplicate in other settings. Variables are identified in these studies that do impact nursing costs, such as nursing turnover, ratio of productive to nonproductive hours, and nursing satisfaction. Russo and Landcaster (1995) evaluated unlicensed assistive personnel models relative to cost-effectiveness, quality patient outcomes, and customer satisfaction. More complex issues emerge for this type of analysis. Relative productivity across discipline levels, recruitment, training, and impact on quality must be added to the equation.

Given the growth of capitation, cost analysis of nursing services will need to take new directions. As critical pathways (benchmark performance tools) evolve as care guides, the costs of pathway changes on nursing delivery, patient outcomes, and case costs must be calculated. What are the most efficient and effective pathways toward resolution of a given health problem? What practice setting is appropriate for patients at each step of the pathway? For example, when is it safe to transfer a fresh open heart patient from critical care to a stepdown environment? (Earliest transfer to a least costly delivery mode saves money.) These calculations may be critical for institutions to secure managed-care contracts in a cost-competitive environment. Determining what activities can be safely eliminated from a pathway without negatively impacting care outcomes will have cost and resource savings as we move to "best demonstrated practices."

Finally, we must move toward a cost-benefit analysis model that incorporates the outcomes of practice. This aspect has been especially elusive, given the "generic" and group nature of nursing practice. With multiple nursing providers impacting a patient's care, how do we separate the relative contributions of each person or each subspecialty of nursing practice that a patient may experience in the course of their care from contributions of other disciplines? Additionally, we need to quantify the costs of increased patient mortality and failure to rescue associated with changes in nurse/patient ratios based on recent landmark studies (Aiken et al., 2002; Cho et al., 2003).

MARY L. FISHER

Critical Care Nursing

In the history of nursing the development of the specialty of critical care is fairly recent, paralleling the growth and development of intensive care units (ICUs) in the 1960s and 1970s. The first ICUs were areas in the hospital designated for the care of patients recovering from anesthesia who required close monitoring during a period of physiological instability. Recognition of the efficiency and effectiveness gained from segregating any patients who required intensive nursing care for a short period of time was spurred by experiences in managing groups of critically ill patients, such as those injured in the Boston Coconut Grove fire of 1942 and victims of the polio epidemics of the 1950s. The development of the mechanical ventilator and advances in coronary care led to recognition of the need for specialized skills and knowledge bases among nurses caring for these patients.

The first specialty organization was formed by nurses working in coronary care. As electrocardiographic monitoring became a routine tool in the care of many patients and critical care broadened to include the care of patients other than postanesthesia and those with cardiac disease, the American Association of Critical-Care Nurses (AACN), originally named the American Association of Cardiovascular Nurses, was formed in 1969 (Lynbaugh & Fairman, 1992). This step was rapidly followed by the development of continuing education programs, formal recommendations for critical care curricular content in undergraduate programs, and a certification program. Today, AACN is the largest specialty nursing organization in the world, with more than 65,000 nurses in the U.S. and 45 other countries.

Heitkemper and Bond (2003) reviewed major advances in nursing research in critical care. Domains of nursing science predicted to emerge as important contenders for research priorities include genetic therapeutics and counseling, infection and emerging infectious epidemics, the aging population, high-risk neonates, health disparities, man-made and natural disasters, and the impact of gender on the mechanism, detection, and management of disease.

From the outset, critical care has been a research intensive discipline, both in medicine and in nursing. The initial narrow focus on maintaining physiological stability of the cardiopulmonary system undoubtedly contributed to the early commitment to research-based practice. Dracup and Bryan-Brown (2003) observed an unprecedented change in the pace of critical care research and practice. Critical care researchers are venturing into multiple areas, including the impact of genomics and molecular biology on disease states. At the same time, there is an increasingly vast amount of published research, coupled with a trend toward specialization. Yet critical care nurse scientists have been extraordinarily productive, creative, and sophisticated in their investigations. A search of grants funded in 2003 by the National Institute of Nursing Research (NINR) yielded 24 federally funded studies of pediatric and adult patients with cardiac problems, four genetically-based studies, and more specifically, critical care research focusing on complex subjects such as heart-rate variability, prone positioning in pediatric patients with acute lung injury, gene expression in cerebral ischemia, the use of acute-care nurse practitioners in improving outcome in patients receiving long-term mechanical ventilation, and an ethnographic study of dying patients in surgical intensive care unit, examining family interactions with clinicians as the goal of care shifts from cure to comfort.

Phenomena of interest can be described as falling into five broad areas: (a) the critical care environment, (b) critical care nurses, (c) monitoring techniques, (d) interventions, and (e) outcomes of critical care. Journal articles published since 2003 in *American Journal of Critical Care, Critical Care Nurse, Heart and Lung, Nursing Research*, and *Biological Research for Nursing* were reviewed for evidence of significant trends and changing patterns of inquiry.

Interest in studying the critical care environment began with observation of postcardiotomy delirium in open heart surgery patients in the 1960s. Efforts to describe this phenomenon and identify causative factors soon broadened to include all forms of delirium and disorientation, grouped under the heading "ICU psychosis." This syndrome is now called delirium, described as a disturbance of consciousness, characterized by inattention and a change in cognition or perceptual disturbance that develop rapidly (Truman & Ely, 2003). Delirium, one of the most common complications in the ICU, has been found to be an independent risk factor for prolonged ICU and hospital stay, and higher mortality rates 6 months after discharge. Delirium may be associated with visual and auditory hallucinations, and sometimes paranoid ideation. It is thought to be related to a variety of physiological, psychological, and environmental factors.

Characteristics of the ICU environment that have been consistently implicated in studies and have been the target of changes in environment and care routines include sleep deprivation, social isolation, and multiple sources of unusual sensory stimulation, such as lighting and noise (Noble, 1982). Predisposing risk factors that are present prior to hospital admission may trigger delirium's onset, including age over 70 years, recent history of alcohol abuse, and transfer from a nursing home (Truman & Ely, 2003). Precipitating risk factors occurring following patient admission have been found to be any noxious stimuli initiated in the ICU setting, such as the administration of benzodiazepines, opiates, the performance of invasive procedures, and the emergence of electrolyte and fluid imbalance. Severe metabolic changes causing imbalances in neurotransmitter concentrations are thought to act as the basic mechanism for delirium, although environmental factors are known to play a role in its development and symptomatic escalation.

Another growing environmental concern is the potentially deleterious effects of light and noise in the neonatal intensive care unit on the growth and development of neonates, a subject that has received increasing attention from nurse scientists and greater funding for nursing research. A third recurring theme in the scientific literature is the need for the ICU environment to appear less threatening to patient family members and to meet family needs. Thus, the subject of ICU visitation has been examined by many investigators, particularly as it affects attitudes of family members and staff nurses alike. The emergency department as an environment of care has also been showcased as an important context of care, as the issue of family presence during patient resuscitation has received considerable attention by nurse researchers over the past several years. The boundaries between the sheltered ICU environment and the rest of the world, however, have become more permeable, given the recent turmoil and changing nature of world events. In response to these changes, Heitkemper and Bond (2003) recommend that nursing broaden its definition of environment to capture the threats of infectious disease, disasters, and health disparities as environmental factors in need of further research.

During the first decade of critical care development, there was considerable interest in studying the practitioners of this new specialty. In general, research projects were aimed at describing characteristics of nurses who chose this area of practice, comparing them with non-ICU nurses. In addition to looking for demographic differences, there was particular interest in the effects of working in the ICU environment on stress levels and the effects of stress, such as burnout and rapid turnover.

Currently, the focus of research on critical care nursing has shifted to a broader recognition of the importance of collaborative, interdisciplinary care and appropriate levels of staffing in order to ensure patient safety, improve patient outcomes, and address the growing nursing shortage due to dissatisfaction with working conditions. In a landmark study of more than 10,000 nurses and 230,000 surgical patients, Aiken and colleagues (2002) reported that when the safe patient-staff ratio exceeded 4 to 1 on a surgical floor, the frequency of patient deaths increased by 7% for each additional patient assignment added to the nurse's workload. This problem is particularly salient in the highly complex critical care environment, where Cullen and colleagues (as cited in Dracup & Bryan-Brown, 2003) found that preventable adverse drug events are twice as frequent when compared with the incidence of medication-related errors outside of the ICU, and where the risk of an adverse event rises by 6% for each day of ICU stay. Proposed solutions evident in the literature include nursing interventions using a teamwork model to improve patient outcomes and the use of acute care nurse practitioners to oversee continuity of patient care.

Physiological monitoring has been the hallmark of critical care since its inception. Until the recent emphasis on reducing the cost of expensive services, the most common reason for ICU admission was either for frequent and close physical assessment by nurses or for monitoring of some physiological parameter that required specialized technology not available on the general hospital ward, such as electrocardiography or intracranial pressure monitoring. It is understandable, then, that studies of monitoring techniques have been so prevalent. In a review of critical care practice research conducted in the decade 1979 to 1988 (VanCott, Tittle, Moody, & Wilson, 1991), the most common content areas were the effect of patient position on hemodynamic parameters (11%), cardiac output measurement (6%), and coagulation studies (5%). In the past decade, the usefulness of physiologic monitoring continues to receive attention, especially in the continuing interest in the accuracy of measurement of cardiac output with position change, temperature, oxygen consumption, work of breathing, neuromuscular blockade, as well as the determination of novel biomarkers of inflammation, rejection of organ transplantation, and sepsis. Greater numbers of critical care nurse researchers are receiving genetic training as well as federal funding for conducting basic laboratory and animal investigations, including such topics as diaphragmatic fatigue, cytokine response to inflammation, and genetic susceptibility to cerebral ischemia following brain injury.

Interventional studies have become more frequent in the recent past. The majority of these studies have focused either on psychosocial interventions, such as teaching, communication techniques, or family support, or on specific nursing procedures, such as suctioning or chest tube drainage procedures. Like much of nursing research in general, many ICU intervention studies have been limited by small sample sizes. In addition, earlier studies have typically used investigator-designed instruments, making comparisons across studies difficult; however, the use of standardized acuity rating systems, such as APACHE or TISS, to describe study populations and control for acuity have become more common. In her year-end review of nursing intervention research, Naylor (2003) noted that between 1999 and 2002, there were 78 nurse-led studies funded by the NINR: several of these projects focused on the critically ill patient, such as measuring changes in cerebral blow flow during suctioning, determination of proper feeding tube placement and detection of aspiration, the provision of ventilator care in patients with Acute Respiratory Distress Syndrome, and meeting the psychosocial needs of the patient following acute myocardial infarction.

One very promising approach to the problem of small sample sizes is the AACN research program of large, multi-site studies coordinated by an AACN research team. These investigations, termed "Thunder Projects," have enabled researchers to conduct large, tightly controlled studies of nursing problems specific to critical care. For example, Thunder Project I was a comparison of the effectiveness of heparinized versus nonheparinized flush solutions for maintaining patency of arterial catheters. This study, which supported the practice of heparinizing flush solutions, had a sample of 5,024 subjects (AACN, 1993). The objectives of Thunder Project II were to describe and compare patients' perceptions of pain and their responses to turning, wound drain removal, tracheal suctioning, femoral line removal, central line insertion, and nonburn wound dressing change (Puntillo, 2003). The sample size consisted of 91 children (ages 4 to 12), 151 adolescents (ages 13 to 17), and 5,959 adults (over 18 years of age). Procedural pain intensity and its associated distress were found to vary depending on the specific procedure performed. Overall, adults and children (ages 4 to 7) reported turning to be the most painful and distressing procedure, while children (8 to 12 years old) rated tracheal suctioning as the worst, and adolescents found wound care to be the most painful and distressing. More than 75% of children did not receive medication prior to and during a painful procedure, and more than 63% of adults did not receive any medication for procedural events. How patients were prepared for the procedure was found to be a key factor; anticipatory preparation should include analgesic administration and information about expected sensations that might occur.

As is occurring in other disciplines, there has been a recent trend toward emphasizing outcomes research in critical care focused particularly on use of quality management tools such as critical pathways; systems of care, such as case management; and alternative environments of care, such as special care units and observation units. It has been estimated that critical care accounts for 15% to 20% of total hospital costs (Berenson, 1984; Rudy & Grenvik, 1992). The high cost of critical care in the context of a national commitment to reducing health care spending will continue to make testing of more cost-effective approaches to care a research priority.

The emphasis for research efforts has also been directed toward establishing best practices for nursing care. It is in this area of research that one can find numerous nursing studies in the scientific literature. Nursing bedside practices of interest have included testing different methods for providing oral care for intubated patients, endotracheal suctioning with saline lavage, skin breakdown in open-heart patients, the beneficial effects of tight glycemic control of preoperative patients, and the success of a weaning protocol for patients receiving mechanical ventilation. Qualitative approaches in research methodologies have flourished, such as focusing on patients living with heart failure, prolonged mechanical ventilation, nurse decision making about hemodynamic status, patient anxiety following cardiac surgery, and end-of-life care. Predictive studies of risk factors have focused on long-term disability posthead injury, transient myocardial ischemia, atrial fibrillation following open-heart surgery, delay in seeking treatment for chest pain, heart failure readmission, heart transplantation, and functional and cognitive status after cardiac surgery and cardiac rehabilitation. Educational nurse-led interventions have targeted compliance as a primary goal in patients with heart failure using telephone counseling and a web-based approach, as well as supporting patients undergoing cardiac rehabilitation,

Critical care research is expected to continue to concentrate in the areas of monitoring techniques, specific procedural interventions, and outcomes research. AACN's research priorities for the 1990s included ventilator weaning procedures, hemodynamic monitoring techniques, measurement of tissue oxygenation, and nutritional support modalities (Lindquist et al., 1993).

Current research priorities (www.aacn.org/research, 6/24/02) include the following:

1. Effective and appropriate use of technology to achieve optimal patient assessment, management, and/or outcomes
2. Creation of a healing, humane environment
3. Processes and systems that foster the optimal contribution of critical care nurses
4. Effective approaches to symptom management
5. Prevention and management of complications.

In addition to the need for more multi-site studies in order to generate adequate sample sizes, there continues to be a need for the development of valid and reliable instruments that can measure outcomes, other than physiological parameters, that are sensitive to nursing interventions. In addition, many of the previously reported intervention studies should be replicated and tested with varying populations. Naylor (2003) pointed out that given the complex nature of effective interventions, the science underlying these interventions often spans knowledge derived from multiple disciplines, requiring the expertise and collaboration of scientists working in the basic, clinical, social, and behavioral sciences. For nurse scientists to succeed in the implementation of programs of research and dissemination of findings, they will need to utilize interdisciplinary collaboration and, ultimately, find ways to effectively transcend traditional disciplinary boundaries for the sake of addressing fundamental health issues and improving the health of individuals, families, communities, and society.

BARBARA J. DALY
UPDATED BY CAROL DIANE EPSTEIN

Cultural/Transcultural Focus

Cultural/transcultural focus is the study of the environment shared by a group seeking meaning for its existence. Nurse investigators pursue this focus to understand the association of culture to health and to provide culturally competent care. Although this focus is growing within research, its impact on patient care has been limited. Culture receives only cursory emphasis in most curricula or practice settings, and few nurses are cultural experts. In light of projections that racial and ethnic minorities will be the majority in the United States by 2030 and the persistence of major health disparities between Euro-Americans and others, more and better nursing research on culture is needed.

Different perspectives on the meaning of cultural/transcultural research (C/TCR) exist. To some, the terms are essentially synonymous and questions of disciplinary origin are unimportant. Researchers in the Leininger tradition regard transcultural nursing as the proper term for a formal, worldwide area of study and practice about culture and caring within nursing.

Cultural/transcultural research is found in a great variety of research and clinical journals. Some C/TCR studies (particularly interventions and randomized controlled trials) may be found in the Cochrane database for evidence-based practice using a keyword search based on such terms as the disease name, nurs* and care, nurs* and intervention, and names of racial or cultural groups. Recent reviews of C/TCR include race and ethnicity as nursing research variables (Drevdahl, Taylor, & Phillips, 2001), health disparities among vulnerable populations as published in *Nursing Research* over five decades (Flaskerud et al., 2002), and application of the Oncology Nursing Society's cultural competence guidelines to published oncology research (Phillips & Weekes, 2002). Searchers are cautioned that (a) the names of racial or ethnic groups are often used only descriptive labels, and findings do not advance true cultural knowledge; (b) race, culture, and ethnicity lack consensual definitions and are often used interchangeably; (c) acceptable names for groups change over time (e. g., Negro, Black, Afro-American, African American); (d) the name of the highest stage of cultural knowledge changes over time, with cultural competence or cultural proficiency being currently preferred; (e) databases on special populations are often nonexistent or inadequate; (f) although reports specify a focus on a cultural group, discussion may not relate findings to that group; and (g) findings ascribed to culture are often not distinguished from the effects of socioeconomic status, history, or political structures.

Most quantitative C/TCR is theory-based. Frequently used frameworks include Leininger's culture care theory, self-care, health-seeking behavior, health belief models, stress and coping, self-efficacy, and transitions. The transtheoretical model of behavior change is becoming popular. Reports are now appearing on the cultural appropriateness of existing frameworks for particular groups. For example health belief models have been criticized for inadequately recognizing real (rather than perceived) barriers to care, spirituality, and the interconnectedness (rather than the individuality) of African-American women. Studies seeking explanatory models of illness are increasing, a welcome trend since this approach, which parallels an intake history and involves all aspects of the disease course and clinical encounter, seems relevant and practical to clinicians as well as researchers. Culture-specific models such as McQuiston and Flaskerud's (2000) model for HIV prevention among Latinos are under development. Studies of model development to promote culturally competent organizations and build culturally diverse workforces, such as the Diversity Competency Model and the Leininger-based Model of Culturally Competent Leadership, are increasingly represented in administrative journals.

Although most data collection strategies, including physiological measurements are used in C/TCR, the most frequently used are focus groups, interviews, ethnographies, participant observation, and written questionnaires. Qualitative approaches have long been recognized as well-suited to C/TCR and are frequently used. However, the realization of their potential depends on the investigator's awareness of or openness to the complexity and pervasiveness of culture in the research encounter (Morse, 2001).

The overwhelming majority of C/TCR has been intracultural, descriptive, small scale, and nonprogrammatic. The typical study is an interview or survey on health knowledge, health beliefs and practices, or a concept like self-efficacy within one designated group conducted by a single investigator. However, cross-national nursing studies, studies with large sample sizes, studies done by interdisciplinary or international teams, and programmatic research are becoming more frequent.

Active C/TCR programs and their principal investigators include diabetes education for Mexican-Americans (Brown), diabetes management in ethnically diverse families (Chesla et al., 2004), HIV risk reduction interventions for impoverished Latina and Asian women (Flaskerud, et al., 2000), cardiovascular health for African-American school children (Harrell, McMurray, Gansky, Bandiwula, & Bradley, 1999), condom use in African-American adolescents (Jemmott, 2000), HIV prevention among Latinos (McQuiston & Flaskerud, 2000, 2003), and health needs of South American, Middle Eastern, and Korean women (Meleis, 1996). The dearth of programmatic nursing research on Native-American health is noteworthy.

Methodological research, including studies of recruiting and retaining subjects and instrumentation, is growing rapidly. The quality of measurement in C/TCR is improving steadily. The standards for rigorous translation are widely recognized, and both the cultural fit of items and the psychometric properties of an instrument for the target group are increasingly being reported and studied. Instrument reading level is receiving considerable attention in recognition of the prevalence of low literacy and low English proficiency in many populations (Weinrich, Boyd, & Herman, 2004). Instruments such as the Cultural Self-Efficacy Scale and the Cultural Awareness Scale are being developed to measure the outcomes of programs to promote multicultural awareness.

There are three major needs in C/TCR. First is the need for more intervention studies (Douglas, 2000). Recent estimates of the proportion of interventions in the C/TCR literature range from 3.6% to 14%. More investigators must move from descriptive studies to interventions to randomized controlled trials. The sheer volume of very similar studies of the health beliefs, family values, sex roles, and the importance of family decision making, folk remedies, or spirituality within certain groups suggests a sufficient base for intervention studies. A second great need is for application of existing guidelines for culturally competent research (Meleis, 1996; Phillips & Weekes, 2002; Porter & Villaruel, 1993; Villaruel, 1996). Research needs to be planned to be culturally competent. Culturally competent research is broader than efforts to select culturally appropriate instruments or to recruit appropriate subjects. Application of these guidelines should mesh nicely with the third great need of C/TCR, which is for research to be planned and conducted with greater community involvement.

More studies, particularly programmatic studies, are needed of Native-American health. Studies of multiracial or multiethnic persons are rare but urgently needed, given the growing numbers of people who identify themselves as having multiple heritages. Studies of rural, occupational, and sexual subcultures (groups not defined by race or ethnicity) are needed, as are comparative explorations of cultural perspectives on ethics. Folk and alternative healing practices and their possible combinations with biomedical approaches, need systematic, sensitive study. Studies of cultural adaptations of care in homes, the development of brief rapid strategies for cultural assessment, and development of the economic case for culturally competent care are needed to insure that culture is considered in this era of managed care, case management, and ever briefer inpatient stays.

Sharol F. Jacobson

Cumulative Index to Nursing and Allied Health Literature

In the late 1940s, although *Index Medicus* existed for the biomedical literature, there was no index to the few nursing journals published at the time. Individual librarians took it upon themselves at particular hospitals or schools of nursing to index the journals they received for their own population. One such librarian in Los Angeles, Ella Crandall, used 3 × 5 index cards to meet the needs of nurses on the staff of White Memorial Hospital and later, Los Angeles County Hospital. This index, which began as an internal project, was published as *The Cumulative Index to Nursing Literature* in 1961, a cumulation of indexing covering the period 1956 to 1960. Seventeen journals were included in this publication—from the *American Journal of Nursing* and *Nursing Research* to the *American Association of Industrial Nurses Journal*. The "red books," as this publication became known, were well received in the nursing community (Raisig, 1964) and became a familiar part of nursing education throughout the United States.

Over the next several decades the *Index* grew and changed, reflecting the changes taking place in the profession itself. As would be expected, many indexing terms are similar or identical to those used in the indexing of biomedical journals. There are some important differences, and many terms added to the thesaurus demonstrate the development and growth of the nursing profession, both as a practice and as a science. Increased emphasis on nursing research, specialty and advanced practice, and managed care has resulted in indexing terms such as phenomenology, survival analysis, family nurse practitioners, case management, and nursing intensity. Research terms describing design, methodology, analysis, and data collection have been added, as have the names of nursing specialties, organizations, and classification systems.

Aside from the terms used, the materials indexed are different from those in indexes of the biomedical and other literature. Books and book chapters, pamphlets and pamphlet chapters, dissertations, audiovisuals, and consumer health and patient education materials are just a few of the other types of materials indexed. Because of the difficulty in obtaining these materials they are often defined as elusive or fugitive literature.

Other changes have taken place over these years. Recognizing that the boundaries of nursing intersect with many other health care disciplines, "Allied Health" was added to the *Index* title in 1977, resulting in *The Cumulative Index to Nursing and Allied Health Literature* (CINAHL®). There are 17 such disciplines covered, including physical therapy, occupational therapy, and communicative disorders. In 1983 the CINAHL® electronic database became part of several online services and was released as a CD-ROM in 1989. Individual access via the Internet is available as well.

Recent years have seen the development of CINAHL-created documents as part of the database. These include research instrument descriptions, clinical innovations, accreditation materials, and legal case descriptions. The database can no longer be viewed as only a bibliographical database, although that continues to be its primary function.

Throughout the nearly 40 years of its existence, the primary goal of the organization has been to connect nursing—and later allied health—professionals with materials written about and for them. The basic premise underlying the existence of the *Index* is that effective and knowledgeable practice depends on access to materials describing or studying that practice. These materials may be present in a variety of formats and from a variety of sources. Whereas indexing began with fewer than 10 journals, the current journal list includes more than 1,000 titles. Content other than that listed above includes practice guidelines, practice acts, standards of practice, critical pathways, and even full text of some journal articles. Searching this material on a regular basis should be a professional obligation of members of all health care disciplines for the duration of their careers.

DIANE SHEA PRAVIKOFF

Current Procedural Terminology-Coded Services

Current procedural terminology-coded services (CPT) include more than 8,000 services listed in the *Physicians' Current Procedural Terminology* manual published annually by the American Medical Association (AMA). Developed by the AMA in 1966, the purpose of the CPT system is to provide a uniform language that describes medical, surgical, and diagnostic services and thereby serves as a method for payment by public (Medicare and Medicaid) and private (commercial insurers) payers. It is used by policy makers in their deliberations on reforming the payment system.

In 1986 Congress created the Physician Payment Review Commission (PPRC) to advise it on reforms of the methods used to pay physicians under the Medicare program (Part B). Nursing groups such as the American Nurses Association lobbied PPRC to consider the contributions of nurses as they engaged in the process of revising the payment system. In its report to Congress, the PPRC stated that nonphysician providers should be paid at a percentage of physician payment levels reflecting differences in physicians' and nonphysicians' resource costs: work as well as practice and malpractice expense. The American Nurses Association (ANA) disagreed, stating that nurses should be paid the same for the same service (Mittelstadt, 1991). The first nurse to serve on the Commission, Carol Lockhart, PhD, RN, FAAN, expressed concern about the lack of nursing data available to the PPRC. She stated:

> Nursing's role in the delivery of Medicare Part B services is undocumented. We have little or no data showing how much of a particular service, now billed by a physician, is done by a nurse, or how many services are delivered by the nurse and billed under the physician's name. (Griffith & Fonteyn, 1989, p. 1051)

In an attempt to identify whether CPT codes might explain nursing work and therefore provide the needed data, studies were conducted to look at how many billable CPT activities were performed by nurses (Griffith, Thomas, & Griffith, 1991; Griffith & Robinson, 1993; Robinson & Griffith, 1997). The *American Journal of Nursing (AJN)* (Griffith & Fonteyn, 1989) published a questionnaire on the performance of CPT-coded procedures by registered nurses; 4,869 RNs returned the questionnaire and 150 made telephone calls or wrote letters. The average number of coded services performed by the respondents was 27, with a range of 0 to 60 (Griffith et al., 1991). Given the large number of currently published codes in the manual, this number appears to be small; however, at the time of the survey, only 107 codes comprised 56.9% of all Medicare procedures (Health Care Financing Administration and Bureau of Data Management and Strategy, 1990). Survey results revealed that associate and baccalaureate degree nurses performed significantly more coded services than nurses with diplomas and masters degrees. The more experienced nurses (practicing more than 10 years) reported performing significantly fewer coded services and, as expected, nurses working in hospital settings performed more services. This exploratory study suggested that nurses often perform CPT-coded services with little or no supervision by physicians.

After realizing that the generalist *AJN* study was clearly supported by nurses, nine nurse specialist groups were surveyed and it was determined that 493 of over 7,000 CPT codes were performed by school nurses, enterostomal nurses, family nurse practitioners, critical care nurses, oncology nurses, rehabilitation nurses, orthopaedic nurses, nephrology nurses, and mid-wives (Griffith & Robinson, 1993; Robinson & Griffith, 1997). The number of CPT codes performed by specialty nurses ranged from 233 for family nurse practitioners to 58 for school nurses. The mean number of coded services performed by individual respondents ranged from 79 for family nurse practitioners to 18 for school nurses; individual respondents performed 0 to 162 codes. Supervision by physicians for these groups of nurses was infrequent. Charges to Medicare in 1988 for the coded services included in the survey were $22,793,427.34 (aggregate allowable charges).

A criticism of the CPT codes is their limitation to describe only physician services and not the full range of health services provided by the entire team. In a study comparing the frequency with which nursing activity terms could be categorized using Nursing Interventions Classification (NIC) and Current Procedural Terminology (CPT) codes, findings revealed evidence that NIC is superior to CPT for categorizing these activities in a study population of 201 AIDS patients hospitalized for pneumocystis carinii pneumonia. Nursing activity terms were categorized into 80 NIC interventions across 22 classes and into 15 CPT codes. All terms in the data set were classifiable using the NIC system and 60% of the terms were classified into 14 NIC intervention categories while only 6% of the terms were classifiable by CPT codes. These findings supported the importance of nursing-specific classifications for categorization of health care interventions in an effort to demonstrate nursing's contribution to quality and cost outcomes (Henry, Holzemer, Randell, Hsieh, & Miller, 1997). However, another way to address the issue is to introduce nursing services into CPT if they are not otherwise described in another CPT code (Sullivan-Marx & Mullinix, 1999).

Recognizing that the CPT system does have deficiencies, the AMA, in 1998, began the task of developing the next generation, the CPT-5. The CPT-5 Project includes six workgroups and an Executive Project Advisory Group (PAG). One of the workgroups, "Nonphysician Practitioners," is reviewing and evaluating weaknesses of the current system for coding the provisions of health services by nonphysician health care professionals (http://www.ama-assn.org/ama/pub/category/3883.html). Efforts are being made to gather information from other provider organizations to determine where and how the CPT system lacks adequate codes for the appropriate description of services of different providers. It is anticipated that the CPT-5 Project will be completed in the near future. ANA, active in dialogues with AMA on inclusion of nursing work in CPT-5, has representatives serving on AMA work groups of the project (Robinson, Griffith, & Sullivan-Marx, 2001).

As we progress further through the 21st century, the public-consumers of care that nurses deliver will become even more interested in cost, accessibility, satisfaction, and quality. Because nurses have the abilities to deliver in all of these areas, they should be directly reimbursed for their services. If nurses want to proceed in this direction, then their challenge must be to accurately document their contribution of nursing practice to patient and program productivity and effectiveness through workload analysis, thereby providing meaningful data to consumers, policy makers, and payers (Robinson et al., 2001).

HURDIS M. GRIFFITH
KAREN R. ROBINSON

D

Data Analysis

Data analysis is a systematic method of examining data gathered for any research investigation to support conclusions or interpretations about the data. Although applicable to both qualitative and quantitative research data analysis is more often associated with quantitative research. Quantitative data analysis involves the application of logic and reasoning through the use of statistics, an applied branch of mathematics, to numeric data. Qualitative data analysis involves the application of logic and reasoning, a branch of philosophy, to nonnumeric data. Both require careful execution and are intended to give meaning to data by organizing disparate pieces of information into understandable and useful aggregates, statements, or hypotheses.

Statistical data analysis is based in probability theory and involves using a number of specific statistical tests, or measures of association between two or more variables. Each of these tests or statistics (e.g., t, F, β, χ^2, ϕ, γ, etc.) has a known distribution that allows the calculation of probability levels for different values of the statistic under different assumptions—that is, the test (or null) hypothesis and the sample size, or degrees of freedom.

Specific tests are selected because they provide the most meaningful representation of the data in response to the research questions or hypotheses posed. The selection of specific tests, however, is restricted to those for which the available data meet certain required assumptions of the tests. For example, some tests are appropriate for (and assume) nominal data, others assume ordinal data, and still others assume an interval level of measurement. Although each test has its own set of mathematical assumptions about the data, all statistical tests assume random sampling.

Several statistical computer programs (e.g., SPSS, SAS, LISREL, EQS) can aid the investigator with the tedious and complex mathematical operations necessary to calculate these test statistics and their sampling distributions. These programs, however, serve only to expedite calculations and ensure accuracy. Because the investigator must understand the computer programs to use them appropriately, there is a hidden danger in the ease with which one may execute such programs. For valid data analysis, the investigator must fully understand the underlying statistical procedures and the implied assumptions of these tests in order to apply them appropriately.

The logic of null hypothesis statistical data analysis is one of *modus tollens*, denying the antecedent by denying the consequent. That is, if the null hypothesis is correct, our findings cannot occur but our findings did occur, so the null hypothesis must be false. However, J. Cohen (1994) and others have convincingly argued that, by making this reasoning probabilistic for null hypothesis statistical testing, the original syllogism is invalidated. Moreover, for decades scientists from different disciplines have questioned the usefulness and triviality of null hypothesis statistical testing (see Labovitz, 1970; LeFort, 1993; Loftus, 1993; Rozeboom, 1960; Walker, A. M., 1986, for examples from sociology, psychology, public health, and nursing). Consequently, increased attention to the factors that contribute to findings of statistical significance is warranted and power, effect sizes (for substantive significance), sample sizes, and confidence intervals are receiving increased attention in quantitative data analysis.

In contrast to quantitative data analysis, which requires that the investigator assign a numeric code to all data prior to beginning the analyses, qualitative data analysis consists of coding words, objects, or events into coherent or meaningful categories or themes as part of the actual data analyses. Also, because qualitative data analysis involves nonnumeric data, there are no statistical probabilistic tests to apply to their coding.

Historically, qualitative data coding has been done manually, but more recently computer programs (e.g., NUDIST) have been developed to aid the investigator in this laborious effort. However, as with the computer programs for quantitative analyses, those for qualitative data analysis are merely aids for the tedious and error-prone tasks of analysis. Using them still requires that the investigator make the relevant and substantive decisions and interpretations about codes, categories, and themes.

Quantitative data analysis allows for statistical probabilistic statements to support the investigator's interpretations and conclusions. Qualitative data analysis depends more exclusively on the strength and logic of the investigator's arguments. Nonetheless, both types of data analysis ultimately rest on the strength of the original study design and the ability of the investigator to appropriately and accurately execute the analytic method selected.

LAUREN S. AARONSON

Data Collection Methods

Nurse researchers use a wide variety of methods for collecting data (the pieces of information used to address a research problem), and these methods vary on a number of important dimensions. One dimension involves whether the data being collected are quantitative or qualitative. Until the 1980s, nurse researchers predominantly used methods of collecting quantitative data (information in numeric form) that could be analyzed by statistical techniques. The collection of quantitative information tends to involve highly structured methods in which exactly the same information is gathered from study participants in a comparable, prespecified way. Although quantitative data collection remains the most frequently used approach, nurse researchers have shown increasing interest in collecting qualitative data (information in narrative form). Researchers collecting qualitative data tend to have a more flexible, unstructured approach to collecting information, relying on ongoing insights during data collection to guide the course of further data gathering.

Another important dimension concerns the basic mode of data collection. The most frequently used modes of data collection by nurse researchers are self-reports, observations, and biophysiological measures. Self-reports involve the collection of data through direct questioning of people about their opinions, characteristics, and experiences. Self-reports can be gathered orally by having interviewers ask study participants a series of questions—in writing by having participants complete a paper-and-pencil task or, less frequently, by having participants engage in some other activity, such as sorting cards. Structured, quantitative self-report data are usually collected by means of a formal, written document or instrument that specifies exactly what questions are to be asked. The instrument is called an interview schedule when the data are collected orally and a questionnaire when the data are collected in writing. Interviews can be conducted either in person or over the telephone. Interviews and questionnaires often incorporate one or more formal scales to measure certain clinical data (e.g., fatigue) or a psychological attribute (e.g., attitudes toward nursing homes). A scale typically yields a composite measure of responses to multiple questions and is designed to assign a numeric score to respondents to place them on a continuum with respect to the attribute being measured (e.g., depression). A less frequently used method of collecting structured self-report data is referred to as a Q-sort, which involves having the participant sort cards with words or phrases on them according to some continuum (e.g., most like me–least like me).

Self-report methods are also used by researchers who are primarily interested in qualitative data. When self-report data are gathered in an unstructured way, the researcher typically does not have a specific set of questions that must be asked in a specific order or worded in a given way. Instead, the researcher starts with some general questions and allows respondents to tell their stories in a natural, conversational fashion. Methods of collecting qualitative self-report data include completely unstructured interviews (conversational discussions on a topic), focused interviews (conversations guided by a broad topic guide), focus group interviews (discussions with small groups), life histories (narrative, chronological self-disclosures about an aspect of the respondent's life experiences), and critical incidents (discussions about an event or behavior that is critical to some outcome of interest). Although most unstructured self-reports are gathered orally, a researcher can also ask respondents to maintain a written diary of their thoughts on a given topic. Projective techniques, although not always considered a form of self-report, encompass a variety of data collection methods that rely on the participant's projection of psychological traits in response to vaguely structured stimuli (e.g., a Rorschach test). Projective techniques almost always solicit qualitative data, but the data can sometimes be quantified. Self-report methods are indispensable as a means of collecting data on human beings, but they are susceptible to errors of reporting, including a variety of response biases.

The second major mode of data collection is through observation. Observational methods are techniques for collecting data through the direct observation of people's behavior, communications, characteristics, and activities, either directly through the human senses or with the aid of observational equipment such as videotape cameras. Researchers who collect qualitative observational data do so with a minimum of researcher-imposed structure and interference with those being observed. People are observed, typically in social settings, engaging in naturalistic behavior. The researcher makes notes of his or her observations in narrative form. A special type of unstructured observation is referred to as participant observation: the researcher gains entry into the social group of interest and participates to varying degrees in its functioning while gathering the observational data.

Structured observational methods dictate what the observer should observe and how to record it. In this approach the observers often use checklists to record the appearance, frequency, or duration of preselected behaviors, events, or characteristics. Alternatively, the observer may use a rating scale to measure dimensions such as the intensity of observed behavior. Observational techniques are an important alternative to self-report techniques, but judgmental errors and other biases can pose a threat to the validity and accuracy of observational data.

Data for nursing studies may also be derived from biophysiological measures, which can be classified as either in vivo measurements (those performed within or on living organisms) or in vitro measurements (those performed outside the organism's body, such as blood tests). Biophysiological measures are quantitative indicators of clinically relevant attributes they require specialized technical instruments and equipment. Qualitative clinical data—for example, descriptions of skin pallor—are gathered not through technical instruments but rather through observations or self-reports. Biophysiological measures have the advantage of being objective, accurate, and precise and are typically not subject to many biases.

Although most nursing research involves the collection of new data through self-report, observation, or biophysiological instrumentation, some research involves the analysis of preexisting data, such as are available through written documents. Clinical records, such as hospital records, nursing charts, and so forth, constitute rich and relatively inexpensive data sources. A variety of other types of documents (e.g., letters, newspaper articles) can be used as data sources for both qualitative researchers (e.g., those conducting historical research) and quantitative ones (e.g., researchers doing a quantified content analysis).

The collection of data is often the most time-consuming and costly activity in the research process. It is also a challenging task that requires creativity, the ability to adequately match the research question with the appropriate approach, and the ability to work within budgetary constraints.

DENISE F. POLIT

Data Management

Data management is generally defined as the procedures taken to ensure the accuracy of data, from data entry through data transformations. Although often a tedious and time-consuming process, data management is absolutely essential for good science.

The first step is data entry. Although this may occur in a variety of ways, from being scanned in to being entered manually, the crucial point is that the accuracy of the data be assessed before any manipulations are performed or statistics produced. Frequency distributions and descriptive statistics are generated. Then each variable is inspected, as appropriate, for out-of-range values, outliers, equality of groups, skewness, and missing data. Decisions must be made about dealing with each of these. Incorrect values must be replaced with correct values or assigned to the missing values category. Outliers must be investigated and dealt with. If a categorical variable is supposed to have four categories but only three have adequate numbers of subjects, one must decide about eliminating the fourth category or combining it with one of the others. If continuous variable are skewed, data transformations may be attempted or nonparametric statistics employed.

Once each variable has been inspected and corrected where necessary, new variables may be created. This might include the development of total scores for a group of items, subscores, and so forth. Each of these new variables also must be checked for outliers, skewness, and out-of-range values. The creation of some new variables may involve the use of sophisticated techniques such as factor and reliability analyses.

Prior to each statistical test, the assumptions underlying the test must be checked. If violated, alternative approaches must be sought. Careful attention to data management must underlie data analysis. It ensures the validity of the data and the appropriateness of the analyses.

BARBARA MUNRO

Data Stewardship

Data and information are the symbolic representation of the phenomena with which nursing is concerned. Data are defined as discrete entities that are objective; information is defined as data that are structured and organized and that have meaning or interpretation. Information that has been synthesized so as to identify and formalize interrelationships is referred to as knowledge. When one term represents all three types of content, it is usually *information*. From this perspective, data are viewed as the raw material on which nursing knowledge and science are developed. Data stewardship refers to the responsibility to manage, administer, attend to, and take charge of the universe of relevant nursing data.

Nursing data issues revolve around several factors. The first relates to identification of the universe of relevant nursing data. Currently, there is no consensus regarding what data elements make up a minimum nursing data set nor what data elements are required to capture nursing diagnoses, interventions, and outcomes. Systems to label or name these elements also are inconsistently defined. Next, the complex nature of nursing phenomena poses measurement difficulties. Measurement is the process of assigning numbers to objects to represent the kind or amount of a character possessed by those objects. It includes qualitative means (assigning objects to categories that are mutually exclusive and exhaustive) and quantitative measures (assigning objects to categories that represent the amount of a characteristic possessed).

Unlike other biological sciences, few nursing phenomena can be measured by using physical instruments with signal processing or monitoring. Measurement difficulties occur because nursing consists of a multiplicity of complex variables that occur in diverse settings. If one is able to identify what significant variables should be measured, then one is challenged with the difficulty of isolating those variables to measure them. Ambiguities and abstract notions must be reduced to develop concrete behavioral indicators if measurement is to be meaningful. Measuring nursing phenomena also requires the acknowledgment of the "fuzzy" and complex nature of nursing phenomena and the richness of the meaning contained in the context of the data. Finally, the value and use of data that are not coded or numeric, such as whole text data, must be studied to understand their benefits and boundaries for representing nursing phenomena. Content analysis of nursing data and their usefulness have to be further explored.

Processing data implies the transfer of data in raw form to a structured, interpreted information form. Information has characteristics of accuracy, timeliness, utility, relevance, quality, and consistency. Data stewardship suggests that attention be paid to these characteristics. For example, accuracy is of concern at the level of judgment in collecting data as well as at the level of the data collected. Quality of data and information is related to the ability and willingness of clients to disclose information as well as to the nurse's ability to observe, collect, and record it. Reliability refers to random measurement errors such as ambiguities in data interpretation. These measurement errors that affect clinically generated data can occur at the point of care delivery, the time of documentation, and when data are retrieved or abstracted for studies (Hays, Norris, Martin, & Androwich, 1994).

With the advent of automated data processing and computerized information systems, decisions about data content, control, and cost need careful consideration. The content and design decisions concern format, standardized languages, level of detail, data entry and retrieval messages, and interfaces with nonclinical data systems. A primary concern of clinicians is the amount of time invested in harvesting data and recording it. Minimum time investment, with maximum clarity and comprehensiveness of data collected and recorded, is needed. Redundancy must be eliminated. Decisions related to content of data demand stewardship to ensure privacy, confidentiality, and security, especially when data are in electronic form. Requirements for legitimate access to data must be managed to facilitate the flow of clinical data while simultaneously restricting inappropriate access. There is a cost associated with the use and development of automated databases; however, accuracy, reliability, and comprehensiveness of information should not be sacrificed because of cost.

Data stewardship poses challenges and responsibilities for nurses in building knowledge bases. Standardization of terms of data is critical, and coordination and synthesis of current efforts are needed. If nurses are to be stewards of their data, then further study should focus on the following areas: (a) the definition and description of the data and information required for patent care, (b) the use of data and knowledge to deliver and manage patient care, and (c) how one acquires and delivers knowledge from and for patient care (National Center for Nursing Research, 1993).

CAROL A. ROMANO

Death and Dying

Death is the cessation of life. The definition of death has changed over time as advances in medicine and technology made it possible to prolong cardiac and respiratory functions by "artificial" means. Today the widely accepted definition of death is the irreversible cessation of circulatory and respiratory functions, or the irreversible sensation of all brain functions, including the brain stem (President's Commission, 1981). Dying is one of the many the transitions we experience in life. It is difficult to determine when dying begins, it occurs at different rates and ways in individuals. The American Geriatrics Society (AGS) offered clinicians some guidance for determining when dying begins with the statement: "people are to be considered to be dying when they have a progressive illness for which there is no treatment that can substantially alter the outcome" (AGS, 1997). Dying has been defined by researchers on the basis of a diagnosis of a terminal illness or one without a cure, physician prognosis, prognostic assessments of patients or family members, and by care settings such as hospice.

Other terms associated with end-of-life care are palliative care and hospice. The World Health Organization (WHO, 1989) defined palliative care as "the active total care of patients whose disease is not responsive to curative treatment when the control of pain and other symptoms and of psychological, social, and spiritual problems is paramount" (p. 152). Hospice refers to a concept of care that can be provided in a variety of settings. The family is the unit of care and a multidisciplinary approach is used to address physical, psychological, and spiritual needs of the dying person and their family. The focus of care is enhancing the quality of remaining life and providing support to the family in the dying process and bereavement.

A number of recent studies of death and dying have identified problems with the care of dying persons and their families (SUPPORT, 1995; Field & Cassel, 1997; Teno et al., 2004). Nurses, as the largest group of health care providers, have the opportunity to change the experience of dying and promote quality end-of-life care. Nursing's contributions to end-of-life care and areas for further research are described in the following sections.

Early studies of death and dying by nurses in the 1960s and early 1970s took place in hospitals and focused on nurses' attitudes toward death and dying and family responses. Benoliel (1983), in a comprehensive review of nursing research on death and dying from 1969 to 1984, noted most nursing studies were descriptive in approach and lacked a central paradigm. She concluded that although the stressful nature of death and dying was well documented, little was known about the nature of support that is helpful to patients and families and the influence of other variables, such as age and culture.

The hospice movement began in the United States in 1974 with the opening of Hospice, Inc. in New Haven, Connecticut. Florence Wald, Dean of Nursing at Yale University Nursing, and a group of volunteers were instrumental in starting the first hospice. Hospice experienced rapid growth due in part to the growing dissatisfaction with medical care of the terminally ill. Studies of hospice began to appear in the literature in the 1980s. Corless (1994) reviewed hospice studies from 1983 to 1992 and noted that researchers examined the impact of hospice as an innovation, family perceptions of hospice care, coping strategies of families in hospice home care, and satisfaction with hospice home care. Studies of the effectiveness of interventions to control symptoms such as pain were lacking. The approaches used in these studies were primarily case studies, Q-sort techniques, and retrospective medical record analysis.

Research on hospice family caregivers has focused on persons with a diagnosis of cancer. The educational needs of caregivers for persons with a diagnosis of cancer were the focus of seven studies (Thiemann, 2000). Both quantitative and qualitative methods were used with similar findings. The most frequent educational needs were for information on the patient's illness, instructions on caregiving techniques, and information on community resources.

Caring for a dying family member is an emotionally intense experience. Hospice family caregivers for persons with a diagnosis of cancer need time for self, time for rest and sleep, spiritual needs, information on how to deal with the patient, and how to maintain independence (Thielemann, 2000; Harrington, Lackey, & Gates, 1996). Studies of family needs and coping are descriptive with small samples and lack diversity of age, diagnosis, and ethnic groups.

Research on the experience of dying is limited and has occurred in acute care hospitals or hospices. The setting of care for older adults has a direct impact on the quality of life at the end of life (Mezey, Dubler, Mitty, & Brody, 2002). The majority of studies are with persons who have a diagnosis of cancer. As people are living longer with chronic illness, there is a need for studies to examine the experience of dying from chronic illnesses, for example heart failure and dementia.

Several large-scale national studies in the 1990s described problems and deficiencies in end-of-life care. The Institute of Medicine studied end-of-life care and identified the following major deficiencies in care: too many people suffer at the end of life; legal, economic, and organizational obstacles obstruct excellent care at the end of life; the education of physicians and other health providers fails to provide them with the knowledge and skills required to care for dying patients, and current knowledge is inadequate to support evidence-based medicine at the end of life (Field & Cassel, 1997).

The Study to Understand Prognoses and Preferences for Outcomes and Risk of Treatment, known by the acronym SUPPORT, was a large-scale controlled clinical research study of more than 9,000 patients in five teaching hospitals. The study was designed to examine end-of-life decision making and test an intervention to improve end-of-life care. The first phase of the study examined decision making and patient outcomes. SUPPORT investigators concluded that physician-patient communication was often unreliable and physicians showed little interest in the patient's preferences for care. The second phase was an intervention designed to improve communication, end-of-life decision making, and pain management. Nurses were an important part of the intervention and worked with patients, families, and physicians. Unfortunately the intervention failed. Communication remained flawed, there was an overuse of aggressive treatment, and patients suffered undue pain at the end of life.

Dying trajectories differ at the end of life with various patterns of functional decline; however there are few studies of functional decline in large populations. Lunney, Lynn, Foley, Lipson, and Guaralnik's study (2003) of 4,190 participants in the Established Populations for Epidemiological Studies (EPES) found that functional decline differs among four types of illness trajectories: sudden death, cancer death, death from organ failure, and frailty. Each of the four groups had different trajectories of dependency and needs.

The Robert Wood Johnson Foundation, the Project Death in America, and the Department of Health and Human Services have made funding available to educate nurses in end-of-life care and support research. Nurse researchers need to conduct research in a variety of settings with diverse population groups in order to influence practice and improve the quality of end-of-life care.

SARAH A. WILSON

Delirium

Delirium is an acute, fluctuating disturbance of consciousness and cognition (American Psychiatric Association [APA], 2000). It frequently accompanies acute physical illness and is found in all care settings. Estimates of the incidence of delirium range from 7% to 80% for all hospitalized patients; 46% for older patients receiving home health care services; and 14% to 39% for residents in long-term care settings. More recently, in a community-based sample, delirium was found to be superimposed on dementia in 13% of the cases.

Previously, delirium was thought to be self-limiting and benign. Recent discoveries indicate that delirium is associated with cognitive and functional impairments persisting for 12 months or more after the index incident of delirium. Moreover, delirium portends poorer outcomes, greater costs of care, and greater chances for dementia and death. Despite these profound negative consequences for patients, families, health care providers, and society, delirium remains understudied. The current state of knowledge of delirium is summarized here.

Delirium is frequently underrecognized and misdiagnosed (although there is disagreement as to whether more patients are misclassified as false positive or false negative) (Inouye, Foreman, Mion, Katz, & Cooney, 2001). Recognition of delirium is especially problematic in elderly patients with an underlying dementia or those with the hypoactive-hypoalert variant of delirium. Explanations for the underrecognition and misdiagnosis of delirium include the fluctuating nature of delirium; the variable presentation of delirium; the similarity among and frequent cooccurrence of delirium, dementia, and depression; and the failure of providers to use standardized methods of detection.

Improving the recognition of delirium requires a complex and dynamic solution. Knowledge of delirium and skill in its detection are necessary starting points for improving the recognition of delirium. However, knowledge and skill alone are insufficient, given the profound impediment to the recognition of delirium posed by negative ageist stereotypes. These conclusions are supported by the work of McCarthy (2003), which also highlights the powerful influence of the practice environment on how providers think about and respond to delirium.

Several instruments have been developed to screen for or diagnose delirium. Such instruments include: Folstein's Mini-Mental State Examination (MMSE), Inouye's Confusion Assessment Method (CAM), Vermeersch's Clinical Assessment of Confusion-Form A (CAC-A), Albert's Delirium Symptom Interview (DSI), Trzepacz's Delirium Rating Scale (DRS), Neelon and Champagne's NEECHAM Confusion Scale (NEECHAM), O'Keefe's Delirium Assessment Scale (DAS), and Breitbart's Memorial Delirium Assessment Scale (MDAS). Each has its advantages and disadvantages; the selection of which instrument to use depends in part on the purpose and patient population. The most frequently used instrument in research and clinical practice is Inouye's CAM. These instruments are reviewed in greater detail elsewhere (Foreman & Vermeersch, 2004; Rapp et al., 2000). Expert opinion recommends the routine use of brief, standardized bedside screening measures as timely, effective, and inexpensive methods for assessing cognitive status and diagnosing delirium. Current standards for surveillance of delirium are to screen for the presence of delirium on admission to the hospital and at a minimum daily. Others recommend brief screening every 8 hours as an element of the standard nursing assessment. Additionally, when there is evidence of new inattention, unusual or inappropriate behavior or speech, or noticeable changes in the way the patient thinks, it is recommended that the assessment be repeated.

A few strategies to prevent and/or treat delirium in hospitalized patients have been tested with various groups of hospitalized adult patients; most have resulted in only modest benefits (Cole, 1999). The prevailing principles guiding prevention and treatment consist of multifactorial interventions that: (a) identify patients at risk, (b) target strategies to minimize or eliminate the occurrence of precipitating factors as primary prevention accomplished through risk reduction, and (c) identify, correct or eliminate the underlying cause(s) while providing symptomatic and supportive care.

Multicomponent interventions targeting several risk factors, rather than targeting a single risk factor for delirium, and interventions with surgical versus medical patients have proved more successful in reducing the incidence, severity, or duration of delirium. However, interventions have had no effect on the recurrence of delirium or on outcomes 6 months after discharge from the hospital.

To better understand why these interventions have not been more successful, some investigators have conducted post-hoc analyses to identify characteristics of patients for whom these interventions have failed. These analyses have indicated that these interventions were less successful with patients who are at greatest risk for delirium: those who are demented, functionally impaired, and frailer. However, it is difficult to determine how to improve these interventions because these studies have been conceptually confused: efficacy has been confused with effectiveness; changing provider behavior has been confused with preventing or treating underlying causal agents for delirium; and primary prevention has been confused with secondary prevention. Moreover, interventions have targeted risk factors rather than the underlying pathogenetic mechanisms (i.e., the metabolic and physiologic deviations that disrupt neurotransmitter synthesis and functioning) (Trzepacz, 1999). Also, these studies have not been designed or powered in such a way as to determine which of the multicomponents actually contributed to the positive outcomes.

To improve the recognition, prevention, and treatment of delirium, the APA (1999), British Geriatrics Society (1999), and University of Iowa Gerontological Nursing Interventions Research Center (Rapp and the Iowa Veterans Affairs Nursing Research Consortium, 1998) have developed practice guidelines. These guidelines tend to be comprehensive and are generally based on expert clinical opinion; few aspects of these guidelines are based on empirical evidence. Moreover, Young and George (2003)—the individuals responsible for compiling the British guidelines—found that the existence of guidelines failed to improve the process and outcomes of care in delirium, indicating that much work remains to improve the care of individuals at risk for or experiencing delirium.

On the basis of this summary of the state of knowledge of delirium, the need for further study of delirium in all care settings is clearly documented. Such study should focus on all aspects of delirium, including the epidemiology and natural history of delirium, to improve our understanding of the duration, severity, persistence, and recurrence of delirium and to better target and time interventions. Greater insight into the underlying pathogenetic mechanism(s) of delirium would enable more rigorous development and testing of the efficacy and effectiveness of interventions to prevent and treat delirium.

MARQUIS D. FOREMAN
PATRICIA E. H. VERMEERSCH

Delphi Technique

The Delphi technique is a research method used to identify key issues, to set priorities, and to improve decision making through aggregating the judgments of a group of individuals. The technique consists of using a series of mailed questionnaires to develop consensus among the participants without face-to-face participation. It provides the opportunity for broad participation and prevents any one member of the group from unduly influencing other members' responses. Feedback is given to panel members on the responses to each of the questionnaires. Thus, panel members communicate indirectly with each other in a limited, goal-directed manner.

The first questionnaire that is mailed asks participants to respond to a broad question. The responses to this questionnaire are then used to develop a more structured questionnaire. Each successive questionnaire is built on the previous one. The second questionnaire requests participants to review the items identified in the first questionnaire and to indicate their degree of agreement or disagreement with the items, to provide a rationale for their judgments, to add items that are missing, and to rank-order the items according to their perceived priority. On return of the second questionnaire the responses are reviewed, items are clarified or added, and the mean degree of agreement and the ranking of each item are computed. In the third questionnaire, participants are asked to review the mean ranking from the second questionnaire and again to indicate their degree of agreement or disagreement and give their rationale if they disagree with the ranking. Additional questionnaires are sent until the group reaches consensus. Many variations of this procedure have been used, the number of questionnaires used ranging from three to seven.

To be eligible to participate as a panelist in a Delphi study the respondent should (a) be personally concerned about the problem being studied, (b) have relevant information to share, (c) place a high priority on completing the Delphi questionnaire on schedule, and (d) believe that the information compiled will be of value to self and others (Delbecq, Van de Ven, & Gustafsen, 1975).

Several disadvantages of the Delphi technique limit its application. First, there must be adequate time for mailing the questionnaires, their return, and their analysis. Second, participants must have a high level of ability in written communication. And third, participants must be highly motivated to complete all the questionnaires.

The Delphi technique was first developed by the Rand Corporation as a forecasting tool in the 1960s, when investigators found that results of a Delphi survey produced better predictions than round-table discussions. The technique was later used to solicit opinions of experts on atomic warfare as a means of defense. It has since been applied in diverse fields, such as industry, social services, and nursing because of its usefulness and accuracy in predicting and in prioritizing.

The Delphi technique has been used in nursing studies to identify priorities for practice and research. The American Nurses Association Center for Nursing Research (1980) used the technique to identify national research priorities for the 1980s; Demi, Meredith, and Gray (1996) used it to identify priorities for urological nursing research; Lewandowski and Kositsky (1983) and Lindquist and colleagues (1993) used it to identify research priorities for critical care nursing; and Lindemann (1981) surveyed members of the American Academy of Nursing to identify and prioritize issues important to nursing in the next decade. In a creative application of the method Demi and Miles (1987) attempted to achieve consensus on the parameters of normal grief by enlisting a panel of experts in the field of grief and mourning.

Alice S. Demi

Denial in Coronary Heart Disease

Coronary heart disease, and the experiences associated with it, precipitate many sudden changes that severely disrupt the balance of psychosocial and environmental factors in an individual's life. Those who experience these changes use various resources such as denial in an attempt to cope with the anxiety caused by the various types of threatened or real losses associated with the disease (Cassem & Hackett, 1971; Ketterer et al., 1998; Robinson, 1988, 1993, 1994, 2003).

Denial is the ability of an individual to mentally ignore or push from one's consciousness the reality of the situation at hand. It is one of the first adaptive behaviors or mechanisms that an individual uses during the stress-producing event of an acute episode of chest pain (Hackett & Cassem, 1982). Through this defense mechanism, the individual attempts to minimize or ignore the significance of the symptoms. For coronary patients, it is not difficult to use denial as a form of coping because once the pain has been alleviated and the person is resting comfortably, there are no other symptoms. As a result, it is easy for the patient to rationalize or deny that anything significant has happened.

Denial can be either healthy or unhealthy. Denial of the fact that a coronary event has occurred can be adaptive behavior during the first few weeks of recovery, enabling the person to cope with the shock and confusion. However, this denial can be maladaptive if it interferes with one's ability to deal with the lifestyle changes needed to recover from the acute phase of the illness (Cassem & Hackett, 1971; Robinson, 1993, 1994). That is, prolonged denial or disbelief might cause the individual to ignore necessary activity restrictions, fail to take prescribed medications, or realize the significance of the illness. The problem then becomes one of understanding when denial is helpful to the coronary patient and when it is harmful.

Given that coronary events result in numerous real and threatened losses, and all loss, whether real, threatened, or perceived, produces a grief response (with denial, shock, and disbelief being the initial response) (Engel, 1962), it becomes necessary to work through the grief process. However, this process should not be prolonged, since movement from denial to the next phase of the grief process might have a long-range effect on one's ability to work through the losses and changes in lifestyle caused by having coronary problems. Since denial does not represent a single, easily understood phenomenon, it is often difficult to determine if denial is adaptive or maladaptive.

The use of denial by coronary clients is described extensively in the literature. However, little attention has been given to measuring it. In addition, clues that coronary clients are using denial may not be recognized through personal interviews or traditional assessment methods. Therefore, the Robinson Self-Appraisal Inventory (RSAI), a self-report assessment instrument, was designed to identify denial in persons with coronary heart disease, quantify it, and aid in its further study (Robinson, 1988, 1994, 2003). It could also assist health care professionals to plan interventions to manage denial.

The RSAI has been under development for approximately 10 years. Earlier studies led to revisions and reconceptualizations (Robinson, 1988), which have resulted in Form D. Even though the Hackett-Cassem Denial Scale was available for measuring denial, the number of items on the scale regarding patients' personality traits and behaviors were not related to coronary heart disease and the general use of denial as a defensive trait. An additional weakness of this measurement was that the nature of several questions in the scale required the interviewer to make inferences when rating denial behavioral characteristics of the participant; it was not a paper-and-pencil self-report (Hackett & Cassem, 1974). Rather than measuring traits, the RSAI directly focuses on the patients' present reactions to illness and it is designed as a paper-and-pencil, self-administered instrument.

Using the RSAI-Form D, Robinson (1994) found a significant decrease in mean denial scores from the 2nd to the 4th hospitalized day of potential or actual myocardial infarction patients. These findings were consistent with those reported by Cassem and Hackett (1971), who stated that feelings of denial are generally mobilized on the 2nd day; however, by the 4th day as the patient's condition stabilizes, denial decreases. Factor analysis indicated that the 20-item RSAI-Form D probably is a multidimensional measure; however, a larger sample is needed with the addition of items to the scale to make the final determination. Four aspects of denial were extracted to include denial of secondary consequences, denial of illness and treatment, denial of anxiety, and denial of impact; thus, providing supportive evidence to the health care professional that using single specific or global criteria does not provide sufficient data for assessing denial. Some individuals may use one type of denial, whereas others may use another type. Each type of denial has its own purpose for the person. Therefore, it is beneficial for the health care professional to observe and listen closely to patients to understand their perspective as well as determine the type of denial that is being utilized (Robinson, 1994).

In summary, denial makes it possible for cardiac patients to block out information with which they cannot cope. It allows them to deal with reality in smaller, more manageable pieces. Denial can be adaptive, so instead of trying to push the patient out of denial before they are ready, one can assist them in adjusting to the loss. The nurse can determine the patient's degree of denial and its effectiveness as a coping strategy, listen closely to the patient, use counseling strategies, provide the patient with opportunities to express any fears, and should not directly confront the patient's denial. However, if the denial is maladaptive, the nurse should not directly confront the patient's denial, but rather focus on establishing a trust relationship with the patient, use reality-focusing techniques, utilize teaching strategies, and provide a psychological professional to meet and discuss the diagnosis with the patient (Robinson, 1993).

KAREN R. ROBINSON

Depression and Cardiovascular Diseases

Over the past 10 years, there has been growing interest in the relationship between depression and cardiovascular diseases. These are two of the most widespread public health problems in the United States, and are among the leading sources of functional impairment and disability. Recent research findings linking depression and cardiac disease will therefore be discussed, along with implications for future research.

In response to the growing awareness of the magnitude of the interaction between depression and adverse cardiac outcomes, several large-scale community-based studies have been conducted. Penninx and others (2001) followed a cohort of 2,847 men and women aged 55 to 85 years for 4 years. These investigators examined the effect of minor depression (i.e., Center for Epidemiologic Studies—Depression scale [CES-D] score of ≥ 16) and major depression (i.e., using DSM-III criteria) on heart disease mortality. They found that patients with major depression had significantly higher risk for cardiac mortality compared with those who had minor depression. These findings suggest that the severity of depression is related to higher cardiac mortality. In another study, Schulz and others (2000) studied a total of 5,201 men and women aged 65 years and older enrolled in the Cardiovascular Health Study. Controlling for sociodemographic variables and common comorbid conditions, individuals with higher scores of depressive symptoms were more likely to die than those who had lower scores. Depressed participants with heart failure at baseline had the highest mortality risk (adjusted RR = 2.44, RR = 1.62 for stroke patients, RR = 1.60 for intermittent claudication, RR = 1.30 for angina pectoris, and RR = 1.15 for myocardial infarction). Further, Cox proportional hazards regression model demonstrated that depressive symptoms were an independent predictor of mortality. In another study of the relationships among depression, coronary heart disease (CHD) incidence, and mortality, Ferketich, Schwartzbaum, Frid, and Moeschberger (2000) found that depressed men and women were at increased risk for incident CHD events, compared with nondepressed counterparts (RR = 1.73 (1.11–2.68), RR = 1.71 (1.14–2.56), correspondingly). Moreover, unlike depressed women, depressed men had an increased risk of cardiac mortality with adjusted RR = 2.34 (1.54–3.56).

Prospective population-based studies of depression also found an increased risk for CHD due to depression. Mendes de Leon and others (1998) conducted a cohort study and found a slight increase in risk for CHD events, RR = 1.03 (1.01–1.05), in fairly healthy older women. However, de Leon failed to find support for depression as an independent risk factor for CHD events in elderly men and women in the aggregate. Another prospective study used data from the Yale Health and Aging Project (Williams, S. A., et al., 2002). The sample consisted of 2,501 men and women, with a mean age of 74 years who were disease-free elders and were followed for up to 14 years. In comparison with nondepressed individuals, depressed individuals demonstrated 69% increase in the risk for incident heart failure. In addition, depressed participants were more likely to be women; consequently, depression was a significant risk factor of heart failure among women but not among men.

Using a randomized clinical trial, Berkman and others (2003) assessed the preventive effect of cognitive behavioral therapy (CBT) on depression in 2,481 myocardial infarction (MI) men and women. Although CBT reduced depression and decreased social isolation, it failed to reduce mortality or recurrent infarction events after a 6-month intervention period.

In short, research findings from community-based studies suggest that depression is a risk factor for cardiac morbidity and mortality. However, interventions that may reduce depression have failed to reduce depression-related cardiac outcomes (e.g., see Berkman et al., 2003). It is essential to note that many of these studies have controlled for demographic variables and medical comorbidity that might otherwise explain the findings reported.

Recognition of the overlap between depression and cardiovascular disease has led to increased interest in finding plausible biobehavioral mechanisms which link them together. In fact, there is evidence to indicate that depression may contribute to increased incidence of cardiovascular events. This effect may be mediated by other behavioral and biological factors that play major roles in the development of negative cardiac outcomes. There are several known behavioral risk factors (e.g., sedentary lifestyle, smoking, high-fat dietary intake) among depressed individuals that may contribute to the development of cardiac disease. In addition, recent research findings suggest that several biomarkers are implicated in both depression and cardiac disease pathogenesis. First, research showed that the hypothalamic-pituitary-adrenocortical (HPA) axis is activated during depression, which increases sympathoadrenal activity. Consequently, some risk markers such as catecholamines, cortisol, and serotonin are elevated in both depression and some cardiac diseases. Second, depressed patients are at increased risk for rhythm disorders. Recent evidence indicates that cardiac patients who are depressed exhibit reduced heart rate variability, a known risk factor for sudden death in patients with CVD (Carney et al., 1995). Third, depressed patients are more likely have platelet dysfunction that may have a negative impact on the development and prognosis of cardiovascular disease such as atherosclerosis, acute coronary syndromes, and thrombosis. Finally, the research demonstrated a close relationship among proinflammatory cytokines, such as IL-6 and TNF-α, depression, and incidents of negative cardiac outcomes. Briefly, any single mechanism will fall short of capturing the underlying pathogenesic processes of depression and cardiac disease. Therefore, several mechanisms are needed to account for the development and progression of the two.

This overview from a biopsychosocial perspective reveals that there is sufficient evidence to support an important association between depression and cardiac disease. It also suggests a number of significant directions for future research. Large, randomized clinical trials are needed to determine whether early detection of depression coupled with early intervention can prevent the development of cardiac disease or reduce the risk for incidents of negative cardiac events. Another research priority is to elucidate the potential mediating factors related to depression, such as failure to comply with medical care, sedentary lifestyle, eating habits, and smoking. Also, biological studies are needed to quantify the latent effect of the alterations in the level of risk biomarkers (e.g., homocysteine, IL-6, TNF-α, IL-2, serotonin, dopamine, cortisol, heart rate variability, and platelet activation), which could have a negative effect on cardiac function. Moreover, depression seems to be more of a problem for women with cardiac disease than for men. Therefore, future studies are needed that focus on whether there is a disproportionate weight of comorbid depression and cardiac outcomes among women.

Designing large-scale clinical trials that test biobehavioral research models, along with considering both physiologic and behavioral outcomes, are essential to better understating of the depression-cardiac disease communication. In addition, studies designed to develop a more clear account of psychosocial risk factors to cardiac disease are urgently needed. Finally, in an era of genetic research, identifying genes or gene expression mechanisms that may link depression and cardiac disease may pave the path for ultimate understanding of the link between depression and cardiovascular diseases.

ALI SALMAN

Depression in Families

Depression is a major mental health problem affecting 25 million Americans and their families. By 2020, depression will be the third leading cause of disability worldwide. Most people suffering from depression live with their families, usually their spouses and children, and the negative impact of depression on families has been well-documented (Coyne et al., 1987; Keitner, Archambault, Ryan, & Miller, 2003; Lee, 2003; Miller et al., 1992). Nursing has long viewed families as a context for caring for the individual with depression, but only recently has focused on the whole family.

Depression is a rather vague descriptive term with a broad and varied meaning ranging from normal sadness and disappointment to a severe incapacitating psychiatric illness. William Styron (1990) describes in *Darkness Visible* the unsatisfactory descriptive nature of the term depression: "a noun with bland tonality and lacking any magisterial presence, used indifferently to describe the economic decline or rut in the ground, a true wimp of a word for such a major illness" (p. 37).

Depression is a universal mood state with all people experiencing a lowered mood or transient feelings of sadness related to negative life events such as loss. For most, the feelings of sadness or disappointment resolve with time and normal functioning resumes. In contrast, the symptoms associated with the psychiatric illness of depression can disrupt normal functioning, influence mortality and morbidity, and can cause a myriad of problems within the family (Badger, 1996a; Bluementhal et al., 2003; Cuijpers & Smit, 2002; Katon, 2003). The psychiatric illness of major depressive disorder (MDD) is diagnosed if five out of the following nine symptoms are present for a minimum of 2 weeks most of the day, nearly every day: (a) depressed mood, (b) loss of interest or pleasure in all activities, (c) decrease or increase in appetite or significant weight change, (d) insomnia or hypersomnia, (e) psychomotor retardation or agitation, (f) fatigue or loss of energy, (g) feelings of worthlessness or excessive guilt, (h) difficulty concentrating or indecisiveness, and (i) recurrent thoughts of death, recurrent suicide ideation or attempt (American Psychiatric Association (APA), 1994). One of the five symptoms must be depressed mood or loss of interest or pleasure. Together, these symptoms cause significant functional impairment. In addition to MDD, depression is further classified in the Diagnostic and Statistical Manual of Mental Disorders (DSM-IV) (APA, 1994) into other diagnostic subtypes such as minor depression or dysthymia by signs and symptoms, onset, course, duration, and outcomes.

Family refers to any group that functions together to perform tasks related to survival, growth, safety, socialization, or health of the family. Family members can be related by marriage, birth, adoption, or can self-identify themselves as family. This definition is sufficiently broad to be inclusive of all types of families; however it is recommended that researchers provide specific definitions of family appropriate to their research.

Genetic-biological research of depression in families includes genetic and biological marker studies (Flaskerud, 2000; Viguera & Rothschild, 1996). The four research approaches to the genetics of mood are: (a) familial loading studies (e.g., comparing families with depression to families without the disease), (b) studies evaluating the inheritability of mood disorders (e.g., twin studies), (c) studies of incidence of the risk for, but not yet ill from, mood disorders to determine biological or psychological antecedents, and (d) in theory, studies using genetic probes to determine which relatives and which phenotypes are associated with the genetic contributants to mood disorders (Suppes & Rush,

1996). The results of the familial loading studies are clear whether the approach used is the "top-down" (i.e., studies of children with depressed parents) or the "bottom-up" approach (i.e., studies of relatives of depressed children) (Birmaher, Ryan, & Williamson, 1996; Jacobs & Johnson, 2001). Children with depressed parents have a significantly greater risk of developing depressive disorders and other psychiatric disorders than do children with parents without depression (Buckwalter, Kerfooot, & Stolley, 1988; Peterson et al., 2003; Nomura, Wickramaratne, Warner, Mufson, & Meissman, 2002). Biological marker studies have focused on growth hormone, serotonergic and other neurotransmitter receptors, sleep, and hypothalamic-pituitary axis (Keltner, 2000; Viguera & Rothschild, 1996). Despite evidence from genetic studies about the strong support for the genetic inheritance of depression, and the fact that abnormalities in biological markers persist throughout the life span, the relationship between genetic-biological predisposition and environment remains unclear.

Psychosocial research of depression in families has focused on communication, marital problems and dissatisfaction, expressed emotion, problem-solving, coping, and family functioning (Beach, Sandeen, & O'Leary, 1990; Biglan et al., 1985; Keitner, Miller, Epstein, Bishop, & Fruzzetti, 1987). The evidence strongly supports that families who contain members with depression have greater impairment in all areas than matched control families, and than families whose members are diagnosed with alcohol dependence, adjustment disorders, schizophrenia, or bipolar disorders (Coyne et al., 1987; Keitner, Miller, & Ryan, 1993). It is not surprising that depression has its most negative impact on families during acute depressive episodes (Miller et al., 1992), yet families with depressed members consistently experience more difficulties than matched control families even 1 year after initial treatment (Billings & Moos, 1985). Family members living with members with depression report greater health problems, with about 40% of adults being sufficiently distressed themselves to require therapeutic intervention (Coyne et al., 1987). The majority of recent studies of families with members with depression have used primarily inpatient samples, have focused on women as the identified patient, have often excluded parents with depression, and have been quantitative in nature (Schwab, Stephenson, & Ice, 1993). Few studies have used qualitative approaches to understand family members' perspectives and treatment needs. Badger (1996a) used a grounded theory method to describe the social psychological process of families living with members with depression. The process, *family transformations*, refers to the cognitive and behavioral changes that occur within the family from the time the member initially exhibits symptoms through recovery and at remission. As family members moved through the three stages (acknowledging the strangers within, fighting the battle, gaining a new perspective), all members are transformed and family functioning forever altered. These results support findings from previous studies and provide perspectives of family members not normally included in depression research.

Despite identifying the multiple problems in these families, the role of the family in the treatment process has received less attention. Systematic family interventions have only begun to be developed and modeled after programs used with people with other psychiatric disorders and their families (Holder & Anderson, 1990; Kietner et al., 2003). For example, Lee (2003) found that in mothers who participated in a program to improve maternal coping skills, these coping skills moderated between depression and negative life events, reducing the negative effects on children. To date, few clinical trials have validated the effectiveness of these interventions. Families have identified the need for information about how to facilitate communication, decrease negative interactions, handle stigma, gain a new perspective, care for self and redesign their relationships (Badger, 1996b). In theory, education, support and partnering could move family members more quickly through the stages to prevent depression from becoming a recurrent and chronic illness for the entire family. Future research should develop and test psychoeducational and support interventions with families. Although a common concern with research with families remains the unit of analysis (individual, dyad, or family as a whole), research representing all perspectives is needed for nursing to more fully understand and treat depression in families.

TERRY A. BADGER

Depression in Older Adults

Depression is the most common mental disorder among older adults in the United States and one of the most disabling conditions among elderly persons worldwide (Sable, Dunn, & Zisook, 2002). More than 6 million Americans age 65 and older representing approximately 15% of U.S. older adults suffer from depression (Sable et al., 2002). The prevalence of clinical depression ranges from about 5% in community samples to 20% in nursing home residents and nearly 30% of older adults seen in primary care settings (Alexopoulos, 2001). About 50% of older adults who are hospitalized for medical illnesses or receiving long-term care experience clinically significant depression (Alexopoulos). Older adults are vulnerable to depression for a number of reasons. Approximately 80% have at least one chronic medical condition that can trigger depression (Sable et al.). In addition, about 6 million older adults need assistance with their daily activities (Sable et al.), and inability to meet one's own personal needs has been associated with increased vulnerability to late-life depression.

While depression is often viewed as a clinical syndrome with specific diagnostic criteria, depression has also been conceptualized as a mood state or as a collection of symptoms (Beck, 1997). Because older adults may not meet the diagnostic criteria for the clinical syndrome, studies of older adults commonly use the term depression to mean depressive symptoms (Futterman, Thompson, Gallagher-Thompson, & Ferris, 1995). Clinical depression is usually qualified by an adjective to specify a particular type or form, including reactive, agitated, and psychotic. In addition, based on etiology, depression is classified as endogenous (due to internal processes) or exogenous (due to external factors). Depression is termed primary when it is not preceded by any physical or psychiatric condition and secondary when preceded by another physical or psychiatric disorder. Finally, depression is classified as acute (less than 2 years duration) or chronic (more than 2 years). Clinical depression consists of characteristic signs and symptoms, as well as type of onset, course, duration, and outcome. The *Diagnostic and Statistical Manual of Mental Disorders* (DSM IV) (American Psychiatric Association, 1994) classifies clinical depression into major, minor, and dysthymic subtypes. Major depression refers to a depression that meets specific diagnostic criteria for duration, impairment of functioning, and the presence of a cluster of physiological and psychological symptoms (American Psychiatric Association). Minor depression includes fewer depressive symptoms than major depression. Dysthymia consists of fewer symptoms than are expressed in major depression but more than in minor depression, and it is more chronic (American Psychiatric Association).

Diagnosing depression in older adults is fraught with challenges. Depressed mood is one of the depressive symptoms that older adults may experience, but others may also experience a range of affective responses (Futterman et al., 1995). Indeed, many studies have reported that in older adults, a predominant depressed mood may not be as prominent as symptoms of irritability, anxiety, or physical or somatic symptoms and changes in functioning (Alexopoulos, 2001; Futterman et al.; Sable et al., 2002). In addition, symptoms of cognitive impairment that may occur in elders with depression may be mistaken for dementia (Sable et al.). It is estimated that about 15% of older adults have depressive symptoms that do not meet diagnostic criteria specified by the *Diagnostic and*

Statistical Manual of Mental Disorders (DSM IV) (American Psychiatric Association, 1994) for diagnosis of major depression (Alexopoulos). Nevertheless, these older adults can experience functional deficits in activities of daily living (ADL) and instrumental activities of daily living (IADL) that compromise their independence and quality of life. Indeed, the symptoms of depression can lead to total inability of the older individual to care for self and to relate to others. There is also a potential for persons with depression to negatively affect family members and others around them.

Not surprisingly, few elders in the community seek mental health services. Most depressed elders are seen by general practitioners for psychosomatic complaints. Part of the symptomatology of depression is a focus on physical problems, and this requires practitioners to carefully assess for depressive symptoms. Suicide is a risk factor for depressed older adults. The suicide rate for individuals aged 80 and over is twice that of the general population and is particularly high in older White males. Interestingly, most suicidal elders recently visited a general practitioner prior to their suicidal act.

Studies of risk factors for late-life depression have examined the effects of gender, age, and race/ethnicity. Like earlier depression, late-life depression more commonly strikes women than men, at approximately a 2:1 ratio (Kockler & Heun, 2002). Recent population-based studies have estimated the prevalence of geriatric depression at 4.4% for women and 2.7% for men, while the estimated lifetime prevalence for clinical depression is about 20% in women and 10% in men (Kockler & Heun; Sable et al., 2002). Although female gender is a risk factor for depression throughout the life span, gender differences decrease with increasing age (Sable et al.), and white men ages 80 to 84 years are at greatest risk for suicide (Kockler & Heun).

Cohort studies have shown that the oldest-old, those over age 85 years, are more likely than the younger-old, those between 65 and 74, to experience depressive symptoms (Blazer, 2003). Depression is thought to afflict older adults of all racial and ethnic backgrounds similarly (Alexopoulos, 2001; Bruce, 2002); however, its symptoms may not be consistent across racial/ethnic groups, making early diagnosis and treatment challenging.

Research on depression among older adults was ignored in the past and is still a neglected area. Clearly, much more nursing research is needed. It is critical that nurses assume leadership in disseminating information about the outcomes of a variety of treatments that can be used for depression in later life. There is a particular need to examine suicide in late life and to develop better assessment instruments for detecting suicidal ideation in elders.

JACLENE A. ZAUSZNIEWSKI
MAY L. WYKLE

Depression in Women

Women seeking help in the general health care sector often are depressed. Studies indicated that between 20% to 45% of women using primary care have major depressive disorder (MDD) (Bixo, Sundström-Poromaa, Björn, & Åström, 2001; Hauenstein, 2003; Kirmayer & Robbins, 1996; Miranda, Azocar, Komaromy & Golding, 1998). In these settings, patients are more likely to report their depressive symptoms as physical problems (Barsky, Peekna, & Borus, 2001; Katon, Sullivan, & Walker, 2001) and physicians less likely to identify and treat the disorder (Freiman & Zuvekas, 2000; Katz et al., 1997; Sundström, Bixo, Björn, & Åström, 2001). Nurses are positioned to detect and manage this major public health problem because of their prominence in the general health sector and their often greater proximity to patients.

MDD remains a significant source of morbidity and disability in women under 65. The physical symptoms of lethargy and sleep and appetite disturbance combine with the cognitive symptoms of disinterest, helplessness, hopelessness, and worthlessness to exact both significant mood disturbances and functional impairments. Unfortunately, MDD is common among women. The population prevalence of MDD in women is 6% to 17% (Kessler et al., 2003). Combined with dysthymia, a milder but more chronic and equally disabling mood disorder, the population prevalence ranges from 12 to 25%, a rate twice that of men (Kessler, 2003). Women's key risk factors for MDD include a family history of the disorder, single parenting, a history of child abuse, impoverishment, and poorer educational achievement (Brown & Moran, 1997; Hanson et al., 2001; Kessler et al., 1994; Kessler et al., 2003; Weiss, Longhurst, & Mazure, 1999). Social discrimination and sexual harassment also contribute to the preponderance of MDD in women. Marginalized women have the highest rates of MDD (Brown, Schulberg, Madonia, Shear, & Houck, 1996; Hauenstein & Peddada, in revision; Miranda et al., 1998).

While MDD is present in elderly women, the highest incidence of the disorder occurs in women 25 to 34, a time when women are developing both their work and family careers. Depressed women have higher rates of unemployment or partial employment, absenteeism, poor work productivity, and fail to progress in their work careers. This translates to an estimated annual cost per employer of almost $10,000 for every depressed woman working in the firm (Birnbaum, Leong, & Greenberg, 2003). Mood disorder also impairs women's family careers (Gotlib, Lewinsohn, & Steely, 1998; Wade & Cairney, 2000). Depressed women are more likely to divorce than are unaffected women, and divorced women tend to be economically disadvantaged. Divorced women often are responsible for young children, and raising these children alone is difficult. These work and family patterns associated with MDD contribute to a cycle of hopelessness, worthlessness, and poverty that promotes a chronic and recurrent course of MDD that is refractory to treatment. This is a global phenomenon; the World Health Organization Global Burden of Disease study showed that MDD was the leading cause of disease related disability in women (NIMH Research on Women's Mental Health—Highlights FY2001–2002).

Maternal depression also has significant effects on children. Research has shown cognitive and social deficits in children of depressed mothers that appear early in infancy (Essex, Klein, Cho, & Kalin, 2002; Field, 1998; Kaplan, Bachorowski, & Zarlengo-Strouse, 1999). These deficits persist into childhood and adolescence and have chronic effects on personal, school, and social functioning (Essex, Klein, Miech, & Smider, 2001; Gotlib et al., 1998; Murray, Sinclair, Cooper, Ducournau, & Turner, 1999; Oyserman, Bybee, & Mowbray, 2002).

A complex interaction of biological, psychological, and social factors contribute to MDD in women. Gender disparities in the occurrence of MDD and its coincidence with women's hormonal changes point to estrogen as a physiological mechanism in women's depression (Shors & Leuner, 2003; Steiner, Dunn, & Born, 2003). Gonadal hormones are thought to alter neurotransmitter functioning and learning resulting in more affective symptoms and nonresponsiveness in stressful circumstances. There is mounting evidence that childhood trauma such as sexual abuse can alter hypothalamic-pituitary-adrenal axis (HPA) functioning and increase vulnerability to future depression (Putnam, 2003).

Hormonal factors alone do not precipitate MDD in women (Kessler, 2003). The unstable HPA system is affected by women's psychological and social environment, which may serve to precipitate physiological events. For example, animal models show that female rats when exposed to uncontrollable stress will fail to respond in subsequent controllable stress situations, a response style not shared by males (Shors & Leuner, 2003). Interpersonal distress is one example of uncontrollable stress. Research has shown that women locked in dysfunctional relationships for economic or other reasons are more likely to have recurrent depressive episodes (Hammen, 2003). Pessimistic thinking arising from low self-esteem also has been associated with depressive symptoms in women (Peden, Hall, Rayens, & Beebe, 2000). Not surprisingly, MDD is more common among women who exhibit dependent personality traits (Widiger & Anderson, 2003). Despite progress in reducing gender discrimination, many women's social environment contributes to MDD by stripping them of personal power. Early victimization contributes to victimization as adults. Low self-esteem increases the likelihood of an early and often unstable marriage that leads to divorce. Divorce is associated with economic hardship and single parenting. Victimization, marital instability, single parenting, and economic hardship have all been associated with often intractable depression (Bauer, Rodríguez, & Pérez-Stable, 2000; Brown & Moran, 1997; Earle, Smith, Harris, & Longino, 1998; Gotlib et al., 1998; Kessler, Walters, & Forthofer, 1998; McCauley, Kern, Kolodner, Derogatis, & Bass, 1998; Petterson & Albers, 2002; Scholle, Rost, & Golding, 1998; Wade & Cairney, 2000). While the evidence for these associations is convincing, the reciprocal relationship between MDD and the social condition of women is far less understood and is an area of needed research.

Evidence-based treatments for MDD include pharmacotherapy and psychotherapy. Minimum treatment includes 2 months of an antidepressant at a dose known to be efficacious in treating MDD or at least eight visits to a specialty mental health provider that last a minimum of 30 minutes each (Kessler et al., 2003; Young, Klap, Sherbourne, & Wells, 2001). The data show that minimum treatment can effect remission in the short-term but the extent to which there are long-term benefits is yet to be determined. There is significant evidence, however, that few receive even this minimum level of care (Kessler et al.; Wang, Berglund, & Kessler, 2000). While there are few large trials focusing specifically on women, three studies using evidence-based treatments have demonstrated modest treatment effects with both urban and rural women attending primary care (Hauenstein, 2003; Miranda, Nakamura, & Bernal, 2003; Pyne et al., 2003).

The multifactorial nature of depression in women, however, may require different or more complex psychological and social interventions than those that meet the minimum standards for depression treatment. Many of the psychotherapies are considered gender neutral but few studies address gender differences in outcome. One example where gender differences in outcome were examined is that by Pyne and his group who used a simple, nurse-managed intervention, which included tailoring known efficacious treatment to the preferences of the patients and regular telephone follow-up. The treatment was cost-effective in women, but not in men, when quality of life was evaluated as the outcome. Gender-specific treatments might target psychological and social factors known to exacerbate depression in women. For example, because of the reciprocal effect of marital instability and MDD, interventions that focus on reducing interpersonal distress and spousal conflict may be especially promising for women (Hammen, 2003; Wade & Kendler, 2000; Worell, 2001). Interventions that stimulate positive life change also may work preferentially in women (Albertine, Oldehinkel, Ormel, & Neeleman, 2000). Treatment for MDD driven by gender-specific theories based on women's own voices and experiences, and the diversities and complexities of women's experience may promote recovery instead of simply remission (Eun-Ok & Afaf-Ibrahim, 2001; Worell, 2001).

Recommendations for needed research on MDD in women have been enumerated by the American Psychological Association and the Office of Women's Health at the National Institutes of Health (Mazure, Keita, & Blehar, 2002; U.S. Department of Health and Human Services, 1999b). Recommendations for research range from bench research to public education. Research focused on treatment approaches is especially relevant to nursing. First, gender-specific treatments for MDD need to be developed and tested. Treatments must be based on the unique biological, psychological, and social conditions of women generally, and tailored to the needs of ethnically diverse women and those in dire social circumstances. The design of treatment programs should target recovery, not simply symptom remission. Second, research on treatment outcome requires evaluation of multiple areas of functioning including marital stability, parenting, and work productivity. From a policy perspective, MDD in women will not become a priority until the impact of MDD at the family and community level is realized and the effects of adequate treatment are determined. Third, attention must be paid to the provision of treatment that is accessible. Health services research in this area should consider novel venues and providers. For example, treatment services for women could be moved to the community in places where women commonly gather, such as churches, schools, and community centers. Because mental health care is a dwindling commodity it is important to consider nonspecialty professional and lay providers. Nurses can be pivotal here, both in providing direct service and in organizing and supervising lay providers. Research paradigms that develop and test alternative health delivery methods will go far in closing the gap between need and treatment.

EMILY J. HAUENSTEIN

Descriptive Research

Descriptive research encompasses a broad range of research activity in nursing and has comprised the majority of nursing studies. Early research efforts were focused on descriptive epidemiological studies. Nightingale's pioneering work is a well-known example of this type of research. Well schooled in mathematics and statistics, Nightingale created elaborate charts demonstrating morbidity and mortality trends of soldiers during and after the Crimean War. Her detailed record keeping and graphic representation of these data convinced officials of the need to improve sanitary conditions for soldiers, which drastically reduced mortality rates (Cohen, L. B.,1984).

The progress in descriptive research activity in nursing has been influenced by several events and movements over the past several decades: advanced degree education in nursing, philosophical debate about the role of nursing and nursing research in the scientific community, establishment of centers for nursing research, and the formation of an agenda for knowledge development in nursing.

With the help of federal traineeship money, the earliest doctorally prepared nurses obtained degrees in basic science programs. The adoption and rejection of the logical positivist view of science helped clarify linkages between philosophy, theory, and method. At one extreme, nurse scientists and theorists argued that the future of nursing knowledge development lay in empirical studies that allowed for repeated observational statements under a variety of conditions. It was believed that one ultimate truth could be found after repeated objective observations, which would eventually lead to discovery of universal laws.

Critics of the logical empiricist approach argued that truth is influenced by history, context, and a chosen methodology and is constantly in a state of flux. What is humanly unobservable one day may be observable with the help of technological innovation another day. Although logical positivism is no longer espoused in nursing theory and science, its role was crucial in initiating dialogue about what nursing knowledge is and how research in nursing should be advanced. These dialogues have helped swing the pendulum from valuing experimental research as the gold standard in nursing to recognizing the important role of descriptive and exploratory research.

Over the years, nursing leaders have struggled to establish which approach to knowledge development is appropriate and necessary for nursing. Dickoff, James, and Wiedenbach's (1968) four levels of theory for nursing included the most basic type, factor-isolating theory, as the product of descriptive studies, with higher level theories built on the necessary base of this first level of theory. Stevenson (1990) depicted a stepwise conceptualization of research in nursing, with exploratory research at the bottom and utilization in practice at the top. Descriptive research was thought to build on exploratory research findings and to provide a foundation of support for intervention studies, with the ultimate goal of utilizing research findings in practice. N. R. Reynolds, Timmerman, Anderson, and Stevenson (1992) encouraged nurse researchers to employ meta-analysis techniques to descriptive research. Meta-analysis is a useful statistical tool that synthesizes extant nursing research, but it has largely been applied only to experimental studies. Application of this technique to descriptive studies can help determine when a phenomenon is ready for testing with intervention studies.

Descriptive studies often are used when little research has been done in an area, to clarify and define new concepts or phenomena, to increase understanding of a phenomenon from another experiential perspective, or to obtain a fresh perspective on a well-researched topic. Also, the formulation and testing of measurement tools (e.g., to measure depression, anxiety, or quality of life) employ descriptive research techniques. The development and refinement of these tools will continue, with increasing emphasis on outcomes research as nurses are required to demonstrate how their interventions make a difference for their patients.

Public and private funding of nursing research has allowed for an expansion of nursing knowledge based in research. Of the many studies funded by National Institute of Nursing Research, Sigma Theta Tau, and private foundations, descriptive research continues to command a large portion of research dollars. Descriptive research can employ quantitative or qualitative (including naturalistic) methodologies. Quantitative descriptive methodologies include surveys, measurement tools, chart or record reviews, physiological measurements, meta-analyses, and secondary data analyses. Qualitative descriptive methodologies include interviews, focus groups, content analyses, reviews of literature, observational studies, case studies, life histories, grounded theory studies, concept analyses, ethnographic studies, and phenomenological studies. Many qualitative methodologies employ exploratory as well as descriptive techniques.

A large portion of descriptive research involves the use of surveys or measurement tools, physiological measurements, and interviews. Other naturalistic or qualitative methodologies (e.g., ethnography, grounded theory, phenomenology) have become more available to nurse researchers in the recent past and continue to add to the descriptive research knowledge base in nursing.

Many nursing organizations and associations have delineated priorities for a nursing research agenda that include clarifying philosophical underpinnings of holism, research on care and caring, health promotion, disease prevention and wellness, development of knowledge about the family and social support networks, and research on minority groups and culturally different views of health and illness. Adding to nursing's knowledge base in these areas will require using descriptive research along with other research methodologies and incorporating the results of these studies into nursing practice and research endeavors.

ANITA J. TARZIAN
MARLENE ZICHI COHEN

Diabetes

According to the Diabetes Research Working Group's recent report *Conquering Diabetes: A Strategic Plan for the 21st Century*, diabetes is the 6th leading cause of death in the U.S., primarily resulting from cardiovascular disease. Diabetes is a disease that affects people of all ages and from every racial background. African, Hispanic, Native, and Asian Americans, the fastest growing segments of the U.S. population, are particularly vulnerable to diabetes and its most severe complications (National Institute of Diabetes and Digestive and Kidney Diseases, 2003). For example, heart disease, stroke, kidney disease, blindness, and death due to diabetes are more common in African-American versus Caucasian adults.

The simplified criteria for diagnosis of diabetes using fasting plasma glucose ≥ 126 mg/dl or casual plasma glucose ≥ 200 mg/dl with classic symptoms confirmed on a subsequent day may be impacting the numbers of persons identified as having diabetes (American Diabetes Association, 2003). The total prevalence of diabetes in the United States is estimated to be 18.2 million: 13 million diagnosed and 5.2 million undiagnosed (Centers for Disease Control, 2003). Along with the tendency for obesity, inactivity, and an ever-aging population, the incidence of diabetes is expected to grow. In pediatric populations, an emerging epidemic of type 2 diabetes is occurring due to higher rates of overweight and sedentary behavior in youth as young as 10 years of age, seen predominantly in ethnic minorities (Fagot-Campagna, 2000).

Given these sobering statistics, there is strong evidence that the United States will face ongoing public health challenges to address the potential burgeoning onslaught of individuals who face declining health status, quality of life (QoL), and lost productivity related to an earlier onset of diabetes. Tighter glycemic control is shown to decrease the progression of diabetes complications in persons with type 1 and type 2 diabetes (Diabetes Control and Complications Trial Research [DCCT], 1993; United Kingdom Prospective Diabetes Group Study [UKPDS], 1998). The conundrum facing nurse researchers is how best to develop interventions that promote effective, individualized self-management in persons diagnosed with diabetes and to implement screening procedures for early detection and prevention in those most at risk for developing diabetes.

The majority of nursing studies focus on adults with diabetes, particularly in African-American women and Mexican and Native Americans with type 2 diabetes. The nurse researchers investigating symptom management, self-management or self-care, and community-based interventions using culturally sensitive approaches include Sharon Brown at the University of Texas at Austin; Felicia Hodge at the University of California, San Francisco; Gail Melkus at Yale University; and Anne Skelly at the University of North Carolina, Chapel Hill. Although each of the principal investigators has developed specific aims for their individual programs of research using quasi-experimental designs, there are some common areas of study. Examples of the diabetes-related outcomes that these investigations are addressing are diabetes knowledge, health beliefs and behaviors, metabolic control of glucose, body mass index, lipid levels, blood pressure, self-efficacy, and QoL. Focus groups with diverse populations are commonly used to gain a more comprehensive understanding of the sociocultural concerns of the study participants regarding diabetes management, to assist with tailoring culturally sensitive and feasible interventions, and to allow for detecting differences in more successful versus less successful results. Most of the studies included longitudinal evaluations of the interventions, which address diabetes education in nutrition, exercise, home glucose monitoring, and coping skills training.

Limited research with adults who have type 2 diabetes was available on the physiological benefits of interventions. Laurie Quinn at the University of Illinois at Chicago has collaborated with James Rimmer, an exercise physiologist, to identify the feasibility of a health promotion intervention with predominantly low-income, low-education, American women with multiple chronic conditions (e.g., obesity, hypertension, joint pain, and depression) in addition to diabetes. The 12-week intervention consisted of health behavior training with peer support, nutrition education, and prescribed exercise based upon personal aerobic capacity (peak $V0_2$). Using a 3 day per week format with transportation provided, subjects had significant improvements in total and LDL cholesterol, cardiovascular fitness, muscular strength, and nutrition knowledge. Thus, there is compelling need to devise interventions that target approaches for individuals with complex sociocultural, economic, and educational backgrounds (Rimmer, Silverman, Braunschweig, Quinn, & Liu, 2002).

Studies of youths with diabetes are addressing the needs of adolescents and their families. The nurse researchers examining issues in this population are Margaret Grey at Yale University, Carol Dashiff at the University of Alabama at Birmingham, and Melissa Faulkner at the University of Illinois at Chicago. Family and developmental perspectives are incorporated into the designs of studies of youths. Key variables are self-care or self-management, self-efficacy, QoL, coping, family adaptation, and autonomy as related to improvement in metabolic control. Grey is conducting a longitudinal study using QoL and metabolic control to evaluate the effects of coping skills training (CST) in youths receiving intensive diabetes management. This investigation is the longest ongoing clinical trial specifically testing the efficacy of an intervention with youths who have type 1 diabetes. Adolescents who received CST and intensive diabetes management had significantly better metabolic control and less impact of diabetes on their QoL than youths receiving intensive diabetes management alone after 1 year. Such evidence lends support for devising interventions to optimize both glycemic control and perceptions of QoL in youths with diabetes. Dashiff is developing a model of influences on the development of adolescent autonomy and family processes for self-care and diabetes control in early and middle adolescence. Her data will reflect the evolutionary development of the parent-adolescent subsystem prospectively over a 2-year period with the goal of identifying factors that improve diabetes control when providing family-based interventions.

Consistent with the overall aim of preventing long-term diabetes-related complications as teens make the transition to adulthood, Faulkner is investigating cardiovascular risks in adolescents with type 1 and type 2 diabetes. The intent is to describe potential sociodemographic, behavioral, or physiological factors that predispose youths with either type of diabetes to subsequent heart disease. This research is partly based upon earlier work that found decreased heart rate variability, a marker for early cardiovascular autonomic disease, associated with having type 1 diabetes and poorer metabolic control (Faulkner, Hathaway, Milstead, & Burghen, 2001).

Improvements in glycemic control through individualized interventions developed and tested through scientific inquiry will increase the odds for minimizing complications of diabetes, which affect personal QoL and productivity and contribute to the economic burden associated with diabetes care. Future research must embrace not only better outcomes, including decreasing health disparities in minorities, but also the enormous need for prevention in those predisposed to the disease. Newer technologies for insulin delivery, continuous glucose sensing, and genetic engineering for individual therapies are on the horizon. Through their leadership in interdisciplinary science, nurse researchers will remain integral to the advancement of evidence-based diabetes care.

MELISSA SPEZIA FAULKNER

Disaster Nursing

Norris et al. (2002) defined a disaster as a sudden event that has the potential to terrify, horrify, or engender substantial losses for many people simultaneously. Disasters are classified by the nature of the event, i.e., natural, technological, and deliberate acts of mass violence (terrorism), and/or by the impact of exposure, i.e. "dose response." Natural disasters are geophysical forces (e.g., earthquakes) or weather forces (e.g., hurricanes, tornadoes). Technological disasters are frequently attributed to human negligence and error and include collapse of structures, environmental catastrophes, and failures of public transportation equipment. Traumatic events are relevant to nursing science and practice for several reasons. First, these events are more common and have more pervasive impacts than previously thought. Norris (1992) in a survey of residents in four Southeastern cities showed a lifetime exposure rate of 69%. Those surveyed had experienced at least one traumatic event. Tragic death, robbery, and serious motor vehicle injuries were the three most frequently reported. The impacts of disasters on individuals and communities are multidimensional and immense, and adaptation to loss is of long rather than short duration (Murphy, 2001; Norris et al.).

Research findings (Hall, Norwood, Ursano, Fallerton, & Levinson, 2002; Murphy, 2001; Norris et al., 2002) resulting from all types of traumatic events suggests five major domains of human responses following exposure to one of these events: (a) Specific psychological problems include shock, terror, guilt, horror, irritability, anxiety, hostility, post traumatic stress disorder (PTSD), and depression; (b) Cognitive responses include inability to concentrate, confusion, self-blame, intrusive thoughts (flashbacks) about the experience, decreased sense of self-efficacy, fear of losing additional control over life events, and fear of reoccurrence of the event; (c) Biological responses include sleep disturbance (insomnia, nightmares), exaggerated startle response, and indicators of stress and immune disorders. Behavioral responses include avoidance, social withdrawal, interpersonal stress (decreased intimacy and lowered trust in others) and substance abuse; (d) Resource losses include losses of income, social support, time for noneffect activities, social embeddedness, optimism, self-efficacy, and perceived control; and (e) Collective responses. Neighborhood and community response studies are rare with assessments generally taking three approaches: Participants have been asked to report community conditions, individual level responses have been aggregated, and archival data have been used to illustrate loss and responses to loss, for example, changes in liquor sales in a given neighborhood or community (Bromet, Parkinson, Schulberg, & Gondek, 1982; Gleser, Green, & Winget, 1981; Norris et al.).

Norris et al. (2002) summarized both the individual and collective outcomes obtained from 160 disaster samples from 29 countries. All three types of disaster, natural, technological, and mass violence events, were examined and analyzed for effect size. The magnitude of severity of negative consequences for the individual level response samples reviewed by Norris et al. was rated by level of impairment: minimal—11%, moderate—51%, severe—21%, and very severe—18%. When the data were assessed by type of event, victims of terrorist attacks (as opposed to natural and technological events) suffered the most severe consequences. Norris et al. reported that women and youths were more severely affected than men and older adults. Rescue and recovery workers were reportedly the most resilient. Examples of U.S. disasters rated as "high impact" by Norris et al. were the Buffalo Creek dam collapse (1972), the Exxon Valdez oil spill (1989), Hurricane Andrew (1992), and the Oklahoma City bombing (1995). Findings emerging from World Trade Center study samples, i.e., Manhattan and nearby areas, showed incidence of symptoms of stress ranging from 20% to 40%, suggesting a high disaster impact (Galea et al., 2002; Schuster et al., 2001).

Disasters and their outcomes are difficult to study. There are several reasons for this and some cannot be overcome. First, "pre-event" data are rarely available. It may be that mental disorders are overestimated in some postdisaster samples. Second, study reports vary widely in their methods. Norris et al. (2002) noted that 68% of the samples in their data set provided single, one-time data frequently by telephone. Initial, postevent data collections ranged from immediately after an event up to 7 years later, making the determination of immediate impact difficult to estimate. Most longitudinal studies have not collected follow-up data for more than a year, leaving long-term outcomes unknown. Thus, study design variability poses a threat to generalizability of findings.

Four suggestions for the study of disasters are to: increase the number of community and family studies, examine the roles of protective factors and lost resources, develop and test evidence-based interventions, and increase nurse researcher involvement. Research is needed in regard to factors that prevent or impede negative consequences, e.g., the roles of social networks and the efficiency of relief agencies. Collective responses interact with individual responses, making outcome measurement a challenge. The measurement and documentation of posttrauma responses has improved over time, but there is a lack of understanding in regard to how to reduce high levels of PTSD. Beaton and Murphy (2002) have made some initial recommendations in regard to the timing of psychosocial interventions following terrorist events. Finally, nurses provide postdisaster emergency services and follow-up treatment, and some have assisted in study data collection, but only a few have been study investigators.

SHIRLEY A. MURPHY

Discourse Analysis

Discourse analysis is a method that has multiple meanings referring to a wide range of analytical procedures. Such methodological diversity has resulted not only from various philosophical traditions that treat discourse differently but also from conceptualization of discourse analysis by diverse disciplines that emphasize different aspects or meanings of discourse. Discourse is viewed as an appropriate subject matter for research by various disciplines, including linguistics, philosophy, anthropology, sociology, psychology, information science, literary criticism, journalism, and practice disciplines such as nursing and medicine.

Although the term *discourse* in relation to discourse analysis is defined and used differently in linguistics and in other disciplines, discourse refers to language-in-use as connected speech or written texts produced in social contexts, rather than in terms of single sentences considered in terms of grammar and syntax. Discourse analysis deals with texts of conversations and written texts produced among individuals, as well as those produced within larger social, historical environments such as journal articles or newspaper accounts, that are not directed to specific individuals as their audiences. Discourse as the object of analysis is usually obtained from natural occurrences rather than from constructions designed solely for the purpose of analysis as either exemplary or ideal cases.

The term *discourse* in discourse analysis is commonly accepted as a mass noun with the above definition. However, the use of "a discourse" or "discourses" can be often found in discourse analysis with the post-structural, critical perspective. But the current literature abounds with both usages of the term (i.e., "discourse" and "a discourse"), not necessarily used consistently within one specific perspective.

Discourse analysis has its historic origin in the ancient Greek differentiation of grammar and rhetoric in language use (van Dijk, T. A., 1985). Although the study of rhetoric was differentiated from the study of grammar in linguistics throughout the centuries, it was not until the middle of the 20th century that a more formal approach to discourse analysis gained its appeal in linguistics. Hence, "pragmatics" in linguistics emphasizing discourse analysis has been separately developed, in contrast to the study of language proper that focuses on formal grammatical, syntactical, and morphological structures. Following this modern revisit in linguistics, many other disciplines have begun to take discourse as the proper subject of their scientific study. Although there are cross-disciplinary discussions of the methodology and application of various approaches of discourse analysis, there is no unified, integrated approach to discourse analysis. The literature across the disciplines suggests that there are at least three general perspectives within discourse analysis: (a) the linguistic perspective, (b) the conversation perspective, and (c) the ideology/critical perspective.

The linguistic perspective takes discourse as text produced by language use in either speech or writing. Thus, discourse text for this perspective can be from interpersonal conversations, written texts, or speech expositions such as testimonies. This perspective encompasses the formal pragmatics in linguistics, sociolinguistics in sociology, and ethnography of communication and ethnopoetics in anthropology. Hence, within this perspective there are several different methodological approaches to discourse analysis. Even within each orientation there are variations in the ways discourse texts are analyzed, depending on the frame within which various contextual features are brought into the analytic schema.

The formal pragmatics that had its beginning with Z. S. Harris (1952) has been recast by speech act theory in the philosophical tradition of Searle (Searle, Kiefer, & Bierwisch, 1980) and J. L. Austin (1975) and also by poetics of the literary study. Discourse analysis from the formal pragmatics orientation addresses such aspects as speech competence with respect to discursive rules, text grammar, discourse comprehension, or discourse organization.

Sociolinguistics as a branch of sociology is a study of language use within the functional paradigm of sociology, which views social life in relation to larger social structures such as gender, status, social class, role, and ethnicity. Sociolinguists are concerned with ways in which people use different linguistic forms according to macrostructural and contextual differences.

Anthropological approaches in the linguistic perspective are ethnopoetics and ethnography of communication. Ethnopoetics is the study of oral discourse as speech art in the tradition of literary analysis and is concerned with the structures of verbal aesthetics. The focus is on the poetic patterning of discourse within different cultures. On the other hand, ethnography of communication, advanced by Hymes (1964), is concerned with general language use as practiced in specific sociocultural context. Ethnography of communication, done either from the cross-cultural, comparative orientation or from the single-culture orientation, is based on the assumption that discourse should be studied, positing it within the dynamics and patterns of discourse events in a given cultural context. In all these branches of the linguistic perspective, the emphasis is on the linguistic forms as used in social life.

The conversation perspective takes discourse as conversational texts; it has been developed from the ethnomethodological tradition of Garfinkel in sociology. In this tradition, Sacks (1967) and others pioneered conversation analysis as a form of discourse analysis. Conversation analysis views discourse as a stream of sequentially organized discursive components that are designed jointly by participants of conversation applying a set of social and conversational rules. Conversation analysis studies rules that participants in conversation use to carry on and accomplish interaction, such as topic organization, turn taking, and use of response tokens. In recent years, however, conversation analysis has extended to include behavioral aspects of interaction (e.g., gesture, gaze, and laughter) as its analytical components. The use of transcripts and transcription symbols has been extensively developed in this perspective.

Discourse analysis in the ideological/critical perspective differs from that in the other two perspectives in its emphasis on the nature of discourse as historically constructed and constrained idea and knowledge. Discourse in this perspective is not considered in terms of linguistic form or interactive patterning. Rather, discourse is not only what is said or written but also the discursive conditions that produce imagined forms of life in given local, historical, and sociocultural junctures and thus is embedded in and with power and ideology.

This perspective was represented by poststructuralists such as Foucault (1972) and Lyotard (1984), who viewed discourse analysis not simply as an analytical process but as a critique and intervention against marginalization and repression of other forms of knowledge and discursive possibilities. Foucault treats discourses in relation to rules tied to specific historical conditions of usage and as power relations. Hence, discourse analysis in this perspective is oriented to revealing sociohistorical functions and power relations embedded in statements of talks and texts as well as what Foucault called "systemic archives," of which statements form a part.

The foregoing discussion indicates that discourse analysis is not a unified approach to studying language use. Although three perspectives are identified for this method, there is a blurring of differences among the perspectives. The method, however, remains multidiscipline-oriented. In nursing, discourse analysis is being applied with all three perspectives. Discourse analysis with the linguistic perspective has been applied to study discourse comprehension in client-nurse interactions or discourse organization of nurses' notes and to analyze various discourses on such topics as abortion, individualized care, and professionalism in the nursing literature related to macrostructural or contextual factors.

On the other hand, discourse analysis with the conversation perspective has been applied to the study of turn taking and topic organization in client-nurse interactions and to examine the dynamics of home visiting. Within the ideological/critical perspective, discourse analysis has been applied to examine nursing documentation as a form of power relations, to analyze discourse of nursing diagnosis in the nursing literature, and to explicate the language of sexuality, menopause, and abortion as power relations and ideology. Written texts produced by clients and nurses and client-nurse conversations, as well as texts in the public domain, are the rich sources for applying discourse analysis to study the language-in-use from these perspectives.

HESOOK SUZIE KIM

Disparities in Minority Mental Health

Disparities in mental health services for racial/ethnic minorities are continuous, ongoing, and persistent (Miranda, Lawson, & Escobar, 2002; Institute of Medicine [I.O.M.], 2003; U.S. Department of Health and Human Services [U.S.D.H.H.S.], 2003; Sue, 2003). Because of the holistic and preventive care attributes found in nursing research, education, and practice, nurses are prepared to address the issues of disparities in minority mental health. Nurses have ethical responsibilities that include doing no harm through the provision of safe patient care (Gastmans, 1998). Practicing within an ethically challenging environment calls for nurses to be aware of and to address the issues of health disparities for racial/ethnic minorities. It is imperative that nurses become culturally competent in the care that they give to all people including racial/ethnic minorities. The Institute of Medicine Committee on understanding and eliminating racial and ethnic disparities in health care (I.O.M.) defines "disparities in healthcare as racial or ethnic differences in the quality of health care that are not due to access-related factors or clinical needs, preferences, and appropriateness of intervention" (pp. 3–4). Racial/ethnic minorities are less likely to receive needed mental health care and when they do it is of poorer quality than whites.

The four major minority groups are both racial—Black, Native Indian/Alaskan Native, and Asian/Pacific Islanders, and ethnic—Hispanic (any race). Miranda, Nakamura, and Bernal (2003) stated that although race is based on an outdated impression of biological origin, race does designate strong social meanings, whereas ethnicity refers to affinity with a group that is believed to share a common lineage. According to the U.S. Census Bureau (2001), from 1900 to 1965, racial/ethnic minorities made up 10% of the U.S. population. By 2000, they were almost 30% of the U.S. population, and by the mid-21st century racial/ethnic minorities will be approximately 40% of the U.S. population. The U.S. Census Bureau reported that of the 281.4 million people that live in the United States, 12.3% are Black, 0.9% are Native Indians/Alaskan Natives, 3.7% are Asian/Pacific Islanders and 12.5% are Hispanic.

Today, racial/ethnic minorities still are affected by long-term legalized racism/discrimination. For Blacks, it was slavery; Native Americans and Japanese—forced relocations; Hispanics—conquest; and Chinese—involuntary noncitizenship. This led to institutionalized racism, with a continued distrust by minorities of organized systems, including the health-care system. Stigma prevents many minorities with mental illness from seeking help. According to the Surgeon General, stigma plays a stronger role in not seeking treatment with racial/ethnic minorities than with whites. As stigma lessens, a change in public attitude should occur and people will be more likely to seek care.

Prevalence of mental disorders are relatively similar across racial/ethnic populations, although there are clear variances within subgroups (Miranda et al., 2002). Blacks in need of mental health care receive only half the care of whites, and the rate of uninsured minorities to whites is 2:1 (U.S.D.H.H.S., 2003). Almost 30% of Hispanics and 20% of Blacks do not have a primary source of health care and many racial/ethnic minorities live in remote and rural areas. People who do not have a primary source of health care or who live in remote and rural locations are less likely to be insured or more likely to be underinsured. Being insured increases the likelihood for accessibility to mental health care.

Mental health disparities for racial/ethnic minority populations are sustained by barriers to cultural competence that include racism/discrimination, stigma, communication, misdiagnosis, treatment, and lack of research (U.S.D.H.H.S., 2003; Miranda et al., 2002; I.O.M., 2003). The Surgeon General in the landmark supplement, *Mental Health: Culture, Race and Ethnicity* (2003) reasoned that racial/ethnic minorities experience (a) less opportunity of entry to and ease of use of mental health services, (b) less potential for receipt of mental health services, (c) poorer quality of mental health treatment, and (d) underrepresentation of racial/ethnic minority clinicians, researchers, and educators in the mental health field.

There are major gaps in empirical data for mental health services for racial/ethnic minorities. Misdiagnosis, treatment, and cultural competence have been studied. Most research has been done with the black population. Misdiagnosis occurs in all groups including whites but it occurs to a more significant degree in minorities (Miranda et al., 2002; I.O.M., 2003). Racial/ethnic minorities were less likely to receive appropriate care for depression or anxiety than were whites. Black patients with affective disorders are more likely to be diagnosed as schizophrenic than are white patients and therefore, less like to receive lithium (Miranda et al.; I.O.M.; U.S.D.H.H.S., 2003).

Misdiagnosis leads to mistreatment in the form of no treatment, inappropriate treatment, or undertreatment. Tardive dyskinesia (a major side effect of major antipsychotic medication), excessive dosing, and as needed medications are complications more likely to occur in racial/ethnic minority groups than in the white population (Miranda et al., 2002; I.O.M., 2003; U.S.D.H.H.S., 2003). Unless a proper diagnosis is made, mindful of the varying presentations of mental health symptoms among racial/ethnic minorities and patient's acceptance of the interview process, which may not be culturally competent, effective treatment is unlikely to occur (I.O.M.).

Other studies indicate that minorities are likely to have untoward effects from treatment because of sensitivity to medication, improper medication, and intermittent or inappropriate treatment (I.O.M., 2003; U.S.D.H.H.S., 2003). Further, a lack of cultural competence among service providers has contributed to a lack of use of mental health services that contributes to the likelihood of minority persons receiving more inappropriate care than whites (I.O.M.; U.S.D.H.H.S.).

Stigma of people with mental illness has existed throughout history (I.O.M., 2003). Over this period of time, the treatment of mental illness has always been separated from the treatment of physical illness. Stigmatization of mental illness leads to the avoidance of and the treatment of persons with mental illness. Stigma is so widespread and such a formidable barrier to seeking mental health services that it is imperative to determine its dynamics and the impact on persons who need and deserve mental health services (U.S.D.H.H.S., 2003).

Significant gaps in nursing literature exist regarding minority mental health. Future research is needed to increase knowledge and ameliorate racism/discrimination, stigma, communication problems, misdiagnosis, and treatment in minority mental health (I.O.M., 2003; U.S.D.H.H.S., 2003). Mental health screening instruments need to demonstrate satisfactory reliability and validity across diverse ethnic minority populations to determine their cultural relevance and sensitivity (Baker & Bell, 1999). Although Baker and Bell addressed instrument appropriateness among mental health care of blacks, the data are generalizable to other racial/ethnic minorities.

The treatment outcomes for racial/ethnic minorities are influenced by the cultural incompetence and bias of providers (I.O.M., 2003; U.S.D.H.H.S., 2003; Sue, 2003). Diagnostic criteria for quantifying mental health symptoms exist, though their use may paradoxically limit the provider from making an appropriate clinical formulation when varying presentations of mental health symptoms in minority ethnic populations exist. An appendix to the DSM-IV TR (2000) features guidelines for the cultural formulation to be putatively incorporated into the clinical interview. These have not been included in the text as an integrated part of multiaxial assessment due to incomplete empirical data to guide practice. Cultural competence needs to be well-defined, evidence-based, and empirically-measured for its impact on outcomes associated with mental health therapies (Sue, 2003).

Cultural influences of both provider and patient potentiate communication difficulties that direct the uninformed provider to underestimate the prevalence of clinically-significant mental health symptoms among racial/ethnic minorities (Baker & Bell, 1999; I.O.M., 2003). After many years of looking at *ethnic* match of provider and client, where both are of a common ethnic background, *cultural* match, where the client regards the provider as culturally-sensitive, flexible, and willing to regard the individual's unique needs, is identified as a better predictor of positive health outcomes, treatment continuity, and function (Maramba & Hall, 2002). Also, studies (Miranda, 2003; Baker & Bell, 1999; I.O.M., 2003; U.S.D.H.H.S., 2003) have recommended that theoretically-based inquiry, culturally-appropriate measurements, and culturally-competent mental health treatment options comprise future scientific studies with racial/ethnic minority populations.

Knowledge development regarding the needs of racial/ethnic minorities is influenced by several factors, including historical and ethical influences, provider cultural incompetence, and the academic and clinical community's lack of consensus guiding inquiry into minority mental health care. Academic and empirical study of minority mental health and related disparities in mental health care are needed to correct the provider's knowledge and decrease prejudice. This is a step toward bringing the best evidence into day-to-day practice.

MARGARET A. WHEATLEY
EVANNE JURATOVAC

Dizziness in the Elderly

Dizziness is a common and perplexing complaint for older adults and their health providers. The many presentations of the symptom and multiple etiologies make diagnosis and treatment difficult. Since it cannot be seen, the symptom may be discounted by health professionals and treatment may be delayed. This elusive symptom effecting balance has been associated with falls, fear of falling, anxiety, functional decline, and a decrease in quality of life (Aggarwal et al., 2000; Yardley, 2000). Because dizziness results from impairments or diseases in multiple systems, Tinetti and colleagues (2000) suggested the best approach to dizziness is to consider it a geriatric syndrome. This designation would lead to a multifactorial approach to evaluation and treatment that has been successful with other geriatric syndromes such as falls and delirium. However, dizziness can often be linked to distinct underlying causes that can be treated (Drachman, 2000).

The prevalence of dizziness has been reported to range from 24% to 34% of older adults living in the community (Boult, Murphy, Sloane, Mor, & Drone, 1991; Tinetti, Williams, & Gill, 2000). Dizziness increases with age and is more common in women (Boult, Murphy, Sloane, & Drone, 1991; Aggarwal et al., 2000). One population-based study in a biracial community found a lower prevalence of 9.6% when defining dizziness as a regular symptom that occurred at least once per month (Aggerwal et al.), and dizziness was not associated with race.

Descriptions of dizziness can range from a sensation of spinning or motion to lightheadedness, fainting or falling, and many variations of these. Balance or the ability to maintain an upright position results from visual, proprioceptive, and vestibular input to the brain. Central integration and motor response are needed. Dizziness results when there is a mismatch between the messages as to our position in space. Aging can cause decreased efficiency or function in any or all of these balance mechanisms, which may explain the increased incidence of dizziness with age. The multiple disease processes which can result in a feeling of dizziness are many, making diagnosis and treatment difficult, and even deciding which specialist to refer a patient to can be challenging. But clinical characteristics usually help the practitioner determine a cause.

Recent efforts have focused on defining the symptom of dizziness and its subtypes so that it can be studied empirically in order to develop guidelines for medical practice. Sloane, Coeytaux, Beck, and Dallara (2001) proposed four subtypes of dizziness: *vertigo* is the feeling that the surroundings or person is moving or spinning, *presyncope* is the sensation of feeling faint or lightheaded, *disequilibrium* is the sense of unsteadiness, and a final category includes *other* sensations. While they note that the elderly may have difficulty placing their dizziness into one of these categories, these subtypes can give clues as to the underlying cause of the dizziness and appropriate treatment.

Vertigo is often caused by benign paroxysmal positional vertigo (BPPV) and may be caused by displaced otoconal crystals in the inner ear. Acute labyrinthitis and Meniere's disease are also common peripheral vestibular causes. Vertebrobasolar insufficiency may interrupt blood flow to the vestibular system. Presyncope is often related to cardiovascular causes including orthostatic hypotension, arrhythmia, transient ischemic attacks, carotid sinus hypersensitivity, and vasovagal syncope and is often associated with lightheadedness or syncope more than vertigo. Disequilibrium can also be due to vestibular causes or balance disorders. Medication effects, anxiety, and neurological conditions should also be explored.

Treatments for dizziness in elderly clients are based on the etiology of the symptom. Symptoms arising from cardiovascular disorders are often resolved through medical management. Postural hypotension may involve ongoing safety measures to avoid dizziness, lightheadedness, or falls. Benign paroxysmal positional vertigo often responds to movement therapy designed to move the displaced otoconia, through a 360° rotation of the head. Medication treatment can decrease the symptoms of Meniere's disease.

Despite medical strides, many must learn to live with ongoing symptoms. Patients can learn to manage their symptoms through an understanding of situations that exacerbate their symptoms and their responses. Yardley tested a nursing educational program including exercises that ameliorated anxiety and physical symptoms (Yardley, Beech, Zander, Evans, & Weinman, 1998). Vestibular rehabilitation using physical therapy can ameliorate symptoms, and one study has shown that older adults do just as well as younger adults in responding to a rehab program (Whitney, Wrisley, Marchetti, & Furman, 2002).

Dizziness has a negative impact on quality of life for older adults, causing feelings of insecurity and anxiety (Mendel, Bergenius, & Langius, 2001). Kao, Nanda, Williams, and Tinetti (2001) found dizziness associated with depression, anxiety, gait and balance disorders, medical conditions, and medications. Others have also found dizziness associated with falls (Lawson et al., 1999), fear of falling, which can lead to avoidance of activity (Yardley, 2000), and functional decline (Aggarwal et al., 2000).

Measures to explore the effects of dizziness have been developed. A vertigo symptoms scale was developed by Yardley, Masson, Verschuur, Haacke, and Luxon (1992) and used to examine the relationship of anxiety and vertigo, and in other studies. Questionnaires were completed by 127 patients from a specialty clinic. Factor analysis identified items for exploring symptoms of vertigo, anxiety, and somatization.

The Inventory for Dizziness (Hazlett, Tusa, & Waranch, 1996) measures symptoms, responses of significant others to the dizzy person, and activity levels. The instrument was an adaptation of a pain inventory, administered to 184 patients presenting to a specialty dizziness clinic. Factor analysis was used for item selection and factor development, and support further investigation of the instrument.

The Dizziness Handicap Inventory (DHI5) (Jacobson & Newman, 1990) was developed to explore the impact of dizziness on everyday life and includes 25 three-level items, and has been used in several studies. Effects were grouped into three categories: functional, emotional, and physical. The scale was tested in 63 patients who complained of dizziness and findings indicated good test-retest reliability as well as homogeneity of the constructs; another study demonstrated good test-retest reliability. A short version was developed by Tesio, Alpini, Cesarani, and Perucca (1999) using item-response methodology for item reduction. Dizziness is common and the difficulties of diagnosis and treatment only increase the patient's challenges in managing this uncomfortable symptom. Some measures have been developed to help understand the problem of dizziness and its impact. Further research is needed to explore the effects of dizziness and interventions to manage the symptoms. As new interventions are available for treatment, additional research into the best ways to educate and deliver information to older adults who suffer its consequences will be needed.

HELEN LACH

Doctoral Education

Doctoral education in nursing includes two general types of programs offering distinctly different types of degrees. The basic differentiation is between research-focused and practice-focused programs. Research-focused doctoral programs comprise the majority of programs. They are designed to prepare the graduate for a lifetime of scholarship and research. Research-focused doctoral programs offer either the academic doctorate (Doctor of Philosophy—PhD) or the professional Doctor of Nursing Science—DNS, DSN, or DNSc) degree; one research-focused program offers the EdD. Practice-focused doctoral programs, which are fewer in number, are designed to prepare the nurse for leadership in practice and for specialized advanced practice and administrative roles. The degree titles that are currently offered by practice-focused programs include the Doctor of Nursing (ND), and the Doctor of Nursing Practice (DNP or DrNP); one practice-focused program awards the DNS. Currently, over 88 institutions offer doctoral programs in nursing and several (7 currently) offer both a research-focused and a practice-focused program. Six programs are offered jointly or collaboratively between two or more institutions.

Over three fourths of existing programs offer the academic doctorate, reflecting the trend in research-oriented programs to offer the PhD rather than the professional degree, because the PhD is universally recognized and accepted and enjoys considerable prestige, particularly in academia. Curricula for programs leading to research-focused doctorates typically contain a core of required courses addressing nursing theory, methodology, theory development strategies, and various aspects of research methodology and statistics. Additionally, students usually are required to develop substantive expertise in a specialized area of nursing knowledge and research by selecting courses in nursing and related disciplines (cognates), becoming involved in hands-on research-related experiences such as research residencies or practica and research assistantships, and conducting a major independent research protect and writing the dissertation. Typically, half or more of the credits focus on research methodology and actual conduct of research. On the average, full-time students complete their doctoral study in 4 years: 2 years to complete the course work and an additional 2 years to complete the dissertation. Although the degree title is different, research-focused programs leading to the professional doctorate (DNS, DNSc, DSN) have curricula that are quite similar to the academic doctoral programs. Theoretically programs offering the DNS are more likely to emphasize research that is applied and relates directly to clinical, administrative, or policy-related practice and leadership. In addition to research preparation, curricula for such programs often include practicum experiences designed to develop a high level of research expertise in a specialized area of nursing practice. The required dissertation is often applied in nature. Graduates of research-focused programs are most likely to assume faculty positions upon graduation, but increasingly are being employed as researchers in clinical environments.

An important trend in nursing is the rapid increase in practice-focused doctoral programs. Although they are not new to nursing, practice-focused doctoral programs have received renewed interest as a viable alternative to the academic doctorate for individuals who wish to attain the highest level of expertise in clinical practice. The curricula differ considerably from those of the research-focused programs, with the major differences being that they typically have fewer credits addressing research and do not require a dissertation. Areas of content that are common to virtually all of the practice-focused doctoral programs include: the scientific underpinnings for practice; advanced practice in a given specialty area of nursing; organization and system leadership, change strategies and quality improvement; analytic methodologies related to the evaluation of practice and the accrual and application of evidence for practice; use of technology and information; development, application and evaluation of health policy; and interdisciplinary collaboration. In addition, programs provide the basis for advanced specialized expertise in at least one area of nursing practice. A dissertation is generally not required; however, most programs include a practice-related project and a residency experience. Some practice-focused doctoral programs limit their specialty areas to those concerned with the direct care of patients as implemented in advanced practice nursing roles (i.e., nurse practitioner, nurse midwife, nurse anesthetist, clinical nurse specialist), while others also include specialty preparation in administration or executive practice. There are several different points of entry into practice-focused doctoral programs; some require students to enter with some specialty preparation at the master's level and others permit post-baccalaureate entry. In all cases, graduates are expected to provide visionary leadership in the practice arena as advanced practice nurses, program managers and evaluators, and nursing service administrators. Graduates of practice-focused doctoral programs frequently assume positions as clinical educators in schools of nursing.

Historically, doctoral nursing education began at Teachers College, Columbia University, and at New York University in the 1920s. After a 30-year hiatus during which no new programs were opened, interest in doctoral education was rekindled; by the end of the 1970s, a total of 18 programs had been initiated. During the 1980s the number of programs more than doubled, and with the rapid increase in programs and enrollments came concern about maintaining high quality. The American Association of Colleges of Nursing took a leadership role in developing indicators of quality regarding student and faculty qualifications, curriculum content, administrative patterns, and support resources. During the 1990s, ideas about the nature of scholarship and doctoral education were refined as the emphasis on establishing and maintaining quality continued. Emphasis expanded from the tools of scholarship to increasingly addressing the growing body of substantive nursing knowledge. The disproportionate focus on process changed to greater emphasis on the content that constitutes the input to and products of the scientific process.

In addition to the growing interest in practice-focused doctoral programs, an important trend is that increasingly students are being encouraged to progress as quickly as possible toward the terminal degree. Fueled in part by a growing faculty shortage and the need to produce more doctoral graduates, programs are increasingly streamlining progression between degree levels and eliminating work experience as prerequisite to admission. As a result the profile of the "typical" doctoral student is changing. The average age of doctoral nursing students is gradually decreasing, and students often enter doctoral study from clinical as well as academic backgrounds.

Doctoral education continues to be an arena of excitement and innovation in nursing education. The need for doctoral graduates continues to escalate, yet the challenge to maintain quality in the face of rapid change is of paramount concern. For individuals, the doctorate is the pinnacle of attainment in nursing education, and for institutions it is the pinnacle of academic attainment. The virtually universal acceptance of the doctorate as the terminal degree signifies nursing's status as a true academic discipline.

ELIZABETH R. LENZ

Drinking and Driving Among Adolescents

Drinking and driving is rooted in the central role that alcohol plays in American life and culture. Alcohol is commonly found at celebrations, parties, and leisure activities. In addition, advertisements on television, magazines, and billboards present messages that shine a positive light on drinking. Given this situation and despite drinking laws, adolescents drink and drive, and adolescents who have been drinking are involved in fatal crashes at twice the rate of adult drivers (National Highway Traffic Safety Administration, 2002). Thirty percent of youth aged 15 to 20 who were killed in automobile accidents had been drinking (National Center on Addiction and Substance Abuse at Columbia University, 2002).

Six articles on drinking/driving were published in the nursing literature from 1995 to 2001. No nursing publications were uncovered on drinking/driving for 2002 and 2003. Only two of the six focused on drinking/driving among adolescents (Kuthy, Grap, Penn, & Henderson, 1995; Shreve, 1998). Kuthy and colleagues evaluated a 20-minute program showing pictures of automobile accidents to determine if there was a change in drinking/driving behavior after the program. One month after the program a telephone interview indicated that the 274 high school driver's education students showed a significant change in drinking/driving behavior. Shreve evaluated a student drinking/driving prevention program with 39 students. Following the program, 40% of the students indicated they would change their behavior. It can be concluded that little has been published in the nursing literature on drinking/driving and there are no studies focusing on intervening in drinking/driving situations. However, health promotion is a major goal of nursing, and investigating intervening as a passenger in drinking/driving situations may offer approaches to change behavior that may prevent the injurious consequences associated with drinking/driving among adolescents.

In a national study of 10,277 drunken driving fatalities, Isaacs, Kennedy, and Graham (1995) found that in 5% to 10% of these cases there were sober passengers who could have intervened. Furthermore, half of the fatalities in persons 16 to 19 years of age had at least one sober passenger in the car who could have intervened. In a study of adolescents in grades 9–12 conducted in 199 schools in 34 states, 30% reported that in the previous 30 days they had ridden with a driver who had been drinking alcohol and 13% had driven a car or other vehicle after drinking alcohol (Grunbaum et al., 2002).

Shore and Compton (2000) describe successful interventions in drinking/driving as forceful statements, clear demands, and concrete actions. These are more effective than requests, pleas, or suggestions. Thus, more assertive interventions tend to be more successful than less assertive interventions. Threatening the drinking driver's competence is less likely to be effective in stopping the drinker from driving (Shore & Compton, 1998). Smart and Stoduto (1997) found that people tend to intervene more with friends than with strangers. Having some familiarity with the intoxicated individual seems to be more conducive to intervening. Smith and colleagues (2004) in a qualitative study on intervening as a passenger in drinking/driving queried 52 youths about drinking/driving situations and interventions. Findings of the study included the following drinking/driving situations where the participants were: entangled with a drinking driver who was determined to drive, endangered while riding in a car with a drinking driver, and stranded because they did not get in the car with a drinking driver and had no one to turn to for a ride. Interventions described by the participants were: to persuade, to interfere, to plan ahead, and to threaten. It can be concluded that if youth passengers intervene and break the link between drinking and driving there is potential for reducing drinking/driving fatalities.

Mary Jane Smith

Drug Abuse

Drug abuse or addiction is a chronic, relapsing, and treatable disease subcategory of psychiatric illnesses called substance-abuse disorders (American Psychiatric Association [APA], 1994). The most common drugs of abuse in the U.S., other than alcohol, nicotine, and caffeine, are cocaine (crack), amphetamines, cannabis (marijuana), hallucinogens, inhalants, opioids, phencyclidine (PCP), sedatives, hypnotics, and anxiolytics (antianxiety agents). Drug abuse interferes with normal brain functioning, usually creating powerful feelings of pleasure or euphoria; however, there are long-term effects on brain metabolism and activity such that physical addiction and craving for more of the drug occurs (http://www.nida.gov/Infofax/understand.html).

The societal economic impact of drug abuse in the U.S. was estimated at $97.7 billion per year in 1992. These costs included crime, medical care, drug addiction treatment, social welfare programs, and lost work. Money spent on illicit drug purchases was found to be $57.3 billion, of which $38 billion was paid for cocaine, $9.6 billion for heroin, $7 billion for marijuana, and the rest for all other illegal drugs or misuse of legal drugs (White House Office of National Drug Control Policy [ONDCP], 1996).

Most drug abusers are men. In 1995 there were 874,000 admissions to publicly funded treatment facilities, with men accounting for 70% and women 30% of admissions. The largest percentage of admissions was for cocaine (38.3%), followed by heroin (25.5%) and marijuana (19.1%). Treatment methods include behavioral therapies (counseling, psychotherapy, support groups, or family therapy), treatment medications (methadone maintenance for heroin addiction), short-term and residential in-patient treatment, drug-free outpatient treatment, and therapeutic communities. In general longer and more comprehensive treatment programs have better results compared to short-term or minimalist treatment programs (http://nida.nih.gov/Infofax/treatmeth.html).

Drug abuse among women often presents different health and treatment challenges compared to men. Up to 70% of drug-abusing women report histories of physical and sexual abuse and drug and alcohol abuse in one or both parents. Case finding and treatment are exceptionally difficult because drug-abusing women are often in relationships with drug-abusing partners and they have well-founded fears of losing the relationship and its economic protection if they seek treatment. Treatment for women often means falling into poverty, homelessness, powerlessness, and losing custody of their children. Furthermore, drug-abusing women were found to have exceptionally low self-esteem, self-confidence, and sense of powerlessness, making the decision to seek drug treatment a daunting experience.

Among both men and women there have been recent increases in illicit use of prescription opiates (oxycodone, hydrocodone), while cocaine/crack use has decreased slightly. Use of PCP and club drugs (MDMA/Ecstasy, GHB/date rape drugs, and Ketamine/Special K/Vitamin K) has increased. The GHB trend is of particular concern as the drug is tasteless and often is put into drinks without the victim being aware of ingesting the drug. Women on college campuses are especially at risk for this scenario.

Areas for future research include prevention research on the special issues facing men versus women and specific to each age group from school-aged youth through the elderly. The major foci of prevention research—the individual, the peer group, or the community all require additional research and theory development and testing. Genetic research is adding new insights every day and young scientists would do well to become trained in this area so as to be on the cutting edge of drug-abuse knowledge development. Better approaches to case finding and referral for treatment are needed. Finally, the realm of drug-abuse treatment is fraught with dropsouts, treatment failures, and relapses. Creative new treatment modalities need to be developed and tested. Rather than one-size-fits-all treatment modalities, perhaps it is time to develop ones that are designed to best match the needs of a specific subpopulation—youth, adolescents, adult women, adult men, or elderly men or women.

JOANNE SABOL STEVENSON

Dysphagia

Dysphagia is a symptom exhibited by either difficulty swallowing or pain on swallowing that is experienced on a continuum from the inability to move food back in the mouth to a total inability to take nourishment. While the prevalence of dysphagia in the general population is unknown, risk has been estimated in adults over 50 from 16% to 22%. The number of nursing home residents requiring extensive to total assistance with eating, sometimes an indicator of swallowing problems, ranges between 17% to 43% depending on the state (Centers for Medicare and Medicaid, 2001; Lindgren & Janzon, 1991). Generally, persons most likely to be at high risk for dysphagia include persons with head injuries, stroke, Parkinson's disease, and malignancy of the head and neck (Lind, 2003). Persons with severe cognitive impairments may simply forget how to eat or may have accompanying neurological compromise affecting the swallow.

Swallowing has both voluntary and involuntary phases; the oral stage, where food is masticated and moved back to the pharynx, is under conscious control, and the pharyngeal and esophageal stages, where food is automatically moved through coordinated reflexive actions, is under involuntary control. Thus, depending on an individual's health problem, such as impairment of the neuromuscular pathways, structural or connective tissue diseases, or mental disorders ranging from Alzheimer's disease to psychogenic dysphagia, dysphagia may occur anywhere along the route food and fluid take to the stomach. While aging has been suggested as a risk factor for dysphagia, there is currently no evidence to substantiate this claim among healthy older adults and the reasons it is seen are more likely related to other factors such as poor oral health or adverse effects of medications.

Identification of persons with dysphagia can be a critical assessment that the nurse needs to make early to prevent further problems and start effective treatment for a potentially occult disease. Accompanying symptoms (Palmer, 2002) associated with all stages of dysphagia include weight loss, dehydration, complaints of food "sticking" in the throat, change in dietary habits, and drooling, while oral and pharyngeal dysphagia includes a change in voice, coughing, difficulty initiating a swallow, and coughing or choking with swallow. Persons with esophageal dysphagia experience recurrent pneumonias. For some individuals, dysphagia may be temporary and with aggressive rehabilitation may reverse, for example in the acute stroke victim. However, for persons with progressive diseases such as dementia and Parkinson's disease, the goal of care is to maintain functional and safe swallowing for as long as possible.

Ethical issues in dysphagia dramatically increased within the past 5 years as results from large studies began to demonstrate the medical futility of tube feeding in persons with severe cognitive impairments. As providers of information and counseling to families and caregivers regarding end-of-life decision making, nurses need to be familiar with these findings. While the ethical arguments of "sanctity of life" versus "quality of life" are often at the core of debates regarding use of tube feeding for persons with dementia, the issue may initially present as a safety problem: should someone with a severe cognitive impairment with an ineffective swallow who is losing weight be tube fed? A review of the literature concerning the use of enteral feeding in persons with severe cognitive impairments by Finucane, Christmas, and Travis (1999) demonstrated that much of the justification for use of tubes was not supported by well designed studies: the prevention of the consequences of malnutrition, improved survival, change in pressure ulcer status, decline in risk of infection, improvement of functional status and comfort. By using a national nursing home database, the Minimum Data Set (MDS), researchers found wide regional variation in use of tube feeding in this impaired population (Aronheim, Mulvihill, Sieger, Park, & Fries, 2001) and that select organizational characteristics, e.g., larger, for-profit homes in urban areas lacking a nurse practitioner, influenced the rate of tube feeding (Mitchell, Teno, Roy, Kabumoto, & Mor, 2003). Several national organizations, including the Hospice and Palliative Nurses Association (HPNA) (2003), developed a position statement on the use of artificial nutrition and hydration in which they addressed the point at the end of life when persons are unable to take foods because of dysphagia or other problems, or resist foods. While not advocating for either using or not using tube feedings, the HPNA recommended counseling patients, families, and caregivers concerning the benefits and burdens of this intervention as well as advocating for advance care planning concerning this issue. Thus, nurses need to consider causes of dysphagia, the individual's capacity for rehabilitation, prior declarations regarding end-of-life care, and put possible treatments into an evidence-based perspective when they consider this issue in persons with severe cognitive impairments (Amella, 2003).

Assessment of dysphagia can be accomplished by the nurse through the use of psychometrically sound instruments; two instruments were developed in the past 5 years, the McGill Ingestive Skills Assessment (MISA) (Lambert, Gisel, Groher, & Wood-Dauphinee, 2003) and the Massey Bedside Swallowing Screen (MBSS) (Massey & Jedlicka, 2002). The MISA addresses a range of criteria—positioning, texture management, feeding skills, liquid and solid ingestion, and has good interrater reliability and internal consistency. However, the testing of the MBSS was criticized for having too broad inclusion criteria, small sample size, and questionable screening criteria (Sasaki & Leder, 2003).

Nurses should not only be assessing who is at risk for dysphagia, but once this is known, who will develop complications. Using MDS data from three states ($n = 102{,}842$), Langmore, Kimberly, Skarupski, Park, and Fries (2002) sought to determine predictors of aspiration pneumonia, one of the assumed consequences of dysphagia. In this descriptive study, the researchers found that of the 3% of the residents who had pneumonia ($n = 3{,}118$), 18 factors predicted aspiration using a logistic regression model: the highest were suctioning, chronic obstructive pulmonary disease (COPD), congestive heart failure (CHF), tube feeding, bedfast, Case mix index, indicators of delirium, weight loss, and dysphagia/swallowing problems, while interestingly, cerebrovascular accident (CVA) was actually protective (OR = .83). Results of this large study support and refute an earlier 5-year study led by the same author (Langmore et al., 1998) that examined predictors of aspiration: tube feeding was found to be a predictor of aspiration in both studies, dysphagia was not found to be a predictor in the earlier study while feeding dependence was the strongest predictor in the earlier study but was only mildly predictive in the larger. Researchers sought to determine if persons who had experienced a stroke were aware of their swallowing problems and would alter their eating patterns, thus decreasing complications. In a descriptive study of 27 persons who were determined to be dysphagic by a speech pathologist, only 3 had awareness of their problem when directly asked (Parker, C., et al., 2004). Poor awareness of swallowing problems also was a predictor at 3 months for persons with more complications. Westergren, Ohlsson, and Rahm Hallberg (2001) found that among patients who were admitted to a facility after stroke with swallowing difficulties ($n = 24$) and received individualized nursing interventions, the level of alertness and the energy level of the patients was most predictive of increased ability to eat and swallow and development of further complications.

It is critical for nurses to examine quality-of-life issues for all persons with impairment in eating and swallowing problems. Several studies (Perry & McLaren, 2003; Mercadante, Casuccio, & Fulfaro, 2000; Sjostrom, Holmberg, & Strang, 2002) showed that among persons with stroke and progressive cancer, dysphagia can be both painful as well as a barrier to the enjoyment of previous activities. Nursing interventions should facilitate the social as well as nutritional aspects of meals so that the one of the critical factors to eating—the pleasure of a good meal and good company—is not lost.

ELAINE J. AMELLA

E

Elder Mistreatment

Elder mistreatment (EM) is a complex syndrome that can lead to morbid or even fatal outcomes for those afflicted. *Mistreatment* is the term used to describe outcomes from such actions as abuse, neglect, exploitation, and abandonment of the elderly, and it affects all socioeconomic, cultural, ethnic, and religious groups. The prevalence of EM is estimated between 700,000 and 1.2 million cases annually in this country (Pillemer & Finkelhor, 1988). The National Elder Abuse Incidence Study documented over 500,000 new cases annually (Tatara, 1993).

The National Research Council (NRC) (2003) convened an expert panel to review prevalence and risk for elder abuse and neglect and concluded that EM is an intentional action that causes harm or creates a serious risk of harm (whether or not harm is intended) to an at-risk elder by a caregiver or other person who stands in a trusting relationship to the elder, or is the failure by a caregiver to satisfy the elder's basic needs or to protect the elder from harm. There are several types of EM described in the NRC report. *Abuse* is generally understood as physical assault inflicted on an older adult resulting in harmful effects. Abusive behavior may include hitting, kicking, punching, and other physical contact. *Neglect* is the refusal or failure to fulfill any part of a caregiver's obligations or duties to an older adult. Neglect may be intentional or unintentional. Self-neglect occurs when an older adult, either knowingly or unknowingly, lives in such a manner that is deleterious to his or her health. *Exploitation* is fraudulent activity in connection with an older adult's property or assets, and *abandonment* is defined as the deliberate and abrupt withdrawal of services in caring for an older adult. *Restriction* as a form of EM has recently been examined in an investigation of caregiver behaviors that have fewer social sanctions but may be equally deleterious to the older person (Fulmer & Gurland, 1996). Evidence suggests that only 1 in 14 EM cases is reported to some public agency. Nurses can do much to help in the screening and detection process of EM by doing a careful history and physical assessment with attention to the subjective complaint of EM, along with any signs or symptoms of the same. Underreporting of EM is a serious concern because older adults may have disease symptoms or age-related changes that imitate or conceal mistreatment symptoms, making the assessment process complex. Few clinicians have been trained in EM assessment and intervention, which has also led to underreporting. With an unprecedented number of individuals living beyond the age of 65 and even beyond the age of 85, nurses must be sensitive to the possibility of EM (Bergeron & Gray, 2003; Capezuti, Brush, & Lawson, 1997; Fulmer et al., 2003; Fulmer, Guadagno, Bitondo Dyer, & Connolly, 2004; Harrell et al., 2002; Heath, Dyer, Kerzner, Mosqueda, & Murphy, 2002).

Theories for EM causality have been posited. The dependency theory refers to the amount of care an elder person requires and is related to stressed caregiver research, which describes overwhelmed caregivers who lose their control or stop providing reasonable care. Conversely, there are data that reflect the caregiver's dependency on the elder (for shelter, money, etc.), which puts the elder at risk. Transgenerational violence theory refers to children who learn violent behavior as normal and then become violent and abusive as they grow older. This might be viewed from a learning theory perspective, although some have looked at it as a retribution act: an adult child may strike back at a parent or caregiver who was once abusive. The psychopathology of the abuser theory refers to any nonnormal caregiver, such as substance abusers (alcohol, drugs), psychiatrically impaired individuals, or mentally retarded caregivers. The number of mentally retarded elders over 65 years of age has grown substantially over the past decade, creating situations where mentally retarded or disabled offspring become caregivers for very elderly parents (National Research Council, 2003).

Early studies looked at the prevalence of EM from a variety of perspectives: acute care, community nursing care, and the nursing home setting. Differences in operational definitions, methodological approaches, and the lack of national prevalence studies have made it difficult to understand the conditions under which EM is likely to occur. Although EM education and training has improved, there is still a great need for more systematic nursing assessment, care planning, and follow-up with the older adult. The need for researchers who can contribute to this area of inquiry is great.

There is no Denver Developmental screen for older adults that enables the clinician to understand what an 80-year-old looks like and what conditions are likely to represent EM. Signs and symptoms of EM might include unexplained bruises, fractures, burns, poor hydration, reports of hitting or any other violent behavior against the older adult, sexually transmitted disease in institutionalized older adults, unexplained loss of money or goods, evidence of fearfulness around a caregiver, or the subjective report of abuse. It is especially difficult to evaluate the demented older adult for EM; a careful and thorough interdisciplinary team approach is required. The American Medical Association's *Diagnostic and Treatment Guidelines on Elder Abuse and Neglect* (American Medical Association, 1992; Aravanis et al., 1993), although over 10 years old, provides excellent guidelines for the assessment of EM, along with flowcharts for assessing and intervening in cases. A summary of EM instruments for screening and assessment is available (Fulmer, Hyex, et al., 2004). Special attention must be given to an older adult who has diminished or absent decision-making capacity. Dementia has been documented as a risk factor for EM and should automatically trigger EM assessment (Lachs, Williams, O'Brien, Hurst, & Horwitz, 1997; Coyne, A. G., Reichman, & Berbig, 1993). Cognitive status can only be determined by rigorous clinical testing and use of validated instruments. Overzealous protection of a competent elder is a form of ageism that infantilizes the older individual and takes away their autonomy. Each state has elder mistreatment reporting laws or requirements that professionals should be familiar with. Interdisciplinary care teams are especially important in the EM assessment process. Each team member is able to use their own expertise to the benefit of older adults (Fulmer et al., 2003). A key practice implication for EM is the inclusion of family violence questions in every history with attention to and documentation of any signs or symptoms of EM.

TERRY FULMER

Electronic Network

In general, a network is composed of a minimum of two connected points. For example, one person talking with another, face-to-face, can constitute a network. Telephone networks connect at least two people using transceivers, wire, switches, and computers. Television networks connect large numbers of people. An electronic network is considered to be the connection or linking of two or more computers to allow data and information exchange. Electronic computer networks may be as small as two computers or as large as the Internet, considered to be a network of networks.

The goal of networks is information exchange and may or may not be bidirectional. Person-to-person conversations, even if using some sort of intermediary like the telephone, are usually bidirectional. Television and some computer network applications may be unidirectional; however, bidirectional computer networks are the most common. Examples include local area networks (LAN), which may serve a department; larger networks called wide area networks (WAN); and the Internet. Intranets, which are the internal deployment of Internet technologies, are becoming more and more common.

Electronic networks are exciting tools for nursing and will be increasingly important in information acquisition and dispersion. Electronic networks, such as the Internet and the World Wide Web (WWW), not only provide a means of communicating but also facilitate collaborative research, promote education regardless of geographic limitations, and allow access and acquisition of needed resources. Electronic networks will continue to affect areas integral to nursing, such as a lifetime electronic health record, nursing research, increased interdisciplinary collaborative research, education without walls for patients and nurses, and nursing knowledge acquisition and information exchange.

Although the essence of nursing has been a network, that is, the nurse-patient relationship, there is limited nursing research on electronic networks. Brennan, Moore, and Smyth (1991) and Ripich, Moore, and Brennan (1992) investigated the use of electronic networks to facilitate nursing support of home care clients and their caregivers. They concluded that a computer network is an excellent tool to facilitate support and information exchange among caregivers and between nurses and caregivers for patients with AIDS and Alzheimer's disease.

There are anecdotal reports and case studies to support nurses' use of electronic networks. Sparks (1993) has been instrumental in her advocacy and promotion of electronic networks and resource availability for nurses. In the early 1990s she championed the Educational Technology Network (E.T.Net). E.T. Net promoted the exchange of information and ideas for nurses, nurse educators, and nursing students. It was the first international electronic network managed by a nurse. Barnsteiner's (1993) and Graves's (1993) work with nursing resource availability (Online Journal of Nursing Knowledge Synthesis and the Virginia Henderson STTI Electronic Library, respectively) and DuBois and Rizzolo's (1994) in the *American Journal of Nursing's* AJN Network to promote continuing education for nurses are additional examples of nursing use of electronic networks.

As information technology increases in use and health care requires increased efficiency, nurses will rely more and more on information technology as one tool for providing the best possible patient care. Local electronic networks, such as clinical information systems, will include other larger networks so that nurses will have the best information resources to assist nursing care. Research concerning the effects of electronic networking on nurses and other health care professionals, as well as on patients and their families, is needed. Electronic networking should be examined as an independent variable through the inclusion of electronic networks in all stages of the research process. This research will promote the advancement of health and patient care by providing the scientific foundation for the appropriate application of electronic networking technologies.

W. Scott Erdley
Susan M. Sparks

Emergency Nursing

Emergency nursing is by its very nature multifaceted. Emergency patients range from newborns to the "old-old" and the nursing and medical diagnoses for which they seek treatment include common illnesses such as flu symptoms to life-threatening injuries or events. Emergency nursing research, then, has many foci. The breadth of emergency nursing care enables emergency nurses to apply evidence-based knowledge from other clinical nursing specialties, but emergency nursing presents challenges that are unique to the emergency or urgent care setting.

While the exact number is unknown, it is estimated that about 80,000 RNs consider emergency nursing to be their clinical specialty. What is known is that in 2003, Americans made 110.2 million visits to hospital emergency departments (National Hospital Ambulatory Medical Care Survey: 2002 Emergency Department Summary, Centers for Disease Control and Prevention [CDC]). This represents a 23% increase in emergency department usage in the past decade. Of note is that while usage of the emergency department has increased, the number of emergency departments in the U.S. has decreased by approximately 15% (National Center for Health Statistics, March, 2004).

In 1991, the Emergency Nurses Association (ENA) Foundation was established as a means to provide funding (and encouragement) for peer reviewed research. In addition, shortly thereafter, a doctorally prepared nurse researcher was hired to be the Director of Research at the Emergency Nurses Association's headquarters. Several multisite studies were developed and conducted by a team of researchers, using practicing emergency nurses as data collectors. The convergence of these factors served to aid in the creation of a "research culture" as a visible component of emergency nursing.

As noted by Bayley, MacLean, Desy, and McMahon (2004), the number of emergency nursing research articles increased from 49 studies in the years between 1982–1991 to 262 published studies between 1992–2002, representing a fivefold increase. They found, however, that emergency nursing research was "scattered across many topics."

As the major source of funding for emergency nursing research, the ENA Foundation established a list of "research initiatives" that would receive preference in funding decisions. The current research initiatives are: (a) mechanisms to assure effective, efficient, and quality emergency nursing care delivery; (b) effective and efficient outcomes of emergency nursing services and procedures; (c) factors affecting emergency nursing practice; (d) influence of health care technologies, facilities, and equipment on emergency nursing practice; (e) factors affecting health care cost, productivity, and market forces to emergency services; (f) ways to enhance health promotion and injury prevention; (g) methods for handling complex ethical issues related to emergency care; and (h) mechanisms to assure quality and cost-effective educational programs for emergency nurses.

While these initiatives gave a sense of direction, in many ways they were considered to be too broad to foster the concerted effort needed to build an emergency nursing knowledge base necessary for evidence-based practice. Excellent studies that have had important consequences for the care of emergency patients and their families have been the direct result of funding provided by the ENA Foundation. One such study involved the issue of family presence during resuscitation. The concept of family members being present at stressful times has received a good deal of attention, not only by and for emergency nurses, but this knowledge base has been extended to use in other areas of nursing.

A review of research presentations and posters displayed at the most recent annual meeting of the Emergency Nurses Association can give an overview of topics of interest in emergency nursing research. Included in oral presentations were topics focusing on blood-drawing techniques, injury prevention, use of the emergency department for nonurgent illnesses, emergency nurse burnout, and aspects of pain management. Some examples of poster presentations included: triage, trauma care, standardized language usage (NIC, NOC, NANDA), pain management protocols, and pediatric issues. It becomes clear that although the research culture in emergency nursing has consistently increased and excellent studies are being conducted, the issue of the research being scattered rather than focused remains a concern.

The Emergency Nurses Association also has worked closely with the U.S. Coast Guard in research funded by the Coast Guard to examine factors related to boating injuries. This is in keeping with a commitment of the Association to engage in injury prevention activities from a number of different perspectives. In addition, the Association has also conducted extensive research funded by the Health Resources and Services Administration's Maternal and Child Health Bureau (HRSA/MCHB) focused on the provision of family-centered care in the emergency department.

In 2002, Bayley, MacLean, Desy, and McMahon, with funding and support from the Emergency Nurses Association and the ENA Foundation, undertook a Delphi study to identify and prioritize "research questions of greatest value to emergency nurses and of highest importance for health care consumers." Participants in the study were highly experienced in emergency nursing and most had advanced degrees. After the round I responses were collapsed into 154 research topics, participants in round II were asked to evaluate each of the topics using two questions: "(1) what is the value of research on this question for practicing emergency nurses, and (2) what is the importance of research on this question for consumers of emergency nursing services?"

Results demonstrated that the answer to the first question about value of the research question to practicing emergency nurses concerned issues related to staffing, holding patients in the emergency department for long periods of time, and the ongoing educational needs of emergency nurses. The second question, having to do with the importance of the research to consumers of emergency care, issues of pain management were of most concern. Other areas of highly ranked research needs for emergency nurses included methods of effective patient education, and the provision of sufficient numbers of adequately prepared professional nurses for the care of persons with emergency health problems.

The authors noted the consistency of the findings with ENA's mission and values, especially the value statement "All individuals have a right to quality emergency care delivered with compassion." They postulated that all of the highly ranked research topics had safety and quality of care as the central organizing principle. The information derived from this important study will be of immense help to future emergency nurse researchers as well as practicing emergency nurses who seek to provide the most relevant, evidence-based practice to their patients. The results of the study can organize and focus future research endeavors as well as establish funding priorities for the ENA Foundation and others. The future for emergency nursing research is brighter because of the Delphi study. Now, emergency nursing researchers will be able to develop the knowledge base essential for effective emergency nursing practice.

Anne Manton

Empathy

Empathy is a dimension of nursing that is central to caring competence, and it is often touted as the essence and art of nursing. Empathy in nursing is the ability of nurses to penetrate the covert thoughts and feelings of the client, to accurately interpret the client's thoughts and feelings as if they were their own, and to verbally and nonverbally convey that interpretation back to the client in forming a positive nurse-client relationship. When empathy is appropriately expressed it is in the form of sincerity, genuine positive regard, and sensitive understanding of the client's private world. Empathic nursing care has been shown to improve physiological and psychological outcomes for clients (Hope-Stone & Mills, 2001).

Carl Rogers (1961) believed that empathy is the ability to perceive the internal frame of reference of another with such exactness as to be one with the other person's frame of reference. Carper (1978) correlated empathy with aesthetic knowing in her description of fundamental patterns of knowing in nursing.

From a historical perspective, the roots of morality are found in empathy. Being able to empathize with potential victims encourages people to act and help others. Empathy underlies many facets of moral judgment and action. An instance when empathy leads to moral action is when a bystander is moved to intervene on behalf of a victim; the more empathy a bystander feels for the victim the more likely it is that the bystander will intervene (Goldman, 1998). The level of empathy felt toward another will shape one's moral judgments and empathic attitudes. Putting oneself in another's place leads people to follow certain moral principles.

Developmentally, there is a natural progression of empathy from infancy onward. At 1 year, children feel distress and will start to cry when they see another child cry. After 1 year, the child will try to sooth another child that is crying. The most advanced level of empathy emerges in late childhood when children begin to feel empathy for the plight of an entire group, such as the poor or the oppressed. During adolescence, empathic understanding can reinforce moral convictions developed earlier in life that center on a desire to alleviate misfortune and injustice (Goldman, 1998).

Early nursing research on empathy indicated that empathy development programs had little to no effect on empathy. However, later studies have shown that by including strategies such as art, nurse educators can enhance basic empathy among nursing students, which may have implications for nurses.

Kunyk and Olson (2001) described the concept of empathy found in the nursing literature between 1992 and 2000. They found five conceptualizations of empathy: (a) empathy as a human trait, (b) empathy as a professional state, (c) empathy as communication process, (d) empathy as caring, and (e) empathy as a special relationship. Nurse authors are approaching empathy from a variety of perspectives, time frames, measurements, and outcomes indicating advancement of the science regarding empathy in nursing.

G. Evans, Wilt, Alligood, and O'Neil (1998) addressed empathy as a multidimensional phenomenon and stressed the importance of understanding two types of empathy: basic and trained. They likened basic empathy to natural, raw, or ordinary feelings for others, such as the innate tendency of a child to cry when recognizing distress in another human. They likened trained empathy to increased empathy as a result of knowledge and education. They used the *Layton Empathy Test* and the *Hogan Empathy Scale* to measure trained and basic empathy in 106 nursing students and found that trained empathy was not sustained over time, causing the researchers to call into question attempts by nursing faculties to teach empathy to students. They emphasized the importance of obtaining a measurement of students' baseline empathy as a way of monitoring changes in basic empathy after exposure to various empathy learning modalities. G. Evans and colleagues (1998) suggested new approaches to facilitate students' discovery of their basic empathy and emphasized that basic empathy can be identified, reinforced, and refined in order to develop expertise in the expression of empathy.

Oz (2001) conducted a quasi-experimental investigation of empathy with 260 nurses who were randomly assigned to intervention and control groups. They utilized *Dokmen's Scale of Empathic Skills*, and the *Empathic Tendency Scale* to measure empathic communication skills and empathic tendency levels. Their intervention consisted of education about empathic communication. Results indicated that nurses gained empathic communication skills as a result of empathy training. However, this training did not significantly change the nurses' basic empathic tendency levels.

Wikstrom (2001) investigated the effect of an intervention program on student nurses' engagement in learning about empathy. The investigator assigned participants to intervention and control groups. The intervention group received empathy exercises involving the use of a reproduction of Edvard Munch's painting, "*The Sick Girl*," to stimulate discussion and account-making regarding interpretations of empathy depicted in the painting. There was a significant improvement in the intervention group members' levels of empathy as compared to the matched control group. The research findings supported the use of art as a complementary strategy to theoretical knowledge on empathy to stimulate nurses' basic empathy.

Kunyk and Olson (2001) found evidence that the concept of empathy is being advanced conceptually and empirically with more depth and breadth in the nursing literature. They, however, insisted that a more mature concept of empathy must emerge before empathy can be fully useful in nursing practice, research, and education.

Alligood (2001) and the Empathy Research Team at the University of Tennessee, Knoxville, developed an implicit middle range theory of empathy to explain how the concept of empathy operates within the context of King's general systems framework of personal, interpersonal, and social systems. A middle range theory of empathy conceptualized within this established nursing framework provides new understandings of basic empathy for nursing. According to Alligood, empathy has been viewed from a behavioral (state) approach; however, the more current view of empathy emanates from a developmental (trait) perspective. Viewing empathy as a state rather than a trait of individuals represents a perspectival shift and opens avenues for research in nursing related to empathy and emphasizes the importance that nurses have to develop and understand their own empathy as a basis for clinical practice (Alligood).

In the past 20 years, empathy has been conceptually and empirically advanced in the nursing literature. Studies have raised critical questions about the nature of empathy and how empathy may or may not be teachable using various educational and experiential strategies. Research findings suggest that baseline measurements of empathy in nurses and nursing students can be a starting point for developing strategies to enhance empathic responding to clients. Nursing as a profession needs more replication of studies to identify basic empathy skills and to discern the differential impact of empathy education versus empathy education combined with experiential exercises in empathic understanding such as art, film, and literature. With continued research and growth in the understanding of empathy, the art of nursing can be enhanced.

Dianna Hutto Douglas

End-of-Life Planning and Choices

End-of-life (EOL) planning and decision-making (i.e., choices) have been explored from myriad perspectives: patient, family, or surrogate decision maker, professional provider, informal or formal caregiver, health system costs, ethics and morality, law and regulation, barriers and facilitators, consumer and professional education needs, culture, sites of care, and organizational characteristics. Research represents virtually all health care clinical and management domains and is widely published in peer-review journals. The nursing research surrounding decision-making capacity, life-sustaining treatment decisions, age and site-specific issues (e.g., pediatrics, nursing homes), clinical issues (e.g., pain, change of condition), and ethicomoral perspectives on choices at the end of life, is presented here.

Clinicians, ethicists, and legal scholars agree that the decision to choose/appoint another to make decisions for one in the event of loss of decision-making capacity (i.e., Durable Power of Attorney for Health Care/ Health Care Proxy [HCP]) is less risky and requires less cognitive capacity than the creation of a list of treatments desired and not desired at some point in the future regarding unknown conditions (i.e., Living Will). There is scant research on how nurses assess a patient's decisional capacity to make choices about life-sustaining treatments. Molloy et al. (1996) assessed individuals living in nursing homes, retirement homes, and homes for the aged for their capacity to create an advance directive (AD). Five different measures of capacity were used, including assessment by a specially trained nurse and by a geriatrician independent of each other. The investigators determined that it was possible to differentiate between those who could learn about and create an AD from those who could not, using the Standardized Mini-Mental Status Examination (SMMSE). Mezey, Teresi, Ramsey, Mitty, and Bobrowitz (2000) developed an instrument ("Guidelines") for determining if a nursing home (NH) resident had the capacity sufficient to create a HCP, that is, to choose a surrogate health care decision maker. The tool demonstrated criterion-related validity and reliability. Data analysis indicated that many cognitively impaired residents had this capacity. Mezey and colleagues suggest that the Guidelines are more predictive than the MMSE in identifying such residents and could be used for that circumscribed purpose.

Schlegel and Shannon's (2000) descriptive study of nurse practitioners (NP) (n = 145) reported that most (but not all) NPs were knowledgeable about the legal guidelines for EOL decision making but few included ACP as part of their practice. To address this, the investigators recommended that formal didactic curricula and role modeling be included in NP education. Lehna (2001) devised and tested a needs assessment for EOL education among NP students. Findings indicated that students were gaining knowledge, competency, and confidence from practice rather than from theory and class discussion. Goodwin, Kiehl, and Peterson (2002) suggest that primary care nurse practitioners should use King's "interacting systems" or transaction model, and goal achievement theory, to facilitate advance care planning. This approach has not been tested although the authors suggest that it would be good only for RNs and NPs who wanted to actively address EOL issues using a nursing model.

For family members of NH residents, decisions about EOL care are easier when staff listen to family's fears and concerns, engage them in ACP well before a crisis or terminal event, and provide relevant information (e.g., what antibiotics can and cannot do) (Wilson, S. A., & Daley, 1999). Qualitative analysis of the investigator-designed interview revealed that staff caring behaviors, family participation in decision making prior to death, knowledge of what the dying process looked like and how long it might take, being present at the time of death, and receiving spiritual support were important for family members making difficult choices. In a review of the research literature about the EOL care provided in NHs and assisted living residences (ALRs), Cartwright (2002) concluded that staff and family differ about the kind and quality of EOL care in these settings.

Hospice care can be provided in ALRs in virtually all states, but the availability of skilled nursing care and oversight is extremely variable (Mitty, 2003). Thus, an older person choosing to remain in an ALR, that is, to age in place and die there, may have to use additional private funds to access the kind of care needed at the end of life. Few states require that ALR residents or staff be educated about ADs but many ALRs want residents to have made a decision about CPR at the time of admission. Most NHs provide "hospicelike" care or have a contract with a hospice provider and all NHs must educate staff and residents about ADs. Some NHs and most ALR—for a variety of reasons—transfer dying residents to the hospital.

Orem's self-care deficit model was used to elicit factors associated with the option for patients with terminal cancer to die at home (Grov, 1999). Self-care deficit of patient and caregiver, availability of nurses and other supports, and resources were key factors in maintaining patient autonomy. The nurse was instrumental in identifying and facilitating patient's choices regarding self-care deficit and symptom relief. Ladd, Pasquarelle, and Smith (2000) used case-based analysis to describe and discuss ethical and legal issues that arise in nursing care of patients dying at home. The authors suggest that the nurse-patient relationship in a home care setting is different, richer, and more nuanced than in the hospital setting. Dying at home means that the family has to be prepared and the nurse has to try to anticipate their disagreement with the patient's AD wishes. Ladd et al. propose a holistic assessment that includes assessment of the patient's decisional authority and relationship with significant others. They also recommend that the nurse work with the patient to define the role of each family member in decision making—with and for the patient.

Many legal scholars and ethicists hold that there is no difference, ethically or legally, between withholding or withdrawing a life-sustaining treatment (LST). To study the decision makers involved in withdrawing or withholding LSTs, Reckling (1997) directly observed and interviewed family members (n = 16) and professional staff (n = 29) of 10 ICU patients. Some items from the Social Context Survey were used to measure attitude toward withdrawing and withholding LSTs. Three basic decision-making roles were identified: advocate (to withhold/withdraw LST), neutral party (will go with any position), and resistor (to withdraw/withhold LSTs). Interrater agreement is reported with regard to the assigned role. More healthcare professionals were advocates than resistors; more family members were resistors than advocates. Nurses were the only professionals who assumed a neutral role. Among Reckling's findings was the feeling that those who made the decision to withdraw a LST did not always carry it out; this often fell to nurses who carried out the action but claimed no responsibility for its consequences. Some respondents felt that it was permissible to withhold a LST but were resistant to withdrawal. Factors associated with advocacy included poor prognosis, patient discomfort, attention to scare resources, and the patient's known preferences. Factors associated with neutrality or resistance were constraints on practice, fear of legal liability, and distrust. Reckling also suggests that situational factors and organizational culture may have influenced nurses' passive role-taking.

Mezey, Kluger, Maislin, and Mittelman (1996) described the decisions made by spouses (n = 50) of patients with Alzheimer's disease to consent to or to forgo LSTs. Presented with two conditions—critical illness and irreversible coma—spouses were asked to rate their agreement with, certainty of, and comfort with four LSTs: CPR, ventilator, feeding tube, and antibiotics. In the face of critical illness, almost equal numbers of spouses would consent to or forgo CPR and a breathing machine; far fewer (n = 5) would forgo antibiotics. Among 50 spouses, 5 chose to forgo all LSTs. In the face of irreversible coma, spouses were more likely to forgo all LSTs and were more certain and comfortable with their decision. Spouses experiencing high burden were more likely to consent to treatment. Few spouses appeared to be acting under the substituted judgment standard of decision making.

In general, there are many limitations to the research regarding EOL planning and choices. Many of the studies we reviewed were based on small and uncontrolled samples. Design weakness can generate misleading and unrepresentative findings. Several studies discussed in this chapter suggest future research that would vary with regard to site, subject, design and methods, questions to be addressed, or interventions to be tested. Baggs and Mick (2000) suggest that collaboration among health care providers, patients, and families could be an effective approach to ACP, given that such collaborative models have support value in community-based care delivery to elders. S. A. Norton and Talerico's (2000) strategies to facilitate EOL decision making include guidelines for communication, such as, clarifying goals and burdens of treatments, and using words such as "death" and "dying" in discussions with patients and families. They suggest assessing patient and family understanding and information needs. Yet, culture studies advise caution in using the "d" words: How should one proceed? Which nursing model, if any, can best guide the nursing strategy? Bosek, Lowry, Lindeman, Barck, and Gwyther (2003) delineate several recommendations to promote a positive death experience that include professional as well as patient and family education about the physiological dying process, comfort interventions, and the utility of ADs for decision making at the end of life. Given the cultural diversity of caregivers and care recipients, understanding the nature, context, and content of EOL care continues to require thoughtful and sensitive research design.

ETHEL L. MITTY
MIA KOBAYASHI

Endotracheal Suctioning

Endotracheal suctioning (ETS) is a common nursing intervention to remove mucus and debris from the tracheobronchial tree by the insertion of a suction catheter through the endotracheal tube and the application of vacuum during catheter withdrawal to aspirate tracheal secretions. Endotracheal suctioning is usually performed every 1–2 hours or as needed to maintain airway patency and arterial oxygenation. There is insufficient research data to identify the most significant clinical indicators to determine the need for ETS. However, clinicians report the following clinical cues: color, breath sounds, respiratory rate and pattern, coughing, presence of secretions in the tubing, saw-toothed flow-volume loops on the mechanical ventilator, and blood oxygen levels to indicate need. The ETS procedure has a number of components including: hyperoxygenation (increased inspired oxygen) which can be delivered either via the ventilator or manual resuscitation bag, hyperinflation (volume of inspired air above baseline tidal volume), open vs. closed ETS through an inline suction catheter to maintain mechanical ventilation, and post-oxygenation. Associated variables include: saline instillation for the purpose of irrigation, suction catheter size, level of negative suction pressure, depth of suction catheter insertion, application of negative pressure either continuously or intermittently, duration of negative pressure application, and number of hyperoxygenation/hyperinflation suction sequences.

Despite almost 80 years of research, controversy continues regarding the most efficacious endotracheal suctioning procedure. While components of the endotracheal suctioning procedure have been well researched, the utilization of research findings has been variable in the clinical setting. The components of the endotracheal suctioning procedure have been developed to prevent the complications associated with the procedure.

The majority of research has been conducted to develop techniques to minimize the most common complication: hypoxemia. Hypoxemia, which is the lowering of blood oxygen levels, may result from the disconnection of the patient from the ventilator during the procedure and/or due to the removal of oxygen from the respiratory tract during the application of vacuum. Researchers have documented other side effects which include: (a) atelectasis, (b) bronchoconstriction and tracheal trauma, (c) alterations in arterial pressure (hypotension and hypertension), (d) increased intracranial pressure, (e) cardiac arrhythmias, (f) cardiac arrest, and (g) death. Atelectasis is due to the insertion of a suction catheter with an outer diameter that is too large for the inner diameter of the endotracheal tube, causing catheter impaction and the removal of respiratory gases from distal alveoli with the application of vacuum. Bronchoconstriction and tracheal trauma are due to the catheter stimulating the bronchial smooth muscle and inner lining of the trachea (Czarnik, Stone, Everhart, & Preusser, 1991; Turner & Loan, 2000).

Hyperoxygenation/hyperinflation is a component of the ETS procedure used to prevent hypoxemia. Hyperoxygenation is the administration of a fraction of inspired oxygen (FiO_2) greater than the patient's baseline FiO_2, either prior to (pre-hyperoxygenation) or following (post-hyperoxygenation) suctioning. Hyperinflation is defined as the delivery of a breath of inspired air greater than the patient's baseline tidal volume. Research has shown that patients who receive no form of hyperoxygenation/hyperinflation with ETS show a significant decline in arterial blood oxygen. A critical evaluation of the research examining the effect of hyperoxygenation/hyperinflation on suction-induced hypoxemia shows variability in the techniques and the results. However, despite the conflicting findings, investigators have documented that three to four hyperoxygenation breaths at 100% oxygen and 135–150% of tidal volume has been effective in preventing suction-induced hypoxemia (Stone & Turner, 1989). A recent survey indicated that the majority of critical care nurses use hyperoxygenation alone ($n = 55/60$) (Paul-Allen & Ostrow, 2000). Researchers have documented that hyperinflation followed by ETS may cause both a decrease or increase in mean arterial pressure and may be due to the number of hyperoxygenation/hyperinflation suction sequences.

Hyperoxygenation/hyperinflation breaths can be delivered using either a manual resuscitation bag (MRB) or a ventilator. Investigators have reported inconsistently on the ability of different MRBs to deliver 100% oxygen. Research has shown that consistency is improved when the MRB has a reservoir of 1,000–2,000 cc attached to an oxygen source at a flow rate of 15 L/min or flush and adequate time is allowed for refill from the reservoir. Recent studies comparing the ventilator and the MRB, which have controlled important intervening variables, have concluded that hyperoxygenation/hyperinflation breaths delivered via the ventilator have resulted in elevated blood oxygen levels which are superior or equivalent to the MRB in preventing suction-induced hypoxemia. Investigators have also determined that the MRB produces a greater increase in airway pressure, arterial pressure, and heart rate when compared to the ventilator. Hence, the ventilator is the preferred mode for delivering hyperoxygenation/hyperinflation breaths (Stone, K. S., 1990; Grap, Glass, Corley, & Parks, 1996).

Closed ETS using an inline suction catheter permits uninterrupted ventilation, oxygenation, and positive end expiratory pressure during ETS. Without hyperoxygenation, blood oxygen levels decline more with open ETS than with closed. With hyperoxygenation, via the ventilator or MRB, the decline in blood oxygen levels is equal or less with closed ETS.While saline instillation prior to ETS is common clinical practice, there is inconclusive research to support any physiological benefit and it may actually cause a decline in blood oxygen levels (Raymond, 1995). The relationship between the outer diameter (OD) of the suction catheter and inner diameter (ID) of the endotracheal tube can be a significant factor in the development of atelectasis during ETS. Researchers recommend an OD/ID ratio of 1:2. This can be achieved with a 14 Fr. catheter and an endotracheal tube of 7, 8, or 9 mm. Since the level of negative pressure or suction applied to the catheter influences the degree of tracheal trauma, negative airway pressure, secretion recovery, and hypoxemia, researchers recommend a suction pressure of 100–120 mm Hg. The suction catheter should be advanced down the endotracheal tube without the application of vacuum until gentle resistance is met to reduce mechanical stimulation of the tracheal tissue that may cause bradycardia, premature atrial contractions, and increased intracranial pressure (Rudy, Turner, Baun, Stone, & Brucia, 1991; Kerr, M. E., Rudy, Brucia, & Stone, 1993). The catheter should be withdrawn a few centimeters prior to the application of vacuum to prevent catheter wedging, the vacuum can be applied either continuously or intermittently with no significant difference in tracheal trauma while withdrawing the catheter in a rotating motion (Czarnik et al., 1991). The duration of suction application should be no more than 10 seconds. The number of hyperoxygenation/hyperinflation suction sequences or catheter passes should be limited to no more than two per episode, as research data indicate that there is a cumulative increase in arterial pressure, heart rate, and intracranial pressure with each pass (Stone, K. S., Bell, & Preusser, 1991; Rudy et al.). If additional suction passes are needed, 5–10 minutes should elapse to allow for the patient's hemodynamic variables to return to baseline. The patient should be assessed for changes in blood pressure, heart rate, arrhythmias, and increased intracranial pressure and the patient's ability to tolerate the procedure should be documented. The lungs should be auscultated to assess airway clearance and the character of secretions (amount, color, and viscosity) should be recorded following ETS.

Kathleen Stone

Endotracheal Suctioning in Newborns: NICU Preterm Infant Care

Neonates with respiratory distress syndrome (RDS) who require endotracheal (ET) tube intubation and mechanical ventilation (MV) are the major population in need of a modern neonatal intensive care unit (NICU). MV is lifesaving to provide adequate oxygen and gas exchange in these neonates. During the period(s) of MV, ET suctioning (ETS) procedure has to be performed by nurses to maintain patent airways to ensure adequate gas exchange. ETS is the only method that can be used to maintain the airway by clearing the airway secretions and debris when the ET tube is inserted, as the ET tube essentially stops the mucociliary transport system and inhibits the infant's capacity to cough and clear out the secretions and debris in the airway. ETS involves steps of inserting a sterile catheter through the ET tube, stopping no more than 1 cm past the end of the ET tube, and using negative pressure while withdrawing the ET catheter to clear out the secretions and debris (Turner & Loan, 2000).

ETS could be one of the most detrimental procedures in NICU care, causing tracheobronchial trauma including mucosal necrosis, tracheal lesions, ulceration, perforation of the trachea and hypopharynx, pneumothorax, and bacteremia (Turner & Loan, 2000). Other complications of ETS include hypoxia and desaturation, bradycardia, and increased intracranial pressure (Shiao, 2002; Skov, Ryding, Pryds, & Greisen, 1992). The trauma to the tracheobronchial tissues can be cumulative over the duration of ET insertion regardless of modes of MV support, including conventional MV and all new forms of high-frequency ventilators, and these traumas cannot be recovered until 28 days after removing the ET tube and discontinuing MV (Turner & Loan). ETS tops all NICU procedures in causing worst desaturation events (Shiao, 2002) and in causing hypoxia lasting 4 minutes or longer (Wrightson, 1999).

Neonates, particularly preterms, who need MV are very sensitive to environmental stimuli and easily develop episodes of desaturation. In addition to RDS, the presence of patent ductus arteriosus and the increased oxygen-hemoglobin affinity of fetal hemoglobin are cardiopulmonary causes of hypoxemia in preterm neonates. Ventilatory weaning, though aggressive, must follow a fine line between oxygen toxicity and hypoxemia. Thus, a better monitoring approach is crucial during MV support in neonates (Shiao, 2002). Significant changes have been demonstrated for ETS procedures with hemodynamic monitoring, cerebral blood flows, autonomic neural responses, and behavioral assessment (Bernert et al., 1997; Segar, Merrill, Chapleau, & Robillard, 1993; Shiao, 2002; Skov et al., 1992).

Since the 1970s, nurse researchers including Turner and the ETS critical care nursing study groups, as well as researchers from medical sciences, have investigated ETS procedures closely, leading to publications with very clear understanding of pathophysiology for the airway system and ETS trauma in neonates (Turner & Loan, 2000). Interventions minimizing the detrimental effects of ETS include preoxygenation, shallow suctioning, sedations, and comforting measures, the nature of catheters and ETS, and the frequencies and duration of ETS procedure.

The summary reviews from Wrightson (1999) supported the use of hyperoxygenation (preoxygenation) for different durations before the ETS procedure, though the most conclusive study on preoxygenation indicated providing 1 minute 100% oxygen before ETS using a manual Ambu bag (Kerem, Yatsiv, & Goitein, 1990). When closed ETS system (insufflation of suction catheter using a special adapter to allow MV to continue while suctioning occurs) is used to cause less interruption of oxygen supply, hyperoxygenation can be supplied using MV (Turner & Loan, 2000). Unlike adults, hyperinflation using peak inspiration pressure is not recommended in neonates because of the potential to cause pneumothorax from excessive pressure due to the infant's poor alveolar compliance. Hyperventilation is commonly used in combination with hyperoxygenation in neonates, and the individual effect has not been documented.

Also supported from the reviews was the use of shallow ETS method (to insert the suction catheter only 1 cm beyond the ET tube) instead of deep ETS method (stopping suction catheter when it meets resistance, indicating that the catheter is touching the tracheal carina or tissue), since this caused less damage to the tracheal tissue (Wrightson, 1999). The newest shallow ETS method, however, suggests advancing the suction catheter to the same length as the ET tube (Ahn & Hwang, 2003) and not beyond the ET tube to prevent trauma to the tracheal tissue.

Saline installation before ETS was not supported by the reviews (Wrightson, 1999). Turning the infant's head sideways for ETS to reach the left lung was not supported either as it only increases the chances of traumatizing the airway with the increased risk of dislocating and removing the ET tube from the airway, without the benefits of removing airway secretions. As the length of the trachea is only about 4 cm in neonates, 3 cm of the tube can be moved in and out of the trachea when the infant's head is turned sideways or extended; thus, turning the head sideways will only increase the risk of ET tube removal and lead to airway trauma from the deep suction method, without any benefits of removing the airway secretions (Turner & Loan, 2000). Chest physical therapy was not supported as it only stimulates afferent vagal nerves to produce aggravating bradycardia and hypoxia in infants without obvious benefits in removing airway secretions (Turner & Loan; Wrightson).

Three additional matters for ETS are suggested from Wrightson's reviews (1999). ETS should only be performed on an as-needed basis by observing and assessing (including auscultation) the signs of secretion in the airway and in the ET tube. ETS procedures should not last longer than 1 minute, with no more than two consecutive ETS passes each time. Also, the monitor readings including oxygen saturation should be examined to prevent hypoxia and to ensure the recovery from ETS procedure before next ETS.

Other recent studies indicated that sedations and music therapy, involving the comforting management of infants with ETS, caused less aggravations and negative afferent vagal stimulation, and attenuated autonomic neural responses for hemodynamic changes in the infants (Burgess, Oh, Brann, Brubakk, & Stonestreet, 2001) and caused less desaturation (Chou, Wang, Chen, & Pai, 2003). ETS catheters are now designed with multiple side holes to prevent abruptly increased suction pressure; thus the trauma to the trachea in neonates is less than using earlier catheters with fewer or a single side hole (Turner & Loan, 2000). Future research could be designed for the following areas in neonates, including more advanced monitoring of tissue oxygenation to prevent hypoxia associated with ETS, comforting interventions in addition to preoxygenation with ETS to prevent detrimental hypoxia and cerebral effects, and ways to eliminate ETS trauma to the airway tissue such as the shallow ETS method.

Shyang-Yun Pamela K. Shiao

Enteral Tube Placement

An enteral tube is defined as any small-bore tube passed through the nose or mouth into the stomach or small intestine for the purpose of decompression, medication instillation, or feeding. Because safety issues related to enteral tubes that can be passed directly through the wall of the stomach or jejunum are different, only the issues surrounding nasogastric/

orogastric (NG/OG) tubes and nasointestinal (NI) tubes will be discussed.

It is estimated that approximately one million enteral tubes are placed in adults and children in the United States annually (Metheny, Spies, & Eisenberg, 1986). Feeding by NG/OG/NI tubes is preferred when the gastrointestinal (GI) system is functional and the need for assisted feeding is expected to be short-term. Enteral feeding is physiologic, achieves a positive nitrogen balance sooner than total parenteral nutrition, enhances gut healing, and reduces bacterial translocation, and also is less costly and is associated with low rates of sepsis. Even in clients maintained primarily by total parenteral nutrition, small amounts of nutrients are fed into the lumen of the gut through enteral tubes to maintain the structure and function of the small intestine. For many clients, feeding by NG/OG/NI tubes remains an essential lifesaving procedure.

Previous studies found NG/OG/NI tube placement errors to be common, with prevalence rates of errors in adults ranging from 1.3% to 89.5% depending on how narrow or broad the definition of error was (McWey, Curry, Schabel, & Reines, 1988; Niv & Abu-Avid, 1988). Studies in children show that between 20.9% and 43.5% of enteral tubes are placed incorrectly when placement error is broadly defined (Ellett & Beckstrand, 1999; Ellett, Maas, & Forsee, 1998). Although estimates of error rates vary, there is no doubt that they are common.

Errors in placement of NG/OG feeding tubes, which include initial erroneous placements as well as displacements over time, can lead to serious complications. If a tube ends in the airway, feeding through the tube will result in pulmonary aspiration or other pulmonary complications. Feeding through a tube ending in the esophagus increases the risk of pulmonary aspiration. When an NG/OG tube erroneously passes into the duodenum and the client is fed formula requiring both gastric and pancreatic enzymes for complete digestion, malabsorption that results in inadequate weight gain (or weight loss), diarrhea, and possibly dumping syndrome may occur. Increasing the safety of NG/OG feeding requires knowledge development in at least two areas—predicting the insertion distance for correct tube placement and determining tube position. The state of the science regarding each of these knowledge needs will be reviewed. At present no methods have been shown empirically to be adequate for predicting correct tube insertion length. The one adult study (Hanson, R. L., 1979) concluded that use of the direct nose-ear-xiphoid (NEX) distance to determine the insertion length, the standard measurement used in practice, was not accurate. Hanson recommended a formula ([NEX − 50 cm]/2 + 50 cm) adapted from his regression equation on NEX, which in his sample was 91.4% accurate for estimating the distance for placing the NG tube tip correctly in the stomach.

Only a few studies have addressed insertion-length estimators in children. Ziemer and Carroll (1978) found at autopsy in infants that an NG tube inserted using the NEX distance almost always reached just past the lower esophageal sphincter and needed to be advanced a few centimeters for correct placement in the stomach. They proposed that a more accurate method would be using the length from the tip of the nose to the lobe of the ear to a point midway between the xiphoid process and the umbilicus (NEMU). Weibley, Adamson, Clinkscales, Curran, and Bramson (1987) found on radiograph that 55.6% of NG/OG tubes in 30 premature infants were incorrectly placed using the NEX distance and 39.3% of NG/OG tubes were incorrectly placed using the NEMU distance. All of these errors involved high placements (which, if in the respiratory tract or the esophagus, often result in serious complications, such as aspiration pneumonia or parenchymal perforation with resulting pneumothorax). Surprisingly, however, in spite of the evidence from these studies, a telephone survey of 113 Level II and III nurseries in five midwestern states found that 98% of nurses continued to use NEX to calculate tube insertion distance (Shiao & DiFiore, 1996).

Beckstrand and colleagues (1990) investigated the methods recommended in the nursing literature for predicting correct placement length for NG/OG tube insertion, including NEX, NEMU, and regression on height. In a sample of 500 children, they found regression on height in three age groups to be the superior predictor of esophageal length. This method, referred to as the age-related, height-based method, was supported by Hanson's (1979) study in adults.

Currently an abdominal radiograph is the only consistently valid and reliable way to verify the position of flexible small-bore NG/OG tubes. Indeed, radiographs have been recommended by many to determine tube placement in patients; however, placement must be checked frequently while a tube is in place, and the summative radiation risk of multiple radiographs as well as their expense makes the development of adequate bedside placement-locating methods imperative.

Several methods of detection have been investigated in adults, including: (a) aspirating gastric contents and measuring the pH, bilirubin, pepsin, and trypsin levels; (b) placing the proximal end of the tube under water and observing for bubbles in synchrony with expirations; (c) auscultating for a gurgling sound over the epigastrium or left upper quadrant of the abdomen; (d) examining the visual characteristics of aspirates; (e) measuring the length from the nose/mouth to the proximal end of the tube; and (f) measuring CO_2 level at the proximal end of the NG/OG tube. Each of these methods has its problems, however. Metheny, Smith, and Stewart (2000) found that the combination of pH, bilirubin, pepsin, and trypsin correctly classified 100% of respiratory placements and 93.4% of GI placements in adults; however, no bedside tests are currently available for measuring pepsin and trypsin, thus limiting their clinical usefulness. Placing the proximal end of the tube under water and observing for bubbles in synchrony with expirations involves risk that clients will aspirate water on inspiration, especially those being mechanically ventilated. Simple auscultation is not a reliable method to assess tube position because injection of air into the tracheobronchial tree or into the pleural space can produce a sound indistinguishable from that produced by injecting air into the GI tract (Metheny, McSweeney, Wehrle, & Wiersema, 1990). Metheny, Reed, Berglund, and Wehrle (1994) showed that visual characteristics improved nurses' predictions of stomach and intestinal placements but reduced discrimination of respiratory placements. Finally, there is evidence that CO_2 monitoring has the potential to differentiate respiratory from GI placement; however, it has yet to be used clinically to detect respiratory placements (Burns, S. M., Carpenter, & Truitt, 2001; Thomas, B. W., & Falcone, 1998). To summarize, in adults pH and bilirubin of aspirate are the only reliable indicators of tube position.

Fluids aspirated from different organs have different mean pH values, and Metheny, Stewart, and coresearchers (1999) suggested that these expected differences might be useful for testing for feeding tube placement errors. Although an advance over auscultation, pH testing alone is an inadequate locator in both adults and children because of overlap in pH between sites, difficulty in obtaining aspirate, and other factors affecting pH readings.

In a study of 800 aspirates collected from 605 fasting adults, Metheny and coresearchers (1999) found that gastric aspirates had significantly lower pH values (mean 3.5) than intestinal aspirates (mean 7.0). About 15% of the gastric aspirates had pH values overlapping with the pH values of intestinal aspirates. In addition, pH values from four tubes inadvertently placed in the respiratory tract overlapped with the range in intestinal placements. Although in the research setting investigators were very successful in obtaining aspirate, in the clinical setting this may be more of a problem. It may be impossible to obtain any fluid if one or more of the orifices are not in a pool of fluid. Furthermore, flexible small-bore tubes tend to collapse when negative pressure is applied with a syringe; therefore, the absence of fluid is not necessarily evidence of improper placement. Another factor that may reduce the usefulness of pH testing is the administration of gastric acid-inhibiting medications resulting in an elevated gastric pH, although the evidence is mixed on this question (Metheny et al., 1993; Metheny, Eikov, Rountree, & Lengettie, 1999).

Metheny, Smith, and Stewart (2000) recommended that the bilirubin level and pH of aspirates be jointly used as tests to help differentiate gastric, intestinal, and respiratory placement of tubes. They measured bilirubin and pH of aspirates from NG and NI tubes as well as tracheobronchial suction and pleural fluid aspirates and found bilirubin levels to differ as predicted. Metheny and Stewart (2002) found bilirubin levels in neonates' gastric fluid comparable to adult levels. Although the pH/bilirubin test correctly identified 100% of actual respiratory aspirates, it correctly identified only 85.9% of nonrespiratory aspirates. Furthermore, only 29.4% of predicted respiratory aspirates were actually respiratory, and 87.7% of nonrespiratory placements were accurately predicted. Metheny and Stewart concluded that a bilirubin concentration of ≥ 5 mg/dL was a good predictor of intestinal tube placement, whereas a bilirubin concentration of < 5 mg/dL was a good predictor of gastric tube placement whether or not the adult was fasting. Bilirubin can be easily measured at the bedside using the method developed by Metheny and Stewart in which reagent strips are compared to a color scale.

In summary, although estimates of tube placement errors vary, there is no doubt that they are common and can lead to serious complications. The direct NEX distance, the standard measurement currently used in practice, has been seen to be inaccurate in both adults and children. The NEMU distance, tested only in children, also seems to be inaccurate. Although the age-related height-based method has some research support, it has never been tested clinically. Because of the overlap in pH values for respiratory, gastric, and intestinal placements; the difficulty in obtaining aspirate to test pH; and the possible effects of acid-inhibiting medications, total parental nutrition, and physiologic immaturity in young infants on the pH of aspirate, it is evident that pH alone is not a reliable method for discriminating among gastric, intestinal, and respiratory placements. Furthermore, these problems may be worse in children than adults. Joint measurement of bilirubin and pH may be a better alternative to the use of pH alone.

MARSHA L. ELLETT

Epilepsy

Epilepsy refers to a chronic condition characterized by recurrent *seizures*. A seizure is a temporary alteration in functioning caused by abnormal discharge of neurons in the central nervous system (Holmes, G. H., 1987). The exact nature of the seizure depends on the function of the brain cells that are affected by the abnormal discharge. Seizures are classified into two major types: *partial* and *generalized*. Partial seizures, which occur when the electrical discharge remains in a circumscribed area of the brain, can be broken down further into elementary or complex divisions. With elementary partial seizures, the person's consciousness is not impaired. With complex partial seizures, there is some impairment of consciousness. In some persons with partial seizures, the abnormal discharge spreads throughout the brain and is referred to as a partial seizure with secondary generalization.

Generalized seizures occur when the discharge affects both brain hemispheres and results in a loss of consciousness. The two most common types of generalized seizures are generalized tonic clonic (grand mal) and absence (petit mal). In generalized tonic clonic seizures, the person typically stiffens all over in the tonic phase, has jerking movements of the arms and legs in the clonic phase, and is incontinent of urine. Following the seizure the person is commonly sleepy. In absence seizures, there are a few seconds of loss of consciousness. The person generally stares blankly and sometimes rotates the eyes upward. An absence seizure begins and ends abruptly (Dreifuss & Nordli, 2001).

Epilepsy affects over 2 million persons in the United States. The cumulative incidence to age 80 years is 1.3% to 3.1%. Incidence rates are highest among those under 20 years of age and over 60 years of age. The trend is for the frequency of epilepsy to be decreasing in children and to be increasing in the elderly. Rates are slightly higher for men than for women. The prevalence of active epilepsy, defined as having had a seizure in the past 5 years or taking daily antiepileptic medication, is between 4.3 and 9.3 per 1,000. In approximately 70% of new cases of epilepsy there is no specific identified cause. In the remaining 30% the risk factors for epilepsy are severe head trauma, infection in the central nervous system, and stroke. In the United States the prevalence of epilepsy is lower in Whites than in non-Whites, although the reasons for these differences are not clear (Hauser & Hesdorffer, 1990).

Remission of epilepsy, defined as 5 years without seizures, is more common among persons with generalized seizures, those with no neurological deficits, and those with a younger age of onset. Approximately 70% of persons with epilepsy can be expected to enter remission (Hauser & Hesdorffer, 1990).

The major treatment of epilepsy is *antiepileptic medication*. Most epilepsy is well controlled with such treatment, but approximately 20% of persons continue to experience seizures despite treatment with medications. When partial seizures originate from a well-defined focus in an area of the brain that could be excised without serious neurological deficits, surgery to remove the affected part of the brain is an option. Other treatments for epilepsy have been tried with some success. The ketogenic diet, which consists of food high in fat and low in carbohydrates, has been used since the 1920s. Recently, there has been increased interest in the ketogenic diet as a treatment. Another recent treatment is the vagus nerve stimulator, which sends electrical energy to the brain via the vagus nerve (Epilepsy Foundation, n.d.).

Most nursing research has been devoted to the impact of epilepsy on the quality of life. Some persons have severe quality-of-life problems that prevent them from engaging in fully productive lives. The exact prevalence of these problems is difficult to establish because most studies have been carried out on clinic samples, that is, on persons with seizures that are more difficult to control. Problems most commonly found in children include anxiety, poor self-concept, social isolation, depression, behavior problems, and academic underachievement (Austin & Dunn, 2000). The most common problems found in adults with epilepsy are unemployment, depression, social isolation, and problems with adjustment. Unemployment may be twice as high in persons with epilepsy as in the general population (Hauser & Hesdorffer, 1990). Factors generally associated with quality-of-life problems are severe and frequent seizures, presence of other conditions or deficits, chronic condition, negative attitudes toward having epilepsy, and lack of a supportive family environment.

Research to guide the nursing care of persons with epilepsy is limited. Research is needed to understand the factors that lead to quality-of-life problems. A recent study with children suggests that behavior problems are already evident at the time of the first recognized seizure (Austin et al., 2001). Moreover, research that tests nursing interventions is needed to guide nursing care designed to prevent and reduce the development of adjustment problems. More nursing research is needed on teaching self-management to persons with epilepsy. DiIorio and colleagues (2003) are studying self-management in adults with epilepsy. Nurses should play a major role in developing knowledge to provide a research base for nursing practice with persons with epilepsy.

JOAN K. AUSTIN

Ethics of Research

The ethics of research—defined as what one morally ought to do in conducting, disseminating, and implementing results from systematic investigation or scholarly inquiry—are determined by both traditional and changing social values. These values vary within and among cultures worldwide; therefore, as international nursing research increases, nurse researchers must be attuned to the ethics of conducting research in other countries (Olsen, 2003). However, within the preceding context, two points cannot be disputed: (a) all research has ethical dimensions, and (b) all research must be ethical.

Rapid advances in science and technology have led to several important policy documents and ethical guidelines for nursing research. The policy documents include the 1980, 1995, and 2003 American Nurses Association's (ANA) *Nursing's social policy statement*. The ethical guidelines for nursing research include the ANA's 1975 and 1985 *Human rights guidelines for nurses in clinical and other research*, as well as part of Provision 7 of the 2001 ANA *Code of ethics for nurses with interpretive statements*.

The conduct of research with humans imposes strong moral obligations on nurse researchers especially in light of genetic advances and the use of human biological materials in nursing research (Jeffers, 2001). Nevertheless, once the ethics of the research have been approved by an institutional review board or its equivalent, subject or participant selection (or human biological materials selection) occurs. The decision of whom or what to include and exclude from a study places the following moral burdens related to the ethical principle of justice on the researcher: (a) how to weigh the ethical pros and cons of using human biological materials or vulnerable persons as subjects, (b) how to avoid consistently selecting human biological materials or subjects based solely or primarily on ease of accessibility or any attribute that is not essential to the study's objectives, and (c) how to avoid overuse or underuse of human biological materials or any group of research subjects.

Once human subjects are selected, they should be given sufficient and unbiased information about all important aspects of the study and their roles in the study before agreeing to participate. In addition, subjects' comprehension of information about the study and the informed consent process should be ascertained initially and throughout the study as indicated. Subjects have the right to stop participation in a study at any time and without fear of retaliation. The preceding steps are based on the ethical principles of autonomy and respect for autonomy. If subjects are not autonomous, proxy consents must be obtained.

The ethical conduct of research also focuses on the ethical principle of nonmaleficence (do no harm). The researcher must understand that the possibility of harm or potential harm can occur to subjects at any time while conducting research. Therefore, the researcher must carefully weigh any benefits against therapeutic harms (i.e., harms that are necessary to produce a greater good in the conduct of the research). However, therapeutic harms always require moral justification, and under no circumstance should the subject be used solely as a means for the advancement of science.

The ethical principle of nonmaleficence also applies to scientific misconduct. Scientific misconduct is viewed as an intended act of deception that deviates from a discipline's ethical norms. It typically takes the form of plagiarism, irresponsible authorship, data falsification, data fabrication, and questionable research practices. Nurse researchers should be familiar with their organization's policies and procedures about scientific misconduct, as well as federal regulations to deter scientific misconduct. In addition, nurse researchers should be aware of three reports authored by the Institute of Medicine on scientific integrity (James, N., Burrage, & Smith, 2003).

When an interdisciplinary team is involved in the conduct of research, the principal investigator should be clearly designated and should assume overall accountability for the study. He or she is responsible for the supervision of all team members, including research assistants. Each team member must not only assume accountability for a part of the research but also must understand how that research builds on that of other team members. Finally, all members of the interdisciplinary research team must come to a common understanding of what the ethics of research means for their study.

The conduct of research with animals also has ethical import because of past and current cruelty to them and because of the increased need for basic research in nursing. The guiding ethical principles for researchers are (a) to use animals for studies only when necessary, (b) to inflict the least amount of harm and suffering to the fewest number of animals while still attaining research objectives, and (c) to obtain the approval of institutional animal care and use committees or their equivalent.

Some scholars and ethicists would argue that significant research of high quality that is not disseminated presents an ethical issue because persons who could benefit from that research are denied that benefit. Furthermore, undisseminated research cannot be implemented into practice. The ethics of the dissemination of research also involves researchers and peer reviewers. Researchers as authors have an ethical obligation to clarify primary and coauthor credits as soon as possible during the preparation of a manuscript; to designate when the manuscript is part of a larger study; to submit a manuscript to only one editor at a time; to present accurate, unbiased, relevant, and appropriately documented information in the manuscript; to notify appropriate persons when scientific misconduct is detected in one's own or other's studies; to avoid the use of retracted or invalid study results; and to understand the ethical issues involved in internet research (Im & Chee, 2003).

Researchers as peer reviewers have an ethical obligation to be objective in their review of research manuscripts and timely in their return of them; to offer constructive critiques that demonstrate respect; to avoid any conflicts of interest; and to maintain anonymity of authors and confidentiality of content until the manuscript is published.

The research literature indicates that many practitioners of nursing lack the education needed to understand research or to use the findings in practice. This lack of knowledge and comprehension diminishes nurses' autonomy and puts them at risk for potentially unsound ethical decision making about research utilization. Therefore, persons responsible for implementation of research into practice must assist practitioners of nursing to critique research for scientific and ethical merit and for clinical applicability. This critique includes the insight that studies typically are replicated before being implemented into practice. Furthermore, persons implementing research into practice must ensure that strong and ethical administrative support exists so that implementation can begin, continue, and terminate if necessary without causing harm to patients, staff, or the organization.

In summary, the most important aspect of research is that it be ethical. Although the ethics of research are complex, nurse researchers should respect these ethics and incorporate them into their studies or scholarly inquiries now and in the future.

MARY CIPRIANO SILVA

Ethnogeriatrics

Ethnogeriatrics is an evolving multidisciplinary subspecialty in geriatrics which examines health and aging issues in the context of cultural beliefs, values, and practices among racial and ethnic minority elders. Demographic effects, heterogeneity, barriers to access and utilization of services, interaction of culture-based practices and formal systems, impact of public policies, and culturally sensitive patient-provider relationships are key concepts in the field (Harper, 1990; McBride, Morioka-Douglas, & Yeo, 1996; Richardson, 1996). They provide useful information to guide health care delivery systems and service providers in reducing health disparities. Because nursing science is deeply rooted in integrative and holistic perspectives, it is well positioned to explore multifaceted conceptual frameworks such as the explanatory model (Kleinman, Eisenberg, & Good, 1978) and transtheoretical models (Plowden & Miller, 2002; McBride et al., 1998), and blend them into established or evolving nursing theories (Chen, 1996; Leininger, M., & McFarland, M., 2002).

A review of literature from 1996–2002 on African-American and Asian-American older adults was summarized according to: what is known about access to community-based health care, issues raised by research findings, and gaps in research (McBride & Lewis, 2004). The limited research on chronic diseases shows variations in type of illness, prevalence of disease, and quality of care (e.g., Baumann, Chang, & Hoebeke, 2002; De la Cruz, McBride, Compas, Calixto, & Van Derveer, 2002; Ness, Nassimiha, Feria, & Aronow, 1999). Information on cohorts of older African Americans are predominantly on individuals born in the United States and descendants of slaves from Africa. In contrast, studies on cohorts of older Asian Americans, whose ethnic origins are from over 50 countries, consist of a mix of recent immigrants, long-stay residents, and U.S. born. Important differences between and within groups (or heterogeneity) in terms of cultural beliefs and historical experiences are seldom measured and examined as factors contributing to disparities in access and utilization of services. Descriptive, exploratory, cross-sectional studies dominate the research effort on African-American and Asian-American older adults to identify unmet needs; few focus on culturally appropriate interventions. In some large databases, health status is often measured by self-reports (McBride & Lewis). However, it is unlikely that the information is verified by clinical data or linked with culture-based practices, particularly for those who are monolingual, low acculturated, or less educated older people.

In view of the projected 12% increase of racial and ethnic minority elders by 2030 and a continuing climate of rapidly diminishing resources, pursuing well-designed longitudinal intervention studies with randomized samples using culturally relevant research designs (e.g., case study designs) which are critical to improving quality of care for racial and ethnic minorities is a serious challenge to current and future nurse scientists.

IRENE DANIELS LEWIS
MELEN R. MCBRIDE

Ethnography

The term *ethnography* translates as "the written description of the folk (people/nation)." However, the term is currently used to refer to both a specific naturalistic research method and the written product of that method. As a research process ethnography is a comparative method for investigating human behavior and patterns of cognition through observations in the natural setting. As a written product, ethnography is a descriptive analysis of the beliefs, behaviors, norms, and patterns of a culture. The focus on culture and cultural processes is central to ethnography and is one of the ways in which ethnography differs from other naturalistic methods, such as grounded theory (the study of basic social processes) and phenomenology (the study of the individual's lived experience).

Ethnography was developed primarily by anthropologists as they sought to understand other cultures and traditions. Although ethnography remains the primary research method in anthropology, it is employed by several other disciplines, most notably sociology, psychology, education, and nursing. As the method was adopted outside anthropology, the focus of study shifted from small-scale or tribal societies to areas more closely linked with the discipline adopting the method. For example, the study of small urban social communities was undertaken by sociologists from the Chicago School, investigations of schools as microcosms of society were addressed by educators, and the health beliefs and lay systems of ethnic groups were targeted by nurse anthropologists.

In the discipline of nursing, ethnography was introduced into the literature primarily by nurse anthropologists beginning in the late

1960s. Two seminal articles appearing in *Nursing Research* by Elizabeth Byerly (1969/1990) and Antoinette Ragucci (1972/1990) laid the foundation for future nurse ethnographers. As doctoral education came to be sponsored through the nurse scientist program, several nurses chose anthropology as a focus of doctoral study. This first generation of nurse anthropologists who conducted ethnographies included pioneers such as Madeleine Leininger, Agnes Aamodt, Pamela Brink, Margarita Kay, Elizabeth Byerly, and Oliver Osborne. A second generation of nurse anthropologists included Juliene Lipson, Evelyn Barbee, JoAnn Glittenberg, Marjorie Muecke, Janice Morse, and Toni Tripp-Reimer. Later, as schools of nursing developed their own doctoral programs, some nurse ethnographers began to be trained within schools of nursing.

There are several different traditions subsumed under the term *ethnography*. Each of these has emerged with its own particular historical context, and each addresses somewhat different elements of culture. However, each of these approaches may be used fruitfully in nursing research, given the appropriate research question. Although there are over a dozen distinct ethnographic traditions, examples of four will be provided to demonstrate the diversity of approaches within ethnography.

An early ethnographic approach developed by Boas around the turn of the century is termed historical particularism. The central tenets of this approach are that each culture has its own long and unique history and that all elements of a culture are worthy of documentation. A typical product of historical particularism is the creation of cultural lists or inventories. This approach has been used in nursing research to identify specific folk treatments used in ethnic groups and to generate items to be used later in the construction of structured instruments.

Functionalism is a second ethnographic tradition. Here, however, the task of ethnography is to describe the structural elements and their interrelated functioning in a culture. This approach historically has been the most widely used in nursing research. A prominent example is that of Leininger's sunrise model.

The goal of ethnoscience, a third ethnographic tradition, is to discover folk systems of classification to determine the ways people perceive and structure their thinking about their world and to identify the rules that guide decision making. The taxonomy known as the Nursing Interventions Classification (NIC) was derived by using the ethnoscience approach.

Symbolic ethnography is a fourth approach, which is rapidly growing in application in nursing research. Here, investigators view culture as a system of shared meanings and symbols. They further believe that cultural knowledge is embedded in "thick descriptions" provided by cultural members. Most nursing research that deals with informants' explanatory models use this ethnographic tradition.

Fieldwork is the hallmark of ethnographic research. Fieldwork involves the investigator's immersion in the target community for long periods of time in order to gain understanding for contextualizing the ethnographic data. Stages of fieldwork include (a) field entry, (b) development of relationships, (c) data collection, (d) data manipulation, (e) data analysis, and (f) termination. Many of these stages, particularly (b)–(e), overlap in time.

In conducting fieldwork an investigator may employ several strategies for data collection, including participant observation, informal interviews, structured interviews, pictures and videotapes, census and other statistical data, historical documents, projective tests, and psychosocial surveys. The variety of research strategies that are appropriately employed is another way in which ethnography differs from most other naturalistic methods. Further, ethnographers may use quantitative data to augment qualitative data. However, the mainstay strategies of ethnography rest in participant observation and informant interviews. If the focus of the ethnography concerns the cognitive realm (attitudes, beliefs, schemata) of the members of the culture, then interviewing is the primary strategy. On the other hand, if the focus of the ethnography involves structural features or patterns of behavior, then observations are the primary strategy. The majority of ethnographies, however, use a combination of strategies.

Methods used for data manipulation include strategies for taking notes and making memos, coding strategies, and indexing systems. More recently, computerized software programs such as ETHNOGRAPH and NUD*IST have been fruitfully employed to aid in the management of data. Methods used in data analysis include matrix, thematic, and domain analysis.

In summary, ethnography is a method designed to describe a culture. The ethnographer seeks to understand another way of life from the perspective of a person inside the culture (emic view). Participant observation and informant interviewing are the major strategies used during fieldwork. The specific ethnographic tradition used by the investigator determines the form of the ethnographic product.

TONI TRIPP-REIMER
JANET ENSLEIN
BARBARA RAKEL
LISA ONEGA
BERNARD SOROFMAN

Evaluation

Evaluation is a method for measuring the effect of some purposeful action on a particular situation. It is often described as an assessment of worth. In evaluation, both anticipated and unanticipated outcomes are important and are included in the discussion of findings and the publication of results. The purpose of evaluation is to provide information for decision makers who usually have some stake in the outcome of the intervention.

Evaluation methods have been categorized along a continuum ranging from simple assessment, in which informal practices are used to look for indication of outcome, to evaluation research, in which research methods are used to allow for generalization to other comparable situations. In actuality, the use of informal practices for determining intervention outcome is never appropriate. Consequently, the term *evaluation* should suffice for all efforts in which a systematic process is used to determine the effect of some intervention on some anticipated outcome. The research component of the term is assumed. No matter what the purpose of the evaluation, the issue of rigor is always foremost, and the methods and measurement approaches used should involve the same level of attention given to any research method.

According to Rossi and Freeman (1985), evaluations serve one of three purposes: (1) to conceptualize and design interventions, (2) to monitor implementation of some intervention, or (3) to assess the utility of some action. In the first type of evaluation, studies focus on (a) the extent of the problem needing intervention, (b) who should be involved in or targeted for the intervention, (c) whether the intervention proposed will address the problem or the needs of individuals, and (d) whether the chance for successful outcome has been maximized.

In the second type of evaluation, studies focus on what is done; they generally are referred to as process evaluation studies. These studies also determine whether the intervention is reaching the targeted population and whether what is done is consistent with what was intended. Process evaluations are essential for determining cause and effect, although they are not sufficient by themselves for measuring impact. That is where evaluation researchers often get into trouble. They stop collecting data once they describe what was done; therefore, process evaluation methods have tended to be viewed with disfavor, which is unfortunate. Although they are insufficient by themselves, they are absolutely necessary for determining whether the intervention caused the outcome and if so, how—and if not, why not.

In the third type, studies determine both the degree to which an intervention has an impact and the benefit of the intervention in relation to the cost. The degree of impact is referred to as the intervention's effectiveness, and the degree of cost is referred to as its efficiency (Rossi & Freeman, 1985).

Recent writings on evaluation focus on the need for theory to guide the investigation and frame the results. Authors have identified theories that range from those targeted solely for the purposes of designing evaluations to those directed at the expected relationships between intervention and outcome. For example, behavioral theories often are used to develop interventions targeted at changing health behaviors; they also are used to select measures for determining impact. Evaluation theories, on the other hand, focus on the purpose of the study—whether it is for determining what goals or outcomes should be examined, how the treatment should be developed and delivered, or under what conditions certain events occur and what their consequences will be. H. T. Chen (1990) has defined these two types of evaluation theory as normative (the first type) and causative (the second). Normative theory is derived from prior knowledge, usual practice, or theory. Causative theory is empirically based and specifies causal relationships between intervention and outcome.

Measuring the true effect of the intervention often is difficult. Evaluation studies are subject to the same measurement and analysis problems associated with other designs. In addition, Ingersoll (1996) has summarized several others that are important to evaluation research. Among these is the need to measure the extent of the intervention introduced, which is frequently absent from reports of evaluation studies. This information assists in demonstrating cause-and-effect relationships and clarifies what magnitude of the intervention is required before an effect is seen. It also helps to prevent the potential for Type III, IV, and V evaluation errors, which affect statistical conclusion validity and generalizability validity.

Type III evaluation error is an error in probability and results in solving the wrong problem instead of the right problem. It usually occurs when the program is not implemented as planned and when insensitive measures are used to determine effect. Type IV error occurs when the evaluator provides information that is useless to stakeholders. Type V error involves confusing statistical significance with practical significance, which ultimately leads to Type IV error (Ingersoll, 1996).

Evaluation is key to measuring intervention magnitude and effect. To assure that evaluations are useful, however, steps must be taken to design them according to some meaningful conceptual framework; and close attention must be paid to maximizing the rigor of the methods, analysis, and rejection of alternative hypotheses. Approaches to quality control recommended for other nonexperimental, quasi-experimental, and experimental designs are appropriate. With attention to these aspects of the evaluation process, evaluations become an effective means for extending nursing science.

GAIL L. INGERSOLL

Evidence-Based Practice

Evidence-based practice (EBP) refers to nursing practice that utilizes research findings as the foundation for nurses' decisions, activities, and interactions with clients. Another term which is often used synonymously but is slightly different is the term "research utilization." Research utilization specifically refers to the practical utilization of findings from one or more scientific studies and is a predecessor of EBP. EBP is broadly conceptualized as a continuum of synthesized information used to improve practice and patient outcomes (Bakken, 2001). These two terms encompass the burgeoning interest in developing a practice in which there is solid evidence from scientific research that explicit nursing actions are clinically relevant, cost-effective, and result in positive quality outcomes for clients. The focus of EBP is its emphasis on integrating the best available research evidence within the clinical, patient, and organizational context of an institution to attain high-quality and cost-effective care.

According to Hewitt-Taylor (2002), evidence-based practice is a process that entails six elements: (a) selecting an area of practice that requires an evidence base, (b) making decisions about what constitutes evidence, (c) conducting a systematic search for evidence, (d) evaluating individual pieces of evidence, (e) synthesizing the findings of these sources into a cohesive whole, and (f) applying this evidence appropriately to patient care situations.

The desire to explore the path and timing of research to practice began in the 1960s and 1970s. N. Caplan and Rich (1975) coined the terms instrumental utilization (changing practice based on empirical evidence) and conceptual utilization (inability to change behavior based on the results, but a new awareness during caregiving). The slow evolution of practice change was called knowledge creep and decision accretion by C. Weiss (1980). Practice changes occur slowly over time as nurses and other health care providers repeatedly come into contact with new knowledge during readings, discussions, and at local and national meetings. Estabrooks (1999) reported three types of research utilization: indirect (changes in nurses' thinking), direct (incorporating findings into patient care), and persuasive (using findings to change decision makers' behaviors and beliefs).

Two formal efforts undertaken in the 1970s to bridge the gap between nursing research and nursing practice were the Western Interstate Commission for Higher Education (WICHE) Regional Program and the Conduct and Utilization of Research in Nursing (CURN) projects. In the WICHE project, although nurses were successful in increasing research utilization, they noted a dearth of scientifically sound nursing research with identifiable nursing implications. The goal of the CURN project was to increase the use of research results in daily practice by disseminating current findings, encouraging collaborative research with relevance to nursing issues, and enhancing administrative and organizational change supportive of implementing new evidence.

The Cochrane Collaboration, which was founded in the United Kingdom in the 1970s, was a foundation of the evidence-based practice movement. British epidemiologist Archie Cochrane, noting the paucity of evidence supporting care, advocated for the availability of clinical summaries upon which health care providers could base their decisions. This led to the formation of the Cochrane Collaboration (www.cochrane.org), whose aim is the preparation and dissemination of systematic reviews of the results of health care interventions. As the Cochrane movement was going on, Dr. David Sackett pioneered evidence-based medicine (EBM) at McMaster Medical School. He conceptualized EBM as "the conscientious, explicit, and judicious use of current best evidence in making decisions about the care of individual patients. The practice of EBM means integrating individual clinical expertise with the best available external evidence from systematic research" (Sackett, Rosenberg, Muir Gray, Haynes, & Richardson, 1996, p. 71).

Rigorous rating systems for evaluating evidence have been developed by Sackett and others (1996), Stetler and others (1998), as well as the AHCPR (2003) (now Agency for Healthcare Research and Quality [AHQR] http://www.ahcpr.gov/new/press/pr2002/strengpr.htm). In general, the rating systems order the types of evidence in the following manner: meta-analyses of randomized, controlled trials (RCT) (strongest evidence); experimental studies (or RCT); quasi-experimental studies (time series, nonequivalent control group) or matched case-control studies; nonexperimental studies (correlational, descriptive); and program evaluations, quality improvement projects, case reports, authoritative opinions (weakest evidence).

Two models (Stetler Model, Iowa Model) that were originally designed for research utilization have been adapted for use in EBP projects. These models have been the inspiration for the following steps to change practice: (a) identify a clinical problem; (b) collect the evidence about clinical issue (literature review, integrative review); (c) review, evaluate, and synthesize available evidence; (d) plan the EBP change; (e) design, implement, and evaluate a pilot EBP project; (f) design, implement, and evaluate a larger EBP project; and finally (g) disseminate the results (Polit & Beck, 2004).

Currently, informatics has become a key contributor to EBP and the promotion of quality patient care (Bakken, Cimino, & Hripcsak, 2004). Although this is not yet the standard, the methodology exists and presents an opportunity to impact quality of care through using up-to-date evidence about best practice tailor-made for an individual patient. For example, a patient is admitted for a specific operative procedure; reminders are sent to the physician and nurses regarding type of antibiotics, changes in care and testing based on laboratory functions, and best educational methodologies for the patient based on his demographics. These care processes are changed based on the most current and best evidence for care and treatment. Computer-based reminders have been demonstrated to decrease errors of omission and enhance adherence to clinical practice guidelines (Overhage, Tierney, Zhou, & McDonald, 1997).

There is some concern by practitioners that the systematic reviews used by clinicians are a watered-down version of the scientific method and raw data. Although Cochrane reviews, summarizations, and metasyntheses of data are used by clinicians in the formation of guidelines, nurses continue to appreciate the scholarly merit of single study or a series of studies—excellently formulated and conducted. In this author's experience, since the nature of nursing problems do not always fit the structure of a randomly controlled trial, evidence in one or a series of studies is evaluated and considered by their scientific soundness and clinical significance.

Polit and Beck (2004) recommend eight strategies for promoting the use of research findings in current practice. Researchers should collaborate with staff nurses to: identify current clinical problems, use rigorous designs, replicate findings, write clear research reports and share the information, report findings that are conducive to meta-analysis, present clinical implications of the research, disseminate findings energetically in multiple media (journals, conferences), and finally, prepare integrative and critical research reviews and make them available to busy practicing nurses.

Polit and Beck (2004) also identify nursing and organizational barriers to the utilization of evidence by practicing nurses. Bedside nurses may not be prepared to critically appraise the evidence. Nurses may not only lack the motivation to make changes, but be resistant to making changes that impact their comfortable practice. For organizations, administrators can foster a climate conducive to innovation. They can offer emotional, moral, and instrumental support for innovation, and can reward nurses for innovative and evidence-based practice at the bedside as well as support organizational initiatives.

Robin Fleschler

Experimental Research

True experiments have the potential to provide strong evidence about the hypothesized causal relationship between independent and dependent variables. Experiments are characterized by manipulation, control, and randomization. The quality of experiments depends on the validity of their design.

Manipulation means the researcher actively initiates, implements, and terminates procedures. In most instances, manipulation is linked to the independent variable(s) under consideration. Essential to manipulation is that the researcher has complete control over the process. The researcher decides what is to be manipulated (e.g., selected nursing intervention protocols), to whom the manipulation applies (e.g., samples and subsamples of subjects), when the manipulation is to occur according to the specification of the research design, and how the manipulation is to be implemented.

Manipulation implies and is impossible without researcher control over extraneous sources that might affect and lead to incorrect scientific conclusions. Control aims "to rule out threats to valid inference." It also adds precision, the "ability to detect true effects of smaller magnitude" (Cook, T., & Campbell, 1979, p. 8). Unlike laboratory studies where total control is often possible, in clinical research control is a relative matter. The researcher has the responsibility for ensuring as much control over extraneous forces as possible.

Control also includes "the ability to determine which units receive a particular treatment at a particular time" (Cook, T., & Campbell, 1979, p. 8). This refers to control over two *processes* that determine who gets what at what time. The first process is the researcher's use of random methods to assign subjects to treatments. This is the preferred method of exerting control over subjects and their treatment as, theoretically, it ensures that known and unknown extraneous forces inherent to subjects are dispersed equally across the different treatment options. This may not always be possible, in which case the second process comes into play—that of structuring the assignment process in such a way that major, known extraneous forces are controlled.

Commonly used design strategies include blocking, matching, and counterbalancing. In blocking the potentially confounding variable is incorporated into the study design as an independent variable. Subjects are then randomly assigned within each block. In matching, a weaker but very common method of control, the researcher identifies one or more extraneous (usually up to three) variables to be controlled. As soon as a subject is recruited for one of the treatment groups, the researcher then tries to find subjects for the other group(s) identical to the first subject on the specified matching variables. Counterbalancing occurs when the researcher is concerned that the order in which treatments are administered influences the results. When counterbalancing is used, all subjects receive all treatments; however, the order of administration of treatments is varied.

Randomization entails two separate processes: (a) random selection of subjects from the population and (b) random assignment of subjects to treatment and control conditions. Random selection is the process of randomly drawing research subjects from the population about which the researcher wants to gain knowledge and to which the researcher hopes to generalize the findings of a study. Random assignment entails allocating sampling units (e.g., patients) to treatment and control conditions by using a decision method that is known to be random (e.g., coin toss, random drawing, use of random tables, computer-generated random sequences of options). Random selection is virtually nonexistent in intervention studies in nursing; moreover, a large proportion (55.3%) of nursing intervention studies do not even use random assignment methods (Abraham, Chalifoux, & Evers, 1992).

T. Cook and Campbell (1979) reviewed four types of validity of research designs, potential threats to each, and strategies to remedy these threats. Statistical conclusion validity addresses the extent to which, at the mathematical/statistical level, covariation is present between the independent and dependent variables (i.e., the extent to which a relationship exists between the independent and dependent variables). Internal validity refers to whether an observed relationship between variables is indeed causal or, in the absence of a relationship, that indeed there is no causal link. Construct validity of putative causes and effects refers to whether the causal relationship between two variables is indeed "the one" and tries to refute the possibility that a confounding variable may explain the presumed causal relationship. External validity refers to the generalizability of an observed causal relationship "across alternate measures of the cause and effect and across different types of persons, settings, and times" (Cook, T., & Campbell, 1979, p. 37). Validity of any type is not a yes/no issue of whether or not it is present. Rather it is a matter of degree, determined by the extent to which the researcher has tried to cope with the various potential threats to each type of validity.

Ivo L. Abraham
Lynn I. Wasserbauer

Exploratory Studies

Exploratory studies are those that investigate little-known phenomena for which a library search fails to reveal any significant examples of prior research. These kinds of studies have been very useful in nursing research in finding out more about nursing-related problems that occur in all areas of clinical practice, administration, and academe. Typically, an exploratory study will use a small sample and will focus on one particular area of interest or on one or two variables. The following are the kinds of research questions that might indicate an exploratory study in nursing: What is it like being a pregnant teenager? What kinds of patients need home care? What health-promoting behaviors do cafeteria workers engage in? What is the lived experience of military widows?

Since the intent of exploratory research is to find out and explore unknown phenomena, it is considered Level I research (designed to elicit descriptions of a single topic or population) and is reflected in many of the early research studies in nursing. An examination of the kind of research designs that were used in nursing just 25 to 30 years ago reveals a predominance of exploratory studies and includes such examples as (a) staff nurse behaviors and patient care improvement (Gorham, 1962), (b) the self-concept of children with hemophilia and family stress (Garlinghouse & Sharp, 1968), and (c) women's beliefs about breast cancer and breast self-examination (Stillman, 1977).

Exploratory studies are still very useful. They can be found in nursing journals and are often thought of as an initial step in the description of a researchable problem. There are many reasons for an exploratory study. Such studies are particularly useful when the investigator seeks to gather baseline information on a particular variable, like loneliness, widowhood, anxiety, or culture. Other researchers may wish to investigate a process about which little is known, such as the types and meanings of caring behaviors among elderly nursing home residents or the meaning of loss of a nursing role. Exploratory research may focus on one concept that has not been described in any great detail in the literature, such as isolation or comfort, or researchers may initiate an exploratory study to determine the feasibility of or need for a more extensive study or to establish baseline information that could lay the groundwork for a future study.

Regardless of the intent of exploratory research, a flexible design that enables the researcher to investigate and examine all aspects of a phenomenon is encouraged. Flexibility in the design allows the researcher to explore all kinds of emerging ideas and to change direction, if needed, as data are collected and analyzed. Thus, exploratory research is not limited to one particular paradigm but may have either a quantitative or qualitative design. Studies that propose a hypothesis and seek to provide a measure of a phenomenon as a description employ a quantitative design. One example of an exploratory study that used a quantitative design is described by Schaefer, Swavely, Rothenberger, Hess, and Williston (1996). In this study the researchers described the nature and frequency of sleep pattern disturbances in patients who were recovering from coronary artery bypass graft (CABG) surgery.

Qualitative or naturalistic designs generally explore phenomena in the natural setting in which they occur and are commonly carried out by using semistructured or open-ended interviewing techniques and by observation. There are multiple approaches associated with qualitative research, but they all focus on those aspects of human behavior that are difficult to measure in numerical terms. One example of an exploratory qualitative study that used a grounded theory approach is that by Fleury, Kimbrell, and Kruszewski (1995). In this study the investigators sought to describe the healing experiences of 13 women who recovered from an acute cardiac event. Verbal transcripts were analyzed to find out more about the important issues and concerns of women during the recovery process.

Any critique of exploratory research would include the facts that these studies are limited in scope and focus, are not generalizable to a larger population, and cannot be used as a basis for prediction. In spite of these limitations, however, exploratory studies are useful to uncover or discover information about little-known phenomena or single concepts, to explore the existence of relationships between and among variables, to find out more about human behavior in a naturalistic setting, to lay the groundwork for more systematic testing of hypotheses, and to determine the feasibility for a more in-depth study.

KATHLEEN HUTTLINGER

F

Factor Analysis

Factor analysis is a multivariate technique for determining the underlying structure and dimensionality of a set of variables. By analyzing intercorrelations among variables, factor analysis shows which variables cluster together to form unidimensional constructs. It is useful in elucidating the underlying meaning of concepts. However, it involves a higher degree of subjective interpretation than is common with most other statistical methods. In nursing research, factor analysis is commonly used for instrument development (Ferketich & Muller, 1990), theory development, and data reduction. Therefore, factor analysis is used for identifying the number, nature, and importance of factors, comparing factor solutions for different groups, estimating scores on factors, and testing theories (Nunnally & Bernstein, 1994).

There are two major types of factor analysis: exploratory and confirmatory. In exploratory factor analysis, the data are described and summarized by grouping together related variables. The variables may or may not be selected with a particular purpose in mind. Exploratory factor analysis is commonly used in the early stages of research, when it provides a method for consolidating variables and generating hypotheses about underlying processes that affect the clustering of the variables. Confirmatory factor analysis is used in later stages of research for theory testing related to latent processes or to examine hypothesized differences in latent processes among groups of subjects. In confirmatory factor analysis, the variables are carefully and specifically selected to reveal underlying processes or associations.

The raw data should be at or applicable to the interval level, such as the data obtained with Likert-type measures. Next, a number of assumptions relating to the sample, variables, and factors should be met. First, the sample size must be sufficiently large to avoid erroneous interpretations of random differences in the magnitude of correlation coefficients. As a rule of thumb, a minimum of five cases for each observed variable is recommended however, Knapp and Brown (1995) reported that ratios as low as three subjects per variable may be acceptable. Others generally recommend that 100 to 200 is advisable (Nunnally & Bernstein, 1994).

Second, the variables should be normally distributed, with no substantial evidence of skewness or kurtosis. Third, scatterplots should indicate that the associations between pairs of variables should be linear. Fourth, outliers among cases should be identified and their influence reduced either by transformation or by arbitrarily replacing the outlying value with a less extreme score. Fifth, instances of multicollinearity and singularity of the variables should be deleted after examining to see if the determinant of the correlation matrix or eigenvalues associated with some factors approach zero. In addition, a squared multiple correlation equal to 1 indicates singularity; and if any of the squared multiple correlations are close to 1, multicollinearity exists. Sixth, outliers among variables, indicated by low squared multiple correlation with all other variables and low correlations with all important factors, suggest the need for cautious interpretation and possible elimination of the variables from the analysis. Seventh, there should be adequate factorability within the correlation matrix, which is indicated by several sizable correlations between pairs of variables that exceed .30. Finally, screening is important for identifying outlying cases among the factors. If such outliers can be identified by large Mahalanobis distances (estimated as chi square values) from the location of the case in the space defined by the factors to the centroid of all cases in the same space, factor analysis is not considered appropriate.

When planning for factor analysis, the first step is to identify a theoretical model that will guide the statistical model (Ferketich & Muller, 1990). The next step is to select the psychometric measurement model, either classic or neoclassic, that will reflect the nature of measurement error. The classic model assumes that all measurement error is random and that all variance is unique to individual variables and not shared with other variables or factors. The neoclassic model recognizes both random and systematic measurement error, which may reflect common variance that is attributable to unmeasured or latent factors. The selection of the classic or neoclassic model influences whether the researcher chooses principal-components analysis or common factor analysis (Ferketich & Muller).

Mathematically speaking, factor analysis generates factors that are linear combinations of variables. The first step in factor analysis is factor extraction, which involves the removal of as much variance as possible through the successive creation of linear combinations that are orthogonal (unrelated) to previously created combinations. The principal-components method of extraction is widely used for analyzing all the variance in the variables. However, other methods of factor extraction, which analyze common factor variance (i.e., variance that is shared with other variables), include the principal-factors method, the alpha method, and the maximum-likelihood method (Nunnally & Bernstein, 1994).

Various criteria have been used to determine how many factors account for a substantial amount of variance in the data set. One criterion is to accept only those factors with an eigenvalue equal to or greater than 1.0 (Guttman, 1954). An eigenvalue is a standardized index of the amount of the variance extracted by each factor. Another approach is to use a scree test to identify sharp discontinuities in the eigenvalues for successive factors (Cattell, 1966).

Factor extraction results in a factor matrix that shows the relationship between the original variables and the factors by means of factor loadings. The factor loadings, when squared, equal the variance in the variable accounted for by the factor. For all of the extracted factors, the sum of the squared loadings for the variables represents the communality (shared variance) of the variables. The sum of a factor's squared loadings for all variables equals that factor's eigenvalue (Nunnally & Bernstein, 1994).

Because the initial factor matrix may be difficult to interpret, factor rotation is commonly used when more than one factor emerges. Factor rotation involves the movement of the reference axes within the factor space so that the variables align with a single factor (Nunnally & Bernstein, 1994). Orthogonal rotation keeps the reference axes at right angles and results in factors that are uncorrelated. Orthogonal rotation is usually performed through a method known as varimax, but other methods (quartimax and equimax) are also available. Oblique rotation allows the reference axes to rotate into acute or oblique angles, thereby resulting in correlated factors (Nunnally & Bernstein). When oblique rotation is used, there are two resulting matrices: a pattern matrix that reveals partial regression coefficients between variables and factors and a structure matrix that shows variable to factor correlations.

Factors are interpreted by examining the pattern and magnitude of the factor loadings in the rotated factor matrix (orthogonal rotation) or pattern matrix (oblique rotation). Ideally, there are one or more marker variables, variables with a very high loading on one and only one factor (Nunnally & Bernstein, 1994), that can help in the interpretation and naming of factors. Generally, factor loadings of .30 and higher are large enough to be meaningful (Nunnally & Bernstein). Once a factor is interpreted and labeled, researchers usually determine factor scores, which are scores on the abstract dimension defined by the factor.

Replication of factor solutions in subsequent analysis with different populations gives increased credibility to the findings. Comparisons between factor-analytic solutions can be made by visual inspection of the factor loadings or by using formal statistical procedures, such as the computation of Cattell's salient similarity index and the use of confirmatory factor analysis (Gorsuch, 1983).

JACLENE A. ZAUSZNIEWSKI

Failure to Thrive (Adult)

Adult failure to thrive (FTT) syndrome is defined as a lower-than-expected level of functioning associated with nutritional deficits, depressed mood state, and social isolation. This definition is derived from numerous theoretic, clinical, and research sources (Newbern & Krowchuk, 1994; Verdery, 1996). Clinically, FTT has been used interchangeably with the terms cachexia, frailty, dwindling, nonspecific presentation of illness, and decompensation. Although it has been discussed primarily in relation to the elderly (Egbert, 1996), based on the above definition, it is likely that the syndrome crosses age boundaries and exists in other chronically ill patient populations, for example, adults with multiple sclerosis, AIDS, or diabetes.

In the International Classification of Diseases, 10th revision (ICD-10), FTT is most frequently classified as a pediatric diagnosis. In children, FTT is very broadly defined as deviation from an expected growth pattern in terms of norms for age and sex (Frank & Zeisel, 1988). Pediatric FTT is generally classified as organic, in which there is a known underlying medical condition; nonorganic, in which the causes are psychosocial; or mixed. Advances in pediatric research also have produced a theoretical framework in which malnutrition is of fundamental importance, either as a primary cause of failure to thrive or a secondary symptom of a chronic illness.

Based on several years of clinical and research experience with the elderly, Verdery (1996) proposed two interesting ideas about the etiology of adult FTT. The first is that the syndrome may occur in response to an event that triggers a more rapid than normal rate of decline. The idea that a trigger event may be a precursor to FTT needs further investigation but it is intuitively believable from both a clinical and research perspective: an event could be physiological in nature (for example, a hip fracture), environmental (for example, a change in residence), psychological (for example, death of a spouse), or a combination of all three. Verdery's second proposition is that there are two categories of adult FTT. This first is *primary* adult FTT, where the reasons for the patient's decline are ambiguous or obscure. In *secondary* adult FTT, the reasons are diagnosable and potentially treatable and there is a wide range of possible underlying factors: (a) medical history and treatment, for example, immune function or polypharmacy; (b) psychological problems, primarily depression; (c) nutritional factors, including eating disorders; and (d) social and/or environmental factors such as isolation or alcohol intake. Although many of the factors in the secondary category of adult FTT have been investigated in relation to health behaviors and outcomes, few have been examined from within a theoretic framework of adult FTT. The framework is in its early stages, and unlike pediatric FTT, there is no consensus on the critical concepts and their relationships, nor are there objective criteria that can be used to evaluate deviation from the norm.

There also is relatively little published research on adult FTT, particularly in the last 5–7 years. Methodological approaches have varied and, without a dominant model of adult FTT, studies have used different definitions of the syndrome, as well as various defining criteria. The following brief summaries of four articles illustrate this feature of our current state of knowledge about adult FTT. In one of the earliest reported studies, Messert, Kurlanzik, and Thorning (1976) identified adult FTT through documentation of a cluster of symptoms in five adult patients diagnosed with neurological disorders (age range = 24–67, mean = 49 years). All of the patients had irreversible weight loss despite high caloric intake, wide variations in body temperature, decreased level of consciousness, unexplained rapid development of decubitus ulcers, and sudden death. A second study examined characteristics of 62 male patients admitted with a medical diagnosis of FTT (Osato, Stone, Phillips, & Winne, 1993), using retrospective chart review. The patients had a wide age range (37–104 years), an average of seven medical diagnoses, required an average of five medications, and 62% had low levels of serum albumin (< 3.5 g/dL). A third study retrospectively examined the medical records of 82 elders admitted with a diagnosis of FTT (Berkman et al., 1986) and used factor analysis to group FTT factors into three categories: patient care management problems, functional problems, and patient coping problems. A fourth study followed 252 subjects for 2 years after new hip fracture (Fox, Hawkes, Magaziner, Zimmerman, & Hebel, 1996). Subjects were generally older (mean = 77 years) and FTT was defined as a decline in walking 6–12 months post-fracture *after* subjects had achieved an initial gain in mobility. Results were mixed: those classified as FTT ($n = 26$) were significantly worse off than the "no decline" group ($n = 226$) in their cognitive decline, number of hospitalizations at 12 months, and self-reported health at 24 months. No statistically significant differences were found between the two groups on the variables of social interaction or depression scores, mortality, physician visits, or nursing home stays.

Although the literature has yet to produce a universally accepted definition, it appears that adult FTT is a multidimensional concept more accurately defined as a syndrome rather than a medical diagnosis (Verdery, 1997). And although it frequently is thought of as a precursor to death, there also is support for the idea that adult failure to thrive is *not* normal aging, the unavoidable result of chronic disease, or a synonym for the terminal stages of dying (Egbert, 1996).

PATRICIA A. HIGGINS

Failure to Thrive (Child)

Failure to thrive is a term used to describe a deceleration in the growth pattern of an infant or child that is directly attributable to undernutrition (Steward, D. K., Ryan-Wenger, & Boyne, 2003). Typically, the deceleration is a growth deficit whereby the rate of the child's weight gain is below the 5th percentile for age, based on the National Center for Health Statistics (NCHS) standardized growth charts. Undernutrition, or caloric inadequacy, and thus a deceleration in a child's growth pattern, can occur for any number of physiological reasons, such as nutrient malabsorption or transient weight loss due to acute illness. When a child's lack of weight gain is attributed to psychosocial factors and developmental concerns rather than organic or disease related factors, the term nonorganic failure to thrive (NOFTT) is used.

Traditionally, the failure to thrive syndrome has been classified into three categories: organic, nonorganic, and mixed. Although the term NOFTT frequently is used in contemporary literature, most researchers agree that the classification is not so clear, especially since all cases of failure to thrive have an organic etiology (i.e., undernutrition). NOFTT is a common problem of infancy and early childhood, and researchers have documented a dramatic increase in its incidence since the late 1970s. NOFTT accounts for 3%–5% of the annual admissions to pediatric hospitals and about 10% of growth failure seen in outpatient pediatrics (Schwartz, I. D., 2002). Infants with NOFTT typically present not only with growth failure, but also with developmental and cognitive delays and signs of emotional and physical deprivation, such as social unresponsiveness, a lack of interactive behaviors, rumination, anorexia, and poor hygiene.

Infant nutrition has long been the focus of pediatric research. Holt (1897) was one of the first to describe marasmus, a significant infant nutrition problem and a condition similar to the failure to thrive syndrome described in contemporary literature. It was in 1915 that the term failure to thrive was first used in the pediatric literature to describe rapid weight loss, listlessness, and subsequent death in institutionalized infants. In the early 1900s, the mortality rate for institutionalized infants was near 100%, and few realized the importance of environmental stimulation and social contact for infant growth and development. It was during this time that the first foster home care program for institutionalized marasmic infants was developed. The home care program involved the identification and training of families, by nurses, to care for the ill infants, and included a significant amount of nursing intervention to monitor the progress of the infants. Unfortunately, this early work was not recognized by the pediatric community, despite a 60% drop in the mortality rate of marasmic infants cared for in the foster homes.

It was not until 1945 that the concept of failure to thrive captured the attention of the psychiatric and pediatric communities. In a classic paper, Spitz (1945) described depression, growth failure, and malnutrition in 61 foundling home infants. He used the term hospitalism to describe the syndrome that he observed, and he proposed that a lack of emotional stimulation and the absence of a mother figure were the main contributors to infant growth failure. Spitz postulated that with adequate love, affection, and stimulation, the infants would grow. Researchers demonstrated weight gain in infants with hospitalism when stimulation and affection were provided. Thus, these findings provided a foundation for a failure to thrive theoretical framework based on maternal deprivation in institutionalized infants.

In the mid-1950s, a number of case reports were published in the psychiatric literature that documented depression, malnutrition, and growth failure in infants living in intact families. These case studies were the first to report feeding and interactional difficulties between the mothers and their infants. Feeding episodes for the mothers were anxiety-provoking, which led the mothers to decrease both the frequency of infant feedings as well as their contact with the infants. Ethnologists and child development experts began studying institutionalized and noninstitutionalized infants to further define the concepts of maternal deprivation and failure to thrive. On the basis of several studies, researchers then concluded that decreased maternal contact directly lead to failure to thrive in the infants. From these works, the maternal deprivation framework for failure to thrive was established, and the mother's role in the infant's well-being became a central focus. Support for this framework grew as data accumulated documenting the association between maternal neglect and failure to thrive in infants.

The maternal deprivation framework dominated the literature until the late 1970s, when a transactional framework was developed to explain the psychosocial correlates of NOFTT. The transactional framework proposes that an infant's growth and development is contingent upon the quality of parental care, the nature of parent and infant interactions, and the ecological conditions impinging on the family. Furthermore, the transactional model recognizes that the quality of the parent-infant interaction reflects infant characteristics as well as parent characteristics (Bithoney & Newberger, 1987). Historically, the emotional deprivation component of NOFTT has been investigated more than the nutritional deprivation component. Although NOFTT experts would agree that undernutrition is the primary biologic insult, systematic studies investigating this element are lacking.

Nutritional deprivation again became the focus of NOFTT research in the early 1970s, when some researchers disputed the hypothesis that maternal deprivation was the principal cause of NOFTT. More recent evidence suggests that the environmental deprivation may occur before the undernutrition. Although the primary cause of NOFTT may never be fully understood, it is apparent that nutritional deficits are dependent on the environmental context in which they occur.

Nurse researchers developed the ecological model to describe parent-child interactions, and the model is used to explain NOFTT (Barnard & Eyres, 1979; Lobo, Barnard, & Coombs, 1992). The ecological model focuses on the three major interaction components of the parent-child relationship: those of the child, the parent, and the environment. These interactions are synchronous and reciprocal. Barnard and her colleagues (1989) emphasized the importance of the parent's and child's physical and emotional characteristics, as well as the supportive or nonsupportive nature of the environment in understanding the interactions.

Researchers have examined parent-child interactions by means of direct, structured observations during feeding and other situations, and found that NOFTT infants demonstrated more difficult behaviors, were less vocal, exhibited negative affect, and had more gaze aversion than infants who were not failing to thrive (Steward, D. K., 2001; Lobo et al., 1992). Furthermore, parents of NOFTT infants were less able to determine their infants' needs, showed a decreased ability to discriminate infant cues, and exhibited less social interactiveness with their infants when compared to parents of healthy infants (Steward, D. K.). These studies supported that interference with the reciprocal process of the parent-child relationship disturbs the opportunity to attain optimal growth and development. Since growth problems, such as NOFTT, in infancy place a child at significant risk for developmental delays as a toddler, it is important to recognize the interactional problems between parents and their infants so that interventions aimed at improving interactions can begin.

HEIDI V. KROWCHUK

Falls

A fall is an unintentional slip, trip, or drop from an upright position resulting in the person landing on the ground or furniture. In older adults, a fall often leads to fear of falling that may contribute to restriction of daily activities or requests for assistance in performing these activities (Howland et al., 1998). The inactivity contributes to deconditioning and disability that place an older adult at an even greater risk for falls. Injury, disability, and death are serious consequences of falls, making this a critical issue for older adults.

Falls are multifactorial in nature and represent the interplay between personal and environmental factors whose pattern of interrelationships varies among individuals and settings. Often falls occur because of a mismatch between these factors. Although being female and over 65 years of age consistently have been found to be risk factors for falls across all settings (community, long-term care, and acute care), these are not sensitive enough for identifying those at greatest risk because all older adults would be considered at risk for a fall. Moreover, these demographic characteristics are not amenable to intervention and provide no direction for interventions to reduce the risk for falls. Although certain diseases and medications have been found to be risk factors, consistency in findings across studies and settings have not been found, and these factors may be of little use in clinical practice to identify those at greatest risk for a fall (Lord, Sherrington, & Menz, 2001) and provide little direction for intervention except for changes to pharmacologic treatments. Although fear of falling has been found to be a risk factor for falls (Harada et al., 1995), this fear may be attributable to poor balance, gait, and muscle strength (Kressig et al., 2001) that also have been related to falls and are more amenable to intervention than demographic characteristics.

Much of the early epidemiological and clinical research on falls focused on environmental factors, while more recent research focuses on personal risk factors. Inconsistencies of findings related to environmental factors among studies and settings abound. Clinical and research interventions targeted to environmental factors were designed to educate older adults about how to eliminate these risks. These environmental interventions and education of older adults were marginally successful at best. In some studies, community-dwelling older adults often were reluctant to make the recommended environmental changes and were more interested in interventions to reduce the risks related to personal factors. In contrast, clinicians and architects used the clinical and research information to design health care facilities and have begun to examine the effects of environmental factors, such as carpeting, on personal factors (Dickinson, Shroyer, & Elias, 2002).

Balance, gait, and muscle strength emerged from more recent research as significant risk factors for falls. The Physiologic Profile Assessment (PPA) consists of physiologic factors associated with balance control (vision, muscle strength, postural sway, reaction time, and peripheral sensation) (Lord, Menz, & Tiedemann, 2003). Using the Internet, the results of the PPA can be compared to a normative sample. Many screening tools contain similar information and have strong sensitivity and specificity in predicting falls (Perell et al., 2001). Consensus regarding the assessment of risk and determination of risk profiles is needed before clinically useful screening tools appropriate for various settings are widely used.

In 1991, the American Geriatrics Society and the American Academy of Orthopedic Surgeons Panel on Falls Panel (2001) put forth an evidence-based tiered approach to screening. The initial screen includes the Get Up and Go test that had good specificity and sensitivity (Perell et al., 2001; Shumway-Cook, Brauer, & Woollacott, 2000) and assesses the older adult for instability or inability in getting up from a chair without using their arms, walking a known distance, and sitting down. If the Get Up and Go (Podsiadlo & Richardson, 1991) is abnormal, the panel recommends a comprehensive assessment that includes medical history, medications, evaluation of balance, gait, vision, and cardiovascular and neurological status. Other measures with good sensitivity and specificity were the Elderly Fall Screening Test (Cwikel, Fried, Biderman, & Galinsky, 1998), and the STRATIFY (Oliver, Britton, Seed, Martin, & Hopper, 1997).

Risk factors for falls are multifactorial, and interventions also must be multidimensional. Interventions must target the deficits of the older person that place them at risk for a fall and compensate for nonmodifiable factors. Consideration of the capabilities of the older adult and the setting are essential in selecting interventions. Comprehensive descriptions for interventions can be found in *Falls in Older People: Risk Factors and Strategies for Prevention* (Lord et al., 2001) and *Falls in Older People: Prevention and Management* (Tideiksaar, 2002).

The American Geriatric Society Panel on Falls Prevention (2001) recommended guidelines for interventions. Reducing medications, exercise, and treatment of disease were most effective in community-based interventions. Reducing environmental hazards in the home, comprehensive assessment of fall risk, and education were not effective. Exercise, aerobic and muscle-strengthening, was the most effective single intervention. The concurrent management of visual impairment and reduction of environmental hazards increased the effects above those attributed to exercise alone (Day et al., 2002). The panel found that staff education, reduction of medications, and comprehensive assessment significantly reduced falls in long-term care facilities. The panel found no significant multifactorial interventions for the hospital setting where shortened hospital stays preclude some interventions (e.g., exercise). Environmental interventions, medication management, and treatment of disease or injury may be the most effective in the hospital setting.

No matter the setting, the acceptability of the intervention to the older adult and their ability to use the intervention are significant factors in adherence. Strategies to increase acceptability and adherence, particularly for exercise interventions, have achieved limited success. The most potent strategies are engaging older adults in the selection of relevant interventions and assisting them to remove barriers and to increase support for using the intervention.

BEVERLY L. ROBERTS

Family Care

Family care is defined in many ways, dependent on the study and approach and how it is applied in health care system policies or regulations affecting support to family members. The role of the family in providing care is considered a normative family role with the obligations and responsibilities that go with such roles. Family care as a normative role includes that of a person caring for a child or the usual role relationships with other members, such as a spouse. Family care however, is also care that goes beyond such a role and takes on the role of a health care provider as the family member assists the individual with the tasks, duties, and responsibilities required of one with a chronic illness, injury, or disability.

Research on family care includes the normal parenting for the growth and development of children, care of children with disabilities, care of children with chronic illness such as cancer or asthma, care of an ill spouse, care of an aging and frail parent, caring for brain damaged adults, caregiving for adults with dementia, and grandparents caring for children. The care role activities and demands on family members vary markedly depending on age, relationship, and patient problems.

The parental care of an infant or child is considered a normative patient role. Research in the normative areas examines mother-infant bonds or father-infant bonds and relationships, parenting, and the role of the parent in growth and development. Recent activities include the father more often, and examine the father-child bonds (Coleman & Garfield, 2004). Some work looks at the role of the single parent with infants and children, and follows the mother across time looking at parenting (Evans, M., 2004; McCreary & Dancy, 2004).

The role that is difficult and assumes the nonnormative role of the parent is caring for a child with low birth weight and infants and children with physical or developmental disabilities. There are also studies of parents with the provision of technological support. Decisions and normalization around children with disabilities and birth defects are also present in the literature. The effort of the patient then is to try to normalize the experience for the whole family (Deatrick, Knafl, & Murphy-Moore, 1999; Sullivan-Bolyai, Knafl, Sadler, & Gilliss, 2004; Sullivan-Bolyai, Sadler, Knafl, & Gilliss, 2003). Consideration of time away from school, social restrictions, fear of exacerbations, and uncertainty about treatment evolve. Child, parent caregiver, and family outcomes in general may be examined. Parental concerns are about time management, child status, finances, and family relations. Family hardiness, family functioning, family stressors, and family need for knowledge to reduce uncertainty, are areas reviewed in family care research.

Formal professional caregivers must work in partnership with family members of a child with a chronic and long-term illness. Much of the research on family care of children with chronic disease is related to the child with asthma, cancer, or diabetes. Health care professionals support the family by providing thorough advice, helping them to cope, assessing perceptions, encouraging expression of feelings, and securing resources (Kurnat & Moore, 1999). The environment, child, family view of health, attitudes toward illness, everyday routines, and social network are important. The chronic illness must be normalized so that both the family and child can have a positive quality of life (Miles, M. S., 2003). Although a lot of the research is related to quality of life of the parent and child, coping, and adjustment, some recent models look at family strengths, assets, and resilience rather than negative dimensions of care. Care responsibilities of parents include managing illness, coordinating resources, maintaining the family unit, and maintaining themselves (Sullivan-Bolyai et al., 2003).

Recent research includes studies on grandparents caring for grandchildren. Many of these studies are descriptive and identify the distress experienced by those who provide care. Grandparents often care for grandchildren with developmental disabilities, chronic illness, or HIV/AIDS. Others care for children from dysfunctional families where a parent is not responsible, abuses substances, abuses or neglects the children, and those whose parents are divorced. Many of the grandparent family caregivers are older and have chronic illnesses themselves, which puts them at risk for additional health problems. In addition, the multiple roles add to their stress and distress. Grandparents who live on fixed incomes may lack support and respite, as well as experience emotional and financial strains (Green, S., 2001; Fuller-Thompson & Minkler, 2001) from their care role.

For the spouse of the adult with chronic illness, literature is limited for the younger spouses, although there is some work in cancer, especially bone marrow transplants and hematological cancers (Langer, Abrams, & Syrjala, 2003). Most of the spouse literature focuses on the female spouse and relates to the older patient with chronic illness. Most of that research relates to dementia, stroke, and degenerative diseases such as multiple sclerosis and Parkinson's disease, with cancer being a more recent focus (Palmer, S., & Glass, 2003; Bakas, Austin, Jessup, Williams, & Oberst, 2004). The definition of this care usually calls the person a family carer, and is defined as one who provides assistance with health-related tasks for someone who is frail or chronically ill. Recent work includes other family relationships, including men who care (Kramer, B., & Lambert, 1999; Kramer, B., & Thompson, 2002). The tasks of care provided by family members sort out those that are direct tasks, and those that are subjective or less direct, such as supervision for patient protection. A variety of conceptual models have been used to examine family care of the adult, but most have been built on the stress and coping literature. There is concern that families may benefit from skill building, which may be more beneficial than information and support (Farran, Loukissa, Perraud, & Pann, 2004).

Literature also includes increasing research on younger family members who care for the older parent or parent-in-law. Most research on family care examines the role of the adult daughter (Chumbler, Grimm, Cody, & Beck, 2003). Few studies exist that look at sons caring for parents (Kramer & Thompson, 2002). The mix of task and care activities and response to that care seem to differ by gender, relationship, and age of the caregiver. Care tasks provided by family members and concerns may center around competency to perform tasks (Farran et al., 2004; Schumacher, Stewart, Archbold, Dodd, & Dibble, 2000). Males may not be comfortable with cooking, cleaning, or community services, but females may find these activities normative. Models for the adult children caring for a parent are likewise built around stress and coping, although a few models look at role theory (Sherwood, P., et al., 2004). The problem with family care literature is that most of the outcomes for all ages to date have been coping, adjustment, and mental health issues such as burden or depression. Only recently has there been research to examine the health practices, health promotion, health status, and skill requirements of the adult family member providing care. Recent research has begun to examine the long-term effect on family members who provide care, and indeed, the mortality rate is higher than for the noncaregiver (Schultz & Beach, 1999). The distress that family members experience for parent care is determined by gender and age. Women more than men and younger persons more than older persons who are involved in family care, report more distress.

Methodologically, most of the early studies of family care are descriptive and cross-sectional, and many still are. Recent studies of families providing health care are beginning to include intervention studies. These studies often do not include a family framework as a guide to the research, but are based on stress, coping, and/or role theory. At times, some family dimensions are added to the studies as the antecedent variable, but not a family focus in general.

Data is collected increasingly from both patients and family members who provide care, even if they are children. Often, however, function and family dynamics are not a part of family care data collection, but data is collected about individuals. Most do not examine the family as a unit. Tools to evaluate family processes after the major insult of these problems are inadequate and need further development. Ethnicity and socioeconomic status are not adequately examined in the family context.

There are many untapped areas for research to help understand how the family as a unit contributes to or hinders family members' health. More work is needed on the areas of family care so that nurses can provide the support to family members that they need to be able to continue their care. The family must be considered as a unit of care since it is essential to the outcomes of the care of individuals or illness—especially in chronic illness at a time of restricted health care resources.

Interventions are needed to relate psychological factors to facilitate coping, family and parent education about disease and treatment to reduce uncertainty, and assist the family member to mobilize resources for the unity of the family.

SUZANNE L. FEETHAM
BARBARA GIVEN

Family Caregiving to Frail Elders

Family caregiving to frail elders refers to the informal caretaking by immediate and extended family of older adults needing assistance due to physical or cognitive impairments. Family caregiving is an important concept for nurses because many older adults will receive some help with activities of daily living and/or in-home care for acute or chronic health problems, including end-of-life care. Such care is frequently provided informally by family members and supplemented by formal care arrangements. The family caregiver does not always live in the same home as the care recipient, and although there is no minimum amount of time that family must provide care to be considered family caregivers, many researchers use 5 hours of care per week as a criterion.

Women are more likely to assume the role of family caregiver to elders, in part due to their traditional caregiving roles in families. Balancing competing responsibilities as a caregiver, employee, spouse, parent, and family and community member is a challenge often faced by midlife women. At what point in one's life caregiving occurs may influence the effects of caregiving (Moen, Robison, & Dempster-McClain, 1995). Some studies suggest that initiating caregiving is especially stressful because it requires many adaptations, but that continued caregiving may be viewed as less difficult as it becomes more routine. Family caregivers often report both burden and reward from the caregiving experience. Whether adult children experience more burden than do spouses is not conclusive. There appear to be ethnic differences in burden from caregiving, with minority caregivers likely to report less burden. Instrumental support from other family members has been associated with less burden.

Family caregiving affects the entire family, regardless of whether the caregiver and care recipient live in the same home. Caregiving requires an investment of resources (time, energy, money) that are diverted from other activities. In one study of caregivers of frail elders (Covinsky et al., 2001), 22% of caregivers either quit a job or reduce work hours. Minority care recipients and those with lower ADL function, dementia, or a history of stroke were more likely to have family who reduced or quit work; daughters and daughters-in-law of the elder were likely to quit working (Covinsky et al.). Minority caregivers were more likely to care for frail elders at home (Cagney & Agree, 1999).

Maintaining the health of family caregivers is a priority, and caregiver health has been the focus of considerable research. Caregivers are often older adults themselves (spouses, siblings, or friends of the care recipient), prone to muscle and back injuries from lifting and other activities, and may neglect their own health in the process of caregiving. Many studies examining the health of older adults have been cross-sectional, and thus evidence about the long-term consequences of caregiving is scanty. In general, caregivers who report greater stress and burden and less mastery tend to report worse health, more health problems, and more depressive symptoms. Most studies have used self-report rather than objective or direct measures. Few studies have followed caregivers after they cease caregiving, although the Canadian Study of Health and Aging Working Group (2002) found that caregivers to healthy elders reported fewer health problems than caregivers to impaired elders, but that death or institutionalization of the elder did not have a consistent impact on caregiver health. Understanding of the consequences of caregiving is complicated by the need to disentangle the effects of caregiver aging from any effects of caregiving burden or activity.

In many situations, formal, paid support services (meal service, home health, respite care) supplement the family's caregiving efforts. Such formal assistance often is associated with less caregiver depression and better self-assessed health, although one longitudinal study (Musil, Morris, Warner, & Saeid, 2003) found that an increase in formal support over 2 years was associated with worsening self-assessed but better muscular-skeletal health. Caregivers may seek outside support from formal services if they need to compensate for their own deficits, but lack of help may cause wear and tear from the physical burdens of caregiving. Current research is examining ethnic differences in the use of services, including formal care and respite services.

Little is known about how the support from the care recipient's health care provider (nurse practitioner, physician) affects family caregiving, although provider support has been shown to influence the perceived rewards of caregiving (Musil et al., 2003). An emerging area of interest involves the types of provider interactions that are viewed as supportive by caregivers, or at what points in the caregiving trajectory various interactions are viewed as beneficial by family caregivers.

Family caregivers to frail elders participate in caregiving not only in-home, but across transitions to other facilities, including hospitals, nursing homes, long-term care, and hospice. Involvement in discharge planning is important for the caregiver and care recipient well-being; caregivers who were more involved in discharge planning for their elder care recipient reported better health and greater acceptance of their caregiving role 2 months post discharge (Bull, Hansen, & Gross, 2000). Recent trends include predicting when families will seek nursing home placement. Coordination of care between informal and formal caregivers with nurse and physician providers is advocated in the literature but often difficult to achieve in practice.

A number of recent studies have looked at interventions to support caregivers' work, maintain or improve caregiver health, or increase caregiver knowledge of the care recipient's disease processes. Intervention studies have examined the effects of support groups, telephone support, computer support, and RN and Advanced Practice Nurse interventions (Dellasega & Zerbe, 2002). In a meta-analysis of 26 intervention studies, Yin, Zhou, and Bashford (2002) found positive effects for group and individual interventions to reduce caregiver burden. Another line of intervention research focuses on interventions to assist caregivers in their daily care of impaired elders. Interventions focus on caregiver activities, such as toileting and feeding impaired elders; maintaining care recipient nutritional status, mobility, and skin integrity; dealing with confusion, verbal outbursts, wandering, and falls; and participation in adult day-care situations.

Increasingly, current research examines family caregiving from different cultural perspectives, including international comparisons of burden, stress, coping, and support. In addition, ethnographic methods illuminate similarities, differences, and the nuances of family caregiving within cultural groups. Such research is increasingly important. Other directions for future family caregiver research include the need for longitudinal perspectives and mixed-method designs incorporating qualitative and quantitative methods to better describe aspects of the family caregiving experience, including gender differences in caregiving. Additional work with interventions aimed at the caregiver and at the care recipient is needed.

CAROL M. MUSIL

Family Caregiving and the Seriously Mentally Ill

Approximately eleven million adults in the United States live with serious mental illness and about three million dependent children suffer from a severe emotional disturbance (Dean, 2003). The United States currently spends over $70 billion per year on mental health treatment. Effective care of the mentally ill and their families requires early community intervention using a variety of integrated approaches including mental health and social service teams. Effective mental health treatment must encompass sick individuals and their families and take into account the complex relationship between mental illness and unemployment, homelessness, drug addiction, and involvement in the criminal justice system.

The importance of alliance building between family caregivers, the mentally ill member and the health care team was described by Kempe (1994). Families are continuing to ask health professionals to communicate with them in a reciprocal way (Biegel, Robinson, & Kennedy, 2000). As mental health care continues to become more community-based, the family is required to assume more responsibility and care of their mentally ill member, yet families are not getting the direction and support that is needed (Levine, 1998). Family caregiving for the mentally ill involves the family steadfastly assisting the mentally ill family member with basic physical and emotional needs as well as maintaining a positive relationship and environment that nurtures a sense of self and belonging and allows the mentally ill person to strive towards educational and vocational goals. The roadblocks facing families attempting to care for their ill family member continue to be: (a) laws, policies, and regulations affecting care, (b) attitudes of health care providers including psychiatrists and nurses, and (c) consumer misinformation and stigma.

From the 1960s through the 1990s caregiving studies identified several negative issues such as burden and related stressors (Maurin & Boyd, 1990). Caregivers were identified as needing much social support. Since 1990, these burdensome issues continued to exist but many positive aspects also have been described. It has now been concluded that health care professionals must develop the theoretical flexibility to accommodate the diverse situations which family caregivers face in caring for their ill members. Encouraging family caregivers to listen to experiences of others in caregiving roles and then learn to think creatively about themselves and their experiences has been a strategy that is helpful (Doornbos, 2002).

Levine (1998) identified that families want information about mental illness and how to cope with the situation. It was also found that family caregivers value a positive relationship with health care providers, which includes respect and nonjudgmental approaches (Rose, K. E., 1998a). In addition, Biegel, Robinson, and Kennedy (2000) found that families also wanted dialogs within groups and individualized whole family support. Those studies reported that families continue to experience difficulties with the mental health system and financial issues.

Chronic mental illness can effect the family in many ways, including changes in familiar roles, changes in subsystems within the family, possible isolation of family members, increased need for problem-solving skills, and adjustments with adaptability to family role changes. Caregivers experience more distress as the number of tasks they must complete increases and the ill member's depression increases. The social support required is really a large affirming social network of support that includes professionals participating in the care of the mentally ill person (Margliano et al., 1998).

More research that focuses on family caregivers of the mentally ill is needed. Researchers need to focus on how to remove barriers that impede access to quality care. Long-standing barriers include: mistaken public policy, insufficient health insurance coverage, money, the attitudes and practices of health care providers, and the attitudes and preferences of health care consumers. One necessary research need is to determine ways to convince the political system of the need for parity in reimbursement for mental illness from insurance providers.

Doornbos (2002) summarized the many difficulties experienced by families as they provide care for their mentally ill members. She found that the issues that families and their mentally ill members must cope with include stress, powerlessness, physical health issues, financial problems, and the enormous burden borne by nonprofessionals attempting to provide care for the mentally ill. Finding a better way to meet the many needs described by family members with a mentally ill member is also an important contribution needed in nursing. Meeting these needs may best be accomplished through research and development of a health care model for all mental health professionals.

ALICE KEMPE

Family Health

No universal definition of family has been adopted by the legal and social systems, family scientists, or the clinical disciplines that work with or study families. How the family is defined determines the factors that will be examined to evaluate the health of individual family members and the family unit. In addition to the biological family, when examining health in the context of the family, the family can be defined as constituting the group of persons acting together to perform functions required for the survival, growth, safety, socialization, and health of family members. These functions include supporting health and caring for ill and disabled members. Research on health has focused primarily at the level of the individual and has demonstrated the interdependence between the health of the individual family members and the family (Feetham, 1999).

Factors influencing family health include (a) genetics; (b) physiological and psychological responses of individual family members; (c) cultural influences; and (d) the physical, social, economic, and political environments, including resources. Researchers have shown that health and risk factors cluster in families because members often have similar diets, activity patterns, and behaviors, such as smoking and alcohol abuse, as well as a common physical environment. Identification of healthy families has focused on family interaction patterns, family problem solving, and patterns of responses to changes in the family system. These definitions and concepts of family health provide a framework for determining measurable outcomes of family health while also accounting for the diversity in family structure (Feetham, 1999, 2000).

In 2003 we entered the genomic era, with findings from genomic research and advances in genetic technologies requiring a reframing of how we think of the continuum of health and illness, and even the concept of disease. The way in which diseases are categorized, and ultimately how they are treated and managed, will change. No longer named by their symptoms (such as asthma), diseases will be more specifically identified by knowing the genetic and environmental causes leading to more focused treatments (Guttmacher & Collins, 2002). Individuals and families will be faced with reframing their concept and experience with diagnosis, treatment, and prevention to include the term "genetically-linked" disorder, with the blurring of the boundary between health and illness (Feetham & Thomson, in press). Genetic information may result in the need to extend the concept of "illness time" phases to include knowledge of a risk state, or in some cases, a presymptomatic phase (Rolland, 1999; Street, E., & Soldan, 1998). The risk state refers to the time before a statistical risk is known or acknowledged or the point in time when symptoms occur. The risk state may require interventions for individuals and families to respond to the increased awareness of risk, new genetic risk information, or even the earliest occurrence of symptoms. Families may need to begin to deal with anticipatory loss, accept increased surveillance, adhere to changes in health behaviors, or accept interventions that may potentially delay the onset or progression of the disease.

Effective interventions with families incorporate an understanding of what health means to individual family members and to the family as a unit, and how the environment influences their health actions. The family has been described as the primary social agent in the promotion of health and well-being; therefore, our knowledge of the family and its relationship to the health of its individual members is central to research related to health promotion and to families responding to risk information and experiencing illness and disability.

SUZANNE L. FEETHAM

Family Satisfaction With End-of-Life Care

The nurse is uniquely positioned to provide the kind of care most needed by patients and families at the end-of-life transition—interventions that not only promote health and healing, but also promote comfort and emotional support for patients and their families. Applying the nursing model, the desired outcome at end-of-life is a *good death*. Given the lack of research available about the needs of dying patients and their families, nurses are not adequately equipped to provide interdisciplinary leadership in establishing evidence-based practice guidelines for caring for patients and families at this critical transition. This review reports on the evidence that exists to guide practice and what knowledge gaps need to be addressed. Specifically, this review focuses on family perspectives regarding end-of-life care: how is the quality of patient care measured and evaluated by the family at end of life; how satisfied are decedents' families with communication and support received at end of life; what are the needs of families and patients and how well are these needs addressed.

Teno and others (2004) evaluated the United States dying experience at home and in institutional settings. A sample of 3,275 was generated from death certificates in 22 states. A total of 1,578 actual telephone interviews resulted to provide national estimates of the dying experience for a target population of 1.97 million deaths in the year 2000. The setting was predominately patients dying in an institution (hospital or nursing facility) (67.1%) but also included patients who died at home (32.9%). Of the group who died at home, 12.5% received nursing services, 38.2% did not receive nursing services, and 49.3% received hospice services. The study concluded that one third of respondents cared for by a home health agency, nursing home, or hospital reported insufficient emotional support for the patient and/or one or more concerns with family emotional support, compared with about one fifth of those receiving home hospice services. Of all categories, nursing home residents were less likely to have been treated with respect at end of life. Of family members of patients who received hospice services, 70.7% rated care as "excellent" compared with less than 50% of family members of those dying in an institution or with home health services. The researchers noted that even within hospice care there is a need for improvement, as 1 in 4 respondents reported unmet needs in the management of dyspnea and in the emotional support provided.

Baker and others (2000) examined family satisfaction regarding patient comfort, communication, and decision making at end of life. The participants were surrogate respondents (97% were family members) for 767 seriously ill hospitalized adults who died. The study design was a prospective cohort study with patients randomized to either usual care or to an intervention that included clinical nurse specialists to assist in symptom control and facilitation of communication and decision making. The intervention was drawn from the Study to Understand Prognoses and Preferences for Outcomes and Risks of Treatments (SUPPORT), which evaluated interventions that increased attention to pain, provided objective estimates of patient prognosis, facilitated communication among medical staff, patients, and their surrogates, and increased patient or surrogate involvement in decision making. The patient settings were five teaching hospitals in urban areas distributed throughout the United States. The study examined family members' ratings of patient comfort and communication/decision making in end-of-life care using telephone interviews conducted 4 to 10 weeks after the date of death. The study found that 84% of family members expressed no dissatisfaction with patient comfort, and 70% expressed no dissatisfaction with communication and decision making. Examination of data revealed that the hospital site was the only factor that was significantly related to both measures of satisfaction. The researchers suggested that because the structure of care and practice affected patient satisfaction, defined quality indicators could be used to improve satisfaction. Also, the study found that satisfaction with patient comfort decreased with increasing impact of the patient's illness on family finances. The findings suggested that those with less financial resources might have received less comfort care. The SUPPORT interventions were significant primarily for those patients who died after their index hospitalization. Respondents for those that died after the index hospitalization and had not received the interventions were significantly less satisfied than those who had received the SUPPORT intervention. The study concluded that male family members were less satisfied, but greater satisfaction was seen when patients were in less pain (Baker et al., 2000).

Steinhauser and others (2000) gathered descriptions of the components of a good death from patients, families, and care providers through focus-group discussions and in-depth interviews. The sample consisted of 75 participants and included physicians, nurses, social workers, chaplains, hospice volunteers, patients, and recently bereaved families. Six broad components of a good death were identified: pain and symptom management, clear decision making, preparation for death, completion, contributing to others, and affirmation of the whole person. The study found that for patients and families, psychosocial and spiritual issues are as important as physiologic concerns. For all categories, professional role distinctions were more influential to attitudes than sex or ethnic differences. Physicians' groups' views differed the most from the other groups and offered the most biomedical approach. A weakness of this study was that researchers did not report specifics about other professional focus groups such as nurses. Also, as the researchers pointed out, although all socioeconomic, educational, and age groups were represented, most patients were recruited from a Veterans Affairs medical center and were mostly men, and as a result, these findings may not generalize to other groups.

This literature review revealed a paucity of research on the topic of family satisfaction and end-of-life care. It was heartening to find that in the study by Baker and others (2000), in many areas family and patient needs are being well met. However, satisfaction levels were not high across the board, and other research pointed to areas where changes in practice are needed. The research by Steinhauser and others (2000) begins to build a consensus of what constitutes a good death, but a more comprehensive random sample of patients and families (as opposed to health care professionals) is needed to truly define this concept. The results from such a study could be incorporated into a subsequent study that evaluates how often a good death is actually experienced by the dying and their families. After evaluating the dying experience against a well-defined universal benchmark of what constitutes a good death, it would make sense to apply various independent variables, such as those that have been touched on in the study by Baker and others. The independent variables might include testing the effect of SUPPORT interventions, examining the differences between structure of care provided by same-type institutions and then versus other types, and then determining precisely which elements of hospice care make it so much more effective in meeting the needs of dying patients and their families. Another variable to be examined is how professionals in various disciplines are educated (or not) to address the needs of the terminally ill. This variable was touched upon in the study by Steinhauser and others, but much more could be done to better understand the impact of this component.

Caring for the terminally ill is an essential aspect of professional nursing, and this review indicates that much research still needs to be done to understand and appropriately care for the dying and their families.

KAREN CORCORAN

Family Theory and Research

Family refers to any group whose members are related to one another through marriage, birth, or adoption. E. Burgess's (1926) description of a family as a unit of interacting personalities is still relevant to how families are viewed today. Because of the variety of family forms, theorists and researchers should provide their own definitions of family.

Nursing has long been interested in families as the context for individual members and has focused more recently on the family as a whole. Families have been a component of studies of psychiatric illness, caregiving, violence, adaptation to chronic illness in both children and adults, and cardiac conditions and other acute illnesses. Family transitions, including grieving, transition to parenthood for adolescent mothers and married couples, and adaptation to divorce, remarriage, and stepfamilies, also have been studied. Nurses have published reports in major family journals as well as in nursing research and specialty journals and the new *Journal of Family Nursing*.

Scholars from various disciplines have studied families, using diverse approaches. Theories presented here (except for stress theory) are based on descriptions provided by Klein and White (1996).

The central focus in exchange theory is on the individual and what motivates his or her actions. Individuals are viewed as rational and self-interested, seeking to maximize rewards and avoid costs. Individuals compare their own situation to others in the same circumstances and to others in different circumstances. In exchange theory the family is viewed as a collection of individuals. The family group is considered to be a source of rewards and costs for individual members. Exchange theory could be used by nurse researchers to investigate the processes of family negotiation and problem solving.

Like exchange theory, conflict theory assumes that individuals are motivated by self-interest. Individuals compete for scarce resources, which include knowledge, skills, techniques, and materials. Resources provide a potential base for the exercise of power. Conflict within the family is seen as the result of inequity of resources among individuals. Because conflict is both endemic and inevitable, a primary focus in the study of families is how they manage conflict.

Concepts of symbolic interactionism include interaction patterns, meanings and definitions, symbols, sense of self, and role expectations. Socialization is the process by which individuals acquire the symbols, beliefs, and attitudes of their culture. Individuals construct a sense of self and meanings for events and things through interactions with other people and with the environment. Role involves each person's adjusting behavior to what he or she thinks the other person is going to do. Children and adults have particularly significant interactions in the context of the family. Likewise, roles that develop within the family are a crucial component of the individual's self-image.

The family as a whole is the focus of family systems theory. All parts of the system are interconnected, and therefore, changes in one part of the system influence all other parts of the system. Subsystems are smaller units of the system, such as individuals and dyads. Boundaries define who participates in the family and who participates in each subsystem. Boundaries exist between family members, between subsystems, and between the family system and the external environment. The degree of permeability of boundaries (open or closed) refers to the extent of impediments to the flow of information and energy. A homeostatic system dynamically maintains equilibrium by feedback and control.

The central concept in the ecological approach is adaptation. The child always develops in the context of family-type relationships, and that development is the outcome of the interaction of the person's genetic environment with the immediate family and eventually with components of the environment. The individual is embedded in four nested systems. The microsystem is the immediate setting in which the person fulfills his or her roles, such as family, school, or place of employment. The mesosystem refers to the interrelations between two or more settings in which the developing person actively participates. The exosystem consists of external settings that do not include the person as an active participant but instead include systems (such as the legal system) that affect the person's immediate settings. Macrosystem refers to culture. Bishop and Ingersoll (1989) used the ecological framework in their research on the effects of marital conflict and family structure on self-concepts of children.

Family development theory focuses on systematic changes experienced by families as they move through stages of their life course. Family stage is an interval of time in which the structure and interactions of role relationships in the family are noticeably distinct from other periods of time. Shifts from one family stage to another are called transitions. Family development theory emphasizes the dimensions of time and change. Using family development theory, Mercer, Ferketich, DeJoseph, May, and Sollid (1988) investigated the effect of stress on family functioning during pregnancy.

The double ABCX model is an extension of R. Hill's (1958) original ABCX family stress model, in which A refers to the stressor event and related hardships, B refers to resources, and C to perception of A (McCubbin & Patterson, 1983). The crisis, X (the amount of disruptiveness or disorganization), emerges from the interaction of the event, resources, and perception of the event. The family's accumulation of life events and added stressors over time (Aa, pileup of demands) influences family adaptation both directly and indirectly through Bb (adaptive resources) and Cc, which is the perception of X, Aa, and Bb. J. Austin's (1996) study of family adaptation to childhood epilepsy is based on a modification of the double ABCX model.

Research on families typically is an effort to test theoretical propositions or to develop theory. Although family research reflects different theoretical orientations, a common concern is the most appropriate unit of analysis. Is the concept of interest a property of the individual, dyad, or the family as a whole? For example, can families as a whole or only individual members perceive? Another recurring issue in family research is how to construct family variables if discrepant reports are provided by different members of the same family. As family scholars address these problems, they can better explain the complexities of family life and ultimately provide guidance for intervention.

LINDA C. HABER

Fatigue

Fatigue is a universal symptom associated with most acute and chronic illnesses. It also is a common complaint among otherwise healthy persons, and often is cited as one of the most prevalent presenting symptoms in primary care practices. Defining fatigue, however, has challenged scientists for years. No clear biological marker of fatigue has been identified and fatigue remains a perplexing symptom for all health care providers.

Not only was fatigue named one of the top four symptoms for study by an expert panel on symptom management convened by the National Institute of Nursing Research (NINR) in the early 1990s, but recently fatigue has been singled out as among the symptoms or health outcomes needing attention for standardized measurement in the National Institutes of Health (NIH) Roadmap for Research initiatives recently released. Because nursing is centrally interested in symptoms and symptom management, fatigue is of major concern for nurse researchers and clinicians alike.

The North American Nursing Diagnosis Association (NANDA) defines fatigue as: "An overwhelming sustained sense of exhaustion and decreased capacity for physical and mental work at usual level" (NANDA, 2003, p. 74). Although a number of nurse researchers have studied fatigue and offered various proposals for categorizing fatigue, most accept the NANDA definition of fatigue. An alternative view of fatigue as: The awareness of a decreased capacity for physical and/or mental activity due to an imbalance in the availability, utilization, and/or restoration of resources needed to perform an activity (Aaronson, L. S., et al., 1999) also has been proposed. This definition is not inconsistent with the NANDA definition; however, it adds a generic understanding of potential causes of fatigue that may differ in different situations, in order to facilitate studying the mechanisms of fatigue in different clinical conditions. This addition also allows for a clearer conception of fatigue as a biobehavioral phenomenon.

With increased recognition of the importance of studying symptoms within nursing, more work on fatigue has emerged. Both investigators and study participants have made distinctions between acute and chronic fatigue. In one qualitative study, participants distinguished acute fatigue from chronic fatigue in terms of origin (specific single event vs. long-term ongoing condition), onset (quick vs. slow), duration (brief vs. continuous), recovery (quick vs. slow) and control (yes over acute, no over chronic) (Aaronson, Pallikkathayil, & Crighton, 2003). These distinctions are similar to those put forth by Piper (1989), who identified acute fatigue as protective, linked to a single cause, of short duration with a rapid onset, perceived as normal, generally occurring in basically healthy persons with minimal impact on the person, and usually relieved by rest; whereas chronic fatigue is identified as being perceived as abnormal, having no known function or purpose, occurring in clinical populations, having many causes, not particularly related to exertion, persisting over time, having an insidious onset, not usually relieved by rest, and having a major impact on the person (see also Potempa, 1993, for a review of chronic fatigue).

In the research and clinical literature, fatigue related to childbearing (see Milligan & Pugh, 1994, for a review) and fatigue related to cancer (see Irvine, Vincent, Bubela, Thompson, & Graydon, 1991; Smets, Garssen, Schuster-Uitterhoeve, & de Haes, 1993; Winningham et al., 1994; and Nail, 2002, for reviews) have received the most attention. Even these areas, however, remain largely understudied and poorly understood. While fatigue has been studied in numerous chronic illnesses, such as AIDS, multiple sclerosis, and rheumatoid arthritis, cancer-related fatigue is somewhat unique in that it is often fatigue associated with the treatment for cancer (both radiation and chemotherapy) that is most troublesome in terms of distress to the individual. In fact, fatigue associated with cancer treatment has been cited as a major reason for prematurely discontinuing treatment.

Fatigue also has been consistently associated with fever and infectious processes, and one of the more puzzling manifestations of fatigue is what is currently called Chronic Fatigue Syndrome (CFS). CFS is a diagnosis used for cases of severe and persistent fatigue for which no specific cause has been identified (see Fukuda et al., 1994, for the current full case definition of CFS and Reeves et al., 2003, for recommended revisions to address the ambiguities in the current case definition). Under varying names (e.g., neurasthenia, myalgic encephalomyelitis, postinfectious or postviral syndrome, and chronic fatigue immune disorder syndrome, CFIDS), a syndrome of unexplained, chronic, persistent fatigue has been documented in the literature since the late 19th century. Preliminary evidence from controlled studies and extensive clinical descriptions point to both a hypothalamic-pituitary-adrenal (HPA) disorder (Demitrack et al., 1991) and an immune system disregulation (Bearn & Wesseley, 1994) as likely central mechanisms operating in CFS.

Difficulty studying, understanding, and consequently, treating fatigue is largely due to its ubiquitous nature and the unknown, but likely multiple, causes of fatigue. Untangling the relationship between fatigue and depression, in particular, further confounds investigations of fatigue. While fatigue is an identified symptom of depression, long-standing chronic fatigue, unrelated to an existing affective disorder, actually may precipitate depression. Evidence that the HPA axis is implicated in both CFS and depression, and that a different pattern of neuroendocrine disturbance in CFS from that seen in depression has been identified in at least one study (Ray, 1991), is encouraging for establishing an important distinction between fatigue that is a symptomatic expression of depression and fatigue due to other causes.

A lack of consistent, valid, and reliable measures of fatigue also contributes to problems studying and understanding fatigue. Early work focused on fatigue in the workplace and was conducted by industrial psychologists, hygienists, and the military. These measures focused on healthy individuals and fatigue experienced at the time of measurement. More recent concern about the debilitating and distressing health effects of fatigue in clinical populations has led to the development of other measures targeting fatigue in ill persons.

There are now a plethora of generic measures of fatigue, as well as a growing list of measures of fatigue in specific illnesses (e.g., cancer, AIDS). However, because there is no known biochemical test or marker for fatigue, and because fatigue is first and foremost a subjective symptom, these measures of fatigue generally rely on self-reports. This also has led to several studies that directly compare measures of fatigue within single samples (e.g., Hwang, Chang, & Kasimis, 2003; Meek et al., 2000).

A major problem with so many different measures of fatigue is that each taps into a somewhat different aspect of fatigue and, consequently, it is not clear whether they are all measuring the same thing. Some focus on the emotional and cognitive expression of fatigue; others include the physical expression of fatigue. Some attempt to quantify the amount of fatigue; others include attention to how fatigue interferes with activities of daily living. When different measures of fatigue are used in different studies, it is difficult to know if discrepant findings are due to real substantive differences in fatigue, or simply to the differences in the measures. This dilemma, in part, is why the NIH Roadmap for Research initiative aimed at patient-reported outcomes is concerned with identifying and standardizing self-report measures, including fatigue. Identifying a set of standardized measures of fatigue with strong psychometric properties that clearly address the different aspects of fatigue and its expression will go far in aiding future research on this elusive symptom.

There may well be many causes of fatigue and each may ultimately be traced to a specific disruption in the HPA axis, in the immune system, or in both. If so, then continued investigations into CFS, in particular, may lead to a better understanding of fatigue in other, more clearly diagnosed clinical problems. Until such work is done that also suggests specific treatments for fatigue, nursing intervention studies that target ameliorating fatigue in different clinical populations must continue. Although rest generally alleviates acute fatigue, currently there are no known methods to eliminate the fatigue that plagues persons with various chronic illnesses or those whose fatigue is secondary to the treatments for their chronic illness. With the use of standardized measures of fatigue, this is a fertile area for nursing research.

LAUREN S. AARONSON

Feminist Research Methodology

Feminist research methodology refers to a perspective that espouses research on women, by women, and for women, with the use of rules for gathering evidence whereby feminist principles are applied to research. Feminist research methodology does not seek merely to be nonsexist, but to take person's lived experience as the methodological starting point for all knowledge-development efforts bearing on girls and women. This means refusing to rely solely on the loosely structured beliefs that pass for "givens" or "common sense" truths about the phenomenon under study.

By refusing to assume beforehand that any beliefs about women's experiences are necessarily true, the expectation is that the researcher is better prepared to *see clearly*, to be critical, and to complete a systematic investigation of their diseases. In women's health research it is difficult to rely on data from earlier studies of the menstrual cycle, exercise, or child rearing because of the many recent changes in the social context. For example, the notion that the "empty nest" is associated with depression in midlife women is a conceptualization that was embedded in a world where the majority of women did not work outside the family.

In the past 3 decades, women's health research as a subset of women's studies has become distinct and with it an emphasis both on conducting nonsexist research (e.g., eschewing traditional biases) and on asserting a new sensibility that positively values women's points of view and a holistic approach to health.

There has been much to critique in traditional research methods. Methods have not distinguished sex differences from gender-related differences (e.g., differences due to lack of opportunity rather than genetic ability) and have overemphasized gender differences when they account for relatively little variance. There has been a systematic preference for the so-called objective perspective of the (usually male) researcher over that of the female subject. The actor-observer effect, disclosed in tests of attribution theory, noted that actors make more use of situational attributions than do observers, so it is not surprising that male researchers have described some single mothers as "overprotective" when those mothers would have emphasized the demands placed on them by an absent father. Because women's behavior has traditionally been explained in terms of male-as-norm theoretical frameworks, female behavior has been pejoratively labeled, describing as dependent the woman whose husband is the breadwinner and not labeling in that way the man whose wife bakes the bread, cleans, and cares for their children. Indeed, research on women has been defined largely in terms of childbearing and child-rearing.

Sometimes sample selection has been biased by using women employed in low-level positions and men employed in high-status professions to represent employed women and men. The possibility that the gender of the experimenter and choice of setting may have differential effects on women and men has been ignored; for example, young male interviewers in a "macho" cardiac rehabilitation setting may not be sensitive to how alien older women feel in such an environment. Inappropriate instruments have been used to evaluate women's behavior, for example, the Masculinity-Femininity (Mf) scale of the Minnesota Multiphasic Personality Inventory to operationalize femininity in women when the validity items for establishing femininity originally involved a criterion group of gay men. Because "main" effects have been sought over "interaction" effects, women have been excluded from research when they acted in unexpected ways.

Feminist research methodology has encouraged some new positive directions. Women have been encouraged to develop research careers. Federal guidelines now require women to be included as subjects in all studies related to their experience, and men are not to be excluded as subjects when the focus is on the traditional concerns of females. Context-stripping methods have been called into question because they ignore the extent to which social integration is associated with lower rates of disease and quality of life; grounded-theory methods have been encouraged because they permit the individual to discuss fully the lived experience. The emphasis is increasingly on doing research *with* women rather than *on* women.

Because one of its basic tenets is the person-environment fit, nursing has long been concerned about the importance of context in understanding health behavior. Nurses were among the first to question a preference for the so-called objective view of the researcher over the subjective view of the patient and to emphasize the lived experience. They took the lead in menstrual cycle research, which underscored the extent to which there is more to midlife women's health than menopause, and in the use of the diary/health journal as a way to analyze the complexity of women's reality. The establishment of the National Center for Nursing Research in 1986, along with the concurrent growth of doctoral nursing programs, meant that there were more women scientists to approach seriously women's health and caregiving (rather than cure-finding) research. Nursing also has extended the notion of a feminist research methodology to include the development of a feminist pedagogy in teaching.

Although nonsexist research methods have gained ground when judged in terms of the most egregious biases, and the concerns of women are no longer automatically given short shrift, the prevailing scientific model still reifies an empiricist, positivist, objective paradigm. Feminist researchers have challenged the very nature of science and how we search for knowledge, but reductionism remains dominant in the sciences. It remains true that context-stripping methods are easier to implement, particularly for the beginning researcher who does not have the skills to handle multifactorial designs.

Matters are complicated by the fact that some qualitative researchers discuss their approach with more enthusiasm for their methods than specificity about why their methods are appropriate to explore a particular phenomenon. Even feminists have tended to treat women as a monolithic group, thus ignoring the special concerns of minority women, who are even more affected by contextual matters (e.g., poverty, violence, and racism) than their White sisters. There remains a significant discrepancy between the methods espoused by feminist researchers and those actually utilized. Nevertheless, the future will increasingly demand that health researchers use biopsychosocial models to frame their programs of study and develop new ways of analyzing human experience within interlocking contexts.

ANGELA BARRON MCBRIDE
SARA CAMPBELL

Fetal Monitoring

Fetal assessment is part of the process of providing prenatal care. It involves early identification of real or potential problems and enables the achievement of the best possible obstetric outcomes. Fetal assessment involves low-tech and high-tech modalities such as fetal movement counting (kick counts), intermittent auscultation (IA), electronic fetal monitoring (EFM), nonstress tests (NST), vibroacoustic stimulation (VAS), auscultated acceleration (AAT), contraction stress tests (CST), amniotic fluid index (AFI), biophysical profiles (BPP), and Doppler velocimetry. The basis for all of these testing modalities is evaluation of certain biophysical parameters related to the developmental and health-related patterns of fetal behavior in utero. Adequate uteroplacental function is necessary for these patterns of healthy behavior. Uteroplacental insufficiency (UPI) has been shown to be the cause of at least two thirds of antepartal fetal deaths (Gegor & Paine, 1992).

Electronic fetal monitoring is the basic intervention used in fetal assessment. Electronic fetal monitoring as an electronic data-gathering and data-processing device was developed during the 1960s. By the end of the 1970s almost all major obstetrical units had at least one monitor, and 70% of all women in labor in the United States were monitored (Bassett, K., 1996). K. R. Simpson (2000) reported that the use of EFM increased from 22.5% of women in labor in 1975 to 84.0% by 1998. In addition to its use in monitoring fetal status during labor, modifications of EFM have been developed for antepartal fetal assessment to determine optimal fetal development and diagnose conditions of actual or potential fetal compromise (e.g., NST, CST, VAS, and BPP).

Controversies still continue over the appropriate place of EFM in obstetric care. It was introduced into clinical practice on the basis of animal studies and became widely used, with no controlled assessment of its effectiveness in improving the outcome of delivery (Smith, M. A., Ruffin, & Green, 1993). It was supposed to provide more accurate fetal assessment with the accompanying prompt identification of fetal compromise. Early retrospective studies suggested that EFM was associated with fewer infants born with low Apgar scores, lower neonatal mortality rates, and better neurological outcomes (Smith et al.).

Schmidt and McCartney (2000) presented a thorough historical review and discussion of the development of fetal heart rate assessment. They found that expectations of the benefits of EFM exceeded and preceded research on outcomes, efficacy and safety. As knowledge accumulated through research and practice, the theories of correlation of causation and intrapartal events has changed. What were once considered to be significant intrapartal events cannot now be linked as conclusively to brain damage in neonates. Current research and improvements continue to report benefits of EFM: a decrease in neonatal seizures and decreased operative intervention for fetal distress, with improved analysis.

The major problem is still the risk of misinterpretation of the EFM tracing. Schmidt and McCartney (2000) included study results that, with a reassuring pattern, EFM can be a sensitive tool for identifying the well-oxygenated fetus. But it is not a specific tool for identifying the compromised fetus when a nonreassuring pattern is seen. Current concerns are focused on the best ways to prevent or reduce inappropriate use of EFM and develop the best ways to assess and monitor fetal development and safety in labor.

McCartney (2000) discussed the proposed benefits of automated EFM assessment (computer analysis): it is objective, standardized, and reproducible. She discusses the use of artificial intelligence (AI) and how it may prove to be of great value along with smart monitors and electronic databases in improving interpretation of EFM. M. L. Porter (2000) reported that the use of fetal pulse oximetry was approved by the FDA for clinical use in May, 2000 to provide more information about fetal oxygen status, especially in cases of nonreassuring fetal heart rate patterns.

The American College of Obstetricians and Gynecologists (ACOG) and the Association of Women's Health, Obstetrical, and Neonatal Nurses (AWHONN) have developed standards and guidelines for practice concerning fetal assessment and the use of EFM and other modalities of fetal heart rate assessment. As cited in Schmidt and McCartney (2000), the ACOG Technical Bulletin No. 207 entitled *Fetal heart rate patterns: Monitoring, interpretation, and management* states that intermittent auscultation is a safe technique for monitoring low-risk births. AWHONN issued *Basic, High Risk and Critical Care Intrapartum Nursing: Clinical Competencies and Education Guide* in 1999 and the 2000 Position Statement entitled *The use of fetal monitoring in support of laboring women*. These standards of practice determine the accepted conduct of antepartal and intrapartal care and provide the core of safe practice. It is the responsibility of all nursing and medical health care providers to be proficient in the use and interpretation of EFM and other intervention modalities employed in perinatal health care delivery. Other recommendations include using EFM as a diagnostic rather than a screening tool and not as a substitute for supportive health care personnel. Additionally, specific indications, such as oxytocin induction or augmentation of labor, an abnormal fetal heart rate by auscultation, twin gestation, hypertension or pre-eclampsia, dysfunctional labor, meconium staining, vaginal breech delivery, diabetes, or prematurity, as noted by Smith and others (1993), are still applicable.

Haggerty (1999) presented an extensive overview of the reliability, validity, and efficacy of EFM. Her work looks at both sides of the controversy, and includes the recommendations of ACOG, the United States Preventive Services Task Force (1996), and AWHONN that EFM and IA both have a place in fetal monitoring. Feinstein (2000) also researched the efficacy of IA, especially with low-risk pregnant women. Miltner (2002) concluded that integrating supportive care provided by labor nurses with other direct and indirect care interventions (such as monitoring modalities) may offer the best model for providing high-quality intrapartum nursing care.

Further prospective studies should be conducted to try to determine the optimal balance of intermittent or continuous EFM and auscultation and the other modalities of fetal assessment and pregnancy management. Rigorous study protocols and close attention to the principles of scientific inquiry are needed so that study results will be reliable and valid. The major concerns of perinatal care should be optimal and cost-effective outcomes for mother and infant, without concern for protection of the caregiver from litigious actions.

SUSAN M. MIOVECH

Fever/Febrile Response

Fever is an abnormally high body temperature that occurs as part of a host response to *pyrogens* (fever producers). An alternate term for fever is *pyrexia*, with *hyperpyrexia* referring to high fever. It is misleading to define fever simply in terms of temperature elevation, however, because it emphasizes only the *thermal* manifestations of the nonspecific systemic host-defense called the *acute phase response* (APR). APR is triggered by endogenous release of *cytokines*, including interleukin-1 (IL-1), IL-6, and tumor necrosis factor (TNF), that cause a cascade of biochemical events, autonomic reactions, and immune responses including heat generation. Some promote immunostimulant properties against infectious disease and tumors.

Pyrogens readjust hypothalamic regulatory centers to a higher set-point range, so that body temperature is maintained at higher levels. In true fever, other cytokines, hormones, and endogenously produced biochemicals act as *cryogens* with antipyretic properties that limit temperature elevation in fever. Controlled temperature elevation and intact thermoregulatory function differentiate fever from *hyperthermia*, a potentially lethal condition in which unregulated thermoregulatory function can produce neurologically damaging high temperatures. Fever occurs in three phases, reflecting rise and fall of circulating pyrogens. Initially, the *chill phase* occurs when thermostatic mechanisms are activated to raise body temperature to the newly elevated set-point range. Vasoconstriction decreases skin perfusion, conserving heat but making skin feel cold. Shivering generates heat and is stimulated by sensory inputs that detect discrepancies between existing temperatures and the new set point. The *plateau phase* follows when body temperature rises to the new set point and warming responses cease. Finally, falling pyrogen levels lead to the *defervescence phase*, with diaphoresis and vasodilation.

Nurses have managed fever throughout history, yet the scientific evidence supporting care decisions is relatively recent. The lag between basic research findings and clinical application is evident in the reluctance of many nurses to change methods of care that have been used for the past century. Early traditions of cooling febrile patients were empirically based on the limited state of scientific knowledge and the erroneous fear that elevated body temperature was the cause, rather than the result, of febrile illness. Intervention was therefore geared toward lowering body temperature. Current knowledge confirms that fever is the host response to illness or invasion. Cooling the body is counterproductive, distressful to patients, and may cause compensatory overwarming. Evidence of fever's host benefits led investigators to focus on methods to reduce distressful febrile symptoms rather than reducing temperature. *Febrile shivering* is among the most distressful and energy-consuming symptoms of fever, particularly in immunosuppressed patients with opportunistic infections or those receiving antigenic drugs or blood products. Vigorous shivering is sometimes described by patients as "bone shaking." Nonpharmacologic nursing interventions are based primarily on thermoregulatory dynamics to: (a) insulate thermosensitive areas of skin from cooling to reduce shivering, (b) facilitate heat loss from less thermosensitive regions without chilling, and (c) restore fluid volume and improve capillary blood flow to skin. Fear of neural damage due to protein denaturation during high fevers is justified at temperatures over 42° C. However, true fevers are usually self-limiting and remain well below this level. Body temperatures of about 39° C may have added immunostimulant and antimicrobial effects. These features make *comfort* the primary reason for treating low-grade fever with antipyretic drugs. Higher set-point levels raise sensitivity to heat loss, causing even mild cooling to stimulate shivering. Aggressive cooling with conductive cooling blankets and ice packs evokes vigorous shivering, raising energy expenditure 3 to 5 times resting values. As the consistent clinical observer of patient body temperatures, nurses find that issues of measurement, febrile patterns, physiological correlates, and sensory responses are of significance to practice and research (see Thermal Balance).

Febrile symptoms are nonspecific responses to both infectious and host defense activities so that many symptoms and interventions are generalizable. Contrasted with studies of fever management in other disciplines that center primarily on pharmacologic control of underlying infection, nursing research focuses on symptom management of fever responses regardless of etiology. Nurse researchers began studying interventions in the early 1970s to cool the body during fever without causing shivering or temperature "drift." By the late 1980s, concern grew about metabolic and cardiorespiratory effects of fever on vulnerable patients with cancer or HIV infection (Holtzclaw, 1998). The "set point" theory of temperature regulation was central to these intervention studies, but as discoveries of the 1990s identified and clarified mechanisms of endogenous pyrogens, cytokines and other biological messengers offered new measurable biomarkers of fever as a host response. Nurse scientists contributed significant scientific information about the febrile response using human and animal models (D. McCarthy, Murray, Galagan, Gern, & Hutson, 1998; Richmond, 2002; Rowsey & Gordon, 2000).

Responsible nursing research on fever draws on principles from physiology, physics, biochemistry, and psychoneuroimmunology. It is often interdisciplinary and diverse in nature, varying from laboratory studies of humans and animals to clinical studies in hospitals and homes. Circadian variations in temperature are well-documented (Bailey & Heitkemper, 2001), but there are few recent studies that confirm that daily temperature screening in hospitals adequately detects fever in persons with abnormal cytokine expression, such as those with HIV/AIDS. A study of febrile-symptom management in patients with cancer tested interventions to suppress drug-induced febrile shivering (Holtzclaw, 1990) showed that insulating thermosensitive skin regions during the chill phase of fever not only reduced shivering (see Shivering) but improved comfort. This preliminary work provided the basis for a comprehensive febrile-symptoms management protocol, tested in hospitalized and home-care HIV-infected persons with febrile illness (Holtzclaw, 1998). In a controlled trial, the intervention of insulative coverings to suppress shivering was shown to be effective. Body water loss and dehydration were monitored by body weight, serum osmolality, and urine specific gravity in hospitalized patients, while a fever diary and home visits reported changes in patients at home. No patients with insulative wraps shivered, while controls experienced both shivering and higher peak temperatures. Systematic oral fluid replacement was not effective in replacing loss despite metabolic, cardiorespiratory, and fever-related fluid expenditures, because fever suppressed thirst. Findings documented the negative effects of fever on hydration and febrile shivering on cardiorespiratory effort. Higher fatigue levels, lower thermal comfort, higher rate pressure product (RPP) and respiratory rate (RR) were experienced by those in the control group who shivered. A growing awareness that cooling measures exert distressful and sometimes harmful effects has stimulated inquiry surrounding procedures commonly used to "cool" patients. The practice of sponge bathing with tepid water to cool down febrile (38.9° C) children was studied in a group of 20 children, ages 5 to 68 months, seen in an emergency room and randomly assigned to acetaminophen alone or acetaminophen with sponge bathing (Sharber, 1997). Although the sponge-bathed children cooled faster during the 1st hour, rapid cooling evoked higher distress and no significant temperature difference between groups over the 2-hour study period. There is evidence that a gradual, less drastic reduction in body temperature evokes fewer adverse responses during aggressive fever treatment with cooling blankets. Warmer settings effectively lower body temperature as well as cooler levels, without inducing shivering (Caruso, Hadley, Shukla, Frame, & Khoury, 1992). Two studies demonstrate that in comparisons of sponge baths, hypothermia cooling blankets, and acetaminophen (Morgan, S., 1990) and of cooling blankets vs. acetaminophen (Henker et al., 2001), no temperature-lowering advantage was seen in the physical cooling treatment, which required more nursing time, caused shivering, and was distressful.

Today's nurse scientist is prepared to investigate many of the questions that remain unanswered in fever care. As investigators acquire skills and resources for these biological measurements, they can be used to quantify and qualify the effects of fever and results of intervention. Research is needed to demonstrate effects of elevated body temperature, cooling interventions, and measures to support natural temperature-stabilizing mechanisms. Fever may provide study variables, with body temperature, cytokines, and biochemical correlates being the outcome of interest. The febrile episode itself may be the *context* of other questions for study. Psychoneuroimmunological factors surrounding sleep, irritability, and tolerance of febrile symptoms remain untapped topics. Likewise, the metabolic toll of fever on nutritional variables, effects of intravenous fluid on endogenous antipyresis, and measures of energy expenditure are important, but relatively untouched, areas of research for nursing.

BARBARA J. HOLTZCLAW

Fitzpatrick's Rhythm Model

Fitzpatrick (1989) presented a rhythm model for the field of inquiry for nursing. Person, environment, health, and nursing are defined and related to the model. All of these elements have been linked to the idea that meaning is essential to life. Meaning is seen as the most crucial piece of the human experience and necessary to enhance and maintain life. Fitzpatrick incorporated Rogers' (1983) postulated correlates of human development as the basis to differentiate, organize, and order life's reality.

Fitzpatrick (1989) recognized the importance of information systems as part of the field of inquiry within her rhythm model for nursing. By asserting that nursing knowledge is fundamentally inseparable from the strategies and structures that represent it and that nursing informatics comprises a new focus to manage the technologies involved in nursing, Fitzpatrick suggested that information systems be linked to nursing knowledge development.

Rogers's (1983) correlates of shorter, higher frequency waves that manifest shorter rhythms and approach a seemingly continuous pattern serve as Fitzpatrick's (1989) foci for hypothesizing the existence of rhythmic patterns. Rogers' position that the human life span approximates transformation with human development aimed toward transcendence has been incorporated within Fitzpatrick's descriptions of life perspective. The developmental correlate whereby time seems timeless represents a beginning of Fitzpatrick's theorizing regarding temporal patterns. Motion patterns have been developed from Rogers' proposal of motion seeming to be continuous with development. Consciousness patterns are aligned with Rogers' idea that one progresses from sleep to wakefulness and from there to a pattern that is beyond waking. The correlates of "visibility" becoming more ethereal in nature and "heaviness" approaching a more weightless phase serve as the basis for Fitzpatrick's perceptual patterns.

Fitzpatrick's (1989) definitions of person and environment are from her interpretations of Rogers' (1983) developmental correlates and explanations of person and environment. Envisioned as patterns within a pattern, or rhythms within a life rhythm, Fitzpatrick's rhythm patterns serve as the specifications for person and environment. Occurring within the context of rhythmical person/environment interaction, indices of holistic human functioning are identified by Fitzpatrick as temporal, motion, consciousness, and perceptual patterns. Fitzpatrick's writings are consistent with Rogers' position regarding person and environment being open systems in continuous interaction.

Fitzpatrick (1989) has asserted that the four indices of human functioning are intricately related to health patterns throughout the life span, and these indices are rhythmic in nature. In a projection of Rogers' (1983) principle regarding the continuous interaction of persons and their environments, Fitzpatrick postulated the dynamic concepts of congruency, consistency, and integrity as complementary with rhythmic patterns. The nonlinear character of patterns noted by Rogers has supported Fitzpatrick's incorporation of Rogers' specifications regarding four-dimensionality. Fitzpatrick stated that health is a basic human dimension undergoing continuous development. She offered heightened awareness of the meaningfulness of life as an example of a more fully developed phase of human health. The ontogenetic and phylogenetic interactions between person and health are regarded as the essence of nursing. Fitzpatrick attended not only to relationships within or between these interactions but also included latent relationships external to person and health. Nursing interventions were interpreted as facilitating the developmental process toward health. Fitzpatrick stated that nursing interventions can be focused on enhancing the developmental process toward health so that individuals might develop their human potential.

Because person and environment are integral with one another and have no real boundaries, environment is applied when the term *person* is used. The human element is treated as an open, holistic, rhythmic system that is described by temporal, motion, consciousness, and perceptual patterns. Fitzpatrick's (1989) conception of person is augmented by awareness of the meaningfulness of life or health. The meaningfulness of life is manifest through a series of life crisis experiences with potential for growth in one's meaning for living. Nursing's central concern is focused on the person in relation to the dimension of meaning within health.

Fitzpatrick's (1989) conceptualizations have been investigated by graduate students in nursing at the master's and doctoral level. Studies looking at temporality in combination with adult and elderly populations, temporality in association with psychiatric clients, temporality in pregnant adolescents, and temporality in relation to terminally ill individuals provide a base for the existence of temporal patterns. However, from a holistic perspective of life span, use of the model is absent in nursing research focused on infants' and children's notions of temporality.

Both younger and elderly groups have been addressed in investigating motion (Roberts & Fitzpatrick, 1983). Nevertheless, patterns of consciousness have been examined exclusively in older age groups (Floyd, 1982).

Different types of perceptual patterns, including for example, perception of color and music, have been investigated. Because one's perception would seem to be dependent on present pattern of consciousness, these studies seem to be related to patterns of consciousness.

Empirical support for the existence of nonlinear temporal patterns emerged from a number of research endeavors and helped to identify the need to generate questions about ways to measure the experience of time. The prevalence of temporal distinctions on the basis of differences in development were apparent in at least one study (Fitzpatrick & Donovan, 1978). A sense of timelessness was described as being characteristic of behaviors identified among the dying.

Pressler, Wells, and Hepworth (1993) investigated methodological issues relevant to very preterm infant (< 30 weeks gestation) outcomes based on the idea of the existence of microrhythms within some larger rhythmic pattern. By applying time series techniques and fuzzy subsets to the analysis of longitudinal data collected in the neonatal intensive care unit (NICU) environment, this study examined single-subject results for generalization across individuals. In general terms, the sequelae and risks associated with the NICU for very preterm neonates indicate that information processing deficits, attention deficit, and hyperactivity disorders are not uncommon during the preschool and school-age years. It is speculated that these problems might reflect these infants' inabilities to cope with stressors or care received while in the NICU environment. Shiao (1993) investigated perceptual patterns of low birth weight infants in neonatal intensive care in terms of routine care interrupting breathing, oxygen saturation, and feeding rhythms. Yarcheski and Mahon (1995) examined human field patterns (as described by Rogers) in relation to perceived health status in healthy adolescents and found results consistent with the life perspective rhythm model. More recently, numerous qualitative researchers have used Fitzpatrick's model to compare and contrast their findings, particularly in phenomenological studies that examine participants' experience of phenomena (see Chiu, 1999; Cowan, C., 1995; Criddle, 1993; Montgomery, 2000, 2001; Moore, S. L., 1997; Pasquali, E. A., 1999; Ross, 1996).

Borrowing from some of her own ideas about temporality, Fitzpatrick (1989) has hypothesized the field of inquiry for nursing knowledge development by outlining nursing inquiry of the past. She has traced major historical milestones of nursing research and identified important events leading up to present-day research in nursing.

In cooperation with two colleagues, Fitzpatrick (Fitzpatrick, Wykle, & Morris, 1990) attempted to specify the field of inquiry for nursing in the area of geriatric mental health. Through the development of collaborative, interdisciplinary teaching, research, and practice relationships, Fitzpatrick and colleagues (1990) described how organizational theory could be used to support the development of a collaboration model for promoting the mental health of elderly persons across care settings. Intervention research with elderly populations was used to determine ways for improving the understanding, treatment, and rehabilitation of the mentally ill. The significance of Fitzpatrick's ideas lies in how rhythmic methodologies might be used to develop nursing knowledge and provide external validity to the model.

Jana L. Pressler
Updated by Kristen S. Montgomery

Formal Nursing Languages

The National Institute of Nursing Research Priority Expert Panel on Nursing Informatics (1993) defined nursing language as

> . . . the universe of written terms and their definition comprising nomenclature or thesauri that are used for purposes such as indexing, sorting, retrieving, and classifying varied nursing data in clinical records, in information systems (for care documentation and/or management), and in literature and research reports. . . . Determining the way that nursing data are represented in automated systems is tantamount in defining a language for nursing. (p. 31)

This report also differentiated between clinical terms, which represent the language of practice, and definition terms, which represent the language of nursing knowledge comprising theory and research. The distinction between language that supports practice versus language that supports theory and research is blurring as the state of the science in this area moves toward definitional, concept representations that can be processed by computer algorithms and shared among heterogeneous information systems (Henry & Mead, 1997).

The research on standardized language to represent nursing concepts reflects four generations of inquiry. Initial research focused on the development of standardized coding and classification systems that represented the phenomena of clinical practice. Testing of systems for multiple clinical and research purposes by persons other than the developers followed. As confidence grew that the nursing-specific systems that had been developed reflected the domain of nursing and the drivers for multidisciplinary care and care systems grew, some investigators evaluated the extent to which terminologies not developed for nursing had utility for nursing practice. Currently, with the increasing sophistication in terminological science and the need for data sharing across heterogeneous information systems, nursing terminology developers, standards experts, and nursing informatics researchers have collaborated to conduct research toward the goal of semantic interoperability, i.e., that data collected in one information system using one terminology can be understood in another information system that uses a different terminology. Also reflective of the current generation is the integration of nursing-specific terminologies into large concept-oriented terminologies such as SNOMED Clinical Terms (CT) (Bakken et al., 2002) and the Logical Observation Identifiers, Names, and Codes (LOINC) database (Matney, Bakken, & Huff, 2003).

Standardized language for nursing developed within the framework of the nursing minimum data set, comprising five data elements specific to nursing: (a) nursing diagnosis, (b) nursing interventions, (c) nursing outcomes, (d) intensity of care, and (e) unique RN provider number (Werley, Devine, & Zorn, 1988). Early research on standardized terminologies focused on the creation of language systems that represented nursing practice in various settings (Table 1). For example, the North American Nursing Diagnosis Association Taxonomy I (NANDA) (NANDA, 2004), Nursing Interventions Classification (NIC) (McCloskey & Bulechek, 2000), and Patient Care Data Set (PCDS) (Ozbolt, 1996) were initially developed for the acute care setting, the Omaha System for the community setting (Martin & Scheet, 1992), and the Home Health Care Classification (HHCC) (now the Clinical Care Classification) for the home care setting (Saba, 1992).

The advent of computer-based nursing documentation systems was only one motivation for standardization of nursing language; others were to document nursing practice, articulate nursing contributions to patient care outcomes, and seek reimbursement for nursing care. Consequently, a number of studies evaluated whether a particular nursing terminology was useful in a particular clinical domain. For example, J. Carter and associates (J. Carter, Moorhead, McCloskey, & Bulechek, 1995) demonstrated the usefulness of NIC in implementing clinical practice guidelines for pain management and pressure ulcer management. Parlocha (Parlocha & Henry, 1998) reported the usefulness of the HHCC for categorizing nursing care activities for home care patients with a diagnosis of major depressive disorder. Several studies demonstrated the capacity of the

TABLE 1 Standardized Terminologies with Utility for Nursing Care

Terminology	Contents	ANA	UMLS	HL7	SNOMED	Availability
Nursing-specific						
Clinical Care Classification[1]	Nursing diagnoses, interventions, outcomes, goals	x	x	x	x	Public domain
Omaha System	Problems, interventions, outcomes	x	x	x	x	Public domain
North American Nursing Diagnosis Association Taxonomy	Nursing diagnoses	x	x	x	x	License
Nursing Interventions Classification	Nursing interventions	x	x	x	x	License
Nursing Outcomes Classification	Patient/client outcomes	x	x	x	x	License
Patient Care Data Set	Patient problems, care goals, care orders	x	x	x		Only at Vanderbilt University
Perioperative Nursing Data Set	Nursing diagnoses, interventions, patient outcomes	x	x	x	x	License
Others						
Current Procedural Terminology Codes	Medical services		x			License
Logical Observation Identifiers, Names, and Codes	V/S, obstetric measurements, clinical assessment scales, research instruments	x	x	x	Laboratory LOINC only	Copyrighted, but free for use
SNOMED Clinical Terms	MD/RN diagnoses, healthcare interventions, procedures, findings, substances, organisms, events	x	x	x	x	5-year federal license

[1]Formerly the Home Health Care Classification
ANA: Recognized by the American Nurses Association
UMLS: Included in Unified Medical Language System
HL7: Registered with Health Level 7
SNOMED: Included in SNOMED Clinical Terms

Omaha system to predict service utilization (Marek, 1996) and outcomes of care (Martin, Scheet, & Stegman, 1993). Moreover, instead of creating new terminologies from scratch, groups such as the Association of Perioperative Registered Nurses (AORN) adopted some terms from existing terminologies and augmented as needed for their specialty practice (Perioperative Nursing Data Set) (AORN, 1997).

Other investigators provided evidence that nursing terminologies were useful to retrospectively abstract and codify patient problems and nursing interventions from sources of research data such as care logs (Naylor, Bowles, & Brooten, 2000) or patient records (Holzemer et al., 1997). In another investigation, Holzemer, Henry, Portillo, and Miramontes (2000) based the documentation of their nursing-delivered adherence intervention on HHCC in order to determine the dose of the nursing intervention in a randomized controlled trial.

Complementary to the research that was being conducted, the American Nurses Association played a significant policy role in "recognizing" nursing language systems (Table 1) that met specific criteria not only related to utility for nursing but scientific rigor (McCormick et al., 1994). This process facilitated the inclusion of selected nursing terminologies into the Unified Medical Language System (UMLS) (Table 1) (Humphreys, Lindberg, Schoolman, & Barnett, 1998).

Several research studies examined whether or not standardized terminologies not designed specifically for nursing were useful for encoding nursing-relevant content such as diagnoses, interventions, goals, and outcomes. The Current Procedural Terminology (CPT) comprises more than 7,000 codes designed for reimbursement of health care services provided by physicians; as such, these terms are present in numerous state and federal databases (American Medical Association, 2000). Studies by Griffith and Robinson (1992, 1993) provided evidence that nurses perform many CPT-coded functions and that some functions are performed multiple times in a single day. Henry, Holzemer, Reilly, and Campbell (1994) demonstrated that the Systematized Nomenclature of Human and Veterinary Medicine (SNOMED) was more comprehensive than NANDA to describe the problems of persons living with HIV/AIDS. In another study, Henry and colleagues (1997) compared the frequencies with which 21,366 nursing activity terms from multiple data sources (patient interviews, nurse interviews, intershift reports, and patient records) could be categorized using NIC and CPT codes. There were significantly ($p < .0001$) greater numbers of nursing activity terms that could be categorized in NIC than in CPT, thus providing evidence for the superiority of NIC in representing nursing activity data.

In recent years, consistent with the state of terminological science and the clear indication that a single terminology could not meet all needs (Cimino, 1998), the focus of inquiry related to nursing language has been on the creation of computable representations of nursing concepts and on the subsequent integration with concept-oriented terminologies with broad coverage for the domain of health care.

The core of a concept-oriented terminology is the reference terminology model. A number of nurse researchers focused on developing and testing models for nursing diagnoses and nursing actions (Bakken, Cashen, Mendonca, O'Brien, & Zieniewicz, 2000; Hardiker & Rector, 1998; Hardiker & Rector, 2001; Henry & Mead, 1997; Moss, Coenen, & Mills, 2003). Under the leadership of the International Council of Nurses and the Nursing Special Interest Group of the International Medical Informatics Association, and with input from many including the Nursing Terminology Summit (Ozbolt, 2000), the International Standards Organization developed an international standard for a reference terminology model for nursing diagnoses and nursing actions (Bakken, Coenen, & Saba, 2004). These models facilitated the integration of selected nursing terminologies (Table 1) into SNOMED CT, a concept-oriented health care terminology that is currently available for free use in the U.S.

SNOMED CT is an evolving national standard for clinical terminology. Selected nursing assessments, goals, outcomes, and standardized measurements have also been integrated into LOINC, a national standard for observation names (Matney et al., 2003). In addition, a number of the nursing terminology developers have registered their terminologies with the Health Level 7 standards organization (Table 1) for use in messaging among information systems (Bakken, Campbell, Cimino, Huff, & Hammond, 2000).

This evolution in nursing language research is important because concept-oriented terminologies are an essential component of the evolving National Health Information Infrastructure (NHII) and to the four goals of the related NHII framework for strategic action: 1) inform clinical practice, 2) interconnect clinicians, 3) personalize care, and 4) improve population health (Thompson, T. G., & Brailer, 2004). Consequently, it is vital that nursing as well as medical terms are included. Moreover, the significant progress through nursing language research has laid the foundation for other types of research including clinical decision support and data mining for nursing knowledge development.

SUZANNE BAKKEN
JEEYAE CHOI

Functional Health

Functional health is a requirement for independent living and is the ability to engage in daily activities related to personal care and socially defined roles. Performance of these activities is integral to quality of life and to living independently and safely. Although functional health represents well-being, most nomenclature reflects deficits in this health. Terms include disability (Nagi, 1991), frailty (Lawton, 1991), functional limitation (Johnson, R. J., & Wolinsky, 1993), and handicap (World Health Organization). Often these terms are used to refer to other concepts that lead to confusion in nomenclature and theoretical definitions. The World Health Organization definition of disability lacks conceptual clarity and theoretical consistency, and this makes operationalization and establishing relationships difficult. In the disablement model (Johnson & Wolinsky), functional limitations are sometimes confused with factors affecting these limitations, and perceived health is used as a proxy for functional limitations. Leidy (1994) proposed nomenclature and definitions of functional status and other concepts related to this status that add to the conceptual confusion in this area.

In spite of the confusion related to nomenclature, Nagi's (1991) model of disability has been supported by an extensive research and is useful to guide research, because disability in this model is conceptually clear, logically consistent, and useful in interpreting current and past research. Disability (poor functional health) is the result of a sequence of factors with temporal relationships. Pathology or lifestyle contributes to functional impairments that are anatomic, physiological, and psychological abnormalities causing functional limitations at the level of the whole person (e.g., poor memory or inability to get up from a chair). Functional limitations then lead to disability, which is the inability to perform daily tasks or roles independently. Risk factors and external and internal factors were added to this model to increase its explanatory capacity (Pope & Tarlov, 1991; Verbrugge & Jette, 1994). Another significant addition to Nagi's model was the notion that upper-extremity limitations were more related to personal care activities of daily living, while lower-extremity limitations were more relevant for instrumental activities of daily living (e.g., shopping, housework, meal preparation) (Verbrugge & Jette). Unique to Nagi's model is the notion of thresholds, where a certain amount of change must occur before change in a subsequent concept is observed. For example, impairments in mobility emerged when the strength of leg muscles was below a certain threshold (Rantanen et al., 1999; Rantanen et al., 2001).

Lacking in these models is the influence of decision making on disability. Persons engage in activities that they believe they have the ability to do without risk of injury or excessive exertion. Evaluative judgments about the environment and personal competencies affect decisions about what activities to participate in and how. Although the congruence between actual and perceived physical competencies is modest at best, little is known about how these affect disability (Roberts, B. L., 1999).

Since functional health is the ability to engage in everyday activities, a plethora of research has focused on daily activities related to personal care (ADLs) and tasks related to providing food and shelter and caring for the home (IADLs), because impairment in these contributes to excessive dependency, morbidity, mortality, and poor quality of life. Health care costs and personal and social resources needed to manage disability are substantial, particularly as the baby-boom generation enters older adulthood when the proportion and number of older adults are expected to increase greatly as well as the associated financial, personal, and societal costs.

In 2000, 41.9% of elders had at least one disability with nearly 60% of them being women (Waldrop & Stern, 2003). While only 9.5% had self-care deficits, 20.4% had difficulty going outside, and women were more disabled in this activity than men (23.0% and 16.8%, respectively). Racial and ethnic differences exist, with only 40.4% of non-Hispanic whites being disabled compared to 52.8% of African Americans. In 1997, 38% of older adults reported severe disability with 14% and 22% requiring assistance with ADLs and IADLs, respectively (Administration on Aging, 2003). In the last year of life, dependency increases (Covinsky, Eng, Lui, Sands, & Yaffe, 2003; Lunney, Lynn, Foley, Lipson, & Guralnik, 2003).

ADLs are hierarchically structured by the complexity of the motor skills required (Spector, Katz, Murphy, & Fulton, 1987). IADLs are dependent on some of the same motor skills as ADLs but are more dependent on cognitive capabilities. ADLs and IADLs are highly related and may represent a continuum of the same construct (Johnson & Wolinsky, 1993; Thomas, V. S., & Hageman, 2003).

Early empirical indicators were self-report, whose accuracy cannot be verified and can be biased by cognitive impairment, social desirability, or minimization of dependency. Although observational measures reflect what a person is able to do, they may not reflect what a person actually does. Gait, dynamic and static postural stability, and muscle strength are physical factors affecting ADLs and IADLs (Guralnik et al., 2000; Roberts, L., 1999). Upper-body function (e.g., muscle strength and range of motion of the arms) was related to ADLs, while lower-body function (e.g., muscle strength of the legs) were associated with IADLs (Lawrence & Jette, 1996). Although the effects of exercise on strength, balance, and mobility are well established, exercise has had little to no effects on ADLs or IADLs (Latham, Bennett, Stretton, & Anderson, 2004).

Recently, biomarkers of increasing dependency associated with frailty have emerged. Biomarkers of catabolic protein metabolism, pro-inflammatory cytokines, and other hormones were related to dependency, frailty, and loss of muscle mass and strength (Chevalier, Gougeon, Nayar, & Morais, 2003; Ferrucci et al., 2002; Roubenoff, 2003). An understanding of their roles may lead to new assessment strategies and interventions.

Relevant psychological factors include cognitive impairment and depression. Certain types of social support are factors that can contribute to dependency in daily activities (Seeman, Bruce, & McAvay, 1996), while men and women use different types of social support in response to limitations in ADLs and IADLs (Roberts, B. L., Anthony, Matejczyk, & Moore, 1994). The role of the environment has not been well established, except for the increase in dependency noted during hospitalization and long-term residence in a nursing home. Although there is beginning evidence that the relationship between actual abilities and perceptions of them is low, how these perceptions influence decisions people make about what activities to perform and how have not been well studied.

More research is needed to identify thresholds in factors related to functional health where declines in this health occur, and to identify factors and processes by which people make decisions about performing daily activities. This knowledge may provide directions for assessment in populations at risk of poor functional health and may lead to more sensitive assessment strategies. A greater understanding of the interplay between environmental and personal factors with functional health may lead to multidimensional interventions that may be more effective than the one-dimensional interventions most often studied.

Beverly L. Roberts

Functional Health Patterns

A functional health pattern (FHP) is a manifestation of an individual's behavior and responses across time. The typology of the 11 functional health patterns identifies and defines each pattern under the following categories: (a) health perception-health management, (b) nutritional metabolic, (c) elimination, (d) activity-exercise, (e) cognitive-perceptual, (f) sleep-rest, (g) self-perception-self-concept, (h) role-relationship, (i) sexuality-reproductive, (j) coping-stress tolerance, and (k) value-belief (Gordon, 1982).

The organization of the FHP assessment framework provides a structure to examine a sequence of behaviors and responses within each pattern area over time. Subjective and objective data obtained during the assessment of each health pattern facilitates pattern construction for the individual, family, or community. Data from all of the functional health patterns' areas are assessed within the context of age and stage of development, culture and ethnic background, current health status, and environment. Each individual functional health pattern reflects a unique response to a particular experience.

A health pattern may be described as functional, potentially dysfunctional, or dysfunctional. A functional health pattern is both mutually exclusive and interactive, reflecting a holistic perspective. Often data obtained about one pattern may be best understood in relation to information assessed in other patterns. Behaviors (cues) obtained during an FHP assessment can be used to generate and support a tentative nursing hypothesis (e.g., nursing diagnosis). To identify a clinical judgment (nursing diagnosis), data from all 11 functional patterns must be obtained and synthesized. Clinical judgments are described as probabilistic and noncausal statements.

Historically, assessment tools were developed to assess clinical populations, frequently duplicating medical information. The lack of a consistent nursing assessment framework resulted in inadequate data and limited information about nursing's judgments and contribution to care outcomes. The National League for Nursing was the first to support a movement away from nursing's task focus to one that was patient-centered and problem-based. Forty schools of nursing participated in a survey that generated a classification list of nursing's 21 problems (Abdellah, 1959). Later, in 1966, Henderson classified 14 basic needs related to patient care. This work identified human needs, articulated nursing functions, and helped direct nursing care toward patient responses.

Gordon's (1982) typology of the 11 functional health patterns provided a structure for organizing and documenting patient behavior over time. The FHP framework offered nurses a consistent framework for identifying human responses that resulted in autonomous nursing interventions and linked evidence-based patient outcomes. This focus continues to be consistent with the Professional Standards of Nursing Practice and Nursing's Social Policy Statement (American Nurses Association, 2003).

The FHP framework provides nurses with an opportunity to know the patient in a unique way. Through a series of semi-structured interview questions, each of the 11 functional health patterns is assessed as the individual's story unfolds. When additional information is required, the nurse uses branching questions to elicit new perceptions. This descriptive approach to data collection is then subjected to analysis where data bits (or cues) are isolated and data are synthesized, leading to the formulation of tentative diagnostic statements that reflect phenomena of concern to nursing.

Many clinical investigations have used the FHP framework as a structure for data collection, patient problem identification, and evaluation of care outcomes. These studies described high-frequency nursing diagnoses and isolated patient responses to phenomena (e.g., eating disorders, sleep disturbances) and linked intervention strategies to specific nursing diagnoses. Other investigations have used the FHP framework to validate cues associated with a particular nursing diagnosis. Nurses working in clinical specialties (e.g. ambulatory surgery, oncology, rehabilitation, and cardiovascular nursing) have used the FHP framework to identify patient responses (nursing diagnoses) throughout illness experience and recovery at home. Nurse administrators, using data from FHP assessments, reported that findings help predict nurse and patient mix, help identify patient problems, link nursing interventions with evidence-based outcomes, and ultimately help cost out care more accurately. Nursing educators have used FHP assessment data to evaluate clinical reasoning skills and diagnostic accuracy (Lunney, 2003).

Currently, research continues to clinically test an assessment screening tool using the 11 functional health patterns to generate screening questions. The Functional Health Pattern Assessment Screening Tool (FHPAST) is a patient-completed, functional health screening instrument (Foster & Jones, 2003). The tool contains 58 items and organizes responses to each item on a 4-point scale. Psychometric properties of the tool have been established with well adult populations. To date, data analysis reveals the emergence of four factors: Interpersonal Perception, Risk/Threat to Function, Health Promoting Behaviors/Beliefs, and Health Protecting Behaviors. The FHPAST is a reliable and valid assessment screening tool. The FHPAST assesses data across all pattern areas and is easily administered. The tool offers a quantitative measure of patient responses and identifies cues that guide further assessment by the nurse.

The FHPAST has been used in the United States with a variety of populations across settings, including same day surgery with patients with congestive heart failure in an outpatient program. The tool has also been used to evaluate health perceptions and behaviors in black Caribbean populations. In addition, the FHPAST has been translated into several languages including Portuguese, Spanish, and Japanese. In clinical practice, it has been used in England with HIV males, and as a screening tool to assess adults in medical inpatient units in Sao Paulo, Brazil. Nurse researchers identified the tool's ease of administration and the ability of the tool to isolate functional health patterns requiring further assessment and evaluation as positive strengths.

Movement toward the use of standardized nursing language and continued refinement of standardized nursing language classifications (NANDA, NIC, NOC, and the International Classification of Nursing Language, ICNP) will promote the use of a consistent database for communicating nursing assessments, diagnoses, interventions, and outcomes across countries. The continued testing and refinement of the FHPAST will improve the use of a valid and reliable instrument to measure patient's functional health over time. The use of the FHP framework can expand nursing knowledge, isolate human experiences in illness and wellness, promote creative interventions, and help articulate evidence that is nurse-sensitive.

Dorothy A. Jones
Frances Foster

Funding

Funding is the provision of money or other resources to carry out a research proposal, usually for a specific period of time. Resources may be money, time, or people to carry out the scientific work. Funding may be intramural (coming from an individual's place of employment, such as a university) or extramural (coming from a source that is external to the recipient or the recipient's place of employment, such as a federal or state agency or a private foundation). Extramural funding almost always is preceded by a scientific or technical review for merit by experts who are considered peers of intended applicants. At times there is also a second-level review made to determine the goodness of fit between the proposed project and the program that will fund it. Many research institutions also have instituted internal peer review of scientific merit for intramural funding.

In addition to scientific merit, proposals are usually reviewed for human subject safety, animal welfare if animal models are proposed, and the reasonableness of the scientific return for the overall cost of the research to be undertaken. This last focus is designed to provide opportunity for consideration of cutting-edge research in comparison to research that may be very well designed but may not provide new knowledge. It also provides opportunity for discussion of new, highly innovative research that may lead to future advances. Organizations that fund research are looking for scientifically superb proposals focused on cutting-edge health problems and issues where the expenditure is reasonable given the complexity of the study.

Funding sources for nursing research are numerous and varied. Such support could be funding for the conduct of research or for research training and career development for nurse scientists interested in a mentored research experience. The National Institute of Nursing Research at the National Institutes of Health (NIH) is the principal federal source. It announces its research interest areas on the NIH homepage and through the literature. However, other NIH institutes and offices that fund clinical research with a specific focus, such as cancer, heart disease, or complementary therapies, are also important resources for nurse investigators. All the institutes at NIH accept and encourage investigator-initiated research. Therefore, it is advisable not to wait for publication of information about an exact topic; if the general topic is related to the institute's mission, contact them to discuss specific ideas. These and similar sources with specific interests should be pursued because their use enlarges the resources available for nursing research.

Information about research interests of the NIH and its institutes can be found through the NIH homepage at http://www.nih.gov. The Centers for Disease Control and Prevention are an important source for prevention and health promotion research and demonstration projects and can be contacted at http://www.cdc.gov. Also, the Agency for Health Care Policy and Research funds research on general health services, care delivery models, outcomes, and health care costs. Information about its research interests can be found at http://www.ahcpr.gov. Generally, federal agencies make their research interests known through their homepages or through contacts with staff listed on the homepages. Also, some agencies provide access to information about funded research. The NIH provides this through the Computer Retrieval of Information on Scientific Projects (CRISP) database, available through the NIH homepage under grants and contracts. Other nonpublic sources of funding are foundations, product and drug companies, and business corporations.

Foundations usually have highly targeted interest areas or specific populations of interest. For example, the W. T. Grant Foundation is interested in children; the Robert Woods Johnson Foundation is interested in end-of-life care, home care, and economics of health care projects, among others. Many foundations have homepages; for example, Robert Woods Johnson's is http://www.rwjf.org. The *Foundation Directory* and various online programs available through libraries are good sources of information on national, regional, and local foundations. Product and drug companies frequently seek clinical investigators to assist with human testing, and nurse investigators have been active in this area. There are research grant programs available for small businesses to test products and to transfer technology into useable health products. The NIH, the Food and Drug Administration, and other federal agencies that fund clinical research are sources for these funds. Funding from entities that may have a vested interest in a particular outcome from the research they support requires special consideration that offices of university-sponsored programs usually can provide.

PATRICIA MORITZ

G

Gastroesophageal Reflux Disease

Gastroesophageal reflux disease (GERD) is a common occurrence affecting 15% to 20% of older adults (Braunwald et al., 2001) and more than 40% of U.S. citizens (Hill, C., 2004), resulting in a lowered quality of living and health complications. Quality-of-life issues stem from esophageal complaints and other symptoms presented in the primary-care setting, including aspiration pneumonia. GERD can result in an overwhelming use of antacids, which often negate the effects of medications used to manage chronic diseases common to older adults (Meiner, 2003).

GERD includes a wide array of illnesses that stem from the retrograde flow of gastric contents into the esophagus. Symptoms of GERD include globus pharyngitis, chronic cough, asthma, hoarseness, laryngitis, chronic sinusitis, dental erosions, dyspepsia, belching, heartburn, regurgitation, and delayed gastric emptying (Sermon et al., 2004; Lackey & Barth, 2003; Williams, J. L., 2003).

The association between GERD and patient's complaints of ear, nose, and throat symptoms has led to several new research studies that look at the phenomenon while attempting to identify a diagnostic feature (Sermon et al., 2004; Vaezi, Hicks, Abelson, & Richter, 2003). These studies include an in-depth look at dental erosions caused by GERD (Lackey & Barth, 2003; Van Roekel, 2003).

Chronic abnormal gastric reflux results in erosive esophagitis in up to 60% of patients diagnosed with GERD. Esophageal stricture, Barrett's esophagus, and esophageal adenocarcinoma are the most serious complications of GERD (Williams, 2003). If unchecked, simple complaints can progress to terminal illness.

Causes of GERD include gastric acid hypersecretion, impaired gastric motility, weakened pressure of the lower esophageal sphincter (LES), transient lower esophageal sphincter relaxations (TLESRs), ineffective esophageal peristalsis, and loss of the integrity of the esophageal mucosa. Increased gastric volume after meals, incorrect positioning that allows gastric contents to remain close to the LES, such as bending over or lying down, and obesity or wearing tight clothing add to the causes of GERD (Storr, Meining, & Allescher, 2000).

Swallowing abnormalities associated with GERD can cause a complex interaction between the various nerves and muscles with involuntary and voluntary patterns of control and the upper airway (Mokhlesi, 2003). These swallowing abnormalities range from dyspepsia to aspiration of esophageal contents resulting in a chronic cough. While the association between GERD and asthma has been previously established (Mujic & Rao, 1999), the relationship between GERD and chronic obstructive pulmonary disease (COPD) is still being studied due to the complex interactions of symptoms, including the use of bronchodilators. Data does indicate that the presence of GERD in patients with COPD is higher than in normal populations (Mokhlesi). Further study is needed to establish the association between the swallowing dysfunction of GERD and stable and acute episodes of COPD.

A progressive increase in the prevalence of severe erosive esophagitis was observed with each decade of life until greater than 37% of patients over age 70 were identified as being affected (Johnson, D. A., & Fennerty, 2004). These researchers found that heartburn is an unreliable indicator of the severity of erosive disease among older adults. This lead to the recommendation that more aggressive investigation and treatment may be needed for older adult patients with or without complaints of heartburn (Johnson, D. A., & Fennerty).

Following the recent establishment of international control values for diagnostic (scintigraphic) gastric emptying assessment, an improvement in the ability to diagnose GERD-associated symptoms from the delay in gastric emptying can be identified (Buckles, Sarosiek, McMillin, & McCallum, 2004). The significance of this research is to identify a subgroup of patients that may have GERD without having the cardinal symptoms, but are at risk for pathophysiology. The "gold standard" study for confirming or excluding the presence of abnormal gastroesophageal reflux that continues to be used most widely across the U.S. is the 24-hour ambulatory esophageal pH monitoring test (Szarka, DeVault, & Murray, 2001). The best marker for the ability to heal erosive esophagitis with any drug is the ability to keep the gastric pH above four. The longer any dose of any drug can keep the pH above four (pH 4), the more likely it is to heal erosive esophagitis (Hatlebakk, 2003).

The introduction of fiberoptic instruments and ambulatory devices for continuous monitoring of esophageal pH (24-hour pH monitoring) has led to great improvement in the ability to diagnose reflux disease and reflux-associated complications. Treatment options include lifestyle changes, medication, and surgery. Polypharmacy and changes in renal, hepatic, and gastrointestinal function can complicate treatment. Due to the large number of medications taken by older adults for comorbidities, drug interactions and treatment responses must be carefully assessed in this population (Ramirez, F. G., 2000).

Lifestyle changes are the cornerstone for effective patient education and an understanding of GERD treatment. Further nursing research is needed to identify behavior modifications that are more likely to be sustained over time. Future nursing studies that may produce long-term lifestyle changes will need to include the following elements that are known to reduce GERD: (a) dietary modifications designed to avoid foods and fluids that lower LES pressure (e.g., tomatoes, peppermint, licorice, alcohol, and caffeine-containing foods and drinks such as coffee, tea, chocolate, and colas); (b) providing a comprehensive history with defining characteristics to the primary health care provider at the onset of ambulatory care; (c) weight loss, when obesity is a factor; (d) elevating the head of the bed 4 to 6 inches with blocks (raising the entire angle of the bed); (e) eliminating all food and fluids for the 2 hours before bedtime; and (f) smoking cessation.

GERD is a chronic problem among many adults. Well-controlled trials are beginning to glean information related to successful lifestyle modifications, improved diagnostic evaluations, and treatment protocols. Nursing research should be undertaken to study ways of improving adults' willingness to make long-term lifestyle and dietary changes. Studies that investigate symptomatic control may provide the foundation for improvement in the quality of life of patients with GERD. Studies that identify drugs and foods that increase inappropriate LES relaxation are needed. Obtaining a thorough past history of illnesses, current symptoms, with past and current medication use including over-the-counter drugs, is a key factor to being able to identify hypotheses for nursing research.

SUE E. MEINER

Gender Research

Gender is an old term used in linguistic discourse to designate whether nouns are masculine, feminine, or neuter. It was not normally used either in the language of social sciences or nursing until after 1955, when the psychologist-sexologist John Money adopted the term to serve as an umbrella concept distinguishing femininity, or womanliness, and masculinity, or manliness, from biological sex (male or female). By using the word *gender* he believed he could avoid continually making qualifying statements about the hermaphrodites he was studying, such as "John was in a male sex role except that his sex organs are not male and his genetic sex is female" (Money, 1955). Sex, in his research, belonged more to reproductive biology than to social science, romance, and nurture, whereas gender belonged to both (Money & Ehrhardt, 1972). By using a new term to describe a variety of phenomena, Money opened up a whole new field of research. It was a field ripe for exploration because it appealed to the increasingly powerful feminist movement (Bullough, 1994).

Even as Money was putting forth his ideas about the influence of sociopsychological factors (nurture) during critical periods of child development, he was strongly criticized by Milton Diamond, another psychologist active in sex research. Diamond (1965) indicated that gender decisions for hermaphrodites, about whom Money had originally drawn his data, were perhaps not as clear-cut as Money implied. Diamond hypothesized that an individual hermaphrodite might be receiving mixed biological signals, which allowed him or her to conform to the assigned gender rather than change it. He charged that Money was in danger of deemphasizing biology, or nature, and overemphasizing nurture.

The argument over nature versus nurture continues although both sides recognize the influence of both factors and it remains an argument over degree. At their scientific best, most biologists and social or behavioral scientists agree that the coding of gender is multivariate, sequential, and developmental, reflecting a complex interaction across the boundaries of disciplines and across biological and social variables.

Ann Constantinople (1973) questioned the assumption that masculinity was the opposite of femininity and suggested that the identification of masculine traits might be independent from, rather than the opposite of, the identification of feminine traits. The "both/and" concept of psychological identification quickly replaced the "either/or" notion that had dominated thinking on the matter since Lewis Terman developed his scales of masculinity and femininity. Sandra Bem (1974) developed a gender identity measure, the Bem Sex Role Inventory, that treated identification with masculine traits independently of identification with feminine traits. Spence and Helmreich (1974) found wide variation in gender traits, although they also found that stereotypical masculine personality traits in males were correlated with self-esteem, which reflects just how much influence society and culture have on self-esteem. However, the difficulty remains because the scales are based on observable patterns without any attempt to evaluate whether there are behaviors that must be distinctly limited to males or to females.

Bonnie Bullough held that the formation of gender identity and sexual preference included three steps: (a) a genetic predisposition, (b) prenatal hormonal stimulation that might follow or interfere with the genetic predisposition, and (c) socialization patterns that shape specific manifestation of the predisposition (Bullough & Bullough, 1993). This theory would allow for wider variations in gender behavior than those of some other theorists. For example, Nancy Chodorow (1978) noted out that infants, both males and females, generally have the most contact with their mothers and initially identify and form intense relationships with their mothers. For girls, this identification is never completely severed, but boys must relinquish their identification with their mothers as they take on masculine roles.

Chodorow maintained that this differing experience produced distinct coping strategies for males and females in dealing with the world. Specifically, women emphasize relationships *with others*, whereas men focus on their own individualism and independence *from others*. Gilligan (1982) pointed out that to hold this view limits personality development. A woman (or for that matter, a man) who views herself only in relationship to others (e.g., wife or mother but not an individual in her own right) may limit her own independent development. The man (or woman) who views himself only in terms of his own achievements and independence (boss, owner, director, sole author) may handicap his capacity for intimate connections with others. Obviously, conceptions of gender influence the way we think about what men and women can accomplish or achieve.

Probably most nursing theorists have followed Gilligan (1982), although a minority have emphasized the unique nature of being a woman. This is particularly true of some of the caring theorists. Dorothy Johnson (1959), who wrote before the concept of gender was fully developed, distinguished between caring and curing, and emphasized the caring aspects of nursing. This influenced Jean Watson in the establishing of caring centers. The concept of caring also became part of the basic educational mission of nursing.

The caring theory fits well into traditional concepts now associated with gender, but the problem is that one faction of nursing interpreted caring as a uniquely feminine quality and in the process ignored most of the mainstream research on gender. Nurses are involved in gender research, but only a few nurses have really done the quantitative studies needed to challenge the persistence of earlier stereotypes both within and outside of the profession.

VERN L. BULLOUGH

Genetics

The genomic era of health care began in April, 2003, with the completion of the sequencing of the Human Genome. The Human Genome uses four proteins: adenosine, cytosine, guanine, and thymine that replicate indefinitely. This double helix is the basis of DNA and, along with RNA, which substitutes uracil for thymine, makes up approximately 20 different amino acids. These proteins constitute just about everything in the body. It is these coded scripts that determine the entire life of an individual (Guttmacher & Collins, 2002). Clinicians can now determine if people will have certain genetic conditions in utero and hereditary conditions can actually be predicted using Mendelian Inheritance Theory. Nurses are understanding the significance of how using the correct questions regarding genetic history during patient admission assessments will assist in preparing a customized treatment and health promotion plan for each patient (Lea, 2003).

Genetic research by nurses is in the infancy stage. Recently multiple opportunities for nurse scientists to conduct biological and behavioral studies in genetics, either individually or in multidisciplinary teams, have become available. The National Institutes of Health (NIH) guide: Opportunities in genetics and nursing research (NIH, 1997) identified the following topics regarding genetics in need of research: holistic and community approaches, role of biopsychosocial factors in health and illness, managing and diagnosing cardinal symptoms of chronic conditions, cognitive decision making and learning skills, family education and counseling, risk behavior symptoms and reduction, and health promotion. Genetics offers nursing multiple research opportunities relating to biological and behavioral studies that could advance nursing science. Nurse clinicians need more research-based evidence to impact practice in every area, especially pharmacology, the neurological and immune systems, genetic testing and screening, and health promotion strategies. Nurse educators must study curriculum program outcomes to insure that Core Competencies in Genetics (National Coalition for Health Professional Education in Genetics [NCHPEG], 2001) are included.

The National Institute of Nursing Research (NINR) and the National Human Genome Research Institute (NHGRI) offer support to nurse scientists studying the clinical implications of human genetics research. Cashion (2002), a nurse faculty member at the University of Tennessee, is studying the effects of genetics and environment on disorders such as obesity, diabetes mellitus, and transplantation. Her study, *Genetic Markers of Acute Pancreas Allograft Rejection*, is funded by NINR and focuses on identifying patients who might experience rejection given their genetic make-up prior to actually manifesting the symptoms. One study about the use of genetic testing (Giarelli, 2003) generated important clinical relevance regarding patients' perceptions that they had gained significant health knowledge about either their own or a family member's genetic illness or predisposition.

Nurses need to become more involved in researching ways to promote health and decrease disease by using genetics, study ethical and legal concerns of genetic health, and become involved in advocating for people with genetic risk factors. Also they should participate in developing evidence-based protocols for identifying genetic risk factors to delay or prevent the onset of chronic illness, and develop methods to positively impact patient and families involved in decisions influenced by genetic conditions by disseminating important information regarding genetics.

RITA MONSEN
JUDITH A. LEWIS
UPDATED BY SHEILA GROSSMAN

Geriatric Interdisciplinary Teams

A recent report from the Institute of Medicine of the National Academies (IOM) challenges all health care professionals to recognize the need for effective interdisciplinary team care (Institute of Medicine, 2001). The sense of urgency implied by the IOM report is related to the growing body of evidence that effective interdisciplinary team care prevents medical errors and leads to improved patient outcomes (Boult et al., 2001; Cohen, H., et al., 2002; Sommers, Marton, Barbaccia, & Randolph, 2000).

Geriatric interdisciplinary team care has been shown to be essential to manage the complex syndromes experienced by frail older adults (Cohen, H., et al., 2002; Regenstein, Meyer, & Bagby, 1998). Providing comprehensive care to geriatric patients with multiple illnesses, disabilities, increased social problems, and fragmented care requires skills that no one individual possesses; therefore, older adults are best cared for by a team of health professionals (Baldwin, 1996; Pfeiffer, 1998; Regenstein et al., 1998). Geriatric interdisciplinary team care improves older adults' functional status (Sommers et al., 2000), perceived well-being (Boult et al., 2001; Knaus, Draper, Wagner, & Zimmerman, 1986), mental status, and depression (Eng, Padulla, Eleazur, McCann, & Fox, 1997). Geriatric interdisciplinary team care has also been shown to be cost effective by reducing patient readmission rates and number of physician office visits (Burns, R., Nichols, & Martindale-Adams, 2000).

The most recent report demonstrating the positive outcomes of team care came from a large, randomized trial of 1,388 frail patients 65 years of age or older who were hospitalized at 11 Veterans Affairs medical centers (Cohen et al., 2002). Participants were randomly assigned according to a two-by-two factorial design to receive either care in an acute inpatient geriatric unit or usual acute inpatient care, followed by either care at an outpatient geriatric clinic or usual outpatient care. The interventions involved teams that provided geriatric assessment and management according to Veterans Affairs standards and published guidelines. The primary outcomes were survival and health-related quality of life, measured with the use of the Medical Outcomes Study 36-Item Short-Form General Health Survey (SF-36), 1 year after randomization. Secondary outcomes were the ability to perform activities of daily living, physical performance, utilization of health services, and costs. The results demonstrated significant improvements in scores for four of the eight SF-36 subscales, activities of daily living ($p < .001$), and physical performance of those patients cared for by a geriatric interdisciplinary health care team as inpatients ($p < .001$). Neither the inpatient nor the outpatient intervention had a significant effect on mortality (21% at 1 year overall), nor were there any synergistic effects between the two interventions. At 1 year, patients cared for by an outpatient geriatric team had better scores on the SF-36 mental health subscale, even after adjustment for the score at discharge, than those assigned to usual outpatient care. Total costs at 1 year were similar for the intervention and usual-care groups. This study suggests the quality-of-life benefits of geriatric interdisciplinary team care. Although geriatric interdisciplinary team care did not have an impact on overall survival at 1 year, preserving function and improving mental health are consistent with the goals of care for frail older adults.

Another randomized clinical control trial demonstrating the positive effects of team care included 128 veterans, age 65 years and older, who were outpatients in a primary care Geriatric Evaluation and Management Unit (GEM) (Burns, R., et al., 2000). This study investigated the outcomes of patients who were randomized to outpatient GEM or usual care (UC). Two-year follow-up analyses were based on the 98 surviving individuals. Study outcome measurements included health status, function, quality of life, affect, cognition, and mortality. The results, after 2 years, demonstrated positive intervention effects for eight outcome measures, five of which attained significance at 1 year. GEM subjects, compared with UC subjects, had significantly greater improvement in health perception ($p < .001$), smaller increases in numbers of clinic visits ($p < .019$), improved instrumental activities of daily living (IADL) ($p < .006$), improved social activity ($p < .001$), greater improvement in Center for Epidemiologic Studies-Depression (CES-D) scores ($p < .003$), improved general well-being ($p < .001$), life satisfaction ($p < .001$), and Mini-Mental State Exam (MMSE) scores ($p < .025$). There were no significant treatment effects in activities of daily living (ADL) scores ($p < .386$), number of hospitalizations ($p < .377$), or mortality ($p < .155$). These findings suggest that a primary care approach that combines an initial geriatric interdisciplinary comprehensive assessment with long-term, interdisciplinary outpatient management may significantly improve outcomes for targeted older adults. In addition, Burns and colleagues have demonstrated the sustainability of positive geriatric interdisciplinary team outcomes over time.

The success of team care has also been demonstrated by investigating service utilization, including rehospitalizations, office visits, emergency department visits, and nursing home admissions (Sommers et al., 2000). A controlled cohort study of 543 patients in 18 private office practices of primary care physicians was conducted to examine the impact of a team intervention involving a primary care physician, a nurse, and a social worker for community-dwelling seniors with chronic illnesses. The intervention group received care from their primary care physician working with a registered nurse and a social worker, while the control group received care as usual from their primary care physician. The outcome measures included changes in number of hospital admissions, readmissions, office visits, emergency department visits, skilled nursing facility admissions, home care visits, and changes in patient self-rated physical, emotional, and social functioning. From 1992 (baseline year) to 1993, the two groups did not differ in service use or in self-reported health status. From 1993 to 1994, the hospitalization rate of the control group increased from 0.34% to 0.52%, while the rate in the intervention group stayed at baseline ($p < .03$). In the intervention group, mean office visits to all physicians fell by 1.5 visits compared with a 0.5-visit increase for the control group ($p < .003$). The patients in the intervention group reported an increase in social activities compared with the control group's decrease ($p < .04$). With fewer hospital admissions, average per-patient savings for 1994 were estimated at $90, inclusive of the intervention's cost but exclusive of savings from fewer office visits. This geriatric interdisciplinary team model of primary care shows potential for reducing the utilization of health care services and maintaining health status for older adults with chronic illnesses.

The effectiveness of geriatric interdisciplinary team care is dependent on the process of team functioning (Drinka & Clark, 2000;

Farrell, M., Schmitt, & Heinemann, 2001). Well-developed team skills are necessary for clinicians to represent their various disciplines when developing a geriatric interdisciplinary care plan (Farrell, M., et al.). Geriatric interdisciplinary team care has been shown to improve patient outcomes through the development of team skills and a willingness to collaborate more effectively (Grant, Finocchio, & the California Primary Care Consortium Subcommittee on Interdisciplinary Collaborative Teams in Primary Care, 1995; Drinka & Clark). The process of team functioning is dependent on the team skills and attitudes of the individual team members, their ability to identify ineffective team behaviors, and their ability to develop an interdisciplinary plan of care (Drinka & Clark; Heinemann, Schmitt, & Farrell, 1994).

In addition to team skills, positive attitudes toward health care teams contribute to effective geriatric interdisciplinary team care (Leipzig et al., 2002; Farrell, M., et al.). Attitudes toward geriatric interdisciplinary team care of nurses, physicians, and social workers have been shown to have an impact on team success, as reflected in, for example, hospital readmission rates (Sommers et al., 2000). Negative attitudes toward geriatric interdisciplinary team care that contribute to sources of team conflict include: (a) differing disciplinary and personal perspectives, (b) role competition and turf issues, (c) differing interprofessional perceptions of roles, (d) variations in professional socialization processes, (e) physician dominance of teams and decision making, and (f) the perception that physicians do not value collaboration with other groups (Abramson & Mizrahi, 1996; Leipzig et al., 2002).

In 1995, the John A. Hartford Foundation of New York City funded the Geriatric Interdisciplinary Team Training (GITT) program, a large multisite national team training program designed to create models to train 2,500 health care professionals in interdisciplinary team care. From 1997 to 2000, the eight GITT sites measured the effectiveness of this training intervention by conducting a prepost training evaluation of the GITT participants. The GITT program was foremost a training model and therefore the core measures that were collected were focused on the trainees, the ultimate unit of analysis. The purpose of the core measures was to evaluate the effectiveness of the intervention, the team training program.

The results from the GITT study demonstrated an overall effect of GITT training at posttest on measures of attitudinal change, change in test of geriatric care planning, and the test of team dynamics (Fulmer, Hyer, et al., 2004). Changes were greatest for attitudinal measures including team skills and modest for knowledge changes in geriatric care planning and test of team dynamics. At the level of the individual variables, significant changes were observed between the pre- and posttest mean scores for overall team skills scale and for the overall attitudes scale and each of its subscales. The GITT program serves as a model for implementing and evaluating geriatric interdisciplinary team training programs.

The need to improve the effectiveness of geriatric interdisciplinary team care has never been more urgent then in today's health care environment. Providing comprehensive care to older adults with multiple illnesses, disabilities, increased social problems, and fragmented care compounds the demographic imperative we face in our aging society. Effective geriatric interdisciplinary team care has been shown to improve patient outcomes by improving functional status (Sommers et al., 2000), perceived well-being (Boult et al., 2001; Knaus et al., 1996), mental status and depression (Eng et al., 1997). In addition, effective geriatric interdisciplinary team care has been shown to reduce medical errors (IOM, 2001).

Ellen Flaherty

Geriatrics

The term *geriatrics* evolved from the Greek word *geras,* "old age," and it refers to the branch of medicine that covers the diagnosis and treatment of the diseases and syndromes that occur primarily among older people. A board-certified medical practitioner of geriatric medicine is called a geriatrician. In the lay press the term has sometimes been overgeneralized to include comprehensive health care and preventive services for older adults, but this blurs the original meaning of the term.

In the specialty of nursing devoted to care of the aged, there has been considerable linguistic confusion and philosophical controversy about what to call the practice specialty. Various attempts were made to clarify and specify terminology and make the terms fit the consensual philosophy and goals of practitioners within the specialty, but no term has been found that pleases everyone.

A specialty referred to as geriatric nursing was first suggested in an anonymous 1925 editorial, "Care of the Aged," in the *American Journal of Nursing,* and the first nursing textbook on the topic was published in 1950. However, the actual birth of the specialty occurred in 1962, when the American Nurses Association (ANA) formed the Conference Group on Geriatric Nursing Practice. In 1966 the ANA officially created the Division of Geriatric Nursing, and in 1976 the name was changed to the Division of Gerontological Nursing (ANA, 1982). The ANA published the first set of *Standards of Practice for Geriatric Nursing* in 1970. The *Journal of Gerontological Nursing* began operation in 1975, and *Geriatric Nursing: Care of the Aged was* first published in 1979. The ANA division's name change and the titles of these two journals reflect the ongoing debate about proper terminology for the nursing specialty.

Many people rejected the term *geriatrics* because it did not properly reflect nursing's interest in the entire continuum of health and disease, including health promotion, disease prevention, care of acute illness, and long-term care. Others rejected it as a medical term that did not convey inclusion of the art of nursing.

Although the ANA division's name change to the Division of Gerontological Nursing pleased some nurses, others said it introduced a new error in terminology. The main criticism about this new label was that gerontology refers to the study of or science-work about the aging processes and the biological, psychological, sociological, and economic experiences of normal aging (Lueckenotte, 1996). Using an "ology" term did not logically lend itself to the name of a clinical specialty in a practice field. This problem led some leaders in the field to lobby for the term *gerontic nursing* to identify the specialty. Gerontic nursing as defined by Gunter and Estes (1979) is more philosophically palatable than geriatric nursing and more linguistically correct than gerontological nursing. Gerontic nursing was defined as a nursing specialty that includes the art and practice of nurturing, caring, and comforting older adults. Supporters of this term maintained that it included both the science and the art of nursing. Detractors argued that it left out health promotion and disease prevention.

A review of the titles of the most popular clinical textbooks in nursing today still shows considerable ambivalence. Nursing textbook titles include: geriatric nursing, gerontological nursing, clinical gerontological nursing, gerontologic nursing, gerontic nursing, and care of the aged; however, the latter three are less in evidence than a decade ago. Interestingly, the National Institute on Aging at NIH (2004) acknowledged the single-term dilemma by naming its clinical research program the "Geriatrics and Clinical Gerontology Program" (GCG). The Geriatrics branch supports research on health issues of the aged, including disease and disability in older persons—both specific conditions and multiples morbidities. The Clinical Gerontology branch sponsors research on clinically related issues regarding aging and research on aging changes over the life span.

An ideal term for the nursing specialty would cover the full range of knowledge needed and services to be provided in this practice field that has age of client as its sole parameter. The specialty is practiced at all levels of the health continuum, with persons who are aged 60+ to 115+, in any and all types of settings where older adults are to be found, and for periods of time that stretch from minutes to decades. Finding a fitting replacement for the term *geriatrics* or *geriatric nursing* has already challenged some of the best minds in the profession for over 40 years. The search for a single ideal term is not likely to end soon.

Even without a clear title for the specialty, nurse researchers have made significant contributions to knowledge about older adults across the spectrum from health promotion through end-of-life care. As genetic knowledge and stem cell research opens new vistas for inquiry, myriad unanswered questions about preventing and arresting the chronic illnesses and disabilities of old age will provide ample fodder for the fertile intellects of present and future nurse scientists for many years to come.

JOANNE SABOL STEVENSON

Gerontological Advanced Practice Nursing

During the last 3 decades, research examining the proliferation of Advanced Practice Nurses (APNs) has demonstrated that APNs improve quality of care, increase patient and staff satisfaction, while being cost effective across health care settings (Feldman, Ventura, Crosby, 1987; Master et al., 1987; Miller, S. K., 1997; Naylor, Brooten, et al., 1999; Ramsay, McKenzie, & Fish, 1982; Sox, 1979; Spitzer et al., 1974).

During the late 1960s to 1970s graduate nursing programs began developing specialties in gerontological nursing. GAPN is an umbrella term refering to Geriatric Nurse Practitioner (GNP) or Gerontological Clinical Nurse Specialist (GCNS). Currently there are near 4,000 certified GNPs and over 1,000 certified GCNSs (American Association of Colleges of Nursing, 2004). GAPN subgroups presently require gerontological-focused graduate education. Traditionally, GCNS roles include educator, researcher, practitioner, manager, and consultant. In addition to the GCNS roles, GNPs have the ability to conduct advanced health histories and physical assessments make diagnosis, and prescribe appropriate medical treatments—including pharmaceuticals within a collaborative agreement with a physician. Scopes of practice for both vary between states. Literature demonstrates more similarities between nurse practitioners (NPs) and clinical nurse specialists (CNSs) than differences. Nursing leaders are currently debating role integration (Fenton & Brykczynski, 1993; Soehren & Schumann, 1994; Lincoln, P. E., 2000).

The literature reported APNs favorably influence health care outcomes such as: mortality, morbidity, length of stay, functional status, mental status, stress level, and patient satisfaction, burden of care, and cost of care. Overall, studies demonstrated consumer acceptance and satisfaction with NPs, physician comparative quality of care, increased productivity, cost savings, saved physician time, effective management of both preventive and chronically ill care, and improved patient education (Feldman et al., 1987; Naylor, Munro, & Brooten, 1991).

The GAPN role impacts the quality of care in long-term care (LTC) populations by decreasing hospitalizations, reducing pharmaceutical usage, and improving patient-family-staff satisfaction. GAPNs hold an essential role in reducing restraints in the nursing home population (Evans, L. K., et al., 1997). Most notably, the GAPNs provide cost-effective quality care. Using a quasi-experimental design, Kane and colleagues (1989) compared data of pre- and post-GNP time periods in 60 nursing homes (30-GNP; 30-control) dispersed throughout eight western states and discovered that GNP provided cost-effective care to residents primarily by reducing hospital utilization. Another study, a 1-year retrospective data analysis for 1,077 LTC residents, compared 414 residents followed by GNP/MD teams and 663 residents followed by MDs alone. Patients of the GNP/MD teams yielded a $72 per resident per month savings (Burl, Bonner, Rao, & Khan, 1998).

GNPs may succeed in nursing home management. Grzeczkowski and Knapp (1988) evaluated a 120-bed nursing home after a

GNP became the Director of Nursing. Their findings demonstrated decreased medication usage, lower rates of urinary/respiratory tract infections, decreased utilization of indwelling urinary catheters, and less decubiti. GNPs' extensive geriatric education and ability to work well within interdisciplinary teams yielded effective patient care.

GAPN education, focused on geriatric issues such as falls, restraint usage, delirium, polypharmacy, and normal versus abnormal physical changes, carves a vital role in acute care management of frail older adults. Often GAPNs anticipate these conditions and provide early intervention. Models of care that have improved hospital care to the elderly include geriatric evaluation teams, Nurses Improving Care to the Hospitalized Elderly (NICHE), Geriatric Resource Nurse (GRN), Case Management (CM), Geriatric Evaluation and Management (GEM) units and Acute Care of the Elderly (ACE) units. GAPNs have been integral members of these models of care.

A retrospective analysis of nursing home patients admitted to an acute care facility demonstrated a mean decrease of 2.78 ($p < 0.05$) days in length of stay when care involved a GNP (Miller, S. K., 1997). Naylor and colleagues (1999) went further than evaluating "in-house" statistics. Their randomized clinical trial included 363 patients (186 control; 177 intervention) with follow-up data collection up to 24 weeks posthospital discharge. In the intervention group, GAPNs were responsible for comprehensive discharge planning and maintaining a home follow-up protocol. Examples of the outcome measures were hospital readmission, recurrence or exacerbation of the index hospitalization diagnostic-related groups (DRG), comorbidity, cumulative days of rehospitalization, functional status, depression, and patient satisfaction. The findings at 24 weeks posthospital discharge demonstrated that GAPN patients experienced fewer hospitalization days, yielding a Medicare savings of almost $600,000. Other findings: functional status, depression scores, and patient satisfaction, were similar in both study groups.

Case studies of older adults living at home describe the accessible, comprehensive, accountable, continual, and collaborative care delivered by GNPs (Burns-Tisdal & Goff, 1989). Alessi and colleagues (1997) studied 414 home care clients (215-intervention and 199-control). The intervention group had GNP-performed geriatric assessments (CGAs) annually for 3 years, along with quarterly follow-up visits. The authors examined the GNP's health care recommendations given to clients and proposed that repetitive reinforcement and the GNP-patient relationship contributed to achieving patient adherence to therapies. This warrants further investigation.

The Program of All-inclusive Care for the Elderly (PACE), developed in San Francisco known as On Lok in 1971, focuses on health and social day services to enable frail older adults to remain in the community. PACE's model requires GAPNs in the interdisciplinary team. PACE programs now exist in nine states providing cost-effective quality care with a reduction in institutional care use (Eng, Pedulla, Eleazer, McCann, & Fox, 1997).

GNPs provide effective ambulatory care. McDowell, Martin, Snustad, and Flynn (1986) performed a retrospective review of 800 patients comparing GNPs' care to two internal medicine board-certified physicians with geriatric experience using polypharmacy and functional status as comparison measurements. GNPs provided high-quality, cost-effective care. Another study (Mahoney, D. F., 1994) compared medication usage of NPs and MDs; three geriatric vignettes designed by GNPs, geriatricians, and geriatric pharmacists were presented to 373 MDs and 118 NPs. Analysis of the MDs and NPs was discussed and it was discovered that NPs utilized fewer drugs. The NP sample was not specifically limited to GNPs; family and adult nurse practitioners were included in the sample. Geriatric experience and prescribing experience proved to be significant factors affecting appropriate prescribing. Mahoney proposed that gerontological education for APNs and Family Nurse Practitioners (FNPs) would ensure proper pharmaceutical usage for the elderly.

Meta-analysis methods have allowed researchers to examine conflicts in the data and deduce clearer and more conclusive findings. Often lacking in the literature is a clear presentation of APN preparation and specialty. Future research needs to be rigorous with attention to (a) conceptual definitions—sensitivity of outcome measures, study of care delivery processes not solely on the provider, relationship between the process and outcomes of care; (b) measurement of variables; (c) APN educational backgrounds; and (d) methodology—more blind randomized trials with attention to internal and external validity (Brown, S. A., & Grimes, 1995).

ANNEMARIE DOWLING-CASTRONOVO

Grandparents Raising Grandchildren

According to the 2000 Census Supplementary Survey, an estimated 6 million or 8.4% of children in the U.S. live with nonparental relatives, a 173% increase since 1970 and a 78% increase since 1990 (U.S. Bureau of the Census, 2001). Of the 6 million children living with nonparental relatives, 75% are being raised by grandparents. Although this phenomenon impacts all racial and economic groups, the most significant rises have been among African Americans and low-income families.

The most common antecedents to children being raised by grandparents—while often interrelated—include child abuse and neglect, substance abuse, mental illness, incarceration, homicide, and HIV/AIDS among parents (Dowdell, 1995; Kelley, Yorker, Whitley, & Sipe, 2001). While some children have been removed from the care of their birth parents by the child protection system and placed with foster parents, many more are with grandparents through informal arrangements among family members (Yorker et al., 1998).

While caregiver burden among those providing for elderly parents or spouses has been studied extensively over the past few decades, only recently has it been examined among older adults raising grandchildren and great-grandchildren. With the dramatic rise in the number of grandparents raising grandchildren in households that do not include either birth parent, research on this population has only recently evolved. Researchers studying this phenomenon represent a number of disciplines including nurses, sociologists, gerontologists, and psychologists. Nurse researchers have made important contributions to empirical knowledge related to the impact of the caregiving role on grandparents raising grandchildren.

Recent research indicates that raising grandchildren was associated with negative consequences for the well-being of grandparents. For instance, numerous studies indicate that grandparents raising grandchildren are at an increased risk for physical health problems, with some health problems serious enough to jeopardize their ability to provide care for their grandchildren (Dowdell, 1995; Whitley, White, Kelley, & Yorker, 1999). Based on a nationally representative sample, researchers found that grandmothers raising grandchildren were more likely than noncaregiving grandmothers to report their health as fair or very poor (Fuller-Thomson & Minkler, 2000). These grandmothers were also more likely to report physical limitations when performing daily living activities. Similarly, Dowdell found that 45% of the custodial grandmothers identified themselves as having a physical health problem or illness that seriously affected their general health, with single grandmothers more likely than married grandmothers to report health problems. In a prospective cohort study as part of the Nurses' Health Study, researchers found that providing high levels of care to grandchildren increases of the risk of coronary heart disease (Lee, S., Colditz, Berkman, & Kawachi, 2003).

In a study involving 102 custodial grandmothers, almost half self-reported their health as only fair or poor (Whitley et al.,

1999). Health assessments by registered nurses indicated that 25% of the participants were diabetic, 54% were hypertensive, and 80% met the criteria for obesity, which is associated with cardiovascular problems. Participants scored significantly worse in the areas of physical functioning, bodily pain, social functioning, role functioning, and general health than national norms on a standardized self-report measure of health.

Researchers consistently have found that assuming full-time parenting responsibilities for grandchildren was associated with increased rates of psychological distress, including depression, in grandparents (Burnette, 1998; Emick & Hayslip, 1999; Force, Botsford, Pisano, & Holbert, 2000; Fuller-Thomson, Minkler, & Driver, 1997; Kelley, Whitley, Sipe, & Yorker, 2000; Szinovacz, DeViney, & Atkinson, 1999). In a study of African-American women raising grandchildren, Minkler and Roe (1993) found that 37% of grandmothers raising grandchildren reported their psychological health had worsened since assuming full-time caregiving responsibilities, with the majority (72%) reporting feeling "depressed" in the week prior to data collection. In another study, researchers found that nearly 30% of grandparents raising grandchildren had psychological distress scores in the clinical range, which is indicative of a need for mental health intervention (Kelley, Whitley, et al.).

Grandparents raising children with special needs or behavioral problems experience even higher rates of psychological distress. In one study, researchers found that grandparents raising special-needs children reported poorer mental health well-being than those raising children without special needs (Brown, D. R., & Boyce-Mathis, 2000). Other studies have found that grandparents raising grandchildren viewed as difficult or as having behavioral problems experienced more negative affects than grandparents raising children viewed as normal (Hayslip, Emick, Henderson, & Elias, 2002; Pruchno & McKenney, 2002).

While many of the studies discussed above involve relatively small and homogeneous populations, researchers analyzing data from the National Survey of Families and Households reported similar findings. For instance, when researchers compared custodial grandparents to noncustodial grandparents, they found that custodial grandparents were almost twice as likely to be categorized as depressed (Fuller-Thomson et al., 1997). Even after controlling for depression that preexisted the onset of caregiving, custodial grandmothers had higher rates of depression. Minkler and Fuller-Thomson (2001) also found that custodial grandmothers were more likely than noncustodial grandmothers to have significant levels of depressive symptomatology.

A number of factors have been identified as contributors to increased psychological distress, including depression, in grandparent caregivers. Some of the most well-documented correlates included poor physical health, social isolation, and financial difficulties. For example, in one study, researchers found that family resources, participants' physical health, and to a lesser extent social support predicted levels of psychological distress in grandparents raising grandchildren (Kelley et al., 2000). Other factors contributing to mental health status that have been identified by researchers include circumstances involved with the onset of assuming full-time parenting responsibilities (e.g., abandonment by, addiction in, incarceration or death of their adult child), changes in role demands, conflict with the children's parents, behavior problems of grandchildren, and legal issues (Caliandro & Hughes, 1998; Dowdell, 1995; Emick & Hayslip, 1999; Yorker et al., 1998).

By assuming full-time parenting responsibilities, grandparents are often faced with increased financial pressures at or near a time in their lives when income is dramatically decreased. This decrease in income is most often related to retirement and living on fixed incomes or from having to leave full-time employment because of the demands of full-time parenting, especially when the grandchildren have special needs. While some families may be entitled to Temporary Assistance to Needy

Families (TANF) cash benefits, the monthly payments are typically nominal and insufficient for adequately housing, clothing, and feeding children. Furthermore, a lack of resources has been found to contribute to increased psychological stress in grandparents raising grandchildren (Kelley et al., 2000).

Findings from several studies portray grandparent caregivers as socially isolated from peers due to demands of raising children at a point in their lives when they would otherwise have few childcare responsibilities (Fuller-Thomson & Minkler, 2000; Hayslip, Shore, Henderson, & Lambert, 1998; Musil, 1998). The social isolation typically reported by grandparents raising grandchildren is important given that social support is a mediator of psychological distress in grandparents raising grandchildren (Kelley et al., 2000).

Further research on the well-being of custodial grandparents is needed. Longitudinal studies would contribute to knowledge of the long-term impact of this type of caregiving. Experimental studies will be necessary to determine which intervention strategies are most effective in improving the physical and mental health of this population. An increase in policy-relevant research is needed to address the health care, financial, and housing needs of grandparents raising grandchildren.

SUSAN J. KELLEY

Grantsmanship

Grantsmanship is the knowledge and skill needed to prepare a grant application. It is the art behind the science. It cannot make bad science fundable, but poor grantsmanship can keep good science from receiving the favorable review needed for funding. Although good science is a necessary prerequisite for success in obtaining funding, good grant writing is what makes the good science shine. Indeed, many characterize good grantsmanship as a type of salesmanship.

Everything a grant writer does to make the grant reviewer's job easier is part of good grantsmanship. The grant writer wants to impress the reviewer with the soundness, importance, and perhaps even the creativity of the science of the proposal. At the same time, the grant writer must stimulate an excitement that turns the reviewer into an advocate or enthusiastic champion of the proposed project.

Achieving a balance between generating such enthusiasm and sticking with a somewhat rigid formula in the actual writing is an artful enterprise. Grant writing itself is not particularly creative. Rather, grant writing can be viewed as a type of formula writing. Good basic writing skills are essential. The grant writer must methodically walk the reader or reviewer through a well-constructed logical argument. The reviewer should have no question about where the grant writer is going. Moreover, a good grant writer anticipates the reviewer's questions and answers them before the question is raised.

Repetition of important content is a key aspect of good grant writing. An important point is worth repeating to ensure that a reviewer does not miss it. Repetition also is essential in the choice of words for key concepts. Once a concept is named and defined, the grant writer should stick with the identified word, term, or phrase. Altering a phrase or using alternative terms in order to provide some variety only serves to confuse a reviewer trying to follow the specific ideas presented.

Good grantsmanship also requires the ability to handle criticism. Many more grants are written and submitted than are actually funded. Therefore, a good grant writer will seek multiple reviews from colleagues before actually submitting a grant to the funding agency. It is wise to seek reviewers for a variety of purposes. Some should be familiar with the content area of the grant application to identify any important errors or gaps in content. Others should be unfamiliar with the specific content area to protect against assumed knowledge by insiders and to determine if the grant is written in a manner that convinces a knowledgeable but otherwise uninformed reviewer about the worthiness of the proposed project. Still others may be used for things such as grammar, editing, and typographical errors not found by computer spell-checks. The ability to handle criticism is needed to request and receive a brutal review and to respond to all concerns and criticisms without defensiveness. It is far better to acknowledge the concern from a colleague and be able to revise the grant application accordingly than to have the very same concern raised in the official review and result in a poor evaluation and no funding.

Although the specific proposal is the heart of the grant, grantsmanship involves much more than just writing the actual proposal. Good grant writers understand other aspects as well. For example, a cardinal rule is to follow the directions. It seems simple enough, but it is surprising how many would-be grant writers neglect to read carefully all instructions for a particular grant application and to follow them faithfully.

Most grant applications come with specific guidelines about such things as eligibility to apply, budget limits, allowable costs, page limits, margins, font sizes, section sequencing, the type of content expected, the number of references allowed, what may go into appendices (if allowed), who must sign where and what, and so on. It is imperative that the grant writer adhere to all the identified specifications. Some funding agencies will return grants unreviewed if the directions are not followed. Not following directions raises questions about the careful attention to detail needed to carry out most projects and thus may reflect poorly on the applicant.

Another basic element of good grantsmanship is to know and understand the goals and mission of the particular funding agency to which one plans to submit the grant. For example, each institute in the National Institutes of Health (NIH) has a specific mandate to fund certain types of research. Further, each institute generally sets priorities identifying specific areas in which they are seeking proposals. Prior to writing a grant, one should investigate and determine what funding agency would be the best match for the intended project.

The grant writer should specifically address the stated priorities and goals of the funding agency or foundation for support of the proposed project. This is particularly true for foundation grants. A helpful strategy when making these arguments is to use the exact language of the program announcement or the foundation's mission statement. It is rarely in the grant writer's best interest to try to convince a foundation or other funding entity of a worthwhile project not clearly within its mandate.

There are a number of references to assist a grant writer. One particularly useful book is the *Grant Application Writer's Handbook* by Liane Reif-Lehrer (1995). In addition to general information about writing and applying for grants, it contains extensive information about the grant programs of the NIH. Over half of the volume is devoted to appendices, with useful resources, references, and information about the NIH, the National Science Foundation, and applying to foundations. Although some of the specific information rapidly becomes dated, much remains valuable and timeless. The NIH also publishes a volume titled *Helpful Hints on Preparing a Research Grant Application to the National Institutes of Health* that contains several useful and informative articles and presentations. It is available free of charge from the NIH website, http://www.nih.gov.

LAUREN S. AARONSON

Grief

Grief is a multifaceted response to the loss of a significant person, object, belief, relationship, body part, or body function. Grief includes the entire range of physical, psychological, cognitive, and behavioral responses to loss. Grief is characterized by intense mental anguish and varies in duration from a few weeks to many years. Three types of grief have been identified: conventional grief, anticipatory grief, and pathological grief. Conventional grief occurs after a loss, while anticipatory grief is the response to an impending loss. Although there is little agreement on the exact nature of anticipatory grief, there is general agreement that anticipatory grief facilitates coping with a loss when the loss actually occurs. Grief that falls outside normal parameters is often labeled pathological grief; however, there are no specific signs or symptoms that differentiate conventional grief from pathological grief.

Loss, bereavement, and mourning are terms related to grief. Loss is the experience of parting with an object, person, belief, or relationship that is valued, wherein the loss necessitates a reorganization of one or more aspects of the person's life. Losses range from minor ones, such as the loss of a wallet which necessitates only minor adjustments, to major ones, such as the death of a loved one or the loss of one's home in a fire or flood which necessitates major adjustments. Bereavement is the state of having experienced a loss, particularly the death of a significant other. Mourning encompasses the socially prescribed behaviors after the death of a significant other. Such behaviors vary from culture to culture. Mourning behaviors are conventional outward signs of grief that are socially constructed and do not necessarily indicate the presence or absence of grief.

Throughout time, nurses have had key roles managing grief. Whether working in the emergency room, a critical care unit, labor and delivery, a psychiatric setting, or any other setting, nurses frequently deal with individuals and families who are experiencing either anticipatory grief or grief following a loss. Despite the importance of nurses in caring for the grieving, little nursing research was conducted on grief until the late 1980s.

In 1983, Jeanne Quint Bonoliel reviewed nursing research on death, dying, and terminal illness at a time when few nurses were conducting research in those areas. Since then, research on grief and bereavement has proliferated. In 1987 Demi and Miles published a review of research on bereavement. Opie, in 1992, published a review on childhood and adolescent bereavement. In 1995 Martinson reviewed research on pediatric hospice care and addressed both anticipatory grief and grief after the death of a pediatric hospice patient. Corless, in 1994, critiqued research on symptom control within hospice care and reviewed research on coping with dying. A number of nurses developed research programs focused on grief, including J. Q. Benoliel, R. Constantino, A. Demi, M. Diamond, N. Hogan, M. Miles, S. Murphy, J. Saunders, and M. Vachon. Hogan and Schmidt (2002) recently developed a model of grief to personal growth through structural equation modeling.

Standardized instruments such as the *Texas Inventory of Grief*, the *Grief Experience Inventory*, and the *Bereavement Experience Questionnaire* have been used to assess grief manifestations. The emotional distress that accompanies grief was often measured with instruments such as the *Brief Symptom Inventory*, the *Profile of Mood States,* the *Impact of Events Questionnaire*, or a depression scale such as the Beck's or Hamilton's. Children's and adolescents' grief was often measured by the *Child Behavior Checklist.* A recent addition is the *Hogan Grief Reaction Checklist* (Hogan, Greenfield, & Schmidt, 2001).

Much nursing research on bereavement has been directed at describing the manifestations of grief among diverse samples: bereaved parents, children, siblings, and widows; suicide survivors; and people facing a life-threatening or terminal illness. Other researchers have described bereaved persons' responses to events such as the loss of a home by fire (Keane, Brennan, & Pickett, 2000) or a spontaneous abortion (Van & Meleis, 2003). Still other researchers have focused on describing nurses' responses to caring for the dying or the bereaved. These descriptive studies have used diverse analytical approaches, such as grounded theory and phenomenology, and diverse data collection methods including participant observation, semistructured interviews, survey questionnaires, structured instruments, and q-sort techniques.

Some nursing research on bereavement has focused on comparing different modes of bereavement (suicide vs. accident, expected vs.

unexpected) or comparing bereaved persons with a nonbereaved group. For example, Murphy, Johnson, Wu, Fan, and Lohan (2003) compared grief manifestations of parents whose child died by suicide, accident, and homicide.

A number of nursing studies have investigated variables related to bereavement outcomes such as self-blame, coping processes, and social support. A few studies have used quasi-experimental designs to investigate the effects of specific interventions to help the bereaved or to help nurses to better meet the needs of the bereaved. For example, researchers have studied the effect of a support group on bereaved parents whose child died from cancer, the effect of a support group on bereaved children and adolescents, and the effect of a grief workshop for pediatric oncology nurses.

Descriptive studies have contributed greatly to our understanding of the grief process and the many forms it may take. Comparative and correlational studies have provided insight into variables related to bereavement outcomes. However, very little research has been done to assess the effects of bereavement interventions. More attention needs to be paid to intervention studies that address what helps people deal with conventional grief and anticipatory grief. Further, most of the participants in the studies reviewed were White Americans. With increasing cultural diversity in the U.S., it is important that research address bereavement responses among diverse cultural groups. Fortunately, a few researchers have addressed cultural differences in bereavement. Lee and Chu (2001) studied the grief of Chinese men who were diagnosed as infertile, and Van and Meleis (2003) studied African-American women's grief after involuntary pregnancy loss; however, much more research is needed on grief of diverse cultural groups. In addition, researchers should work on developing culturally relevant instruments to assess bereavement outcomes.

Grieving people are vulnerable and need special attention to protect them from studies that could increase their vulnerability. Although many grieving people find that participating in research that focuses on their grief provides them an opportunity to express their thoughts and feelings to a nonjudgmental researcher, there is the potential of increasing the participant's pain and distress. The researcher must have the skills to provide immediate support if this occurs and also should be prepared to refer participants for counseling if they need further support.

Alice S. Demi

Grounded Theory

Grounded theory refers to a method of qualitative research which seeks to explain variations in social interactional and social structural problems and processes. The goal is to generate theory from the data and resultant conceptual schema. The grounded theory approach presumes the possibility of discovering fundamental patterns in all of social life, called core variables or basic social processes (Hutchinson, 1993; Wilson, H., 1993). According to its sociologist originators, Barney Glaser and Anselm Strauss (1967), grounded theories should be relevant and work to explain, predict, and be modified by social phenomena under study. Data are not forced to fit existing theories but rather are used to develop rich, dense, complex analytic frameworks.

Grounded theory as an original mode of inquiry oriented to the discovery of meaning emerged from the social philosophy of symbolic interactionism and an intellectual tradition in social science called pragmatism. Both emphasize (a) the importance of qualitative fieldwork in data collection in order to ground theory in reality, (b) the nature of experience as a process of continuous change, and (c) the interrelationships among conditions, interpretive meaning, and action. Knowledge is viewed as relative to particular contextual circumstances. Such a worldview was in contrast to the dominant paradigm that emphasized stability and regularities in social life.

Grounded theory, as a qualitative, nonmathematical analytic process is particularly well suited to nursing studies that are conducted to uncover the nature of clinically relevant phenomena such as chronic illness, caregiving, and dying in real-world rather than laboratory conditions. The resulting theoretical formulation not only explains human experience and associated meanings but also can provide a basis for nursing intervention research and nursing practice.

The influence of grounded theory methods has been particularly striking in the evolution of nursing research because Glaser and Strauss, who developed the method, were professors in the School of Nursing at the University of California, San Francisco, starting in the 1960s. Consequently, many of the seminal methodological references and landmark publications of findings in the nursing literature can be traced to nursing doctoral students who studied and collaborated with them in the 1970s and 1980s. Subsequently, those early colleagues mentored cohorts of other nurse researchers. Several nurse researchers, including Jeanne Benoliel, Juliet Corbin, Sally Hutchinson, and Holly Wilson, have been leaders in the application, articulation, and dissemination of the use of grounded theory methods by nursing and other disciplines.

Grounded theories are focused on what may be unarticulated social-psychological and social-structural problems and are integrated around the basic social process that is discovered in observational, interview, and document data (Wilson, H. S., & Hutchinson, 1996). The researcher does not begin with a preconceived theory and experimentally prove it. Rather, the researcher begins by studying an area under natural conditions. Data are usually derived from qualitative data sources—interviews, participant observation (fieldwork), and document analysis—although quantitative data can also inform the emerging analysis. Sensitizing questions are asked to learn what is relevant in the situation under study. Sampling is not conducted according to conventions of probability, nor is sample size predetermined. Instead, purposive, theoretical sampling is used so that concepts emerging from the data guide additional data collection.

Doing grounded theory research departs from the typically linear sequence of theory verifying research because data collection and analysis go on simultaneously. As soon as data are available, an orderly, rigorous, constant comparative method of data analysis is initiated. Analysis proceeds through stages of in vivo (or substantive) coding in which themes and patterns are identified in the words of participants themselves, coding for categories in which in vivo codes are clustered together in conceptual categories, and theoretical coding in which relationships among concepts are developed. Memos are written detailing each of the codes and categories and linking them to exemplars from the data. Concepts and propositions that emerge from the data direct subsequent data collection.

The sample is considered complete when saturation is achieved. Saturation refers to the point at which no new themes, patterns, or concepts appear in the data. Sorting memos (conceptual notes about codes and categories and their data exemplars) into an integrative schema provides an outline for integrating and then reporting the grounded theory discovered.

The outcome of analysis is a dense, parsimonious, integrative schema that explains most of the variation in a social psychological situation. Properties, dimensions, categories, strategies, and phases of the theory are inextricably related to the basic social process. Grounded theory may be context-bound to a specific substantive area (substantive theory) or may be at a more conceptual level and applicable to diverse settings and experiences (formal theory) (Glaser, B., 1978).

The grounded theory approach has resonated with a wide variety of social scientists and professional practitioners interested in human experiences with health and illness. In their book, *Discovery of Grounded Theory*, B. Glaser and Strauss (1967) acknowledged that it was a "beginning venture" and did not offer "clearcut procedures and definitions" (p. 1). Over time, grounded theory, as an approach to the generation of theory from data has undergone some major transformations. Some of the changes that were designed to promote rigor in the method have been criticized as diverting the research from generating theory directly from data, for risking theoretical sensitivity in the investigator, and for eroding the method. Others are of the opinion that assuming that grounded theory was taught and conducted from a single unified perspective is erroneous and that the ongoing discourse among qualitative researchers is part of an intellectual movement essential to grounded theory's refinement and evolution. The hallmarks, however, continue to be data-theory interplay, making constant comparisons, asking theoretically oriented questions, conceptual and theoretical coding, and the development of theory.

Holly Skodol Wilson
Sally A. Hutchinson
Updated by Deborah F. Lindell

H

Health Care Communication

Health care communication remains at the core of nursing practice providing the groundwork for relationships with patients, family members, and health care colleagues; and the medium for teaching and caring. Verbal communication includes "all behavior conveying messages with language" (Caris-Verhallen, Kerkstra, & Bensing, 1997, p. 916). Nonverbal communication includes any behavior that imparts information without the use of verbal language, including body movement, physical appearance, conversation timing, voice qualities, personal space, and touch (Oliver, S., & Redfern, 1991). Sustained programs of research in health care communication remain scarce. S. Brown's (1999) review of the research literature on patient-centered communication in the *Annual Review of Nursing Research* contained only 15 nursing journal references out of 69 references. The majority of health care communication research has been conducted in psychology and medicine. The following review highlights contributions that nursing research has made to health care communication.

The development of expertise in communication has been examined in the clinical setting and with educational interventions. Kotechi (2002) conducted a grounded theory study of baccalaureate nursing student communication and found that the students moved through a four-stage process to develop a "personal communication repertoire" (p. 63). Stage one, affirming the self, involved self-talk to bolster confidence in communicating with patients and to evaluate their own communication. Stage two, engaging the patient, moved beyond feeling like an intruder to establishing acceptable boundaries, and developing a relationship and rapport with patients. To engage the patient, students used social talk (superficial conversation), professional talk (communication strategies learned in school), and personal talk (communication used on special occasions to share a common experience). During stage three, students experienced communication breakdowns when they worked with more challenging patients, but learned to keep going by using additional communication strategies. Students relied heavily on how the staff nurses talked with more challenging patients and incorporated the helpful communication strategies into their repertoire. During stage four, refining the repertoire, students became more facile in selecting or switching to more effective communication strategies, and did so with greater confidence in order to persevere through more challenging patient-care situations.

The majority of nursing research in health care communication has focused on describing how nurses communicate with patients across a variety of clinical contexts. In some studies communication has been conceptualized as either affective (providing social or emotional support) or instrumental (completing a necessary task). Caris-Verhallen and colleagues (1997) examined nurses' communication with older adults in both the community and extended care setting. Nurses, nursing assistants, and older adults were videotaped and Roter's Interactional Analysis system was used to score the interactions. A total of 44% to 72% of the communication was socioemotional. Most of the older adults had received care for a year or more, which may have facilitated the increased interpersonal nature of the communication (Caris-Verhallen, Kerkstra, van der Heijden, & Bensing, 1998).

A different pattern of verbal communication was found in an experiment in which nurses were videotaped admitting a simulated cancer patient. A total of 62% of the verbal communication was instrumental. Few of the verbalizations encouraged patient input such as asking if patients understood (Kruijver, Kerkstra, Bensing, & van de Weil, 2001). The simulated conditions of the study might have decreased the usual efforts that nurses make to provide emotional support and involve patients during admission interviews. Home care nurses initiated talk about compliance with the medical regimen, an instrumental focus, approximately 60% of the time (Vivian & Wilcox, 2000), suggesting that an instrumental focus might predominate in nursing communication with patients. Studies testing the effects of socioemotional/instrumental communication and patient involvement on patient outcomes might guide the use of more effective communication strategies.

The context for the communication has generally not been directly examined, with the exception of Caris-Verhallen et al. (1998). Studies that have examined nurse and patient communication across different populations and settings provided some insight into the effect of context. For example, while nurses initiated most of the child-health topics with parents during a well-child visit, nurses invited questions from parents in 66% of the visits (Baggens, 2001), a finding contrary to Kruijver and colleagues (2001). It would be helpful to more closely examine the impact of context in future communication studies.

Therapeutic use of communication provides a helpful area for nursing research and shifts the focus to the patient and health care provider interaction. Nurses and patients were found to encourage optimism in a constructive, realistic manner during cancer-care communication. Nurses and patients developed positive statements by elaborating on more positive points. Conversations were generally ended on a positive note, often with the patient spontaneously providing the comment (Jarrett & Payne, 2000). Listening in order to understand what has been said is an essential part of therapeutic communication. Listening involves focusing on the patient, and providing patients the opportunity to talk and find their own interpretation of their experience (Fredriksson, 1999). Research is needed to translate descriptive findings about therapeutic communication into effective interventions.

Supporting patients to communicate effectively has reemerged as a nursing research focus, moving beyond testing the effects of communication boards. Augmentative and alternative communication (AAC) devices improve or supplement talking and writing, and include devices such as computer-generated speech. Uncovering the meaning of using AAC devices might encourage nurses to value and support use of such devices. Patients' experience of using AAC devices to communicate was found to enable humanness. Use of AAC devices helped communicate thoughts but was less effective in communicating emotion (Dickerson, Stone, Panchura, & Usiak, 2002). A less technical means of supporting patient communication was tested by teaching pain-communication skills via videotape to older adults awaiting surgery. Older adults who were taught the communication skills reported greater pain relief on the 1st day after the operation (McDonald, D., & Molony, in press). The study did not directly measure patient communication and did not clarify which specific communication strategies or combinations were most helpful.

Nursing research in health care communication continues to be widely dispersed. Approaches that microanalyze segments of conversation provide some description of the content of the communication, but they do not capture the context, motivations, or consequences. Naturalistic studies (e.g., Jarrett & Payne, 2000; Kotechi, 2002) have provided some helpful insights, suggesting the need to further explore aspects of health care communication from the naturalistic approach, for example, conducting a grounded theory study to identify the basic process by which expert nurses effectively communicate with patients. The majority of the research has focused on how nurses communicate with patients. Future research must include patient contributions to the communication, testing ways to support patients to effectively communicate with health care providers. Ways of enhancing patient communication must be linked to positive patient outcomes such as increased self-care and decreased pain, and must be obtainable within the constraints of current health care systems.

DEBORAH DILLON MCDONALD

Health Conceptualization

The concept of health is a critical concept for nursing as it informs the profession's goals, scope, and outcomes of practice. The goals of nursing are to restore, maintain, and promote health; the scope of nursing's concern is with problems of health. When nursing practice assists people back to a healthy condition, successful outcomes are correctly declared. To be effective, nurses must have an understanding of health.

Health has been conceptualized in many ways in our society, including physical, emotional, mental, spiritual, and social well-being; what people in a culture value or desire; maximization of potential; high-level wellness; fulfillment of personal goals; successful performance of social roles; successful interaction with the environment; and proper functioning. Health has also been viewed as subjective or relative (self-report), object ive (measured against an agreed-upon standard), comparative (a more-or-less condition viewed as a continuum or gradation), classificatory (a dichotomy), holistic (indivisible), a state (condition), and a process (continuous change over time). Thus, with such multiple, sometimes overlapping, sometimes redundant, sometimes contradictory conceptions of health, the term has to be understood in terms of the purposes to which it is being applied.

What is the meaning of health for nursing science, that is, for human responses to actual and potential health problems? The concept of health has been dominated by two broad approaches: (a) descriptive analysis, and (b) visioning the goals and practice of nursing for the future. In this context, the intention of the descriptive analysis is to understand the aims, goals, and criteria of success in current nursing practice. Investigators are trying to understand, systematize, and render coherent what nurses understand themselves to be doing and to clarify the different forms that disease or failures of health can take. Assessing the results of this approach amounts to determining which conception makes better sense of nursing practice and how the different parts of nursing practice fit together.

To most nursing clinicians and researchers, regardless of specialty area, the conception of health most applicable to practice is health as the absence of signs and symptoms of physiological malady and disability. Most nurses spend their careers observing, administering, modifying therapies, interpreting conditions, and treating people who are sick and need to be restored to health or teaching them how to stay free of those signs and symptoms. There are many theories that illustrate this approach. These include Nightingale's conceptualization of health as an innate process that could be influenced by education, lifestyle changes, and improvement of environment (Nightingale, 1885). Smith's (née Baigis) clinical, role-performance, and adaptive models of health (Smith, J. A., 1981) also illustrates this approach as do the conceptual models, including the self-care framework (Orem, 2001). Orem identified health as the state of being whole and sound, where sound means strength and absence of disease, and whole means nothing is missing. She conceptualized health as an outcome of self-care and as an influencing factor on both self-care agency and self-care demand. Finally, theories focused on stability, balance, and adaptation (e.g., Johnson, 1990; Roy & Andrews, 1999) also illustrates this approach clearly. D. E. Johnson (1961) identified health as a constantly moving equilibrium during the health change process whereas Roy's model of health emphasizes well-being rather than illness.

The second approach visions the goals and practice of nursing for the future. What currently passes for nursing is fundamentally inadequate; only by articulating a proper conception of health can we clearly explain what nurses should be doing. Assessing the results of this approach is much more difficult and controversial. In part, this is because some of the particular proposals reflect specific theories of human nature or philosophical orientations, like existential phenomenology, that have assessments that are a matter of dispute. In addition, these nondescriptive approaches disagree not only in their proposals for what nursing should be but also in what they identify as fundamentally wrong with current nursing practice.

Holistic theories of health are one type illustrating this second approach. Some of these are based on M. E. Rogers' (1990) science of unitary human beings. They are attempts to operationalize what Rogers meant by health as a state of continuous human evolution to ever higher levels. Examples are health as a process of becoming as experienced and described by the person (Pase, 1992), and as the totality of the life process, which is evolving toward expanded consciousness (Newman, 1990a). In Fitzpatrick's life-perspective rhythm model, health is identified as a basic human dimension in continuous development (Pressler & Montgomery, 2005).

The concept of health as self-actualization is another type illustrating this approach, as in Smith's (née Baigis) eudaimonistic model (Smith, J. A., 1981) and Pender's (1996) definition of health in her health-promotion behavior model.

How are these theories applicable to practice? Within the context of these theories of health, there can be something wrong with a person even though the standard clinical concepts are not at issue. There are cases in the second approach where success in practice has not been achieved, yet success in practice implicitly determines what health is. If someone does not have any signs and symptoms of malady or disability and is still not actualized, the nurse has not done her job. Does this make the nurse's job unbounded? Is the nurse being set up for burnout? Does nursing practically and theoretically want to claim that its domain covers all of the actual and potential health problems inherent in all of these meanings of health? The profession must be clear about what a health problem is so that it can determine who has the problem and who does not.

Nursing is not the only profession analyzing the idea of health. Much work is also being done in the philosophy of medicine, public health, and public policy. For example, some theories of health care allocation rest on specific conceptions of health and disease—why there might be a right to adequate health care but not necessarily a right to convenient transportation (e.g., having a car) gets explained in terms of the details of what is health and why it is important. Nursing researchers should try to integrate these concerns into current theories or at least explore common themes in this work.

JUDITH A. BAIGIS
UPDATED BY MARY T. QUINN GRIFFIN

Health Disparities

The term health disparity has been widely used to refer to both inequalities, or differences, and also inequities, differences that imply unfairness or injustices. Health disparities have been discussed in relation to health care access and quality, health status, burden of disease, and excess deaths (Carter-Pokras & Baquet, 2002). Health disparities in the United States have been associated with age, gender, income, educational level, sexual orientation, disability, geographic location, and racial and ethnic minority status. Recognizing these categories are not mutually exclusive, the focus on this section will be on health disparities of racial and ethnic minority groups.

In the 1980s, the U.S. Department of Health and Human Services (DHHS) created the Task Force on Black and Minority Health. It was convened "in response to a national paradox of phenomenal scientific achievement and steady improvement in overall health status, while at the same time, persistent, significant health inequities exist for minority Americans" (U.S. DHHS, 1985, p. 2). The Task Force examined mortality data between minority groups and nonminority groups to determine excess deaths. Six causes of death accounted for more that 80% of the mortality among minority populations. The causes of excess deaths in minority populations included cancer, cardiovascular disease and stroke, cirrhosis (attributed to chemical dependency), diabetes, homicide and unintentional injuries, and infant mortality.

Since that time, there have been numerous national policy initiatives to address health disparities. Healthy People 2000, for example, called for a reduction in health disparities, while Healthy People 2010 set as a national priority the elimination of health disparities among racial and ethnic groups. President Clinton in 1998 focused attention on six health disparities confronted by racial and ethnic minority groups, which were remarkably similar to those identified in 1985. These areas included cardiovascular disease, diabetes, cancer, HIV/AIDS, infant mortality, and pneumonia and influenza. Finally, the creation of the National Center for Minority Health and Health Disparities within the National Institutes of Health helps to focus research priorities and resources towards eliminating health disparities.

While there is no denying that health disparities exist for racial and ethnic minorities, the cause of disparities and therefore the design of appropriate strategies and interventions to eliminate disparities is the subject of many debates. Causes of disparities range from individual influences, including genetic predisposition and behavioral choices, to broader social determinants including living in hazardous environments, limited opportunities for education, and finally barriers to health care including limited access, cultural and linguistic barriers, and institutional racism in health care and other settings.

Nursing groups have provided direction for research needed to address racial and ethnic disparities in health. For example, the National Coalition of Ethnic Minority Nursing Associations (NCEMNA) partnered with the National Institute of Nursing Research (NINR) to develop recommendations for a nursing research agenda for minority health. Basic research, epidemiological, clinical, and community studies, as well as health services research were identified as being needed to address the top 10 causes of death for each ethnic minority group. Specific research areas identified in the areas of health promotion and illness management included the need for descriptive research to identify health-promotion and disease-management behaviors, the development of culturally and linguistically appropriate instruments and interventions, consideration of spiritual dimensions, and the integration of mental health with illness management. In considering health disparities, NCEMNA called for an accounting of social justice and parity. Further, there was emphasis on focusing on positive aspects of racial and ethnic minority populations such as resilience, cultural strengths, and family and community supports. The need to identify vulnerable points across the life span also was identified.

The challenge for nurses in addressing racial and ethnic disparities in health and health care are many. First, there is an insufficient breadth and depth of nursing research with racial and ethnic minority populations that is adequate to guide practice. Certainly the lack of research in this area is not unique to nursing. As Zambrana (2001) pointed out, there is a tendency to attribute culture and language as influences on health outcomes because they are easier to talk about rather than the more powerful influences of socioeconomic status, literacy, poverty, and inequity.

The lack of an adequate science base to direct nursing practice with racial and ethnic minority populations is a critical barrier in guiding the delivery of culturally competent care. Both are also compounded by the limited racial and ethnic diversity within nursing.

It is critical that nurses increase their leadership in eliminating health disparities among racial and ethnic minorities as well as other segments of the population. In order to do this, we need to consider the role that nurses play in contributing to these disparities. Recognizing the influence of social determinants on health and health care, acknowledging and working toward the elimination of institutional racism and discrimination in health care settings and schools, increasing the racial and ethnic diversity within the nursing workforce, and the need for true partnerships with racial and ethnic minority communities are several of the needed strategies that nursing must take.

ANTONIA M. VILLARRUEL

Health Indicators

Health indicators are defined as the means by which one can describe either quantitatively or qualitatively an individual's state of health or those factors that influence the health of a health system, population, or community (Atlas of Canada, 2001). Health indicators are "constructs of public health surveillance that define a measure of health (i.e., health status or other risk factor) among a specified population" (Lengerich, 1999).

In 1870, Farr, founder of modern concepts of surveillance, depicted statistics by developing graphic displays that took into account age at death (Lengerich, 1999). In so doing, Farr initiated a focus on health descriptions and analyses based on mortality and survival measures. In 1979, the U.S. Surgeon General's Report established measurable improvement targets to be achieved by 1990 for individuals at each of the five major life stages (U.S. Department of Health and Human Services [HHS], 1998). Instead of being called health indicators, they were referred to as goals. Subsequent publications (*Healthy People 2000* & *Healthy People 2010*) were more comprehensive in terms of objectives and in priority areas for research and improving health. Each of these documents can be used to draw attention to benchmarks related to the health of the nation. Today, the challenge that HHS has to address is the identification of the indicators that are not only priorities, but also are reasonable in number. Additionally, more extensive work was directed to listing of leading indicators and extending the reach of HHS beyond the health community to opinion leaders, the public, and nonhealth professionals (U.S. Department of Health and Human Services).

In 1998, the Canadian Institute for Health Information (CIHI) and Statistics Canada were instrumental in launching a collaborative effort in order to ultimately share the resulting health indicators report with Canadians from province to province. More than 500 health-related individuals (providers and consumers) met to identify health information needs. A priority for this group was to establish a list of health indicators for health and health services that could be used as comparable data (Statistics Canada, 2004). The list of indicators was relevant to Canadian health goals, based on standard or comparable definitions and methods, and available electronically throughout Canada. As in the United States, Canada has as a primary goal of the Health Indicators project "to support health regions in monitoring progress in improving and maintaining the health of the population and the functioning of the health system for which they are responsible . . . " (Statistics Canada).

Key aspects of health indicators are that they are measurable, credible, and valid, based on data that are relatively easy and economical to collect, easily understood, and capable of providing information either for communities that are geographically defined or for populations or subpopulations that are well-defined (Atlas of Canada, 2001). Ten items were listed by *Healthy People 2010* as leading health indicators. Leading health indicators represent the important determinants of health for the full range of issues in the 28 focus areas of *Healthy People 2010* (Office of Disease Prevention and Health Promotion, 2002). These indicators are: physical activity, overweight and obesity, tobacco use, substance abuse, responsible sexual behavior, mental health, injury and violence, environmental quality, immunization, and access to health care (Office of Disease Prevention and Health Promotion).

The Canadian Health Indicators project resulted in the identification of the following: health status (well-being, health conditions, human function, and deaths); nonmedical determinants of health (health behaviors, living and working conditions, personal resources, and environmental factors); health system performance (acceptability, accessibility, appropriateness, competence, continuity, effectiveness, efficiency, and safety); and community and health system characteristics (community, health system, and resources) (Statistics Canada, 2004).

Health status indicators include mortality indicators (deaths and types of deaths), infectious disease indicators, maternal and infant health indicators, and community health status indicators (risk factors, access to care, preventive services use, death rates, birth measures, summary measures of health, leading causes of death, vulnerable populations, and environmental health). Other indicators are the health determinants and health outcome indicators (physical environment, poverty, high school graduation, tobacco use, weight, physical activity, health insurance, early detection of cancer, preventable deaths from injury, and disability), life course determinants (tobacco use, health care access, low birth weight, physical activity, poverty, cognitive development, substance abuse, violence, and disability), and prevention-oriented indicators (disability, preventable deaths from injury, poverty, tobacco use, childhood immunizations, cancer screening, hypertension screening, diabetes management, and health care access) (Public Health Foundation, 1999).

Several models have been set forth to reflect different but overlapping approaches to the development of health indicators. They include the Mortality Model, Health Status Model, Disparities Model, Leading Contributors Model, Focus Area Model, Summary Measures Model, Social Indicators Model, Environmental Model, Report Card Model, Index Model, Single Parameter Model, Sentinel Model, Prevention Model, Human Development (or Life Stage) Model, and Change Theory Model. Of these models, the ones that help advance the initiative of *Healthy People 2010* focus on areas that need more attention (lifestyle, disparities in health, social and environmental factors that influence health) (Office of Disease Prevention and Health Promotion, 2002).

Data gathered related to the health indicators provide a basis for comparison of health status locally, regionally, and nationally. Changes in the health status should be readily available and appropriate interventions can be initiated accordingly. Naturally, care must be taken to ensure that data that are compiled can be verified. With verified data, responsible decisions can be made in terms of health policy, health care delivery, health system management, and public awareness of health concerns.

The overarching goals for *Healthy People 2010* are to increase the quality and years of healthy life and to eliminate health disparities (Office of Disease Prevention and Health Promotion, 2002). Interdisciplinary or multidisciplinary collaboration can lead to comprehensive plans to ensure that any deficits in health status are addressed in a timely manner. Data gathered may support current health care efforts or identify areas for improvement at home, in communities, at worksites, businesses, or beyond.

In summary, health indicators serve as measures for spatial and/or temporal comparisons, help health care professionals assess health conditions, provide empirical evidence that could be used to support health programs and policies, clarify starting and end points for interventions, and identify extent of gaps in population or community health and well-being (Atlas of Canada, 2001). Health indicators are useful in charting progress, forecasting trends, and directing programmatic attention and resources to areas that require attention (Office of Disease Prevention and Health Promotion, 2002).

Access to quality health services is a major concern, especially for those who are uninsured or underinsured. Health promotion and disease prevention are important foci that relate directly to health indicators. Ensuring appropriate care for individuals who are diagnosed with chronic disease or who have a predisposition to chronic disease is imperative. Health care education directed to diverse individuals requires heightened awareness of potential barriers in communication. Also, cultural sensitivity issues must be addressed in order to develop strategies that will overcome such barriers.

Research areas are many and varied from health care delivery issues to health policy to health awareness. Identifying the most significant health indicators and asking researchable and meaningful questions is essential if health care providers wish to support the goals and objectives set forth by *Healthy People 2010*. Clearly, priorities that need attention include those that could be improved by changes in lifestyle such as smoking and obesity. Education and intervention research are major activities that could result in improved outcomes. Nurses and other health care providers need to keep these health indicators in mind and seek to incorporate a variety of sources when integrating and applying interventions that will potentially improve individual, population, or community health and well-being.

KAREN L. ELBERSON

Health Policy

Health policy is what governments or private institutions choose to do, or not to do, in regard to health. If a choice is made to take action, a formal plan for a course of action is adopted—this is the realm of health policy. Health policy in the public governmental sector mainly focuses on legislative proposals, policy implementation (writing and publishing regulations), and judicial review of policy decisions. In the private sector, policy decisions are made that lay out operational principles to guide action and behavior within an institution. Achieving understanding of current health issues and finding suitable solutions to policy problems have fueled a distinct field of policy research that includes two subfields, that of health services research and that of policy analysis.

Health services research examines how people get access to health care, how much care costs, and what happens to patients as a result of this care. Today's issues drive the investigations. For example, how will the nation identify and address the most effective ways to organize, manage, finance, and deliver high-quality care for all, and at the same time, reduce medical errors and improve patient safety?

Policy analysis uses a comparative methodology that examines how current policy proposals compare favorably or unfavorably with selected criteria. Criteria are drawn from previous research and a thorough review of the literature on the policy issue. Legislative proposals, in particular, lend themselves to this type of analysis.

The need for policy research has grown in importance as the nation confronts the rising costs and inadequacies of present day health care. It has been demonstrated that health policy research can assist in a number of areas, including: the elimination of health disparities; the closure of the gap between the "haves" and "have-nots" in health care; the protection of communities from avoidable health hazards; and the shift from a purely biomedical model, that accorded priority to science and services to treat the diseases of the individual, to one that focuses on population health and the many determinants of health and disease (Boufford & Lee, 2001, p. 1).

As governments and the private sector explore suitable policy solutions to the nation's health care woes, the call for credible health policy is greater than ever. In the past, both health services research and health policy analysis have been concerned with issues, such as access, quality, and cost of health care, with more emphasis on cost than access and quality. Today, there are perceptible changes, principally because consumers of health care are increasingly more vocal and more prominent players. Health care consumers are assisting in moving the health care industry toward increased accountability through evidence-based practice and the elimination of medical errors.

As health care problems increase in complexity, it has become obvious that no one health professional can address all of the issues and find all of the appropriate solutions. Within this context, research efforts have become increasingly grounded in the multidisciplinary investigations of complex policy problems.

As the largest group of health care professionals, nurses are in an ideal position to collaborate with and lead health policy researchers in the exploration of significant areas of concern. To do this, nursing must develop a new dialogue with other health professions and all those who participate in health policy decision making by developing greater flexibility and enhanced collaborative behaviors (Dickenson-Hazard, 1999). Furthermore, many health policy decisions directly influence the practice of nursing. These include: defining the scope of practice, regulation of practice environments, cost of malpractice insurance, government subsidization of nursing education and research, and securing direct and indirect reimbursement for services. Examples of federal agencies within the Department of Health and Human Services (DHHS) that directly impact nurses are: the Health Services and Resource Administration (HRSA) and, in particular, the Division of Nursing; the Centers for Medicare and Medicaid Services (CMS); and the National Institute for Nursing Research (NINR).

Four interrelated characteristics of present-day health care systems have significantly shaped health policy and will continue to influence the practice of nursing now and in the near future. These characteristics are: systemic change, interdependence, financial viability, and the changing face of the health professions. The ability to adapt to systemic change within the health care system, the movement toward the interdependence of all health care providers (along with the changing face of the health professions), and the realization that financial viability drives and determines which health care institutions and systems of care survive and flourish (Jennings, C. P., 2000). Taken as a whole these characteristics provide the context for nursing education, practice, and research.

Participation of nurses in the shaping of health policy and public health policy is critical for the future of the profession and the well-being of all citizens (Algase, Beel-Bates, & Ziemba, 2004). Political participation goes hand in hand with policy development. Political participation or action is not new to nurses. For many years nurses have advocated for issues that promote the profession—money for education and research, scope of practice concerns, reimbursement for services by third-party payers, and more recently the passage of the Nurse Reinvestment Act (a federal effort to combat the nursing shortage). Today, nurses are lobbying to secure "a place at the table." They are active participants in setting the broader health policy agenda. Nurses have been influential in developing protocols for first responders in bioterrorist attacks; they have challenged some of the key provisions in the Medicare Prescription Drug Benefit legislation; they have fought to expand access to primary care services in rural and underserved areas; and they are strong proponents for universal health care.

Health policy is a worthy and exciting arena for nursing practice. It includes the political imperative to participate in all phases of the policy and political cycle. Achieving "political maturity" is a goal that requires that each and every nurse have the proper education and skill development to effectively intervene in the policy process in order to achieve professional and national goals for long-term health and well-being. Nursing organizations, such as the American Nurses Association (ANA), lobby on behalf of all nurses. Often, organizations such as the ANA are able to directly interface with policymaking bodies at the local, state, and federal level. It is important that nurses develop effective channels for communicating with policy decision makers.

In closing, nurses must remember that the relationship between nursing and health policy is reciprocal and mutually reinforcing—herein lies the greatest hope for the future of nursing and the nation's health care.

CAROLE P. JENNINGS

Health Services Administration

Health services administration (HSA) research is multidisciplinary and focuses on factors and issues effecting delivery of health services in a wide variety of settings from a systems perspective. HSA also focuses on the effect of health care processes on the health and well-being of clients and populations. Issues such as access to care, development of tools to measure health status, effectiveness of treatment modalities, health policy, delivery systems, professional practice, impact of magnet hospitals, outcomes of care, impact of managed care, financing of health care, and organizational change only partially represent the vast diversity of foci for HSA research. A breadth of issues, and intent to affect care delivery, are the hallmarks of HSA research.

Health services administration research, by its multidisciplinary nature, must address nursing issues for full impact on systems affecting care delivery. Nurses, as the largest health care delivery professional discipline, are integrally involved in all aspects of the health care system. Nurse researchers in nursing administration, practice specialties, nursing health policy, and community health can lead or participate in HSA research. These types of research reflect the team concept by including all disciplines involved in a specific project and by reflecting those disciplines' perspectives in the study design and findings.

If quality of services is to be assured and improved, this type of research is necessary for improving care systems. Whether the research focus is smoking cessation or health policy, the HSA approach would be to investigate preferred systems for optimal client outcomes. Nurse researchers must shift their focus from studying individual adaptation to illness or disease to investigating the systems that facilitate maximizing such adaptation if they are participating in HSA research. The relevance to nursing comes in the ability to replicate such systems across practice settings and to extend the influence of research knowledge in practice. Magnet hospital research is attempting to do this by linking magnet characteristics to lower mortality rates and increased patient satisfaction as well as other outcome markers (Scott, J., Sochalski, & Aiken, 1999).

In this age of multidisciplinary emphasis, nurses' participation in HSA research places them in a position to influence client outcomes on a larger scale than in the past. Many nursing research efforts have been hampered by not accounting for the influence of other disciplines on client outcomes. The contribution of nursing to those outcomes is difficult to measure in isolation from medical and allied health treatments. There is tremendous potential for nursing's effects on client outcomes to be showcased by involvement in HSA research. Such research is presented in national and international multidisciplinary forums that have potential to influence health policy beyond the discipline of nursing.

Donabedian's (1980) model of using a "structure, process, and outcome" framework for evaluating the quality of medical care has been widely adopted for many HSA studies. Structure relates to the physical and organizational framework of the setting where care is delivered. Process refers to the "dynamic exchange" between provider and client that includes all interchanges that occur in support of care events. Outcomes are the dependent variables, the "measurable events" that occur as a result of the structure and process of care (Scott, J. D., 1996). The Joint Commission on Accreditation of

Healthcare Organizations (JCAHO) has used this framework to evaluate health care organizations for decades. In 1997, JCAHO shifted emphasis, through its Agenda for Change, to stress outcomes and to develop performance indicators that are less reliant on structure and process. Beginning in 2002, JCAHO has the ability for "rigorous comparison of the actual results of care across hospitals" (JCAHO, 2003b).

Health care delivery systems routinely engage in action research aimed at improving the quality of care. Quality improvement research has become ingrained in the very process of care delivery, and nurses are integrally involved in these studies. Although often not theoretically based, such studies have a direct impact on quality of care in our country and have potential to improve care broadly if the results are disseminated more widely, rather than serving solely as the basis for internal, proprietary improvement processes.

Insurers are using the results of treatment effectiveness studies to determine which procedures to cover. Health Maintenance Organizations (HMO) practices are evaluating the effect of their wellness plans on subsequent client illness patterns. Many of these studies examine cost-effectiveness.

The federal government routinely invests in HSA research. Agencies such as the Agency for Healthcare Research and Quality (AHRQ), the Center for Medical Effectiveness Research, the Health Care Financing Administration, the National Institutes for Health, the Health Resources and Services Administration, and the National Institutes for Nursing Research, to name a few, are all engaged in funding and directing HSA research. The Medical Treatment Effectiveness Program was begun in 1989 by the Agency for Health Care Policy and Research (now AHRQ) to investigate clinical conditions that are costly, have high incidence, evidence variation in clinical outcomes, and affect Medicare or Medicaid programs. There are, at present, 19 Clinical Practice Guidelines that review best practices for these clinical conditions. Government support for HSA research directly influences health policy by making study results available to policymakers, caregivers and the public. Information is available at governmental web sites. At its Research in Action site (AHRQ, 2003b), AHRQ-sponsored studies in the categories of cost, disease-related, elderly, pharmaceuticals, and quality of care are synthesized for the purpose of making them generally available for the improvement of care. A similar AHRQ page highlighting the National Quality Measures Clearinghouse provides "evidence-based quality measures and measure sets" (AHRQ, 2003a).

Private foundations actively fund HSA research. The Robert Wood Johnson Foundation is notable for its efforts to improve nursing care delivery. The Commonwealth Fund, the Henry J. Kaiser Foundation, and the Pew Charitable Trusts are among the most notable organizations that support HSA research on an ongoing basis.

Health Services Administration research can be found in almost every health care-related journal. Journals that concentrate on this multidisciplinary focus include the following: *Advances in Health Economics, American Journal of Public Health, Frontiers of Health Services Management, Health Care Financing Review, Health Care Forum Journal, Health Policy, Health Services Research, Inquiry, International Journal of Health Services, Journal of Health Economics, Journal of Health Politics, Policy and Law,* and *Quality Review Bulletin.*

HSA research is engaged in investigating improvement of health care delivery and in discovering ways to provide more effective and efficient care, both of which can have a great impact on the health care system. Scarce resources can be more effectively utilized if we improve care delivery to "best demonstrated practices" levels. Of course, these levels continue to evolve and to be refined as knowledge expands. Thus, HSA research must continually expand understanding to maximize the potential of an evolving health care system.

HSA research can provide a valuable check to the financial emphasis of our current managed care system. An emphasis on the population's needs and how they might influence health care systems and health policy to maximize public health would be a welcome change from the financial emphasis of the past (Ingersoll, Spitzer, & Cook, 1999). Outcomes research can demonstrate unanticipated effects of limiting access to care, treatment options, and care provider choice. Long-term outcomes can be monitored through systematic longitudinal studies to determine relative health status of client populations based on payer system, for-profit status, demographic variables, and treatment options. HSA research is needed to investigate these larger issues and to influence health policy for years to come.

Mary L. Fisher

Health Services Research

Health services research is a part of a broad scientific continuum which addresses fundamental mechanisms of health and disease including prevention, diagnosis, treatment, and the evaluation of health care services and the system in which they are delivered. It is described by the Institute of Medicine as "the interdisciplinary field that investigates the structure, processes, and effects of health care services" (Institute of Medicine, 1995). It is different from biomedical research; however, the boundaries between the two are not distinct, nor should they be. Domains along the research continuum overlap, thereby reducing the gaps that would occur if they were totally separate (Eisenberg, 1998).

Health services research addresses issues of health care organization, delivery, financing, and utilization, as well as patient and provider behavior and the quality, outcomes, effectiveness, and cost of health care. It appraises both clinical services and the system in which these services are provided. It evaluates information about the cost of care and its effectiveness, efficiency, quality, and outcomes and it includes studies of the structure, process, and effects of health services for individuals and populations. Both basic and applied research questions are addressed, including aspects of individual and system behavior and the application of interventions in practice settings (Eisenberg, 1998).

The health care environment is changing rapidly and is characterized by consolidation of health plans and movement of patients and providers into managed care settings. Efforts to contain rising health care costs are coupled with fears that cost-containment measures will lower the quality of care. Problems related to access to health care and health insurance coverage persist for many Americans. This market-driven health care system cannot function efficiently without better information for all decision makers in health care. Purchasers are looking for value at low cost, patients want to make informed decisions about care, clinicians need information about evidence-based treatments, health plans must determine which services to cover, and institutional providers need to make organizational and management decisions. Health services research addresses the information needs of all of these groups at the clinical, system, and policy decision level (Agency for Healthcare Research and Quality, 2004).

Outcomes and effectiveness research is a type of health services research that studies the impact of interventions on patients and the effectiveness of treatments in noncontrolled settings. The terms "outcomes research" and "effectiveness research" have been used to refer to a range of studies, and no single definition for either has gained wide acceptance (Stryer, Tunis, Hubbard, & Clancy, 2000). Effectiveness research is often contrasted with efficacy research. Effectiveness research is conducted in typical practice settings with diverse patient populations; efficacy research is carried out in more controlled research settings, often with a less diverse population (Hubbard, Walker, Clancy, & Stryer, 2002). Outcomes research seeks to understand the end results of particular health care practices and interventions. In this context, end results include effects that people experience and care about, such as change in the ability to function.

Health services research is heavily invested in issues of quality, patient safety, and disparities in health care. Evidence is needed to inform practice. Health services research provides that information on interventions related to benefits, risks, and results so that both clinicians and patients can make informed choices about care. Propelled by the Institute of Medicine report *To Err Is Human* (Institute of Medicine, 2000), there is growing recognition of the need for research into better methods of safeguarding health care services and delivery (Hubbard et al., 2002). An important end result of health services research is the translation or transformation of the findings into practice and policy and the utilization of evidence-based care. Health services research will continue to improve science-based information on health disparities so that the health of minorities, women, and children is enhanced.

Health services research is germane to nurses. Understanding the impact of nursing interventions is an important component of health services research because enhanced nursing care is critical for the growing number of elderly and chronically ill people. Nurses play a large and significant role in the interdisciplinary team, and many of the outcomes critical to health services research function (e.g., improved health status and satisfaction) are measures that are usually dependent on the collective practice of the entire health care team (Hubbard et al., 2002). Nurses have always been involved in patient outcomes, and the outcome measures noted above are important components of current nursing education. Nurses' high degree of interaction with patients makes them likely candidates as health services researchers or members of the health service research team. The Agency for Healthcare Research and Quality, a major funder of health services research, encourages nurse scientists to apply for grant support. Funding opportunities can be found at AHRQ's nursing web site: www.ahrq.gov/about/nursing.

Investigating the various components of nursing care and how they influence patient outcomes represents an essential area of research needing further development. As prime observers of and participants in health care delivery, nurses can make important and valuable contributions to health services research (Hubbard et al., 2002).

**Disclaimer:*
The views expressed in this article are those of the author and do not necessarily reflect those of the Agency for Healthcare Research and Quality or the U.S. Department of Health and Human Services.

HEDDY BISHOP HUBBARD

Health Systems Delivery

Health systems delivery is a global term used to define the structures and processes by which health care is provided to individuals and populations. The term generally refers to the collective availability of services rather than to an individual organization by itself, although larger organizations such as academic health science centers may use the term to reflect the extent of their capacity. The features that distinguish health systems from other connected services are their level of differentiation, their extent of centralization, and their degree of integration (Bazzoli, Shortell, Dubbs, Chan, & Kralovec, 1999). Health systems have a single owner and some type of decision-making oversight group, whereas health networks (which also provide an array of services) are more loosely linked and each participating organization maintains its original ownership (Bazzoli et al.).

Probably the most significant influence on health systems delivery has been the introduction of managed care, which places restrictions on access and consumption of services and has prompted delivery systems to identify ways to provide a variety of services more efficiently and at a lower cost (Cook, J. A.,

Ingersoll, & Spitzer, 1999). Investigations of managed care delivery systems have identified five characteristics common to the service delivery processes associated with these systems—the use of population-based strategies for cost containment, a focus on wellness rather than illness care, the increased influence of consumers on services offered and selected, the interdependence of professionals involved in care, and the use of delivery systems reengineering to improve services (Ingersoll, Spitzer, & Cook, 1999). Comprehensive studies of these processes are limited, with even less information available concerning the impact of systems delivery models on care delivery outcome.

Subsumed within the broader classification of *health services research*, studies pertaining to health systems delivery focus on which collection of services are most effective and efficient for achieving maximum care delivery outcome. Few large-scale investigations of delivery systems are available, however, with most studies examining specific types of organizations (e.g., hospitals, long-term care, hospice care). Although these studies are not focused on health delivery systems, per se, they provide useful information about the structures and processes that may achieve favorable outcomes in individual or linked organizations.

The organizational characteristics investigated in prior research were examined recently in a comprehensive analysis of the ways in which care delivery systems influence patient safety. The state of the science was reviewed by an Institute of Medicine (IOM) expert panel, which identified four environmental factors that consistently contribute to the quality of care delivered and the patient outcomes seen (Page, 2003). The IOM expert panel described these systems characteristics as sources of threats and labeled them management, workforce, work processes, and organizational culture. Using the literature available, they proposed several safeguards for addressing these systems components and improving patient safety. Included in the recommendations were: developing governing boards that focus on safety, introducing evidence-based management of organizational structures and processes, assuring high levels of leadership ability, providing sufficient staffing, promoting ongoing learning and decision support at the point of care, encouraging interdisciplinary collaboration, creating work designs that promote safety, and achieving an organizational culture that continuously addresses patient safety (pp. 16–17).

Multisite studies supporting the IOM expert panel's recommendations have been drawn from acute care, long-term care, and home care settings. Among the studies providing data to support these recommendations were several multisite investigations conducted by nurse researchers—four of which are summarized here. The studies included in this description were selected because of the variables they investigated, their inclusion of institutions from a variety of locations, and their potential application to health delivery systems regardless of size or type of services delivered.

The most commonly measured structure variable in health delivery systems research is *nurse resources*, with several large-scale investigations exploring the impact of nurse staffing mix and nursing care hours on employee, organizational, and patient outcome. Three studies of hospitals drawn from across the U.S. have demonstrated consistent evidence of the beneficial effect of registered nurse (RN) care hours on length of stay (Kovner & Gergen, 1998; Needleman, Buerhaus, Mattke, Stewart, & Zelevinsky, 2002), mortality (Aiken, Clarke, Sloane, Sochalski, & Silber, 2002), and adverse events (Aiken, Clarke, Sloane, et al.; Kovner & Green; Needleman et al., 2002).

Comparable findings were seen in a multisite investigation of the best and worst performing nursing homes, although the investigators of this study defined nurse resource variables as an indicator of care delivery process, rather than organizational structure (Anderson, R. A., Hsieh, & Su, 1998). Although a case can be built for defining nurse resources as both a structure and a process variable, simply identifying skill mix or percent of RN hours does little to clarify what actually occurs during the delivery (or process) of care by one type of provider (RN) versus another (licensed practical nurse [LPN] or patient technician). Nonetheless, in this study the greater the number of RNs, the better the patient outcome. Structure variables associated with type of ownership, size of nursing home, and percentage of private-pay residents were not associated with any of the outcomes measured.

Few studies have explored the impact of processes of care on care delivery outcome, primarily because this variable is difficult and costly to assess. Care delivery processes evolve over time and change in response to work-group makeup, leader vision, standards used to guide care delivery, and types of patients served. Monitoring what transpires during the interactions that take place among care providers and between care providers and patients and families requires an understanding of group relationships, individual motivation and need, and the ways in which work gets done. Consequently, studies of organizational processes are inherently complex and difficult to carry out. As a result, employee perceptions are often used as proxy indicators for work-group or leadership behaviors and the processes they use to get work done. For example, nurses are commonly surveyed about their perceptions of ideal and actual nurse leaders or work groups. Favorable perceptions of both are frequently related to nurse satisfaction and retention (Page, 2003). What processes nurse leaders and work groups use to produce these favorable or unfavorable perceptions are less clear, with most reports describing general categories of behaviors (e.g., inclusiveness, cohesiveness) to denote the characteristics of ideal leaders and group members. How they go about creating an inclusive and cohesive process is unknown.

One area of increasing interest in health systems delivery research is the impact of health care teams and team functioning on care delivery outcome. This interest is generated by evidence linking poor interpersonal interactions among team members with health care errors (Ingersoll & Schmitt, 2003). Because the number and makeup of teams varies significantly even within a single institution, measuring the effect of team performance on care delivery outcome is troublesome. Moreover, the structure of the team, including its hierarchical nature, its placement within the organizational system, and its mission and purpose all contribute to its potential for effectiveness and ultimate impact on care. Consequently, measuring one team's performance will not necessarily help with understanding what processes result in favorable care delivery outcomes. Ideally, a variety of teams should be monitored to identify differences in the ways the team members work together to achieve a good effect.

Studies of comprehensive health delivery systems are in their infancy, with limited information available from comprehensive multisite investigations of health care organizations. Additional research is needed that focuses on both the structures and the processes that promote favorable outcomes for employees, patients, and organizations. A combination of approaches will be required to achieve this goal, with qualitative methods used for understanding care delivery processes and expectations of providers and quantitative methods for examining causal relationships between organizational structures, processes, and outcomes seen.

GAIL L. INGERSOLL

Hemodynamic Monitoring

Hemodynamic monitoring is the use of advanced technology and application of physiological principles to clinically assess the cardiac function and circulatory system in critically ill patients. The pulmonary artery catheter was first introduced in 1970 by Dr. Jeremy Swan (Swan et al., 1970), and continues to be a frequently used tool in the critical care setting. The catheter tip is positioned in the distal pulmonary artery and is used to monitor pulmonary artery systolic, diastolic, and mean pressures, and to obtain blood samples to determine mixed venous oxygenation. The distal balloon port is used to measure the pulmonary artery wedge pressure (PAWP) when the balloon port is inflated with 1.5 cc of air. Additional hemodynamic parameters and data are obtained from other ports and lumens of the catheter, such as right atrial pressure, cardiac output measurements, blood (core) temperature, and saturation of venous oxygenation (SvO_2).

Using data obtained at the bedside from the pulmonary artery catheter and other physiologic indices such as cardiac output, heart rate, preload, afterload, and contractility, critical care nurses and physicians are able to make rapid assessments and determinations about the clinical status of the critically ill patients. The catheter enables clinicians to assess ventricular function, diagnose complications following acute myocardial infarction, differentiate shock states, cardiac and pulmonary disorders, manage high-risk cardiac surgical patients, and monitor unstable patients with complexities such as sepsis and multiple organ dysfunction. The original balloon-tipped, flow-directed thermodilution catheter has evolved since 1970 and has added enhancements such as saturation of venous oxygenation (SVO_2), right ventricular volumes and ejection fraction, continuous monitoring of cardiac output, and intracardiac atrioventricular sequential pacing.

Newer technologies to monitor cardiac output using noninvasive methodology include the Esophageal Doppler monitor and the Exhaled Carbon Dioxide (CO_2) monitor. The Esophageal Doppler monitor measures cardiac output via a probe placed within a naso-gastric tube that measures aortic blood flow, enabling the clinician to assess stroke volume and heart rate adjusted cardiac output. A second technology, Exhaled CO_2, is a noninvasive method of cardiac output monitoring that measures blood flow from exhaled CO_2 using a modified Fick Equation. Its clinical application is limited to the operating room setting since the technology requires measurement of blood flow from exhaled CO_2 under controlled ventilation, but it has great potential for the future when the technology can be used for different modes of mechanical ventilation with or without spontaneous breathing. Examining the impact these new technologies may have on patient outcomes is an important area for future nursing research.

Hemodynamic monitoring has great relevance to nurses in critical care because of the important role it plays in the care of critically ill patients. Critical care nurses are responsible for continuous monitoring, interpretation, and trending of hemodynamic indices and for communicating critical information to physician colleagues. Understanding the implications of subtle changes in pressures and parameters will directly impact a patient's response to complex therapeutic interventions such as fluid administration and manipulation of vasoactive drips. Utilizing research to examine existing practices and to change practice is vital to ensure research-based practice and positive patient outcomes.

The majority of nursing research on hemodynamic monitoring has been focused on the technical and clinical variables affecting accuracy of pulmonary artery pressure monitoring. Because many variables affect accuracy, this topic is particularly relevant for nurses caring for critically ill patients. The standard in critical care has traditionally been to reference (level the air/fluid interface stopcock at the phlebostatic axis) and zero the catheter system a minimum of once per shift and at times more often, to offset zero drift, and to ensure accuracy. The results of one nursing study suggested that zeroing disposable transducers may be required only once during hemodynamic monitoring, before initial readings are obtained (Ahrens, Pennick, & Tucker, 1995). These findings encourage practitioners to reevaluate a long-held critical care nursing standard and demonstrate the value of keeping pace with new technology. Replication studies are needed in this area to validate this practice.

A major focus in recent nursing research has been to study hemodynamic pressures in various backrest elevations. There is considerable nursing research supporting accurate and reliable measurement of hemodynamic pressures in backrest elevations from 0° to 60° if the air/fluid interface (zeroing stopcock) is leveled or referenced at the phlebostatic axis. Lateral positioning may be used if the air/fluid interface is leveled at the phlebostatic axis, but the patient must be at a 90° side position with the backrest flat to ensure accuracy. The phlebostatic axis in the right lateral 90° position is the fourth intercostal space at midsternum, compared to the fourth intercostal space at the left sternal border in the left lateral 90° position (Paolella, Dorfman, Cronan, & Hasan, 1988). The question of accuracy and reliability of measurements in lateral positioning other than 90° has been the subject of two recent nursing studies. In one study, pulmonary artery (PA) pressures were obtained with patients in the 60° lateral position (Aitken, 2000). The dependent midclavicular line at the level of the fourth intercostal space was used as the zero reference level. Statistically significant differences were found and the author concluded that PA pressures cannot be obtained with patients in the 60° lateral position. Another group of researchers studied the effect of 30° lateral recumbent position on PA and PAWP pressures (Bridges, Woods, Brengelmann, Mitchell, & Laurent-Bopp, 2000). Using an angle-specific left atrial reference point, the investigators found a statistically significant difference between measurements of PA pressures with the patient supine and those obtained in 30° lateral position. Mean differences were small and the author considered the measures clinically equivalent to those of patients in supine position. The optimal reference point for lateral positions other than 90° with backrest flat continues to be an area that will require further study and validation in future research studies.

Recent studies have examined cardiac output technology in patients with low cardiac output. Continuous cardiac output technology was found to be more precise than measurements using the bolus technique in one study of patients with low-cardiac output (Albert, Spear, & Hammel, 1999). The practice of using room-temperature injectate versus iced solution was supported in another study examining traditional thermodilution methods of cardiac output in patients with low cardiac output (Kiely, Byers, Greenwood, Carroll, & Carroll, 1998).

To ensure accuracy and reliability, all hemodynamic pressures are read at end expiration in ventilated patients as well as those breathing spontaneously. Numerous studies continue to support the use of a strip chart recorder to provide more reliable and accurate hemodynamic readings than do digital data (directly off the monitor) in both ventilated and spontaneously breathing patients.

Since the advent of the pulmonary artery catheter, technology in hemodynamic monitoring has advanced at a rapid pace. Future studies must continue to keep pace with the ever-changing technology. Technical difficulties in measurement, as seen in patients with severe respiratory variation, in ventilated patients on high levels of positive end expiratory pressure (PEEP), and in the presence of large "v" waves on the hemodynamic waveform, are examples of clinical issues that continue to confound critical care nurses. Critically evaluating the use of both new and traditional technology is essential to the provision of good patient care.

The potential risk versus benefit of pulmonary artery catheterization is an important ethical consideration in hemodynamic monitoring. Questions have been raised within major medical journals and the media about the safety and efficacy of pulmonary artery catheterization. As a result of the controversy, organizations such as the Society of Critical Care Medicine have intensified efforts to conduct large randomized controlled trials to evaluate critically the safety and effectiveness of PA catheters in critically ill patients.

The results of studies on the clinical competency of critical care nurses' knowledge of PA catheters have been less than impressive, and underscore the need to provide ongoing training and competency assessments of nursing staff to ensure safe and quality patient care. Hemodynamic monitoring is a valuable tool if used judiciously by specially trained and competent medical and nursing professionals.

MAUREEN KECKEISEN

Henderson's Model

Since 1960 when the International Council of Nurses (ICN) first published *Basic Principles of Nursing Care*, a work their Nursing Service Committee commissioned, Virginia Henderson's description of nursing and the unique function of the nurse has been used throughout the world to standardize nursing practice. *Basic Principles of Nursing Care* was written just after the 1955 publication of Harmer & Henderson's *Textbook of the Principles and Practice of Nursing*, 5th edition (Henderson, 1955), which until 1975 was the most widely used nursing textbook in English and Spanish speaking worlds. A third book, *The Nature of Nursing* (Henderson, 1966, 1991), included implications for how nursing could provide direction for four essential functions of a profession: service, education, research, and leadership. Henderson's model of nursing is most succinctly presented in the ICN's *Basic Principles of Nursing Care*, a work available in 30 of the world's languages. She says:

> The unique function of the nurse is to assist the individual, sick or well, in the performance of those activities contributing to health or its recovery (or to a peaceful death) that the person would perform unaided given the necessary strength, will or knowledge. And to do this in such a way as to help the individual gain independence as rapidly as possible. (Henderson, 2004, p. 12)

Basic nursing care means helping patients with activities such as eating and drinking adequately, eliminating body wastes, and moving and maintaining desirable postures or providing conditions under which he can perform them unaided.

Henderson also described conditions in persons that always affect basic needs such as nursing care of newborn or the dying. There are also pathological states (as contrasted with specific diseases) that modify basic need, such as marked disturbances of fluid and electrolyte balance including starvation states, pernicious vomiting, and diarrhea, acute oxygen want, and shock (including "collapse" and hemorrhage).

According to Henderson's model, the nurse is temporarily the consciousness of the unconscious, the love of life for the suicidal, the leg of the amputee, the eyes of the newly blind, a means of locomotion for the infant, knowledge and confidence for the young mother, a "voice" for those too weak to speak, and so on. (Henderson, 1997, pp. 23–24)

That this model was first authored in 1950 when Henderson was preparing the 5th edition of her textbook is noteworthy. The era of the antibiotic made much of what Nightingale wrote in *Notes on Nursing* about the importance of nature obsolete. Needed was a description of nurses' functions that built on Nightingale's intervention-focused book and extended it into the era of science and biotechnology. *Basic Principles of Nursing Care* [BPNC] and *Notes on Nursing* [NN] are remarkably similar in content. Eat and drink adequately in BPNC became the modern version of the "Taking food" and "What food?" sections of NN, for example. Henderson continued the emphasis on interventions but shifted the ideal performer of procedures from nurses to nurse-educated and nurse-supported patients, encouraging independence, especially important in chronic illness. Neither doctors nor hospitals are required to practice nursing under this model.

Gladys Nite (Nite & Willis, 1964) explicitly tested the Henderson model of nursing in clinical experiments of effective nursing care for cardiac patients. Brooten (Brooten & Naylor, 1995) and Naylor (Naylor et al., 1999) implicitly examined this model in clinical research. The "nurse dose" which they seek to measure may indeed be some quantified measure of this unique function. Similarly, other researchers seem to be addressing the universality of this unique nurses' function in their examination of the effectiveness of nurses in different roles and in different settings (S. Douglas et al., 1995; Landefeld, Palmer, Kresevic, Fortinsky, & Kowal, 1995; Olds et al., 1997, 2002).

Henderson went on from this work to prepare a critique of nursing research and an index of the English-language nursing literature written between 1900 and 1960. When finished, she revised the textbook which she had twice previously redone. Remarkably, the textbook incorporated countless citations from the professional literature synthesizing what was known about the nursing profession up to its 1978 publication date. *Principles and Practice of Nursing*, 6th edition (Henderson & Nite, 1978), organized a disparate literature around her model of nursing which had not appreciably altered in the nearly 20 years since it first appeared. Rather than changing her mind based on her close reading of the literature, Henderson synthesized the citations into a coherent reference document, an evidence-based text as it were.

Three of Henderson's papers extend her model; two by validation, the other by contradiction. *The Concept of Nursing* (Henderson, 1978) specifically addressed her work as a model. *Preserving the Essence of Nursing in a Technological Age* (Halloran, 1995, p. 96) extended her ideas to include services nurses provide in intensive care units and was organized using the four essential professional functions first depicted in *The Nature of Nursing*: practice, education, research, and leadership. In *Nursing Process—Is the Title Right?*, Henderson (Halloran, p. 199) contradicted what had become the accepted alternative to the use of the word "nursing" by arguing that the word "process" unnecessarily constrained professional vision and precluded experience, logic, expert opinion, and research as bases for practice.

The most complete exposition of Henderson's model of nurses' function and nursing practice is contained in the 6th edition of *Principles and Practice of Nursing*. This reference text is a modern book largely unknown to the American nurses who today struggle with many of the issues of professional practice elaborated on in the documents related to the Henderson model.

EDWARD J. HALLORAN

Hermeneutics

Historically, hermeneutics described the art or theory of interpretation (predominantly that of texts) and was prevalent in disciplines such as theology and law. German philosopher Wilhelm Dilthey (1833–1911) redefined hermeneutics as a science of historical understanding and sought a method for deriving objectively valid interpretations. Martin Heidegger (1889–1976) recast hermeneutics from being based on the interpretation of historical consciousness to revealing the temporality of self-understandings (Palmer, R., 1969).

Hermeneutics is an approach to scholarship that acknowledges the temporal situatedness of both the researcher and the participants. Time as it advenes, or time-as-lived, is central to the work of hermeneutics. The centrality of time is what differentiates hermeneutics from traditional forms of Husserlian phenomenology. The hermeneutic scholar works to uncover how humans are "always already" given *as* time. Hermeneutics has no beginning or end that can be concretely defined but is a *continuing* experience for all who participate.

Interpretation presupposes a threefold structure of understanding, which Heidegger called the fore-structure. The premise of the fore-structure is that all interpretations are based on background practices that grant us practical familiarity with phenomena. Heidegger called this sense of phenomena fore-having. Our background practices also form the perspective from which we approach understanding. Our interpretive lens, termed fore-sight, is constituted by background practices. Fore-conception describes our anticipated sense of what our interpreting will reveal. This too is shaped and framed by our background practices. Understanding is circular, and humans as self-interpreting beings are always already within this interpretive (hermeneutic) circle of understanding. Thus, "interpretation is never a resuppositionless grasping of something previously given" (Heidegger, 1927/1996, p. 141). Hermeneutic researchers do not attempt to isolate or "bracket" their presuppositions but rather to make them explicit. Hans-Georg Gadamer (1989), a student of Heidegger's, has extended hermeneutical research in this area. The essence of hermeneutics lies not in some kind of mystic relativism but in an attitude of respect for the impossibility of bringing the understanding of "Being" to some kind of final or ultimate closure. The way of hermeneutics is to allow oneself to be drawn into the complexity of the simple and overlooked (Heidegger, 1977/1993).

The work of interpretive phenomenologists moves beyond traditional logical structures to reveal and explicate otherwise hidden relationships. Calling attention to human practices and experiences, hermeneutics is closely related to critical social theory, feminism, and postmodernism. Unlike them, however, hermeneutics does not posit politically or psychologically determined frameworks as the modus operandi of the method, nor does the interpretive phenomenologist attempt to posit, explain, or reconcile an underlying cause of a particular experience. Rather, the description of the common practices and shared meanings is intended to reveal, enhance, or extend understandings of the human situation as it is lived.

The thinking that accompanies hermeneutical scholarship is reflective, reflexive, and circular in nature. However, describing the process of hermeneutical research may suggest a linearity and structure that belies the seamless, fluid nature of this approach to inquiry. On the other hand, not describing the process implies a thoughtless or haphazard approach that does not reflect the scholarliness of hermeneutical research. Therefore, although a brief summary of hermeneutical analysis is given here, the reader is referred to several authors (Benner, 1994; Gadamer, 1960, 1989; Grondin, 1995; Palmer, 1969) who discuss hermeneutical methodology in more detail.

Commonly, hermeneutical researchers work in teams and study areas of personal interest and expertise. Each interview, as text analogue, is read by team members to obtain an overall understanding. Members of the research team identify common themes within each interview and share their written interpretations, including excerpts from each interview, with the team. Dialogue among team members clarifies the analyses. As the team analyzes subsequent interviews, they read each text against those that preceded it. This enables new themes to emerge and previous themes to be continuously refined, expanded, or overcome. Team members clarify any discrepancies in their interpretations by referring to the interview text or reinterviewing participants. This is not to say that hermeneutic researchers reduce phenomena to differences or similarities. Rather, through dialogue, the team members explicate the practices of identifying the seemingly simple and overlooked.

Team members identify and explore themes that cut across interview texts. They reread and study interpretations generated previously to see if similar or contradictory interpretations are present in the various interviews. Though an underlying assumption of hermeneutical analysis is that no single correct interpretation exists, the team's continuous examination of the whole and the parts of the texts with constant reference to the participants ensures that interpretations are focused and reflected in the text. Whenever conflicts arise among the various interpretations of the interviews, team members provide extensive documentation to support their interpretations.

Reading across postpositivist, feminist, critical, and postmodern texts, team members hold open and problematic the identification and interpretation of common practices. Team members read across all texts and write critiques of the interpretations. The purpose is to conduct critical scholarship using other interpretive approaches to extend, support, or overcome the themes and patterns identified by hermeneutics. In this way analysis proceeds in "cycles of understanding, interpretation, and critique" (Benner, 1994, p. 116). Like the hermeneutic circle, interpretations are complete but never ending.

During the interpretive sessions, patterns may emerge. A pattern is constitutive, present in all the interviews, and expresses the relationships of the themes. Patterns are the highest level of hermeneutical analysis. The hermeneutic approach provides an opportunity for team members and researchers not on the team to review the entire analysis for plausibility, coherence, and comprehensiveness. In addition, participants in the study may be asked to read interpretations of their interviews as well as the interviews of other participants to confirm, extend, or challenge the analysis. Others, not included in the analysis but likely to be readers of this study, may review the written interpretations. This review process exposes unsubstantiated and unwarranted interpretations that are not supported by the texts. The purpose of the research report is to provide a wide range of explicated text so that the reader can recognize common practices and shared experiences. The researcher writes the final report using sufficient excerpts from the interviews to allow the reader to participate in the analysis.

Hermeneutical research that draws on interpretive phenomenology was introduced to nursing by Patricia Benner in *Expertise in Nursing Practice: Caring, Clinical Judgment, and Ethics*. This study revealed nursing as a interpretive practice with skills, expertise, and practical knowledge (Benner, Panner, & Chesla, 1996). Viewing nursing as a practice rather than as an applied science presents a new approach to understanding that has implications for practice, research, and education. Hermeneutics deconstructs the corresponding relationship between theory and practice and reveals the practical knowledge and expertise that evolves over time.

Following the Benner study, hermeneutics emerged as a significant area of scholarship in nursing. Christine Tanner, through hermeneutical analyses of the narratives of nurses, has recast clinical judgment making and clinical thinking as interpretive practices. Nancy Diekelmann is utilizing hermeneutics to describe the concernful practices of teaching and learning. These shared practices of students, teachers, and clinicians offer a view of schooling, teaching, and learning as interpretive practices to transform conventional nursing education.

NANCY DIEKELMANN
PAMELA MAGNUSSEN IRONSIDE

History of Nursing Research

The first public health policy act was signed on July 16, 1798, by President John Adams. A public health service organization, later named the U.S. Public Health Service (USPHS), would operate hospitals and rest homes for sick merchant seamen. The act was expanded in 1877 as a result of a yellow fever epidemic in New Orleans that required the passage of the Quarantine Act of 1878.

In 1879 a national Board of Health was established to monitor public health regularly, especially in the area of sanitation. A weekly report that later became the *Public Health Reports* was published. The board had the authority to intervene in case of an epidemic. In the late 19th century, Robert Koch and Louis Pasteur made important discoveries about the nature of infectious diseases that explained the transmission of such diseases and aided in controlling their spread. In this control, government had a significant role.

Although the role of the federal government became significant in 1938 through grants-in-aid to universities under a research grants program, it is generally held that nursing research began after World War II, even though the work of Florence Nightingale (1820–1910) introduced the use of statistics in analyzing nursing data. Beginning in 1920, the Goldmark study was the first of the landmark studies of nursing. Research developed into nursing education, time studies, salaries, supply and demand, employment conditions, costs, status of nurses, job satisfaction, needs, and resources. In 1955 the Nursing Research Grants and Fellowship Program of the Division of Nursing, USPHS, was established; it awarded grants for nursing research projects, nursing research fellowships, and nurse-scientist graduate training. In 1978 the Division of Manpower Analysis was established within the Division of Nursing in the Bureau of Health Manpower to conduct research on manpower.

In the 19th century, Florence Nightingale, a founder of modern nursing, was the first nurse to do research in connection with nursing, when she used statistics in the analysis of her data. She was the first biostatician in nursing. Nightingale did her work alone and not until after World War II was there an organized, continuing effort to conduct further nursing research. Nursing care research is defined as research directed to understanding the nursing care of individuals and groups and the biological, physiological, social, behavioral, and environmental mechanisms influencing health and disease that are relevant to nursing care. Nursing research develops knowledge about health and the promotion of health over the life span, care of persons with health problems and disabilities, and nursing actions that enhance the ability of individuals to respond effectively to actual or potential health problems. The following is a summary of major hallmarks in the history of nursing research:

1920. Josephine Goldmark, under the direction of Haven Emerson, conducted a comprehensive survey that identified the inadequacies of housing and instructional facilities for nursing students.

1922. In a time study of institutional nursing, the New York Academy of Medicine, showed wide discrepancies in the costs of nursing education and services.

1923. The Committee for the Study of Nursing Education conducted the first comprehensive study of nursing schools and public health agencies. The final report was published as *Nursing and Nursing Education the United States.*

1924. The first nursing doctoral program was established at Teacher's College, Columbia University.

1926. May Ayres Burgess was commissioned by the Committee on the Grading of Nursing Schools to ensure that nursing service provided adequate patient care. The result was the classic report, *Nurses, Patients, and Pocketbooks.*

1934. The second project of the Committee on the Grading of Nursing Schools was a job analysis reported in *An Activity Analysis of Nursing.* The grading of nursing schools was not realized until the establishment of the National Nursing Accrediting Service in 1950.

1935. The American Nurses Association (ANA) published *Some Facts About Nursing: A Handbook for Speakers and Others,* which contained yearly compilations of statistical data about registered nurses.

1936. The ANA scrutinized the economic situation of nurses by studying incomes, salaries, and employment conditions; it excluded public health nurses.

1940. Pfefferkorn and Rovetta compiled basic data on the costs of nursing service and nursing education.

1941. The United States Public Health Service (USPHS) conducted a national census on nursing resources in cooperation with state nursing associations as World War II loomed.

1943. The National Organization of Public Health Nursing surveyed needs and resources for home care in 16 communities. The work was reported in *Public Health Nursing Care of the Sick.*

1948. The publication of the Brown Report identified issues facing nursing education and nursing services for the first half of the century. The recommendations led to much research during the next 10 years, for example: studies on nursing functions, nursing teams, practical nurses, role and attitude studies, nurse technicians, and nurse-patient relationships. Other studies rooted in the Brown report were on the hospital environment and economic security as well as the report *Nursing Schools at Mid-Century,* from the National Committee for the Improvement of Nursing Services. The Division of Nursing Resources (now the Division of Nursing) of the USPHS conducted statewide surveys and developed manuals and tools for nursing research. Major breakthroughs in nursing research were made by such studies as: (a) patient satisfaction, (b) patient classification studies, (c) problem-oriented record. These studies laid the ground-work for nursing research for the next 2 decades.

1949. The ANA conducted its first national inventory of Professional Registered Nurses in the United States and Puerto Rico. An Interim Classification of Schools of Nursing Offering Basic Programs was prepared with classifications I, II, and III according to specific criteria.

1950. The National Nursing Accrediting Service, established a system for accrediting schools of nursing.

1952. The journal *Nursing Research* was published in June 1952. It was the ANA's first official journal for reporting nursing and health research.

1953. Leo Simmons and Virginia Henderson published a survey and assessment of nursing research which classified and evaluated research in nursing during the precious decade. Teachers College, Columbia University, established the Institute of Research and Service in Nursing Education under Helen Bunge.

1954. The ANA established a Committee on Research and Studies to plan, promote, and guide research and studies relating to the functions of the ANA (1968 published) ANA Guidelines in Ethical Values.

1955. The ANA established the American Nurses' Foundation (ANF), a center for research to receive and administer funds and grants for nursing research. The foundation conducts its own programs of research and provides consultation to nursing students, research facilities, and others engaged in nursing research. *Twenty Thousand Nurses Tell Their Story* was published. The Nursing Research Grants and Fellowship Programs of the Division of Nursing, USPHS, were established to stimulate and provide financial support for research investigators and nursing research education.

1956. The study of *Patient Care and Patient Satisfaction in 60 Hospitals* was published.

1957. The Department of Nursing, established at Walter Reed Army Institute of Research, provided opportunities for growth in military nursing research. The Western Interstate Commission for Higher Education (WICHE) sponsored the Western Interstate Council on Higher Education for Nursing (WICHEN) to improve the quality of higher education for nursing in the western U.S., focus on preparing nurses for research, and develop new scientific knowledge and communicate research findings. Other such groups were the Southern Regional Education Board (SREB), New England Board of Higher Education (NEBHE), Midwest Alliance in Nursing (MAIN), and Mid-Atlantic Regional Nurses Association (MAR NA).

1959. The National League for Nursing (NLN) Research and Studies (later the Division of Research) was established to conduct research, provide consultations to NLN staff, and maintain information about NLN research products.

1960. Faye Abdellah developed the first *federally* tested Coronary Care Unit and published *Patient Centered Approaches to Nursing*, which altered nursing theory and practice.

1963. The Surgeon General's Consultant Group on Nursing reported on the nursing situation in the U.S. and recommended increased federal support for nursing research and education of researchers. Nursing Studies Index, Volume IV, 1957–1959, was completed as a guide to analytical and historical literature on nursing in English from 1900–1959. Volume I, 1900–1929, was published in 1972; Volume II, 1930–1949, was published in 1970; and Volume III, 1950–1956, was published in 1966.

1964. Nursing Research: A Survey and Assessment provided a review and assessment of research in areas of occupational health, career dynamics, and nursing care.

1965. ANA Nursing Research Conferences (1965 through the 1980s) provided a forum for critiquing nursing research and opportunities for nurse researchers to examine critical issues.

1966. International Nursing Index was published. One of the first textbooks on nursing research was published by Abdellah and Levine: *Better Patient Care Through Nursing Research.*

1968. The ANA *Blueprint for Research in Nursing* and *The Nurse in Research*, ANA guidelines in ethical values were published.

1970. ANA Commission on Nursing Research was established and prepared position papers on human rights in research. Papers included: *Human rights guidelines for nurses in clinical and other research* (1974), *Research in nursing: Toward a science of health care* (1976), *Preparation of nurses for participation in research* (1976), and *Priorities for nursing research* (1976). An abstract for action made recommendations for changes in nursing such as increased practice research, improved education, role clarification and practice, and increased financial support for nursing. Overview of Nursing was supported by the Department of Health, Education, and Welfare, 1955–1968, to assess nursing research, knowledge, gaps, and future needs.

1971. The ANA Council of Nurse Researchers was established by the ANA Commission on Nursing Research to advance research activities and published issues in research: *Social, Professional, and Methodology* (1973). The Secretary's Commission, Department of Health, Education and Welfare (DHEW) published *Extending the Scope of Nursing Practice* as a position of the health professions to support the expansion of the functions and responsibilities of nurse practitioners.

1973. The American Academy of Nursing was founded with 36 charter fellows to advance new concepts in nursing and health care, to explore issues in health care, the profession and society as directed by nursing, to examine dynamics of nursing, and to propose resolutions for issues and problems in nursing and health.

1977. *Nursing Research* became the first nursing journal to be included in Medline, the computerized information retrieval service.

1979. *Healthy People*, the Surgeon General's report on health promotion and disease prevention, was published. *Clinical content of nursing proceedings Forum on Doctoral Education in Nursing* defined the content of nursing research at the doctoral level.

1980. *Promoting Health, Preventing Disease: Objectives for the Nation* was published. ANA published a social policy statement, which defined the nature and scope of nursing practice and characteristics of specialization in nursing.

1981. *Strategies for Promoting Health for Specific Populations* was published by the Department of Health and Human Services (formerly Department of Health, Education, and Welfare). DRGs (Diagnostic Related Groups) were mandated by Health Care Financing Administration for Medicare regarding reimbursement. This stimulated the importance of evidence-based practical nursing.

1983. *The 1981 White House conference on aging: Executive summary of technical committee on health maintenance and health promotion* and *Report of the mini conference on long-term care: Report of the technical committee on health services: Nursing and nurse education-Public policies and private actions.* Report of the Institute of Medicine, National Academy of Sciences defined nursing research and delineated its direction. *Magnet Hospitals: Attraction and Retention of Professional Nurses* was published by the American Academy of Nursing. *Report of the Task Force on Nursing Practice in Hospitals.* New legislation established reimbursement policies for hospitals based on prospective payment of Diagnosis Related Groups (DRGs) the determined amount paid for Medicare patients.

1983. The first volume of the *Annual Review of Nursing Research* series was published by Springer Publishing Company.

1984. The ANA formed the ANA Council on Computer Applications in Nursing to focus on computer technology pertinent to nursing practice, education, administration, and research. The ANA Cabinet on Nursing Research published *Directions for Nursing Research: Toward the Twenty First Century.*

1985. The National Center for Nursing Research (NCNR) was established in the PHS. Programs would work to enlarge scientific knowledge underlying nursing services, administration, and education. The Center was initially located in the Division of Nursing, Bureau of Health Manpower, Health Resources, and Services Administration, but in 1986 it became part of the National Institutes of Health (NIH). In 1993, the NCNR was renamed the National Institute of Nursing Research.

1988. The Agency for Health Care Policy and Research (AHCPR) within the Department of Health and Human Services (DHHS) was established to focus on the development of clinical practice guidelines, outcome measures, and effectiveness research. (The name was changed to Agency for Health Care Research and Quality).

Thirty years after the idea was first proposed by the National Institute of Health's National Advisory Council, the National Center for Nursing Research (NCNR) was established in 1986. Its mandate was "to advance science to strengthen nursing practice and health care that promotes health, prevents disease, and ameliorates the effects of illness and disability." The placement of NCNR at the National Institute of Health (NIH) moved nursing research into a broader based biomedical research environment and facilitated the collaboration between nursing and other research disciplines. On June 9, 1993, the NCNR was renamed and became the National Institute of Nursing Research, which placed nursing on an equal footing with other NIH institutes.

The National Institute of Nursing Research (NINR) is the key organ for funding nursing research grants and contracts and has approved priority areas for research as determined by its National Advisory Council for Nursing Research. NINR provides a scientific base for patient care and is used by many disciplines among health care professionals—especially by the nation's 2.5 million nurses. NINR-supported research spans both health and illness and deals with individuals of all age groups. Nursing research addresses the issues that examine the core of patients' and families' personal encounters with illness, disability, treatment, and disease prevention. In addition, nursing research addresses issues with a community or public health focus. NINR's primary activity is clinical research, and most of the studies directly involve patients. The basic science is linked to patient problems.

The nursing programs of the USPHS stimulated the postwar expansion of nursing services through pilot studies, nursing research, and community health services. The Division of Nursing Resources, with a modest budget of $95,000 and a small staff, was able to undertake a number of landmark studies to find solutions to postwar nursing problems in hospitals and health agencies. During the years 1949 to 1955, a number of state surveys of nursing needs and resources were conducted in almost all states.

In 1954, among the many studies and tools developed by the USPHS Division of Nursing Resources, (now the Division of Nursing) was a cooperative study carried out with the Commission on Nursing of Cleveland, Ohio, to discover the reasons for the understaffing of nursing departments. A by-product of the study was that it produced the outcome measure satisfaction study. Another study involved the use of disease classification for nursing planning. The diagnoses were then coded and classified into 58 groups representing discrete nursing problems. A similar methodological approach was followed in the development of the problem-oriented medical record more than a decade later and in the development of Diagnostic Related Groups. In 1955, Congress earmarked $625,000 for nursing research and fellowships that were awarded directly to universities, hospitals, health agencies, and professional associations.

The Army Nurse Corps initiated nursing research in the military and has been a major contributor to the evolution of both military and civilian nursing research. The army developed a program designed to concentrate on clinical nursing research in addition to fostering participation in the collaborative studies of other disciplines.

The history of nursing research in the navy (primarily unpublished master's theses) covers research topics that are broad and focus on various aspects of the organization and administration of nursing service. Further work to incorporate nursing research into the Navy Nurse Corps became prominent in 1987, when the navy conducted a review of billets and identified the need for doctorally prepared nurses.

The history of nursing research in the air force is found primarily through the review of unpublished mimeographed documents covering research at the School of Aerospace Medicine at Brooks Air Force Base, Texas. Among the research topics reported are the development of equipment for aeromedical evacuation (such as examination lamps, oxygen and humidity apparatus, hand disinfection devices, patient monitoring and blood pressure measurement, litter lift, and transportable airborne stations). Physiological and psychological changes experienced by air force nurses associated with flying duty on jet and propeller aircraft and ways to evaluate patient care in flight are other areas of research.

In the Fall of 1990, representatives from the army, navy, and air force met to discuss collaborative research among the services. This group formed the Federal Nursing Research Interest Group, which later became the Tri-Service Nursing Research Group (TSNR Group). The TSNR Group was made responsible for finding ways to promote military nursing research both collectively and individually, within and across the services. The initial appropriation for the TSNR program under S.R. 102-154 was $1 million for fiscal year (FY) 1992 and it increased to $5 million in FY 1996, $6 million thereafter, authorizing the TSNR program as part of the Department of Defense Health Care Program, administered by the TSNR Group and established at the Uniformed Services University of the Health Sciences. In 2000, the Council for the Advancement of Nursing Science (CANS) created the research policy and facilitation arm of the American Academy of Nursing.

FAYE G. ABDELLAH

HIV Risk Behavior

By the end of 2003, an estimated 40 million people throughout the world were living with HIV/AIDS (United Nations Program on AIDS/HIV [UNAIDS], 2004a). With the highest incidence rate in any one single year since the commencement of the pandemic, 5 million people worldwide become newly HIV infected in 2003 (UNAIDS, 2004b). This increasing rate of HIV/AIDS infection is a critical public health crisis and highlights the need to continually advocate for the reduction of HIV risk behaviors. Since an effective vaccine or cure for HIV/AIDS infection has not been invented yet, developing effective intervention programs to prevent or reduce the risk of becoming HIV/AIDS infected is extremely important. Nurses, with an obligatory role in providing quality health care for all, are cooperating with other professional disciplines and contributing to the prevention of HIV/AIDS infection.

Studies to date have identified that unprotected sexual intercourse, having multiple sexual partners, and injection drug uses are the main risk behaviors for HIV transmission. Sexual contact is the major exposure to the HIV transmission in most reported AIDS-infected cases. Therefore, HIV risk behaviors generally imply sexual activities in which the likelihood of having HIV infection is increased. Unsafe sexual behavior, risky sexual behavior, or sexual risk-taking behaviors are the terms commonly and widely used by scientists and researchers to represent sexual activity that increases the risk of getting sexually transmitted diseases, including HIV/AIDS infection, or becoming pregnant. Since the tragedy of the HIV/AIDS epidemic is spreading gravely, these terms in most studies specifically refer to HIV/AIDS-related sexual behavior.

Many psychosocial, biological, and sociologic circumstances or cofactors have been recognized as impacting the likelihood of HIV risks as well. The personal factors, including age, gender, race, developmental stage, early age of initiation of intercourse, HIV/AIDS-related sexual knowledge, sexual identity, self-esteem, self-efficacy, alcohol uses, and the use of illicit drugs, are associated with HIV infection-related risks. Interpersonal factors such as discussing safe sex with sexual partners and asking sexual partners about his/her sexual history may also be correlated with reduced risk of HIV infection. Environmental factors, such as social economic status, peer, school, family, and gender role, cultural norms, religious beliefs, and social isolation, were also found to influence the likelihood of becoming HIV infected.

Many behavioral contributors that increase or decrease the risk of HIV infection have been explored and identified; however, the contextual risk factors and their casual relationships with HIV risk behaviors are still not well understood. This limited understanding is an obstacle for developing effective interventions to prevent or reduce HIV risk–associated behaviors.

Several health behavior theories, such as Social Cognitive Theory (Bandura, 1994), Health Belief Model (Rosenstock, 1974), and the Theory of Reasoned Action (Fishbein & Ajzen, 1975), have suggested possible mechanisms and been popularly employed in the understanding and prevention of HIV-related risk behaviors. Most of the cognitive-behavioral interventions that stem from these theories report effectiveness in reducing risk of HIV infection. Strong evidences have shown that human's cognitive functions, such as self-efficacy, uniquely contribute to the rationale of the safer sexual behaviors, and especially in the domain of condom use. For example, a cross-sectional survey tested the social cognitive-based model for condom use in a randomly selected sample of 1,380 participants with ages 18 to 25 years who were single and reported initiation of sexual intercourse (DiIorio, Dudley, Soet, Watkins, & Maibach, 2001). Self-efficacy was found to be directly related to condom-use behaviors and indirectly through its effect on outcome expectancies.

Thousands of experts have contributed to research in this field since the beginning of the HIV epidemic. Research related to HIV risk behaviors has significantly moved toward interventional studies. Ongoing research is also being conducted on the contextual factors that increase HIV risk behaviors. Successful programs for reducing HIV risk-related sexual behaviors are targeted toward different populations (e.g., based on race/ethnicity, sexual orientation, drug use).

When examining the effectiveness of an intervention, measurement issues regarding the indications of the HIV risk behaviors are especially important. Because of its complex nature, HIV risk behaviors are measured variously by researchers in terms of content and form. In most of the existing correlational studies, HIV risk behaviors were measured using "relative frequency" data collected through Likert scales or "count data" which provided the accurate number of behavioral events used in interventional studies (2003). The "condom use" measure is the most frequently used indicator for HIV risk behaviors in many related behavioral studies. Many interventional programs also focus on improving the constant condom use. Besides the single item or several questions asked to measure risk behaviors, a small number of questionnaires for measuring HIV risk-related sexual behaviors are also available, such as the Safe Sex Behavior Questionnaire (SSBQ) (Dilorio et al., 1992).

Research is urgently needed to involve women and young people, especially adolescents, because these groups have increasingly high HIV risks (UNAIDS, 2004b). It is important to track emerging behavioral risks to identify the settings, subpopulations, or areas at particular risk for HIV infection so that preventive interventions can take these factors into consideration. For example, drug users, men who have sex with men, homeless people, HIV-positive individuals, and people affected with psychiatric disorders have diverse potential risks and disparate abilities to reduce their HIV risk-related behaviors. Moreover, intervening factors of HIV risk behaviors, such as culture, race, age, and gender among the target populations as mentioned earlier in this section, should be identified and considered in order to design effective HIV prevention programs.

To understand and evaluate the maintenance of behavior change for reducing the risk of HIV infection, longitudinal and multivariate studies are necessary to detect causal relationships and the changing patterns of HIV risk behaviors. Moreover, methodological issues, including criterion measures, validity of self-report risk behaviors, comparability and generalizability of studies, need special consideration. Future nursing studies in this field are encouraged to include biological markers that can bolster the validity of the studies, because risk behaviors and factors are complex and not easily measured. It is expected that future studies on the effectiveness of prevention programs and change of HIV risk behaviors utilize randomized controlled trial designs, as these are the most powerful designs for intervention studies. Meta-analysis research that integrates the results from various individual HIV risk-behavioral studies is also needed to provide multiperspective views for future direction of nursing practice. Developing a specific HIV risk-behavioral reduction theory from the nursing perspective may be useful and efficacious for nurses to apply to the reduction of HIV risk behaviors.

Effective interventions that prevent or reduce HIV risk behaviors must be disseminated to successfully contain the HIV/AIDS epidemic. Bridges between research, practice, and policy, as well as with other disciplines, must be built. This includes releasing research findings to the public and translating them into community-based practices.

Yi-Hui Lee

HIV Symptom Management and Quality of Life

Since the advent of highly active antiretroviral therapy, persons with human immunodeficiency virus (HIV) are generally living longer. Viral loads have diminished to undetectable levels, $CD4^{+}$ cell counts have increased, and opportunistic infections have become more manageable. However, persons with HIV frequently reported increased medical and disease-related symptomatology (Kirksey et al., 2002). Therefore, client-initiated or provider-directed symptom management has become an increasingly important component of care. The primary objective of nursing interventions is to enhance health-related quality of life (HRQOL) for persons with HIV.

Symptoms are primary reasons why individuals seek health care (Lee, K., & Carrieri, 2003). A symptom is "any condition accompanying or resulting from a disease or physical disorder and serving as an aid in diagnosis" (Webster's New World College Dictionary, 2001, p. 1451). Symptoms are subjective phenomena that indicate a departure from normal functioning, sensation, or appearance. These entities are a person's perception of abnormal physical, emotional, or cognitive states. I. B. Wilson and Cleary (1995) described symptom reporting as an expression of subjective experiences that summarize and integrate data from an array of different sources. Several authors have noted that when symptom control is not achieved, quality of life can be adversely affected (Holzemer, Spicer, Wilson, Kemppainen, & Coleman, 1998; Lee, K., & Carrieri).

The University of California, San Francisco, School of Nursing Symptom Management Faculty Group (1994) defined symptoms as subjective experiences based upon cognitive changes, sensation, or biopsychosocial function. The model is comprised of three interrelated dimensions: symptom experience, management strategies, and outcomes. The first category reflects an individual's perception of a symptom. The second category, management strategies, includes self-care behaviors. And the last category, symptom outcomes, may include entities like HRQOL.

The University of California, San Francisco (UCSF) International HIV Nursing Research Network has conducted a number of multisite studies in order to identify the pervasive symptoms and self-care management strategies used by persons with HIV. Among the most frequently reported symptoms were: anxiety, depression, fatigue, and neuropathy. The following sections contain brief summaries of recent scientific studies related to each of these symptoms.

According to Kemppainen and others (2003), anxiety is one of the most prevalent symptoms experienced by persons with HIV. Dew and colleagues (1997) noted that clients with a prior history of an anxiety disorder prior to being diagnosed with HIV were at greater risk of recurrence of symptoms. Precipitating factors may include lack of partner support and inability to master or control life events. J. G. Johnson, Williams, Rabkin, Goetz, and Remien (1995) found a relationship between preexisting personality disorder and the onset of HIV-related anxiety. The researchers compared 52 HIV-negative and 110 HIV-positive men, 19% of whom had a preexisting personality disorder. Participants in the HIV-positive group displayed greater levels of anxiety than those persons in the HIV-negative group. In another study with a similar premise, Ferrando and colleagues (1998) noted a relationship among depression, substance use, and prevalence of anxiety in an ethnically-diverse sample of 267 HIV-negative and HIV-positive males. HIV-positive participants ($n = 183$) who continued to use illegal substances reported higher levels of emotional stress.

Neidig, Smith, and Brashers (2003) postulated that aerobic training may assist in reducing or preventing depression symptoms experienced by persons living with HIV. Sixty HIV-infected adults participated in a randomized controlled trial where clients were subjected to a 12-week aerobic exercise training program. When compared with the control group, participants in the exercise group showed significant reductions in depressive symptoms.

In another study using a telephone support group for HIV-positive persons over the age of 50 years, Nokes, Chew, and Altman (2003) determined that identifying symptoms and exploring the use of effective medications and treatments aided in reducing depression.

Fatigue is a common symptom of HIV and is associated with impaired physical functioning and poor HRQOL (Breitbart et al., 1998). Piper, Lindsey, and Dodd (1987) defined fatigue as "a subjective feeling of tiredness that is influenced by circadian rhythm. It can vary in unpleasantness, duration and intensity" (p. 19). Some researchers (Capaldini, 1998; Perkins, D. O., et al., 1995; Walker, K., McGowan, Jantos, & Anson, 1997) have postulated that there is a correlation between depression and fatigue in persons with HIV infection.

However, others (Breitbart et al., 1998; Ferrando et al., 1998) disagreed and observed that although it is associated with depression, fatigue makes a separate contribution to morbidity in HIV-infected persons.

Nicholas and colleagues (2002) stated that peripheral neuropathy is "the most common neurological complication in HIV disease" (p. 763). These investigators noted that neuropathy was the third most frequently reported symptom in a convenience sample of 422 persons living with HIV. Forty-four percent of the self-care management strategies were categorized as complementary or alternative therapies; however, there was lack of consensus about the efficacy of these interventions.

Quality of life is a perception of circumstances which is dependent upon psychological makeup. The central assumption is that individuals are the best sources of judgment about HRQOL, and it cannot be assumed that everyone will value life circumstances in the same way. Burgoyne and Saunders (2001) stated that quality-of-life assessment involves an appraisal of one's current state against some ideal. Goal attainment, coping, decision-making assessment, and value systems are examples of predictors of HRQOL.

Kemppainen (2001) examined whether or not variables relating to sociodemographic attributes, illness severity, and psychological status predict quality of life in persons with HIV. Using a convenience sample ($n = 162$), the author found that the strongest predictor of decreased HRQOL scores was depression. Additionally, the investigator noted that the number of symptoms also had a profound effect on HRQOL.

In another study, Sousa, Holzemer, Henry, and Slaughter (1999) performed a secondary analysis ($n = 142$) to empirically test the influence of symptom status, functional status, and general health perceptions on overall HRQOL in persons living with HIV. Analysis suggested that these variables were key dimensions of HRQOL. The investigators concluded that focusing nursing interventions on decreasing symptoms or assisting the client in identifying self-care management strategies positively affects general health perceptions and enhances overall HRQOL. Douaihy and Singh (2001) noted that "physical manifestations, antiretroviral therapy, psychological well-being, social support systems, coping strategies, spiritual well-being, and psychiatric comorbidities are important predictors of QOL . . . " (p. 1).

This review presented select articles addressing symptom identification and management as correlates to HRQOL in persons with HIV infection. Scholarly endeavors concerning quality of life have helped shape standards of care by broadening conceptualizations of outcome measures. However, additional scientific studies designed to explore the efficacy of complementary and alternative therapies, as well as public discourse on symptom management strategies related to quality-of-life enhancement, are still needed.

Kenn M. Kirksey
Danielle Deveau

HIV/AIDS Care and Treatment

There has been a major shift in the nursing of persons with HIV/AIDS in resource rich countries after 1996. With the introduction of highly active antiretroviral medications targeting different phases of the host/virus interaction, HIV rapidly changed from an acute, often terminal, infection to a chronic illness with a long disease trajectory. Symptom management and identification of strategies to promote treatment adherence emerged as important foci of nursing research. In communities like the United States where medications are readily available through government-supported medication access programs, nursing research moved its area of concentration from the needs of tertiary-care patients to community-living clients and their support systems.

Goldrick, Baigis, Larsen, and Lemert (2000) reviewed the nursing research literature (1986 to 1997) and found that, although many descriptive and/or correlational studies described clinical problems experienced by

HIV positive persons, they believed that future studies should focus more on clinical interventions. The Delphi technique was used with expert members of the Association of Nurses in AIDS Care (Sowell, 2000) to identify HIV/AIDS research priorities into the 21st century. Five categories were identified: (a) HIV community-level education and prevention, (b) development of more tolerable drugs, (c) prevention focusing on individual or specific group behavior, (d) vaccine development, and (e) development of new and more effective drugs. Hare (2003) identified the six major categories of National Institute of Nursing Research funded research as: (a) biobehavioral and sociocultural research in HIV prevention and intervention, (b) risk reduction, (c) interventions to improve adherence to drug regimens, (d) end-of-life care, (e) symptoms, and (f) shifting trends including informal caregiving.

Symptoms can emerge from the disease pathology, treatment strategies, and comorbidities. Nurse researchers have examined individual symptoms such as diarrhea (Anastasi & McMahon, 2003), but through descriptive studies that used instruments such as the SSC-HIV (rev) (Holzemer, Hudson, Kirksey, Hamilton, & Bakken, 2001), it was found that HIV positive persons usually report more than one symptom. The UCSF International HIV/AIDS Nursing Research Network identified six commonly reported symptoms: anxiety, depression, diarrhea, fatigue, nausea, and neuropathy. Identification of self-care symptom management strategies were described for anxiety and fear (Kemppainen et al., 2002), neuropathy (Nicholas et al., 2002), and fatigue (Corless et al., 2002).

In order to suppress the HIV viral load, adherence with prescribed medications must be almost perfect. Research with chronically ill populations has demonstrated medication adherence rates as low as 30%. Therefore, nurse researchers have developed many different protocols to examine strategies that promote treatment adherence and informed decision making since incomplete viral suppression cannot only harm the infected person but promote viral mutation and resistance. Other interventions tested by nurse researchers have focused on health promotion behaviors such as regular aerobic exercise (Baigis et al., 2002).

The two major routes of HIV transmission are sexual and sharing blood products often, through injection drug use. Populations living with HIV/AIDS vary vastly in ethnicity, socioeconomic, and educational status. Physical comorbidities such as hepatitis, especially hepatitis C, must also be considered. Differences must be addressed in the development of intervention protocols. Recruitment issues, especially the use of incentives, must be carefully considered to avoid situations where the incentive becomes such an important benefit that the potential study participant minimizes the risk. Retention is a major issue when the study population is not in stable housing and does not have regular access to phones or mailing addresses.

Depending upon the nature of the intervention, the setting may be the home, primary care setting, hospital unit, or community-based organization. Some nurse researchers have conceptualized their interventions using principles of models from other disciplines, such as the Stages of Change model, while others used nursing theorists such as the Personalized Nursing LIGHT model based on Martha Roger's science of nursing (Anderson et al., 2003). Many of the intervention studies require multiple points of contact over time, which can be difficult to achieve in a highly mobile, resource-poor population. Findings emerging from these behavioral intervention studies may seem disappointing since there is often not a significant statistical improvement in the outcome variable after the intervention. This lack of significant findings may be due more to the lack of sensitivity in the instruments being used than in the effectiveness of the intervention. Nursing interventions are usually noninvasive and care is used to avoid harm. Rather than being discouraged by a lack of significant improvement, nurse researchers are using these findings to refine their interventions and choose more sensitive instruments to measure change over a relatively short period of time.

KATHLEEN M. NOKES

Home Care Technologies

The Office of Technology Assessment, in a 1987 memorandum to the U.S. Congress, described a technology-dependent person as one who needs both ongoing nursing care and a medical device to compensate for loss of a vital body function. Home care technologies include mechanical ventilation; apnea detection monitoring; oxygen assist; continuous positive airway pressure (CPAP); nutrition or hydration via central venous infusion; hemodialysis and peritoneal dialysis' spinal infusion for pain; infusion for chemotherapy, insulin, or antibiotics; automatic internal defibrillation; and other systems that avert death or further disability. With home care technology a family member provides nursing care, makes complex decisions, and learns skills in managing machines without inadvertently causing harm. Studies verify the additive length, quality of life, and cost-effective outcomes from use of various home care technologies (Smith, O. E., 1995).

A common requirement for placing complex technological equipment in the home is that a competent and willing caregiver is available to manage the equipment before treatment (such as home parenteral nutrition therapy) will be authorized (Ireton-Jones, 1998; Steiger & Ireton-Jones, 2001). Problems to be studied included the impact on family caregiver quality of life (Smith, C. E., 1994), ethical decision making in use of technologies, costs of safety regulations for manufacturers, and quality control measures for home care.

Technology caregiving resembles a miniature, urgent care center where families provide complex, direct patient care, maintain equipment and supply inventories, obtain needed home services, negotiate for reimbursement, and manage caregiver problems (Cohen, 2003; Noddings, 1994). Nursing research has contributed to study findings in several areas. C. E. Smith (1995, 1996) has a series of studies on families, caregivers, and patients dependent on technology for lifelong survival (Smith et al., 2002). The ethical issues in technological home care were summarized and research questions posed in a Hastings Center report (Arras, 1995). Family members reported being ill-prepared for technology caregiving (McNeal, 2000; Scott, L. O., 2001) and little has been done to support caregivers with their long-term daily technology care (Gorski, 1995).

Research with home care technologies should be systems-oriented on a variety of levels: machine reliability and safety, compensated physiological systems, family caregiving, community support, health care providers, and third-party payers' reimbursement. The most extensive research has been at the machine level, where manufacturers' studies of the mechanical system has led to Food and Drug Administration's (FDA) approval for clinical trials conducted by nurses. Government regulation also has called for research on the manuals accompanying devices to determine readability and effectiveness of instructions for laypersons. In 1996, the National Academy of Science presented a report to Congress from manufacturers, regulators, health professionals, families, and patients regarding findings from research on safety and issues of home technologies and family care. Problems to be studied included the impact of family caregiver quality of life (Smith, 1996), ethical decision making in use of technologies, costs of safety regulations for manufacturers, and quality control measurers for home care.

Major conclusions from research are that home care technologies enhance and extend quality of life for those who would otherwise succumb to illness, frailty, or disability. Further, family members are very capable and desirous of home care for their technology-dependent loved one. Direct physical care and indirect costs (reduced income, innumerable expenses, and transportation fees) are shifted to the family (Gaskamp, 2004) and evidence of emotional and physical strain occurs in family caregivers. Delivery of technology services in home care is costly and uncoordinated, although cost-savings and quality improvements occurred when models of comprehensive care were followed. In some communities and states and in some populations of patients (e.g., ventilator-dependent), coordinated services do exist (Naylor et al., 2004).

Future directions for research include the need for continued study of informatics that can support safe, optimal technology care. A variation of the word 'technology' is technogenesis, which is used in educational technology where health care students, practitioners, and faculty nurture new technologies while preserving safety equipment. For instance, Healthy People 2010 goals for supporting those persons requiring restorative technology devices (ANA, 2002) and the Library of Medicine Quality Chasm report have a goal for safe use of infusion pumps. Effective interventions (such as step-by-step algorithms, videoscene illustrations of equipment assembly, use, cleaning, and trouble shooting) delivered over modern informatics technology will achieve the Picker Institutes' 1998 Health Care Quality Improvement goal from the patient's perspective of "establishing access to information to overcome the discontinuity between inpatient and home care setting" (Picker Institutes, 2005). Effectiveness of the informatics interventions themselves and the technology devices must be tested.

Study of interventions for technology home care in culturally diverse populations is still needed (Smith, 1994). In addition, policy, ethical, professional, and interdisciplinary areas of authority issues should be studied to reduce duplication and enhance resource availability. Predicting cost and outcomes of care should be compared to patients' and families' desired quality of life. Consumer demand and technological advances will continue, one hopes, with nursing research verifying theoretical frameworks that guide effective home technology.

Carol E. Smith
Helen A. Schaag

Home Health Care Classification (HHCC) System

The Home Health Care Classification (HHCC) system is a decision-support system designed to assess, document, and code home health care, using two interrelated terminologies. Its documentation method tracks home health care over time, across settings, and geographical locations, whereas the terminologies are used to code and classify the care. The HHCC system is based on a conceptual framework using the nursing process to assess, document, and evaluate a patient holistically.

The HHCC system was developed by Saba and colleagues at Georgetown University School of Nursing, Washington, DC. It was developed from the Home Care Project research study (1988–1991) funded by the Health Care Financing Administration (HCFA; Cooperative Agreement No. 17009 8983/3) "to develop a method to assess and classify home health Medicare patients in order to predict their need for nursing and other home care services as well as measure their outcomes of care." A national sample of 646 home health agencies (HHAs) randomly stratified by size, type of ownership, and geographic location participated in the study. The HHAs collected retrospective data on 8,961 newly discharged cases for the entire episode of home health care, from admission to discharge. This landmark study, which represents the largest sample of HHA data in the United States, provided new knowledge for the home health care industry.

The Home Care Project produced several materials, including the *HHCC of Nursing Diagnoses and Outcomes* and the *HHCC of Nursing Interventions and Actions*. The HHCC terminologies were created empirically from computer processing of approximately 40,000 textual phrases representing nursing diagnoses and/or patient problems and 72,000 phrases depicting patient care services and/or actions collected on the study cases. The textual phrases were processed by computer, using keyword sorts from which the standardized coded labels were developed. The coded labels were also grouped into 20 Care Components providing the framework for classifying, coding, and indexing the textual phrases for the two terminologies.

The HHCC terminologies are used to assess, document, and code the six steps of the nursing process, its conceptual framework for documenting nursing practice. The standards of nursing practice recommended by the American Nurses Association in 1991 comprise these six steps of nursing process, namely: assessment, diagnosis, outcome identification, planning, implementation, and evaluation.

The coding framework for the two HHCC terminologies—*HHCC of Nursing Diagnoses* and *HHCC of Nursing Interventions* is structured according to the 21 Care Components. Each is structured hierarchically and coded according to International Classification of Diseases Version 10 developed by the World Health Organization. Each term uses a five-character alphanumeric code: (a) first position: an alphabetic character for the care component; (b) second and third positions: a two-digit code for a core data element (major category) followed by a decimal point; (c) fourth position: a one-digit code for a subcategory (if needed); and (d) fifth position: a one-digit code for a modifier.

This structure facilitates the design of clinical care pathways as well as other applications that make the terminologies useful. It is also critical for the development of decision support and/or expert systems. The *HHCC of Nursing Diagnoses* and *HHCC of Nursing Interventions* have been "recognized" by the ANA as providing a valid and useful nursing language that can be used not only to classify nursing practice but also to document nursing care of patients in the electronic health record (EHR). Additionally, the two HHCC terminologies have been incorporated in the Metathesaurus developed by the National Library of Medicine for its Unified Medical Language System (UMLS), indexed in the Cumulative Index of Nursing and Allied Health Literature (CINAHL). They are registered as an HL7 language, are integrated into Logical Observations Identifiers Names and Codes (LOINC), and the Systematized Nomenclature of Human and Veterinary Medicine Combined Terminology (SNOMED CT). Further, they are translated into Dutch, Portuguese, Spanish, Finnish, Korean, and Chinese, and they are being translated into other languages. The original 20 Care Components were adapted by Ozbolt for her development of the Patient Care Data Set (PCDS).

The system provides the coding strategy and methodology for tracking clinical care for decision support, offers standardized assessment data for mapping and predicting health care resources, and provides information for quality management and evaluation of various clinical care pathways. The clinical information allows for the aggregation of data to provide meaningful cross-population comparisons as well as administrative decisions for allocating human resources. Further, the HHCC System can be used in home health, community health, ambulatory care settings as well as hospitals and long-term care settings.

The HHCC System consisting of two terminologies makes it possible not only to assess and document but also to code, index, and classify the nursing care according to the 21 Care Components. This innovative system provides the structure and coding strategy for the EHR, can identify a nursing minimum data set, and track the nursing care process across time, different settings, and geographic locations. The HHCC System facilitates the documentation of patient care electronically at the point of care instead of by the traditional paper-based method. The data once collected can be used many times, which allows for better documentation and more efficient analysis. The HHCC system is freestanding and can be integrated into any home health system and linked electronically to any system designed to collect the data required for professional and/or federal home health care reporting. It can be used to (a) improve the efficiency of assessing and documenting home health nursing care, (b) develop clinical care protocols and/or pathways, (c) provide the strategy for evaluating quality and measuring outcomes of care, and (d) develop a method for costing patient care.

A complete description of the *HHCC of Nursing Diagnoses* and *HHCC of Nursing Interventions*, classified by the 21 Care Components including their definitions, is available on the Internet at http://www.sabacare.com

VIRGINIA K. SABA

Home Health Systems

Home health systems are computer-based information systems designed to support care of the sick in the home. Home health systems primarily support home health and hospice programs provided by home health agencies (HHAs). Home health is more than "care in the home." It focuses on the continuity of care from the hospital to the community, public health concepts of disease prevention and health promotion, and out-of-hospital acute illness services.

Home care is the oldest form of health care and yet the newest. Home health nursing, previously called care of the sick in the home, is one of the earliest developments in the field of public and community health. Care of the sick at home traditionally has been provided by voluntary nonprofit agencies, such as visiting nurse associations (VNAs), organized to provide out-of-hospital services (Saba & McCormick, 1996).

In 1966, with the introduction of Medicare and Medicaid legislation, home health programs emerged from hospital-based ambulatory care, health maintenance organizations, and proprietary home health agencies. The programs and providers increased in number and size. They increased faster than all other organized providers in the health care industry because Medicare primarily addressed the health care needs of the aging population. As this population grew, more health services were required, resulting in an increase of health care costs that required cost containment. As a result, health care began to shift from acute short-term hospital care to community home-based and chronic long-term care. Patients began to be discharged "sicker and quicker" and required more health care services in the home.

Home health systems were initially introduced as management information systems designed to manage the flow of information in the proper time frame and to assist in the decision-making process. The early home health systems were introduced in large visiting nurse associations and other nonprofit HHAs as billing and financial systems. They were developed for the sole purpose of improving cash flow, holding down costs, and addressing the federal regulatory needs for HHAs. They were designed to furnish the information required for payment by Medicare, Medicaid, and other third-party payers for reimbursement for services.

Home health systems were generally developed by commercial vendors who obtained the computer system hardware and developed the software to process the services data provided by the HHAs. The computer vendors owned the home health system and were responsible for maintaining and updating them. Home health computer vendors were usually contracted by the HHAs to provide billing services and financial management, without the HHAs having to develop their own system. With the introduction of the microcomputer and online communication systems, local area networks (LANs) and wide area networks (WANs) were introduced, designed to advance and enhance the home health systems. They were used to link state and local units, to share hardware and software, and to integrate data (Saba & McCormick, 1996).

Home health systems are designed not only to collect and process home health data required by the federal government and third-party payers for reimbursement of services but also for the efficient management of the HHA. They focus on billing and financial applications, such as general ledger, accounts receivable, accounts payable, billing, reimbursement management, and cash management. They also may include other management applications, such as scheduling, patient census, visit tracking, cost statistics, utilization reports, accounting statements, and discharge summaries.

Newer home health systems have emerged that are designed to focus on the patient encounter and visit during an episode of care. They include clinical applications used to assess and document the care process, to generate care plans, and to prepare critical pathways or protocols that outline the critical events. These newer systems are using the electronic information superhighway to communicate patient information for continuity of care from hospital to the home, to the community, and back to the hospital. The systems also offer other applications that focus on decision support, evaluation of care, and measurement of outcomes across settings, time, and geographic locations. The systems are considered part of the lifelong longitudinal record containing patient-specific health-related data.

HHCC systems are being used to identify care needs in terms of care components and their respective nursing diagnoses and interventions and to determine resource use in terms of nursing and other health providers. They are being designed to document the clinical care pathways and record protocols for an entire episode of care. Further, they are being used to determine care costs and provide a payment method for managed care organizations offering home health care services.

VIRGINIA K. SABA

Homeless Health

Ongoing armed conflicts and poor economic conditions are daily increasing the ranks of the homeless in the world through the creation of refugees and immigrants. The level of increase in the homeless population worldwide can only be estimated because of the continuous fluctuation of this population. However, the World Health Organization as well as nongovernmental agencies managing the homeless around the world confirm that there are greater numbers each year.

In the United States, the increase in the number of homeless became a subject of local, state, and national concern in the 1980s, with the profile of the homeless changing from that of an older male with alcohol addiction to that of young men and women (21–39 years) who often entered homelessness accompanied by their young children (National Coalition for the Homeless, 2002). In 1987 the federal government, in the Stewart B. McKinney Act, initially enacted legislation providing limited funding for health care for the homeless via the federally funded community health centers.

Since the number of homeless continued to increase, this funding was reapproved in 1994. In this act a homeless person is defined as one who

> lacks a fixed, regular, and adequate nighttime residence; and . . . has a primary night time residency that is (a) a supervised publicly or privately operated shelter designated to provide temporary living accommodations . . . (b) an institution that provides a temporary residence for individuals intended to be institutionalized, or (c) a public or private place not designated for, or ordinarily used as, a regular sleeping accommodation for human beings. This definition does not include individuals incarcerated by federal or state governments. (42 U.S.C. § 11302(c)

Currently the Urban Institute estimates that in the U.S. the number of individuals experiencing homelessness at some time within a given year is 3.5 million, with 39% (1.5 million) of this group being children (Urban Institute, 2000). This estimate is flawed and minimal as it reflects only the homeless counted by agencies servicing the homeless. The homeless who are not included in this estimate are those who do not seek services from homeless shelters and reside outside, in abandoned buildings or autos, or with relatives or friends.

Homelessness and health are interrelated in three major ways: health issues may lead to homelessness; being homeless may predispose an individual to health threats; and homelessness can impact health by limiting one's access to health care. Health status can easily lead to homelessness. When an individual with physical or mental illness or drug/alcohol addiction is unable to maintain employment and housing—homelessness results. Being homeless in a shelter setting exposes the individual to health threats (communicable diseases) from living in close quarters with others (primarily respiratory, gastrointestinal, and dermatological health threats) and exacerbates common health problems (colds, extremity swelling, foot lesions, etc.) due to shelter restrictions which require residents to rise early and leave the premises. Being homeless also makes access to health care more difficult since most homeless individuals do not have health insurance, and most shelters do not have onsite health care providers or access to cost-free medications. Consequently, the homeless seek care for acute episodes of illness at their peak and do not seek preventive care.

Nurses and nurse researchers around the world have been in the forefront studying the health care needs of the incoming homeless (refugees and immigrants). The U.S. nursing literature focuses primarily on the health of homeless U.S. citizens who have descended into homelessness for various reasons (eviction, substance abuse, release from prison, domestic abuse, etc.). Early research in this area was directed primarily at gathering demographic information related to the homeless, such as age, sex, reason(s) for homelessness, health care needs, etc. (Lindsey, 1995) and providing reports of the health care needs of this population from newly developed nurse-managed clinics.

Although reporting of demographic information has continued, in the last 5 years nursing research in this area has evolved in new directions. Qualitative studies to better understand the lives of the homeless and the homeless experience have been published (Rew, 2003; Huang & Menke, 2001; Morrell-Bellai, Goering, & Boydell, 2000). New research instruments have been developed and validated with various subgroups of this population, and new theoretical frameworks have been offered to better explain the phenomenon of homelessness in particular homeless subgroups (veterans, single mothers, substance abusers, domestic violence victims, adolescents, etc.).

These research studies have expanded the base of nursing knowledge through examining areas unique to this population, such as the relationship of early childhood trauma and abuse to adult homelessness; identification of the stressors and coping behaviors of individuals (adults, mothers, and children) who are homeless; identification of the personal strengths of the homeless; and identification of the meaning and value of pets for the homeless. Through these studies unique factors impacting the physical, mental, and spiritual health of subsets of the homeless have been identified and nursing interventions proposed to utilize this new knowledge in addressing their health issues. Nurse researchers have also been active in developing mechanisms to include the homeless and their nursing care needs in nursing school curricula through service learning projects, faculty-managed care centers, and clinical homeless shelter rotations (Wilk, 1999).

New research instruments have also been used in studies with the homeless. Some have been adapted and validated for use with the general homeless population and others developed and validated specifically for use with subgroups of this population, such as homeless sheltered women (Hogenmiller, 2004).

In the future, nursing research related to the health of the homeless will expand on current new directions to include: (a) identification of how to incorporate preventive health activities for individuals in the homeless state, (b) empowering the homeless to become competent health care consumers, (c) identification of the unique elements and health care needs of second-generation homeless, (d) identification of a continuum of health care strategies for individuals with recurrent homeless episodes, and (e) development of cost-analyses and cost sharing models with other health care institutions to provide needed health care that is cost effective.

MARY J. MCNAMEE

Homelessness

The phenomenon of homelessness is multidimensional with macro (health policy), meso (health care systems), and micro (individual) structural mechanisms. Homelessness is not a random event that occurs to families and individuals outside the context of their lives and personal history. Epidemiological medicine and social researchers continue to amass a body of literature whose focus is the identification and description of individual risk factors that are correlated with homelessness. These studies have documented the rates of mental illness, substance abuse, experiences of childhood physical and sexual violence, and experiences of abuse and neglect (Bauman, 1993). This work has promoted the humanization of homeless people through its descriptive distinctions between the various subgroups within this population. However, focusing on individual-level risk factors, in describing who is at risk for becoming or remaining homeless is only part of the picture.

Contemporary analyses have looked at the interaction of individual and structural factors that contribute to homelessness. This approach continues to be informed by a simple, sequential causal relationship. What needs to be considered at this point in time is a model that stresses the myriad ways in which factors on the macro, meso, and micro levels interact in the formation of various pathways into homelessness. Researchers have pointed out that structural factors are heightened when there are fewer housing subsidies and the gap between median rents and median income is relatively wide. These structural factors in conjunction with individual factors such as gender, race, history of childhood or adult abuse, substance abuse, and the level of social support, contribute to a complex interplay exerting a dominant effect on homelessness (Ringwalt, Greene, Robertson, & McPheetes, 1998).

The life of a homeless person holds more uncertainty than its poverty. Homeless people are marginalized within the marginalization of poverty (Hall, J. M., Stevens, & Meleis, 1994). There are more labels for homeless people than for segments of mainstream America. There is fringe homeless, long-term homeless, temporary homeless, emergency homeless, visibly homeless, and invisibly homeless. Within all of these categories there are different groups of homeless: single women never married without children, single women who are pregnant and underage, divorced women with children, single unmarried women with children, single men, divorced men with children, divorced men without children, families with children, runaways (minor children), adolescents, throwaways (children whose parents have told them to leave home and never return), lesbian and gay youth, transgender youth and adults, elderly, disabled, handicapped, veterans homeless, impoverished, immigrants, and illegal aliens. In addition to the aforementioned categories, there are homeless who have been evicted or those who are addicted to substances; there are homeless who are mentally ill; those who are homeless because of domestic violence and/or abusive family situations; and those who are homeless because of release from incarceration without transitional support mechanisms in place. When considering all of the above categories of homelessness, how then does a generally accepted definition of "homeless" result? The National Coalition for the Homeless (2002) reports a definition according to the Stewart B. McKinney Act, 42 U.S.C. § 11301, et seq. (1994),

> . . . a person is considered homeless who "lacks a fixed, regular, and adequate nighttime residence, and has a primary nighttime residency that is: (a) a supervised publicly or privately operated shelter designed to provide temporary living accommodations . . . (b) an institution that provides a temporary residence for individuals in-

> tended to be institutionalized, or (c) a public or private place not designed for, or ordinarily used as, a regular sleeping accommodation for human beings." 42 U.S.C. § 11302(a) The term "homeless individual' does not include any individual imprisoned or otherwise detained pursuant to an Act of Congress or a state law." 42 U.S.C. § 11302(c).

People experiencing homelessness in rural areas are less likely to live on the street or in shelters, and more likely to be "couch surfing," living with relatives or friends in overcrowded or substandard housing. Although homeless people are heterogeneous, while experiencing homelessness they do have certain shared basic biopsychosocial needs, such as affordable housing, adequate incomes, mental and physical health care, and possible substance abuse treatment. All of these needs must be met to prevent and end homelessness.

An ongoing dilemma is estimating how many people are homeless. There are several national estimates, many of which are based on dated information. No one estimate is a definitive representation of an accurate count but only the best approximation. In 2000, the Urban Institute found that there were approximately 3.5 million people, 1.35 million of them children, who probably have or will experience homelessness in any given year (O'Sullivan, 2003).

Baumann (1993) reported that the research on homelessness could be divided into three levels of analysis. The first focus was on the individual with numerous biopsychosocial issues, disaffiliated, disabled, mentally ill and addicted, and living in a shelter. The second level focused on homelessness in the context of the person's environment and the third level of inquiry defined homelessness as economic dislocation related to housing shortages. A significant amount of research focused on specific homeless populations such as those with mental illnesses and disaffiliated by society (McCarthy, D., Argeriou, Huebner, & Lubran, 1991).

Within the rise of the trajectory into homelessness there is a rapidly growing increase in the number of homeless elders. This can be attributed to their vulnerability to poverty and undertreated mental illness, accelerating a course of nursing home placement and/or early death. Women have become a major segment of the homeless population, with access to health care a major issue. Lim and colleagues (2001) conducted a study interviewing 974 homeless women in 78 homeless shelters and soup lines in Los Angeles County. Using multivariate analyses, the key enabling factors associated with improved health care access were having health insurance and a regular source of health care.

Families are the fastest-growing segment of the homeless population representing diverse backgrounds. Most are female-headed single-parent households with mounting incidences of violence, abuse, and neglect. Numerous researchers reported the intense stress and adverse effects that homelessness has on a child's development, health, behavior, and academic success.

Research pertaining to homeless adolescents incorporated biopsychosocial, cultural, and spiritual health problems in addition to the homeless adolescent's propensity for engaging in delinquent or maladaptive social and health behaviors. Concepts such as risk, resiliency, and connectedness were found to be critical for survival, supported by the creation of peer communities or street families (Ensign & Gittelsohn, 1998; Jezewski, 1995; O'Sullivan, 2003; Rew, Taylor-Seehafter, Thomas, & Yockey, 2001).

Nursing research, education, and practice have philosophical foundations in advocating and facilitating health care for marginalized and vulnerable populations. In light of the increasing number of groups of homeless people and the known biopsychosocial outcomes of homelessness, intervention research is needed not only to prevent the trajectory of homelessness but also to develop programs and educate health care providers to the specific concerns of the homeless. Nursing research and advocacy as a course of action is essential on the macro, meso, and micro levels.

JOANNE O'SULLIVAN

Homelessness and Related Mood Disorders

The causes of homelessness are complex, and mental illness and related mood disorders add additional layers of difficulties. Approximately 25% of the homeless population suffers from some serious mental illness (Kusmer, 2002). Many homeless suffer from common mental illnesses such as depression, psychotic disorders, substance abuse, and personality disorders. In addition, the population of homeless is very diverse including all ethnic groups, usually ranging in age between 30 to 50 years of age, unmarried, unemployed, with the largest segment of the population being women (Martens, 2002).

Two growing trends are increasingly responsible for the rise in homelessness over the past 20 years: the growing shortage of affordable rental housing and a simultaneous increase in poverty (National Coalition for Homeless, 2005). In 1998, the U.S. Conference of Mayor's survey of homelessness in 30 cities found that children under the age of 18 years accounted for 25% of the urban homeless population. This same study found that unaccompanied minors comprised 3% of the urban homeless. Most studies of the homeless show that single adults are more likely to be male and comprise 45%, while 14% are single women (U.S. Conference of Mayors, 1998). Families with children are among the fastest-growing segments of the homeless population representing approximately 40% of people who become homeless (Shinn & Weitzman, 1996).

The homeless population varies demographically according to location. The U.S. Conference of Mayors (1998) found that 49% are African Americans, 32% Caucasian American, 12% Hispanic, 4% Native American, and 3% Asian American. Approximately 22% of the homeless population left their last place of residence because of domestic violence (Homes for the Homeless, 1998).

The homeless population commonly identified the usual signs of mood disorders such as: ongoing sadness, anxiety, lack of energy, loss of interest in ordinary activities, sleep problems, excessive weight loss or gain, physical aches and pains, difficulty concentrating, hopelessness, and thoughts of suicide and death (McMurray-Avila, 1997). One of the identified mood disorders, depression, is the most treatable of all mental illnesses. About 60%–80% of depressed people can be successfully treated outside the hospital with psychotherapy alone or with specific drugs. Unfortunately, most drug therapies, if needed, take at least 6 to 19 weeks before there are real signs of improvement. There is a reluctance to receive drug treatment due to side effects of the drugs (McMurray-Avila) and the continuing stigma of mental illness in our society.

Advocacy is critical to ending homelessness. Advocacy means working with the homeless to bring about positive changes in policies and programs on the local, state, and federal levels. Breaking the cycle of homelessness and related mood disorders also requires eliminating some of the obstacles to receiving medical care that the homeless face. Obstacles for the homeless include: a lack of awareness of services available, lack of financial resources and health insurance, language or cultural barriers, poor attitudes of some providers of services, lack of transportation, difficulty scheduling and keeping appointments, fear and distrust of institutions, and fragmented community services (Kusmer, 2002).

On the bright side, organizations which offer information and assistance with depression and treatment include: The National Institute of Mental Health Depression Awareness, Recognition, and Treatment Program (2003); the National Depressive and Manic-

Depressive Association (2003); the National Alliance for the Mentally Ill (2003) and its branch organizations available in each state; and the National Mental Health Association (2003) which publishes information on a variety of mental health issues. In addition, the President's New Freedom Commission on Mental Health (2003) clearly identified goals needed to transform mental health care in the United States, which in turn should decrease the number of homeless with mental illness when implemented.

There is a paucity of nursing research linking the role that professional nurses play as advocates in improving the care for homeless with mental illness and related mood disorders. Because primary health care for the homeless population is often provided by nurses, there is an excellent nursing opportunity to initiate helpful research in this area as well as assist those with mental illness to get care so that they may function at a higher level in our society.

Interventions are those successful actions taken to attempt to break the cycle of homelessness. Project Achieve (www.homelessness.net, 2003) attacked the cycle of homelessness for families and individuals with information resources described on their web site. This web site lists access to social services and emergency shelters to meet basic needs, services to prepare individuals for successful independent living, and case-management services sites to provide counseling, assistance with employment, and housing placement. This kind of web site assistance could be provided regionally throughout the country, educating health professionals and others who lack the knowledge of available resources. Another valuable resource is a listing of available grant money on this web site that can be used to develop additional programs to better meet the needs of the homeless.

The strengthening of the family unit of individuals with chronic mental illness is an important need revealed by community-based case management programs. This was a longitudinal study of family support among homeless mentally ill in community-based housing programs (Wood, P., Harbert, Hough, & Hotstetter, 1998). This study was one of the first to look at the strength of homeless family relationships over time. As contact with family members increased, so did their mental health as did greater satisfaction in their relationships and housing.

The most useful strategies for professionals working with homeless mentally ill individuals and families include: setting a tone of respect using observational, listening, and interviewing skills that quickly identify problems; locating existing resources; making timely and appropriate referrals; and functioning as an advocate when needed (Williams, 1994).

There has been a slow increase in research targeting the problems and needs of the homeless over the past decade. However, in the field of nursing there continues to be a paucity of research related to the important roles that professional nurses can play and the interventions they could use to provide care for the homeless chronically mentally ill. Research is needed on the nature of the relationship between homelessness and related mental disorders such as depression and related mood disorders. The etiology of homelessness needs studies which include demographics comparing national, cultural, psychosocial, genetic, and neurobiological determinants of specific homeless populations. Other studies might explore the impact of urban versus rural environments on person vulnerable to homelessness. Both qualitative and quantitative nursing research cojoined with the research done by other disciplines is essential to clearly document the important role and interventions already used in practice by the professional nurse in providing care to the mentally ill individuals and their families.

ALICE R. KEMPE

Hospice

Hospice research in the United States began with studies of the differences between hospice care and care received in traditional settings for the terminally ill. Although these studies examined the impact of care provided by hospice, largely nursing care, such studies were not nursing research. In Canada, Mary Vachon, a U.S.-trained nurse, was invited by the palliative care team at the Royal Victoria Hospital in Montreal, Canada, to investigate stress in the caregivers who composed the palliative care team. Other researchers examined pain pathways, medications for pain, and the impact of music therapy. In England, Dame Cicely Saunders, trained as a physician, social worker, and nurse, and others examined the impact of medications for symptom relief. These early studies had as their focus the improvement of care of the dying and, in the United States, the evaluation of whether hospice care improved such care and was fiscally sound so as to be worthy of a new benefit to fund such care. These studies were conducted by researchers from a number of disciplines.

Nursing research about hospice has been conducted using a variety of methodological approaches including qualitative ones: ethnography, observations, semi-structured interviews, and interviews; and quantitative ones: quasi-experimental, questionnaires/surveys, and audit; as well as a combination of methods. Research about hospice covers an array of topics. Topics include organizational methodologies, demographic data, social support, physiological, psychosocial, and spiritual issues, self-care, how patients spend their time, grief, bereavement, studies of nurses and their knowledge, and the impact of hospice care. Some of these topics use hospice for a setting for research but are not about hospice per se. Topics for such studies include an examination of cancer pain in home hospice patients, a comparison of nurses' knowledge about AIDS by practice setting, training, and educational programs where the focus is the program and not the hospice patients and nurses, and the grief experience of older women. In this case, the husbands had received hospice care but that was not the focus of the study. Indeed the researcher suggested that a future study might compare the experience of women whose husbands had received such care and those who had not (Jacob, 1996). A similar study in Finland examined the adjustment of relatives after the death of a hospice patient. Again the focus was on the adjustment and not the differential impact of the hospice program on such adjustment.

In an attempt to validate the impact of a hospice palliative-care unit on perceived family satisfaction, and to examine the demographics of patients, Kellar, Martinez, Finis, Bolgar, and von Gunten (1996) surveyed 240 families of patients of the program. The most frequent response to an opened-ended question about the advantage of the program was the professional nursing care. Few remarks were made about disadvantages and these had to do with parking-facility expenses, the distance families had to travel, and the potential for patient transfer due to the facility's designation as an acute-care facility. Of the 92 eligible surveys returned, the researchers found that 88% (81/92) considered the hospice to be very helpful to the patient, 9% (8/92) found the program to be helpful, and 1% (1/92) were neutral. This type of study is representative of a host of studies conducted by hospice programs to assess their audience and the satisfaction with the program.

Hospice referral remains crucial to the viability of such programs. While interest is usually expressed in the attitudes of physicians, Schim, Jackson, Seely, Gruinow, and Baker (2000) examined the attitudes of home care nurses to hospice referral. Attitudes of 160 nurses were assessed with a 15 item survey. Surveys were completed by 75 nurses for a response rate of 46.9%. Home care nurses saw little difference between home care and hospice services. Many (42.6%) of the respondents thought insurance with a hospice benefit was necessary for referral. These and other misperceptions underscored the importance of home care nurses understanding the requirements and components of hospice care.

The importance of attitudes as well as knowledge was underscored by a study investigating the factors that increased the likelihood that nurses would discuss terminal illness care and hospice care with patients and families. Cramer, McCorkle, Cherlin, Johnson-Hurzeler, and Bradley (2003) found that prior experience with hospice, greater knowledge, and religiosity, as well as greater comfort in initiating such discussions, were related to their initiation by nurses.

Another example of program-related research is a study on patient-focused menu planning (Fairtlough & Closs, 1996). Over a 4-week period, 108 interviews were conducted related to specific meals. Foods not liked included those difficult to swallow, tough or fried foods, or those with bones. Patients indicated they wanted seafood including salmon and prawns, beef, Yorkshire puddings, yoghurt, eggs, fruit juices, and beer. Three major comments concerned the size of the portions (too large), foods not the right temperature (not hot enough), and the time of food service (preferred later in the day). This study, although used to help nurses understand the research process, had an impact on patient care in the facility where the research was conducted. Although not commented on by the authors, it would be helpful in future research if a larger sample of patients were included in the study where closeness to death was taken into account in examining food preferences of hospice care recipients.

The needs of family caregivers also have been of concern to hospice providers. V. Harrington, Lackey, and Gates (1996) studied the needs of caregivers of both hospice and clinic patients. Results indicated that the top information need required by caregivers of clinic patients was for honest and updated information and specifically information regarding treatment side effects. In contrast, the information needs of hospice caregivers concerned the symptoms to be expected. These represent the differences in the point in the illness trajectory of the two sets of patients. Spiritual needs were the second most frequently noted for both groups. Personal needs included the need for adequate rest for both groups of family caregivers, but these were not considered to be as important by the family caregivers as the needs for care of the patient. The authors recommend a longitudinal study on this subject.

The congruence between patient and caregiver reports of symptom intensity was examined by McMillan and Moody (2003). The symptom intensity of pain, dyspnea, and constipation were evaluated by both patients and their family caregivers. Symptom intensity of all three symptoms were significantly overestimated by caregivers ($p = .000$). This overestimation is the basis upon which hospice nurses base their clinical decisions. The authors note that this study has implications for the education of hospice family caregivers.

Perceptions of the intensity of symptoms by nurses might be expected to be closer to those of their patients than was true for family caregivers. In a study by Rhodes, McDaniel, and Matthews (1998), 53 hospice patients, mean age 69 years, were queried about their symptom experience with the Adapted Symptom Distress Scale Form 2 (ASDS-2). The nurses were also questioned about their patients' symptom experience. Like the informal caregivers, the nurses in this study overestimated the symptom intensity of their patients. The authors note that this is congruent with some other findings of overestimation but conflicted with findings of underestimation, particularly with regard to perceptions of pain. Indeed, McMillan (1996) demonstrated that pain was still not well managed in cancer patients. The importance of the instrument as a reliable means of assessing symptoms resulted in the incorporation of the ASDS-2 into the clinical practice of the nurses.

Quality of life (QOL) is an important concept in health care. N. Hill (2002) examined both the measurement of QOL and how it might be improved in hospice patients. This study, like the previous one, underscored the importance of nurses understanding how the patient assessed aspects of QOL. This knowledge was a guide to the reflective practice of the nurse and assured clinically significant improvements of care for the patient.

In an exploration of the context for care, Rasmussen and Sandman (1998) investigated how patients in an oncology unit and in hospice spend their time. It was found that family members and nurses spend more time with patients in hospice than in oncology units but the time nurses spend is concerned with "tasks." If hospice nurses increased their time with patients due to the increased need for tasks, then the context has had little effect on the type of caregiving. The authors note the importance of time spent "being with" patients, not only in "doing for" patients.

The time devoted solely to tasks raises the question of whether death anxiety is a significant factor in hospice nurses. Payne, Dean, and Kalus (1998) examined death anxiety in hospice and emergency nurses and found that the latter had higher death anxiety and less support from their peers and supervisors. In another study, support was also deemed to be significant for hospice nurses if they were not engaging in blocking behaviors when confronted with the emotions of patients (Booth, Maguire, Behir, Butterworth, & Hillier, 1996). Research demonstrating the interest and need for advanced education for hospice nurses had the additional benefit of providing information to nurses interested in hospice as a career (Wright, D., 2001). Death anxiety can be reduced for student nurses through educational experiences, as Mallory (2003) demonstrated.

The bottom line question for patients and families is whether hospice has a positive impact on quality of life. Using the Hospice Care Performance Inventory, Yeung, French, and Leung (1999) identified six issues in which patient expectations and effectiveness of care were not congruent. Maximization of self-care and mobility were the two issues with the greatest discrepancy. Patients preferred to do their own self-care rather than have it done to them. Another patient priority included dispelling fear of death which, given that this was investigated with a Chinese population where it is considered a forbidden topic of conversation, is a challenge. Other patient priorities identified included gaining enough sleep, willingness to listen and give reassurances, and providing a satisfying diet. Interestingly, pain relief was not a high priority for patients. Not only does an approach such as this measure the discrepancy between patient expectations and effectiveness of care, it also has the potential to evaluate the impact of hospice care for patients.

Another example of research that examined the impact of hospice care was that by Kabel and Roberts (2003), who examined how the philosophy of hospice providers influences their perceptions of patient personhood. Specifically, this qualitative study examined how hospice staff at two hospice facilities in northwest England approached "normalizing" the symptoms of terminal illness. "Special" patients were found to be related to support of personhood of all patients although the "special patients" were perceived to receive no preferential treatment. In fact, "special" patients were found to have a positive impact on the caregivers.

As noted, much hospice research has examined the impact of hospice on costs, an early concern of government officials when the development of a hospice benefit was being considered. The coming of age of hospice is indicated by the focus on enhancing hospice access and focusing on the quality of remaining life of hospice patients as well as the quality of care received. Research is crucial to assuring that hospice care is all that it purports to be.

INGE B. CORLESS

Hydration and Dehydration in Older Adults

Hydration is the chemical combination of a substance with water, the addition of water to a substance or tissue (Taber's Cyclopedic Medical Dictionary, 1997, p. 920). Water is essential to sustain all cellular function (Chernoff, 1999). The percentage of water in older adults is approximately 60%. Clinicians contend that by promoting sufficient quantity and quality of fluids, especially water, fluid balance will more likely be achieved. Dehydration is the rapid weight loss of greater than 3% of body weight (Weinberg, A. D., &

Minaker, 1995, p. 1553). Clinical symptoms of dehydration may be absent in older adults, until the condition warrants immediate hospitalization and intravenous replacement fluids (Weinberg & Minaker). Symptoms include change in mental status, confusion, lethargy, tachycardia, and syncope. Assessing skin turgor and dry mouth, a diagnostic marker of dehydration in middle-aged adults, is unreliable for detection of dehydration in older adults because of common age-related changes. Skin turgor may already be poor because of decreased subcutaneous tissue, while dry mouth may be due to mouth-breathing or lack of oral care.

Dehydration is one of the top 10 reasons for hospitalization of older adults (Centers for Disease Control [CDC], 2002). In 1996, the hospitalization of older people with the primary diagnosis of dehydration cost $1.36 billion Medicare dollars (Burger, Kayser-Jones, & Bell, 2000). Older adults with a primary hospital admission diagnosis of dehydration are three times more likely to die within 30 days of admission compared to those with a primary admission diagnosis of a hip fracture (CDC). Managing hydration status to increase oral fluid intake in older people may reduce the number of hospitalizations and deaths associated with dehydration (Burger, Kayser-Jones, & Bell).

The prevalence of dehydration in the nursing home is not easily tracked, but it is thought to be significantly higher than among community-dwellers because of nursing home residents' comorbidites, polypharmacy, declining functional and cognitive status, insufficient oral fluid intake (OFI), and dependence on scarce staff and the institutional food delivery system. Estimated prevalence of dehydration among Skilled Nursing Facility (SNF) residents is 35% or higher (Weinberg & Minaker, 1995). Of those SNF residents with dehydration, mortality rates are as high as 50% (Wakefield, Mentes, Diggelmann, & Culp, 2002). Yet, in many cases, dehydration of nursing home residents is reversible and preventable.

Across all settings, older adults are at risk for insufficient hydration and for dehydration for the following major reasons:

1. Older adults sustain lower *baseline* TBW (total body water). Episodic illnesses such as diarrhea, nausea accompanied by vomiting, and fever result in even lower TBW. Depletion of as little as 1 to 2 liters of water can create a state of dehydration in an older adult. Infants and young children dehydrate for the same reason—lower baseline TBW. With decreased TBW, hypernatremia or hyponatremia become a potential electrolyte problem.
2. Thirst response is diminished in older adults. As TBW drops below 1 liter, older adults may not experience thirst as a prompt to drink fluids due to changes in baroreceptors, decreases in vasopressin, and antidiuretic hormone (ADH) (Phillips, P. A., et al., 1984).
3. Decreased reserve capacity, especially in renal function and creatinine clearance, and slower response to illness and stressors create a more delicate homeostatic balance. Thus, it takes a lesser body stressor to fuel a crisis in an older adult than would be necessary to similarly affect a middle-aged adult. The older adult's ability to recover is also extended beyond that which would be expected in a middle-aged adult.
4. Older adults limit their fluid intake for convenience, especially if incontinence is present (Gaspar, 1999). For some individuals, the embarrassment of incontinence may outweigh the health benefit of drinking water or other fluids. In addition, disease states, such as diabetes or congestive heart failure, could place the older adult's fluid balance at risk for imbalance (Weinberg & Minaker, 1995).

Preventively, evaluating OFI and laboratory values over time may be useful in detecting insufficient hydration in older adults. Older people generally fail to drink sufficient amounts of fluids. The recommended older adult OFI is a minimum of 1.5 L of liquid over 24 hours (Chernoff, 1999). Thirty milliliters per kilogram of body weight has also been used as a parameter to estimate the adequacy of daily fluid intake (Chernoff). Laboratory tests include: blood urea nitrogen/creatinine ratio (BUN/Cr), sodium, plasma specific gravity, and serum osmolality (Weinberg & Minaker, 1995). Bioelectric impedance analysis (BIA), a noninvasive method using electrodes to measure body compartments including intracellular, extracellular, and TBW, has been used to detect fluid balance (Chumlea & Guo, 1994; Robinson, S. B., & Rosher, 2002). Urine color charts have also been used and show correlation with some laboratory tests (Wakefield et al., 2002). Yet further research needs to be conducted to study sensitivity and specificity of tests to detect varying degrees of hydration status, from adequate hydration to mild-moderate-acute dehydration.

Prevention of dehydration in the most vulnerable group—nursing home residents—needs to be studied empirically. Two recent evidence-based studies provide findings to support specific effective protocols.

S. F. Simmons, Alessi, and Schnelle (2001) tested a three-phase 8-month intervention on 63 nursing home residents. They used three behavioral approaches to improve residents' hydration status: (a) prompting (four times/day for 16 weeks), (b) increased prompting (eight times/day for 8 weeks), and (c) increased prompting plus offering choice of beverage each day for 8 weeks. Eighty-eight percent of the sample was mildly or moderately dehydrated at baseline. OFI, serum osmolality, and BUN/cr ratio laboratory tests were measured before, during, and after each phase of the intervention. Eighty-one percent of the intervention group showed significant increases in between-meal oral fluid intake (OFI). Serum osmolality and BUN/Cr ratios in dehydrated residents significantly improved compared with the control group. A behavioral approach that combines consistent and frequent prompting and giving nursing home residents choices of beverage can support an effective hydration program which may improve hydration status.

Robinson and Rosher (2002) demonstrated that using a beverage cart in nursing home residents ($N = 51$) improved OFI and was associated with reduced use of laxatives, improved bowel function, and fewer falls. They based their hydration program on suggestions of Zembrzuski (1997) and T. Welch (1998) to use beverage carts, provide appealing fluids, offer choice of beverage, and use containers with visual appeal. Four types of between-meal fluids were displayed on a beverage cart along with colorful glassware and seasonal decorations. Nursing home residents were assisted by two hired Certified Nurses Aides (CNAs) to consume an additional 480 cc daily over 5 weeks. Use of BIA showed that at the end of the intervention, the residents' TBW increased significantly ($p = .001$), laxative use decreased significantly ($p = .05$), falls declined ($p = .05$), and number of bowel movements increased ($p = .04$). Robinson and Rosher concluded by recommending beverage cart service at mid-morning and mid-afternoon. Application of this research suggests that offering 480 cc total of between-meal fluids to nursing home residents can make a clinical as well as statistically significant difference in their hydration status.

Increasing OFI of older adults can prevent dehydration and unnecessary hospitalizations. Assessment and early-detection screening tools and empirically supported hydration programs are needed.

Cora D. Zembrzuski

Hypertension

Hypertension is the term applied to sustained and elevated levels of systolic and/or diastolic blood pressure. The exact level at which hypertension poses a health risk has been arbitrarily and continually redefined; however, the importance of hypertension is based on a rational association between sustained, elevated levels of arterial pressure and the probability of increased risk for morbidity and mortality from cardiovascular disease. The Joint National Committee on Prevention, Detection, Evaluation, and Treatment of High Blood Pressure defined hypertension as systolic blood pressure ≥ 140 mm Hg and/or diastolic blood pressure ≥ 90 mm Hg or taking antihypertensive medication (Chobanian et al., 2003). The committee classified blood pressure into three categories and introduced the prehypertensive category for use in medical diagnosis, evaluation, and treatment (see Table 1).

Sustained and elevated systolic blood pressure is now considered to be as crucial a measure as the diastolic level in evaluating the risks for cardiovascular disease. Elevated systolic blood pressure accompanied by normal diastolic levels, known as isolated systolic hypertension, is common in older populations. Primary hypertension, formerly known as essential hypertension, occurs in as many as 95% of all individuals with high blood pressure, as opposed to secondary hypertension, which is due to an identifiable and usually treatable cause (Kaplan, N. M., 1994).

Hypertension affects approximately 50 million Americans, a major portion of the U.S. adult population. In the 1999–2000 National Health and Nutrition Examination Survey (NHANES III), 33.5% of non-Hispanic Blacks, 28.9% of non-Hispanic Whites, and 20.7% of Mexican Americans had hypertension (Hajjar & Kotchen, 2003). Two thirds of hypertensive individuals were aware of their condition, and 58.4% reported being on drug therapy. Among Mexican Americans, 40.3% of the hypertensive individuals were under treatment, but only 17.7% of all Mexican-American hypertensive individuals had controlled blood pressures, compared to 28.1% and 33.4% of the non-Hispanic Black and White populations, respectively, with controlled blood pressures. Given equal access to therapy, Black Americans, who are among the most affected population group, achieve less blood pressure reductions.

TABLE 1 Classification of Blood Pressure for Adults Age 18 Years and Older

Category	Systolic (mm Hg)	Diastolic (mm Hg)
Normal	< 120	and < 80
Prehypertenisve	120–139	or 80–89
Hypertension		
Stage 1	140–159	or 90–99
Stage 2	≥ 160	or ≥ 100

Hypertension increases with age, is more common in Blacks, and is more prevalent among lower socioeconomic populations. Hypertension has a higher prevalence in men throughout young adulthood to middle age. Thereafter, the prevalence in women rises above that of men. The highest rates among women are found in non-Hispanic Black women and among men in non-Hispanic Black men.

In the 2003 report, the Joint National Committee (JNC) on Prevention, Detection, and Evaluation of High Blood Pressure amended the standards for clinical classification of adult patients with high blood pressure. The new classification (Table 1) differs in several ways from that published in 1997. A new clinical category has been added: prehypertension which is not a disease category; also there are now two instead of three stages in the hypertension category.

Hypertension seldom exists in isolation but most often occurs with other risk factors that increase the probability for cardiovascular disease. Factors commonly associated with hypertension that are nonmodifiable include low birth weight, older age, family history of high blood pressure, and history of diabetes mellitus, coronary heart disease, stroke, or end-stage renal disease. Modifiable confounders include smoking, alcohol consumption, high saturated dietary fats, excess dietary sodium, adiposity, and a sedentary lifestyle, as well as recreational and over-the-counter drugs. In addition, psychosocial and environmental factors create life stressors that may influence hypertension as well as care and management. Target-organ disease as a consequence of sustained, uncontrolled elevated blood pressure includes arteriosclerosis, heart failure, transient ischemic attacks (TIA), stroke, peripheral vascular disease, aneurysm, and end-stage renal disease. Currently, researchers have identified several emerging cardiovascular risk markers such as high-sensitivity C-reactive protein (Blake, Rifai, Buring, & Ridker, 2003) and homocysteine (Lim & Cassano, 2002).

Hypertension is a major independent risk factor for coronary artery disease and stroke, the first and third causes of mortality in the United States, respectively, yet its importance is not emphasized satisfactorily in research and practice. The individuals hardest to reach and at the highest risk are often not in care or are uninsured. Medical and behavioral intervention approaches lack cohesiveness and cultural relevance, therefore failing to achieve the strength of their impact as a combined intervention. Additional research is required to evaluate multidisciplinary strategies with a team approach to increase entry into care, remaining in care, and long-term compliance with prevention and treatment recommendations. Research also is needed to increase understanding of cost-benefit of interventions and the effects of self-monitoring and titration, including pharmacological vacations. Identifying markers for early detection continues to be a challenge, and research should focus on exploring biochemical and genotypic methods to define and classify the population at risk.

The ultimate goal for treatment is to prevent morbidity and mortality by the least intrusive means. The treatment regimen is determined by evaluating the severity of the blood pressure elevation, the presence of target-organ disease, and the effects of other coexisting risk factors. The inability to adhere to treatment recommendations is a major barrier in attaining and maintaining goal blood pressure levels in long-term management, evidencing the need for planned patient education programs. Traditional treatment strategies targeted to the general population lack cultural sensitivity, neglect active involvement of the patient in decision making, and fail to motivate and keep the patient in care. More individually oriented treatment methodologies that address the patients' concerns, including their social support system, employment status, health insurance, and barriers in daily life to meeting compliance goals, are required. Nursing can provide the training, education, and support to design planned health programs to increase the efficacy of interventions and improve overall compliance.

Lifestyle modification, formerly termed nonpharmacological therapy, includes interventions targeted toward healthier lifestyles and reducing the risks for cardiovascular complications at the family, community, and population levels. Lifestyle modifications for blood pressure control include reduction in weight, adoption of the Dietary Approaches to Stop Hypertension (DASH) eating plan, adequate physical activity, dietary decreases in sodium, and moderation of alcohol consumption. Smoking, although not directly related to hypertension, is a major cardiovascular risk and should be avoided.

Nonpharmacological therapy for treatment of hypertension is an evolving strategy in line with the objectives of *Healthy People 2010* (Healthy People 2010). It represents a prevention area ideally suited for nursing practice and research. Public-health prevention strategies focusing on lifestyle modification at the community and practice setting will help achieve an overall downward shift in the distribution of blood pressure levels in the general population. Interventions should target high dietary sodium, fats, alcohol, and low intake of potassium, as well as physical inactivity. Although these intervention strategies show promise in prevention of high blood pressure, societal barriers, such as the lack of satisfactory food substitutes, lack of access to care, and absence of economic resources, constrain compliance and achievement of intervention goals. Moreover, further research should focus on patient-oriented outcomes that affect patients' well-being such as sexual functioning, ability to sustain family and social tasks, and ability to carry out activity of daily livings.

Martha N. Hill
Susan Dale Tannenbaum
Updated by Ali Salman

I

Immigrant Women

Immigration is a process of movement of people from one country to another. Immigrants experience a transition that begins with preparation for immigration and includes the act of immigrating, the process of settling in, and over time, identity transformation. Throughout this transition process, individuals and families experience both euphoric and highly stressed responses. These experiences increase the vulnerability of immigrating populations to health risks. The effects of marginalization and barriers to health care access, resources, and support are magnified for immigrant women.

The uniqueness of women's health care needs is well established and has led to several women's health care centers. Immigrant women share unique characteristics that require special gender-sensitive research and clinical efforts. Immigrant women share the vulnerabilities and the marginalization of minority women in general. Immigrant women face constraints associated with being new in the United States, such as language, transportation, and role overload. Another constraint is maintaining home country heritage and developing new values and beliefs to integrate themselves and their families into the host culture. Although most studies of immigrant women focus on groups with gender inequality, there is some evidence that even women from groups without gender inequality experience more psychological distress and have different sources of distress than their male counterparts (Aroian, Norris, & Chiang, 2003). These variables influence immigrant women's health and health care, and many of the variables have not been adequately studied.

Foreign-born or immigrant women tend to work in environments that increase their health risks. They are more likely to work at home or in family businesses that provide them with limited benefits. When employed outside the home, they often work in low-income jobs such as work in garment shops or domestic work. Women often accompany male family members in immigrating to the United States rather than obtaining their own visas. Therefore, their status is insecure, and they are more vulnerable and less likely to disclose battering, harassment, or abuse.

A nursing perspective focusing on immigrant women and their health includes research on gender and health, culturally influenced explanatory models of illness, transitions and health, and marginalization and health (Aroian, 2001; Meleis, 1995; Meleis, Lipson, Muecke, & Smith, 1998). Immigrant women's gender relates to their ability to access and receive quality care. They are expected not only to cook, do housework, care for children, and often to contribute income but also to act as family mediators and culture brokers. Health care professionals have limited knowledge of the demands and the nature of immigrant women's multiple roles and their health care needs, nor has research adequately uncovered the contextual conditions that influence their health-seeking strategies, the nature of their illnesses, and compliance with treatment (Anderson, J., 1991b). How immigrant women express their symptoms and what meaning they attach to health care encounters also determine their health outcomes. Describing their explanatory models of illness may improve provision of care and ultimately their health (Reizian & Meleis, 1987).

Conceptualization of immigration as a transition allows researchers to focus on the process, timing, and critical points in the process of becoming an American. Lipson (1993) described the traumatic experiences of Afghan refugees before leaving Afghanistan, during transit, and while settling in the United States. Knowledge of the traumatic experiences of the immigrants and refugees helped to explain their responses to the immigration transition and provided a context in which to identify their health care needs. During transitions there is loss of support and networks. In addition to these stressors, women in particular are expected to take responsibility for family health and to mediate between the demands of the new social structure and members of their families for health care, schools, and social services.

Several strategies have been developed to provide care for immigrant women. Some of the most effective models are groups that focus on women's strengths (Meleis, Omidian, & Lipson, 1993; Shepard & Faust, 1994), the use of cultural interpreters (Jezewski, 1993), and feminist participatory models, such as group discussion of dreams to deal with psychosocial issues (Thompson, J., 1991). However, there is a need for further research to capture the transition experiences of such neglected populations as women immigrants from South America, Eastern Europe, and the Middle East, as well as studies that address issues of language, symbolic interpretation, and cultural competence in health care. In particular, there is need to develop and test nursing interventions that decrease structural barriers to health care as well as those that support culturally appropriate preventive and health-promoting behaviors (Lipson & Meleis, 1999).

Future areas for scholarship include methods for defining populations, developing culturally competent research tools, using appropriate theoretical frameworks, and uncovering the critical markers in the transition process that render immigrants more vulnerable. Developing and testing culturally competent models of care is of top priority with the increasing diversity of populations and the backlash against women and immigrants.

AFAF IBRAHIM MELEIS
JULIENE G. LIPSON
UPDATED BY KAREN J. AROIAN

Individual Nursing Therapy

Nursing practice is becoming increasingly complex and diverse, and many changes have been noted by authors in psychiatric mental health nursing in recent years (Jones, 2003). Increasingly, mental health services are taking place in the community rather than in inpatient settings. As a result, contact time between nurses and clients has become limited. In discussing individual nursing therapy and nursing interventions on a one-to-one basis, one must move beyond the traditional parameters of individual therapy as first described by Peplau and consider brief psychotherapy and crisis intervention, case management, and even family interventions as crucial aspects of the nurse-client relationships. Today, with the emphasis on psychobiology in the cause and treatment of mental illness, the importance and relevance of individual nursing therapy is in question (Kraus, 2000; McCabe, S., 2002; Raingruber, 2003).

The cornerstone of psychiatric mental health nursing today is the therapeutic relationship. Peplau defined the therapeutic nurse-client relationship as the interpersonal process between professional nurse and the client (Peplau, H. E., 1952). In this process the nurse needs to establish trust, strive toward mutually established goals of the relationship, and focus the movement of the interpersonal process toward growth for the client (Gelazis & Coombe-Moore, 1993). Peplau described the nurse as the basic tool or resource for the betterment of the client.

Researchers have studied various aspects of Peplau's theory, including the phases of the nurse-client relationship (Forchuk, 1995), the various roles of the nurse studied by Morrison (1992) and concepts and constructs identified as important to nurses by Peplau (O'Toole & Welt, 1989). Forchuk et al., (2000) studied Peplau's theory and clarifies many aspects of the theory, including the assumptions, basic definitions, and relationships between the concepts. Future researchers need to continue the study of Peplau's interpersonal paradigm, for it is a rich source of knowledge about the therapeutic individual nurse-patient relationship and the interpersonal process as it is used and is relevant today.

Other nurse theorists based their own ideas and frameworks on Peplau's nurse-client relationship theory (Orlando, 1961; Travelbee, 1972). Theorists, such as King, have communication and interpersonal process as central to the theory (King, 1992). Some have studied aspects of therapeutic process, such as empathy (Evans, G., Wilt, Alligood, & O'Neil, 1998). Individual one-to-one nurse-client relationships continue to be highly important in psychiatric mental-health nursing. Much of nursing, both inpatient and outpatient, involves the nurse's ability to engage the client in interpersonal interactions. In recent years, however, as care is more profit-driven, the nurse-client relationship has undergone some changes. The fact that the client has much shorter contact with the nurse in inpatient settings due to short hospital stays means that the phases of the nurse-client relationship, which in the past had more time to develop, now must solidify within brief periods of time. Sometimes there are only a few days available and at times only hours for contact between nurse and patients (Vaughn, Webster, Orahood, & Young, 1995). The relevance of individual nursing therapy has been called into question by those who claim that giving the appropriate medication to the mentally ill person is the most important feature of care, thereby calling forth serious discussion of how psychiatric nurse clinical specialists should use their time (Raingruber, 2003). Complex mental illness seems to require more than a medical approach with medication. The recent success of dialectical behavioral therapy, DBT, with patients having this disorder suggests that more complex treatments are in order which blend various paradigms in treatment of mental illness (Perseius et al., 2003).

Brief therapies or short-term psychotherapies are time limited, have limited goals, and generally cost less than longer forms of therapy. Psychiatric nurses and particularly psychiatric nurse clinical specialists are well suited and prepared to use a brief psychotherapy model because their education and clinical experience prepares them well to use this form of therapy (Shires & Tappan, 1992). Brief therapy usually lasts for six to twelve sessions, but for clients with chronic problems the sessions may be spaced over a 3 to 6-month period (Wells, R., & Gionnetti, 1990). Visits tend to be shorter and may be from 15 to 30 minutes (Budman & Gurman, 1988). In brief therapy the therapist is usually quite active and can use techniques such as homework assignments to extend treatment (Shires & Tappan). Frequently therapeutic experiences occur in the community setting (Budman & Gurman). Nurses are usually knowledgeable regarding community resources and may work for community-based agencies.

The psychiatric mental-health nurse practicing in the community setting deals with chronically mentally ill clients both in long-term therapeutic relationships and in crisis situations. In this setting communication skills are even more important because trust needs to be established in a relatively short period of time. The nurse applying crisis intervention uses her assessment skills to the utmost and builds trust to have clients confide important information. For example, if the client is suicidal, trust is a highly important element to buy time for the client so that emergency services can be sent (Wheeler, 1993).

Another use of crisis intervention in individual nursing therapy is by the triage nurse in community mental-health nursing, who frequently deals with suicidal clients or clients who may be dangerous or threatening to others due to exacerbation of psychiatric symptoms (Wheeler, 1993). The nurse not only must communicate therapeutically with clients, but also with distraught families. The principles of individual therapy as outlined by Peplau must therefore be expanded to include family members and clients, all of whom may be in crisis at the time of contact (Gilliss, 1991). Some work has been done in this area, but nurse researchers need to continue to systematically study how the interpersonal process can be expanded to include family and others and how this process is therapeutic.

The psychiatric mental-health nurse is part of the community mental-health system and is able to help coordinate care of clients through the use of case management. Often the criticism of the care of the chronically mentally ill in the community is that care is fragmented and uncoordinated (Anthony, W. A., Cohen, Farkas, & Cohen, 2000). Research has shown that care-management services may be available to clients in the community, but that clients rarely take advantage of such services due to lack of knowledge or other reasons (Parson, 1999). Some researchers pointed out that case management can be the key to adjusting to the community for the chronically mentally ill because it provides a link for the client to the support services he or she needs (Forchuk & Brown, 1989). Forchuk recommends that an essential component of a case-management model is the establishment of a one-to-one relationship, which can be the basis for continued long-term care in the community. Thus Peplau's theory comes into play through its use in case management. The Peplau case-management model provides a framework for delivering nursing care and comprehensive care for the chronically mentally ill client (Forchuk & Brown).

In the demanding environment in which psychiatric mental-health nursing takes place today, the nurse must use basic skills in new applications. The individual therapy that nurses use is based on Peplau's interpersonal framework. This theory is still relevant and can be used in various forms of individual therapy, which include brief psychotherapy, crisis intervention, and case management. All of these frequently occur in community settings. Nurse researchers need to study the therapeutic process in various settings and time frames to establish the effectiveness of the nurse's interactions and interventions. The interpersonal framework and theory itself also would benefit from continued study and research, particularly because of the extreme emphasis today on the psychobiological aspects in the care of the mentally ill.

RAUDA GELAZIS

Infant Injury

Injuries are defined in two ways: (a) the physical damage to the body caused by the transfer of mechanical, chemical, or thermal energy (e.g., a broken bone, salicylate-related poisoning, or frostbite to a toe); and (b) as the event that caused the damage (e.g., motor vehicle crash, aspirin ingestion, or prolonged exposure to cold). When talking about unintentional injuries, it is still common to use the word accident as if unexpectedness or lack of intent were the primary feature of the injurious process. However, although the moment of occurrence of an injury may not be precisely known, its likelihood of occurring is usually predictable. If events are predictable, they are not called accidents; rather, the term injury is used.

It is crucial that those who study injury and collect injury data recognize that the term injury can refer both to the physical damage caused to the body and to the predictable causative event. In fact, the International Classification of Disease (ICD-10-CM) uses two separate systems to classify injuries. One is a set of physical damage codes (N-codes; e.g., humerus fracture); the other is a set of event codes (E-codes or External Cause of Injury Codes; e.g., fall on stairs). Together these two systems of classification provide a fuller picture of an injury episode than does either alone (knowing that an infant fell on stairs is important; knowing that the fall resulted in head trauma provides a more complete description.

Unintentional injuries are the principal cause of death in the United States for individuals from the newborn period, 29 days, to age 44 years. For infants in particular they represent the predominant cause of nonbirth-related death. Fatal injuries are usually recorded according to the events that cause them, such as the number of deaths from motor vehicle crashes or house fires; whereas nonfatal injuries usually have been reported by physical damage groups. This is because fatality data are derived from death certificates, which classify cause of death by circumstances and facilitate E-coding. Morbidity data generally are gathered from medical records and often are derived from N-coding.

National mortality data are routinely available from death certificate reviews. These vital statistics mortality data from 2001 show the principal causes of infant (under 1 year) injury death as suffocation, 16.41 deaths/100,000; homicide, 4.07 deaths/100,000; motor vehicle, 3.45 deaths/100,000; drowning, 1.69 deaths/100,000; fire and burns, 1.24 deaths/100,000; and other, 5.63 deaths/100,000 (Centers for Disease Control, 2003). Hospital discharge data from the State of California found that for infants 0 to 2 months of age the most frequent injury cause was falls from heights, not from furniture; for 3 to 5 months, battering; for 6 to 8 months, falls from furniture; and for 9 to 11 months, nonairway foreign bodies (Agran et al., 2003).

National data are not routinely available regarding the incidence of and associated risk factors for nonfatal injuries in infants, which means that most morbidity data by type of injury event are generated only by special studies. Siegel and colleagues (1996), investigating the association between maternal age and other risk factors for infants deaths in the state of Colorado from 1986 to 1992, found that rates peaked at a maternal age of 22 years for unintentional infant injury deaths. Among the unintentional injury deaths, more mothers had inadequate education, higher proportion of low-birthweight infants, more siblings in the family, and a higher proportion of interpartum intervals or less than 2 years.

Data from studies by Jordan, Dugan, and Hardy (1993) and O'Sullivan and Schwarz (2000) documented the nonfatal injury rate specifically for infants (< 15 months) of adolescent mothers as 15.7 and 16.3 per 100 children, respectively. Falls and burns were the two leading causes of injury in both studies. Additional studies on injury rates for infants through age 18 months of life also documented falls, burns, and ingestions as the leading causes of nonfatal injuries, as shown by the work of O'Sullivan and Schwarz with infants of teenage mothers and Schwarz and coworkers (Schwarz, Grisso, Holmes et al., 1994) in an urban African-American population.

The most recent explorations of infant injuries have generally been event-specific, for instance Banever and colleagues' description of infant hand burns caused by touching home treadmills (Banever et al., 2003); foreign body ingestions, particularly coins and batteries (Wahbeh, Wyllie, & Kay, 2002); or the large body of work on infant injuries caused by sitting in the front seat of a motor vehicle with a passenger-side air bag (Arbogast, Cornejo, Kallan, Winston, & Durbin, 2002). Suffocation in adult beds and sofas or chairs has also recently become more widely recognized as an important cause of injury to infants, with a 20-fold increase reported since 1980 (Sheers, Rutherford, & Kemp, 2003).

Injury researchers bemoan the flaws in studies of external causes in fatal injuries and the fact that existing mortality data do not give a good picture of how injuries occur. To target intervention efforts, nurses must know how injuries are occurring. These data do not exist because fatal injuries are relatively infrequent events. The few studies on injury risk factors usually use data on nonfatal and minor injuries (which are relatively more frequent) to identify risk factors for injury. Unfortunately, whether or not nonfatal and fatal injuries involved the same causative factors and sequence of injury is not known (Peterson & Brown, 1994, for review).

In addition to these data-specific barriers to effective injury prevention, there are others. Many injuries occur because of an interaction between environmental and behavioral risk; for example, burns from hot water could not occur if water heaters were all set at a safe temperature (below 125°). Environmental change strategies that avoid change in behavior have been favored by injury prevention professionals (e.g., air bags in cars, sprinkler systems in buildings). For many infant injuries, the behavioral piece in injury prevention must be addressed with parents, but there is sparse information about changing parental behavior with regard to injury or most other infant health-promoting activities. Unfortunately, injury often has no meaning to families until after an injury has already affected a child. Moreover, parents can often repeatedly behave in a relatively risky fashion without injury occurring. This leads to complacency and denial of risk. In fact, as parents obtain more experience with the environment around the infant, there is evidence that their expectations of severity of injury decreases. They become more willing to take risks. This adds to the difficulty of undertaking successful behavior change with parents to improve infant safety.

To provide a framework for injury prevention strategies, Haddon and Baker (1980) described the occurrence of injuries through the interaction of three factors: an agent that can do harm, a vector or vehicle that conveys the agents, and a host. Knowledge exists on how to change the agents, vehicles, and hosts to prevent death and disability. The value of these options for nurses is that they specify the various stages in the injury process in which intervention could be considered, and they address both behavioral and environmental approaches.

At present, other than for motor vehicle injuries, where passenger restraints, drunk-driving laws, and road and automotive safety standards have been shown to reduce infant injury and death, there are few supported injury-prevention interventions for infants. Much more work is needed by nurses and other researchers to define and evaluate injury-control strategies. In the meantime, research to understand injury etiology and better data collection systems are urgently needed.

ANN L. O'SULLIVAN
DONALD F. SCHWARZ

Infection Control

The infectious process depends on the interaction between an infectious agent, a susceptible host, and the environment. Essential to this interaction is a means of transmission of the agent from an infected host to a susceptible host. This occurs through direct contact, airborne droplet transmission, and indirect contact. Airborne transmission involves the dissemination of particles suspended in air that contain infectious microorganisms. When replication of the infectious agent occurs in the tissues of the host, causing local cellular injury, secretion of toxins, and/or an antigen-antibody reaction that produces signs and symptoms, infectious disease is present. Communicable diseases are infectious diseases that may be transmitted from one person (or animal) to another. Not all infectious diseases are communicable.

Infection control occurs both in the community and within institutions. However, since 1980 increasing emphasis has been placed on hospital-acquired infections.

The CDC has long been involved in the development of guidelines for infection control programs. The Joint Commission on Accreditation of Healthcare Organizations (JCAHO) sets standards for practice and requires infection control committees to recommend and approve surveillance programs based on previous nosocomial infection statistics. In addition, the Occupational Safety and Health Administration (OSHA) has published a regulatory document titled *The OSHA Bloodborne Pathogen Standard*. This document requires that all employers of health care workers provide employees with an environment safe from exposure to bloodborne pathogens (U.S. Department of Labor, 1991). The American Public Health Association has published a classification system for reporting communicable diseases that is used by state and national public health services. The National Nosocomial Infection Surveillance system collects data from a variety of hospitals nationwide. Reports of findings are published periodically.

The purpose of infection control surveillance is to establish and maintain a database that describes the endemic rates of nosocomial infections. Knowledge of endemic rates allows recognition of increased rates of nosocomial infection resulting in clusters or outbreaks. These data also can be used to prioritize infection control activities and identify trends such as shifts in prevalent pathogens or outcomes of hospital-acquired infections. The surveillance process includes definition of nosocomial infections, systematic gathering of case findings, and tabulation, analysis, interpretation, and reporting of relevant data to individuals or groups for appropriate action.

There are three major types of surveillance. Total house surveillance detects and records all nosocomial infections that occur anywhere in the hospital. It is expensive because of the time and personnel required. Priority-directed or targeted surveillance concentrates on specific areas, patient populations, or procedures, depending on the characteristics of the hospital. Problem-oriented surveillance is conducted to measure the occurrence of specific infection problems, such as outbreaks in specific areas of the hospital. Other surveillance programs may include prevalence surveys or a focus on the identification of risk factors associated with nosocomial infections.

Control of infectious diseases depends on interrupting the interaction between an infectious pathogenic agent, a susceptible person, and the characteristics of the environment. The characteristics of transmission of the organism through direct contact, airborne droplets, and indirect contact are important considerations. Nosocomial infections are iatrogenic, costly complications of hospitalization. In order of incidence, the top four nosocomial infections are urinary tract infections, pneumonia, surgical wound infections, and bacteremia. Preventive interventions for high-risk patients are the most effective measures to prevent morbidity and mortality.

GAIL A. HARKNESS

Informed Consent

Informed consent is the process by which a potential subject or a legal representative is given explanations about the purpose of the research and the risks, inconveniences, costs, potential benefits, and right to withdraw from the study without repercussions. This must occur prior to obtaining written or verbal consent for enrollment. The use of informed consent for research and the process for obtaining it have evolved over the past 50 years. The major impetus for increased attention to the issues of informed consent was a series of studies involving unethical actions on the part of researchers toward their subjects. These studies involved human rights violations in which subjects were neither informed nor had the ability to refuse participation. Highly publicized examples included experiments conducted on Nazi prisoners in concentration camps; withholding treatment for a group of poor Black men with syphilis in Tuskeegee, Alabama, to determine the course of the untreated disease; and not informing elderly patients at the Jewish Chronic Disease Hospital in New York that they were injected with live cancer cells (National Commission for the Protection of Human Subjects, 1979).

The Nuremberg Code, which outlined ethical standards for research, was adopted in response to the human rights violations in Nazi prison camps. This was followed by the Declaration of Helsinki, adopted by the World Medical Assembly in 1964. In the United States the National Commission for the Protection of Human Subjects of Biomedical and Behavioral Research (1979) developed a code of ethics for the protection of human subjects, specifying guidelines for research sponsored by the federal government. The basic principles of beneficence, justice, and respect for persons were the guiding ethical principles. This was followed by federal regulations, specifying in greater detail the conditions under which humans could be used in research sponsored by the federal government. Professional organizations then issued their own guidelines. In 1975, the American Nurses Association published *Human Rights Guidelines for Nurses in Clinical and Other Research*.

Today research involving human subjects requires that, prior to giving consent, the subject or legal representative be informed of the purpose, duration, and procedures of the study; risks or discomforts; potential benefits; alternatives to participation; confidentiality; compensation; person to contact for questions; and a statement that participation is voluntary. There are special provisions when subjects are fetuses (in and ex utero), children, pregnant women, or prisoners (USDHHS, 1983).

Not all research involving humans requires informed consent. The local institutional review board (IRB) is the authority for determining the need for informed consent. Issues about informed consent debated in the literature include understandability of the consent form, research in emergency or critical care situations, genetic research, and use of blood cell line development.

Understandability of the consent form has two components: the subject's ability to understand the information in the consent form and the reading level. The subject must be legally competent to give informed consent. Competency to give consent can be affected by the age of the potential subjects (child vs. adult); mental ability (Alzheimer's patients or mentally retarded adults); medical condition (unconsciousness, sedated, incubated); or ability to read, speak, and understand English. The researcher has to ensure that the consent form is written at a level that can be understood by the subject.

Until the fall of 1996 the ability of researchers to conduct studies in emergency and critical care situations, when the potential subject was not able to give informed consent and the legal representative was not available, was severely limited. A change in federal regulations (USDHHS, 1996) allows the exemption from informed consent requirements for emergency research under very specific conditions: (a) the subject's condition is life-threatening, (b) available treatments are unproved or unsatisfactory, (c) consent cannot reasonably be obtained prior to the initiation of the intervention, (d) there is the potential for direct benefit to the subject, and (e) the community is aware of the research prior to the initiation of the study.

Nursing research on informed consent primarily has addressed the issue of patient advocacy, with emphasis on the patient's ability to understand the informed consent document. Susman, Dorn, and Fletcher (1992) investigated how much information 44 subjects, aged 7 to 20 years, retained about the research protocol in which they were enrolled. They found that over 50% of the subjects understood that they could ask questions about the research study, knew how long they would be in the study and what the benefit of the study would be, and were aware that they could withdraw at any time. However, less than 3% knew the purpose of the study, 9% knew the risks associated with the study, and 14% knew what procedures were associated with the study.

A second study focused on what subjects understood of the words used in research consent forms. Lawson and Adamson (1995) interviewed 86 adults on research protocols and found that over 80% understood the following commonly used terms: *efficacy*, *lesion*, *orally*, *benefits*, *adverse reactions*, *placebo*, *compensation*, *ineligible*, and *withdrawal of consent*. Conversely, less than 50% of the subjects understood words such as *protocol*, *open label*, and *nonsteroidal antiinflammatory drugs*.

Techniques for improving subject understanding of the research include giving a copy of the informed consent form to the subject, viewing a videotape of the research procedure, and calling subjects after they have signed the consent to answer questions or concerns. Additional research is needed in the area of informed consent.

BARBARA S. TURNER

Instrumentation

Instrumentation is a general term for the activities involved in developing, testing, and revising measures of concepts important to nursing. The term is usually applied to these processes as they relate to psychosocial or self-report measures of attitudes and behaviors. However, instrumentation also refers to the validating of measures for physiological parameters or laboratory devices. The goal of instrumentation is to create measures that reduce error in research through consistency, accuracy, and sensitivity of measurement. For self-report instruments, consistency is analogous to reliability, and accuracy is analogous to validity. With laboratory instruments, validity is also used to describe the accuracy of the measures, but precision refers to the instrument's consistency in measurement. Sensitivity is directly applicable to both types of measurement and refers to the instrument's ability to finely discriminate in individual differences and changes in the concept under study. Control of measurement error is achieved by assuring that as much response variability as possible is due to the subject's relationship to the concept under study rather than to inconsistent or systematic extraneous factors.

The term *psychometrics* is often used to refer to the results of testing self-report measures and to the statistics that are utilized in that examination. Self-report measures generally fall into the categories of norm-referenced and criterion-referenced. With norm-referenced instruments the goal is to obtain a spread of scores across a wide range for the purpose of discriminating between subjects. Criterion-referenced measures are constructed for the purpose of determining whether a subject has or has not achieved a predetermined set of target behaviors. Steps in instrumentation for these two categories differ; however, the majority of attitudinal and behavioral measures applicable to nursing are norm-referenced, and their construction and testing is emphasized.

Instrumentation for self-report measures involves three general phases: development, testing, and revision. Instrument development involves concept clarification, developing a theoretical definition, operationalizing the concept, and generating items. Concept analysis involves a careful review of literature with attention to consistencies and inconsistencies in the use of the concept. Concept synthesis uses clinical observations to explore the phenomenon of interest. Concept derivation consists of moving a concept from one field or discipline to another. After the concept to be measured is clarified, a theoretical definition is formulated that delineates the dimensions of the concept to be measured based on the result of concept clarification. Operationalization is the process of moving to an operational variable that is isomorphic with the theoretical definition. Item generation involves decisions about concept dimensionality and scaling methodology.

When the phenomenon of interest is a highly abstract concept, the theoretical definition will include a number of conceptual aspects. Less abstract concepts can often be indexed with items that tap only one, more finite aspect. For each aspect of the concept, items must be developed in a manner that assures homogeneity within that conceptual dimension. Thus, the instrument may have to be multidimensional or unidimensional, depending on the concept of interest. Typically, multidimensional concepts will be measured with instruments that have a subscale that relates to each dimension.

Decisions about scaling involve whether the model is meant to scale stimuli or people. Methods used for scaling stimuli are paired comparisons, constant stimuli, successive categories, and psychophysical methods. Common approaches to scaling people are cumulative (e.g., Guttman-type), differential (e.g.,

Thurstone-like), and summated (e.g., Likert-type) instruments. Nunnally (1978) provided an excellent overview of these scaling procedures. Other decisions in item generation include factors involved with instrument formatting. These factors relate to levels of measurement, scaling responses, and the appearance of the scale to the respondent.

Instrument testing for self-report measures involves two aspects. Initially, the content of the instrument is examined to assure its relationship to the theoretical definition of the concept. The procedures include estimates of whether the concept has been sufficiently indexed by the instrument's items and whether the format is clear and promotes response consistency. Evaluation of the link between the concept and items is primarily performed by a panel of content and instrument experts. Once it is determined that the concept is adequately indexed, a second phase of testing involves the use of the instrument with a sample from the target population. This testing results in a quantitative examination of reliability and validity measures (see "Reliability" and "Validity").

Instrument revision for self-report measures includes a critical examination of testing results and individual items. Options for items are (a) inclusion as is, (b) alteration to clarify or meet theory, and (c) elimination. Once the instrument has been revised, it must be tested again with another sample from the target population.

Instrumentation for laboratory measures involves the similar phases of development and testing. However, the development phase typically focuses on the establishment of procedures for the use of the device. Testing evaluates the precision, accuracy, and sensitivity of the device, given the procedures established. Examination of precision must include calibration of the device and evaluation for inconsistency in readings, given repetitive use. Assessment for accuracy includes not only the meeting of established standards but appraisal of appropriate theoretical specification of results to the concept of interest. Revision of procedures may be needed when results of testing do not meet established standards for precision and accuracy.

Joyce A. Verran
Paula M. Meek

International Classification for Nursing Practice (ICNP®)

The International Classification for Nursing Practice (ICNP®) is a program of the International Council of Nurses (ICN). The ICNP® is intended to be used to represent nursing phenomena (diagnoses), nursing interventions, and nursing outcomes in documentation in the health care record. As a combinatorial terminology, the ICNP® facilitates cross-mapping of local terms or terms from other standardized classifications and serves as a unified nursing language system. As a unifying framework or unified nursing language system, the ICNP® enables comparison of nursing data across recognized nursing classifications, across organizations, across sectors within health care systems, and among countries. In addition to promoting comparable nursing data, the ICNP® is intended to facilitate comparison of nursing data with data from other health disciplines

Use of standardized terminologies can support the electronic capture of clinical data by nurses at the source of care delivery. This data can be reused for many purposes, including communication, clinical decision-support, policy making, and knowledge generation. In order to represent nursing practice worldwide, the ICNP® needs to be broad enough to capture the domain of nursing practice globally and sensitive enough to represent the diversity of nursing practice across countries and cultures. The benefits of the ICNP® are to:

- Establish a common language for describing nursing practice in order to improve communication among nurses, and between nurses and others;
- Represent concepts used in local practice, across languages and specialty area;

- Describe the nursing care of people (individuals, families, and communities) worldwide;
- Enable comparison of nursing data across client populations, settings, geographical areas, and time;
- Stimulate nursing research through links to data available in nursing and health information systems;
- Provide data about nursing practice in order to influence nursing education and health policy making;
- Project trends in patient needs, provision of nursing treatments, resource utilization, and outcomes of nursing care.

ICN, representing member associations in over 120 countries, has provided an infrastructure to enhance the development of an ICNP®. Along with the ICNP® member associations, additional partners, such as informatics experts, researchers, governments/health ministries, and industry, are needed to realize the vision of the ICNP®. The vision of ICNP® is to have nursing data readily available and used in health care systems worldwide.

In 1989, based on the concern that there was no common language to describe nursing's contribution to health, the ICN approved the resolution that launched the ICNP® project. The ICNP® Development Team was organised in 1990 and facilitated the work of many nurses around the world, which resulted in the ICNP® Alpha Version, published in 1996 and followed then by the ICNP® Beta Version in 1999. The Beta 2 Version was released in 2000.

Although the ICNP® has been a project of the ICN since 1989, it was only in 2000 that a formal ICNP® Program was established. As a program the ICN's commitment to the ICNP® is strengthened. The objectives and plans of the ICNP® program are identified and reviewed annually and organized into three activity clusters:

- communication and marketing,
- research and development,
- coordination and program management.

The ICNP® Program facilitates participation of individuals and groups in the ongoing development and maintenance of the ICNP®. Recent research and development efforts have focused on testing the ICNP® Beta Version and preparing ICNP® Version 1.

It is important to understand that the ICNP® will always be dynamic. Just as nursing science and technology evolve, the terminology that represents nursing practice must evolve. In addition, the ICNP® must continue to meet international criteria set by standards organizations and to work in harmony with other informatics and terminology initiatives. The ongoing development and revision of the ICNP® continue to be complementary to efforts already underway in nursing, building on and unifying the existing work in nursing classifications.

As a program of ICN, there is a major emphasis on worldwide participation of nurses in the development of the ICNP®. Through the European Union-funded Telenurse Project and the support of many ICN member National Nurses Associations, over 25 translations of the ICNP® Beta Version have been completed. The translations expanded opportunities for nurses to participate in research and development in their own language.

A number of ICNP® program activities and mechanisms facilitate research and development; for example the ICNP® Evaluation Committee was formed to provide formal review, consultation, and recommendations for the purpose of revising the ICNP®. Evaluation Committee members have already established the *ICNP® Review Process*, to facilitate submission of new terms and other recommendations to ICN for review and consideration. Currently, there are more than 150 Nursing Practice Expert Reviewers, representing more than 25 countries, participating in the ICNP® review process. To date, hundreds of recommendations have been submitted to ICN and more that 100 reviews for new terms and definitions have been completed. Some examples of new terms submitted to ICNP® include: homelessness (South Africa), gender violence (Swaziland), family crisis

(Chile), informal settlements (South Africa), community development (Botswana and Colombia), and newborn care (Portugal).

To facilitate networking among researchers, a reference list and a database of ICNP® development and evaluation projects are published on the ICN web site. Examples of types of ICNP® research projects include (a) concept validation studies, (b) computer-based information system demonstration projects, (c) evaluation studies, and (d) cross-mapping projects.

In a study by Hyun and Park (2002), terms from other nursing classifications were cross-mapped to the ICNP® and demonstrated that the ICNP® was able to describe many of the existing terms in these systems. One effort underway to support the ICNP® as a unified nursing language system is the development of ICNP® catalogues (or subsets) of nursing diagnoses, interventions, and outcomes. Projects are underway to create a number of catalogues, including for example, work with specialty nursing areas such as maternal-child and perioperative nursing.

Partnerships are a priority for the ICNP® Program. ICN already has a strong infrastructure, including collaborative relationships with the member national nurses associations and other established nursing, health care, and governmental organizations. A new ICN initiative to facilitate collaboration is the establishment of ICN Research and Development Centers. The initial ICN Centers will focus on ICNP® Research and Development. The first ICN Center is the German-language ICNP® Users Group, including participants from Germany, Austria, and Switzerland. Ongoing efforts such as these will continue to promote open partnerships and the use of ICNP® as a unifying framework.

ICN plans to launch the release of the ICNP® Version 1 in 2005, at the ICN Congress in Taipei. ICNP® Version 1 will include revision to comply with relevant international standards.

MADELINE MUSANTE WAKE
UPDATED BY AMY COENEN

International Nursing Research

International nursing research represents comparative research on nursing phenomena and on nursing issues conducted in more than one country. This includes research that is conducted cross-nationally to examine issues of global interest to nurses and to test and develop theories. The research is usually conducted by a nurse who resides in one country and studies phenomena in another country. The purpose is to compare the findings with the results of similar research obtained in other countries. Such research provides opportunities to clarify scientific values, explore assumptions, and develop shared frameworks.

International research in nursing is growing with the increased opportunities for travel, networking, and collaboration. The increasing abilities of nurses to study abroad, to attend international conferences, to visit international institutions, and to communicate through electronic mail systems, enhance comparative and collaborative research projects. International scholarship has focused on the use of U.S. nursing theories and the evaluation and testing of their utilities and appropriateness to the different nursing cultures. There are many descriptive and analytical dialogues related to theory in the international literature. These dialogues have resulted in scholarly publications related to the introduction and analysis of U.S. theories in many countries.

Human resources analyses and investigations led to several international projects. Questions related to the image and status of nursing, shortage of nurses, and distributions of nurses in urban and rural settings were examined. The results were compared and contrasted among and between countries and regions. There is general agreement among researchers in many countries on the perception of nursing and the difficulty in recruitment of students and retention of nurses in the workforce.

There are commonalities in nurses' reasons for leaving the countries and seeking employment in other countries or regions. Nurses emigrate to seek better job opportunities, to secure a better future for their children, to improve their skills, and to complete their graduate education.

Other research areas that received the attention of international nurses were the caring practices of nurses and the relationship between nurses' cultural heritage and language and patients' cultural heritage and their primary language of communication. There is beginning evidence that nurses of multicultural heritage who speak more than one language tend to provide more culturally competent care.

Other areas of comparative and collaborative research were focused on women's health and quality of life. Questions about women's health were considered within a sociopolitical context, with attention to health and health care in the overall development of women through better options, more education, and higher status. Other research examples were in ethical and clinical decision making, pain management, and the management of the care of the elderly.

Future international research requires the development of culturally competent methods, analysis of ethical issues in conducting collaborative international research, development of guidelines for international collaboration, and a framework for decisions related to data ownership, authorship, and culturally sensitive rules for data dissemination.

The International Council of Nursing, in collaboration with the U.S. Institute for Nursing Research, developed a list of priorities for international research, which addressed the urgency for preparing researchers internationally and providing international strategies to support nursing research. A future direction for priorities in substantive research questions has to be identified to enhance international collaboration and provide nurses with shared goals.

Afaf Ibrahim Meleis

Interpersonal Communication: Nurse-Patient

Interpersonal communication is defined as verbal interactions between nurses and patients or patient companions for the purpose of sharing relevant health information. Interpersonal communication is one of many skills nurses use when caring for patients. It is central to the work of a profession that depends on interpersonal expertise as much as clinical expertise. Effective delivery of health care frequently depends to a great extent on the quality of communication between health care providers and their patients. Communication can encompass the verbal, nonverbal, vocal, content, and process aspects of the interaction as well as the social, cultural, relational, behavioral, and interactional characteristics of participants. The majority of health-related research has been on the verbal communication styles of providers during patient interactions.

Interpersonal communication is the primary means by which patients learn about their particular health problems, appropriate prevention and treatment strategies, and the roles both nurses and patients play in achieving health outcomes. Such communication is likely to influence patients' willingness to share information, adhere to treatment plans, and participate in follow-up. Interpersonal communication in health care is often complex—influenced by personal characteristics and interaction styles of nurses, patients, or patient companions as well as contextual factors. Despite the complexity and importance of such interactions, studies of nurses' communication and its impact on the processes and outcomes of care are few.

The majority of research on provider-patient communication has occurred over the past 30 years. The focus of this research has been on communication styles and strategies that occur within the provider-patient relationship. Physicians' verbal communication has been studied far longer and more frequently than that of any other type of health care provider. Medical researchers have largely ignored the role of nonphysician providers and have excluded them from communication analysis. Much of what is known from this research is limited to what is said by white male primary-care physicians during initial acute-care visits (Roter, 2003). Nurse-patient communication has also been examined during this time period and has provided a basis upon which to describe the types of communication styles used by nurses in practice. Important issues have been raised regarding the communication styles nurses most frequently employ and their effect on patient responses and health outcomes (Courtney & Rice, 1997; Jarrett & Payne, 1995; Lawson, M. T., 2002). The communication patterns studied have been mainly those of white female advanced practice nurses in primary-care settings or basic clinical nurses in acute-care settings. Until recently, little attempt has been made to disentangle the independent effects on communication of key provider, patient, and contextual characteristics. This has resulted in diminished attention to the important role these characteristics may play in shaping the nature and dynamics of communication. Critical methodological issues are also raised about limitations in the ways provider-patient communication research has been studied.

Effective communication does not just depend on the acquisition of the right skills. A variety of characteristics have been identified that affect the quality and quantity of provider-patient communication (Wilkinson, S., Roberts, & Aldridge, 1998; Roter, 2003).

Provider characteristics. Provider communication has been studied more than patient communication; however, provider characteristics were studied less than patient characteristics. Provider characteristics include role, gender, race, specialty training, level of education, practice experience, and communication styles. Most communication studies enlisted small numbers of providers and meaningful individual differences in providers were difficult to find. There may also be assumptions that only patients' attitudes, emotions, and characteristics influence the interpersonal communication. Since nurses are human beings, it is important to discern how their specific characteristics are reflected in the care provided and the outcomes of that care. It would be important to discover if there are behavioral differences in the communication styles of male and female nurses and if they produce corresponding gender differences in patients' behavior directed back to them. Discerning whether relationships exist between specific provider characteristics and their ability to pay attention, give comfort, use feedback behaviors, and adjust communication styles to various individual patients would be important. A better understanding of the effects of nurse characteristics on communication behaviors and clinical judgment is needed.

Patient characteristics. Researchers have been mostly concerned with one direction of causality—how providers influence patients. Little work has been done to determine if patient characteristics impact a nurse's communication style. Patient characteristics include race, gender, age, health status, diagnosis, communications styles, role of patient companion, and values. What research has been done frequently showed no significant correlations or unexpected relationships (Caris-Verhallen, de Gruijter, Kerkstra, & Bensing, 1999). Because the relationship is both reciprocal and dynamic there is a pressing need to capture the contribution of both participants. Not only can a nurse be influenced by his or her own attributes and attitudes, but by those of the patient.

Contextual characteristics. Interpersonal exchange does not occur out of context. Most communication research has been focused almost exclusively on the verbal interchange between nurse and patient without taking into consideration the setting and context in which it occurred. Contextual characteristics comprise environmental and situational factors such as site of interaction, initial or established relationship, type of care provided, time constraints, stressors for participants, and role of participants. Research on nurse practitioner-patient communication occurs mainly in the context of initial or episodic encounters, although in practice the majority of dialogue occurs in the context of established relationships (Lawson, 2002). Most research between basic clinical nurses and patients occurs during the provision of physical care with the focus on providing instructions and explanations (Jarrett & Payne, 1995). This restricted view has limited the discovery of relevant factors and their implications for clinical practice. To obtain a more reflective view of the real contributions of nurse-patient communication to health outcomes, the context in which the interpersonal exchange is studied must be broadened.

Nurse leaders developed conceptual models that focused on describing aspects of nurse-patient communication and the intricacies of the nurse-patient relationship; these leaders are known as "interactionist" theorists (Orlando, 1990; Peplau, H. T., 1952; Travelbee, 1971). Most communication research remains atheoretical, exploratory, and descriptive and appears to be driven by available methodology rather than application of dedicated theories. Discoveries in knowledge about the presumed mechanisms behind the effects of communication will occur when theory-driven questions and hypotheses are systematically asked and tested. Other issues to consider are the realistic selection of subjects (patients or providers), studying subjects in various contexts, and use of simulated patients and contexts; the use of multiple research methods (experimental, observational, survey, ethnographic); the development of valid and reliable instruments; data collection methods; and the inclusion of other research designs to track the patterns and possible changes in nurse and patient communication over time. In addition to being studied as a process, communication may serve as an outcome, a predictor, a mediator of process, or a moderator of relationships among other variables. When these issues begin to be addressed the profession will be better able to determine how the findings on nurse-patient communication research can be used to impact the clinical and educational aspects of nursing.

MARJORIE THOMAS LAWSON

Intimate Partner Violence

Intimate partner violence refers to physical, sexual, and psychological abuse and stalking committed by one partner against the other in a relationship. Although relationship violence affects both sexes, women are victimized more and they sustain the most severe injuries. Data reported by the Bureau of Justice Statistics show that almost 700,000 events of nonfatal intimate partner violence were documented in 2001 (Bureau of Justice Statistics, 2003). Federal Bureau of Investigation data show that in the last 25 years, 57,000 individuals have been killed in domestic violence situations. The problem is a significant one for the health care community and society at large. Health-related costs of rape, physical assault, stalking, and homicide by intimate partners exceed $5.8 billion each year. Of this total, nearly $4.1 billion are for direct medical and mental health care services.

Nurse researchers have conducted many investigations regarding the physical and mental health of adult victims of intimate partner or domestic violence. Representative nursing research conducted since 1998 is included here. Campbell (2002) and her colleagues compared selected physical health problems of abused and never-abused women with similar access to health care. Employing a case-control study of enrollees in a multisite metropolitan health maintenance organization, they sampled 2,535 women enrollees aged 21 to 55 years, and found that abused women have a 50% to 70% increase in gynecological, central nervous system, and stress-related problems, with women who were sexually and physically abused most likely to report problems. Glass, Dearwater, and Campbell (2001) surveyed all women (N = 4,641) aged 18 years or older who came to the emergency department in 11 mid-sized community-level hospital emergency departments in Pennsylvania and California. They found that more than a third of women who had recently been abused and 76% of women who acknowledged experiencing physical or sexual intimate partner violence within the past year reported that they did not come to the emergency department for treatment of an injury. The majority of women (76% to 90%) agreed with the concept of health care providers reporting intimate partner violence to police. Dienemann and colleagues (2000) surveyed 82 women to determine the extent to which domestic violence was part of the history of women diagnosed with depression. They found a 61.0% lifetime prevalence of domestic violence, and that abused women were less healthy. Prevalence of headaches, chronic pain, rape including marital rape, and sleep problems or nightmares were significantly higher. Severity of abuse was significantly correlated to severity of depression. In a similar vein, Torres and Han (2000) examined psychological distress in a sample of 62 White and an equal number of Hispanic women who had been abused. They found that White women experienced a higher prevalence of psychological distress than Hispanic women. Japanese nurse researchers (Weingourt, Maruyama, Sawada, & Yoshino, 2001) also found that women who experienced abuse had significant clinical symptoms of depression and anxiety.

Researchers also conducted research on safety and assessment issues and educational protocols. Mohr, Fantuzzo, and Abdul-Kabir (2001) studied the ingenious ways in which women keep themselves and their children safe in the face of intimate partner and community violence, while R. E. Davis (2002) documented the phenomena of leaving the abusive situation. Employing specific educational protocols, McFarlane, Parker, Soeken, Silva, and Reel (1998) found that pregnant women who were abused and were offered an intervention protocol report a significant increase in safety behavior adoption during and after pregnancy. In a randomized controlled study, McFarlane et al. (2002) tested the efficacy of an intervention administered to abused women in order to increase safety-seeking behaviors. They demonstrated that such an intervention is highly effective when offered following an abusive incident and remains effective for 6 months.

Other noteworthy research conducted by nurses on women exposed to intimate partner violence include findings by McFarlane, Soeken, et al. (1998), who investigated the relationship between abuse to pregnant women and gun access, finding that women who reported gun access by their abusers also reported higher levels of abuse. Nurse researchers also studied nurses' attitudes and behaviors toward abused women (Henderson, A., 2001), tensions between service providers and victims (Peckover, 2002), and stereotypical thinking focusing on "physical problems" among nurses that precluded assessment of danger and safety issues of victims (Varcoe, 2001).

In sum, studies of the abused adult victim constitute a well-developed and developing body of research. Not only are nurses exploring aspects of safety, education, and assessment, but they are also carrying out intervention studies.

WANDA K. MOHR
SARA TORRES

J

Job Satisfaction

Job satisfaction is the degree to which individuals like their jobs. As a general attitudinal construct, job satisfaction reflects a positive affective orientation toward work and the organization, whereas job dissatisfaction reflects a negative affective orientation.

Job satisfaction has been studied extensively in nursing, psychology, sociology, management, and organizational development. Most commonly, researchers have studied job satisfaction as a dependent variable in assessing the impact of organizational changes and innovations, or as an intervening variable with multi-staged models of employee turnover, retention, or absenteeism. Currently, nurses' job satisfaction is being studied as a part of the organizational context, in conjunction with variables such as nurse staffing, autonomy, control over nursing practice, burnout, and emotional exhaustion to determine effects on outcomes such as patient satisfaction, quality of care, adverse events, morbidity, mortality, length of stay, and costs. Registered nurse (RN) staff in acute care hospitals has been the population of greatest interest in studies of nurses' job satisfaction. Less is known about job satisfaction among RNs who work in other settings or about licensed practical/vocational nurses in any setting.

In early studies of organizations, workers' liking or disliking their jobs usually was labeled morale. Midway through the 20th century, researchers began to develop both general and dimension-specific measures of satisfaction-dissatisfaction. General or global measures estimate an individual's overall feelings about the job. In dimension-specific measures, subconstructs distinguish satisfaction about specific facets of the job, such as the work or task, pay and benefits, administration, and, for nurses, dimensions such as professional status, nurse-physician relationships, and quality of care. As work on job satisfaction continued, debate arose about whether job satisfaction and dissatisfaction were opposite ends of a single continuum or were two separate constructs. Although job satisfaction currently is reported most often in the research literature, the one-or-two-constructs issue has not been resolved. The terms are used inconsistently and sometimes interchangeably. A more recent concern is the possibility that positive and negative affectivity, which are mood-dispositional personality traits, contaminate effects of determinants (e.g., autonomy, stress, burnout) on strain-related variables such as job satisfaction. In a meta-analysis of affective underpinnings of job perceptions, Thoresen, Kaplan, Barsky, Warren, and de Chermont (2003) found that both positive and negative affect uniquely contributed to the prediction of job satisfaction, organizational commitment, emotional exhaustion, and personal accomplishment.

Commonly used measures of job satisfaction have been influenced by or adapted from instruments developed in the organizational research field. Subsets of the Brayfield and Rothe (1951) items have been used frequently as general measures of job satisfaction. Prominent in the measurement of dimension-specific job satisfaction among nurses are the *Index of Work Satisfaction (IWS)* (Stamps,

1997), the *McCloskey-Mueller Satisfaction Scale (MMSS)* (Mueller & McCloskey, 1990), and the *Nursing Work Index (NWI)/ Revised Nursing Work Index (NWI-R)* (Aiken & Patrician, 2000; Kramer & Hafner, 1989). These measures all estimate job satisfaction at the individual level. Recently, Taunton et al. (in press) adapted the Stamps *IWS* for use in the *National Database of Nursing Quality Indicators (NDNQI)*. The adaptation included changing the wording of items to a unit-level referent so that satisfaction data could be aggregated to the unit level and analyzed with other unit-level indicators (e.g., nursing care hours per patient day, nurse staffing mix, pressure ulcers, patient falls, and patient satisfaction) as part of the American Nurses Association *Safety and Quality* initiative.

Researchers choose measures of job satisfaction based on the nature of the study and the response burden for subjects. For instance, a short, general job satisfaction measure would impose less subject burden in a multisite study that includes multiple measures of organizational and clinical variables or when assessing the overall relationship of job satisfaction to behavior. In contrast, researchers focused on the impact of a specific nursing practice innovation in one setting might be interested in nurse satisfaction about professional status, nurse-physician relationships, quality of care, or other dimension-specific facets. Also, as more researchers study job satisfaction as part of the unit organizational context, it will be important to use a measure that is reliable and valid at the aggregated unit or hospital level, such as the *NDNQI-Adapted IWS* (Taunton et al., in press).

Researchers (Blegan, 1993; Irvine & Evans, 1995) conducting meta-analyses of accumulated nursing job satisfaction research have found that autonomy, stress, commitment to the organization, and intent to stay in the job demonstrate the strongest, most consistent correlations with job satisfaction; autonomy and stress usually are antecedents of job satisfaction, whereas commitment and intent to stay are outcomes. Other variables with more moderate correlations are communication with supervisor, recognition, routinization, communication with peers, fairness, and locus of control. In general, variables measuring job characteristics (e.g., routinization, autonomy) and work environment (e.g., leadership, stress) have stronger relationships than economic (e.g., pay, opportunity elsewhere) or individual difference (e.g., age, experience, organizational tenure) variables. More recently, researchers of the organizational context for nursing have found higher nurse-to-patient ratios are associated with lower job satisfaction and higher emotional exhaustion, as well as higher patient risk-adjusted mortality and failure-to-rescue (Aiken, Clarke, Sloane, Sochalski, & Silber, 2002).

A high priority for current and future research is examining the relationship between nurses' job satisfaction and outcomes of care, such as quality of care, patient satisfaction, adverse events (e.g., falls, pressure ulcers, failure-to-rescue, infections), mortality, and the like. These relationships need to be studied not only in acute care settings, but also in the community, in home care, and in long-term care facilities—which will allow improvement of outcomes across all health care settings. Issues that still need more elucidation are first, the degree to which nurses' positive and negative affectivity confound relationships between job satisfaction and variables such as autonomy, job stress, burnout, and emotional exhaustion. Second, the association between patient positive and negative affectivity and patient satisfaction with nursing care is not clear. Here again, associations between nurse satisfaction and patient satisfaction could be confounded by underlying affectivity. Last, the unresolved issue about whether job satisfaction and dissatisfaction are separate constructs warrants further attention. Nurses' satisfaction and dissatisfaction may associate differently with outcomes of care.

ROMA LEE TAUNTON
UPDATED BY DIANE K. BOYLE
PEGGY A. MILLER

Job Stress

Results of a 1995 survey conducted by the American Nurses Association indicated that nurses considered stress to be their number-one occupational hazard. The nursing literature is replete with opinion articles on factors in the work setting that make situations conductive to stress for nurses; however, few articles report research results. It was during the 1970s that nurse researchers as well as sociologists and psychologists became interested in studying job stress for nurses. Early research on job stress for nurses centered on the disruptive effects of changing shifts on circadian rhythms and subjective sense of well-being. In large measure as a result of research on the effects of frequent shift changes, the practice of changing shifts more frequently than every 2 weeks ceased during the 1980s. Research to identify other factors that contributed to job stress focused on intensive care nurses, neonatal intensive care nurses, and hospice nurses.

One of the first studies concerning the experience of stress by staff nurses was conducted by Gray-Toft and Anderson (1981). They developed a measure of stress for nurses called the Nursing Stress Scale (NSS). The commonly used NSS contains 34 potentially stressful events divided into seven categories: death and dying, workload, uncertainty concerning treatment, conflict with physicians, conflict with other nurses, lack of staff support, and inadequate preparation to deal with emotional needs of patients. In 1983, Jacobson and McGraw published *Nurses Under Stress*, which included a summary of their research on stress experienced by neonatal intensive care nurses as well as the work of other nurse researchers on stress experienced by nurses. During the 1980s through early 2004, much of the research on nurses and stress has been as conducted by nurse researchers in European and Asian countries.

Among the studies focused on nurses and stress there have been consistent findings that the following factors make situations conductive to stress for nurses: work overload, staff shortages, lack of autonomy, equipment failures, conflict with physicians, conflict with administration or perceived lack of support from administration, lack of communication, ethical issues concerning patients on life support, high personal expectations for performance, and caring for high-acuity patients. Several factors have been examined as possible buffers to job stress experienced by nurses, including hardiness (Wright, Blache, Ralph, & Luterman, 1993) and social support (Cronin-Stubbs & Rooks, 1985). There is a fairly consistent finding in research reports that social support acts as a buffer to stress experienced by nurses in all settings.

Consistent with previous findings, a critical review and meta-analysis of the research that focused on strategies to help nurses with work-related stress (McVicar, 2003) found that " . . . work overload, leadership/management style, professional conflict and the emotional cost of caring have been the main sources of distress for many years . . . " (p. 633). Importantly, McVicar also found that although there were common themes across studies, it is apparent that stress perceptions are subjective and individualized, making it difficult to generalize from one clinical area to another. Therefore, it is critical to examine the personal factors that influence the perception of stress.

According to Mimura and Griffiths (2003), based on an extensive search of databases including CINAHL, Medline, and the Cochrane Library, there were only seven randomized controlled trials and three prospective cohort studies assessing the effectiveness of stress management interventions to assist nurses to either prevent or manage stress effectively at work. Although the use of cognitive techniques and social support has demonstrated more effectiveness than exercise, music, and relaxation training, the results of the ten studies reviewed cannot be interpreted with confidence due to small sample sizes and methodological problems.

Given the growing shortage of nurses in the United States over the last decade, it is very surprising that the issue of work-related stress for nurses in the U.S. has not become a significant focus of nurse researchers. Future directions for nursing job stress research should include: (a) studies to evaluate the person-environment fit model (French, Rodgers, & Cobb, 1974) or the job demand model (Karasek & Theorell, 1990) to explain factors that contribute to job stress for nurses; (b) identification of personal factors that put a nurse at risk for job stress; (c) intervention studies to evaluate the effectiveness of stress management strategies, including cognitive restructuring to bolster resistance resources such as hardiness and use of social support; and (d) longitudinal studies to evaluate the effectiveness of stress prevention and stress management strategies taught to students in nursing by following them to job sites.

BRENDA L. LYON

(Dorothy) Johnson's Behavioral System Model

Johnson's Behavioral System model consists of two major components, nursing and person. Nursing is a function of actions and goals while person is described as a behavioral system (Johnson, D. E., 1980). As a behavioral system, the person is made up of interrelated subsystems that influence one another and are influenced by the environment. The seven subsystems are open and linked. While equilibrium is the goal of the behavioral system, maturation causes each subsystem to continuously change which results in temporary disturbances in equilibrium. Greater disequilibrium occurs due to environmental stimuli or internal forces, and nursing is an external regulatory force that assists the person to regain equilibrium. The seven subsystems have requirements of protection, nurturance, and stimulation from the environment. Without the existence of those requirements, the subsystems are unable to perform their function. Behavioral actions of the subsystem are also driven by a particular goal, the individual's "set" which is a predisposition to respond in a particular way, and the choices that the individual may make.

The function of the attachment/affiliative subsystem is security. Social inclusion, intimacy, and social bonding are part of that security. The dependency subsystem evolves developmentally from total dependence on others to independence that continues to provide nurturance in terms of approval, attention, or recognition as well as physical assistance. The achievement subsystem is concerned with mastery or control of some aspect of self or environment. Proposed consequences include physical, creative, mechanical, and social skills.

Behavioral, rather than biological, aspects are the focus of the ingestive and eliminative subsystems. Therefore, appetite satisfaction is identified as the function of the ingestive subsystem and behavioral excretion of wastes as that of the eliminative subsystem. The emphasis is on when, where, how, what, how much, and under what conditions individuals eat or eliminate wastes. Social and psychological factors are major influences on these subsystems.

Procreation and gratification are the dual functions of the sexual subsystem. Cultural norms and values as well as biological sex influence this subsystem. Consequences of this subsystem include gender identity, courting, and mating. The function of the aggressive subsystem is defined as self-protection and preservation, and is not viewed as a learned, negative response.

The Behavioral System model leads the researcher to problems and solutions. Researchers have investigated behavioral system distresses that are connected to illness or major environmental stimuli. In clinical practice, the usefulness of Johnson's model has been demonstrated, particularly with the nursing process and assessment of outcomes. Using this model, nursing assessments are based on patterns that individuals have for meeting their needs. Johnson's model has also been used as a framework for nursing interventions that are personalized for individual patients (Cox, M., 1994; Derdiarian, 1990; Holaday, 1997), and patient classification systems have been developed based on the subsystems identified in this model (Poster, Dee, & Randell, 1997).

With the goal of maintaining or restoring balance to an individual's behavioral system, nurses can develop precise measurements for evaluating the efficacy of nursing actions. Majesky, Brester, and Nishio (1978) developed patient indicators of nursing care. This tool is considered one measure of quality nursing care. W. Reynolds and Cormack (1991) have been able to evaluate outcomes of nursing interventions with psychiatric patients. Numerous other studies have demonstrated the usefulness of the Behavioral System model in nursing practice in a variety of settings (Raudonis & Acton, 1997; Stuifbergen, Becker, Rogers, Timmerman, & Kulberg, 1999). Thus the ultimate goals of research using the Behavioral System model are to study the effects of nursing action on the behavioral system equilibrium and to foster changes as appropriate.

JACQUELINE FAWCETT
UPDATED BY SHARON A. WILKERSON

K

Kangaroo Care

Most nurses working in an intensive care nursery have witnessed parents expressing intense need to hold their ill preterm infants. A new method of care addressing this need is "kangaroo care," a term derived from its similarity to the way marsupials mother their immature young. During kangaroo care (KC), mothers simply hold their diaper-clad infant underneath their clothing, skin-to-skin, and upright between their breasts; if needed for warmth, a cap and a blanket *across* the infant's back may be added. In complete kangaroo care mothers allow self-regulatory breast-feeding. In developing countries the method is called kangaroo mother care (KMC), because mothers are usually the central figure responsible for care and they breast-feed exclusively. Kangaroo care, also known as skin-to-skin contact (SSC), is widespread in Scandinavia and Africa and is proliferating elsewhere. The method, which originated in Bogotá, Colombia, represents a blend of technology and natural care. Full-term infants also are vulnerable during the physiologically demanding intrauterine-extrauterine transition following birth and therefore benefit from kangaroo care (Anderson, G. C., Moore, Hepworth, & Bergman, 2003).

Relevant theoretical paradigms include stress, mutual caregiving, and self-regulation (Anderson, G. C., 1977, 1989, 1999), programming, inappropriate stress responsivity, and allostatic load, all of which are physiological/developmental and life span in nature; and Fitzpatrick's Rhythm Model, Levine's Energy Principles, Nightingale's Model, Orem's Self-Care Model, Rogers' Energy Fields, and Roy's Adaptation Model (Fitzpatrick, J. J., & Whall, 1989).

There are five categories of kangaroo care, based primarily on how soon kangaroo care begins (Anderson, G. C., 1995). Late Kangaroo Care, still the most common category in the U.S., begins when infants are stable in room air and approaching discharge. Infants given Intermediate Kangaroo Care have completed the early intensive care phase, but usually still need oxygen and probably have some apnea and bradycardia. Also included in this category are infants who are stabilized with mechanical ventilation and infants who, although too weak to nurse, are placed at the breast during gavage feedings, a method that facilitates lactation. Early Kangaroo Care is used for infants who are easily stabilized and begins as soon as infants become stable, usually during the 1st week and perhaps even the 1st day postbirth. The idea is that mothers can help maintain stability by giving kangaroo care. Very Early Kangaroo Care begins in the delivery or recovery room between 15 and 60 minutes postbirth. With Birth Kangaroo Care the infant is returned to the mother immediately following birth. The rationale in these last two categories is that the mother can help to stabilize her infant.

Numerous important extensions of kangaroo care have been reported as separate case studies, mostly in *MCN, The American Journal of Maternal-Child Nursing*; examples are with twins, triplets, an intubated preterm infant, full-term infants having breast-feeding difficulties, a near-term infant with gastric reflux, adoptive parents, and a mother who felt depressed during early postpartum (Anderson, G. C., Dombrowski, & Swinth, 2001). Other journals that frequently carry kangaroo care articles include *Acta Paediatrica* (formerly *Acta Paediatrica Scandinavica*); *Journal of Obstetric, Gynecologic, and Neonatal Nursing (JOGNN)*; and *Neonatal Network, the Journal of Neonatal Nursing.*

Kangaroo care is safe and has health benefits based on evidence (Anderson, G. C., 1991, 1995, 1999). In the United States nurses have done most of this research. Findings included adequate warmth, energy conservation, regular heart rate and respirations, fourfold decrease in apnea, adequate oxygenation, more deep sleep and alert inactivity, less crying, less cranial deformity, no increase in infections, fewer days in incubators, greater weight gain, and earlier discharge; lactation and breast-feeding increase and last longer. Kangaroo care, especially during breast-feeding, was analgesic for infants, *provided mothers feel relaxed.* Fathers also gave kangaroo care effectively, as do grandparents, young siblings, and selected important others. Parents feel more fulfilled, become deeply attached to their infants, and feel confident about caring for them even at home. Cost-effectiveness and improved long-term outcomes exist but are not yet evidence-based.

The National Institute of Nursing Research has funded nurses to conduct six randomized trials with preterm infants in which kangaroo care was the intervention. Five trials have been conducted by Ludington; three completed trials were with infants in open-air cribs, in incubators, and on mechanical ventilation (e.g., Ludington et al., 2003). Two trials are in progress: one on sleep and brain development measured by electroencephalogram and the other on blunting of pain measured by heart rate variability. The sixth trial was with 32–36 week healthy infants beginning kangaroo care on average 4.5 hours postbirth (e.g., Anderson, G. C., Chiu, et al., 2003). In a pilot trial for the funded trial, 34–36 week infants began almost continuous kangaroo care by 30 minutes postbirth, had remarkable behavioral organization, began breast-feeding exclusively by 2 hours, and were breast-feeding competently within 24 hours. Importantly, two infants had developed respiratory distress (grunting) by the time kangaroo care began, but this disappeared quickly while the infants stayed in kangaroo care and received warmed humidified oxygen via oxyhood; the warmth and humidity are essential (Anderson, G. C., 1999). Seven randomized trials done in developing countries, numerous others in Europe, and two in Taiwan have led to additional publications.

Although fully implemented in some hospitals, use of the kangaroo care method generally remains scattered. The method is not allowed in some hospitals and may not last in others due to resistance from some hospital staff with resultant variable support for parents. An elegant model for introducing the method and effecting desired change and implementation is described by Bell and McGrath (1996). Because kangaroo care benefits are dose-related, parental burdens such as time required, fatigue, discomfort, home-related responsibilities, stress, and anxiety warrant creative initiatives including broad social services to facilitate relaxation and extend caregiving (Anderson, G. C., Chiu, et al., 2003).

Other trends in kangaroo care include increasingly rigorous research, federal funding, publication of detailed guidelines (e.g., by WHO [2003a], available online), conferences devoted to kangaroo care, kangaroo care for sicker infants and for full-term infants, kangaroo care provided by selected family members or friends, consumer awareness of and desire for kangaroo care, and increased use of kangaroo care to facilitate lactation and breast-feeding especially for dyads having breast-feeding difficulties. The new realization that very early kangaroo care can help stabilize some preterm infants and prevent NICU admission has increased interest in giving kangaroo care as soon as possible postbirth, as often as possible thereafter, and for as long as possible each time. Nursing research is needed to document the great potential that kangaroo care in its various forms has for quality care, mutual relaxation and stress reduction, improved outcomes, parental satisfaction, and cost reduction.

GENE CRANSTON ANDERSON

(Imogene) King's Conceptual System and Theory of Goal Attainment

Imogene King's initial interest in theory was to develop a conceptual frame of reference to focus and organize nursing knowledge with the goal of identifying a systems theory for nursing (King, 1981). Introduced in 1981, King's theory focused on individuals as personal systems, two or more individuals as interpersonal systems, and organized boundary systems that regulate roles, behaviors, values, and roles as social systems. Interactions within and across systems influence human acts, or behavior, and subsequently, health outcomes. According to King, systems, and interactions are best understood by concepts, the building blocks of theory. Concepts for understanding personal systems are perception, self, growth and development, body image, learning, time, personal space, and coping. Concepts important for understanding interpersonal systems are interaction, communication, role stress/stressors, and transaction. Concepts useful for understanding social systems are organization, authority, power, status, and decision making. King identified that concepts and relationships are interrelated both within and between systems, which is consistent with general systems theory. Interpersonal systems are composed of personal systems, and interactions with social systems influence both interpersonal and personal. Interactions influence behavior, attitudes, beliefs, values, and customs.

Perception, interaction, and organization are comprehensive concepts for personal, interpersonal, and social systems, respectively. Perception is a process of organizing, interpreting, and transforming information from sense data and memory (King, 1981, p. 24). Interaction is defined as two or more persons in mutual presence and includes a sequence of goal-directed behaviors (King, p. 85). Organization is a system whose continuous activities are conducted to achieve goals (King, p. 119). The metaparadigm concepts of person, health, environment, and nursing are well-defined and explicitly linked: "The focus of nursing is human beings interacting with their environments leading to a state of health for individuals, which is the ability to function in social roles" (King, p. 143). There have been few changes to the conceptual system since it was first published. King has, however, provided clarification, explanation, and expansion of concepts through multiple publications; addressed concerns and questions raised by others; and explicated the philosophical and ethical basis of the conceptual system (Frey, 2004).

As a grand level theory, King's Conceptual System provides a distinct focus for the discipline, the process of nursing, and a framework for deriving middle-range theories. The first middle-range theory derived from the conceptual system was King's Theory of Goal Attainment (King, 1981). The Theory of Goal Attainment was derived from personal and interpersonal system concepts and focused on nurse-client interactions that lead to transactions and goal attainment. A descriptive study of nurse-client interactions by King resulted in the Model of Transactions and a classification system of behaviors in nurse-patient interactions that lead to transactions and goal attainment. Key behaviors in the process of transactions include mutual goal setting, exploration of means to achieve goals, and agreement on means to achieve goals. The theory of goal attainment specifies the process of nursing. In addition, it clearly reflects King's historical emphasis on nursing outcomes. Outcomes are defined as goals achieved and can be used to evaluate the effectiveness of nursing care.

In the past 2 decades there has been a considerable extension and application of King's Conceptual System and Theory of Goal Attainment (Frey & Sieloff, 1995; Sieloff, Frey, & Killeen, in press). Sieloff, Frey, and Killeen present a state-of-the-art perspective by reviewing application of the conceptual system and theory of goal attainment across systems, client concerns, patient populations, nursing specialties, and work settings; implementation in hospitals and community settings; the fit of the conceptual system and theory of goal attainment with evidence-based practice, nursing process, standardized nursing languages, performance improvement, and technology; and middle-range theories derived from the conceptual system. In addition to King's theory of goal attainment, middle-range theories derived by others address family (Doornbos, 2000; Wicks, 1995), health outcomes in children with chronic conditions (Frey, 1995), empathy (Alligood, 1995), and nursing department power (Sieloff, 2003). Each theory represents an ongoing program of research.

Imogene King is a strong advocate for theory-based education and practice for nursing. Her conceptual system for nursing provides a broad and enduring framework to guide nursing practice, derive middle-range theories, and integrate ongoing changes in nursing and the health care system.

MAUREEN A. FREY

L

Leininger's Theory of Culture Care Diversity and Universality

The Theory of Culture Care Diversity and Universality is derived from the disciplines of nursing and anthropology. Madeline Leininger conceptualized the theory in the mid-1950s while working as a clinical nurse specialist with disturbed children and their families (George, 2001). Troubled by the lack of knowledge available to help nurses understand the variations in care required for people from different cultures, Leininger set out to establish a new direction for nursing and to bridge the knowledge gap between nursing care and culture (Leininger, 2001a).

Leininger was the first professional nurse to earn a doctorate in anthropology. She is credited with establishing transcultural nursing and coining the term "culturally congruent care" (Leininger, 2001a). According to Leininger, culture care is the broadest holistic means of knowing, explaining, interpreting, and predicting nursing care phenomena to guide nursing practices. Culturally congruent care is beneficial care and occurs only when the culture care values, expressions, or patterns of the client (individual, group, family, or community) are known and used in appropriate and meaningful ways by the nurse. Thus, transcultural nursing focuses on comparative care knowledge of specific and diverse cultures that helps clients regain and maintain their well-being, and face death, disabilities, or chronic illnesses in ways that are beneficial to them and fit with their beliefs, values, and lifeways (Leininger, 1995, 2001b).

Leininger established the theory of culture care to account for and explain much of the phenomena related to transcultural nursing. The purpose of the theory is to discover human care diversities and universalities while the goal of the theory is to improve and provide culturally congruent care. Leininger first published the theory in 1985 with subsequent publications of revisions in 1988, 1991, 1995, and 2001 (Leininger, 2001a). With each publication of the theory, the conceptual definitions have evolved to higher levels of clarity, as has the nature of the underlying theoretical assumptions and statements.

The components of the theory are depicted in the Sunrise Model. The Sunrise Model is designed to function as a cognitive map for the study of culturally congruent care. Even though Leininger provides orientational definitions for the concepts in the model, she discourages the use of operational definitions in the study of culture care (Leininger, 2001a). Leininger supports exploring and discovering the essence of care for a particular culture, and puts forth the theory of culture care worldwide as necessary research for epistemic knowledge for the profession of nursing. The theory has three theoretical modes: cultural care preservation and/or maintenance, cultural care accommodation and/or negotiation, and cultural care repatterning or restructuring (Leininger). The three modes were developed based on Leininger's experiences with using culture care knowledge to assist clients in several Western and non-Western cultures. According to Leininger, the modes are care centered and use both emic (generic or folk care) and etic (professional care) knowledge.

In Leininger's theory, culture care diversity points to the differences in meanings, values, patterns, and lifeways that are related to assistive, supportive, or enabling human care expressions within or between collectives, while culture care universality points to the common, similar, or dominant uniform care meanings (Leininger, 1995, 2001a). Worldview is the way people look at the world and form a picture about their lives and the world. According to the tenets of the theory, this worldview is defined by cultural and social structure dimensions that involve dynamic patterns of a particular culture that include technological, religious, philosophical, kinship, social, political, economic, and educational interrelated factors as well as culture values and lifeways. The environmental context is the totality of an event or experience and gives meaning to human expressions, social interactions, and interpretations in particular physical, sociopolitical, ecological, and/or cultural settings. Ethnohistory refers to past facts, experiences, and events that are primarily people-centered and describe, explain, and interpret human lifeways within a particular cultural context. Generic care system refers to folk or lay knowledge and skills that are culturally learned and transmitted and used to provide assistive, supportive, or enabling acts for another individual. Professional care system refers to health, illness, and wellness-related knowledge and practice skills that are formally taught, learned, and transmitted.

In the Theory of Culture Care Diversity and Universality, Leininger orientationally defines health as "a state of well-being that is culturally defined, valued, and practiced, and which reflects the ability of individuals (or groups) to perform their daily role activities in culturally expressed, beneficial, and patterned lifeways" (Leininger, 2001a, p. 48). Care is described as being essential to curing, healing, health, well-being, and survival. Care is also presented as the dominant and unifying feature of nursing, and one of the most important concepts of transcultural nursing (Leininger, 1985a, 1995, 2001a). Nursing is presented as a transcultural humanistic and scientific profession and discipline whose central purpose is to serve human beings worldwide. Leininger asserts that even though the concepts of health, person, nursing, and environment are supported by nursing theorists as the major elements under consideration in the practice of nursing, care is the essence of nursing and includes "concrete phenomena related to assisting, supporting, or enabling experiences or behaviors toward or for others with evident or anticipated needs to ameliorate or improve a human condition or lifeway" (Leininger, 2001a, p. 46).

The Theory of Culture Care Diversity and Universality is broad, comprehensive, and worldwide in scope, demonstrating the criterion of generality, and addressing nursing care from a multicultural and worldview perspective. The ethnonursing research method was designed to systematically explore the purpose, goal, and tenets of the theory through a naturalistic and predominantly emic open-inquiry discovery approach (Leininger, 2001a). Ethnonursing focuses on the study of nursing care beliefs, practices, and values, cognitively perceived and known by a particular culture through their experiences, beliefs, and value systems. Over the past 40 years, Leininger's theory of culture care has become well-known and valued; studies have been conducted in approximately 100 cultures using the culture care theory (Leininger, 2001b). Leininger has published approximately 27 books and 250 articles on transcultural nursing and human caring, and the *Journal of Transcultural Nursing,* which was founded by Leininger, has been a major source for dissemination of caring constructs and culture care information. The knowledge gap between nursing care and culture has narrowed and clients worldwide are realizing the benefits of culturally congruent care. There is a wealth of new generic and professional culture care knowledge available to guide transcultural nursing teaching and practices. The theory has contributed significantly to soundly establishing the field of transcultural nursing as a formal area of study, research, and practice, and Leininger predicts that "by the year 2010, transcultural nursing with a human care diversity and universality focus will become the arching framework of nursing" (Leininger, 2001a, p. 414).

SANDRA C. GARMON BIBB

Longitudinal Survey

In longitudinal study designs the variables of interest are measured at several points in time for the same individuals. A value of longitudinal designs is the ability to shed light on trends and the temporal sequencing of phenomena. Most health-related phenomena of interest in nursing science are dynamic in nature. Describing patterns of change in phenomena and evaluating the outcomes of nursing interventions over time often are the focus of nursing research. Topics such as sense of well-being, family coping in chronic illness, adaptation to parenthood, and recovery from life-threatening illness are appropriate for longitudinal investigation. Nursing intervention outcomes are often measured during the course of the intervention and at several follow-up points—for example, changes in quality of life following a telecommunications nursing intervention or improvement in parents' ability to discipline children after participating in a series of parenting classes. A variety of longitudinal designs are employed in nursing research, such as time series design with repeated measures on a single entity or a number of entities at a relatively large number of time points. Panel designs may be used for making observations on many entities but at relatively few times. Although the relationship of the selected variables to the appropriate timing of measurement is critical in longitudinal research, nurturing a longitudinal sample is an art that researchers often underestimate.

Attrition of the sample is a serious compromise to meaningful study outcomes. Despite a precise sampling strategy, the population of interest will be represented inadequately if a large proportion of the sample fails to respond to the questions. Once a sample is accrued, retention is essential because attrition is financially costly and threatens the internal and external validity of results. There are many reasons for sample attrition, including loss of interest, loss to follow-up due to address changes, burden of participation, and exacerbation of the illness.

Obtaining an adequate response rate for cross-sectional surveys requires careful attention. A more challenging task is maintaining the response rate from participants who are repeatedly answering the same set of questions over several test points, extending for months or even years. Dillman (1978) established techniques that have been shown to facilitate the process of engaging respondents and enhancing the quality and quantity of responses. The total design method (Dillman) is based on the process of getting potential participants to complete questionnaires honestly and return them. The process can be viewed as a special case of social exchange. Classic social exchange theory asserts that the actions of individuals are motivated by the return these actions are expected to bring (Blau, 1964; Homans, 1961). The assumptions are that (a) people engage in any activity because of the rewards they hope to reap, (b) any activity incurs some costs, and (c) individuals attempt to keep their costs below the rewards they expect to receive. In the case of research there are three things that mush be done to maximize survey response: minimize the costs of responding, maximize the rewards, and establish trust that rewards will be delivered (Dillman).

Costs to participants in survey research include tangible costs, such as envelopes and postage, which can be easily addressed by the researcher. The intangible costs of time and effort take more creativity and thoughtfulness. A questionnaire that is attractive, distinctively identified with the project, easy to read and complete, reduces perceived cost. Techniques for reducing the effort in completing the questionnaire include (a) stapling the booklet in the centerfold, thus allowing it to open out flat; (b) using clip art throughout the booklet to reduce boredom; (c) constructing response choices so that a simple mark is required, thus reducing error and mental effort; and (d) using adequate "white space" to give the image of being easy to complete.

Thibaut and Kelley (1959) noted that being regarded positively by another person has reward value. Techniques to increase intangible rewards include (a) frequent expressions of positive regard in all correspondence; (b) expressions of the importance of participation; (c) personal salutations and real signatures; (d) a consultative approach, including an open-ended question asking for information that the respondent thinks would be important for the study; (e) holiday greetings and birthday cards; (f) newsletter every 6 months; and (g) handwritten notes in response to those who share personal information. Tangible rewards such as money or gifts should be carefully considered.

Identification of the research with an agency with a good reputation may increase the sense of trust. Respondents may return their questionnaires to the researcher, not so much because of any feelings of obligation to the researcher but because they feel that they have received past benefits from the university or health care agency (Dillman, 1978). Over the course of a longitudinal study, carrying out promises for a newsletter with updates on the progress of the study and brief reports of results is critical for engendering trust. Sensitivity to the needs of particular groups may also increase trust. For example, calling the post office in a small rural town before sending a mass mailing, to express concern about the additional workload, can engender trust with a key person in the community. This trust and interest in the study will be translated to the community at large. Exchange relationships must be nurtured throughout the course of the study. For example, as the project unfolds, members of the research team often come to be viewed as experts. When phone calls are received asking for advice about a specific disease or a new treatment or requesting information about the availability of support groups or educational programs, the response should be friendly and accurate; and a referral is made when appropriate. Dealing with phone calls and mail in a manner that is respectful and helpful is critical to the maintenance of the study sample.

Attention to follow-up is critical to a good response rate. The total design method contains a detailed routine for prompting nonresponders that has been very effective. An important aspect of follow-up is a personalized, signed thank-you letter after the return of the questionnaire. In a 5-year study in which questionnaires were completed annually, a systematic follow-up routine was used. A response rate of 89% for usable data for the 5th year was reported (Weinert & Catanzaro, 1994).

Undertaking longitudinal research requires a skillful and creative research team. Attention to issues related to costs and rewards, engendering trust, and maintaining interest are essential elements of success. Nonresponse and loss to the study cannot be totally eliminated, but careful attention must be paid to techniques designed to increase response rates and engage participants in the activities of the research project. Successful longitudinal research is truly an art form. Although careful attention to minor points may appear to be overly labor-intensive, they can lead to sustaining the sample for long periods of time and obtaining higher quantity and quality of data.

Clarann Weinert

M

Managed Care

The health care industry has experienced a dramatic transformation over the last 50 years. After World War II, American health care witnessed an unprecedented growth. With the advent of social programs such as Medicare and Medicaid, the number of Americans with access to health care increased as did the number of health care professionals and hospitals. The demand for health care with a traditional payment fee-for-service resulted in insurers passively reimbursing for what was charged. This fact, coupled with emerging technology, resulted in increased health care utilization and cost of care (Light, 1991; Robinson, J. C., 1995).

The term managed care has been broadly defined as a system that provides health care at an acceptable level of quality and cost (Kirk, 1997). Specifically, it is the combining of a prepaid, capitalized payment for health insurance with group medical practice as the means of delivery of services (Newbrander & Eichler, 2001). Physician and hospital payments are made through an agreed-upon capitated reimbursement. The benefits of managed care include the spreading of risks, since premiums are prepaid by large populations; a focus on prevention with a wide range of services; and the performance of case management (preauthorization, utilization services, and discharge planning). Four basic forms of managed care organizations (MCO) exist. These include health maintenance organizations (HMO), preferred provider organizations (PPO), exclusive provider organizations (EPO), and point-of-service (POS).

Prior to the 1960s only a few MCOs existed, such as Community Hospital Association of Elk City, Oklahoma (1929) and Kaiser Foundation Health Plan in California (1942). MCOs became prominent in the 1970s to inhibit cost inflation. Peer review, rate setting, and passage of certification-of-need legislation was also instituted to decrease costs. Today purchases of health care have become active price setters of health services and surveyors of quality care instead of passive negotiators. By 1996, over 25% of the U.S. population, 67 million people, were enrolled in some form of managed care. Today more than 50% of insured individuals are enrolled in a MCO.

As MCOs have proliferated so has the type and amount of related research. Initially research efforts focused on variations in health services provided throughout the United States (Wennberg & Cooper, 1999). Currently managed care researchers explore such issues as cost, quality, and the impact of MCOs on the health care environment. Theories such as the principle/agent theory (Buchanan, A., 1988), and social exchange theory (Blare, 1964) are used to explain the behaviors and outcomes of individuals in the health care system. The emerging work environment will include a continued focus on quality and decreased costs. Managed care will heighten the need for preventative services offered in community agencies. Additional research should be conducted that substantiates the positive cost/quality ratio.

Susan Houston

Maternal Anxiety and Adaptation During Pregnancy

Pregnancy, as a period of substantial biological and psychosocial change, can be expected to raise anxiety about the future. Anxiety is the psychological consequence of exposure to stressful circumstances that challenge one's capacity to cope. Patterns of maternal anxiety may be adaptive or maladaptive from psychosocial and psychophysiological perspectives. Maladaptive psychosocial prenatal responses have been associated with postpartal maternal adaptive difficulty, marital disturbance, and infant and childhood development problems.

Psychophysiological responses to anxiety involve neuroendocrine pathways. The sympathetic autonomic nervous system, through catecholamine release, may alter uterine contractile activity in pregnancy and labor and, by arterial vasoconstriction, may restrict uteroplacental perfusion and fetal growth. Also, the hypothalamic-pituitary-adrenal (HPA) axis and corticotropin-releasing hormone production during pregnancy may control the timing of birth and influence preterm birth. Adrenocorticotropic hormone also is a sensitive indicator of maternal psychological stress. Another HPA axis pathway may alter immune system response, rendering the expectant mother less resistant to infection. While such disregulation is associated with maladaptive responses, other factors can modify stress responses. The magnitude and duration of the stressor, the timing of a critical event, the genetic vulnerability of the mother and fetus, and social environment factors, may foster homeostasis and offset disregulation.

In general, pregnant women have higher anxiety in all trimesters of pregnancy than nonpregnant women (Singh & Saxena, 1991). Studies of maternal anxiety cite psychosocial factors as the most frequent and significant influences on pregnancy adaptation, birth outcomes, and subsequent postpartal maternal/infant adaptation. Two different and complementary conceptual frameworks of maternal prenatal adaptation have been presented by Rubin (1975) and by Lederman (1996). Rubin posited trimester tasks concerning binding-in and binding-out of pregnancy. Lederman identified seven dimensions of maternal development based on studies of prenatal health outcomes and postpartum adaptation:

- *Acceptance of Pregnancy*: Planning and wanting the pregnancy, happiness, tolerance of discomforts, ambivalence.
- *Identification with a Motherhood Role*: Motivation and preparation for motherhood.
- *Relationship to Mother*: Availability of the gravida's mother, her (mother's) reactions to the pregnancy, respect for the gravida's autonomy, willingness to reminisce; the gravida's empathy with the mother.
- *Relationship to Husband/Partner*: Mutual concern for each other's needs as expectant parents; effect of pregnancy on the relationship.
- *Preparation for Labor*: Practical steps; maternal thought processes.
- *Fears Pertaining to Pain, Helplessness, and Loss of Control in Labor*: Stress, pain, self-estimated coping ability.
- *Concern about Well-Being of Self and Infant in Labor*: Regarding deviations from the norm.

These seven dimensions are measurable using questionnaire and interview instruments, both showing high reliabilities for each dimension.

Significant differences have been found in the outcomes of pregnancy for women experiencing high prenatal-state anxiety and psychosocial or developmental conflict. In several studies (summarized in Lederman, 1995a, 1995b, 1996), the personality dimensions on adaptation to pregnancy showed that higher maternal anxiety in pregnancy and labor were correlated with higher plasma catecholamines during labor, decreased uterine contractility, fetal heart rate deceleration, and prolonged labor. Recently, results of another study (Lederman, Weis, Brandon, &

Mian, 2002) showed that anxiety, as measured by the different personality dimensions, predicted length of gestation (preterm labor), gestational age at first prenatal visit, and antepartal and labor complications. Of particular interest were findings that none of the demographic dimensions, such as age, education, and income, when entered into a multiple regression analysis with the personality dimensions, retained predictive significance. These novel results build on earlier findings, suggesting that the mother's psychosocial history and her perception of the meaning, challenges, and expectations of pregnancy are of paramount importance in the adaptation to pregnancy, and they carry greater weight than demographic factors in predicting birth outcomes.

Although they are conceptually and clinically related, research results suggested a distinction may be warranted between preterm delivery and newborn birthweight. Significant relationships have been reported between life-event stress and infant birthweight, and between a measure of pregnancy-related anxiety (adapted from Lederman's dimension measures, 1996) and gestational age at birth; both results occurred independent of subjects' biomedical risk (Wadwha, Sandman, Porto, Dunkel-Schetter, & Garite, 1993). Socially stressful factors, such as single marital status, little contact with neighbors (Peacock, Bland, & Anderson, 1995), not cohabitating with a partner or having a confidante, and highly stressful major life events (Nordentoft et al., 1996), have been associated with preterm delivery. Paarlberg, Vingerhoets, Passchier, Dekker, and van Geijn (1995) likewise concluded that the most consistent finding in the literature was the relationship between preterm birth and taxing situations.

Low birthweight appears to have a greater association with altered biophysical states. Smoking, hypertension, prenatal hospitalization, and prior preterm birth have been associated with low birthweight (Orr et al., 1996). Paarlberg and colleagues (1999) found that first-trimester smoking and maternal height, weight, and educational level were significant risk factors for low birthweight. M. S. Kramer (1998) found that the strongest predictors of intrauterine growth restriction were smoking and low gestational weight gain. Thus, prior studies suggested that maternal anxiety (pregnancy-specific anxiety, psychosocial adaptive anxiety, and major life-event stress) and maternal coping responses have more associations with preterm labor, whereas chronic stress, smoking, and other physical factors (height, weight, hypertension) may be more consistently related to infants that have restricted growth in utero or are low birthweight. The aggregate of findings suggest different modes of preventive intervention for the two disorders.

Decisions regarding *wantedness* and *acceptance of pregnancy* remain relatively stable or constant throughout pregnancy (Lederman, 1996). Not wanting pregnancy is associated with inadequate maternal prenatal care (Albrecht, Miller, & Clarke, 1994) and physical violence (Gazmararian et al., 1995). Women who report an unwanted pregnancy were more likely to have lower birthweight newborns, higher infant mortality rates (Myhrman, 1988), a more than twofold-increased risk of neonatal death (Bustan & Coker, 1994), and children who later developed psychopathology (Ward, 1991).

Studies of *motherhood role identification* indicate that maternal attachment and parenting confidence showed consistent and stable responses across prenatal and postpartum periods (Deutsch, Ruble, Fleming, Brooks-Gunn, & Stangor, 1988; Fonagy, Steele, & Steele, 1991; Lederman, 1996). Deutsch and colleagues also found that the woman's relationship with her mother during pregnancy strongly correlated with self-definition of her maternal role.

Kin relationships of the gravida with her husband/partner and mother have relationships to pregnancy outcomes. A lack of social stability, social participation, and emotional and instrumental support increased the mother's likelihood of giving birth to a small-for-gestational-age infant (Dejin-Karlsson et al., 2000). As in the study by Lederman and colleagues (2002), these results occurred independent of background, lifestyle, and biological risk factors, attesting to the significance of kin relationships, particularly the husband/partner relationship. Lederman (1996) reported high intercorrelations among the developmental dimensions in all trimesters, indicating that early anxiety measures were stable predictors of later anxiety. This suggested that prenatal assessment can identify women who would benefit from early counseling.

Socially supportive community intervention during pregnancy may have near-term and long-term beneficial effects for mother and child. A registered nurse home visit program for African-American gravidas with inadequate social support substantially reduced low birthweight (Norbeck, DeJoseph, & Smith, 1996). Pregnant women who received social support from midwives had fewer low birthweight infants, and at a 7-year follow-up still showed significant benefits for mothers and children (Oakley, Hickey, Rajan, & Rigby, 1996). Another supportive prenatal nurse home-visitation program (Olds et al., 1998) yielded beneficial maternal-child results as much as 15 years later, including improvement in women's health behaviors and the quality of child caregiving.

In summary, maternal anxiety and specific prenatal personality dimensions, operating through neuroendocrine pathways, influence maternal and fetal/newborn birth outcomes as well as longer-term outcomes. Many adverse outcomes may be modified or prevented by supportive prenatal nurse-visitation programs.

REGINA PLACZEK LEDERMAN

Measurement and Scales

The focus of measurement is the quantification of a characteristic or attribute of a person, object, or event. Measurement provides for a consistent and meaningful interpretation of the nature of an attribute when the same measurement process or instrument is used. The results of measurement are usually expressed in the form of numbers. Measurement is a systematic process that uses rules to assign numbers to persons, objects, or events which represent the amount or kind of a specified attribute. However, measurement also involves identifying and specifying common aspects of attributes for meaningful interpretation and categorization, using a common conceptual perspective. Ambiguity, confusion, and disagreement will surround the meaning of any measurement when it is undefined. The measurement relevancy can be determined only when an explicit or implicit theory structures the meaning of the phenomenon to be studied. Qualitative assessments apply measurement principles by providing meaning and interpretation of qualitative data through description and categorization of phenomena. Thus, measurement may not result in scores per se but may categorize phenomena into meaningful and interpretable attributes. Therefore, measurement is also basic to qualitative analysis.

Measurement is a crucial part of all nursing settings. Nurses depend on measuring instruments to determine the amount or kind of attributes of patients and use the results of measurements such as laboratory and physical examination results to determine patient needs and their plan of care. Nurse researchers use a large array of clinical laboratory, observational, and questionnaire measures to study phenomena of interest. Nurse educators depend on measurement instruments and test scores to help determine a student's mastery. Measurement is central to all that nurses do.

The rules used for assigning numbers to objects to represent the amount or kind of an attribute studied have been categorized as nominal, ordinal, interval, and ratio. These types of measurement scales are common in nursing. Measurements that result in nominal-scale data place attributes into defined categories according to a defined property. Numbers assigned to nominal-level data have no hierarchical meaning but represent an object's membership in one of a set of mutually exclusive, exhaustive, and unorderable categories. For example, categorizing persons in a study as either female or male is measurement on the nominal measurement scale. In ordinal-scale measurement, rules are used to assign rank order on a particular attribute that characterizes a person, object, or event.

Ordinal-scale measurement may be regarded as the rank-ordering of objects into hierarchical quantitative categories according to relative amounts of the attribute studied. The categorization of heart murmurs in grades from 1 through 6 is an example. In this ordinal measure, a Grade 1 murmur is less intense than a Grade 2, a Grade 2 less intense than a Grade 3, and so forth. The rankings in ordinal-level measurement merely mean that the ranking of 1 (for first) has ranked higher than 2 (for second) and so on. Rankings do not imply that the categories are equally spaced nor that the intervals between rank categories are equal.

Interval-scale measurement is a form of continuous measurement and implies equal numerical distances between adjacent scores that represent equal amounts with respect to the attribute that is the focus of measurement. Therefore, numbers assigned in interval-scale-measurement represent an attribute's placement in one of a set of mutually exclusive, exhaustive categories that can be ordered and are equally spaced in terms of the magnitude of the attribute under consideration. However, the absolute amount of the attribute is not known for a particular object because the zero point is arbitrary in an interval scale. The measurement of temperature is a good example of an interval-level measure because there is no true zero point. For example, the zero point is different based on whether the Fahrenheit or Centigrade measurement approach is used, and one cannot say that an object with a temperature of 0° F or 0° C has no temperature at all. Ratio-level measures provide the same information as interval-level measures; in addition they have absolute zero points for which zero actually represents absence of the attribute under study. Volume, length, and weight are commonly measured by ratio scales.

There is controversy about the level of measurement scales and the type of statistical procedures that may be appropriately used for data analysis. There are researchers and statisticians who believe that only nonparametric statistical procedures can be used for data analysis when data are nominal or ordinal and that inferential statistics can be properly applied only with interval and ratio data. There is controversy about whether Likert scaling (which is often used in nursing with measures of attitude or opinion) is in actuality ordinal-level measurement for which only nonparametric statistics should be used. Likert scaling involves having subjects rank their responses to a set of items on a range of numbers, such as "1" to represent lack of agreement to "5" to represent complete agreement. It has been the accepted practice for investigators to use scores generated with Likert-type scales as interval-level data.

Nurses have typically borrowed many measures from other disciplines. This reflects the fact that nursing is a field that considers the biological and psychosocial aspects of care and is based on knowledge generated by many fields of inquiry. Therefore, many instruments developed by other disciplines are consistent with nurses' measurement needs. However, the heavy dependence on borrowing instruments from other disciplines reflects the trend in the 1970s for nurses to pursue doctoral education in related fields, such as education, psychology, sociology, and physiology. Nurses became familiar with instruments from other fields during their graduate studies and were encouraged to use them in the nursing context.

By the mid 1970s nurses became more cognizant of some of the limitations in borrowing certain instruments from other disciplines. It is not unusual for instruments developed to measure psychosocial variables in other fields to be cumbersome and inefficient for use in the clinical settings of nurse researchers. Often the instruments needed by nurses to measure attributes in populations such as children, frail patients, the elderly, and the culturally diverse, instruments that measure important variables from the nursing perspective, do not exist. Nursing studies of families, communities, and organizations and systems have been hampered by the lack of effective measures to address group and system variables from the nursing perspective (Strickland, 1995).

The movement in nursing to develop more rigor in the use and development of measurement instruments gained prominence in the 1970s. In June 1974, a contract was awarded to the Western Interstate Commission for Higher Education by the Division of Nursing, Bureau of Health Manpower, and Health Resources Administration to prepare a compilation of nursing research instruments and other measuring devices for publication. With Doris Bloch as project officer, a two-volume compilation of instruments, titled *Instruments for Measuring Nursing Practice and Other Health Care Variables*, was published in 1978. Priority was placed on compiling instruments dealing with nursing practice and with patient variables rather than nurse variables. This was an important milestone for nursing measurement because it was the first effort that placed a large number of clinically focused instruments developed or used by nurses in the public domain.

During the late 1970s and early 1980s, two groups of nurse scientists focused their work on developing measurement as an area of special emphasis in nursing. At the University of Arizona–Tucson, Ada Sue Hinshaw and Jan Atwood focused their efforts on refining and further developing instruments for clinical settings and for clinically focused research. The first postdoctoral program in nursing instrumentation and measurement evolved at the University of Arizona, and annual national conferences on nursing measurement were offered. These conferences provided nurses a forum in which to discuss measurement issues and problems and to present information on instruments used in studies.

Ora Strickland and Caroyln Waltz at the University of Maryland at Baltimore focused on defining measurement principles and practices to build rigor in nursing research. Careful assessments of nursing research published in professional journals were conducted. The assessments revealed that nurse investigators were not giving adequate attention to reliability and validity issues when selecting and developing instruments. In addition, nurse investigators tended to rely too heavily on paper-and-pencil self-report measures and did not give adequate attention to selecting biological measures as indicated by the conceptual frameworks of the studies (Strickland & Waltz, 1986). The Maryland group published the first measurement textbook for nurses, *Measurement in Nursing Research*, and developed and implemented a measurement project funded by the Division of Nursing of the Department of Health and Human Services. This project prepared over 200 nurse researchers in clinical or educational settings to develop and test instruments for use in nursing and resulted in an award-winning four-volume series of books, *Measurement of Nursing Outcomes*, which compiled instruments developed by project participants.

In 1993, Ora Strickland initiated and edited the *Journal of Nursing Measurement* with Ada Sue Hinshaw as coeditor. This journal brought nursing measurement to a new level of focus, responding to the need for continuing development and dissemination of nursing measurement instruments and providing an identifiable forum for the discussion and debate of measurement concerns and issues of interest.

The nursing profession has developed nursing measurement to a great degree between the late 1970s and the present. Nurses have developed and tested instruments for use in a variety of settings. In addition to creating new instruments, nurses have further developed instruments designed in other disciplines for use in nursing studies. Although much has been done, much remains to be done in nursing measurement.

Ora L. Strickland

Medications in Older Persons

Due to increased life expectancy, older age is associated with the prevalence of multiple comorbidities (e.g., congestive heart failure, chronic obstructive pulmonary disease, diabetes mellitus), which often necessitate lifelong and multiple medication intake. Consequently, older persons are the largest consummers of medication. Polypharmacy is worrisome in the elderly because of the increased risk for adverse events. Moreover, polypharmacy may result in nonadherence to the therapeutic regimen, a factor found to be associated with poor outcomes in view of physical and psychological health. Adherence needs to be monitored as a clinical parameter during each clinical encounter. Evaluating older person's capabilities and risk-factors for successful management of the medication regimen should be part of a thorough geriatric assessment as a cornerstone of chronic illness management. Nurses play an important role in this assessment and assist older persons and their families in the management of and adherence to their medication regimen.

Older persons are the largest per capita consumers of medications. Several international studies show that persons older than 65 years account for 15%–18% of the population, but consume 40%–50% of prescribed drugs (Klauber, 1996; Linjakumpu et al., 2002; Swafford, 1997). Prevalence of polypharmacy increases with higher age and number of concomitant comorbidities (Linjakumpu et al., 2002; U.S. Agency for Healthcare Research and Quality, 1996). In two recent large-scale studies, it was noted that 11%–25% of older persons use five or more medications simultaneously (Chen, Dewey, & Avery, 2001; Linjakumpu et al., 2002).

Polypharmacy is worrisome in view of the increased risk for adverse events as this may be associated with poor outcomes in view of poor physical and psychological health. It has to be noted that, secondary to higher age or multiple chronic diseases, older persons are most vulnerable to pharmacokinetic, pharmacodynamic, and homeostatic changes (Raik, 2001). These changes make them particularly sensitive to adverse events, interactions, and toxicity of medications. Older persons are also at greater risk for inappropriate prescribing. The average clinician often lacks sufficient knowledge regarding possible drug-drug interactions. In addition, a lack of information regarding medication prescriptions ordered by other providers serves as a significant factor in increasing the complexity of the therapeutic regimen. Every new drug added to the medication regimen will increase the risk for adverse outcomes (Raik).

Suboptimal use of prescribed medications is often associated with unplanned hospitalizations among the chronically ill: 28.1% of visits in an emergency department were due to medication-related visits, and 63.35% of hospital admissions due to drug reactions could have been prevented (Mc Donnell & Jacobs, 2003). Furthermore, the risk of medication mishaps is higher in the older population due to errors in self-administration, caused in part by visual and cognitive impairment, illiteracy, high medication costs, the complexity of the medication regimen, duration of treatment, and/or side effects of the medications (Raik, 2001).

Adherence is defined as the extent to which a person's behavior (taking medications, following a recommended diet, and/or executing lifestyle changes) corresponds with the agreed recommendations of a health care provider (Haynes, McDonald, Garg, & Montague, 2003). In persons aged 60 years or older, nonadherence with medication regimens varies from 26% to 59% (Van Eijken, Tsang, Wensing, de Smet, & Grol, 2003), numbers that are very similar to those of younger populations. Nonadherence with drug treatment is highly prevalent in all chronic patient populations among different age groups and is *not* more prevalent in older normally aging persons, as is sometimes wrongly stated.

Because nonadherence has been found to be associated with poor outcomes, adherence needs to be monitored as a relevant clinical parameter during each clinical encounter. Clinicians can use direct as well as indirect methods to assess adherence with medication regimens. Direct methods refer to assay of medication, medication by-products or tracers in bodily substances (e.g., digoxin, phenobarbital), and observation of medication administration. Indirect measurement methods are self-report, collateral report, prescription refills, pill-count, and electronic event monitoring. Yet there is no gold standard to evaluate adherence with a medication regimen, as all methods have specific drawbacks in view of underestimating of nonadherence or the lack of revealing medication-taking dynamics. Electronic event monitoring (EEM) has emerged as the most valid and reliable method to date. EEM consists of a pill bottle fitted with a cap that contains a microelectronic circuit. The date and time of each bottle opening and closing are recorded as a presumptive dose. Recorded data can be downloaded to a computer that lists and graphically depicts individual medication-taking dynamics. Indirect, electronic event monitoring has superior sensitivity compared to other direct and indirect methods, as it allows assessment of noncompliance at a continuous level and in a multidimensional manner (De Geest, Abraham, & Dunbar-Jacob, 1996).

A number of processes associated with aging may negatively influence older persons' ability for independent and correct medication management and prevent adherence. Knowledge of risk-factors for nonadherence will allow identification of older patients at risk for inadequate medication management. Modifiable factors can be targeted for adherence-enhancing interventions. A selection of factors with special relevance for the older population will be discussed next.

Aging is associated with decline in auditory, visual, cognitive, and functional capacities. It can be more difficult for older persons to handle childproof caps, blister packages, or nebulizers, or to swallow large pills. Adherence to medication regimens requires, among other abilities, reading labels and distinguishing tablets according to their color. Nineteen percent of persons aged 70 years and older have visual impairments, including blindness; one third have hearing impairments (Desai, Pratt, Lentzner, & Robinson, 2001). Labels may be misread and colors of pills may not be recognized. Reading difficulties with regard to prescription labeling was not significantly related to nonadherence in seniors, although 38.8% were not able to read all the prescriptions labels and 67.1% did not fully understand all information (Maison, Gaudet, Gregorie, & Bouchard, 2002), admittedly restricting options for adequate medication management. Older persons have to be aware of the intended effect of the medication, how to administer it, possible side effects, and other relevant aspects of the medication regimen. A significant proportion of the older population has inadequate or marginal functional health literacy, making it difficult to process the health information and instructions given to them.

Although cognitive decline is associated with aging, in the absence of pathophysiological decline such as Alzheimer disease, cognitive functioning of older persons is normally sufficient to independently manage their own medication regimen (Park et al., 1999). Forgetfulness is a common reason for nonadherence in older persons; however, severe cognitive impairment most compromises patients' abilities to independently manage their treatment regimen. Cognitively impaired persons are more likely to receive assistance with medication management compared to cognitively intact subjects (Conn, Taylor, & Miller, 1994).

Treatment-related factors such as duration, complexity, and cost of medication regimens can also negatively affect adherence. Medication restriction, i.e., taking less medications than prescribed, is common in seniors who lack prescription coverage, particularly among certain vulnerable groups (Steinman, Sands, & Covinsky, 2001). The fact that many older persons live alone and are relatively socially isolated deprives them of necessary social support and places them at risk for depression, both of which are known risk factors for medication nonadherence (De Geest, von Renteln-Kruse, Steeman, Degraeve, & Abraham, 1998).

Compliance-enhancing interventions should be built on the available empirical evidence of modifiable risk-factors and intervention studies. Evidence shows that compared with single, generalized, and short interventions, multifaceted, tailored, and continuous interventions result in improved medication adherence (Haynes, McDonald, Garg, & Montague, 2003; Peterson, Takiya, & Finley,

2003; Roter et al., 1998; Van Eijken, Tsang, Wensing, de Smet, & Grol, 2003). This implies a combination of educational, behavioral, and social support strategies tailored to the specific situation of each individual older person and his family within a biopsychological care paradigm. Moreover, it is important that older patients and their families are seen as partners in the development of tailored and multifaceted medication management interventions.

Successful management of medication regimens in older persons requires an understanding of the risks associated with polypharmacy and specific factors associated with the aging process that put patients at risk for nonadherence. Interventions aiming at supporting older persons and their families with regard to medication-taking further should be multifaceted and tailored along the continuum of chronic illness management.

Sabina De Geest
Fabienne Dobbels
Els Steeman
Koen Milisen

Menstrual Cycle

The menstrual cycle is a truly gender-specific process that has a profound effect on women's lives. When viewed in the general context of biological rhythms, the menstrual cycle requires a complex sequence of physiological events coordinated by the hypothalamus in conjunction with the pituitary glands, ovaries, and uterus, along with the adrenal and thyroid systems, and that adapts to environmental phenomena.

Derived from the Latin *mensis* (month), the menstrual cycle is marked by the shedding of the uterine lining—menstruation, or a menstrual "period." We start menstruating at 11–12 years of age (menarche) and have our last menstruation at about 51 years (menopause). With a few interruptions, such as pregnancy or taking the Pill, women will have about 400 periods during their lifetime.

Menstrual period and menstrual cycle are not one and the same: menstrual period refers to the days that a woman bleeds. An average length of a period is 5 days; about half of all women bleed for 3–4 days and another 35% bleed for 5–6 days (Voda, Morgan, Root, & Smith, 1991). The term menstrual cycle (or menstrual cycle interval) refers to the span of time from the start of one period to the start of the next. The length of a menstrual cycle can range from 21 to 35 days, with 29 days as the average.

The basic facts about the cyclical changes in hormonal levels and in the reproductive organs are well-known and appear in many medical and nursing textbooks (Fogel & Woods, 1995; Speroff, Glass, & Kase, 1999). The neuroendocrine mechanisms which control the reproductive cycle are by no means completely understood. Most interest has focused on the ovarian hormones estrogen and progesterone, and on their influence on the release of follicle stimulating hormone (FSH) and luteinizing hormone (LH) from the pituitary gland at the base of the brain. Not only a physiologic process, menstruation is associated with feminine role development and feelings of health and well-being, and it is embedded in the sociocultural context of women's experience.

Nursing scholarship and science focused on menstrual-cycle phenomena can be traced to the care our profession provided to women and their children beginning with Lillian Wald's work among the poor women of New York, Margaret Sanger's efforts to help women control their fertility, and Mary Breckenridge's efforts to provide maternity care in the rural Kentucky Hills.

Since the late 1970s, nursing research has contributed in unique ways to understanding menstrual cycle events—menarche, menstruation, and menopause—as normative experiences and symptoms related to the menstrual cycle and menopause as illness experiences. In contrast, during the same period, biomedical research has focused on understanding the problems related to menstruation and menopause as disease or risk factors for disease with little attention to the interaction of psychosocial, behavioral, cultural, or health factors. Nursing science and scholarship have contributed new conceptual models, advanced research methods, and new interventions that link therapeutics with advocacy.

Nurse investigators have explored phenomena such as beliefs and attitudes among menarcheal girls, menstrual cycle characteristics and premenstrual changes among adult women, experiences typical of menopausal transition among midlife women, as well as examining the menstrual cycle experiences in populations seldom studied, such as disabled women, athletes, shift workers, toxic exposures in oncology nurses, diabetic women, and beyond those of gynecology clinic populations to the broader spectrum of healthy community samples. They have contributed to work complementing biomedical research in describing physiologic patterns across the menstrual cycle, developing diagnostic categories and criteria for phenomena such as dysmenorrhea, premenstrual syndrome, premenstrual dysphoric disorder, and therapies for problems related to menstruation and menopause.

Nurses with a concern for women's health have historically included feminist approaches in their clinical practice as well as their research. Angela McBride (McBride & McBride, 1981) was one of the first nurse scholars to embrace feminist theory as a research paradigm, calling for a reframing of gynecological disease within the greater context of a woman's everyday life. The early nursing literature related to the menstrual cycle reflects a definition of health grounded in everyday life (gyn-ecology) and not just clinical definitions of health such as risk factors and diseases (gynecology) (McBride, 1993). Nurses have focused their study on biopsychosocial response patterns, normative or developmental transitions, functional status, role performance, adaptation to environmental demands, and high-level wellness (Woods, 1988). Nursing research has helped to focus women's development and normative transitions (menarche and menopause) as normal rather than deficiency conditions that need medical treatment (Andrist & MacPherson, 2002). Feminist methods of inquiry have been expanded by nurse researchers to provide information "for" women rather than merely "about" women. For example, nurse investigators' use of methods such as researcher-in-relation, reflexivity, and social transformation to understand women's perimenstrual and menopausal symptom experiences provides the basis for women-centered therapeutics.

In the past decade, multidisciplinary efforts have increased our power to institute change in women's health status through cross-disciplinary research, building on the wisdom of early pioneers. For example, the Society for Menstrual Cycle Research (SMCR), a multidisciplinary organization with strong nursing leadership, has been the vanguard of the movement away from a reductionist perspective to a more comprehensive approach to the study of women's health (SMCR web site). Since 1977, the Society's published research conference proceedings have provided an invaluable chronology of research on the menstrual cycle and advanced thinking across several disciplines: nursing, psychology, sociology, epidemiology, anthropology, biostatistics, physiology, medicine, and literature (SMCR web site). Instead of a circumscribed phenomenon peculiar to sex hormones, the Society defined the menstrual cycle in the context of other biorhythms of human variability or a sociocultural network of meanings, and of a new understanding of how the endocrine system interacts with other functions.

Nursing research has been at the forefront in the study of normative experiences of menstrual cycle events. Menarche presents nurses with a unique opportunity to address health promotion issues, particularly those related to reproductive and sexual health of school-age girls. In a review of nursing research contributions to menstrual cycle research (Woods, Mitchell, & Taylor, 1999), investigators addressed images of menstruation presented to menarcheal girls, menstrual attitudes, symptoms, and the relationship of recalled menarcheal experiences and attitudes to adult women's subsequent experiences of symptoms. Since the last *Encyclopedia of Nursing Research* review by Reame, Medline and CINAHL searches yielded 34 published papers related to menstrual function and alterations related to daily activities, menstrual attitudes and knowledge, and preparation for menarche across multiple cultures. In contrast to the last review, the cultural and ethnic context is addressed by nurse researchers more than by other disciplines. These studies of menarcheal experiences and programs for menarcheal preparation in 12 cultures, including African-American girls, provides an expansive understanding of the developmental opportunity presented by menarche. More recently, nurses have been at the forefront of translating research to practice in the development of menstrual health advocacy groups (Red Web Foundation) and internet-based education (www.redspot.org).

Early efforts to understand the normative experience of menstruation and menstrual symptoms as illness experiences have included studies of healthy community-based populations of women. From these studies, we have been able to estimate the normative experiences of women and identify some that are idiosyncratic.

The Tremin Trust Database, first administered by Ann Voda at the University of Utah and now at Pennsylvania State University, represents a national resource of information about women's menstrual cycles that includes data from over 5,000 women spanning four generations (Voda, 1991). From the Tremin Trust Database it is possible to follow women from menarche through menopause and in some instances to do so for three generations. This database has provided important information about menstrual cyclicity across the reproductive years, length of cycles and bleeding episodes, regularity, and estimates of menopause.

Since the early 1980s, nurse researchers have expanded the scope of explanatory models and methods for menstrual cycle research. Woods and colleagues have systematically examined how symptoms synchronized to the menstrual cycle are influenced by the context of social class, education, race, marital status, self-esteem, occupation, and menstrual attitudes (Woods, Most, & Longenecker, 1985). They have documented the dynamic nature of symptom formation across and within individuals in response to their changing social environments (Taylor, Woods, Lentz, & Mitchell, 1991).

A by-product of nursing studies has been the development of improved designs and methods for the biobehavioral assessment of menstrual cycle phenomena (Woods, Most, & Dery, 1982; Shaver & Woods, 1986; Taylor, D., 1990; Mitchell, Lentz, & Woods, 1991; Reame, Kelch, Beitins, Yu, Zawacki, & Padmanabhan, 1996; Woods, Mitchell, & Lentz, 1999; Mitchell, Woods, & Mariella, 2000; Woods, Mitchell, & Mariella, 2002). Such methods have included the measurement of menstrual flow absorbency, assessment of perimenstrual symptom patterns and cluster types, statistical methods for handling the detection of LH pulsatile secretion, and comparison of daily menstrual symptoms across cycles of the same individual. The Washington Women's Daily Health Diary includes a menstrual symptom severity list of positive and negative experiences. It has been used by several nurse researchers to define a variety of menstrual cycle symptom patterns, including menarcheal and menopausal experiences.

Nursing research on menopause, like that on the menstrual cycle, has emphasized studies of normative experiences. A review of the literature contains rich descriptions of symptoms associated with menopause, including studies of hot flashes, sleep problems, and depression (Woods, Mitchell, & Taylor, 1999). In addition, nurses have focused on the meanings of menopause, women's attitudes toward the experience, and the social context in which it occurs and how the social context modifies the experience. In a recent review of nursing research on the menopausal transition, Andrist and MacPherson (2002) demonstrated that nursing research has helped to refocus women's development and developmental transitions as normal rather than deficiency conditions that need medical treatment. Nursing scholars have also focused on the experience of menopause across cultures (George, 1996; Punyahotra & Street, 1998; Meleis & Park, 1999; Berg & Taylor, 1999), studies of decision processes women use in arriving at a commitment to use (or not use) hormone therapy (Rothert & O'Connor, 2002), and more recently on nonhormonal symptom management strategies (Cohen, Rousseau, & Carey, 2003).

Nursing research results reflect a wide range of studies with women seeking care in clinical settings as well as community-based populations of women. Comorbidity in these samples remains a challenge, as does accounting for the influences of oral contraceptives, other drugs, psychiatric history, age, ovulatory status, and characteristics of the menstrual cycle. Encouraging is the promotion of the menstrual cycle as the "fifth vital sign" to be incorporated into all women's health assessment.

There is only beginning work focusing on biological changes surrounding menarche and in relation to symptoms. More studies of menarcheal preparation are needed to provide young girls with optimum preparation for healthy experiences of menstruation and their sexuality. The type of information girls need, beyond how to cope with the hygienic challenge of menstruating, is yet to be defined. Psychoeducational interventions for school-age girls provided by school nurses is an area for continuing study.

What is needed for future menopause-related research are studies of health education interventions, such as those designed to reduce women's uncertainty about the experience. In addition, primary care models of therapeutics for menopause are needed. There is an acute need to find nonpharmacological and culturally-appropriate options for symptom management for symptoms such as hot flashes and sleep disturbances.

DIANA L. TAYLOR

Mental Disorders Prevention

The prevention of mental disorders is based on a science that examines the incidence, prevalence, causes, and consequences of public health problems and the development, evaluation, refinement, and dissemination of interventions intended to prevent the occurrence or reoccurrence of those problems (Coie et al., 1993; Institute of Medicine [IOM], 1994). Among the tenets underlying the science of prevention is that many mental disorders result from environmental stressors that place individuals and communities at risk. Moreover, dysfunctional intra- and interpersonal patterns that evolve from social and health disparities contribute toward the development of mental health problems (Albee, 1996). However, behavioral strategies can be powerful preventive interventions that block the onset or recurrences of mental disorders.

The goal of preventive intervention is to reduce malleable risk factors and/or enhance protective processes. Risk factors are those attributes or circumstances that contribute to an individual's vulnerability (National Institute of Mental Health [NIMH], 1998a). The likelihood of developing a mental disorder increases for adults with each additional risk factor that they possess or encounter. Among children, each additional risk exponentially raises their susceptibility to mental disorders (Reiss, D., & Price, 1996). Protective processes, on the other hand, are the compensatory resources that moderate or even mollify the negative consequences of adversity (IOM, 1994). Protective factors include individual attributes such as an easy temperament, above-average intelligence, competency skills, and a supportive family environment. The resiliency of children is enhanced by effective parenting and the involvement of other caring adults. For adults, a supportive marital relationship can be protective.

Two major classifications of mental health preventive intervention exist. The first evolved from a public health perspective (IOM, 1994). Primary prevention is intended for individuals who do not have mental health problems, but who wish to gain greater competence. Secondary prevention is intended for individuals and families who are at risk for developing mental disorders because they live in communities with more than one environmental stressor. Appropriate participants in secondary preventive intervention include those individuals who are experiencing mild or moderate psychological symptoms, but who are not in crisis. Tertiary prevention is directed at those who are in crisis. The goal of such intervention is to prevent psychiatric hospitalization or incarceration. Once the crisis is past, such individuals and families should be directed to primary or secondary intervention programs to sustain or enhance their adaptational outcomes.

Another classification is derived primarily from the mental health field (IOM, 1994). Universal preventive interventions are directed at populations of individuals. McClowry (2003) used a translational approach to provide low-risk consumers with a self-help parenting manual. Selective prevention is intended for individuals, families, and communities who are at risk for the development of mental disorders. Nies, Chrusical, and Hepworth (in press) engaged inner-city women in a walking exercise program to enhance their health and reduce their level of stress. Indicated interventions are for those high-risk individuals who have biological markers or who have experienced early psychological symptoms of a mental disorder that has not reached a DSM-IV diagnostic level. Schepp and colleagues (1999) reported on an indicated intervention for adolescents who are diagnosed with schizophrenia.

Preventive science is an expansive multidisciplinary field comprised of researchers and clinicians who often work in teams to capitalize on their various types of expertise. Moreover, prevention scientists employ a wide range of qualitative and quantitative strategies to examine the multiple and interacting causes related to prevention issues. Epidemiological and other descriptive studies identify how risk factors and protective processes are related to mental disorders. The results from such studies subsequently inform interventionists about the mechanisms that are related to the disorder that they are trying to prevent. Interventionists also need to be aware of the cultural implications of the problem or disorder. Partnership with the relevant stakeholders is critical to assess the cultural appropriateness of the program (McClowry, Mayberry, Snow, & Tamis-LeMonda, 2004).

The timing of prevention programs is essential for maximizing effectiveness. The optimal time is before dysfunctional behaviors are established (Coie et al., 1993). Transitional times that occur during the life course are particular periods during which individuals and families are vulnerable. The birth of a child or the death of a family member are just two examples of such normative experiences that are transitional and thus lend themselves to preventive intervention.

Prevention science and its related interventions are consistent with the nursing profession. Nurses have a history of being engaged in prevention activities, often labeling them "anticipatory guidance" or "health promotion" (McClowry et al., 2004). Examples of such clinical services include suicide, domestic violence, or drug-abuse prevention, HIV education, pregnancy prevention, and bereavement support. Other prevention programs include parenting programs aimed at reducing child neglect or abuse and those aimed at supporting caregivers of chronically ill or elderly family members.

Nurses engaged in preventive services, however, are unfortunately experiencing the same challenges that face other disciplines in the field. The time restraints imposed by the current health care system compromises the amount of time many health care providers can spend with their clients. Since most types of preventive services are not reimbursable from third-party payers, a danger exists that preventive intervention will be further reduced due to the current health care environment. As patient advocates, nurses will need to work diligently to make sure preventive services remain accessible to health care consumers.

A recent report on prevention science (NIMH, 1998a) identified recommendations for future initiatives that will advance the field. A higher level of funding dedicated to preventive intervention and the related basic prevention science topics is essential. The prevention field especially needs to strengthen its epidemiologic foundations and expand the number of interventions that have been evaluated empirically. Preventive intervention programs often lack standardization and, too frequently, have been inadequately tested to determine whether they are achieving their intended outcomes. Demonstration of the efficacy of prevention programs supports the fact that this type of research is valuable and worthy of additional funding.

Challenges, however, are embedded in expansion of the field. Coordination across federal, state, and private agencies will be difficult to achieve, but necessary to assure that duplication of services is avoided and that the highest quality of programs are developed and tested. Findings should be disseminated so that constituents, funding agencies, and policy makers are kept informed of the developments of the field.

Although the prevention field has expanded rapidly over the last decade, highly qualified researchers and interventionists are still needed. Nurses are particularly well prepared to contribute toward a recent emphasis on the comorbidities between mental and physical disorders. The ideal way to prepare nurses to engage in such research and to be prevention interventionists is the same as for other professions—interdisciplinary courses, mentoring, and opportunities for collaboration.

SANDRA GRAHAM McCLOWRY

Mental Health in Public Sector Primary Care

Primary care was first comprehensively defined by the World Health Assembly following a seminal conference in Alma-Ata in 1977 (Health for All by the Year 2000). Building upon the key aspects of Alma-Ata, the 1978 World Health Organization emphasized the defining aspects of primary care as essential, first-level health care embedded in the community, available to all, evidence-based, socially acceptable, and affordable. In the U.S., this optimistic vision for high-quality primary care has been only partially achieved. Ongoing challenges to high-quality primary care services are especially pronounced for public sector primary care. Public sector primary care services serve disproportionate of numbers health care users who have limited ability to pay for health services and experience significant health disparities. Both economic barriers to care and health disparities—inequalities in health care related to race and ethnicity (Institute of Medicine, 2003b)—are key priorities for research on improving health services. These issues cut across all areas of public health need, including mental health services.

Also in the late 1970s, the primary care setting became formally recognized as the *de facto* mental health services system in the U.S. Of the minority of individuals who receive needed mental health services, most receive their services in primary care instead of the mental health specialty sector. Many people seen in primary care for medical problems have significant clinical comorbid mental health conditions (Miranda, Hohmann, Attkinson, & Larson, 1994), especially anxiety, depression, and substance-misuse disorders. The burden of unmet mental health needs is higher for racial and ethic minorities compared to whites (U.S. Department of Health and Human Services, 2001b). Significant barriers exist to accessing public sector health services, including the affordability of care, social stigma associated with mental illness, and fragmented care delivery systems acting as barriers to care when care is sought (U.S. Department of Health and Human Services). Recent changes in the financing of public health care services for cost-containment reasons may have further exacerbated health disparities by creating heightened barriers to effective community-based care (Leigh, Lillie-Blanton, Martinez, & Collins, 1999), including primary care services. These issues in the quality and access to primary health care services are particularly problematic in public sector primary care mental health.

A central goal of contemporary mental health services research is to generate new knowledge directed to the transformation of mental health services to achieve high-quality, accessible, recovery-oriented care for all (President's New Freedom Commission on Mental Health, 2003). Some significant progress toward this goal has been achieved over the past decade. Tests of interventions for primary care mental health care have been evolving in recent years from primarily efficacy assessments to effectiveness assessments. In effectiveness assessments, understanding what approaches work for which populations and individuals under what set of circumstances becomes of central importance. Effectiveness research also involves testing interventions in populations that experience significant health disparities and other barriers to high-quality health care. Examples of primary care research topics funded by the National Institute of Mental Health (NIMH) include incorporating sociocultural aspects of mental health care delivery, managing complex comorbid conditions, access to and acceptance of mental health services, effectiveness of mental health care delivered in "usual care" primary care settings, and quality of mental health care processes in relation to treatment guidelines and outcomes (NIMH, 2003).

As primary care research continues to evolve to better address issues of health disparities and mental health care delivery models for primary care settings, there are key opportunities for nurse researchers. Nurse researchers have the potential to make significant contributions to mental health services and interventions research for redesigned primary care mental health services in two key areas. The first area concerns testing models of care for common mental health issues within the primary care setting that are tailored in ways acceptable for various high-need patients populations and which can be shown to be both effective and cost-effective. In general, consistent with other bodies of clinical literature in medicine and other fields, the nursing literature on managing mental health issues in primary care (especially depression) has burgeoned over the past decade. However, there are still very few tests of nursing interventions using advanced practice nurses (such as nurse practitioners and mental health clinical nurse specialists) to manage mental health issues in "usual care" primary care and community-based settings. This is especially so for public sector primary care with populations that are most underserved and which experience health disparities. Recent examples of research with underserved populations include the work of Hauenstein (1996) to test a nursing intervention for managing major depression in rural women, and Torrisi and McDanel (2003) on the participation of two urban nurse-managed centers in a depression collaborative to improve care for depression.

The second area of research opportunity concerns evaluations of now rapidly evolving "blended roles" for advanced practice nursing, nursing roles in which medical and mental health skills are available in the same primary care provider (Williams, C. A., et al., 1998). Advanced practice nurses who effectively "blend" medical and mental health training are well-positioned to manage the holistic needs of the patients they see in primary care settings. For example, Lyles and others (2003) reported on the use of nurse practitioners trained to manage the medical and mental health needs of primary care patients with medically unexplained symptoms. These types of blended roles need additional research testing for combinations of comorbid health conditions most commonly seen in primary care settings.

Emily J. Hauenstein
Updated by Celia E. Wills

Mental Health Services Research

Mental Health Services Research (MHSR) is a relatively new, evolving area of health services research that focuses on access to, costs of, and quality of mental health care services within diverse health care delivery systems and socio-politico-cultural contexts (National Institute of Mental Health [NIMH], 2003). The importance of MHSR to inform improvements to public health services has become increasingly recognized in recent years, especially as mental disorders recently have been shown to be a leading cause of disability in the U.S. and worldwide (Office of the Surgeon General, 1999; World Health Organization, 2001). MHSR generates new knowledge directed to the transformation of mental health services to achieve high-quality, accessible, recovery-oriented care for all (President's New Freedom Commission on Mental Health, 2003). In MHSR, the methods of general health services research are applied to examining a diverse range of topics such as: sociocultural aspects of mental health care delivery; access to and acceptance of mental health services; effectiveness of mental health care delivered in "usual care" settings; economics and financing of mental health services; and, quality of mental health care processes in relation to treatment guidelines and outcomes (NIMH).

MHSR is interdisciplinary and integrative of the expertise of researchers in diverse fields, including psychiatric-mental health nursing, psychology, psychiatry, social work, anthropology, sociology, economics, biostatistics, health administration, and public policy. Broad interdisciplinary research expertise is needed for the diverse range of health services research topics that require the integration of literature from multiple fields, construction of complex research designs and data collection protocols, and the use of sophisticated approaches to data analysis. Research funding for MHSR is supported by multiple sources, including local, state, and federal. At the federal level MHSR is especially supported by the NIMH Division of Services and Intervention Research (DSIR). Most academically-based federally-funded research centers for mental health services research are led by nonnurse researchers. An exception is the Southeastern Rural Mental Health Research Center (SRMHRC) at the University of Virginia School of Nursing, which began in 1992 supported by NIMH funding and continues its focus on unmet mental health needs in rural settings.

Distinctions between interventions (treatment) and services research are somewhat vague (see NIMH's Bridging Science and Service report, 1998b). However, during the past decade, nurse researchers have most often focused on mental health interventions (treatment efficacy and effectiveness) research as opposed to broader service systems research. MHSR programs led by nurses remain uncommon, in parallel with the small number of nurses entering psychiatric nursing (Delaney, K., Chisholm, Clement, & Merwin, 1999) and the very limited numbers of nurses with doctoral and postdoctoral training in mental health services research. Relatively few doctoral programs in nursing prepare students to conduct MHSR. In 2001, in recognition of the need to increase the numbers of mental health services researchers, the American Psychiatric Nurses Association (APNA) facilitated the initiation of a postdoctoral mental health mentorship program, "Building the Capacity of Psychiatric Mental Health Nurse Researchers," cosponsored by the National Institute of Nursing Research and the National Institute of Mental Health (Cochrane, 2001). This program included a Phase I technical workshop on knowledge and skills for preparing grant applications, and a follow-up phase in which a concept paper was prepared and a mentoring plan developed to prepare a full grant application for review by NINR or NIMH. The current supply of mental health services researchers remains low in relation to present and projected future needs. There remains an urgent need to increase the supply of doctorally-trained nurses with funded MHSR research programs to improve the key contribution of nursing to this growing field.

Results of MHSR appear in journals publishing mental health services research, such as the *Archives of Psychiatric Nursing*, *Issues in Mental Health Nursing*, the *Journal of the American Psychiatric Nurses Association*, the *Journal of Psychosocial Nursing and Mental Health Services*, *Mental Health Services Research*, and *Psychiatric Services*, as well as many other journals not specifically focused on mental health or health services research. Pullen, Tuck, and Wallace (1999) concluded that quality outcomes and mental health delivery systems are among mental health nursing research priorities, based on a review of literature published in the mid-1990s in mental health nursing journals. Merwin and Mauck (1995) concluded that few psychiatric nursing studies were published in major nursing journals and that there was a lack of programmatic research upon which to base rigorous evaluation of outcomes. A review of the nursing literature done for this *Encyclopedia of Nursing Research* manuscript a decade later obtained results that remained consistent with the earlier conclusions of Merwin and Mauck. Some representative examples of MHSR appearing in nursing journals over the past 5 years include the work of Baradell and Bordeaux (2001) on outcomes and satisfaction of patients of psychiatric clinical nurse specialists, and Merwin, Hinton, Dembling, and Stern (2003) on shortages of rural mental health professionals.

JEANNE C. FOX
UPDATED BY CELIA E. WILLS

Mental Status Measurement: The Mini-Mental State Examination

Individualized assessment of cognitive status is necessary for the planning and evaluation of nursing care to determine the patient's capacity to understand instructions, be an active participant in his/her care, make health care decisions, and detect changes that will determine subsequent nursing actions. It is especially important to assess the cognitive status of elders who may have an undetected mild cognitive impairment or delirium; for example, assessing baseline cognitive status of hospitalized elders would allow early detection of side effects from receiving a new medication or of postoperative delirium. The Mini-Mental State Examination (MMSE) (Folstein, Folstein, & McHugh, 1975) is frequently used as a clinical assessment in a variety of settings and for preliminary screening of elders for neurodegenerative disorders such as Alzheimer's disease (AD).

The MMSE was developed over 30 years ago for serial testing of the cognitive mental state of patients on a neurogeriatric ward. The MMSE was specifically developed to be a formal and relatively thorough clinical evaluation tool that is brief and easy to administer, and consists of eleven tasks of cognition: (1) *orientation* to time and place, (2) *registration* assessed by ability to learn the names of three unrelated objects, (3) *attention and calculation* by performing serial sevens or spelling the word "world" backwards, (4) *recall* by naming the three objects previously learned, (5) *language* assessed by six items of naming objects, following verbal and written commands, writing a sentence spontaneously, and (6) *visual-spatial ability* by copying two intersecting pentagons. The tester asks the patient to respond to items and records the score for each. Item scores are added to provide the MMSE score, which can range from 30 (all correct) to 0 (no correct) responses.

Before conducting an MMSE assessment, the nurse should make the patient comfortable and establish rapport. The test is not timed but usually takes 5–10 minutes. During the testing, the nurse should praise success and attempt to enhance cooperation by not pressing on items the patient finds difficult. The testing situation may be an embarrassment for patients who are aware that they are "missing" some of the items (Mahoney, Volicer, & Hurley, 2000) and the nurse needs to be sensitive to this phenomenon and protect the self-esteem of such patients while preserving the integrity of the testing procedures to assure administration accuracy.

The degree to which the MMSE is reliable and valid is critical to the interpretation of scores. The tester needs to follow the administration procedures exactly. The MMSE is considered to have satisfactory psychometric properties. Initial reliability and accuracy by measuring consistency in the items and different raters were adequate for interrater agreement and retest stability when two samples of patients and several test administrators were compared (Folstein, Folstein, & McHugh, 1975). Validity, the degree to which the MMSE measures the construct of cognitive impairment, was supported by convergent and discriminant validity comparing hypothesized similarities/differences between scores from three groups of participants: normal, demented, and depressed subjects with and without cognitive symptoms. Age and education may influence test scores (Butler, S. M., Ashford, & Snowdon, 1996) in that elders and persons with low education may score slightly lower yet have higher cognitive capacity, so there are MMSE test norms based on these variables (Crum, Anthony, Bassett, & Folstein, 1993). After many years of use in several studies, a score of 23 points or less is considered to be *preliminary* evidence of cognitive impairment and *grounds for further evaluation* (Cockrell & Folstein, 1988).

Clinically, scores on the MMSE should be considered with other assessment data to provide clinicians with an estimate of patients' cognitive capacity to make treatment and research decisions. MMSE scores are one of several neuropsychological test results used to assess the need for and/or efficacy of cognitive enhancing medications for persons with AD. In the research arena, the MMSE is used both as an enrollment criterion as well as to describe project participants, enabling comparisons across studies.

At least reliability and if possible validity estimates of instruments used in particular studies should be reported each time the instrument is used in a study. Over 30 years use of the MMSE in reported studies illustrates the stability of the initially reported psychometrics. The MMSE has been translated into several languages and modifications have been made for versions that are culturally and linguistically appropriate (Folstein, 1998).

Our research team has used the MMSE in all our studies conducted since 1990 with persons who have AD and found measurement properties of interrater reliability to be adequate by rater agreement (Volicer, Hurley, Lathi, & Kowall, 1994) and internal consistency to be acceptable by examination of Cronbach's alpha (Hurley, Volicer, Hanrahan, Houde, & Volicer, 1992; Mahoney, E. K., et al., 1999; Camberg et al., 1999). Our experience shows that research assistants can easily learn to administer the MMSE, are accurate and consistent in its administration to patients following training, and do not upset patients when using it. Because the MMSE is used in so many studies, it is almost incumbent on researchers to include the MMSE to characterize subjects so that consumers of research have a benchmark of cognitive capacity for comparing results across studies.

The MMSE is a brief scale that can be administered to patients who have very different levels of cognitive impairment, from no impairment to being quite impaired. However, once a patient scores "0," the MMSE does not quantify the cognitive differences that can exist between patients who all score "0." If it is important to clearly characterize research participants in an AD project, another scale such as the Bedford Alzheimer Nursing Subscale (BANS) (Volicer et al., 1994) does allow additional discrimination of dementia severity for subjects who "bottom" on the MMSE. Because the MMSE does not measure executive function, the MMSE alone should not be used as an enrollment criterion in AD research, but should be combined with additional neuropsychological tests.

The lack of complexity in administration leads to high levels of rater reliability—a very important feature. The MMSE can be scored without need for a calculator or computing scores and the total can be entered onto the patient's record or data. Despite ease of administration and scoring of the MMSE, reliability checks need to be in place and testers should periodically be observed for accuracy. For example, one item asks the patient to follow a standardized 3-stage command, not three sequential single commands. During rater training for our research projects, we have found that some testers wanted the patient to do well and needed to be corrected for imprecisely administering (giving three sequential commands versus one 3-stage command) and scoring ("It was so close").

The MMSE is a brief screening test and scores were never intended to be a proxy for AD severity or to provide a cut score rule for determining when an individual has the capacity to provide informed consent. MMSE scores provide a useful and objective assessment for nurses in a wide range of clinical situations.

ANN HURLEY
LADISLOV VOLICER

Mentoring

A formal definition of mentoring is a spontaneous pairing by two individuals or a grouping of two or more individuals who feel they can assist each other in professional and sometimes personal growth. The mentor–mentee relationship tends to evolve and endure for the rest of one's career and consists of counseling, teaching, networking, and coaching. Vance and Olson (1998) described mentoring as a developmental and caring support or connection between two people which assists with socialization at each stage of a mentee's career.

More and more nurses are seeing the benefits of having an expert-to-novice relationship both as an expert as well as a novice. Certainly the advantages to the novice are clear. Mentors see the experience as an extremely positive opportunity to expand their own vision, and at the same time, impact the profession by assisting in shaping future nurse leaders. The health care organizations employing the mentors view the experiences as a favorable and cost-effective recruitment and retention tool, which ultimately improves job satisfaction and morale. With the current interest in acquiring Magnet Status for hospitals and health care organizations, the concept of providing staff and new graduates with ongoing mentoring relationships will flourish. Professional organizations such as the American Association of Critical Care Nurses and Sigma Theta Tau International also encourage their experienced and new members to pair up in a variety of activities such as: starting new local chapters, developing evidence-based protocols, preparing for a leadership role, and conducting clinical research. Higher education uses mentoring models to connect their students to practicing and experienced alumni and to friends or partners of the university.

Most mentees see the person who eventually becomes their mentor as a role model. Role modeling has been used in nursing pedagogy to improve interpersonal skills and impact change as well as with clinical skills (Kolb, 1982). Whether the experience is labeled an internship, externship, apprenticeship, fellowship, preceptorship, or mentorship, the fact remains that an experienced person is facilitating the role transition of an inexperienced individual to some extent. The degree of success of this growth is influenced by many variables including: the selection method of mentors, the way the assignment of mentees is determined, the readiness of the mentee to assume the formal as well as the informal knowledge from the mentor, and the organizational culture that surrounds the mentor–mentee relationship.

The process of an experienced individual coaching, guiding, or mentoring a novice has frequently been cited in nursing as a mechanism of building leadership skills (Vance & Olson, 1998; Grossman & Valiga, 2000; Bennetts, 2000; Peluchette & Jenaquart, 2000). Many of these labeled mentorships are actually preceptorships since they are an assigned relationship that is part of a course assignment or a component of job orientation. There are multiple peer, professional, and faculty mentorship publications in the literature that focus on specific skill acquisition over a set, prescribed time frame (Suen & Chow, 2001; Price & Balogh, 2001; Lloyd Jones, & Walters, 2001). Some of the skills include acquiring: new communication strategies for success as a nurse, methods to enhance creative abilities, all types of clinical skill building, and mechanisms to facilitate research and publications. In nursing it is also accepted that nurses can have different mentors during the various stages of their careers.

Due to our tumultuous health care environment it is more imperative than ever that nurses gain self-confidence, a goal that can be achieved by becoming competent not only with clinical skills but also with leadership skills such as negotiation, creative thinking, communication, and collaboration. In order to achieve this confidence nurses need to be mentored or guided by experienced nurses who can provide clinical knowledge and skills, practice with leadership and management skills, as well as psychosocial support. Having a mentor can assist a nurse to gain insight into their ability to impact change, think creatively, empower themselves and others, and acquire various skills to prepare themselves for a successful career as well as to strengthen the nursing profession (Grossman & Valiga, 2000).

Nursing students need to be socialized into the profession in order to adjust to the new graduate role. The nursing profession often uses preceptors to orient new staff and to assist them in gaining competency-based skills as well as to increase clinical decision-making ability before being deemed safe to practice independently. In fact, having a mentor is extremely important as a developmental tool for the progression of a nurse's career, for it can influence one's confidence and self-esteem in assisting with preparing people for leadership roles (Vance & Olson, 1998).

The mentor–mentee dyad does not include the aspect of formal evaluative feedback. When two people are assigned to work together by faculty or administration it is considered a form of mentoring called a preceptor–preceptee relationship and involves evaluation (Flynn, 1997). Historically, precepting has been a tried and true method of assisting new graduates and inexperienced nurses in acquiring the supervised practice of working with patients requiring specific nurse competencies. This one-to-one assigned expert and novice relationship allows the novice to gain skills and decision-making experience, while receiving instant feedback from the expert, and still provide safe patient care. It is important for longitudinal research studies to be conducted which track a mentoring relationship from the beginning to its current status. It would be interesting to assess how many assigned preceptor–preceptee relationships evolve into mentoring dyads and to identify patterns which may predict a successful match between experienced nurses and novices. More databased outcome studies measuring a mentee's leadership skills, assessing a mentee's career status, and identifying the mentee's mentoring of others are needed. Noe, Greenberger, and Wang (2002) cite several ideas for conducting future research studies which have clear significance to the nursing profession. If having a mentoring experience as a beginning nurse clinician, educator, researcher, and/or administrator is found to be a reliable predictor for success, an evidence-based protocol of mentoring could be established.

As for specific studies regarding mentoring in nursing research, Byrne (2003, 2002), Zambroski (2004), Records (2003), and Morrison-Beedy (2001) describe strategies for assisting faculty and students to participate in research. Jacelon (2003) describes mentoring for new faculty that includes suggestions on succeeding with the scholarship aspect of the tensure process and Olson (1995) and K. Roberts (1997) present ideas for increasing faculty scholarship productivity through mentoring in predoctoral fellowships. No studies were found depicting measurable outcomes of how mentoring assisted faculty and students with research.

CONNIE VANCE
UPDATED BY SHEILA GROSSMAN

Meta-Analysis

Meta-analysis is a quantitative approach that permits the synthesis and integration of results from multiple individual studies focused on a specific research question. Meta-analysis was first introduced in 1976 by Glass, who referred to it as an analysis of analyses. A meta-analysis is a rigorous alternative to the traditional narrative review of the literature. It involves the application of the research process to a collection of studies in a specific area. The individual studies are considered the sample. The findings from each study are transformed into a common statistic called an effect size. An effect size is a measure of the magnitude of the experimental effect on outcome variables.

Once the results from each study have been converted to a common metric, these findings can be pooled together and synthesized. The most common effect size indicator is *r*, which is the Pearson product moment correlation. Another effect size indicator is the *d* index. Cohen's *d* is the difference between the means of the experimental and control groups divided by the standard deviation. Cohen (1988) has provided guidelines for interpreting the magnitude of both the *r* and *d* effect size indicators. For the *r* index, Cohen has defined small, medium, and large effect sizes as .10, .30, and .50 or more, respectively. For the *d* indicator an effect size of .2 is considered small, .5 is medium, and .8 or more is large.

Approaches are available to examine and reduce bias from operating within a meta-analysis. Some ways that biased conclusions can occur in a meta-analysis are effects of a bias toward publishing positive but not negative results, giving each study an equal weight in the meta-analysis despite the fact they differ in sample size or quality, inclusion of multiple tests of a hypothesis from an individual study, and not ensuring an acceptable level of agreement or reliability among raters in coding the study characteristics.

The possibility that unknown, unpublished studies may exist, whose results fail to support the pattern illustrated by the published findings, is referred to as the file drawer problem (Rosenthal, 1979). The conclusions of the meta-analysis can be distorted if the retrieval of studies yielded only published studies in which a publication bias in favor of significant results may occur. R. Rosenthal developed a technique to assess the magnitude of the file drawer problem by calculating the minimum number of unpublished studies with nonsignificant results that would be necessary to change the conclusion reached by the meta-analysis.

It can be argued that not all studies synthesized in a meta-analysis should be given equal weight. Some studies may be poorly designed and have small unrepresentative samples, whereas other studies use randomized control group designs with large sample sizes. To remedy this problem, studies can be evaluated and assigned a quality score. The meta-analysis can then be calculated with studies weighted by their quality scores.

A source of nonindependence in a meta-analysis can result from using multiple hypothesis tests based on multiple variable measurements obtained from a single study (Strube & Hartman, 1983). One suggested remedy when selecting findings obtained from multiple measures of the hypothesis tests located within a single study is to collapse the various findings into a single, global hypothesis test.

One assumption that should be met before specific studies are quantitatively combined in one meta-analysis is that each study provides sample estimates of the effect sizes that are representative of the population effect size. Homogeneity tests can be calculated to identify any outlier studies. If outliers are identified, they can be removed.

Meta-analysis first appeared in the nursing literature in 1982, when O'Flynn published her article describing meta-analysis in the "Methodology Corner" of *Nursing Research*. A meta-analysis of the effects of psychoeducational interventions on length of postsurgical hospital stay (Devine & Cook, 1983) was the first meta-study analysis published in nursing. Since then meta-analyses have been conducted and published in a wide variety of areas, such as patient outcomes of nurse-practitioners and nurse-midwives, job satisfaction and turnover among nurses, relationship between postpartum depression and maternal-infant interaction, effects of educational interventions in diabetes care, quality of life in cardiac patients, and nonnutritive sucking in preterm infants.

The outcome of this quantitative approach for reviewing the literature has tremendous potential for a practice-based discipline such as nursing. One example of a meta-analysis that has consequences for nursing practice integrated the research on predictors of postpartum depression. C. T. Beck's (1996) meta-analysis of 44 studies helped to clarify which variables were significantly related to postpartum depression; there had been conflicting findings reported in the literature. The following eight variables were revealed to be significant predictors: prenatal depression, history of previous depression, social support, life stress, child care stress, maternity blues, marital satisfaction, and prenatal anxiety. An instrument based on the findings of this meta-analysis can be designed to help detect women at risk for developing postpartum depression.

Meta-analysis of the abundance of research being conducted can benefit nursing practice. Not only will the use of meta-analysis further knowledge development in the discipline of nursing, but it also can help nurses in the clinical setting to decide whether to apply research findings to their practice based on the size of the difference an intervention makes. Meta-analysis can resolve issues in nursing where there are multiple studies with conflicting findings. In addition, meta-analysis highlights gaps in nursing research for future studies.

CHERYL TATANO BECK

Middle-Range Theories

Middle-range theories are described by Merton (1968, p. 9) as those "that lie between the minor but necessary working hypotheses that evolve in abundance during day-to-day research and the all-inclusive systematic efforts to develop unified theory." He goes on to say that the principal ideas of middle-range theories are relatively simple. Simple here means rudimentary, straightforward ideas that stem from the focus of the discipline. Thus middle-range theory is a basic, usable structure of ideas, less abstract than grand theory and more abstract than empirical generalizations or micro-range theory. Middle-range theory is a set of related ideas that are focused on a limited dimension of the reality of nursing. These theories are composed of concepts and suggested relationships among the concepts that can be depicted in a model. Middle-range theories are developed and grown at the intersection of practice and research to provide guidance for everyday practice and scholarly research rooted in the discipline of nursing.

In 1999, a review of a decade of nursing literature identified the existing foundation of middle-range nursing theory (Liehr & Smith, 1999). To locate this literature, the Cumulative Index to Nursing and Allied Health Literature (CINAHL) was searched using the terms "middle-range theory," "mid-range theory," and "nursing." All papers written in English were evaluated according to four inclusion criteria: 1) the theory's author identified it as middle-range in the paper, 2) the theory name was accessible in the paper, 3) concepts of the theory were explicitly or implicitly identified, and 4) the development of the theory was the major focus of the paper (Liehr & Smith, p. 83).

Twenty-two theories, published from 1988 to 1998, met these criteria and were addressed. Seven were published between 1988 and 1992, and 15 were published between 1994 and 1998 (Liehr & Smith, 1999). The 22 middle-range theories were grouped as high, middle, and low relative to each other based on the generality or scope of the theory as determined by the name of the theory. Six of the 22 were high-middle, 7 were at the middle range, and 9 were grouped as low-middle (Liehr & Smith). It was recommended that persons creating middle-range theory: (a) describe clearly the theory name and how it was generated, (b) clarify conceptual linkages with a model, (c) articulate the research-practice links, and (d) tie the theory to the disciplinary perspective of nursing.

A 2001 CINAHL search using the same search terms and the same criteria for inclusion resulted in identification of 14 new middle-range theories published from 1998 through 2001. Two of the theories on the list of 14 (Precarious Ordering: Theory of Women's Caring and Experiencing Transitions) are referred to as "emerging" by their authors, indicating that they are in early stages of development (Smith, M. J., & Liehr, 2003). Four of the theories (Enlightenment, Family Health, Urine Control, and Pathway to Chemical Dependency in Nurses) were derived from grand theories of nursing or other middle-range theories (Smith, M. J., & Liehr).

The 14 middle-range theories were grouped as high, middle, and low relative to each other based on the generality or scope of the theory as determined by the name of the theory. One theory (Enlightenment) was high-middle; 7 were at the middle range (Attentively Embracing Story, Comfort, Cultural Negotiation, Experiencing Transitions, Family Health, Investing in Self-Care, and Truthful Self-Nurturing); and 6 were grouped as low-middle (Caring Through Relation and Dialogue for Patient Education, Family Dynamics of Persons with Chronic Pain, Pathway to Chemical Dependency in Nurses, Precarious Ordering: Theory of Women's Caring, Prevention as Intervention, and Urine Control Theory) (Smith, M. J., & Liehr, 2003, pp. 11–17).

All middle-range theories are works in progress. It is to be expected that middle-range theories change over time as they are applied to guide practice and research. Theories are published so that others can critique, test, revise, and use them as a source of scholarly productivity in research and practice. The 8 middle-range theories that follow cover a broad spectrum, including ones that were proposed decades ago and have been used extensively, to those that are newly developed and just beginning to be used. Some of the theories were originated by nurses and some were originally created by persons outside of nursing. Middle-range theories are offered as starting points for nurses wishing to structure their practice and research. With these theories comes a challenge to stretch the boundaries of thinking, consider the rub between each theory and what is known from experience, and apply the theories so that the body of nursing knowledge remains a vibrant, relevant foundation for guiding practice and research.

Community Empowerment Middle-Range Theory

The middle-range theory of community empowerment was developed by Cynthia Armstrong Persily and Eugenie Hildebrandt (2003). This theory evolved from participatory action research (Hildebrandt, 1994, 1996) and is an amalgamation of theories related to community development and empowerment. It is based on the premise that improving the health of people rests in programs that enable active participation of members of the community to take responsibility for their own health (Persily & Hildebrandt). Community development is embedded in models advocating the development of strength and confidence of community people while they are working on problems they have identified (Persily & Hildebrandt).

The purpose of the theory is to provide a framework for interventions at individual and community levels; it "explicates for nursing the direct transfer of knowledge and expertise from nurse professionals to lay people to promote health" (Persily & Hildebrandt, 2003, p. 111). The theory offers a community involvement process to augment the knowledge and health care decision-making potential of persons living in the community.

There are three major concepts in the theory. The concepts are: involvement, "a linking of people in the community to identify needs, resources and barriers;" lay workers, "trained persons who share backgrounds with persons in the community;" and reciprocal health, "actualization of inherent and acquired human potential" (Persily & Hildebrandt, 2003, pp. 113–114).

A model of the middle-range theory of community empowerment is depicted as the involvement of lay workers in the promotion of health (Persily & Hildebrandt, 2003, p. 117). When considered together, the concepts explain the potential for empowerment of community people through the involvement of lay workers in promoting reciprocal health. Lay workers in the community work with health care professionals to increase access and extend opportunities to promote health. This partnership of lay community members with professional providers offers opportunities to facilitate community involvement and attain reciprocal health.

Hildebrandt (1994) applied the theory in participatory action studies in South Africa with an exploratory descriptive design aimed at meeting the health needs of black South Africans in a township setting. Indigenous lay workers diminished the barriers of distrust, race, and language. Identified needs were: health knowledge, diagnostic screening, literacy training, and food through gardening. Findings of the study revealed that lay workers and health care personnel effectively responded to basic human health needs with all age groups in the community; it took a considerable investment of time and resources to introduce community involvement; and it was fitting to empower lay people in the promotion of community health.

Application of the theory of community empowerment in advanced practice nursing offers widespread opportunities to promote health. Some applications include: organizing lay community members to become involved in strategies to provide access to health care clinics to empower persons who have difficulty with transportation in rural areas, educating lay resource mothers to be involved in the care of empowering pregnant women during and after delivery, and involving older lay members of the community in different community roles to empower frail elder persons who live alone (Persily & Hildebrandt, 2003, p. 121). Each of these applications of the theory offers the potential to increase community competence and empower the community through the process of structuring community participation with lay workers to promote reciprocal health.

This theory offers a beginning foundation for future development through practice and research. Use of the theory in advanced practice nursing provides opportunities to develop the potential of a community by realizing achievement of outcomes that empower reciprocal health for individuals and groups. Identifying research questions related to the theory can structure the design of studies that will test and refine the theory.

This theory should be a part of the education of undergraduate and graduate students to enhance the awareness of community empowerment. Teaching students to apply theory in practice will give direction to their care and advance their understanding of theory-based practice.

Family Stress and Adaptation Middle-Range Theory

Family Stress and Adaptation theory is derived from a framework known as the Double ABCX Model of family adaptation (McCubbin, H. I., & Patterson, 1982). This middle-range theory, which has its roots in sociology, developed over decades beginning with the study of family response to war following World War II (LoBiondo-Wood, 2003). The original theory included the concepts of stressor event, family existing resources, and family perception of the stressor contributing to a crisis; additions to the theory over time included postcrisis variables, such as pile-up, coping, and adaptation; most recently the model has been configured to include resiliency (LoBiondo-Wood). "All of these conceptualizations add important pieces to the puzzle of what the family is and how it functions and adapts in periods of tranquility as well as upheaval" (LoBiondo-Wood, p. 93). LoBiondo-Wood notes five underpinning assumptions which address: (1) hardships as natural aspects of family life; (2) basic family strengths that protect the family unit and foster growth when families are faced with change; (3) basic and unique competencies to protect the family unit and foster recovery in the face of unexpected stress; (4) connection with communities to give and receive resources during stress and crisis; (5) work to restore order and harmony when families are faced with crisis demanding change. The assumptions and concepts of this theory make it applicable to nursing, when nurses are seeking a structure for guiding practice and research focused on family stress and adaptation.

The key concepts of the middle-range theory of family stress and coping are stressor, existing resources, perception of the stressor, crisis, pile-up, existing and new resources, family perception of the stressor, coping and adaptation (LoBiondo-Wood, 2003). Stressors are family hardships; existing resources include intrafamilial and community sources of support; perception of the stressor is the meaning assigned to the hardship by the family; crisis is the demand for family change; pile-up is the effect experienced when change is confronted over time; existing and new resources refer to evolving opportunities for facing the hardship; family perception of the stressor is the meaning assigned to the total experience of facing the hardship; coping is an active process of using resources; and adaptation is the outcome of this middle-range theory, suggesting that the family has accommodated (LoBiondo-Wood).

LoBiondo-Wood (2003) notes strengths and weaknesses of this middle-range theory. Central strengths are that the theory focuses on the family as a whole and has multiple instruments developed to address the concepts of the theory. Family Stress and Adaptation theory is unique in this way because the instruments have been specifically created to measure the ideas of the theory and psychometric data are available for the existing instruments. From a negative perspective, the theory has a large number of concepts and sometimes the concepts are not well distinguished from each other (LoBiondo-Wood). For instance, the reader may have noticed that in the listing and description of the concepts, perception of the stressor appears twice with little to distinguish one concept from the other. Examination of the model indicates that the first appearance of "perception of the stressor" occurs precrisis while the second appearance, entitled "family perception of the stressor," occurs postcrisis. This pre- to postcrisis view is another strength of the theory. Even though the pre- to postcrisis view contributes to complexity and a cumbersome structure, it provides a longitudinal perspective, enabling application to situations which are changing over time, as most health problems are. "The model calls upon nurses not only to be able to understand the processes and stages of the illness, but also how families respond to the illness trajectory" (LoBiondo-Wood, p. 106).

In spite of this strength of providing a longitudinal perspective, when the theory is used for research the researcher often selects specific variables from the model rather than using the whole model (LoBiondo-Wood, 2003). LoBiondo-Wood (2003) and colleagues have used the model to study children undergoing liver transplant, employing the Family Inventory of Life Events & Changes (FILE) to address pile-up; the Family Inventory of Resource Management (FIRM) to address existing and new resources; the Coping Health Inventory for Parents (CHIP) to address coping; the Family Coping Coherence Index (FCCI) to address perception of the stressor; and the Family Adaptation Device (FAD) to address adaptation. It is apparent from this list of instruments which operationalize theory concepts that the theory of Family Stress and Adaptation is very amenable to use by researchers. The theory has provided a

> wealth of instruments for testing family response to chronic illness. The model, extensions, and conceptual distinctions may seem cumbersome, but when the model is broken down and the elements that are consistent with a problem are delineated, the measurement and testing of hypotheses can be accomplished. (LoBiondo-Wood, p. 107)

In spite of years of research and continued development of the Family Stress and Adaptation theory, LoBiondo-Wood (2003) has identified several areas for continued study, such as examination of the fit of ethnicity and culture and consideration of new definitions of family, where parents may be same-gender individuals or individuals from two generations who come together to coparent a child. The middle-range theory of Family Stress and Adaptation is a valuable structure for guiding nursing research and practice and it could be an asset to undergraduate and graduate students learning to care for families in crisis. Further, nursing research could effectively contribute to the areas in need of further development, making this middle-range theory even more relevant for the sociocultural context of today's families.

Middle-Range Theory of Meaning

The middle-range theory of meaning evolved out of the work of Victor E. Frankl (1984) who used the theory to administer to persons with problems of a psychological nature. Patricia L. Starck (2003) used the theory for application to average human beings who are coping with the stresses of everyday life and significant life-changing events. The theory can also be applied with groups and communities.

There are three major concepts in the theory. These concepts are life purpose, freedom to choose, and human suffering. Life purpose is defined as "that to which one may feel called to and to which one is dedicated" (Starck, 2003, p. 129). Finding a purpose is related to the changing meaning in life. Freedom to choose is "the process of selecting among options over which one has control" (Starck, p. 132). Human suffering is "a subjective experience that is unique to an individual and varies from simple discomfort to anguish and despair" (Starck, p. 133). The relationship among the concepts "suggests that meaning is a journey toward life purpose with the freedom to choose one's path in spite of inevitable suffering" (Starck, p. 134).

Starck (2003) identifies four instruments that have been used in research and practice to quantify meaning. These instruments are: the Purpose in Life Test, Seeking of Noetic Goals Test, Meaning in Suffering Test, and the List of Values. Research has been conducted with hospice patients and families, breast cancer patients, persons with HIV/AIDS, a physically disabled population with people who had a permanent spinal cord injury, and with persons in a nursing home (Starck, pp. 135–138). These research studies focused on how the experience of intense suffering is related to the search for meaning and finding purpose in life.

Logotherapy is described as a method "to help persons separate themselves from their symptoms, to tap into the resources of their noetic dimension, and to arouse the dynamic power of the human spirit" and is a contrast to psychotherapy (Starck, 2003, p. 139). Three logotherapeutic approaches are identified by Starck as useful for application of the theory of meaning to nursing practice. These are dereflection, paradoxical intention, and Socratic dialogue. Dereflection is the "act of de-emphasizing or ceasing to focus on a troublesome phenomenon, issue, or problem; it is putting this issue aside" (Starck, p. 139). It is believed that dereflection strengthens one's capacity for transcending the problem and finding a greater purpose. Paradoxical intention is "intentionally acting the opposite to one's desired ends, thereby confronting one's fears and anxieties" (Starck, p. 140). Paradoxical intention distances one from the triggers of the problem, thus neutralizing the triggers and breaking the cycle of fear. Socratic dialogue is a "conversation of questions and answers, probing deeply into existential issues such as one's values. It is a rhetorical debate to trigger a change in attitude, behavior or both" (Starck, p. 141). In the dialogue, there is a conversation punctuated by probing questions to facilitate a deeper level of awareness.

This theory should be a part of the education of undergraduate and graduate students to enhance the awareness of the importance of finding meaning and purpose in one's suffering. Teaching students to apply theory in practice will give direction to their care and advance their understanding of theory-based practice.

Self-Efficacy Middle-Range Theory

The theory of self-efficacy, which was originally developed by Bandura (1977), is based on social cognitive theory. The theory

> conceptualizes person-behavior-environment interaction as triadic reciprocality, the foundation for reciprocal determinism. . . . Triadic reciprocality is the interrelationship among person, behavior and environment; reciprocal determinism is the belief that behavior, cognitive and other personal factors and environmental influences all operate interactively as determinants of each other. (Resnick, 2003, p. 49)

Early work by Bandura and colleagues attempted manipulation of the level and strength of an individual's self-efficacy to effect behavioral change (Resnick). Self-efficacy theory is at the middle range of abstraction, appealing to nurses who are interested in a conceptual structure which will guide practice and research focused on behavioral change. To say the theory is at the middle range means that it is more complex than simple hypotheses and yet targeted enough to be applicable. Self-efficacy is defined as "an individual's judgment of his or her capabilities to organize and execute courses of action" (Resnick). The major concepts of self-efficacy theory are self-efficacy expectations and outcome expectations. Resnick describes self-efficacy expectations as judgments about one's own ability to accomplish a particular task; outcome expectations are judgments about what will transpire if a particular task is successfully accomplished. "Self-efficacy and outcome expectations were differentiated because individuals can believe that a certain behavior will result in a specific outcome; however, they may not believe that they are capable of performing the behavior required for the outcome to occur" (Resnick, p. 51). For instance a smoker might believe that her frequent bouts of bronchitis would diminish if she would stop smoking; however, she may not believe that she is able to stop. In this instance, expected outcomes are dependent on self-efficacy judgments. Resnick also describes times when outcome expectations are dissociated from self-efficacy expectations (behavior change is loosely linked or not linked to outcomes). For example, dissociated expectations would occur if the smoker previously discussed believed that her bronchitis was related to the geographic area where she lived. In this instance, smoking is not firmly linked to bronchitis symptoms in the mind of the smoker, influencing likelihood of attempting behavior change.

Resnick (2003) discusses four information sources which influence judgment about one's self-efficacy: (1) enactive attainment—actual performance of the desired behavior, (2) vicarious experience—watching others who are similar to self perform the desired behavior, (3) verbal persuasion—encouragement by others, noting the individual's capability for performing the desired behavior, and (4) physiological feedback—bodily experience while performing the desired behavior. Each of these information sources becomes an avenue for nursing intervention to affect behavior change in practice or to study behavior change in research. In addition to information sources which may influence self-efficacy, experience interacts with individual characteristics and environment to affect self-efficacy and outcome expectations.

Resnick (2003) reports that within the decade more than 400 articles in nursing journals incorporate self-efficacy theory when addressing behavior change. These articles cover a broad range of topics including the education of nurses and parental training, but the majority of these articles have been related to chronic health problems and participation in health-promoting activities, such as exercise, smoking cessation, and weight loss. Resnick herself has used self-efficacy theory to develop interventions such as the WALC (Walk, Address unpleasant symptoms, Learn about exercise, Cueing to exercise) intervention, the Exercise Plus Program, and the Seven Step Approach to Developing and Implementing an Exercise Program. She has used the theory to guide research intended to influence elders' participation in functional activities and exercise (Resnick). When measuring self-efficacy, scale items query respondents' confidence (0 = not confident; 10 = very confident) regarding specific factors that might affect behavior change. "The development of appropriate self-efficacy and outcome expectation measures enables the testing of interventions designed to help participants believe in the benefits and overcome the challenges of performing selected activities" (Resnick, p. 60).

In less than 30 years since Bandura introduced self-efficacy theory, it has been widely used by professionals from many disciplines. Its usefulness for nursing stems from its relevance for health promotion through behavioral change. The theory could offer valuable guidance for undergraduate and graduate students who wish to teach patients about changing health behaviors; it would provide an evidence-based framework for selecting potentially effective teaching strategies. Self-efficacy is a mature middle-range theory, which has been tested through research and has demonstrated application for practice. Since most of the research on the theory has focused on self-efficacy expectations (Resnick, 2003), there continues to be a need for studying outcome expectations and the relationship between self-efficacy and outcome expectations. Nursing is well positioned to lead the way with continuing development of this middle-range theory to promote further understanding of factors influencing health-promoting behavior change.

Self-Transcendence Middle-Range Theory

The middle-range theory of self-transcendence was developed by Pamela G. Reed (1991, 1996, 2003) to provide an understanding about enhancing well-being for any person in a life situation where there is an increase in the awareness of vulnerability and mortality. The two assumptions underpinning the theory of self transcendence are that human beings are integral with their environment and capable of an awareness that extends beyond temporal/spatial dimensions, and that self-transcendence is an innate human characteristic that necessitates expression and the realization of full potential (Reed, 2003).

Reed (2003) makes the case that the theory is grounded in research and theories on postformal thinking, which is reasoning about life situations that is more pragmatic, spiritual, and tolerant of ambiguity. When engaging in postformal thinking, a person integrates experience as an expanded awareness of the moral, social, and historical context of life. There is an enhanced appreciation of self and life.

There are three concepts that make up the theory. These concepts are self-transcendence, well-being, and vulnerability. Self-transcendence, a major concept of the theory, is defined as

> the capacity to expand self boundaries intrapersonally (toward greater awareness of one's philosophy, values, and dreams), interpersonally (to relate to others and one's environment), temporally (to integrate one's past and future in a way that has meaning for the present), and transpersonally (to connect with dimensions beyond the typically discernible world). (Reed, 2003, p. 147)

Well-being is defined as a "sense of feeling whole and healthy, in accord with one's own criteria for wholeness and health" (Reed, p. 148). Vulnerability is defined as "awareness of personal mortality" (Reed, p. 149). The relationship between self-transcendence and vulnerability is nonlinear in that very low and very high levels of vulnerability are unrelated to increased transcendence. The relationship between self-transcendence and well-being is direct and positive when the outcome indicator of well-being is positive.

The Self-Transcendence Scale developed by Reed (1991) has been used in research related to the theory. Reed (2003) reports research focused on well elders, elders who were hospitalized for treatment of depression, the oldest-old (80 to 100 years of age), healthy adults, and adults facing end-of-life experiences with advanced breast cancer and AIDS (Reed, 2003, pp. 152–156). These studies demonstrated the consistent finding that transcendence was related to outcome indicators of well-being. In addition, Reed (2003) cites several dissertation studies on self-transcendence. It can be concluded that there is significant research providing support that self-transcendence is related to well-being across a diversity of human health experiences.

The theory has been used in nursing practice that aims to facilitate self-transcendence in bereavement, in caregivers of adults with dementia, sobriety, and in primary care situations (Reed, 2003, pp. 158–161). Intrapersonal strategies, interpersonal strategies, and transpersonal strategies for enhancing self-esteem are proposed (Reed). Intrapersonal strategies include: meditation, prayer, visualization, life review, and journaling. It is believed that these strategies assist a person to look inward to clarify and expand an understanding about self and the meaning of a situation. Positive self-talk and involving oneself in challenging activities can help a person to heal, grow, and transcend beyond an illness experience (Reed). Interpersonal strategies include support groups, altruistic activities, and group psychotherapy. Support groups enable people to connect with each other around a challenging life event and enhance self-transcendence through sharing experiences and reaching out to help and be helped by others. Transpersonal strategies include facilitating the connection with a power greater than self (Reed). Providing an environment where a person can look beyond self toward a higher power for help can promote self-transcendence.

Self-transcendence is a theory at the middle range of abstraction, appealing to nurses who are interested in a conceptual structure which will guide practice and research focusing on enhancing well-being. This theory should be a part of the education of undergraduate and graduate students to enhance an awareness of self-transcendence. Teaching students to apply theory in practice will give direction to their care and advance their understanding of theory-based practice.

Story Middle-Range Theory

Story theory, which was originally titled "Attentively Embracing Story" (Smith, M. J., & Liehr, 1999), proposes that story is a narrative happening of connecting with self-in-relation through nurse-person intentional dialogue to create ease. The authors of this middle-range theory recognize story as a fundamental dimension of human experience and nursing practice (Smith, M. J., & Liehr, 2003b). All nursing encounters occur within the context of story. The stories of the nurse, patient, family, and other health care providers are woven together to create the tapestry of the moment—the unfolding story about a complicating health challenge. The idea of story is not new to nursing but has been explicitly or implicitly incorporated into theories, used as an intervention, or as a source of research data (Smith, M. J., & Liehr, 2003b). Story theory calls attention to the human story as a health story in the broadest sense, structuring concepts to provide one perspective of the place of story in health promotion. The theory is based on three assumptions which underpin the conceptual structure. The assumptions state that people: (a) change as they interrelate with their world in a vast array of flowing connected dimensions, (b) live in an expanded present moment where past and future events are transformed in the here and now, and (c) experience meaning as a resonating awareness in the creative unfolding of human potential (Smith, M. J., & Liehr, 2003b). The three concepts of the theory are connecting with self-in-relation, intentional dialogue, and creating ease. Intentional dialogue is the central activity between nurse and person which brings story to life as a health-promoting endeavor.

Intentional dialogue is querying emergence of a health challenge story in true presence. It is purposeful engagement with another to summon the story of a complicating health challenge (Smith, M. J., & Liehr,

2003b). Intentional dialogue demands that the nurse come to the other with full attention to learn the meaning of a complicating health challenge through abandoning pre-existing assumptions, respecting the storyteller as the expert who knows the meaning, and querying vague story directions to clarify what is being shared.

Connecting with self-in-relation occurs as reflective awareness on personal history. It is an active process of recognizing self as related with others in a developing story plot uncovered through intentional dialogue (Smith, M. J., & Liehr, 2003b). To connect with self-in-relation, people see themselves not as isolated individuals but as existing and growing in a context, which includes awareness of other people and times, sensitivity to bodily expression, and a sense of history and future in the present moment.

> In following the story path, the nurse encourages reckoning with a personal history by traveling to the past to arrive at the story beginning, moving through the middle, and into the future all in the present, thus going into the depths of the story to find unique meanings that often lie hidden in the ambiguity of puzzling dilemmas. (Smith, M. J., & Liehr, p. 171)

Creating ease is re-membering disjointed story moments to experience flow in the midst of anchoring (Smith, M. J., & Liehr, 2003b). The re-membering creates a space of fit where one can anchor even for only a moment. Paradoxically, anchoring is accompanied by flowing as energy surfaces with the coming together of story moments into a comprehensible whole and there is movement toward resolving the complicating health challenge.

Story theory comes to life in research and practice through complicating, developmental, and resolving processes, essential elements of all stories.

> When gathering health story data, the complicating process focuses on a health challenge that arises when there is a change in the person's life; the developmental process is composed of the story-plot that links to the health challenge and suffuses it with meaning; and the resolving process is a shift in view that enables progressing with new understanding. (Smith, M. J., & Liehr, 2003b, p. 173)

Each time a nurse engages a patient to learn about what matters, story theory is applicable. By abandoning preexisting assumptions, respecting the storyteller as the expert, and querying vague story directions, the nurse intentionally engages the other, enabling connecting with self-in-relation to create ease. When the foremost intention of the nurse is caring-healing, the nurse queries the story about "what matters" to a unique individual culminating in a distinct story of how one person is living a presenting health challenge. The distinct story enables nursing care which is fine-tuned to uniqueness, addressing what is most important from the perspective of the patient.

A health story gathered for the purpose of scholarly inquiry represents a different foremost intention. When scholarly inquiry is the intention, the nurse has posed a research question about a particular health challenge and the participant is queried to understand how the health challenge has been lived. Regardless of the intention, caring-healing or scholarly inquiry, stories are gathered with a focus on essential story processes: complicating health challenge, developing story-plot, movement toward resolving. The only quality that distinguishes the caring-healing from the scholarly inquiry intention is where the intentional dialogue begins—either with what matters most as identified by the patient or with a phenomenon addressed in the research question developed by the nurse. Regardless of intention, story-plot can be pursued by drawing structures like a family tree or story path (Smith, M. J., & Liehr, 2003b, p. 175). Likewise, with either intention, movement toward resolving is possible as the storyteller is immersed in sharing a health challenge experience with someone who really cares to listen. "Finding a center of stillness and letting go of busyness and distractions energizes mindful attention to the story and propels movement toward resolving" (Smith, M. J., & Liehr, p. 176).

A story of a health challenge gathered for the purpose of scholarly inquiry demands a research strategy based on a research question. M. J. Smith and Liehr (2003b) propose approaches for qualitative and quantitative analyses of story data. They are pioneering the dual analyses (qualitative and quantitative) of a single set of stories, suggesting that dual analyses may provide the most meaningful direction for practice, further theory development, and continued research. Qualitative approaches for use in dual analyses include any qualitative method in which stories have been gathered and audio-recorded for transcription. Quantitative analysis is accomplished with narrative analysis software, Linguistic Inquiry and Word Count (LIWC), using the transcriptions prepared for qualitative analysis (Smith, M. J., & Liehr).

Research and practice have contributed to the development of story theory, establishing the middle-range foundation for the theory. Since the theory's publication in 1999, the authors have been developing methods guided by the theory. The real test of any theory, especially a middle-range theory, occurs as it is used to guide practice and research. By this criterion, story theory is in early stages of growth, but the theory is well-positioned for use by nurses who share a belief about the central place of story for the discipline of nursing and it is well-positioned for use with undergraduate and graduate students who are seeking guidance about engaging patients to talk about a health challenge.

Uncertainty in Illness Middle-Range Theories

Two middle-range theories of uncertainty in illness were developed by Merle Mishel. The original uncertainty in illness theory (Mishel, 1988) addressed the diagnostic and treatment phases of illness and the reconceptualized uncertainty in illness theory (Mishel, 1990) addressed living with continuous uncertainty, be it a chronic illness or an illness that may reoccur. Mishel refers to these theories as UIT for the uncertainty in illness theory and RUIT for the reconceptualized uncertainty in illness theory (Mishel & Clayton, 2003). The theories can be applied to the experience of ill persons, caregivers, and parents of children who are ill as well as to all age groups.

Uncertainty is defined as "the inability to determine the meaning of illness-related events occurring when the decision maker is unable to assign definite value to objects or events and/or is unable to accurately predict outcomes" (Mishel & Clayton, 2003, p. 29). They identify three major themes in the UIT. These themes are: antecedents of uncertainty, appraisal of uncertainty, and coping with uncertainty. The antecedent theme is composed of stimuli frame (symptom pattern, event familiarity, and event congruence), cognitive capacity (information processing ability), and structure providers (resources available). The appraisal of uncertainty is composed of inference (based on personality dispositions, experience, knowledge, and context), and illusion (beliefs that have a positive outlook). Coping with uncertainty is composed of danger (possibility of a harmful outcome), opportunity (possibility of a positive outcome), coping (reducing and managing uncertainty), and adaptation (usual range of biopsychosocial behavior). The proposed health outcome related to the UIT is adaptation and the regaining of personal control of one's life. Mishel's model of the UIT (Mishel & Clayton, p. 30) shows linear relationships among the themes with no feedback loops. The model depicts uncertainty resulting from antecedents with the major pathway going through the stimuli frame variables that have been influenced by cognitive capacities.

The RUIT "includes the antecedent theme in the UIT and adds the two concepts of self-organization and probabilistic thinking" (Mishel & Clayton, 2003, p. 31). Mishel and Clayton describe self-organization as the structuring of a new sense of order that comes from the acceptance of uncertainty as a natural life rhythm. Probabilistic thinking is a pattern of thinking incorporating a conditional view of the world. The RUIT sets forward "four factors that influence the formation of a new life perspective. These are prior life experience, physiological status, social resources, and health care providers" (Mishel & Clayton, p. 31). On the basis of this theory it can be concluded that a person comes to a different view of the continuous experience of uncertainty in illness that goes on through time. The health outcome of the RUIT is the expansion of consciousness. Mishel's model of the RUIT (Mishel & Clayton, p. 33) shows a spherical configuration over time representing repatterning and reorganization resulting in a different view of uncertainty in illness.

Mishel published an Uncertainty in Illness Scale in 1981 and the scale has been frequently used to study the experience of uncertainty for persons in acute or chronic illness situations. Mishel and Clayton (2003, pp. 34–38) report research that directly supports elements of the UIT, such as symptom pattern, event congruence, event familiarity, social support, credible authority, appraisal, coping, and adjustment to uncertainty. They note that the RUIT has less frequently been used for research and support, for the RUIT has come from qualitative studies of people with chronic illness (Mishel & Clayton, p. 38).

Within the last decade, an uncertainty management intervention was evaluated in four clinical trials with persons with breast cancer and prostate cancer (Mishel & Clayton, 2003). The intervention was based on the UIT and implemented with weekly telephone calls. The intervention demonstrated effectiveness for teaching skills to manage uncertainty, teaching problem solving, improving cognitive reframing, enhancing patient-provider communication, and improving the management of the side effects of cancer treatment (Mishel & Clayton).

Mishel and Clayton (2003) propose substantive direction for practice guided by the theories and tested in research. Use of the two theories in practice offers opportunities for nurses to understand, address, and manage sources of uncertainty in illness for patients. Providing well thought out information directly related to uncertainty is a way of providing structure to the stimuli frame. Communication with patients experiencing uncertainty by providing contextual cues, such as what will be heard and felt during procedures, is a way to reduce ambiguity and increase understanding. Uncertainty is a human response to the illness experience that is found in the frontlines of nursing practice. These theories directly relate to the planning of care to reduce or prevent uncertainty for persons with acute or chronic illness.

These theories can enhance the education of undergraduate and graduate students by bringing awareness of uncertainty in illness to routine care planning. Teaching students to apply theory in practice will give direction to their care and advance their understanding of theory-based practice.

Unpleasant Symptoms Middle-Range Theory

The middle-range theory of unpleasant symptoms was created for application with a broad range of diseases whenever unpleasant symptoms demand nursing attention. The original theory was published nearly a decade ago (Lenz, Suppe, Gift, Pugh, & Milligan, 1995) as a result of collaboration between faculty and graduates of the doctoral program at the University of Maryland School of Nursing. Each of the graduates had studied an unpleasant symptom for dissertation research. Gift had studied dyspnea; both Milligan and Pugh had studied fatigue (Lenz & Pugh, 2003). The individuals who developed the theory

had collaborated in dyads or triads on various empirical studies and theoretical articles. They shared geographic proximity, which facilitated collaboration, and, by virtue of their common association with one PhD program in nursing, they also shared exposure to the same philosophical and metatheoretical perspectives regarding the de-

> velopment and substance of nursing science. (Lenz & Pugh, p. 70)

A philosopher of science who taught in the doctoral program at the University of Maryland, Frederick Suppe, coauthored the manuscript which introduced the theory. Two years after its first publication, a refined version of the theory, which emphasized the reciprocity between the concepts of the theory, was introduced into the nursing literature (Lenz, Pugh, Milligan, Gift, & Suppe, 1997).

The theory of unpleasant symptoms has three major concepts: symptoms, influencing factors (physiological, psychological, and situational), and performance outcomes (Lenz & Pugh, 2003). A symptom is defined as an individually perceived indicator of aberration in normal function, which may occur in isolation or in combination with other symptoms and is characterized by intensity, distress, duration/frequency, and quality, which refers to the nature of the symptom or how it is manifested (Lenz & Pugh). Influencing factors are physiological (e.g., anatomic/structural, genetic, bodily processes), psychological (affective and cognitive), or situational (social and physical environment) qualities that can influence and be influenced by symptom experience. In addition, the theory suggests that when more than one symptom is experienced, the symptom experiences influence each other, emphasizing a reciprocal nature depicted by the model. The authors (Lenz & Pugh) give the example of nipple pain and fatigue, common symptoms for nursing moms which can exacerbate each other and lead to premature termination of breast-feeding, an undesirable performance outcome. Performance outcomes are the consequences of the symptom experience. "Quite simply, the theory asserts that the experience of symptoms can have an impact on the individual's ability to function, with function including motor skills, social behaviors and cognition" (Lenz & Pugh, p. 78).

Lenz and Pugh (2003) report that research related to the middle-range theory of unpleasant symptoms is just recently beginning to be reported in the literature, with much of the research being done by the developers of the theory themselves. Some of this research has examined interventions to diminish symptoms and therefore improve performance outcomes; some has examined the relationship between influencing factors which impact symptom experience. Some of the unpleasant symptom research completed by people other than the developers of the theory has examined symptoms in cancer patients undergoing chemotherapy, people with heart-lung transplants, end-stage renal disease patients, and people with Alzheimer's disease (Lenz & Pugh). Use of the theory for research has resulted in critique of the theory which was considered and applied when the developers refined the theory (Lenz et al., 1997).

Lenz and Pugh (2003) note that published reports of use of the theory in practice are few. This is surprising given the fact that unpleasant symptoms are a common experience for most patients whom nurses encounter. Unlike theories at a lower level of abstraction which focus on one symptom, such as pain, the more generic theory of unpleasant symptoms guides approaches for more complex symptom combinations, as often occur in real-world practice situations. For instance, the theory emphasizes the importance of in-depth assessment of symptoms which considers the contribution of influencing factors.

> It suggests that multiple management strategies may need to be applied simultaneously, given the multivariate nature of the factors influencing symptoms. It also emphasizes the importance of considering the effect of several symptoms, occurring together, on patient's functioning, and encourages assessment of functional patient outcomes. (Lenz & Pugh, pp. 85–86)

Thus far, the research guided by the middle-range theory of unpleasant symptoms has addressed the symptoms of pain, dyspnea, nausea, vomiting, and fatigue (Lenz & Pugh, 2003). Clearly, there are more symptoms to be explored. Likewise, there is need for further elaboration of the relationship between the influencing factors and how the factors relate with the symptom experience. Finally, Lenz and Pugh note the potential for further development of the performance component of the model, suggesting the consideration of primary and secondary outcomes as well as temporally proximal and distal outcomes. There is no question that the middle-range theory of unpleasant symptoms is a work in progress, which could benefit practicing nurses, undergraduate and graduate students, and researchers if used as a guiding framework. Likewise, the theory could benefit from use in practice and research so that continued empirically based development would further enhance the usefulness of the theory.

PATRICIA LIEHR
MARY JANE SMITH

Middle-Range Theories of Dementia Care

Nursing has developed and synthesized a number of approaches to guide research and practice for the care of people with dementia. Primarily middle-range theory in nature, these approaches drew upon theoretical propositions developed within and outside nursing that were modified via experiential observations. Nursing knowledge concerning dementia care has grown tremendously during the past decade. Utilizing the criteria of publication and dissemination within nursing, the following middle-range theories were selected (listed alphabetically) : Cognitive Developmental (CD) Model (Matteson, Linton, & Barnes, 1996), Individualized Care for Frail Elders Model (Happ, Williams, Strumpf, & Burger, 1996), the Need-Driven Dementia-Compromised Behavior Model (Algase et al., 1996), and the Progressively Lowered Stress Threshold Model (Hall, G. R., & Buckwalter, 1987).

The CD Model (Matteson, Linton, & Barnes, 1996) posits in part that loss of cognitive abilities in dementia follows a reverse order from acquisition. Piagetian theory determines the order in which skills are affected, e.g., at first, formal operational skills are lost, followed by concrete operational tasks, and lastly, sensorimotor abilities which include speech and motor dysfunction. Propositions derived from the model are based on an assessment of the appropriate cognitive level and problem behaviors associated with it. Behavioral management, environmental modification, and caregiver interactions are then determined according to the appropriate developmental stage. Preliminary results of model testing indicate that it was possible to manage behaviors while reducing the number of psychotropic medications (Matteson, Linton, Barnes, Cleary, & Lichtenstein, 1995). Instrument development to assess earlier periods of cognitive function and the combination of this approach with other staging and assessment models have been suggested.

Individualized Care for Frail Elders (ICFE) Model

The ICFE Model (Happ et al., 1996) embodies an interdisciplinary approach to care and emphasizes four points. These are: (1) knowing the person (life story and patterns of response), (2) the relationship (staff continuity and reciprocity), (3) choice (decision-making and risk-taking), and (4) resident participation (daily planning). Evan's cross-cultural observations in four European countries supported related propositions and delineated three factors that contributed to individualized care: (1) congruent societal and health care values, (2) commonalities of patient needs in all settings, and (3) primacy of caring through knowing the person. Rowles & Dallas (1996) found that family involvement in nursing home decision making served to individualize care and provided a continuing link to the person's personal history and preferences. Several studies supported cost-effectiveness linked to lowered medication costs and staff turnover. Further research on outcomes and refinements in definitions, goals, and critical attributes is ongoing.

Need-Driven Dementia-Compromised Behavior (NDB) Model

The NDB approach views the person with dementia as experiencing an unmet need or goal that results in need-driven behaviors such as aggression, wandering, problematic vocalizations, and a recent addition, passive behaviors. Behaviors reflect the interaction of salient background and proximal factors found either within the person or in the environment or both. Background variables include neurological, cognitive, health status, and psychosocial factors. Proximal factors include physiological and psychosocial need states and the physical and social environment. NDBs are evaluated on dimensions of frequency and duration. Nursing's role is to identify those at risk and to intervene with strategies under various sets of environmental circumstances. Collective programs of research on the model were highlighted in a special issue of the *Journal of Gerontological Nursing* (Overview of NDB Model, 1999). Multiple methods for deriving practice interventions from the model were also published in a subsequent special focus section of this journal (NDB Intervention, 2002). A special section in *Aging and Mental Health* was devoted to model-derived measurement and intervention strategies (Behavioral Symptoms, 2004). Current research efforts are focused on the identification of variables common to and different from each of the behaviors and on the application of linear modeling to further build the theory.

Progressively Lowered Stress Threshold (PLST) Model

The PLST Model (Hall, G. R., & Buckwalter, 1987) views the person with dementia as experiencing baseline anxieties and dysfunctional states throughout the course of the disease. Anxious behavior occurs during stress, and if stress continues, dysfunctional states such as panic occur. Six principles guide nursing: (1) maximize the level of safe function by supporting all areas of loss in a prosthetic manner, (2) provide unconditional positive regard, (3) use behaviors indicating anxiety to determine limits of stimuli and activity, (4) teach caregivers to listen and evaluate verbal and nonverbal responses, (5) modify environment to support losses and enhance safety, and (6) provide education, support, care, and problem-solving for caregivers. The PLST Model has been used to investigate caregiver education effects on caregiving consequences. Training decreased the impact of caregiving (Garand et al., 2002), and improved caregivers' mood (Buckwalter et al., 1999). The model has been tested in regard to interventions centered on music, touch, pain, nonnutritive sucking, and sleep. Continued research will test the main assumptions of the model.

Examples of other approaches from the last decade (organized chronologically) include: the Sensoristasis Model (Kovach, 2000), the Cognition-Sensitive Approach (Barnes & Adair, 2002), the Implicit Memory and Familiarity Framework (Son, Therrien, & Whall, 2002), and the Comprehensive Model of Psychiatric Symptoms of Progressive Degenerative Dementias (Volicer & Hurley, 2003). Algorithmic frameworks (Beck, Heacock, Rapp, & Mercer, 1993) and decision trees (Richie, 1996) have addressed strategies to determine level of assistance and nursing interventions.

A number of other approaches explicated selected aspects of middle-range theory work for dementia and produced instruments which assess model variables. These include the modification as an observational tool of the Cohen-Mansfield Agitation Inventory by Whall (Chrisman, Tabar, Whall, & Booth, 1991), the Ryden Aggression Scale (Ryden, Bossenmaier, & McLachlen, 1991), Hurley's Discomfort Scale (Hurley, Volicer, Hanrahan, Houde, & Volicer, 1992), the Modified Interaction Behavior Measure (Burgener, Jirovec, Murrell, & Barton, 1992), the Dementia Mood Picture Test (Tappen & Barry, 1995), and the Algase Wandering Scale (Algase, Beattie, Bogue, & Yao, 2001).

The past decade has been characterized by a resurgence of interest in the development and testing of middle-range theories of dementia care. As these efforts continue to be supported by programs of research, they hold great promise for more effective care in the years ahead.

KATHY COLLING
ANN WHALL

Minority Women Offenders

To date, criminal justice programs are based on the male experience because of the preponderance of men prisoners. However, criminal justice statistics indicate female detainees are increasing in numbers more rapidly than the male detainee population (Haywood, Kravitz, Goldman, & Freeman, 2000). Additionally, because minority women are disproportionately represented in the numbers of incarcerated women, there is a need for cultural-specific, gender-responsive programs.

Although the majority of federal female offenders are under community supervision, there is very little information available on their characteristics and needs. There is even less known about supervision issues and strategies, treatment approaches, and characteristics that enhance effective programs and successful outcomes for female offenders. The effectiveness of rehabilitation programs for the general offender population has received much attention; however, there is a paucity of research dedicated to the female offender population (Koons, Burrow, Marash, & Bynum, 1997).

Many of these women offenders are supervised by a probation agency and are considered as low risk and therefore have very little contact with their probation officer. There is, however, indication that this lack of contact with their supervising agent leads to higher rate of failure on community supervision (Chesney-Lind, 2000).

The rationale for women committing a crime is generally different than for their male counterpart. For instance, a woman may have been coerced into drug offenses or other criminal behavior because of an abusive spouse or boyfriend. This type of influence is referred to as gender entrapment (Ritchie, 1996).

Probation and parole periods were initially intended to afford the opportunity of gradual reintegration into the community, eliminating the social stigma in due time; however, this hoped-for pattern of reintegration into a healthy life pattern generally does not occur (Simon, 1993). There is a lack of opportunities for reintegration and acceptance by society. The stigma remains, marking the ex-felon and often creating angry and defiant responses to the related feelings of shame and rejection (Scheff & Retzinger, 1991).

Female offenders have several unique needs and concerns different from their male counterparts. According to Greenfield and Snell (1999), women offenders have different needs than men, probably due to their disproportionate victimization from sexual or physical abuse. They have histories of trauma and substance abuse, and their pathways to crime are based on survival of abuse and poverty (Bloom, 2000). They begin to use alcohol and other drugs at an early age, and there is indication that there is a link between their addiction and physical and sexual abuse (Covington, 1998).

When they are besieged with problems of low self-esteem and the stigma and shame of incarceration, the separation from their children and/or the potential to lose their children will present their probation officer with supervision difficulties. Multiple studies indicate that they present with more complicated and severe mental health problems (DeCostanzo, 1998).

Criminal justice supervision, programs, and services have been based on the male experience, mostly due to the higher number of men in the criminal justice system as compared to women. Therefore, many of the supervision and program needs of women have been ignored. Thus there is very little empirical evidence indicating what works for female offenders to prevent relapse and recidivism (Bloom, 2000). Programs dominated by men result in women's issues being minimized and they are less likely to be adequately addressed. Women have been socialized to value relationships and connectedness; thus developing a support system for them is congruent with their orientation. To prevent relapse and recidivism, strategies that are gender-responsive need to be developed and implemented.

Although the Federal Court system in San Antonio has recently adopted the Level of Service Inventory—Revised (LSI-R) for use as the risk/need assessment tool for all persons who are in the probation phase, the tool has not been evaluated for validity and clarity with minority women. This pilot represented the first step in a series of pilot studies preliminary for development of a mentoring support program directed to decrease recidivism among minority women offenders.

The Level of Service Inventory—Revised (LSI-R) is an instrument designed to provide a basis for correctional intervention programming that is both appropriate to the level of need for service and to the level of risk for recidivism (Andrews & Bonta, 1995). It was unknown if the major and minor criminogenic targets reflected in the LSI-R were appropriate for minority women or if these women's recidivism risk can be accurately assessed.

The psychometric properties of the Level of Service Inventory—Revised (LSI-R) were found to be reliable, had content validity, and were understood by the majority of participants. This assessment tool will be effective in assessing the recidivism risk of minority female offenders who are in the community supervision phase of their federal sentencing.

Norma Martinez Rogers
Susan K. Moore
Yolanda Narvaez-Edwards

Moral Distress

Moral distress describes a feeling that occurs in relation to a particular type of morally troubling experience. The term *moral* represents judgments about good or bad (right or wrong) actions, thoughts, or character of people, particularly in relation to human responsibilities. The term *distress* signifies a profoundly negative outcome demonstrated in affective, physical, and relationship domains. Moral distress is the pain or anguish affecting the mind, body, or relationships in response to a situation in which the person is aware of a moral problem, acknowledges moral responsibility, and makes a moral judgment about the correct action, yet, because of real or perceived constraints, participates in perceived moral wrongdoing (Nathaniel, 2004).

Virtually absent from common language usage, the term *moral distress* originated when ethicist Andrew Jameton (1984) recognized that nurses' stories about moral dilemmas were inconsistent with the definition of *dilemma*. In a moral dilemma, one struggles to decide between two or more mutually exclusive courses of action with equal moral weight. Jameton asked nurses to talk about moral dilemmas in practice. Consistently, the nurses talked about moral problems for which they felt they clearly knew the morally correct action, but believed they were constrained from following their convictions (Jameton, 1993). Jameton concluded that nurses were compelled to tell these stories because of their profound suffering and the importance of the situations. Jameton defined moral distress as follows: "Moral distress arises when one knows the right thing to do, but institutional constraints make it nearly impossible to pursue the right course of action" (Jameton, 1984, p. 6). Further refining the concept in 1993, Jameton stipulated that, in cases of moral distress, nurses participate in the action that they have judged to be morally wrong. Based upon Jameton's work, J. M. Wilkinson (1987–88) defined moral distress as "the psychological disequilibrium and negative feeling state experienced when a person makes a moral decision but does not follow through by performing the moral behavior indicated by that decision" (p. 16). Further refining the definitions and offering examples for clarification, nearly every subsequent source relies on Jameton and/or Wilkinson's definition of moral distress.

Situations involving moral distress may be the most difficult problems facing nurses. Moral distress results in unfavorable outcomes for both nurses and patients. Because of moral distress, nurses experience physical and psychological problems, sometimes for many years (Nathaniel, 2004; Wilkinson, J. M., 1987–88; Fenton, 1988). Reports of the number of nurses who experience moral distress vary slightly. Between 43% and 50% of nurses leave their units or leave nursing altogether after experiencing moral distress (Wilkinson; Millette, 1994; Nathaniel).

Moral distress requires a complex interplay of human relationships, institutional factors, personal attributes, and a morally troubling situation. Moral distress occurs in high-stress situations or with vulnerable patients. Areas that engender high overall stress levels, such as critical care or other areas with very vulnerable patients, harbor a greater proportion of moral problems (Bassett, C. C., 1995; Corley, 1995; Rodney, 1988; Fenton, 1988; Hefferman & Heilig, 1999; Millette, 1994). Moral distress has been documented in the following specific situations: prolonging the suffering of dying patients through the use of aggressive/heroic measures; performing unnecessary tests and treatments; lying to patients, failing to involve nurses, patients, or family in decisions; and incompetent or inadequate treatment by a physician (Wilkinson, 1987–88; Bassett, C. C.; Hefferman & Heilig; Rodney; Corley; Nathaniel, 2004).

Individual nurse's sense of moral responsibility is an integral part of the moral distress process (Wilkinson, 1987–88; Jameton, 1984). The level of nurses' moral distress may be influenced by their perceptions of the degree to which they are responsible for what happens to their patients and the degree to which they are able to say, " 'it is my decision to make' " (Wilkinson; Hefferman & Heilig, 1999; Jameton, 1993).

Moral judgment is also a factor in moral distress. Moral distress is not a response to a violation of what is unquestionably right, but rather a violation of what the individual nurse judges to be right. Nurses respond differently to moral problems in terms of their moral awareness, their orientation toward consequences rather than rules, or their orientation toward justice rather than caring (Wilkinson, 1987–88; Millette, 1994).

Institutional setting also contributes to moral distress. Many nurses view themselves as powerless within hierarchical systems (Wilkinson, 1987–88; Rodney, 1988). They perceive little support from nursing and hospital administrations (Fenton, 1988). Nurses may experience moral distress as a result of having been socialized to follow orders, remembering the futility of past actions, or fearing job loss. Other organizational factors contributing to nurses' moral distress include their views concerning the quality of nursing and medical care, organizational ethics resources, their satisfaction with the practice environment, and the law and/or lawsuits (Wilkinson).

Since conflicting moral judgment is a central theme in moral distress, relationships between nurses and physicians are the most frequently mentioned institutional constraints (Wilkinson, 1987–88; Bassett, 1995; Corley, 1995). Nurses experience moral distress because physicians and nurses have different moral orientations, different decision-making perspectives, and an adversarial relationship (Wilkinson; Bassett; Corley).

Psychological and physical sequelae and changes of behavior may be indicative of moral distress. Psychosocial indicators of moral distress include blaming self or others, excusing one's actions, self-criticism, anger, sarcasm, guilt, remorse, frustration, sadness, withdrawal, avoidance behavior, powerlessness, burnout, betrayal of personal values, sense of insecurity, and low self-worth (Wilkinson, 1987–88; Fenton, 1998). Nurses describe a need to detach themselves emotionally or withdraw from the situation when they are no longer able to deal with the stress, and may leave the unit for a less stressful area or leave nursing altogether (Fenton; Hefferman & Heilig, 1999). Nurses' somatic complaints related to moral distress include weeping, palpitations, headaches, diarrhea, and sleep disturbances (Fenton; Wilkinson; Nathaniel, 2004). In addition, empirical evidence suggests that prolonged or repeated moral distress leads to loss of nurses' moral integrity (Wilkinson).

Moral distress also affects the quality of patient care. Some nurses lose their capacity for caring, avoid patient contact, and fail to provide good physical care because of moral distress. Nurses may physically withdraw from the bedside, barely meeting patients' basic physical needs (Hefferman & Heilig, 1999; Wilkinson, 1987–88; Millette, 1994; Corley, 1995, Nathaniel, 2004).

Moral distress is a serious problem in nursing. It affects the individual nurse, the patient, and the health care system. It also offers important implications for nursing practice, education, and administration, and in the face of a nursing shortage of crisis proportions, presents urgent and unique opportunities for further investigation.

ALVITA NATHANIEL

Moral Reckoning

The Grounded Theory of Moral Reckoning in Nursing identifies a process that nurses move through when they have experienced moral distress in the workplace. Moral reckoning includes a critical juncture in nurses' lives and explains a process that includes motivation and conflict, resolution, and reflection (Nathaniel, 2003). Moral Reckoning is a three-stage process that offers important implications for nursing practice, education, and administration. Distinct stages include the Stage of Ease, the Stage of Resolution, and the Stage of Reflection.

Stage of Ease. During the Stage of Ease, nurses are motivated by core beliefs and values to uphold congruent professional and institutional norms. They are comfortable: they have technical skills and feel satisfied to practice within the boundaries of self, profession, and institution. They know what is expected of them and experience a sense of flow and at-homeness. The Stage of Ease continues as long as the nurse is fulfilled with the work of nursing and comfortable with the integration of core beliefs and professional and institutional norms. For some, though, a morally troubling event will challenge the integration of core beliefs with professional and institutional norms. Nurses find themselves in *situational binds* that herald a critical juncture in their professional lives.

Situational Binds. A situational bind interrupts the Stage of Ease and places the nurse in turmoil when core beliefs and other claims conflict. Situational binds force nurses to make difficult decisions and give rise to critical junctures in their lives. Binds involve serious and complex conflicts within individuals and tacit or overt conflicts between nurses and others—all having moral/ethical overtones. Inner dialogue leads the nurse to make critical decisions—choosing one value or belief over another. Types of situational binds include (a) conflicts between core values and professional or institutional norms, (b) moral disagreement in the face of power imbalance, and (c) workplace deficiencies. These binds lead to consequences for nurses and patients.

Stage of Resolution. Situational binds constitute crises of intolerable internal conflict. The move to set things right signifies the beginning of the Stage of Resolution. For most, this stage is a critical juncture that alters professional trajectory. There are two foundational choices in the Stage of Resolution: making a stand or giving up. These choices are not mutually exclusive. In fact, many nurses give up initially, regroup, and make a stand. Others make an unsuccessful stand and later give up.

Stage of Reflection. Moving from the Stage of Resolution, nurses reflect as they reckon with their behavior and actions. The Stage of Reflection may last a lifetime. In most cases, the incidents nurses recall occurred early in their careers. The Stage of Reflection raises questions about prior judgments, particular acts, and the essential self. The properties of the Stage of Reflection include remembering, telling the story, examining conflicts, and living with consequences. These properties are interrelated and seem to occur in every instance of moral reckoning.

ALVITA NATHANIEL

Mother-Infant/Toddler Relationships

The study of mother-infant/toddler relationships centers on knowledge related to the health and development of the mother-child dyad from birth to 3 years. This focus of inquiry is necessarily large because the mother-child system is an open one, responsive to genetic, biological, environmental, cognitive, and psychological influences (Institute of Medicine, 2000).

The mother-infant/toddler relationship is influenced by genetic factors such as the child's temperament. Temperament is an inborn constellation of traits that affect the individual's behavioral reactions to environmental stimuli. Temperamental qualities such as high-intensity reactions, low adaptability to change, or shyness, influence children's abilities to regulate emotions in stressful situations, relate to other people, and adjust to changes in daily routines. Similar temperamental qualities in the mother are likely to affect her ability to adjust her parenting behaviors to accommodate an unpredictable infant or a defiant 2-year-old (Gross & Conrad, 1995). A poor fit between parent and infant/toddler temperamental styles has been associated with more child behavior problems and increases in physiological indices of stress (Bugental, Olster, & Martorell, 2003).

Biological factors can influence the child's developmental trajectory, making parenting more stressful and altering the quality of the mother-infant/toddler relationship. For example, low birthweight infants with neonatal medical complications are at greater risk for later developmental, visual, physical, and behavioral disabilities (Boyce, G. C., Smith, & Casto, 1999). Even in the absence of medical complications, mothers of low birthweight infants experience greater stress and caregiver burden than mothers of normal birthweight infants (May & Hu, 2000). Such early biological risk can have significant effects on the quality of the mother-infant/toddler relationship.

The relationship between parenting environment and the mother-infant/toddler relationship has been extensively studied, although the theory underlying cause-and-effect relationships remains poorly understood. For example, there are many hypotheses to account for the significant associations found between parenting in low-income environments and poorer outcomes in very young children (Duncan & Brooks-Gunn, 1997; Mistry, Vandewater, Huston, & McLloyd, 2002). As a result, interventions for promoting healthy parent-child relationships among low-income families simultaneously target many environmental risk factors (e.g., support, psychological guidance, education, nutrition, and facilitating access to community-based services). The complexity of the parenting environment and understanding how social contexts in early life affect young children and parents is an important but underdeveloped area of inquiry (Boyce, W. T., et al., 1998).

The psychological health of the mother and child has received much attention. Maternal stress, low social support, marital discord, and maternal depression have been viewed as important factors placing young children at risk for poor developmental outcomes (Gross, Sambrook, & Fogg, 1999; Petterson & Albers, 2001). Recently, researchers have shifted the focus away from unidirectional to bidirectional effects. For example, depressed mothers who are sad, preoccupied, and irritable may be unable to attend to their infant's needs or to deal calmly and effectively with their toddler's demands for attention. However, it is also possible that behaviorally demanding children cause mothers to feel ineffective, fatigued, and ultimately depressed. The clinical implications of viewing problems in the mother-infant/toddler relationship as bidirectional is that effective nursing interventions should focus on the mother-child dyad or the family unit rather than on the mother or child alone.

In the past 10 years, greater attention has been placed on the role of race/ethnicity in the development of the mother-infant/toddler relationship. Demographic trends toward greater multiculturalism and expectations for researchers to understand how parenting processes may differ across racial/ethnic groups have led to more thoughtful examinations of parenting processes among families of color (Garcia Coll et al., 1996; McLloyd, Cauce, Takeuchi, & Wilson, 2000). Different family structures and childrearing values will affect how parents socialize their infants and toddlers. While all children thrive under the care of a loving and responsive parent, research has shown that there is no single way that love and attention need to be expressed. Indeed, research has shown that some parenting strategies that negatively affect behavioral outcomes in European-American children appear to have no such affect on African-American children (Whaley, 2000).

Finally, maternal cognitions affect how mothers interpret and respond to their children's behavior. For example, a mother's belief that using corporal punishment with her defiant 2-year-old may be based on a series of cognitions related to her values about child defiance and physical punishment, cultural expectations, perceived environmental dangers, how she was raised, and her knowledge of alternative discipline strategies (Garvey, Gross, Delaney, & Fogg, 2000; Goodnow & Collins, 1990).

Although many investigators have understandably narrowed their research to one or two conceptual areas of inquiry, the dyad is dynamically affected by all of these influences. That is, mothers identify parenting goals and devise child-rearing strategies that are consistent with their temperaments, biology, child-rearing environments, cognitions, and psychological capacities (Gross, 1996). Likewise, children's responses to parents are similarly tied to these same factors. Future research should refine how these influences transact within the parent-child relationship so that research methods can be clarified and cost-effective nursing interventions disseminated to populations in need.

DEBORAH GROSS

Music Therapy

Music therapy is the use of music for the purpose of improving physiological and psychological health and well-being. For music to be therapeutic, there must be an interaction between the music and the person who desires a health outcome from the music (Meyer, 1956). This implies that there are individual, age, culture, and situation-related differences in choice and effect. The saying that music is a universal language gives the false impression that everyone appreciates and is helped by the same music. Although all cultures of the world use music in some form and derive meaning from it, different cultures and different generations are accustomed to listening to widely divergent kinds of music. There may be large differences in volume, pitch, rhythm, tempo, harmony, disharmony, words, and meaning (Cross, 2003). In addition, there is variation within age and cultural groups (Good, Picot, Salem, Picot, & Lane, 2000).

Music therapy may be provided by a registered music therapist who has been taught to use music in many therapeutic ways. However, any member of the health care team may suggest to patients that soft music can be helpful for stress, pain, and mood, and can use stimulating music to encourage socialization, expression, and exercise. Nurses can assess musical preferences, offer a choice of selections, and encourage patient involvement in the music with the goal of achieving specific health outcomes.

Throughout history, music has been used for a variety of therapeutic purposes by primitive people to ward off evil spirits, prevent or cure illnesses, relieve depression, modify emotions, and achieve inner harmony. Early cultures had little means to treat disease, so music and spirituality were used to provide comfort and help people cope. During the

Renaissance, physicians became interested in the therapeutic value of music and incorporated it in their training and practice. From the 17th century onward, physicians studied the effect of music on physiology and psychology, and debated whether to focus on the type of music that was effective versus the type of person who responds positively to music. Nightingale used music with injured soldiers in the Crimea. She had recreation areas where recovering men could go to listen to singing or playing of musical instruments.

At the beginning of the 20th century, the first laboratory studies of the physiological effects of music were conducted on animals and humans. These experiments demonstrated changes in vital signs and body secretions in response to various types of music. They are rejected by most investigators today because of the poor quality of measurement, analysis, and control. In the 1930s music began to be used in patients' hospital rooms, in surgery prior to general anesthesia, and during local anesthesia. Music was used in obstetrics and gynecology to reduce the side effects of inhalation anesthetics.

Nursing reviews of research on the effect of music on health outcomes can be found in chapters by Good (1996), Guzzetta (1988, 1997), Standley and Hanser (1995), and Snyder and Chlan (1999). The American Music Therapy Association and two journals, the *Journal of Music Therapy* and *Music Therapy Perspectives*, are excellent resources.

Music can transport patients' thoughts to a new place, give them new perspectives, lift their mood, provide comfort, familiarity and pleasure to patients, and stimulate memories, meanings, and self-insight. In addition, studies have shown that music reduces pain and anxiety, reduces muscle tension, raises levels of beta-endorphins, and lowers adrenocorticotropic stress hormones. Music has been found to improve the immune system, salivary cortisol, postoperative and cancer pain, sleep, nausea and vomiting of chemotherapy, mood during stem cell transplantation, pain of osteoarthritis, and cardiac anxiety and autonomic balance. It has also been effective for acute and chronic pain and during stressful or painful procedures (e.g., injections, gastrointestinal endoscopy, and lumbar punctures). Music has been generally found to reduce anxiety before, during, and after surgery, during burn debridement, in chronically ill patients, and after myocardial infarction. It has been studied for circumcision pain in infants, for injection pain in children and adults, for disturbances in psychiatric, demented, and agitated patients, in the critically ill, in dyslexic children, in postanesthesia patients, in the emergency department, and in those who are comatose or dying. Lullabies have shown beneficial effects on preterm infants. A double-blind study of music during surgery showed effects on recovery. In mice, music reduced stress and metastasis and improved immune factors.

Music has been categorized into stimulative and sedative types. Stimulative music has strong rhythms, volume, dissonance, and disconnected notes, whereas sedative music has a sustained melody without strong rhythmic or percussive elements. Stimulative music enhances bodily action and stimulates skeletal muscles, emotions, and subcortical reactions in humans. Sedative music results in physical sedation and responses of an intellectual and contemplative nature (Gaston, 1951). Precategorization by the nurse, however, does not consider the kind of subject response. Other ways of categorizing are slow and fast music, or by type of music or instrument.

To choose music that is therapeutic, the nurse should consider the nature of the music, the patient preferences, and the health state. Nurses can assess patients' sex, cultural background, musical preferences, music training, participation in music, degree of auditory discrepancy, time available, and, most of all, degree of liking for the music under consideration. Variations in the nature of the health state determine whether music will be used to cheer, encourage, soothe, relax, distract the mind, stimulate exercise, or evoke emotions of joy, triumph, resolve, or peace. Studies have indicated that different kinds of music result in positive or negative feelings and differences in serotonin. Music is economical for patient use. Tapes, compact discs, and players are relatively inexpensive, and a small library can be maintained on any nursing unit. Music piped into patients' rooms also may be available. Nurses can suggest that patients and their families bring in favorite music from home that is likely to invoke healthy responses. They can refer patients to a music therapist if one is available.

There are some contraindications and considerations when using music for patients. Contraindications include hypersensitivity to sound, tone deafness, musicogenic epilepsy, and inability to recognize music in some stroke patients. Nurses should consider any patient dislike for any particular selection or type of music, their inability to turn it off when desired, cochlear implants, and culturally incongruent music. In addition, those with hearing loss may or may not find that listening to music is beneficial. Future research in music may include studies that determine the kinds of music that are effective for health outcomes in countries around the world and between cultures in each country. More work on comparing symptomatic response with physiological response is needed to generate theories of conditions in which music is effective, how it affects body processes, and what effect it has on recovery, immune function, and health.

Music brings an air of normalcy, entertainment, pleasure, and escape into a world where illness is often the enemy and both patients and caregivers are fighting back. Music is an integral part of most people's normal lives and should not be forgotten when they go to hospitals and other health care facilities. With the increased reliance on technology in health care today, music can add a humanistic touch. Beyond the humanistic value of music is the therapeutic value in reducing stress, pain, anxiety, and depression and promoting movement, socialization, and sleep.

MARION GOOD

N

Narrative Analysis

Narrative analysis is gaining popularity among nurse researchers as one of the representative modes of studying human experiences, of both clients and nurses, especially from the perspective of interpretivism. Narrative analysis is being used in many different disciplines: literary studies, linguistics, anthropology, psychology, sociology, theology, history, and practice disciplines such as nursing, medicine, occupational therapy, and social work.

All sorts of oral and written representations are considered narratives—fables, folktales, short stories, case histories, exemplars, news reports, personal stories, historiography, interview data, and so forth. Although there are controversies, the term *narrative* in narrative analysis refers to a story that contains two or more sequentially ordered units, with a beginning, middle, and ending, and represents structured meaning. Narratives are structured about a story plot or plots illustrated by characters (actors) and events. Narratives as stories are characterized by a sense of internal chronology (either temporal or thematic) and connectedness that brings about coherence and sense making. Narratives differ from discourse in that narratives contain descriptions of chronologically articulated events along with sketches of characters of that story.

As narratives are human linguistic products, their construction is closely tied to "storytelling," that is, the processes involved in producing them. Storytelling is often the object of analysis, along with narratives themselves, in narrative analysis.

The heterogeneity of narratives, representative disciplinary plurality, and the varieties in narrative theories have evidenced in various approaches and orientations in narrative analysis. There are at least three diverse orientations within narrative analysis: (a) structural orientation, (b) storytelling orientation, and (c) interpretive orientation (for other ways of categorizing narrative analysis and a typology of models, see Mishler, 1995).

Structural orientation can be identified with structuralists such as Barthes (1974) and sociolinguists such as Labov (1972) and Gee (1991). In this orientation, narratives are thought to be organized about a specific set of structural units that bring about coherence and connectivity in the narratives. Attention to narrative structures is analytically juxtaposed to such aspects as functions that different structural units perform—sense making in story, or narrativity.

Narrative analysis in the structuralist tradition within literary studies and linguistics focuses on structural-functional connections, as in Propp's (1968) morphology in relation to internal patterning and narrative genre and in Genette's (1988) three specific aspects of a story's temporal articulation (i.e., order, frequency, and duration). In this tradition, narratives subjected to analysis tend to be public material such as folktales, novels, short stories, and case histories.

Sociolinguists attend to "natural" or "situated" narratives, which are constructions produced in specific situations of social life. Labov (1972) identified six structural units for fully formed narratives: abstract, orientation, complicating action, evaluation, resolution, and coda. He suggested that these structural units are related to two functions in narrative: the referential function and the evaluative function. Gee (1991), on the other hand, identified structural properties of narrative as poetic structures of lines, stanzas, or strophes, which organize meaning constructions in telling a story. The structural orientation is primarily an examination of structural elements of story in relation to the narrative's form, function, and meaning.

In storytelling, narratives are not viewed simply as products that can be taken out of the context of narrating but as process-oriented constructions that are enmeshed with linguistic materialization of cognition and memory, interactive structuring between the teller and listener, and contextually and culturally constrained shaping of experiences and ideas. From this standpoint, narrative analysis is closely aligned with discourse analysis, as in ethnography of communication in anthropology and ethnomethodology in sociology.

Narrative analysis in this orientation is differentiated into two schools: linguistic/cognitive and sociocultural. The linguistic/cognitive version focuses on how narratives are materialized in language from ideas and experiences. This construction is viewed to be accomplished by applying communicative and interactive functions of language and through scripting and schematizing of yet unorganized information into connected storytelling. In this version, storytelling is considered as the processing of nonlinguistic ideas, events, and actions into a series of connected and coherent representation of meanings.

On the other hand, narrative analysis in the sociological version within the ethnomethodological tradition is concerned with the interactive process of narrative making. Conversational narratives are of prime interest. The listener is an active part of storytelling as an interactive participant in the making of a story. From an anthropological perspective, storytelling is viewed as bounded by cultural conditions and cultural categories. Narrative analysis in this orientation carries out an analysis of narrative texts in terms of form and content, along with an analysis of the flow of storytelling, with the assumption that the nature of narrative text is integrally connected to the processes of construction.

Narratives in the interpretive orientation are chronological in a double sense: chronology in terms of temporal serialization of events and chronology in terms of temporality of story itself. Ricoeur (1984) specified episodic and configurational dimensions as the temporal dialectics that integrated plot in narrative. Hence, narratives are stories of individuals etched within the communal stories of the time and context. Narrative analysis thus involves interpretation of representation posed within the contexts in which the story is shaped and the storytelling occurs, reflecting on the worldviews that provide a larger contextual understanding. In this sense, the interpretative orientation is more concerned with meaning of narratives than with either the structure or the process.

Riessman (1993) offers five levels of representation in the research process of narrative analysis: attending, telling, transcribing, analyzing, and reading. Interpretation occurs at the levels of transcribing and analyzing by the researcher, whereas the level of reading implies additional interpretation that occurs in the readers of research reports. Riessman favors the use of poetic structures as the mode of structuring narratives as interpretive; however, the use of any specific structuring model is less critical for the analysis than interpretation.

Although there are distinct differences among these orientations, there are many hybrid forms of narrative analysis used in actual research practice. Hybrid forms often combine analysis of process or meaning with structural analysis. In nursing research, narrative analysis has been applied with various orientations and in different hybrid forms. Narratives of clients' personal experiences, such as suffering, being diagnosed with cancer, isolation, and dying, have been studied by applying Labov or Gee as well as within the storytelling orientation. Narratives of practice by nurses have been subjected to analyses in the interpretive orientation for understanding the meanings of their practice and their value orientations. In addition, the interpretive orientation from the feminist perspective has been used to study women's experiences, such as health care seeking, pregnancy with the history of drug abuse, and recovery. Research of narrative accounts of clients and nurses, as well as their interactions, can produce deep understanding of human experiences that are fundamental to nursing practice.

HESOOK SUZIE KIM

National Institute of Nursing Research

The National Institute of Nursing Research (NINR) is one of 24 institutes, centers, and divisions that comprise the National Institutes of Health (NIH). The NIH is one of eight health agencies of the Public Health Service in the U.S. Department of Health and Human Services. Headquartered in 75 buildings on more than 300 acres in Bethesda, Maryland, the NIH is the steward of biomedical and behavioral research for the nation. Its mission is to improve the health of the American people through increased understanding of the processes underlying human health and the acquisition of new knowledge to help prevent, detect, diagnose, and treat disease. Approximately 80% of the annual NIH investment is made through grants and contracts to support extramural research and training in more than 1,700 universities; medical, dental, and nursing schools; hospitals; and other research institutions throughout the United States and abroad. About 10% of its budget goes to the more than 2,000 projects conducted in its own intramural laboratories.

In 1996 the NINR celebrated the 10th anniversary of its establishment at the NIH. Originally designated as the National Center for Nursing Research by Public Law 99-158 in 1986, it attained institute status through the NIH Revitalization Act of 1993. Its budget of $16 million in 1986 had grown to $139 million in 2005. The original staff of 9 members has increased to over 50 people, including scientists, administrators, and support staff.

Nursing research is a relative newcomer to the scientific community. Unlike other health-related disciplines, nursing began as an occupation in hospital settings, not as a discipline in academic institutions. Although there is a history of nurses receiving advanced degrees in many different academic fields, it has been only within the past 25 years that doctoral preparation has been available in the field of nursing, paving the way of nursing research to grow and flourish at universities and research centers.

The mission of the NINR supports basic and clinical research to establish a scientific basis for the care of individuals across the life span—from management of patients during illness and recovery to the reduction of risks for disease and disability and the promotion of healthy lifestyles. With this broad mandate, the institute seeks to understand and ease the symptoms of acute and chronic illness, to prevent or delay the onset of disease or slow its progression, to find effective approaches to promoting good health, and to improve the clinical settings in which care is provided. The NINR supports research on problems encountered by patients' families and caregivers. It also emphasizes the special needs of at-risk and underserved populations. These efforts are crucial in translating scientific advances into cost-effective health care that does not compromise quality.

The first NINR director, Dr. Ada Sue Hinshaw, who held the position from 1987 to 1994, is widely recognized for her contributions to teaching, nursing research, and academic administration. Under her leadership the institute was established as an active participant within the federal research community and achieved national recognition for nursing research. The current director, Dr. Patricia A. Grady, an internationally recognized stroke researcher, was appointed in 1995, following positions as deputy director and acting director of the National Institute of Neurological Disorders and Stroke.

The NIH employs a two-level system for reviewing grant applications. In the first level, panels of extramural experts evaluate the scientific merit of the proposed research. The second level of review is carried out by national advisory councils, which consider scientific merit as determined in the first level of review, program relevance, and appropriate allocation of resources. Councils also advise on policy development, program implementation, evaluation, and other matters of importance to the missions and goals of the NIH institutes and centers. Advisory councils are composed of scientific and lay representatives who are noted for their expertise or interest in issues related to the missions of the institutes and centers they serve.

The NINR's advisory council—the National Advisory Council for Nursing Research—is composed of 15 members. Ten are leaders in the health and scientific disciplines relevant to the activities of the NINR, and five public members are leaders in health care, public policy, law, and economics. The advisory council also includes six ex officio members: the secretary of the Department of Health and Human Services (DHHS), the NIH director, the chief nursing officer of the Department of Veterans Affairs, the assistant secretary for health affairs of the Department of Defense, and the director of the Division of Nursing, Health Resources and Services Administration, DHHS.

NIH award mechanisms are divided into three categories: grants, contracts, and cooperative agreements. The primary mechanism used by the NINR is the investigator-initiated grant. This mechanism supports research and research training projects for which the applicant develops the protocol, concept, method, and approach. It includes research projects (R01s), First Independent Research Support and Transition (FIRST) awards (R29s), and Research Scientist Development awards (K01s). In certain instances, the NINR may solicit applications for special mechanisms such as core center grants (P30s) and small research grants (R03s). The NINR uses the cooperative agreement mechanism, which supports the recipient's activities and provides for substantial involvement of the funding agency during the period of performance. The NINR also supports research training through individual and institutional National Research Service awards (F31s, F32s, F33s, and T32s).

As the NINR identifies new opportunities for research, nursing researchers are moving to the forefront of many innovative areas of scientific exploration. For example, the NINR is responding to the clinical implications of genetics discoveries with research programs in the clinical management of conditions associated with genetic disorders, including genetic screening and counseling, clinical decision making, and bioethical considerations. Nursing researchers are also taking the lead in the remediation of cognitive impairment, the prevention and control of pain, and the management of side effects associated with medical treatment. In addition, nursing research focuses on methods to stem microbial threats to health through improved approaches to prevention and adherence to treatment. NINR-funded research also links biological and behavioral approaches to health care. A further area of research interest is the role of cultural sensitivity as a factor in health research and health care.

The NINR research portfolio is broad, invites collaboration among many disciplines, and is cosponsored by most of the other NIH research institutes and centers. The NINR supports research across six major areas: (1) neurofunction and sensory conditions; (2) reproductive and infant health; (3) immune, infectious, and neoplastic diseases; (4) cardiopulmonary and acute illnesses; (5) metabolic and other chronic illnesses; and (6) human development and health risk behaviors. Individuals who are interested in submitting applications for grants to conduct research in areas of interest to the institute are encouraged to contact the NINR program staff at the following address and telephone number to discuss research opportunities and proposed areas of investigation before embarking on the application process. Division of Extramural Activities, National Institute of Nursing Research, NIH, Building 45,

Room 3AN-12, 45 Center Drive, MSC 6300, Bethesda, MD 20892-6300; telephone: (301) 594-6906. General questions regarding the NINR may be addressed to Office of Science Policy and Information, National Institute of Nursing Research, NIH, Building 31, Room 5B13, 31 Center Drive, MSC 2178, Bethesda, MD 20892-2178; telephone: (301) 496-0207.

PATRICIA A. GRADY

National Institutes of Health

Begun as the one-room Laboratory of Hygiene in 1887, the National Institutes of Health (NIH) today is one of the world's foremost biomedical research centers. Although the institution's roots extend back over a century, the "modern" NIH dates from the years following World War II, when growing awareness of public health needs converged with new scientific capabilities and an increased national investment in health-related science. As the federal focal point for health research, the NIH is one of eight health agencies of the Public Health Service, which, in turn, is part of the U.S. Department of Health and Human Services. The NIH is composed of 24 separate institutes, centers, and divisions, each focused on a particular aspect of health research. The NIH has 75 buildings on more than 300 acres in Bethesda, Maryland. From about $300 in 1887, the NIH budget has grown to nearly $28 billion as of 2005.

Since its inception the NIH has had 14 directors. The first was Joseph James Kinyoun, who was the founder and director of the Laboratory of Hygiene that later grew to become the NIH. The current director is Elias Z. Zernouni, a well-respected leader in radiology and medicine.

NIH Institutes, Centers, and Divisions

National Cancer Institute (NCI)
National Eye Institute (NEI)
National Heart, Lung, and Blood Institute (NHLBI)
National Institute on Aging (NIA)
National Institute on Alcohol Abuse and Alcoholism (NIAAA)
National Institute of Allergy and Infectious Diseases (NIAID)
National Institute of Arthritis and Musculoskeletal and Skin Diseases (NIAMS)
National Institute of Child Health and Human Development (NICHD)
National Institute on Deafness and Other Communication Disorders (NIDCD)
National Institute of Dental Research (NIDR)
National Institute of Diabetes and Digestive and Kidney Diseases (NIDDK)
National Institute on Drug Abuse (NIDA)
National Institute of Environmental Health Sciences (NIEHS)
National Institute of General Medical Sciences (NIGMS)
National Institute of Mental Health (NIMH)
National Institute of Neurological Disorders and Stroke (NINDS)
National Institute of Nursing Research (NINR)
National Human Genome Research Institute (NHGRI)
National Library of Medicine (NLM)
National Center for Research Resources (NCRR)
John E. Fogarty International Center (FIC)
Warren Grant Magnuson Clinical Center (CC)
Division of Computer Research and Technology (DCRT)
Division of Research Grants (DRG)

The NIH website at http://www.nih.gov contains links to each of the above organizations' websites, which contain information on their missions and activities in support of research (Office of Communications, 1996).

The NIH Mission, Goals, and Research Support

The NIH is the steward of biomedical and behavior research for the nation. Its mission is science in pursuit of fundamental knowledge about the nature and behavior of living systems and the application of that knowledge to extend healthy life and reduce the burdens of illness and disability. The NIH works toward that mission by conducting clinical and basic research in its own laboratories, supporting research institutions throughout the country and abroad, helping in the training of research investigators, and fostering communication of information on health improvement.

The goals of the agency are as follows: (a) to foster fundamental creative discoveries, innovative research strategies, and their applications as a basis to advance significantly the nation's capacity to protect and improve health; (b) to develop, maintain, and renew scientific human and physical resources that will assure the nation's capability to prevent disease; (c) to expand the knowledge base in biomedical and associated sciences in order to enhance the nation's economic well-being and ensure a continued high return on the public investment in research; and (d) to exemplify and promote the highest level of scientific integrity, public accountability, and social responsibility in the conduct of science.

In realizing these goals the NIH provides leadership and direction to programs designed to improve the health of the nation by conducting and supporting research in the causes, diagnosis, prevention, and cure of human diseases; in the processes of human growth and development; in the biological effects of environmental contaminants; and in the understanding of mental, addictive, and physical disorders. The NIH also directs programs for the collection, dissemination, and exchange of information in medicine, nursing, and health, including the development and support of medical libraries and the training of medical librarians and other health information specialists (National Institutes of Health, 1996).

NIH Impact on the Health of the Nation

NIH research played a major role in making possible the following achievements of the past few decades.

1. Mortality from heart disease, the number-1 killer in the United States, dropped by 41% between 1971 and 1991.
2. Death rates from strokes decreased by 59% during the same period.
3. Improved treatments and detection methods increased the relative 5-year survival rate for people with cancer to 52%. At present, the survival gain over the rate that existed in the 1960s represents more than 80,000 additional cancer survivors each year.
4. Paralysis from spinal cord injury is significantly reduced by rapid treatment with high doses of a steroid. Treatment given within the first 8 hours after injury increases recovery in severely injured patients who have lost sensation or mobility below the point of injury.
5. Long-term treatment with anticlotting medicines cuts stroke risk by 80% from a common heart condition known as atrial fibrillation.
6. In schizophrenia, where suicide is always a potential danger, new medications have reduced troublesome symptoms such as delusions and hallucinations in 80% of patients.
7. Chances for survival have increased for infants with respiratory distress syndrome, an immaturity of the lungs, because of development of a substance to prevent the lungs from collapsing. In general, life expectancy for a baby born today is almost three decades longer than one born at the beginning of the century.
8. Those suffering from depression now look forward to returning to work and leisure activities, thanks to treatments that have given them an 80% chance to resume a full life in a matter of weeks.
9. Vaccines protect against infectious diseases that once killed and disabled millions of children and adults.
10. Dental sealants have proved 100% effective in protecting the chewing surfaces of children's molars and

premolars, where most cavities occur.

11. Molecular genetics and genomics research has revolutionized biomedical science. In the 1980s and 1990s researchers performed the first trial of gene therapy in humans and were able to locate, identify, and describe the function of many of the genes in the human genome. Scientists predict this new knowledge will lead to genetic tests to diagnose diseases such as colon, breast, and other cancers and to the eventual development of preventive drug treatments for individuals in families known to be at risk. The ultimate goal is to develop screening tools and gene therapies for the general population, not only for cancer but for many other diseases.

PATRICIA A. GRADY

Neuman Systems Model

The Neuman Systems Model (NSM) provides a broad, comprehensive, systems approach as a framework for the profession of nursing to organize care, educate future providers, and conduct research. The model offers a holistic approach, a wellness orientation, client perception, and motivation with a systems perspective of variable interaction with the environment (Neuman, 2001, p. 12). The model's philosophical and theoretical underpinnings include: von Bertalanffy's (1968) general systems theory, De Chardin's (1955) philosophical views of the wholeness of life, gestalt theory and its focus on perception (Pearls, 1973) and field theory (Edelson, 1970), and the typology of prevention interventions (Caplan, G., 1964). Additionally, Seyle's (1950) theory of stress and adaptation and Lazarus and Folkman's (1984) theory of stress and coping were foundational to the development of the NSM. Consequently, two components undergird much of the focus of the model: exploring the client's response to stressors, and identifying the nurse's preventive interventions that assist the client in responding to these stressors. The ultimate goal of the unique profession of nursing is to assist the client in achieving the goals of an optimum state of wellness.

Betty Neuman first developed the Neuman Systems Model to assist graduate students at the University of California, Los Angeles, to conceptualize a systems approach to health care. It is based on Neuman's personal philosophy shaped by the philosophical and theoretical tenets mentioned previously, and her experience as a consultant in public health and community mental health nursing (Walker, P. H., 2004). It was developed in 1970 and is used by practitioners, educators, and increasingly by researchers nationally and internationally.

The main concepts of the NSM are consistent with those of the nursing metaparadigm which undergird most of the other grand theories in nursing: person, environment, health, and nursing. Within the context of the nursing metaparadigm, the primary components of the NSM include: stressors, lines of defense and resistance, levels of prevention, the five client systems variables (basic structure, interventions, internal and external environment, and reconstitution). All concepts have been defined by Neuman in each of her texts (Neuman, 1982, 1989, 1995, 2001).

Neuman describes nursing as a "unique profession"—concerned with the interrelationship of "all variables affecting a client's possible or actual response to stressors. Thus, nursing uniqueness is related to the way the discipline organizes and utilizes its knowledge (Neuman, 1989, p. 24). The nurse is an intervener who uses *three levels of prevention (primary, secondary, and tertiary)* to achieve the goal of reducing the client's encounter with stressors and/or mitigating the impact of the stressor. The ultimate goal is to help the client system retain stability.

The client or client system is the term Neuman uses for *person*, because the focus of the model is wellness and fostering a collaborative relationship between the client and the caregiver (the nurse, in this case). The client or client system may be an individual, group, family, and/or community and is composed of five interrelated variables (*physiological, psychological, sociocultural, developmental, and spiritual*). The spiritual variable was added to the model in 1989 to be more consistent with Neuman's holistic belief about humans (Neuman, 1989). These variables are surrounded by various lines of defense and resistance. According to Neuman, a client's normal *line of defense* is dynamic, evolves over time, and contains the client's normal range of responses to stressors, thereby reflecting his or her usual wellness level (Neuman, 2001, p. 18). Further, the client or client system has *internal lines of resistance* which function to protect the client's basic structure or system integrity which, if ineffective, will result in system energy depletion and eventually death (Neuman, 2001, p. 18).

Environment, according to Neuman consists of *internal, external and created environment(s)*. The internal environment is composed of forces within the client identified by Neuman as intrapersonal stressors. Other stressors (interpersonal and extrapersonal) make up the external environment. The concept of a created environment was also added in 1989, again to reflect Neuman's holistic perspective and beliefs. The created environment is considered to be unconsciously developed by the client in order to protect the client from *intra-, inter-, and extrapersonal stressors* and maintain system stability (Neuman, 1989, p. 12).

Health, according to Neuman is equated with living energy, determined by the degree of harmony among the five client variables and basic structure factors, on a continuum from wellness to illness. The degree of wellness is determined by the amount of energy required to retain, attain, or maintain system stability (Neuman, 2001, p. 12).

Although the NSM has been used widely in practice and education, it is increasingly being utilized in the research community, particularly by students in masters and doctoral programs. An integrative review of NSM-based research conducted by Fawcett and Giangrande (2001) found 200 research reports with an analysis focused on general information, scientific merit, and the NSM. The majority of the 200 studies were related to clinical nursing topics (75%), followed by nursing administration (14%), nursing education (9%), with the least on continuing education (2%). The fact that much of the research is related to practice-oriented questions hopefully begins to address concerns by P. H. Walker and Redman (1999) that evidence-based practice may be threatening the foundation of nursing's disciplinary perspective on theory-guided practice. Analysis of the scientific merit revealed the following: 37% were descriptive studies, 32% were experimental studies, 25% were correlation studies, and approximately 4% were designed to develop and test instruments (Fawcett & Giangrande, 2001, p. 124). A summary of the analysis of elements related to the NSM indicated: most frequently, development of testing of prevention as intervention; next, 24% explored perception of stressors; 9% were studies involving client variables; and only a few studies (1% to 5%) were on lines of defense and/or resistance.

In reference to use of instrumentation, Gigliotti and Fawcett (2001) reviewed 212 research reports and identified different instruments explicitly linked to the NSM—sometimes more than once, and for different purposes. These instruments included: Beck Depression Inventory, State Trait Anxiety Inventory, the Norbeck Social Support Questionnaire, the Dynamap, the Carter Center Institute Health Risk Appraisal, and the Health Status Questionnaire. In an important evaluation of instrumentation related to middle-range theory, Gigliotti and Fawcett found that 26 instruments measured concepts related to stressors, 24 measured concepts related to lines of defense, and 22 measured prevention interventions. Other NSM-related concepts (middle-range) were measured by the remaining 16 instruments. Of those instruments, 59 were classified as standardized (having sufficient evidence of validity and reliability testing) and 62 were considered nonstandardized (Gigliotti & Fawcett, pp. 153–154).

To enhance and facilitate future research related to the NSM, Neuman and Fawcett (2001) have established a set of guidelines for NSM-based research. Additionally, Fawcett and Giangrande (2001, pp. 136–137) encourage collaborative research and cluster studies which would look at related phenomena. For example, one researcher might explore the impact of inter- or extrapersonal stressors on some of the five variables while another researcher could study the impact of intra- or interpersonal stressors on the same variables using the same sample of study participants. Finally, Gigliotti and Fawcett (2001, pp. 166–169) concluded that more attention should be paid to validity of existing instrumentation and to the examination of the utility of instruments used in NSM-based clinical practice with an eye to the research potential of clinical and educational tools.

PATRICIA HINTON WALKER

Neurobehavioral Development and Nutritive Sucking

Neurobehavioral development is a genetically determined process by which the primitive central nervous system (CNS) achieves maturity in form and function. Neurodevelopment also depends on the environment since CNS development occurs through an "experience expectant" process in which normal species-typical experiences enable the CNS to make the structural and functional changes necessary for the next stages of development (Greenough, Black, & Wallace, 1987). In order to balance the needs of the present developmental stage and the anticipated needs of subsequent stages, this process is somewhat plastic (Oppenheim, 1981). When an infant is placed in an atypical environment such as a neonatal intensive care unit, ontogenetic adaptation is affected. Although the infant may initially adapt successfully, changes in the trajectory of the infant's neurobehavioral development may be maladaptive at older ages. The effects of this disturbance vary depending on the timing and severity of environmental stresses, individual genetic background, the interaction of genetic background and prenatal history, adaptations made to uterine stresses, and specific neurological insults. Infants probably develop normally when neural plasticity—the process by which the brain develops new connections after neural damage—compensates for abnormalities due to any atypical ontogenetic adaptation and neurological insults. Infants exhibit abnormal neurobehavioral development when neural plasticity is not able to compensate, or when compensatory processes result in structural or functional changes that are maladaptive at later ages.

The Synactive Model of Neonatal Behavioral Organization provides a framework for exploring the concept of neurobehavioral development. Als (1991) has proposed a dynamic model for assessing infant behavioral organization. She proposed that the behavioral organization displayed by an infant is a reflection of the infant's central nervous system integrity, defined as the potential for the brain to develop normally. The infant's behaviors reflect subsystems of functioning, which include the autonomic, motor, state, attentional or interactive, and regulatory systems. The autonomic system controls physiologic functions that are basic for survival, such as respiration and heart rate. The motor system involves muscle tone, infant movements, and posture. State organization encompasses clarity of states and the pattern of transition from one state to another. The attentional or interactional system can be observed only in the alert state and is indicative of an infant's ability to respond to visual and auditory stimulation. An infant's regulatory system reflects the presence and success of an infant's efforts to achieve and maintain a balance of these other subsystems.

Another framework used is the perspective of developmental science, a multidisciplinary field that brings together researchers and theorists from psychology, biology, nursing, and other disciplines (Cairns, Elder, & Costello, 1996; Miles & Holditch-Davis, 2003). In this perspective, infants are viewed as developing in a continuously ongoing, reciprocal process of interaction with the environment. Infants and their environments form a complex system, consisting of elements that are themselves systems, such as mother and child, interacting together so that the total system shows less variability than the individual elements. Moreover, plasticity is assumed to be inherent in infants, their families, and the environment. Infants are active participants in their families and the greater environment, constantly changing them at the same time that they are influencing the infant. Interactions, rather than causation, are the focus of this perspective. No action of one element can be said to cause the action of another since interactions between elements are simultaneous and bidirectional. The interactions affecting development of infants are too complex to ever be totally identified, and infants can achieve the same developmental outcomes through different processes.

Newborn behavior, which includes sucking, sleeping, and waking, is the infant's primary expression of brain functioning and the critical route for communication with adults. Investigation of these behaviors and their central mechanisms is essential for nursing understanding of the needs of infants and in planning interventions to improve their neurodevelopmental status.

The idea of evaluating the vitality and central nervous system integrity of a neonate by assessing sucking is not new. Nutritive sucking is initiated in utero and continues to develop in an organized pattern in the early weeks after birth. It involves the integration of multiple sensory and motor central nervous system functions (Wolff, 1968). Sucking behaviors are thought to be an excellent barometer of central nervous system organization. They can be quantified in detailed analysis and are disturbed to various degrees by neurologic problems. Wolff describes the study of sucking rhythms to investigate serial order in behavior and development, which has remained among the most resistant to empirical investigation.

The work of Medoff-Cooper and colleagues (Medoff-Cooper, 1991; Medoff-Cooper, McGrath, & Bilker, 2000; McGrath & Medoff-Cooper, 2001) demonstrated that changes in the pattern of nutritive sucking behaviors can be described as a function of gestational age in healthy preterm and full-term infants. They reported a systematic pattern of gestational related change in sucking behavior that was reflected at each level of temporal analysis, with a strong correlation between increasing maturation and more organized sucking patterns (Medoff-Cooper, 2002). When comparing sucking behaviors at term of 213 extremely early born infants (gestational age ≤ 29 weeks), more mature preterm infants (30–32 weeks gestational age) and newly born full-term infants, feeding behaviors were noted to be a function of gestational age at birth as well as the interaction of maturation and experience. Extremely early born preterm infants were found to demonstrate less competent feeding behaviors than either more mature preterm infants or newly born full-term infants.

Lau, Smith, and Schandler (2003) also found that with increasing postconceptual age (PCA), preterm infants demonstrated significant improvement in feeding performance. They reported a significant relationship between average bolus size and sucking pressures and sucking frequency. Tolerating as well as adapting to increasing bolus size serves as an indicator of maturation in feeding behaviors.

Gewolb, Bosma, Reynolds, and Vice (2003) used increasing rhythmic stability as the index of maturation of sucking or feeding behaviors. In their comparison of healthy preterm infants and preterm infants with bronchopulmonary dysplasia (BPD), an increase in stability of rhythm and uniformity of waveform morphology was correlated with feeding efficiency and increasing PCA in healthy preterm infants. This relationship was not found to be true in the BPD cohort. They concluded that the poor feeding efficiency may be related to decreased respiratory reserves or may be secondary to nonspecific neurologic impairment.

The potential link between nutritive sucking and future developmental problems has been identified throughout the feeding literature. One early study by Burns and colleagues (1987) showed that infants with significant intraventricular hemorrhage were delayed in their ability to achieve a nutritive suck reflex.

At week 40 only 75% of the 110 infants demonstrated mature nutritive sucking patterns. Medoff-Cooper and Gennaro (1996) reported that sucking organization or rhythmicity was a far better predictor than neonatal morbidity of developmental outcome at 6 months of age. At 12 months of age, organized feeding patterns at 40 week PCA were significantly correlated with both Mental Developmental and Psychomotor Developmental Index (Medoff-Cooper, 2002).

Sleeping and waking states are clusters of behaviors that tend to occur together and represent the infant's level of arousal, responsivity to external stimulation, and central nervous system activation. Three states have been identified in adults: wakefulness, non-REM (rapid eye movement) sleep, and REM sleep. In infants, it is also possible to identify states within waking and states that are transitional between waking and sleeping. Because the electrophysiological patterns associated with sleep in infants are different than those in adults, infant sleep states are usually designated as active and quiet sleep.

Because of infants' neurological immaturity, EEG and behavioral scoring of states in preterm and full-term infants provide quite similar results. Sleeping and waking states in infants can be validly scored either by EEG or by directly observing infant behaviors. Four standardized systems for scoring behavioral observations of sleep-wake states are currently being used by nurse researchers: the 6 state system developed by T. Berry Brazelton, the 10 state system of Evelyn Thoman, the 12 state system from Heideliese Als's Assessment of Preterm Infant's Behavior (APIB), and 12 state scoring system based on the Anderson Behavioral State Scale (ABSS) developed by Gene Anderson (see Holditch-Davis, Blackburn, & Vandenberg, 2003). These systems define states in very similar ways and are probably equally useful for clinical purposes. However, the Brazelton system is the most limited for research as it can only be used with infants between 36 and 44 week PCA, and Thoman's is the most flexible as it has been used with 27 week PCA preterm infants through 1-year-olds.

Sleeping and waking states have widespread physiological effects. The functioning of cardiovascular, respiratory, neurological, endocrine, and gastrointestinal systems differs in different states. Sleeping and waking also affect the infant's ability to respond to stimulation. Thus, infant responses to nurses and parents depend to a great deal on the state the infant is in when the stimulation is begun. Timing routine interventions to occur when the infant is most responsive is an important aspect of current systems of individualized nursing care.

Studies have indicated that sleep and waking patterns are closely related to neurological status (Thoman, 1982; Halpern, Maclean, & Baumeister, 1995). State patterns of infants with neurological insults differ markedly from those of healthy infants. Abnormal neonatal EEG patterns are associated with severe neurological abnormalities and major neurodevelopmental sequelae during childhood. Also, preterm infants with severe medical illnesses exhibit patterns of sleep-wake states that differ from those of healthier preterms, although most of these differences disappear when infants recover (see Holditch-Davis et al., 2003b for references).

Sleep and wakefulness may be directly related to brain development. For example, because active sleep is less common in adults than non-REM sleep but is much more common in infants, it has been hypothesized to be necessary for brain development (Roffwarg, Mazio, & Dement, 1966). Also, EEG changes over age in sleep architecture, increasing spectral energies, and greater spectral EEG coherence probably indicate maturational changes in the brain, including synaptogenesis, evolution of neurotransmitter pools, and myelination.

Sleep-wake patterns can also be used to predict developmental outcome. Measures of sleep–wake states during the preterm period (amount of crying, quality of state organization, sleep cycle length, and amount of night sleep) predict Bayley scores during the 1st year. Developmental changes in the amounts of specific sleep behaviors during the 1st year are related to developmental and health outcomes in the 2nd year. Further, the stability of behavioral sleep-wake patterns in the late fetal period and in the 1st month predicts later development. EEG sleep measures in preterm infants have been related to developmental outcome at up to 8 years. Acoustic characteristics of infant cries have been used to predict developmental outcome in preterm infants and infants exposed to drugs prenatally (see Holditch-Davis et al., 2003b for references).

In summary, nutritive sucking, a noninvasive and easily measured behavior, appears to be an excellent index of neurodevelopment in preterm infants. Sleeping and waking patterns appear to provide an excellent index of neurodevelopmental status in preterm and full-term infants that can be either scored behaviorally or by EEG.

BARBARA MEDOFF-COOPER

Neuroleptic Use in Nursing Homes

Psychiatric illnesses, particularly dementia, are common diagnoses in nursing home residents. Often they are the main reason for nursing home placement (Stoudemire & Smith, 1996). It has been reported that dementia, mostly Alzheimer's disease (AD), may be present in over 70% of residents in nursing homes and 24% of those residents may exhibit psychotic features (Stoudemire & Smith). Primary care providers, including advance practice nurses (APNs), are treating a growing population of older adults with dementia and many cases will be complicated with behavioral problems such as agitation. In addition to the complexities of the illness the clinician must frequently practice in an environment of fiscal constraints, staff shortages, and concerns about meeting federal standards.

Treatment can be divided into pharmacological and nonpharmacological interventions. Psychotropic medications are the mainstay of pharmacological treatment. Lasser and Sunderland (1998) did a retrospective chart review involving 298 residents in seven nursing homes. They found that 70% of the subjects took at least one psychotropic, 32% were taking benzodiazepines, and 42% were on neuroleptics. Within the AD group 54% were taking neuroleptics, 27% were taking benzodiazepines, and 13% took both. Another study involving a secondary analysis of a clinical trial with 446 subjects in three nursing homes yielded lower but still significant results. Between 14% and 19% of the subjects were taking neuroleptics in the three groups studied (Siegler et al., 1997). Although neuroleptics are commonly used to treat disruptive or psychotic features of dementia, the potential for anticholinergic and extrapyramidal side effects requires careful weighing of risks and benefits.

"Chemical restraints" is a term used to describe the excessive or inappropriate use of psychotropic medications, particularly sedatives and neuroleptics, in residents who do not have a psychiatric diagnosis or behavioral symptoms that justify their use (Siegler et al., 1997). Another description is a drug that is used to limit the physical movement of the patient (Fletcher, 1996). In an effort to protect the residents of nursing homes from overreliance on psychotropics and their adverse reactions, the federal government passed legislation restricting their use. This legislation was part of the Omnibus Budget Reconciliation Act of 1987 (OBRA 1987). In 1990, the Health Care Financing Administration (HCFA) issued guidelines based on OBRA 1987 regulations (Gurvich & Cunningham, 2000).

The first step in the guidelines requires clinicians to rule out medical or environmental causes of a problem behavior. This is essential in avoiding the misdiagnosis of delirium, which would dictate a different course of treatment possibly targeting an underlying medical cause. To justify the use of a neuroleptic the target behavior must be diagnosed and documented. The resident with delirium must be reevaluated at set intervals with a goal of reducing or eliminating the medication. Ideally the smallest effective dose will be used for the shortest period necessary

(Gurvich & Cunningham, 2000). Behaviors that may be inconvenient to the staff but not dangerous to the resident or others are not considered appropriate for neuroleptic use. Residents diagnosed as having psychosis or certain medical conditions are not included in these restrictions. Short-acting benzodiazepines may also be used to treat dementia with agitation. They also have restrictions that seek to limit adverse reactions and long-term use.

Research done by Siegler and colleagues (1997) indicated a decrease in use of neuroleptics after the OBRA '87 legislation. In 1998, a panel consisting of the American Psychiatric Association and the American Association for Geriatric Psychiatry reported that there had been decreased use of psychotropic medications in nursing facilities in response to OBRA '87 (Colenda, Streim, Greene, Meyers, Beckwith, & Rabins, 1999). The panel also reported that there might be uncertain or negative outcomes related to OBRA '87. The focus on eliminating "chemical restraints" from nursing homes may have led to a tense atmosphere between clinicians who feel they are making sound clinical decisions and state surveyors (Colenda et al.). It is uncertain whether these regulations have affected quality of life for the nursing home residents (Colenda et al.).

Research involving neuroleptics for treatment of agitation shows modest improvement at best; however, consensus statements recommends their use (Bartels et al., 2002). Overall, evidence that psychoactive medications are effective was inconclusive. The adverse reactions such as sedation and anticholinergic effects are known to be a risk for this frail population. The atypical neuroleptics may offer a lower side-effect profile, but still carry risks such as extrapyramidal side effects. Herrmann (2001) reported that there is emerging evidence that antidepressants and anticonvulsants are effective in reducing noncognitive symptoms of dementia. These classes of medications may be better choices for some patients depending on comorbidities present.

According to Bartels and colleagues (2002), research suggested that nonpharmacological interventions have been effective in reducing behavioral problems, and evidence-based practice recommends their use. They should be instituted before psychotropic medications, when possible, and continued after medications are prescribed. Some of the interventions for behavioral symptoms include light exercise, music, and environmental modifications (Bartels et al.). The National Guideline Clearinghouse has similar evidence-based practice guidelines for AD, including specific interventions to reduce wandering and to treat problem behaviors.

The guidelines issued by HCFA seem to concur with evidence-based practice guidelines. The clinician is expected to assess the cause of a problem behavior and weigh the risks and benefits of prescribing a neuroleptic to a person with dementia. Nonpharmacologic interventions should be considered first line and may be used in conjunction with psychotropics.

One randomized controlled trial comparing psychotropics, behavior management techniques, and a placebo found no significant differences in efficacy for treatment of agitation (Teri et al., 2000). Future research should be directed at comparing the effectiveness of combining pharmacological and nonpharmacological interventions. Randomized control studies comparing anticonvulsants with neuroleptics in subjects with dementia may also be of benefit. As the population continues to age, APNs will be providing care for a growing number of patients with dementia. Knowledge of the treatment options and their effectiveness is essential and will apply to all practice settings that encounter older adults.

MICHELE FREEMAN IRWIN

Newman's Theory of Health

Margaret Newman is an eminent, visionary nurse theorist whose contributions to nursing science and nursing practice span 30 years of sustained scholarship on the theory of health as expanding consciousness. Newman's theory of health exemplifies her focus on a unitary-transformative paradigm for the discipline of nursing and on research as praxis methodology.

Newman's conceptual framework of health was introduced in her book *Theory Development in Nursing* (1979) and was expanded and refined in two editions of her book *Health as Expanding Consciousness* (1986, 1994). Her work was published at a time when less-abstract theories of nursing based on current practice were emphasized. Rather than being viewed as visionary with a creative and futuristic conceptualization of health, Newman's highly abstract grand theory as well as other grand theories of nursing was dismissed by the majority of nurses as far removed from the real world of everyday practice. As scientists in other disciplines revolutionized their former mechanistic worldviews to align more closely with a unitary-transformative paradigm, Newman's theory of health has achieved greater acceptance by nurse scientists and practitioners, particularly transcultural nurses and holistic nurses.

Newman's (1986, 1994) theory of health was inspired by her own nursing experiences, grounded in Rogers' science of unitary human beings and later expanded to include premises from Bentov's life process as expanding consciousness and Prigogine's theory of dissipative structures. She reconceptualized health as a manifestation of an underlying unitary field pattern rather than as a health-disease dichotomy. Health was defined as *a unitary pattern of the whole*, reflecting the dynamic, evolving human-environment process of expanding consciousness which occurs within a multidimensional matrix of movement, time, and space. Consciousness was defined as the informational capacity of the whole. She utilized Bohm's theory of undivided wholeness of reality and Young's theory of human evolution to support the concept of unitary field pattern and the pivotal influence of human choice. Nursing practice was defined as a mutual process of attunement during which the underlying patterns of the client and nurse are identified and both individuals are transformed.

Newman was an early eloquent advocate for nursing to identify, develop, and differentiate a paradigm that addressed the unique knowledge of nursing embodied in practice and in scholarly inquiry. In collaboration with Sime and Corcoran-Perry (Newman, Sime, & Corcoran-Perry, 1991, p. 3), she defined the focus of nursing as "caring in the human health experience." Differences between (a) the prevailing particulate-deterministic and interactive-integrative paradigms that had previously shaped nursing education, research, and practice and (b) a unitary-transformative paradigm for the discipline of nursing in the future were discussed. In the unitary-transformative paradigm, "a phenomenon is viewed as a unitary, self-organizing field embedded in a larger self-organizing field" (Newman et al., p. 4) and is identified by its pattern and its interaction with the larger whole. Change is unidirectional and unpredictable, with systems moving through stages of organization and disorganization to increasingly complex levels. Knowledge, which is personal and involves pattern recognition, is seen as a function of both the viewer and the phenomenon viewed.

In accordance with the unitary-transformative paradigm, Newman (1990b) described a model of differentiated nursing practice having three levels based on education, with advanced practice nurses having graduate preparation in the unitary-transformative paradigm. Newman proposed using nursing diagnoses that recognize patterns of person-environment interaction, rather than the North American Nursing Diagnosis Association diagnoses which reflect a static client in isolation from the environment. Her work subsequently moved away from conventional assessment and diagnosis as part of the nursing process toward nursing practice and research using her model of *research as praxis*, in which nursing interventions may be viewed as inherent in the mutual process of client and nurse pattern recognition.

Newman (1990a) identified the lack of conceptual fit between conventional quantitative research methods and the unitary-transformative paradigm of her theory of health. She posited that nurse scientists should use research as praxis methodology, a hermeneutic method of inquiry in which the client and nurse are coresearchers in identifying, describing, and verifying the client's pattern of expanding consciousness from narrative data about the most meaningful events in the client's life. Nurse scientists identified patterns of individual study participants in their practice, with qualitative comparison of patterns across study participants. Research as praxis is therefore both a research method and a transformative intervention.

Early quantitative research using conventional methods emphasized testing propositions derived from Newman's (1979) conceptual framework of health, focusing on the concepts of movement, time, space, and consciousness (Engle, 1996). Nurse scientists included Engle, Guadiano, Mentzer, Newman, Schorr, and Tompkins. Healthy adults were studied in community and laboratory settings with predominantly small, nonprobability samples of male college students, female college students, older adults, and older women.

Subsequent elaboration and refinement of Newman's (1986, 1994) theory of health shifted the focus of research to health as expanding consciousness, recognition of unitary field pattern, and research as praxis methodology (Engle, 1996). Nurse scientists included Lamendola, Moch, Newman, Schorr, and Schroeder. Small convenience samples of adults with and without health problems were studied in community and health care settings, including adults who exercised regularly, women with rheumatoid arthritis, women with breast cancer, adults with cancer, adults with coronary heart disease, and persons with HIV/AIDS. Much of the current research has demonstrated a transcultural theory application. International nurse scientists include Connor and Litchfield in New Zealand, Endo in Japan, Jonsdottir in Iceland, and Yamashita in Canada. The preceding studies have demonstrated the congruency of Newman's theory of health and of the research as praxis methodology for pattern identification with different cultures (Engle & Fox-Hill, 2005).

Newman's theory of health exemplifies the relationship between theory, research, and practice. The mutual process of evolving pattern recognition by the client and nurse using research as praxis informs nursing practice. As pattern recognition occurs, clients gain insights that create the opportunity for action. This practice approach exemplifies the participatory paradigm (Litchfield, 1999) emphasized by current health care systems that values shared decision making, collaboration, and partnering with multicultural clients, families, and interdisciplinary health care providers.

VERONICA F. ENGLE
EMILY J. FOX-HILL

(Florence) Nightingale

Florence Nightingale was born on May 12, 1820, in Florence, Italy, and died on August 13, 1910, in London, England. She is widely considered to be the founder of contemporary nursing and nursing education, as well as an early expert on health care statistics, hospital design and construction, and military health care. Nightingale's remarkable success at decreasing the death rates during the Crimean War gave birth to legends of the Lady with the Lamp. Her personal fame was critical to her ability to gain attention for her ideas, including those about the value of female, well-trained, nurses. Nightingale's birthday is remembered each year as International Nurses' Day, and it is the anchor date for Nurses' Week in the U.S.

Nightingale did NOT found the first nursing school: religious orders had been training nursing nuns for centuries, and the Kaiserwerth Institute opened its training school in 1836. Nightingale was much impressed by both the training techniques and quality of care evident at Kaiserwerth (Nightingale, 1851/1956), and later recommended some of the same strategies for the Training School at St. Thomas. Nightingale's contribution was the attention she brought to nursing education and in developing a system for nursing education that was secular and could be replicated in many different places. By the time she died, "Nightingale schools" could be found in 24 countries on five continents (Donahue, 1996).

Nightingale has further contributed to nursing by identifying what has become known as the meta-paradigm of nursing: person, environment, health, and nursing (Fawcett, 1978). She also established a firm tradition of basing nursing practice on carefully collected and analyzed data, the forerunner of today's evidence-based practice emphasis. Nightingale's most widely circulated work, *Notes on Nursing: What it is and What it is Not* (Nightingale, 1859/1969), was written not only for trained nurses, but for all women who would have the charge of another's health, and explicated how all persons were able to learn the laws of health through observation, experience, and reflection. This is reflective of her view of nursing as part of a larger whole, an opportunity for all women to become useful citizens and develop their spirituality. Nursing was also meant to be a part of social progress, and Nightingale (1892) encouraged all women to use their influence to improve life for everyone.

Nightingale did not set out to develop a conceptual model for nursing, yet her writings contain the elements needed for nursing theories, a clear conceptualization of the client, nursing goals, and nursing interventions (Meleis, A. I., 2004). The essential concepts she considered were the patient, the patient's environment, and nursing. She defined nursing as putting "the patient in the best condition for nature to act upon him" (Nightingale, 1859/1969, p. 133) through scrupulous attention to "fresh air, light, warmth, cleanliness, [and] quiet, and the proper selection and administration of diet" (p. 8). Health was defined as being "able to use well every power we have to use" (Nightingale, 1885, p. 1043). Health was affected by environmental factors, as well as by dietary choices and adequate amounts of exercise (Nightingale, 1863a).

Nightingale's most far-reaching ideas may have been her conceptualizations of persons, their environments, and the interaction between them that affected health. She identified persons as having physical, intellectual, social, emotional, and spiritual components (Nightingale, 1859/1969). This holistic understanding was a unique one, distinct from that of other scholars of her day (Welch, M., 1986). Her holistic view of human beings continues to be a hallmark of nursing, differentiating it from other health care professions.

Nightingale's insistence on the role of the environment in the health of individuals was also extremely innovative. She was adamant that deficiencies of light, fresh air, space, and sanitation were the chief culprits in disease, and she was fearful that the emphasis on antisepsis and disinfection would divert attention from the "dirt, drink, diet, damp, draughts, and drains" that needed to be addressed (Nightingale, 1859/1969, 1893/1949). She initially came to her beliefs about the environment's role in health in Scutari, where she was greeted by filthy conditions and a hospital mortality rate of 57% (Cohen, I. B., 1984). Conscientious application of her principles of sanitation soon reduced the mortality rate to 2% and gave her access to the military medical chiefs. She refined her thoughts about environmental impacts on disease by studying the mortality rates and locations of English hospitals. She noted that hospitals in the congested city of London had mortality rates of 90.84%, while those in small country towns were much more successful at discharging their patients alive (Nightingale, 1863b). Healthy hospitals provided sufficient fresh air, light, and space, and subdivided the sick into separate buildings or pavilions. Using these data, Nightingale laid out detailed plans for the construction of hospitals, including site selection, and hospitals for special populations such as children. A careful reading of her principles of hospital construction demonstrates that her ideas are as salient now as when they were written.

A liberally educated woman, Nightingale brought the skills of a classical scholar to her study of nursing and health, and she was passionate about the use of data and statistics (Grier & Grier, 1978). She laid a strong foundation for nursing research and evidence-based practice, and strove for the use of knowledge in patient care, writing "What then? Shall we have less theory? God forbid. We shall not work better for ignorance" (Nightingale, 1851/1956, p. 6). It is a curiosity that over 100 years lapsed between her initial enunciation of these ideas and their general acceptance by the nursing profession. Too many nurses equate Nightingale with outdated notions of etiquette and deportment, rather than with the volumes of data and statistics she produced. Even fewer are aware of her phenomenal grasp of politics and the use of personal power, tenacity, and shrewdness to achieve her goals (Baly, 1988). Professional nursing has made tremendous strides since Nightingale set out to establish the school at St. Thomas'. It is almost mind-boggling to think where the profession (and discipline) might be today without that 100 year gap.

TAMARA L. ZURAKOWSKI

Nosocomial Infections

Approximately two million nosocomial (hospital-associated) infections occur annually in the United States, resulting in increased morbidity, mortality, and cost (U.S. Department of Health & Human Services, 2000). Despite a decrease in the average length of hospital stay in the United States from 7.9 days in 1975 to 5.3 days in 1995, the rate of nosocomial infections rose from 7.2 per 1,000 patient-days to 9.8 per 1,000 patient-days, respectively; an increase of 36%. Hospital surveillance data indicate a 5% nosocomial infection rate, or an incidence of 5 infections per 1,000 patient-days; however, the infection rate may be closer to 10% in larger institutions (Wenzel & Edmond, 2001). The length of hospital stay due to nosocomial infection can increase up to 4 days for a urinary tract infection (UTI), 8 days for a surgical-site infection (SSI), 21 days for a bloodstream infection, and up to 30 days for pneumonia. The overall mortality rates associated with nosocomial bloodstream infections and pneumonia can be as high as 50% and 71%, respectively. In addition, these infections have attributable mortality rates of 16% to 35% (Jarvis, 1996). Serious nosocomial bloodstream infections are associated with central venous catheters (CVCs) placed in patients in intensive care units (ICUs), and it has been estimated that approximately 80,000 CVC-associated bloodstream infections occur in ICUs each year in the United States (O'Grady et al., 2002).

Pneumonia is the second most common nosocomial infection in the United States, following UTIs, which can add 7 to 30 days to a hospital stay at an average cost of $4,947 (Jarvis, 1996). Nosocomial pneumonias are mostly bacterial, with gram-negative bacilli generally the predominant organisms. However, *Staphylococcus aureus* (especially methicillin-resistant *S. aureus,* MRSA) and *Streptococcus pneumoniae* have emerged as significant pneumonia pathogens. Also, outbreaks of *Aspergillus* pneumonia have been reported in granulocytopenic bone-marrow transplant patients. Although patients with mechanical ventilation are not a major proportion of patients with nosocomial pneumonia, they have the highest risk of developing an infection (Tablan et al., 1994).

Surgical-site infections rank third among reported nosocomial infections, accounting for 14% to 16% of all infections (Mangram, Horan, Pearson, Silver, & Jarvis, 1999). According to Jarvis (1996), hospital stays increased 7 to 8 days for each SSI, at a cost of $2,734. The main criterion for an SSI is that it occurs within 30 days after surgery (or within 1 year with an implant). Studies show that most SSIs occur within 21 days of surgery, and 12% to 84% of all SSIs are diagnosed after patients are discharged from the hospital. Declines in average length of hospital stays and increasing numbers of outpatient surgical procedures place limitations on surveillance to identify SSIs (Mangram et al.). Avato and Lai (2002) found that 72% of post-coronary artery bypass graft SSIs were identified after discharge, compared to 28% before patients were discharged. Without postdischarge data, including surveillance data for SSIs by nurses and other health care providers in clinics and ambulatory care settings, meaningful comparisons cannot be made, making it difficult to identify best practices to improve patient safety (Goldrick, 2003).

The total cost of nosocomial infections to society is unclear; however, it is estimated that they are the fifth leading cause of death in the United States, with approximately 90,000 deaths attributed to such infections annually (Haley, Culver, White, Morgan, & Emori, 1985). In 1992, the total cost of nosocomial infections in the United States was estimated to exceed $4.5 billion (CDC, 1992), which converted to $5.7 billion in 2001 dollars (Stone, P. W., Larson, & Kawar, 2002). In prospective payment systems based on diagnosis-related groups, Jarvis (1996) estimated that the average cost to the health care system for nosocomial infections in 1996 ranged from $576 for each UTI to $22,000 for each bloodstream infection.

In an audit of 72 distinct results in published studies, P. W. Stone and colleagues (2002) found that 40% of the infection control interventions studied were cost-saving interventions. For example, Papia and colleagues (1999) found screening high-risk patients for MRSA colonization on admission prevented nosocomial transmission and was cost-effective. Kotilainen and Keroack (1997) found that extending ventilator circuit changes from 72 hours to 7 days was cost-effective and did not increase rates of nosocomial pneumonia in ICU patients.

Handwashing is considered to be the most important infection control practice to prevent the transmission of pathogenic microorganisms, and studies demonstrate a relationship between improved hand hygiene and reduced infection rates (CDC, 2002c; F. Pittet, 2001). However, observational studies indicate that adherence to recommended hand-hygiene procedures among health care providers had an overall average of 40%, with rates ranging from 5% to 81% (CDC). Pittet reported that alcohol-based hand rubs may be better than traditional handwashing because they require less time, contribute to sustained improvement in compliance, and are associated with decreased infection rates. A study comparing the efficacy of an alcohol-based hand rub versus conventional handwashing using an antiseptic soap found that the alcohol-based hand rub was significantly more efficient in reducing hand contamination (Girou, Loyeau, Legrand, Oppein, & Brun-Buisson, 2002). Another study found that the introduction of easily accessible dispensers with a waterless alcohol-based antiseptic led to significantly higher handwashing rates among health care providers (Bischoff, Reynolds, Sessler, Edmond, & Wenzel, 2000). The CDC's revised hand hygiene guidelines strongly recommend an alcohol-based hand rub for routine decontamination of hands in certain clinical situations; however, the CDC also emphasizes that hands must still be washed with soap or an antimicrobial product and water when visibly soiled or contaminated with blood or other body fluids.

Nurses play an important role in the prevention of nosocomial infections, and represent the first line of defense for such adverse outcomes. In a study, the American Nurses Association (2000b) identified five adverse outcomes related to nurse staffing: length of stay, pneumonia, postoperative infections, pressure ulcers, and UTIs. Multiple regression analyses found statistically significant inverse relationships between nurse staffing and all five outcome measures. A recent study reported that a higher proportion of hours of care provided by registered nurses (RNs) was associated with lower rates of nosocomial infections (Needleman, Buerhaus, Mattke, Stewart, & Zelevinsky, 2002). Other studies have shown that health care facilities with appropriate levels of nursing staff can prevent infections. For example, Cho, Ketefian, Barkauskas, and Smith (2003) showed that a 10% increase in RN staffing decreased the odds of a patient acquiring nosocomial pneumonia by 9.5%. Kovner, Jones, Zhan, Gergen, and Basu (2002) found an inverse relationship between RN staffing and post-surgical adverse events. A study of the effect of nurses' educational level on surgical patient mortality found, after controlling for all other risk factors, that surgical patients who were cared for in hospitals where a higher proportion of direct-care RNs held bachelor's degrees had a better survival rate over those treated in hospitals where a lower proportion of staff nurses held bachelor's degrees (Aiken, Clarke, Cheung, Sloane, & Silber, 2003). Although these studies do not imply causation, nurses who incorporate evidence-based infection prevention and control recommendations into their practice can decrease infectious adverse events and the odds of failure to rescue while reducing health care costs.

BARBARA A. GOLDRICK

Nurse-Patient Interaction

Nurse-patient interaction refers to the dyadic reciprocal interactions that occur between nurses and patients in the context of providing and receiving nursing care. Early nursing theorists such as Peplau, Orlando, Travelbee, and Widenbach, who drew attention to the process of interaction in nursing practice, prompted researchers to describe, operationalize, and measure the efficacy of nursing interactions. In 1977, Diets and Schmidt classified the rapidly expanding research on nurse-patient interaction as descriptive or correlational studies, studies that measure the indices of nursing by using hypothetical interactions, and studies that describe or evaluate nursing interactions using conception or interaction frameworks borrowed from other disciplines (e.g., counseling psychology). These initial research efforts were largely focused on single channels of communication (e.g., nurse conversation or touch) and produced only partial information about the interaction. Resulting failures to capture relevant clinical data prompted the redesign of instruments and studies specifically for examining nurse-patient interactions. As one example, the Nurse Orientation System developed by Diets was used by researchers to examine the effect of nursing on patient experiences of pain (Diets, Schmidt, McBride, & Davis, 1972).

Researchers continued to study those aspects of the nurse-patient interaction that were quantifiable, using predominantly deductive approaches; and despite the use of increasingly sophisticated techniques, the results of many studies raised concern about the quality of nurse-patient interactions. Some researchers attempted to explain their findings in terms of nurses' lack of communication skills or their busy workloads; others pointed to problems inherent in the research, citing a lack of attention to the patient's role in nurse-patient interaction, unsubstantiated assumptions about the nature of nurse-patient interactions, and failure to take into consideration important contextual factors that influence nurse-patient interactions as major issues. In addition, in the absence of adequate definitions of nurse-patient interaction or its components (e.g., touch) researchers used narrow and simplistic conceptualizations. As a result, in deciding a priori what behaviors were important to study, researchers risked missing important behaviors or focusing on insignificant behaviors; as a consequence, they ended up with incomplete or invalid descriptions.

As support for "caring" in nursing developed in the 1980s, theorists drew attention to the complexities inherent in the process of providing nursing care, stimulating a resurgence of interest in examining nurse-patient interactions with a variety of new approaches, such as grounded theory, conversational analysis, ethology, and discourse analysis. By using inductive approaches, researchers identified nurse and patient behaviors that were important to study (rather than deciding this a priori), explored interaction patterns from the perspective of the nurse and patients, and considered important factors of context and relationship. Studies completed by researchers such as Carl May, Maura

Hunt, Jocalyn Lawler, and Janice Morse are representative examples. Using these new approaches, researchers identified exceptional nursing interaction skills, such as "tactics," "comfort talk," "minifisms," and other previously unrecognized interaction strategies that nurses typically used in clinical settings—skills that were rarely part of communication courses and often devalued.

One of the most important developments in the study of nurse-patient interactions is the use of video technology. Videotaping observations preserves the observational context, verbal content, nonverbal behaviors, and interactive processes for analysis and coding. Of particular advantage is the ability to repeatedly review videotapes, both in real time and in slow motion. This facilitates in-depth study of a wide range of simultaneous behaviors, including rarely occurring events and subtle or rapid changes in behavior. Videotaped observations are particularly useful when studying interactions with patients who are preverbal, unconscious, or otherwise unable to recall interactions with sufficient detail.

Although new lines of research show promise and appear to be unraveling some of the unique complexities inherent in nurse-patient interaction, much work remains to understand nursing interactions as they occur in health care settings, including patients' homes or other community settings. Far more attention has been given to identifying and describing components and patterns of nurse-patient interaction than studying the efficacy of different types of interactions in relation to patient outcomes. It appears that some patterns of interaction may be powerful therapeutic tools, yet more systematic investigation is needed to demonstrate these effects. Furthermore, negative or undesirable psychological and physiological sequalae associated with interaction patterns should be documented.

Although the definition of nurse-patient interaction has not received careful attention, the focus has been on the verbal and nonverbal behaviors of the nurse. Yet increasingly, patients are being encouraged to take an active role in decision making and their nursing care. To develop innovative and supportive strategies to foster collaboration in care and involvement in decision making, a sound understanding of the nature of interactions between nurses and patient, with a strong focus on the role of patient behavior in these interactions, is necessary. In addition, the links between nurse-patient interaction and types of nurse-patient relationships must be explored.

JOAN L. BOTTORFF

Nurse-Patient Relationship

The interpersonal relationship between nurses and patients has become an important subject of discussion, theorizing, and research since Peplau and Orlando introduced the concept of the nurse-patient relationship as an essential component of nursing practice. Recognition of the need for individualized nursing care, the introduction of new approaches to care delivery (e.g., primary nursing), increasing concerns about dehumanization related to advances in technology, and the emergence of theories delineating caring as a pivotal concept in nursing have reinforced the centrality of the nurse-patient relationship in contemporary practice. The nurse-patient relationship is now viewed as essential content in nursing curricula, and clinicians value the development of therapeutic relationships with patients as a significant part of their work. Yet despite the overwhelming endorsement of the importance of the nurse-patient relationship, the practical difficulties associated with developing relationships remain unresolved. Of importance are issues related to balancing personal involvement and professional detachment. Other important issues concern building relationships in contexts where the organization of nurses' work limits involvement or where reporting practices undermine the development of trust. Issues also arise from challenges related to renegotiating relationships in response to changes in patient dependence and vulnerability.

Nurses have attempted to identify the unique characteristics of the nurse-patient relationship through their conceptualizations, although to date there is little evidence to support this assumption. The nurse-patient relationship has been described as a therapeutic instrument with levels or types of involvement and as an interactive process requiring the active participation of both patients and nurses. Important components of the nurse-patient relationship include concepts such as empathy, trust, respect, knowing the patient, commitment, advocacy, and social control. Nursing writers critiquing current conceptualizations of the nurse-patient relationship have pointed out the failure to consider the collective nature of nursing work and other realities of everyday practice such as the provision of bodily comforts. Theorists such as Sally Gadow and Jean Watson have attempted to explain the nature of the links between nurse-patient relationships and positive health care outcomes, and there is some empirical evidence that supports these assertions.

Although researchers have begun to explore the complex dynamics involved in nurse-patient interactions and their therapeutic potential, there is relatively little empirical data related to what takes place in everyday clinical settings to support current conceptualizations of the nurse-patient relationship. Early investigations of nurse-patient relationships were influenced by definitions from the social sciences and the traditions of logical positivism. However, explanations of the relationship proved difficult to quantify. With increasing acceptance of qualitative research methods in nursing, researchers have turned to a variety of new approaches to examine patterns of relationships in nursing, including grounded theory and narrative analysis. These studies have revealed important new information about nurse-patient relationships, some of which has contradicted professional rhetoric surrounding the development of these relationships.

The complexities inherent in the nurse-patient relationship demand that the research agenda be augmented by micro-level approaches (such as sociolinguistics, ethnomethodology, and in-depth videotape analysis), advances in interpretive methodology (e.g., using a feminist perspective), and triangulation (e.g., triangulating conversational analysis with data from ethnographic research), as well as by taking advantage of constructionist, critical, and postmodern theory to understand the dynamics of nurse-patient relationships. For example, observational studies of the development of nurse-patient relationships as they occur in everyday clinical settings would augment nurses' narratives of memorable relationships. Some researchers are exploring the potential value of using video recorders to capture the development of relationships over time. Detailed analysis of videotaped patient and nurse behaviors at the interaction level have produced some encouraging results.

For the most part, researchers have focused on the affective dimensions of nurse-patient relationships by interviewing nurses, particularly those who were able to provide exemplar cases. Other dimensions of the nurse-patient relationship should be examined, as well as outcomes, as they relate to different phases and types of relationships. Attention must be given to the patient's perspective and role in shaping relationships.

JOAN L. BOTTORFF

Nurse Researcher in the Clinical Setting

The term *nurse researcher in the clinical setting* is used to denote nurses who have research as one of their responsibilities or their sole responsibility and are at least partly supported by salary from a clinical setting, inclusive of hospitals, clinics, and other agencies providing health care to patients. Such nurses are usually prepared at the doctoral level but sometimes at the master's level. The additional responsibilities of these individuals may include education, quality improvement, evaluation in the clinical facility, and the requisite administration accompanying those duties. The position in the clinical setting can be either line or staff. The individual also may be jointly appointed to a school or college of nursing or another health-related institution for a percentage of their time.

The specific responsibilities for these individuals include conducting research and assisting others in conducting, applying, and utilizing research. Although those are the explicit role responsibilities, the nurse researcher in a clinical setting is expected to affect the nursing staff positively in several indirect ways. The nurse researcher is an educator, teaching about the research process, guiding critiques of completed research for application and utilization, and developing research days for sharing of research. The researcher is involved in the professional development of staff, facilitating staff to present and publish their databased projects under the tutelage of the researcher. Nurse researchers in clinical agencies usually have the responsibility to represent the agency with outside researchers using the agency as a data collection site. In the role of change agent, the researcher helps to make practice research-based. The change agent role and the researcher role are often combined with the quality control role, where pre- and postmonitoring or longitudinal monitoring around a change are needed.

To carry out these responsibilities, the researcher must possess several attributes. Knowledge and skills in the research are the most obvious, but equally important are people skills (e.g., motivating, confirming, guiding professional development) and conceptual skills. The latter set of skills comes into play in several ways, for example, identifying a researchable problem and reworking complaints and questions into a basis for finding solutions.

A major difference between the academic researcher and the nurse researcher in the clinical setting is the mission of the employer. The university has a societal responsibility for knowledge advancement. The health care institution has a responsibility for health care. Mission is a key work environment characteristic, and the work environment has a profound impact on the outcomes of one's work. This is especially true for nurse researchers in clinical settings, whose outcomes are influenced by their environment. Within clinical agencies the following have been associated with research productivity: (a) research culture (policies and procedures indicative of a consistent commitment to nursing research, such as the presence of research in the agency's mission); (b) resources for research activities (e.g., library holdings, funding of research activities, presence of other nurses with advanced nursing education); (c) attitudes (e.g., belief that the public and other professional colleagues value nursing research; and (d) esprit, a positive group work morale. Clearly, these nurse researcher roles are complex and not an insignificant addition to any staff.

One of the first tasks for the nurse researcher new to a setting is to assess the work environment, including the resources available. In particular, the nurse researcher cannot function well if isolated from others with research skills. Baccalaureate graduates with a foundation in research, master's-prepared nurses who have completed a thesis or have had strong intermediate research instruction, and doctorally prepared nurses with advanced research preparation are important resources. The last may not be part of the researcher's organization but available through an affiliated university. The availability of university-educated nurses is both an indication of the education programming needed and whether the environment has a "critical mass" of nurses for research activities.

KARIN T. KIRCHHOFF
PATRICIA A. MARTIN

Nurse Staffing

Nurse staffing is the number and type of workers employed by an agency to provide nursing care to the persons served by the agency. Nurse staffing numbers are typically given in full-time equivalents [FTE] that represent fifty-two 40-hour work weeks of five 8-hour days, or 2,080 hours, the typical annual paid work time for a full-time employee. The hours that individuals actually work would be fewer and depend on paid benefit hours (vacation, holiday, sick, etc.) that are included in each FTE-paid 2,080 hours. The advent of 12-hour shift schedules has either reduced the full-time work week to three 12-hour shifts, 36 hours, or has extended the work week by 2 hours to 42, typically three 12-hour shifts one week and four 12-hour shifts the next, averaging 42 hours per week. Hours are reported by the type of worker used or needed and staff are classified as registered nurses [R], licensed practical (or vocational) nurses [L], and aides [A], variously called attendants, technicians, or assistants.

Nightingale (1863b) identified ward size as a contributor to variation in hospital nurse staffing. Smaller wards (like intensive care units or ICUs) have high fixed costs, suggesting both the relevance of new applications for studies of ward design and use, and/or controlling for ward size and use in staffing studies.

After the publication of the Institute of Medicine report, *Nursing Staff in Hospitals and Nursing Homes: Is it Adequate?*, research on nurse staffing has been advanced by reports that have employed large data sets where variations in staff numbers and composition have been used to explain differences in end results of hospital care. Prominent among the studies are those reported in medical journals by Aiken, Needleman, and their colleagues who analyzed abstracted patient records and hospital characteristics and reported structure-outcome associations (Aiken, Clarke, Cheung, Sloane, & Silber, 2003; Aiken, Clarke, Sloan, Sochalski, & Silber, 2002; Needleman, J., Buerhaus, Mattke, Stewart, & Zelevinsky, 2002). The definition of nurse was refined to incorporate consideration of basic nursing education, and hospital outcomes were extended beyond mortality to include complication rates and rates of failure-to-rescue (Aiken et al., 2003, 2002; Needleman et al.). Results reported in these newer, aggregated staffing studies have yielded nurse-to-patient ratios and have provided health policy with a metric that may replace the standardized nursing hours per patient day (NHPD). Studies of this type, while important, have problems associated with standardization, selection of variables, and multicollinearity (Silber, Rosenbaum, & Ross, 1995). Mark and Saylor (1999) outlined the methodological issues associated with large samples of hospitals or patients that employ existing data for secondary analyses or study specific prospective data.

Analyses of nurse staffing are performed retrospectively (essentially a count of the workers who were present and cared for the patients who were present) and prospectively. While nurse staffing research has been prospective, in that studies attempt to predict the number and type of worker needed to care for specified patient (or person) groups, the more influential quantitative research reports have looked back on the nurse staffing that was in place when patient samples were drawn and used regression analyses to both explain and predict.

Implicit in the study of nurse staffing is an expectation that research will yield results that are generalizable—that is, others in the specified universe can safely apply the findings from valid and reliable studies and experience comparable results. It may be unreasonable to expect a high degree of standardization among the individuals (patients) who use nursing services, those (nurses) who provide them, and the agencies that enroll the patients and employ the nurses. Yet it seems worthwhile to understand the reasons for the one consistent finding in nurse staffing analyses: some hospitals (where nurse staffing has been studied most) provide twice as much nursing care for their patients as other similar institutions (Dartmouth Medical School, 1998).

The three traditional perspectives from which to study nurse staffing are: (a) task, procedure, intervention, or work analysis; (b) by disease and treatment; and (c) through nursing viewpoints.

Nurse staffing studies based on task or work analysis emanate from F. W. Taylor's

Principles of Scientific Management (1911). These were first applied to hospital work in the 1920s and have been in use since that time. The most important development of work-analysis methods applied to hospitals was the linkage J. Connor (1960) established between nurse staffing and variability in patient types and numbers. Patients are classified based on the type of work they generate, and the classifications are mapped to an unstandardized number and mix of nursing staff. It is uncommon to find reports that compare patient classification done in one institution to that of another.

A great deal of attention has been directed to the reliability of patient classification techniques, and few reports validate patient classification beyond the face validity established in the agency using the instrument. Two nurses classifying the same patient, at the same time, in the same way, achieve perfect reliability. Because of differences in nurses, it is not infrequent that ratings of the same patient differ. To bypass this reliability concern, prototype patient classification instruments have been developed. Prototype instruments cumulate weighted factors (items from a list of procedures done or a list of patient conditions for which interventions are needed) into scores that two nurses can agree on, but which may have been derived from different factors. The result is to refer to the classified patient as a member of class I, II, III, or IV, rather than as a patient who needs assistance with toileting, feeding, and/or ambulating. Further validity is lost because psychosocial aspects of care, long described as essential to effective care, have never been associated with weights reflecting the time nurses spend with patients.

Failure to specify intended results and measure the capacity of different patterns of work and worker to achieve those results is the most common problem with work-analysis techniques for the study of nurse staffing. Few have studied the appropriateness of either the task or the performer in achieving a specified end result. Work-analysis methods are criticized because they result in standards of care that are inconsistent with clinical research results, qualitative studies of nursing care, and nearly all concepts or theories of nursing. In one concept of nursing work, nurses assist individuals to perform their own tasks/procedures/interventions through encouragement and education as a means to their independence (Henderson & Nite, 1997).

Nurse staffing research has been linked to the diseases and treatments afforded patients on hospital specialty units. Most hospital inpatient wards care for specific patient groups organized by the physicians who admit the patients. Common groupings include orthopedics, cardiology, oncology, neurology, respiratory, gynecology, psychiatry, obstetrics, pediatrics, geriatrics, and many others. The earliest nurse staffing studies differentiated medical from surgical units, and many recent reports are addressed to even more specific physician and patient disease groupings, for example, HIV-AIDS.

The assumption that underlies this representation of patients' disease as the basis for nurse staffing is that the care rendered is homogeneous for the members of the patient group and different from other groups and that it is associated with a specific mix and number of nursing staff. Also implicit in the use of disease and treatment classification for the assignment of nursing staff is that nursing care is prescribed by physicians. The diagnosis related group (DRG) is the most common representation of medicine applied to nurse staffing. Medical methods for computing staff needs should be used with caution as much nursing literature addresses the differences in individual human beings, even if they should be suffering from the same disease (Henderson & Nite, 1997). Staffing methods based on medical diagnoses and treatment are inconsistent with clinical nursing research results, qualitative studies of nursing care, and nearly all concepts or theories of nursing.

A clear exposition for the representation of time in nurse staffing research is needed. In nurse staffing research, time can be represented in three ways: by nurse (or nursing) hours per patient-day, by nursing hours per case, and by length of hospital stay (LOS).

The association between nurses' time and length of patients' stays raises questions of causality. Are physicians and medical care responsible for variability of length of stay (and thus nursing hours per case)? Development and use of LOS norms established by physicians suggests that doctors control LOS and nursing hours per case. DRGs are a poor predictor of LOS. Further, LOS variability within DRGs has been explained and predicted from nurses' classifications of patients (Rosenthal, Halloran, Kiley, Pinkley, & Landefeld, 1992; Rosenthal, Halloran, Kiley, & Landefeld, 1995). If the discharge decisions made by physicians are more optimally made (in terms of care quality and cost) by nurses, ineffectiveness and inefficiency results.

Research on staffing should be intrinsically linked to concepts and theories of nursing as well as to the scientific and expert opinion literature on nursing. Existing methods for studying nurse staffing that employ work measurement methods, or that assume nursing care is derived from medical care, should be viewed with caution. Much more study of nurse staffing is required for generalization. Needed research should take place on two levels. First and foremost, differences in nursing care and their effects on patients should be examined at the bedside. Second, comparisons should be made among institutions using standardized methods that capture valid, reliable, and retrievable data from nurses about patients. These institutional comparisons should also incorporate data about nurses (education, experience, assignments, etc.) so that inference can be drawn about nurses' contributions to the end results of patient care.

EDWARD J. HALLORAN

Nursing Assessment

Assessment is widely recognized as the first step in the nursing process. Nurses use assessment to determine patients' actual and potential needs, the assistance patients require, and the desired outcomes to evaluate the care provided. There is consensus that nursing assessment is crucial as the starting point for establishing relationships and for determining how patients and nurses will subsequently interact. Assessment begins with the initial nurse-patient encounter; it involves collecting information to plan care and is an important basis for determining which interventions can be delegated to other providers. Information collected includes social and health history data, which come directly from patients, or physical assessment data, which are derived from physical assessment techniques and diagnostic studies.

The purposes of assessment are to begin to establish a therapeutic relationship and to identify the patients' strengths and problems in order to determine appropriate interventions. Both the process and content of assessment are important. Process includes using communication and physical assessment skills to establish a relationship and to gather needed information. The important content will vary with the patient but generally includes physical assessment, other diagnostic data, assessment of the meaning of the health experience, quality of life, symptoms, and cultural factors that may affect health.

Florence Nightingale was among the first to discuss nursing assessment (Nightingale, 1860/1969). She believed that observation was essential, and provided specific guidance about nursing assessments. Nightingale noted that the best process for interactions (including assessment) was to: "Always sit down when a sick person is talking business to you, show no signs of hurry, give complete attention and full consideration . . . Always sit within the patients' view" (pp. 48–49).

Assessments must be complete and detailed. Nightingale noted that "leading questions" are "useless or misleading" (p. 107). Rather than asking for evaluation (e.g., asking if a night's sleep was good), details should be asked for (e.g., the number of hours the person slept). These details need to be reported rather than just the opinions derived from them. Nightingale attributed physicians' not believing nurses' assessments to nurses' failing to provide these details (p.

123). Nightingale also gave examples of information that was misleading because it was incomplete or based on incomplete observations (e.g., the difference between "how often the bowels acted" and the number of times the "utensil" was emptied, p. 107).

Nightingale discussed the content needed in assessment, which included the importance of individualizing assessment, as "taking averages" is misleading (p. 120). She noted the need to understand "all the conditions in which the patient lives" (p. 121), including lifestyle factors, social conditions, and hygiene. Among the areas that ought to be observed were patients' dietary intake, symptoms and their meaning, changes in patterns (such as physical abilities), and "idiosyncracies" of patients. She noted that "peculiarities might be observed and indulged much more than they are" (p. 117).

Assessment begins the nurse-patient relationship and determines how they will work together. Considerable research has been conducted on factors that influence interpersonal relationships. Several classic works in nursing have dealt with the process of establishing these relationships, including the roles in nursing at various phases in relationships and the importance of observation and communication, including use of self-disclosure and empathy, in establishing relationships (e.g., Peplau, 1952).

Communication is essential in assessment, and is both the means for nurses and patients to influence each other and the process that leads to therapeutic and supportive influences on patients' health. Patients' successful communication of their needs to nurses is vital to individualized care. Individualized patient care has been found to produce more favorable outcomes and to reduce the cost of health care (Attree, 2001).

Although assessment and communication skills have been taught for decades, many studies have found that nurses had difficulty facilitating communication and that the patients' analysis of communication is often omitted. A variety of factors have been related to low facilitation of communication, including management in some health care settings, increased patient volume, the value placed on tasks, and not having the attitudes, desires, and skills needed to effectively communicate (Kruijver, Kerkstra, Bensing, & van de Wiel, 2000). Nurses have also been found to be confused about the purpose of nursing assessment. Observations have found that nurse-patient interactions are superficial, routinized, and task-related, and that nurses create barriers in communication.

Surveys of nurses revealed that most had received training in communication skills, felt they were fairly effective in using these skills, and felt that the skills are important to their jobs. However, they also thought they needed and were willing to receive additional training. Communication training programs have had mixed results, including that benefits did not persist, that changes were limited, and that nurses taught communication skills did not improve in their ability to elicit and identify patient concerns despite increased use of the skills learned. The Study to Understand Prognoses and Preference for Outcomes and Risks of Treatment (SUPPORT) was a striking example of a communication intervention that did not improve outcomes (Lynn, J., et al., 2000).

Physical assessment skills are routinely included in nursing curricula. They include (a) a general survey of patients' appearance and behaviors; (b) assessment of vital signs, temperature, pulse, respiration rates, and blood pressure; (c) assessment of height and weight; and (d) physical examination to assess patients' structures, organs, and body systems. Physical assessment can be complete, assessing all of the persons' organs and body systems, or modified to focus only on areas suggested by the persons' health history or symptoms.

Perceptions of symptoms and quality of life are important areas for assessment. Both symptoms and quality of life are primarily subjective experiences, influenced by many factors but knowable primarily through patients' descriptions of their experiences. Moreover, symptoms that are not properly managed can be life-threatening.

Nurses need to explore the meaning of illness from patients' perspectives in order to help patients mediate between the medical role of fighting disease and the patients' perspectives (Steeves, Cohen, & Wise, 1994). The link between meaning making and the experience of illness and treatment may help elucidate important nursing interventions that can assist patients in meaning making in ways that are helpful to coping with their experiences and symptoms (Kleinman, 1988).

Understanding experiences of illnesses and treatments of members of diverse cultures is important but currently limited. Many have argued for the need to understand clients' lived experiences and their interactions in order to provide quality nursing care (Cohen, M. Z., & Palos, 2001). Producing unbiased and culturally appropriate knowledge is both important and complex (Cohen, M. Z., Phillips, & Palos, 2001). This knowledge is important because those from diverse cultures may differ in ways that profoundly affect their health, what we need to assess, and the interventions that will be effective.

Despite consensus about the importance of understanding patients' perspectives, patients' descriptions show a consistent and persistent discrepancy between their views of their health care experiences and professionals' understandings of these experiences. The meanings that patients attribute to their experiences help determine what needs they have and how these needs can best be met. Since action is based on meanings, common meanings between nurses and patients will provide the most effective base for helpful nurse-patient relationships. Research indicates that nurses need to understand the patients' perspective in order to deliver effective nursing care, but that often nurses assume they know what their patients need without eliciting actual patient concerns. Effective assessment is the essential basis for providing effective nursing care.

MARLENE ZICHI COHEN

Nursing Centers

Nursing centers, also known as nurse-managed centers (NMCs), nurse-managed health centers, or community nursing organizations, provide nursing services to individuals, families, and communities and serve as unique sites for linking nursing research, education, service, and faculty practice. Types of services provided range from health teaching, assessment, and referral to increasingly full primary-care services including health promotion, risk reduction, and management of health-related issues common to primary care including prenatal care.

Historically, the nursing center idea originated in the early 1900s with the establishment of district and public health nursing. Later examples were Kentucky Frontier Nursing Services and the New York City Loeb Center. During the 1970, storefront clinics, independent nursing practices, and community nursing center demonstration sites represented the nursing center concept. During the 1980s, many schools and colleges of nursing, as well as hospitals, clinics, and public health agencies, established nursing clinics. With increasing emphasis on primary, managed, and interdisciplinary care in the 1990s, nursing centers entered into partnerships and business agreements.

Based on a national survey of academic nurse-managed centers, there are close to 200 such centers across more than 90 schools of nursing (Sebastian, Barkauskas, Stanhope, Pohl, & Vonderheid, 2004). In addition, 22 reported closing in the past 5 years, the primary reason being financial. There has been increasing emphasis on financial sustainability of these centers as reported in the literature (Vonderheid, Pohl, Barkauskas, Gift, & Hughes-Cromwick, 2003; Vonderheid et al., 2004). In addition, in the past 5 years there has been an increased effort to bring NMCs into the health care system through credentialing practitioners, obtaining federal funding for community health centers, and other reimbursement efforts. With increasing emphasis on full primary-care services, nursing centers are developing more sophisticated business plans and entering into partnerships and business contracts with a broad range of consumers. Sound fiscal management has emerged as a critical skill for sustainability (Frenn, Lundeen, Martin, Riesch, & Wilson,

1996; Vonderheid et al., 2003; Vonderheid et al., 2004). Although many nursing centers do provide a safety net function in the current health system, others do this in combination with strong commercial and government contracts including managed care (Pohl, Vonderheid, Barkauskas, & Nagelkerk, 2004).

Nursing centers may be classified by the types of services they provide as well as by their sponsors. Many nursing centers are affiliated with schools of nursing and essentially serve as academic centers in which the tripartite mission of the university is modeled (e.g. Michigan Academic Consortium and the Midwest Nursing Center Consortium). Others are freestanding and do not have formal connections with academia. The first model is full primary-care community-based nursing centers. A recent survey (Sebastian et al., 2004) indicates that 94% of the nursing centers associated with academic units are located in either fully or partially medically underserved areas. Funding for these centers is diverse and includes patient revenues including managed care contracts (such as Michigan State University's contract with the Veterans Administration), grants, school of nursing/university support, and other contributions (Vonderheid et al., 2003; Pohl et al., 2004). Many centers partner with their communities and also have community advisory boards.

Nursing centers based on wellness and health promotion are the second type of model and commonly are located where people gather—in workplaces, schools, meal sites, neighborhoods, and homeless shelters. Services provided are based on aggregate needs. Creative use of private and public funding sources is necessary to establish and maintain these services. The following are examples of wellness and health promotion models: the Pine Street Inn of Boston, supported by city and county funds and servicing homeless persons; and the Minnesota Block Nurse Program funded as a community nursing organization (CN) demonstration project of the federal Health Care Financing Administration (HCFA) and servicing Medicare beneficiaries who are homebound elders.

Faculty practice, independent nursing practices, and entrepreneurship are the third type of model. Whether these practices are linked with nursing centers or set up as part of a network of practices within a school of nursing, they often serve a specific population or need in the community.

Research on and in nursing centers is both quantitative and qualitative. Research utilization is evident in the development of standards of care and protocols. Research in centers has been descriptive of patient/clients, services provided, patient/client satisfaction, differentiation of nurse practitioners (NPs) versus physician roles, and student experiences and satisfaction with those experiences. In addition, outcomes of care, using the Health Plan Employer Data and Information Set (HEDIS) and other national benchmarks, as well as cost of care in nursing centers have been more recently documented along with intervention studies and their outcomes. Positive outcomes with chronic disease (e.g., hypertension, diabetes, asthma) have been documented (Barkauskas, Pohl, Breer, Benkert, & Wells, in press).

Patients and families who receive care in nursing centers report an extraordinary high level of satisfaction with their care (Benkert, Barkauskas, Pohl, Tanner, & Nagelkerk, 2002). Findings from focus groups report that the NP spends more time with patients, prevents emergency room visits, provides patient-centered care, and provides this care in the community close to their work, home, or school. Findings indicate that nursing centers are located in community settings such as public schools, public housing, churches, mobile vans, other community agencies, and small community settings. Patient volume per clinic is relatively small but large enough to be sustainable. Although reimbursement and credentialing of NPs continue to be issues, there are increasing contracts with managed care organizations.

The Midwest Nursing Center Consortium has been funded by the Agency for Healthcare Research and Quality as a Research Network Group (University of Wisconsin, Milwaukee) as has the Yale School of Nursing. This funding facilitates the infrastructure for research in nursing centers. In addition the creation of a data warehouse for nursing centers that is funded by the W.K. Kellogg foundation advances the research agenda for nursing centers.

The use of electronic health records (EHRs) and electronic practice management systems are changing the way nursing centers do business. Although EHRs are still relatively rare, it is expected that these will be critical to creating the national database and warehouse on nursing centers.

Development of a national database and warehouse is critical for nursing centers to continue to move into the main health care area. The National Network for Nurse Managed Health Centers (http://www.nnnmhc.org) is developing such a database and warehouse. The standardization of nursing language diagnoses, interventions, and outcomes contributes to understanding the process of care in these centers. Nursing centers offer an excellent choice for cost-effective, high-quality care with high patient/client satisfaction. Nursing centers provide a very rich resource for student experiences that is congruent with the model of care learned in the classroom (Tanner, Pohl, Ward, & Dontje, 2003), service to the community, research for faculty and students, and faculty practice. They provide a model of care that might be replicated on a larger scale and inform policy as health care costs and health care systems are reexamined.

Susan K. Riesch
Updated by Joanne M. Pohl

Nursing Diagnosis

The nursing diagnosis movement began in 1972 in a meeting of a group of nurses discussing the need for better nursing documentation. Those nurses were concerned that nursing information was not being valued nor was it being used to demonstrate the effectiveness of nursing care. Something was missing. The patients' life situations and problems that nurses were dealing with on a regular basis were not well described by the patient's medical diagnoses. It was apparent to them that nursing needed a standard set of nursing-specific terms or names for the patient situations and problems they were treating independently. And thus began the effort to develop nursing "diagnoses" that would describe the responses patients were having to their illnesses, life transitions, and lifestyle changes. That work eventually evolved into an organization (the North American Nursing Diagnosis Association, now NANDA, International) of nurses interested in developing names for nursing-specific diagnoses and later for nursing interventions and outcomes as well.

Although interest in nursing diagnosis waned in the late 1980s and early 1990s, it began to revive as the move toward electronic health records accelerated. Nurses began to realize that the only way to be sure nursing information was available, retrievable, and usable in an electronic system was if it was coded so the computers could read it. "Free text" such as that in nurses' paper notes cannot be used or retrieved in an electronic database. So if nurses wanted to have their own information available and reusable for determining patient outcomes or staffing, for example, that nursing information needed to be captured using a standardized language that could be coded and used by nurses in any system. Thus the interest in nursing diagnoses, nursing interventions, and nursing outcomes has been increasing steadily.

With the emphasis today on evidence-based practice and monitoring patient outcomes, reliable nursing data is imperative. Nurses are being asked to prove they are effective. The best way to do that is to use standardized languages to document the patients' responses to their illness and to their nursing care in such a way that outcomes can be demonstrated and even compared across settings.

Nursing diagnosis is the second step in the nursing process. It is the judgment made about the meaning of a cluster of signs and symptoms (defining characteristics) found in the nursing assessment of the patient. Without a nursing diagnosis, a nurse is left rudderless to determine what goals should be set for the patient, what outcomes are desired, or what interventions to choose to meet the goals and resolve the nursing diagnosis.

NANDA, International (2003) defines a nursing diagnosis as a "clinical judgment about individual, family, or community responses to actual or potential health conditions/problems/life processes. A nursing diagnosis provides the basis for selection of nursing interventions to achieve outcomes for which the nurse is accountable" (p. 263). There are three types of nursing diagnoses: actual, risk, and wellness.

An actual nursing diagnosis is a human response to health conditions/problems/life processes that exist in individuals, families, or communities. An actual nursing diagnosis is "supported by defining characteristics (manifestations, signs, symptoms) that cluster in patterns of related cues or inferences" (NANDA, 2003, p. 263). An example of an actual nursing diagnosis is 'impaired skin integrity" defined as "altered epidermis and/or dermis" with the defining characteristics of "invasion of body structures, destruction of skin layers (dermis), disruption of skin surface (epidermis)" and supported by related external and internal factors such as shearing forces, pressure, restraint, altered fluid status, skeletal prominence, altered sensations, etc. (NANDA, p. 166).

A risk nursing diagnosis describes a human response that may develop in vulnerable individuals, families, or communities. It is "supported by risk factors that contribute to increased vulnerability" (NANDA, 2003, p. 263). An example of a risk diagnosis is "risk for impaired skin integrity" defined as "at risk for skin being adversely altered" and supported by risk factors such as radiation, moisture, extremes of age, medications, alterations in nutritional state, etc. (NANDA, p. 167).

A wellness nursing diagnosis describes a human response that indicates a readiness for enhancement in levels of wellness in the individual, family, or community (NANDA, 2003). An example of a wellness diagnosis is "readiness for enhanced therapeutic regimen management" defined as "a pattern of regulating and integrating into daily living a program(s) for treatment of illness and its sequelae that is sufficient for meeting health-related goals and can be strengthened" and supported by defining characteristics such as "expresses desire to manage the treatment of illness and prevention of sequelae" and "choices of daily living are appropriate for meeting the goals of treatment or prevention," etc. (NANDA, p. 190).

NANDA does not develop diagnoses. Its mission is to foster development and to provide mentorship and publish the new lists every 2 years. All diagnoses are developed by real working nurses and then submitted to NANDA. Revisions and deletions of diagnostic terms are handled in the same way. Submission guidelines are available online at http://www.nanda.org.

By the early 1980s there were a sufficient number of diagnoses to require some way to organize them. Taxonomy 1 was developed by a group of nursing theorists based on patterns of unitary human beings. It remained in place until it became clear that it was hindering instead of helping classify the new diagnoses. Work began on a new taxonomy in 1994 and Taxonomy II was adopted in 2000.

Kay C. Avant
Updated By Mary E. Kerr

Nursing Education

In 1873 three hospital training programs, modeled on Florence Nightingale's work in the United Kingdom, were established in the United States. In 1907 a Department of Nursing and Health was initiated at Teachers College, Columbia University, to provide graduate-level leadership for the preparation of nurse tutors, faculty, and administrators (Dock, 1912). Not until 1923 did nursing education enter the university with the establishment of programs at Yale University and at Western Reserve University. These were the country's first schools of nursing to have an independent status among the schools and colleges of a university. These early developments led to nursing education both as a training program controlled by the hospitals and an academic program within the university setting.

As early as 1915 the National League of Nursing Education called for university-level education, a demand reinforced by the Committee for the Study of Nursing Education, in the Goldmark (1923) report and other important reports on nursing education (Brown, 1948). However, Mildred L. Montag's (1959) writing on the potential role of nursing education at the community college level has had the greatest impact on nursing education today. From these early writings arose the distinction between the professional nurse, educated at the baccalaureate level or above, and the technical nurse educated at the community college level. In 1951 the first nursing program at a community college opened in Middletown, New York. Today community colleges prepare the largest number of nurses for practice.

From the turn of the century until the 1960s nursing leaders often obtained their graduate preparation in schools of education. Consequently, most major developments that took place in schools of education were rather quickly transferred to nursing curricula. The University of Chicago's influence, through Ralph Tyler, had a major impact on nursing education, with focuses on learner objectives and curricular structure. However, in the 1980s there was a backlash against the objectives-based curriculum and a renewed focus on the nursing curriculum as a humanistic endeavor, where "caring" and not behavioral objectives formed the core of the content (Watson, 1988).

Licensure is required to practice nursing in each state, and until 1944 each state developed its own testing mechanism to license nurses. Today the National Council of State Boards of Nursing (NCSBN) has jurisdiction throughout the United States and its territories. The NCSBN sets standards for requirements and regulations for schools of nursing and licensure of new graduates. However, authority for requirements and regulations rests at the state level. All the states have agreed to use the same licensing examination to facilitate the mobility of the nursing work force in the United States.

Currently there are three types of educational programs to prepare students for licensure as registered nurses (RN): baccalaureate degree (BSN), associate degree (ADN), and diploma programs. BSN programs, including accelerated options for second-degree seekers, are currently offered at 673 schools in the United States. On the graduate level, 400 master's programs and 88 doctoral programs are available nationwide. In 2003, there were 126,981 nursing students enrolled in baccalaureate programs, 37,241 in master's programs, and 3,299 in doctoral programs (AACN, 2004a). As of 2002, there were 700 ADN programs and only a small number of diploma programs operating in the U.S. (BLS, 2004).

In 2003, there were 10,167 full-time faculty in nursing programs offered in four-year colleges and universities. The faculty in these programs were 9.4% minority and 4.5% male (AACN, 2004b).

As of 2000, there were 2,694,540 RNs in the United States, and these nurses were 94.6% female, 86.6% white (non-Hispanic), and 81.7% were employed in nursing (HRSA, 2000). Their level of education is as follows: 22.3% diploma, 34.3% associate degree, 32.7% baccalaureate, 9.6% master's degree, and 0.6% doctorate (U.S. DHHS, HRSA 2000).

Nursing has many professional organizations, yet it has successfully developed a unified position in dealing with federal issues that affect nursing education and patient care. The vehicle for cooperation is the Tri-Council, made up of representatives from three major nursing organizations: the American Nurses Association (ANA), the National League for Nursing (NLN), and the American Association of Colleges of Nursing (AACN). The AACN, headquartered in Washington, DC, is an organization composed of collegiate schools of nursing. It conducts annual surveys of faculty salaries, faculty workload, and similar topics of primary interest to deans and directors of programs.

The ANA provides a voluntary credentialing mechanism that recognizes both RNs who are involved in advanced practice and those who are generalists practicing in a specialty area.

E. Smith (1979) defined continuing education as postregistered learning activity designed to increase knowledge or skill or to challenge attitudes. Several states now require varying amounts of additional education for relicensure. Moreover, some states (including Michigan, Idaho, Utah, and Minnesota) require competency-based continuing education.

Research on topics related to nursing education has been comprehensive and have examined many different areas, including quality of education, care planning, clinical judgment, clinical decision making, clinical teaching, learning styles, performance on licensure examination, faculty productivity, computer-assisted instruction, socialization processes, teaching learning processes, competencies, and others.

William L. Holzemer
Updated by Jeanne Novotny

Nursing Informatics

Nursing informatics is a branch of informatics concerned with all aspects of the nursing profession's use of computer technology. It can be viewed as the use of computer technology to support nursing (Hebda, Czar, & Mascara, 2001). Nursing informatics enhances and facilitates the legitimate access to and use of data, information, and knowledge. It is integrated in nursing practice, administration, education, and research programs and activities. It is incorporated in the design and development of computer-based patient records and other health-related systems (Saba & McCormick, 2001).

In 1992 the American Nurses Association (ANA) designated nursing informatics as a new nursing specialty. In 2001 the definition of nursing informatics evolved to incorporate the core elements considered to be key, namely: nurse, patient, health, environment, decision making, and nursing data, information, knowledge, information structures, and information technology. Nursing informatics is defined as a

> specialty that integrates nursing science, computer science, and information science to manage and communicate data, information, and knowledge to support patients, nurses, and other providers in their decision-making in all roles and settings. This support is accomplished through the use of information structures, information processes, and information technology (ANA, 2001, p. 17).

Informatics is derived from the French word *informatique*, which refers to all aspects of the computer milieu. Informatics emerged in the 1960s with the introduction of computers in the health care industry. As the industry advanced and expanded, computer applications and information systems emerged for health care facilities, specialties, and professions. During the past 3 decades, several nursing initiatives also have advanced the progress of nursing informatics for the profession. This period included several ANA recommendations designed not only to advance the development of nursing practice but also nursing data standards for computer-based systems.

As early as 1970 the ANA recommended that the nursing process be used as the standard for documenting clinical nursing practice. In 1988 the ANA recognized the Nursing Minimum Data Set (NMDS) as those 16 minimum data elements designed to document nursing care of patients and their families in any delivery setting. Four nursing care data elements in the NMDS—nursing diagnoses, nursing interventions, nursing outcomes, and intensity of nursing care—were envisioned as essential to be incorporated into computer systems with the idea of comparing nursing data across health care facilities, clinical population groups, and geographic areas (Werley & Lang, 1988).

Since 1992 the ANA, through the Committee on Nursing Practice and Information Infrastructure (CNPII), has recognized several vocabulary classification schemes or terminologies as meeting nursing data standards and clinical practice standards. These include the NANDA Taxonomy, the Home Health Care Classification (HHCC) System, the Omaha System, the Nursing Intervention Classification (NIC), the Nursing Outcomes Classification (NOC), the Nursing Minimum Data Set (NMDS), the Nursing Management Minimum Data Set (NMMDS), the International Classification for Nursing Practice (ICNP), the Patient Care Data Set (PCDS), the Perioperative Nursing Data Set (PNDS), SNOMED-CT, and Clinical LOINC. Each of these schemes addresses one or more of the data elements in the NMDS, and they are professionally recognized as the data standards essential for computer-based nursing information systems. Many of these terminologies are included in the National Library of Medicine's (NLM) Unified Medical Language System (McCormick et al., 1994; Saba & McCormick, 2001).

Another national nursing initiative, an expert panel in Nursing Informatics, was convened in 1988 by the National Institute for Nursing Research (NINR), National Institutes of Health (NIH), Public Health Service (PHS), and Department of Health and Human Services (DHHS) to investigate the scope of nursing informatics. The panel indicated that research was needed to determine the data and information needed by nurses for the computer-based patient record systems that affect nursing practice. They also recommended that efforts be focused on designing decision support systems, evaluating nursing information systems, and developing other applications to improve patient care.

Since 1999, annual Nursing Terminology Summit Conferences have been held with representation from national and international nursing informatics experts. The work from these conferences, combined with the efforts of the International Council of Nurses, the Nursing Informatics Special Interest Group of the International Medical Informatics Association, and others, has resulted in the first proposed nursing international standard.

The nursing informatics specialist, a nurse with formal education and practical experience using computers to support the information needs of all facets of nursing practice (Hebda, Czar, & Mascara, 2001), has the goal of improving the health of individuals, families, communities, and populations by optimizing information and communication (ANA, 2003). This is accomplished by incorporating theories, principles, and concepts from appropriate sciences into the use of technology in direct patient care, in the establishment of effective administration systems, in managing and delivering educational experiences, and in supporting nursing research (ANA). Nursing informatics focuses on the information management and processing of nursing data. It provides the framework for nursing data, information, and knowledge processed by the computer. Nursing informatics concepts require nursing classification schemes and vocabularies to provide the structure and framework for the data. Applications of nursing informatics are needed to standardize nursing documentation, to improve communication, to support the decision-making process, and to develop and disseminate new knowledge. They also are needed to enhance the quality, effectiveness, and efficiency of health care; empower clients to make health care choices; and advance the science of nursing (ANA).

Basic to the understanding of nursing informatics is an understanding of nursing data, data standards, and practice standards. Nursing data form the basis and foundation of nursing informatics. They are essential for the documentation of nursing care and management of clinical nursing practice. Nursing data refers to the atomic-level data elements or the unstructured raw facts. These data, once processed with other data elements, are transformed by the computer into information, and information, once aggregated and synthesized, creates new knowledge. Nursing knowledge forms the basis of knowledge-based systems, expert systems, and decision support systems that advance the science of nursing (Saba & McCormick, 2001).

Nursing informatics is critical to the conduct of research of nursing practice problems. Computer hardware and software are being used to design research tools, collect and process research data, and analyze and retrieve research information. The nursing vocabularies and data standards are being used to research the critical data elements for the computer-based patient record (CPR) systems, including the lifelong longitudinal health care record. The data elements also are being used for nursing information systems designed to document patient care, measure outcomes, and determine quality indicators. Nursing informatics is becoming an integral component in nursing administration, practice, education, and research as well as the nursing profession and health care industry.

Virginia K. Saba
Updated by Ida Androwich

Nursing Information Systems

Saba and McCormick (2001) described nursing information systems as the use of technology and/or computer systems to collect, store, process, display, retrieve, and communicate timely data and information in and across health care facilities that:

- administer nursing services and resources,
- manage the delivery of patient and nursing care,
- link research resources and findings to nursing practice, and
- apply educational resources to nursing education.

Nursing information systems are used to support nursing education, nursing practice, and nursing research. A nursing information system (NIS) is an information system that supports the use and documentation of nursing processes and provides tools for managing the delivery of nursing care (Hebda, Czar, & Mascara, 2001).

Early information systems focused on financial transactions models and were designed primarily to support charge capture, administrative, and operational transactions. With the increased introduction of computer technology in the health care industry, computer developers of the early hospital, medical, and patient care information systems began to expand their systems to include subsystems that addressed the documentation of nursing care. Then, as now, the challenge remains as to how to best computerize the existing paper-based methods of documenting nursing in health care facilities to support nursing and patient care. Developers began by computerizing the standardized nursing care protocols or plans that focused on medical diagnoses, surgical procedures, or disease conditions. With the introduction of the microcomputer, NISs emerged as stand-alone systems for a specific nursing application for different aspects of nursing administration, practice, education, research, and community health. Such systems were designed by nurses who were becoming proficient in their design.

In 1996, the American Nurses Association (ANA) established the Nursing Information and Data Set Evaluation Center (NIDSEC) to develop and disseminate standards pertaining to information systems that support nursing practice, and to evaluate voluntarily submitted information systems against those standards.

A number of models for viewing information systems have been proposed. One model, developed by Graves and Corcoran, focuses on the design of an NIS as the framework that represents the management processing of data, information, and knowledge. Zielsdorff, Hudgings, and Grobe (1993) identified design criteria for systems supporting the nursing process that included system capabilities, such as performance, flexibility, and connectivity, as well as user-machine interface, hardware, and data security and integrity requirements. They also believed it essential that the system would promote efficiency and effectiveness of care by supporting decision-making by the nurse. Androwich et al. (2003) emphasize that the information systems of the future must go beyond meeting basic information needs to support practice. They envision data, information, and knowledge available to the nurse as needed to inform every present clinical encounter and to provide and generate new knowledge to improve future encounters. NIDSEC identified four dimensions of nursing data sets and the systems that contain them: nomenclature (the terms used), clinical content (the "linkages" among terms), clinical data repository (how the data are stored and made available), and general systems characteristics.

Nursing information systems can be found in all areas where nurses function and in all settings where nurses provide patient care: hospitals, community health agencies, managed care organizations, ambulatory care facilities, and other settings where services are provided.

NIS in nursing administration are used primarily for the administration of nursing services and the management of nursing units. For the administration of nursing services, these information systems are designed to generate information focusing on budget, personnel, and resource management. The focus is on the specific applications needed to run a nursing department effectively and efficiently, such as staffing, scheduling, utilization, productivity, quality assurance, and discharge planning. Systems designed for the management of nursing units focus on the patient care services and address nursing intensity, patient classification, acuity, decision support, and patient outcomes. These systems are used to track the care process during an episode of illness as well as measure the impact and outcomes of the care.

In the area of nursing practice, NIS are used to document care planning and patient care services and comprise the computer-based patient record (CPR). The major applications are order entry, results reporting, medication protocols, care planning protocols, patient education, quality assurance, and discharge planning systems. The system utilizes the point-of-care computer terminals to capture direct patient care and can support the care process with decision support systems. Well-designed systems focus on the integration of information and care by all providers and can be used for discharge planning and referral to community health agencies and home health care services for follow-up.

In the area of nursing education, NIS form the technology that support the education process, such as computer-assisted instruction (CAI), interactive video (IVD) programs, and web-based courseware for synchronous or asynchronous learning. They use a wide range of educational strategies that enhance and integrate nursing informatics into the educational process (Saba & McCormick, 2001).

In nursing research, NIS support the research process. Without such systems, nursing research cannot be accomplished on large-scale databases and population groups. NIS are needed to process and analyze research data that only a computer application can perform. Nursing research applications include searching the literature by using bibliographic retrieval systems containing nursing-related material. Other applications include classification systems needed to code, classify, process, and analyze nursing research data, as well as the instruments and tools used to conduct research: database management systems, file managers, spreadsheets, and statistical software designed to process research data. Other applications, such as graphic displays, text preparation, and editors, are designed to disseminate and communicate research findings and conclusions via online databases or the Internet.

Nursing information systems represent the nursing informatics applications. They are described by the focus of the specific application, which varies according to the focus of the nursing activities supported. NIS are used in all major areas of nursing, namely, nursing administration, practice, education, research, and community health.

VIRGINIA K. SABA
UPDATED BY IDA ANDROWICH

Nursing Intensity

The concept of nursing intensity relates to the amount of nursing care provided to one or more patients. While there is not yet a universally accepted definition or measure of nursing intensity, all sources agree that it is partly a function of average hours of care provided to patients in a particular setting in a specific time frame. In the research literature, nursing intensity has often been operationally defined as patient acuity.

The first controlled clinical trial that varied nursing intensity levels in a patient care unit was done by New, Nite, and Callahan in 1959. In an attempt to determine optimal staffing, they varied nursing hours per patient day from the usual 4.5 to as high as 7.9 hours of care per day. They discovered that chronic overstaffing had deleterious effects on morale. New, Nite, and Callahan did not measure or address patient acuity as part of their study.

Patient acuity was first measured as a predictor of nursing care needs by Robert Connor in 1960. Connor's research demonstrated that need for nursing hours was not predictable from census alone, but by a combination of census and illness level of the patients. Connor developed the first patient acuity measure and concurrently developed a plan for allocating nursing resources by patient requirements. A serious problem with matching nursing intensity to patient care needs is the reality that patient care needs are not constant. Connor found that providing a fixed number of nurses in a particular patient care unit guaranteed that there would be frequent incongruity between nursing resources and care requirements. Connor found and other researchers confirmed that patient care workload varied randomly from day to day and concluded that nursing resources must be able to be varied since care requirements varied (Connor, R., 1960).

Patient acuity is readily measured through use of a set of patient care requirements. There are algorithms that allow patient care needs to be translated into required hours of nursing care. There are two major problems with using patient acuity as a measure of nursing intensity. First, there is no guarantee that the number of nursing hours called for by the patient acuity system will be the same as the number of nurses available to provide care. Second, the approach assumes no differences between nurses with different education or different experience. In a report submitted to the American Nurses Association's Database Steering Committee, M. McHugh (1994) recommended that a measure of nursing intensity have at least the following six critical attributes: A time frame in which the care is delivered, hours of nursing care provided in that time frame, educational level of the nurses providing the care, years of experience of the nurses, years of experience in the particular clinical specialty, and years of experience in the particular setting in which the care is delivered. Recent studies have greatly increased the interest in the effects of educational levels of the nurses due to findings that this variable may have significant effects on patient outcomes.

More recently, a variety of studies examined the relationship between Magnet Hospital Status and patient outcomes. A key characteristic of Magnet Hospitals is professional nursing, and studies of nursing in Magnet Hospitals set the stage for later studies of nursing intensity and patient outcomes. Aiken, Smith, and Lake (1994) reported a lower mortality rate in Magnet Hospitals and related that to nursing autonomy and adequate staffing. In a review of research related to Magnet Hospitals (Scott, Sochalski, & Aiken, 1999), nursing intensity was not specifically addressed, but their discussion of primary nursing, nursing control of practice, and nursing autonomy as characteristics of Magnet Hospitals clearly relates to professional nurses rather than to Licensed Practical Nurses or unlicensed assistive personnel. There are several major issues that require study in nursing intensity. First is the total number of care hours provided relative to patient care needs. That was the focus of the studies from the 1960s through the early 1990s. However, beginning with Aiken, Smith, and Lake's study in 1994, the focus shifted from simply matching nursing resources to measured patient care requirements to studying patient care outcomes related to nursing care.

The first research concerns the relation of RN skill mix to patient outcomes. The second concerns the relation of educational level of the RNs to patient outcomes. Blegen, Goode, and Reed (1998) studied RN skill mix and patient outcomes. In that study and others, a higher RN skill mix means that of the staff, more are RNs than LPNs or unlicensed assistive personnel. This study found that a higher skill mix was associated with a lower rate of adverse patient occurrences such as falls, medication errors, and decubitus ulcer formation. Other studies confirmed the relationship between RN care and positive quality and patient outcomes. In a secondary analysis of a survey of over 11,547 Pennsylvania nurses, Sochalski (2001) found that intensity of nursing care (defined as workload) was significantly associated with quality of care. Aiken, Clarke, Sloan, Sochalski, and Silber (2002) reported that in hospitals with high patient-to-nurse ratios (lower nursing intensity), surgical patients experienced higher risk-adjusted 30-day mortality and failure-to-rescue rates, and nurses were more likely to experience burnout and job dissatisfaction.

Lichtig, Knauf, and Milholland (1999) conducted a study of hospitals in California and New York. Their most consistent finding was that more nursing hours and a higher skill mix of nurses were both associated with reduced hospital length of stay. They also found that a higher nursing skill mix was associated with a lower rate of decubitus ulcers—each additional percentage point of personnel who were RNs was associated with a reduction in pressure ulcers of between .79% and 1.77%. In the California hospitals, a higher percentage of RNs was also associated with lower rates of pneumonia and lower postoperative infection rates.

Given the repeated findings of lower lengths of stay, lower complication rates, and lower mortality rates associated with a higher RN skill mix, there can no longer be any question that a nursing staff that includes a high percentage of RNs produces more positive patient outcomes and lower lengths of hospital stay. To date, only two studies were found that examined the relationship of educational level of nurses to patient care outcomes.

Blegen, Vaughn, and Goode (2001) found that experience of professional nurses, but not education, was associated with lower rates of falls and medication errors. In fact, in units with a higher percentage of BSNs there was a slightly higher medication error rate. However, in a landmark study in 2003, Aiken, Clarke, Cheung, Sloane, and Silber found that even after adjusting for a wide variety of patient and hospital characteristics, a 10% increase in the proportion of nurses holding a bachelor's degree was associated with a 5% decrease in both the likelihood of patients dying within 30 days of admission and the odds of failure to rescue. Aiken did not study mediation error rates as did Blegen, Vaughn, and Good. Therefore, the difference in the results may be related to the different dependent variables, to different patient populations (all Aiken and colleagues' subjects were in Pennsylvania hospitals while Blegen and colleagues studied hospitalized patients in the Midwest). Also the two researchers used very different methodologies.

In summary, much has been learned about the positive outcomes of having sufficient staff to provide patient care. Research has demonstrated that a higher percentage of RNs is associated with more positive patient outcomes. However, the research on the effects of nursing experience and of BSN versus non-BSN prepared nurses is limited and the results are not yet sufficiently confirmed so as to draw definitive conclusions. Ultimately, an index of nursing intensity that includes nursing time, nurses' experience and nurses' educational level would greatly facilitate further studies of the effects of management decisions about nurse staffing on patient care outcomes.

Mary L. McHugh

Nursing Interventions Classification (NIC)

The Nursing Interventions Classification (NIC) is a comprehensive standardized classification of interventions that nurses perform. It is useful for clinical documentation, communication of care across settings, integration of data across systems and settings, effectiveness research, productivity measurement, competency evaluation, reimbursement, and curricular design. The Classification includes the interventions that nurses do on behalf of patients, both independent and collaborative interventions, both direct and indirect care. An *intervention* is defined as "any treatment, based upon clinical judgment and knowledge, that a nurse performs to enhance patient/client outcomes" (Dochterman & Bulechek, 2004, p. xxiii). Although an individual nurse will have expertise in only a limited number of interventions reflecting her or his specialty, the entire classification captures the expertise of all nurses. NIC can be used in all settings (from acute care intensive care units, to home care, to hospice care, to primary care) and all specialties (from critical care to ambulatory care and long-term care). The entire classification describes the domain of nursing; however, some of the interventions in the classification are also done by other providers.

The first edition of NIC was published in 1992 with 336 interventions; the second edition was published in 1996 with 433 interventions; the third edition in 2000 with 486 interventions; and the fourth edition in 2004 with 514 interventions. NIC interventions include both the physiological (e.g., Acid-Base Management) and the psychosocial (e.g., Anxiety Reduction). Interventions are included for illness treatment (e.g., Hyperglycemia Management), illness prevention (e.g., Fall Prevention), and health promotion (e.g., Exercise Promotion). Most of the interventions are for use with individuals, but many are for use with families (e.g., Family Integrity Promotion) and some are for use with entire communities (e.g., Environmental Management: Community). Indirect care interventions (e.g., Supply Management) are also included. Each intervention as it appears in the classification is listed with a label name, a definition, a set of activities to carry out the intervention, and background readings.

The portions of the intervention that are standardized are the intervention labels and the definitions—these *should not* be changed when they are used. This allows for communication across settings and comparison of outcomes. Care can be individualized, however, through the activities. From a list of approximately 10 to 30 activities per intervention, the provider selects the activities that are appropriate for the specific individual or family and then can add new activities if desired. All modifications or additions in activities should be congruent with the definition of the intervention. For each intervention, the activities are listed in logical order, from what a nurse would do first to what s/he would do last. The short lists of background readings at the end of each intervention are those found most helpful in developing the intervention or supporting some of the activities in the intervention. They are a "beginning" place to start reading if one is new to the intervention, but they are by no means a complete reference list, nor are they inclusive of all the research on the intervention.

The interventions are grouped into 30 classes and seven domains for ease of use. The seven domains are: Physiological: Basic, Physiological: Complex, Behavioral, Safety, Family, Health System, and Community. A few interventions are located in more than one class, but each intervention has a unique number (code) that identifies the primary class and is not used for any other intervention. In the fourth edition the interventions are also grouped into a second organizing structure, the Taxonomy of Nursing Practice, developed by a collaborative group working toward a common structure for NANDA diagnoses, NIC interventions and NOC outcomes (Dochterman & Jones, 2003).

NIC interventions have been linked with North American Nursing Diagnosis Association (NANDA) nursing diagnoses, Omaha System problems, Nursing Outcomes Classification (NOC) outcomes, resident assessment protocols (RAP) used in nursing homes, and OASIS (Outcome and Assessment Information Set) used for collection for Medicare/Medicaid-covered patients receiving skilled home care. The research to develop NIC began in 1987 and has progressed through four phases, each with some overlap in time:

Phase I: Construction of the Classification (1987–1992)
Phase II: Construction of the Taxonomy (1990–1995)
Phase III: Clinical Testing and Refinement (1993–1997)
Phase IV: Use and Maintenance (1996–ongoing)

The research was begun with 7 years of funding from the National Institutes of Health, National Institute of Nursing. Multiple research methods have been used in the development of NIC. An inductive approach was used in phase I to build the classification based on existing practice. Original sources were current textbooks, care planning guides, and nursing information systems. Content analysis, focus group review, and questionnaires to experts in specialty areas of practice were used to augment the clinical practice expertise of team members. Phase II was characterized by deductive methods. Methods to construct the taxonomy included similarity analysis, hierarchical clustering, and multidimensional scaling. Through clinical field-testing, steps for implementation were developed and tested and the need for linkages between NANDA, NIC, and NOC were identified. Over time, more than 1,000 nurses have completed questionnaires and approximately 50 professional associations have provided input about the classification.

Several tools are available that assist in the implementation of the Classification. Included are the taxonomic structure to assist a user to find the intervention of choice, linkages with NANDA diagnoses to facilitate decision support with these diagnostic languages, the core intervention lists for areas of specialty practice, as well as the amount of time and level of education need to perform each intervention.

NIC is recognized by the American Nurses Association (ANA) and is included as one data set that will meet the uniform guidelines for information system vendors in the ANA's Nursing Information and Data Set Evaluation Center (NIDSEC). NIC is included in the National Library of Medicine's *Metathesaurus for a Unified Medical Language.* The *Cumulative Index to Nursing Literature (CINAHL)* includes NIC interventions in its indexes. NIC is included in the Joint Commission on Accreditation for Health Care Organization's (JCAHO) accreditation requirements as one nursing classification system that can be used to meet the standard on uniform data. Alternative Link Systems (2001) has included NIC in its ABC codes for reimbursement for alternative providers. NIC is registered in HL 7 (Health Level 7), the U.S. standards organization for health care. NIC is also licensed for inclusion in SNOMED (Systematized Nomenclature of Medicine). Interest in NIC has been demonstrated in several other countries, and translations into Chinese, Dutch, French, Icelandic, German, Japanese, Korean, Spanish, and Portuguese are completed or underway.

Many health care agencies have adopted NIC for use in standards, care plans, competency evaluation, and nursing information systems; nursing education programs are using NIC to structure curriculum and identify competencies for nursing students; vendors of information systems are incorporating NIC in their software; authors of major texts are using NIC to discuss nursing treatments; and researchers are using NIC to study the effectiveness of nursing care.

JOANNE MCCLOSKEY DOCHTERMAN

Nursing Occupational Injury and Stress

According to the Bureau of Labor Statistics (BLS, 2000), there were approximately 11 million workers employed in the health services sector in 1999 representing nearly 9% of employed U.S. workers. Health care workers face numerous work-related hazardous exposures that can result in injury and illness. Health care workers can include nurses, physicians, physical therapists, aides, physician assistants, laboratory workers, and the like.

As reported by BLS (2000), an estimated 606,000 cases of health services worker injury or illness occurred in 1998, with an incidence rate of 7.7 injuries or illnesses per 100 full-time workers. The rate compared with an overall rate of 5.2 injuries or illnesses per 100 full-time workers in all service industries (including health care) and a rate for private industry in general of 6.7 per 100 full-time workers. Of the 606,000 cases, 279,700 involved days away from work and days of restricted work activity. This rate of 3.6 cases per 100 full-time workers exceeded that for all service industries at 2.4 cases per 100 full-time workers and for private industry at 3.1 cases per 100 full-time workers.

Occupational health hazards include:

1. Biologic and infectious hazards: infectious and biologic agents, such as bacteria, viruses, fungi, or parasites, that may be transmitted through contact with infected individuals or with contaminated body secretions or fluids.
2. Chemical hazards: various forms of chemicals that are potentially toxic or irritating to the body system, including medications, solutions, and gasses.
3. Enviromechanical hazards: factors encountered in the work environment that cause or potentiate accidents, injuries, strain, or discomfort (e.g., poor equipment of lifting devices, slippery floors).
4. Physical hazards: agents within the work environment, such as radiation, electricity, extreme temperatures, and noise, that can cause tissue damage.
5. Psychosocial hazards: factors and situations encountered or associated with one's job or work environment that create or potentiate stress, emotional strain, or interpersonal problems.

Exposure to biologic agents and subsequent diseases that can develop are the most familiar risk faced by health care workers (Rogers, 1997). While there are many biological agents of importance, most notably HIV and hepatitis B and C are of most concern. Each year an estimated 600,000 to 800,000 needlestick or sharps injuries occur among health care workers (Twitchell, 2003a, 2003b). As of 1999, the Centers for Disease Control and Prevention (CDC) (2000a) has documented 56 cases of occupationally acquired HIV infection or AIDS among health care workers and, of these, exposures included 49 percutaneous, 5 mucotaneous, 2 with both percutaneous and mucotaneous, and 1 had an unknown exposure route. The CDC is also aware of a possible 138 additional occupationally acquired HIV infections or AIDS.

In 1989, the CDC estimated that approximately 12,000 health care workers were annually occupationally infected with hepatitis B virus (HBV) and that approximately 250 would die. As a result of the Occupational Safety and Health Administration's Bloodborne Pathogen Standard in 1991, the standard compelled employers to offer cost-free HBV vaccine to at-risk employees. This has resulted in a steady decline in the number of infections of HBV to an estimated 400 cases annually in 1995 (Mahoney et al., 1997). This change is attributed to immunization and use of standard precautions.

Hepatitis C virus (HCV) infection is the most common blood-borne infection, with nearly 4 million persons estimated to have chronic infection worldwide. In the U.S. an estimated 3.9 million people are infected with HCV, resulting in 8,000 to 10,000 deaths annually from acute and chronic liver disease (CDC, 1998). Among health care workers the prevalence of HCV infections is about 1%–3% (Alter et al., 1998).

Chemical agent exposures in the health care work environment can be irritating and toxic to tissues, mostly through inhalation or skin contact exposures. The most common exposures include disinfectants, sterilizing agents, inhaled anesthetics, aerosolized pharmaceuticals, chemotherapeutic agents, and latex. Disinfectants can result in airway symptoms and skin problems, while ethylene oxide, used to sterilize equipment, has mutagenic and carcinogenic properties, as demonstrated in animal studies (Rogers, 1997).

Glutaraldehyde is an extremely effective microbiocide used for cold sterilization of endoscopes and bronchoscopes. While technical personnel bear the brunt of the exposure, nurses and physicians also have significant contact if fumes are not vented or scopes are not adequately rinsed. Skin, eye, and respiratory tract irritation is the result along with the possibility to develop allergic dermatitis and asthma.

The principal hazardous drugs of concern for occupational exposure are the antineoplastic agents. Pharmacists and nurses who handle and administer the agents are at significant exposure risk. As a result health care workers exposed to antineoplastic agents have been found to have a significantly greater risk of urine mutagenicity and adverse symptoms common to specific agents including lightheadedness, nasal sores, nausea, hair loss, depressed leukocytes, skin rash, and higher fetal loss (Rogers & Emmett, 1987; Valanis, Vollmer, & Steele, 1999). Those most at risk for toxicologic effects will have regular cumulative exposure in practice settings such as hospital oncology floors, oncology units, private physicians' offices, and outpatient clinics.

Latex allergy is a growing problem for health care workers with some reports of more than 17% prevalence (NIOSH, 1997). Latex is ubiquitous in home and health care environments to which nurses are exposed. The allergen is usually a protein which binds to the glove powder as part of the manufacturing process (Kurup et al., 1996; Posch et al., 1997). Inhalation occurs when the powder is expelled into the air during glove donning or removal. Reactions can range from contact dermatitis, systemic reactions, and/or anaphylaxis.

Enviromechanical agents relate to exposures resulting from poorly designed or inadequate equipment or devices, work stations, or situations that can result in worker injury. There is a high prevalence of low-back pain and injury among nursing personnel (Nelson, Fragala, & Menzel, 2003), and back injuries are cited as the most costly worker's compensation problem today. While back injuries are highly prevalent in the health care industry, the actual incidence is thought to be underestimated. Several studies implicate lifting techniques, poor staffing, lack of ergonomic design, and constitutional factors as contributory (Nelson et al., 2003). In addition to the aforementioned factors the authors cited lack of accessibility, physical stress, lack of skill and training, and increased patient transfer activities, lack of use of assistive devices, and solo lifting as etiologic factors. Nurses' aides are at higher risk for back injuries than construction workers and laborers (NIOSH, 2001). The impact of these injuries is enormous in terms of worker pain and safety, disability, lost work time, absenteeism, medical care costs, personnel replacement costs, and decreased productivity. Better use of equipment, training, and improved work conditions and staffing could help prevent this disabling problem.

Physical agents are probably the least important hazard in health care environments; however, exposures do occur. Radiation is a common hazard used in medical therapeutics, and exposure can occur during diagnostic x-rays, radioactive implants, and from patient body fluids with metabolized therapeutic nuclear radiation. Obviously developmental anomalies can occur from exposure during pregnancy (Wagner, Lester, & Saldano, 1997). Lasers emit non-ionizing radiation and can cause eye or skin injury from a point of impact. "Laser" is an acronym for "light amplification by stimulated emission of radiation." Exposures to lasers can result in skin thermal burns and corneal damage as a result of poor use of protective wear. In addition, air contaminants may be generated when a specific laser beam (class 3b or 4) interacts with matter (NIOSH, 1999), which may produce toxic and noxious vapors, the presence of dead and live cellular materials and viruses, and metal or plastic fumes to which health care workers are exposed.

Psychosocial agents or stressors and their effects are often reported in nursing literature

(Rogers, 1997). While many areas in nursing have been studied and are highly stressful, intensive care nursing, hospice, emergency nursing, and oncology nursing have been studied the most. Factors cited most frequently as contributory to workplace stress in nursing include death and dying, inadequate staffing and resources, interpersonal conflicts, dealing with family needs, work overload, organizational politics, and poor communications. Issues related to quality concerns have created job stress, resulting in increased depressive symptomology, increased role conflict, and decreased job satisfaction (NIOSH, 2002).

Burnout continues to be a serious problem and has been found to be associated with shift work, lack of autonomy, floating, and lack of administrative support. Many of the same factors that contribute to stress also lead to burnout, resulting in decreased job satisfaction, increased absenteeism, and turnover.

Health care workers are at continual and increased risk for injury and death from workplace violence (Drury, 1997; Boyd, 1998; NIOSH, 2001). This includes both threatening behavior and physical assaults. Homicide is the second leading cause of occupational fatality in the U.S. and victims of workplace violence account for 15% or almost 1 million violent acts experienced. Health care institutions mirror society and increasingly nurses are called to manage potentially harmful situations at work (Drury).

The Emergency Nurses Association (ENA) identified that the most important workplace factors determining violence in the emergency room were the presence or absence of security personnel, presence or absence of safety equipment, work norms, policies, staffing patters, staff training, and physical design of the work area. They also concluded that the nurse's size, gender, and work experience mattered. Though some studies have identified gender as a factor that increases vulnerability to assault, most experts agree that male and female health care workers are equally vulnerable to assault (ENA, 1994).

In summary, work-related hazards are ubiquitous and becoming more problematic in the health care environment. Recognition of the events and those at potential risk is critical as is developing strategies to prevent and control the exposure and the risk.

BONNIE ROGERS

Nursing Outcomes Classification

The Nursing Outcomes Classification (NOC) is a comprehensive, research-based standardized classification of patient/client, family, and community outcomes developed to evaluate the effects of nursing interventions across the continuum of care. An outcome is stated as a variable concept representing an individual, family, or community condition that is measurable along a continuum and responsive to nursing interventions. The definition of a nursing-sensitive patient outcome is

> an individual, family or community state, behavior, or perception that is measured along a continuum in response to a nursing intervention(s). Each outcome has an associated group of indicators that are used to determine patient status in relation to the outcome. (Moorhead, Johnson, & Maas, 2004, p. 26)

Each outcome has a label name, definition, set of specific indicators, and a 5-point scale to measure the concept and indicators. The outcomes are developed for use in all specialties and with all patient populations and have been used in interdisciplinary care plans and care maps. Since the outcomes describe patient/client status, other disciplines may find them useful for the evaluation of their interventions. An important characteristic of the classification is that NOC outcomes can be used across the care continuum to follow patient outcomes throughout an illness episode or over an extended period of care.

The first edition of NOC was published in 1997 with 196 outcomes (Johnson, M., &

Maas, 1997) and is the first classification focused on outcomes of nursing care. The second edition, published in 2000, contained 260 outcomes (Johnson, M., Maas, & Moorhead, 2000) and the third edition contained 330 outcomes (Moorhead, Johnson, & Maas, 2004). The classification is on a 4-year publication cycle. In the third edition, 76 outcomes have a new 2-scale format. This format uses two scales to measure the indicators of the outcome. The second scale is used to measure symptoms that previously were difficult to state using the primary scale. For example the outcome "Endurance" defined as the "capacity to sustain activity" uses the severely compromised scale to rate the majority of the indicators such as "performance of usual routine," "activity," and "concentration." This scale has the following anchors: severely compromised, substantially compromised, moderately compromised, mildly compromised, and not compromised. The second scale measures severity of symptoms using endpoints of severe, substantial, moderate, mild, and none. Three symptoms are measured using this scale: exhaustion, lethargy, and fatigue. The overall outcome is measured on the compromised scale.

New to the third edition is the ability to set a *target outcome rating* that allows the nurse to determine if the goal of nursing intervention is to maintain the outcome at a desired rating or to increase the rating to a higher score. In some circumstances the main goal of nursing intervention is to prevent decline in the outcome. An example of this situation is often seen when elderly patients are admitted to a nursing home. The nursing staff focuses on preventing deterioration in outcomes such as mobility and endurance.

The classification was developed using inductive and deductive methods as well as quantitative and qualitative approaches. Nursing outcome statements were extracted from nursing textbooks, clinical information systems, and research studies as a first step in building the classification. Most of these statements were goal statements that were evaluated as "met" or "unmet." A series of sorting exercises was used where team members clustered like concepts into grouping for further refinement by eight focus groups. Each focus group then developed each outcome with its definition and indicators from this sorting process for review by the research team. The focus group chairs were doctorally prepared investigators on the research team, and focus group members included research team members and practicing clinicians. Focus groups used a modified concept analysis to establish face validity as outcomes were developed for the classification. Each outcome was reviewed by the entire team, suggestions for revision were offered by members, and the final draft was approved by the research team prior to placement in the taxonomy.

The outcomes in the classification are grouped into seven domains: Functional Health, Physiologic Health, Psychosocial Health, Health Knowledge and Behavior, Perceived Health, Family Health, and Community Health. Within each domain are several classes that contain the outcomes specific to that class. For example the domain Functional Health has the classes Energy Maintenance, Growth and Development, Mobility, and Self-Care. Examples of outcomes under Energy Maintenance are Activity Tolerance, Endurance, Energy Conservation, and Sleep. The classification has 29 classes under these seven domains to assist nurses in finding the outcomes that they use in practice. Each domain and class is defined to facilitate the placement of outcomes in the taxonomy as they are developed. The entire taxonomy (outcomes, indicators, and measurement scales) is coded for implementation in computerized clinical information systems and for the manipulation of data to answer questions about nursing care quality and effectiveness.

The original taxonomy was developed using hierarchical cluster analysis, a technique used previously by the Nursing Interventions Classification research team in the development of their initial taxonomy (Moorhead, Head, Johnson, & Maas, 1998). Building on their procedures, three groups of nurse experts sorted the developed outcomes into categories. Following these sorts by individual team members, the outcomes were grouped into 5, 10, 15, and 25 tentative categories using hierarchical clustering techniques. Using the 25-category structure, the original taxonomy had 24 classes identified and names and definitions were created for each class. The domain level of the taxonomy was created in the same way using the classes, and the original structure had six domains. Community Health was added as community-level outcomes were developed.

Initial phases of the research tested content validity of the outcomes by using survey research methods and master's prepared nurse experts. Questionnaires were developed by team members that asked respondents to rate the importance of each indicator for determining the outcome on a 5-point scale, from "never important" to "always important." In addition the research team was interested in the sensitivity of the outcomes to nursing interventions. Each respondent was asked to rate each indicator on a five-point scale, from "no contribution" to "contribution is mainly nursing." Fehring's methodology (1987), using ratios identified by Sparks and Lien-Gieschen (1994), was the basis of evaluation of the importance and sensitivity of the indicators and outcomes. These surveys reinforced the importance of the indicators. There was more variation in the nursing contributions of the outcomes surveys and this was especially true for physiological indicators. During the work with these surveys, there was a major shift in practice to a more interdisciplinary model. On some outcomes respondents suggested additional indicators which the team reviewed and added as appropriate. Following the survey work, the outcomes were piloted in a tertiary care setting, a community hospital, and a nursing home with favorable results.

The research team realized that a more thorough study of the outcomes use in practice was needed and determined that a grant focused on measurement was the next step needed in the refinement of the classification. A 10-site study was funded by the National Institute of Nursing Research to test the reliability and sensitivity of NOC outcomes as well as their feasibility in practice settings. This study focused on testing the classification across the continuum of care in the United States. Clinical sites participating in the study include two academic teaching hospitals, three community hospitals, one nursing home, one parish nursing organization, two visiting nurse associations, and one nurse practitioner clinic.

This study focused on testing the 190 outcomes from the first edition of the classification. Data were collected on over 2,300 patients with a total of over 12,500 outcome ratings. Methods used were inter-rater reliability, construct validity using criterion tools, and an evaluation of the sensitivity of the outcome measures to capture change in outcome ratings over time. The measurement scales used in the NOC have been shown to be sensitive to nursing interventions with patients in a variety of care settings and have been able to capture change in patient status even during short admissions in acute care. This research produced important data for the revisions made to the classification for the third edition. Many nurses have contributed to this important work in outcome language development for nursing.

Refinement of the outcomes and outcome development are still a large part of the work of the research team. New outcomes are being developed to meet the needs of practicing nurses, and beginning work on the identification of core outcomes by specialty organizations was published in the third edition. More work in the identification of core outcomes is needed as nurses shift their practice from goals to outcomes. Linkage work with the North American Nursing Diagnosis Association (NANDA) International diagnoses is included in the book, and an additional book identifying linkages among diagnoses, interventions, and outcomes was published in 2001 (Johnson, M., Bulechek, Dochterman, Maas, & Moorhead, 2001). More recently the need for a common taxonomic structure for NANDA, NIC, and NOC led to an invitational conference that developed an initial common structure known as Taxonomy of Nursing Practice, published in 2003 by the

American Nurses Association (Dochterman & Jones, 2003). The importance of effectiveness research using standardized languages is becoming a reality, as hospitals and other agencies where nurse work begin to gather the needed data to evaluate in more detail the effectiveness of nursing interventions on the problems nurses face with patients, families, and communities. Accurate measurement of outcomes using NOC is an important piece of effectiveness studies.

The NOC is endorsed by the American Nurses Association as a classification for use by nurses to capture the outcomes of care. This recognition occurred in 1998 as did the inclusion of NOC in the National Library of Medicine's Metathesaurus. In 2001 NOC was registered in Health Level 7. NOC was also licensed for inclusion in the Systematized Nomenclature of Medicine (SNOMED) in 2002 and content was added in 2003. NOC has been translated into Dutch, French, German, Japanese, Korean, and Spanish. A Portuguese translation of the second edition of NOC is forthcoming. Endorsement of NOC by the international community has been important to its development.

NOC is an important classification for the implementation of the Nursing Minimum Data Set (Werley & Lang, 1988). It has been used with other standardized languages such as the NANDA International Nursing Diagnoses (NANDA, 2003), Nursing Interventions Classification (Dochterman & Bulechek, 2004), and the Omaha System (Martin, 1982), and it has been linked to the Long-Term Care Minimum Data Set Resident Assessment Instruments (RAI), the Resident Assessment Protocols (RAPs), and the Outcome and Assessment Information Set (OASIS).

Standardized languages for nursing practice are essential to capture the nursing problems, interventions, and outcomes of nursing care. They are also essential for today's health care system focused on quality outcomes in a cost-conscious environment. We need data about outcomes of care to influence policy and policy makers focused on changing the health care system. The Nursing Outcomes Classification is the most comprehensive classification of nursing-sensitive patient outcomes currently available for nurses to use with individuals, families, and communities across the care continuum and in specialty practice.

MARION JOHNSON
MERIDEAN MAAS
UPDATED BY SUE MOORHEAD

Nursing Practice Models

A nursing practice model can be described as a guide, a road map, or a framework that provides a structure for the organization and the delivery of care. Practice models have been developed by administrators and managers in response to changes in health care. Over the years, practice models used within organizations have resulted in various outcomes, including decreased cost and increased quality of care. Several practice models have incorporated dimensions such as interdisciplinary practice, differentiated practice, and communication as integral components of the framework.

The goal of most nursing practice models focuses on decreasing cost, improving quality outcomes, increasing nurse satisfaction, autonomy, financial compensation, and impact on patient satisfaction with care. Models developed during the past decade have focused on shared governance, professional practice, collaborative governance, theory-based practice, and transitional models of care.

Shared governance is designed to increase nursing's presence in the health care system by differentiating responsibilities of providers based on education and experience while compensating expert practitioners financially. This model provides opportunities for shared decision making and organizational participation through committee work. Evaluation of successful implementation of the model has varied. Cost and commitment to the governance process have became issues, although evaluation reports indicate satisfaction with staff participation in decision making and teamwork. Some continue to use the model, whereas others have abandoned it for other structures.

Use of professional practice models and collaborative governance is a more recent practice model and builds on some aspects of shared governance. The model focuses on the contribution of all professionals within the organization, including nurses and other providers. Collaborative governance is used to implement many of the components of the professional practice model. A committee structure is developed to involve staff from across disciplines to participate in the leadership of patient care services. Interdisciplinary team building is used to bring about change. Emphasis is placed on communication among caregivers and respect for each discipline's contribution to quality patient care. The model offers individuals who deliver patient care at all levels a voice in decision making through a committee structure and open forums. The goal of the model is to work toward increased recognition of all providers and as a result improve the work environment and patient care outcomes.

Theory-based practice models incorporate nursing, and theoretical perspectives outside the discipline to guide practice. Other models have implemented midrange theories (e.g., pain and stress) to direct practice. Community-based practices have focused on prevention and risk reduction to decrease mortality related to smoking. Nursing theories also have been used as practice frameworks. For example, advanced practice nurses in managed care setting structured nursing practice around the Neuman system model. Nursing practice models have been found successful in directing resource utilization and staffing. In addition, nursing models have been used with high-risk populations in rural communities to demonstrate the impact of nursing interventions (e.g., teaching) on decreasing cost while improving and maintaining health across populations and settings.

Transitional models of care have been developed to focus on care outcomes such as cost, length of stay, and patient satisfaction. Models using advanced practice nurses as case managers or clinical specialists enable patients to move rapidly from the acute care settings to a less costly care site, such as the home.

Use of various models to guide nursing practice helps to foster the philosophy, values, and beliefs of an organization. A nursing practice model can serve as a structure for the planning and direction of nursing and health care and help guide resource distribution. Strategic planning is improved as participation from all providers in organizational decisions can occur when nurses have a shared vision about health care. Through the use of nursing practice models, practitioners from beginner to expert can be recognized for unique contributions to care and for their educational and clinical expertise.

Organizing care around a nursing practice model also can create a stronger patient-centered environment, where providers can come to know the patient and use nursing knowledge to improve care outcomes. A professional practice model can help to expand nursing's leadership for patient care and foster those behaviors associated with patient, family, and community health. Through practice models, new strategies and nursing interventions can be generated and tested to expand nursing knowledge and inform clinical practice.

With the continued emphasis on health care reform, cost savings, and quality, it is essential that practice be implemented within a framework that is realistic and useful. Within nursing, the continued creation of practice models will promote quality care and facilitate the articulation of nursing's contribution to care outcomes. Emerging practice models that are patient-centered and respectful of the contribution of all providers will foster quality health care for all and initiate creative approaches to practice that can maintain and sustain individuals in less costly environments. Through teamwork, cooperative planning, and increased participation in decision making, system members can move the organization toward a shared vision and new directions in care delivery.

DOROTHY A. JONES

Nursing Process

Nearly all authors define the nursing process as a problem-solving process composed of the elements of assessment, planning, implementation, and evaluation. Many a priori assumptions have been identified and studied concerning the nursing-process approach to patient care that includes decision making as a characteristic of the process. These assumptions are that the nursing process is a holistic, scientific, individualized, problem-solving approach with an emphasis on diagnosing. The concept emerged as early as the 1950s from Lydia Hall and was more directly described by Orlando (1961).

Interest in the type of systematic identification of a nursing process spread rapidly, as evidenced in many proceedings, position statements, and policies from groups as influential as the American Nurses Association and the Joint Commission on the Accreditation of Hospitals. By the mid 1970s there was widespread implementation underway. Early writings began to emerge in the literature at this time. Although little research appeared in publications, writings in journals and textbooks were abundant, promoting the process as a useful tool for teaching and understanding nursing. It was commonly held that full implementation of the nursing process would bring about radical changes in nursing education and nursing practice. In the late 1970s the World Health Organization (WHO, 1977) endorsed the use of the nursing process. With this support the United Kingdom quickly adopted the approach throughout nursing.

A review of the research on nursing process in the past 15 years has focused less on the merits, processes, and structure of the nursing process and more on the study of the implementation of the nursing process. A large amount of the research conducted on this concept has come from the United Kingdom. However, studies on the implementation of the nursing process in both the United States and the United Kingdom reveal that nursing process has not been implemented. Researchers have attempted to identify and study what barriers exist to the full use of the nursing process as identified by educators and clinicians in both countries. Studies focused on the attitudes of nurses, environmental factors, educational preparation, strategies to promote and encourage use, and instrument development to measure the concept more empirically. The reports were very consistent in finding that nurses placed a high value on the nursing process as a vehicle to provide quality, individualized, patient care, although they did not implement the nursing process regardless of their preparation and knowledge of the process or their educational level or years of experience. The data indicate that even those novice nurses recently educated within the nursing process did not use it in actual patient situations when providing independent nursing care.

There are problems with the evaluation and study of such a multidimensional concept as the nursing process. A review of the literature reveals few objective indicators or criteria to measure this concept. A variety of research designs and methodologies have been described in the literature primarily aimed at investigating the implementation or lack of implementation. Instrument development to measure the nursing process has been reported in the literature. Authors have designed quantitative studies using such strategies as attitudinal questionnaires with complex analyses, intervention studies intended to compare group outcomes, retrospective studies, and questionnaires assessing documentation. Other research strategies to study implementation issues have been inductive in nature. Researchers have used extensive literature analyses on the subject, grounded theory approaches, action research, direct observation with field recording, and cooperative inquiry to describe and understand these phenomena.

There is a considerable amount of unpublished dissertation work in the United States addressing issues and concerns about educational variations, environmental impact, and barriers in attitude and structure to the full implementation of the nursing process. Intervention studies have attempted to influence attitude and behavior with motivational therapy, increased education through innovative teaching strategies and on-site inservice, and skills-reinforcement strategies.

Throughout the reported studies a clear theme emerges. The profession of nursing holds a high value for the nursing process. There seems to be a convergence of thinking that it is the best vehicle to individualize patient care. Nurses verbally articulate this commitment and value on behalf of the profession and practice of nursing, but consistently the data support the reality that nurses do not use the nursing process in practice and that the assumptions and characteristics of the nursing process are not supported as tested in a myriad of research approaches.

Researchers interested in this field in the future might take some direction from this review as well as from clinical judgment. There are strong indications that a scientific, analytical, systematic approach to patient care is of value to the novice student who experiences the complexities of the human condition in early training. However, equally supportive research indicates that more advanced students and practicing nurses revise and adapt the nursing process within the realities of practice. Some nursing process researchers, as well as those that study clinical judgment (decision making), call for a new model that reflects a more holistic approach to analyzing patient situations and arriving at individualized care that is open to multiple ways of knowing and the evolving contexts of the environment and the patient. One future direction might be generating theory-based practice models for individualized patient care and testing the effectiveness of these new process models. This research may contribute greatly to the new outcomes-focused initiatives shaping nursing for the 21st century.

SALLY PHILLIPS

Nursing Studies Index

The *Nursing Studies Index* is a four-volume, annotated, guide to literature on nursing as published in English from 1900 through 1959. The literature indexed was cumulated in a broad and systematic search of periodical and nonperiodical sources and the indexing of everything in those journals, books, and pamphlets of an analytical or historical nature that involved nursing or nurses. The Index was designed to serve a public with widely different interests and educational backgrounds, and as such the indexing staff developed an inclusive policy. Historical and biographical articles and monographs were included as were articles believed to involve nurses or nursing. No effort was made to index publications of interest to nurses and the Index did not supplant *Index Medicus*, *Hospital Literature Index*, the *Education Index* or other essential library tools.

Computer technology has stimulated renewed interest in bibliographic searches but at the same time has relegated non-digital documents such as the *Nursing Studies Index* to remote corners of health science libraries if they are retained at all. The *Nursing Studies Index* was as important when published in 1963 as the Internet is today. Both have made it possible to access professional literature and became indispensable library tools in their day.

The *Nursing Studies Index* filled a void in the development of the modern nursing profession. The professional literature was scattered and inaccessible to those who desired to systematically review a topic. This was especially true of nurses involved in research, but it also concerned practitioners and teachers. Virginia Henderson, director of the indexing project, was aware of the challenge in accessing nursing literature because of her involvement in two related activities: textbook writing, and review and critique of nursing research. The latter project was performed under the direction of Leo Simmons and together they published a volume entitled *Nursing Research: A Survey and Assessment* (Simmons & Henderson, 1964). Henderson had previously prepared two editions of the textbook, *Principles and Practice of Nursing* (Harmer & Henderson, 1939, 1955).

The index is organized chronologically, with volume I covering the years 1900 through 1929; II, 1930 through 1949; III, 1950 through 1956; and IV, 1957 through 1959. They were published inversely, volume IV first in 1963 followed by volumes III, II, and I in 1966, 1970, and 1972, respectively. The entries are arranged using the first edition of *Medical Subjects Headings* (MeSH, 1960). MeSH was employed in the hope that both doctors and nurses would access each other's professional literature when searching topics of mutual interest. Contemporary, automated, library database literature searches make this hope more remote as a keystroke now divides the medical and nursing literature, even when the topics generate results applicable to both fields. Most thorough database searches on nurses and nursing now require the use of at least two databases: *Cumulative Index to Nursing and Allied Health Literature* (CINAHL), and *Index Medicus* (Medline and PubMed) as some nurse-written and nursing publications appear in medical journals only.

Volume IV of the Index contains a classification system for nursing studies that was not used in the work. The classification scheme is instructive and timely now that the proliferation of professional literature has made it challenging to place articles and studies in context and into mutually exclusive and exhaustive categories. Organizing entries for the *Encyclopedia of Nursing Research* is one possible use for the *Classification for Nursing Studies* (Henderson et al., 1963, p. xii).

The *Nursing Studies Index* was the direct forerunner of the *International Nursing Index* (*American Journal of Nursing,* 1966), once the standard reference to nursing literature. The 6-year gap between the Index and the 1966 beginning of the *International Nursing Index* was filled by the *Cumulative Index to Nursing Literature*. CINAHL is now the primary source for digital searches of professional nursing literature (Seventh Day Adventist Hospital Association, 1961, 1967) while the nursing journals subset of *Index Medicus* is a close second. The *International Nursing Index* was discontinued by Lippincott, Williams, & Wilkins after the *American Journal of Nursing* was sold to them by the American Nurses Association.

The four-volume Index is now used primarily for historical research. It is still the only source of citation information about the profession cumulated before 1961. Henderson went on from the Indexing project to write a sixth edition of her text, *Principles and Practice of Nursing*, coauthored with Gladys Nite (1978). It is the only edition that capitalized on her exhaustive knowledge of the professional literature, and as such, is perhaps the first evidence-based nursing textbook and the most important book written on nursing in the 20th century.

EDWARD J. HALLORAN

Nursing Workload Measurement Systems

Nursing workload systems refer to the array of methods and procedures designed for the determination and allocation of nursing personnel in both inpatient and community settings. Some of the systems are based on the concept of patient classification, yielding an average number of hours of care for each patient category. Others identify a unique care-time requirement for each patient. In general, the systems have become a major component of the management of nursing resources.

Nursing resource management is not a new concept. Florence Nightingale not only addressed the question of how many nurses were needed for her many exploits but gave serious thought to the larger question of human resource planning. From a historical perspective, Giovannetti (1994) identified three major perspectives for addressing the questions related to nurse staffing. First, staffing decisions were made primarily on the basis of the perceived requirements of recognized leaders in the field, employing both personal and professional sources of power. This approach was employed by Nightingale and remained dominant until about the mid-1930s. The second perspective, in part driven by rapid growth in both the size and complexity of institutional care and the demand for a less variable assessment, led to the development of global staffing standards. Fixed staff-to-patient ratios in terms of hours per patient-day became the norm. This approach assumed that the basis for staffing was the number of occupied beds, and thus the staff required was a function of the number of occupied beds multiplied by the global standard hours per patient-day.

The work of Connor, conducted at the Johns Hopkins Hospital in the 1960s, was instrumental in bringing about a more scientific perspective, that involved the concept of classification theory coupled with use of time studies to determine the average amount of care time for each patient category. In contrast to global standards, the focus of the measurement model attended to the variable needs of patients who occupied the beds (Connor, Flagle, Hseih, Preston, & Singer, 1961). This was the beginning of the third stage, the development of workload measurement systems. Connor developed a three-category patient classification scheme using criteria from observational studies of the direct nursing care time provided to patients. The criteria for assigning patients to categories included physical needs (based on activities of daily living), emotional needs, selected treatment needs such as oxygen and suctioning, and certain patient states such as unconsciousness and impaired vision. Following the work of Connor, there was a proliferation of nursing workload measurement systems, developed by individual nurse investigators, institutions, and vendors. A number of sources are available for the reader interested in the historical development in the United States, Canada, and the United Kingdom (Baar, Moores, & Rhys-Hearn, 1973; Giovannetti, 1978).

The terminology employed in reference to nursing workload measurement systems varies widely, and according to Edwardson and Giovannetti (1994), has contributed to both misunderstanding and misuse. The term *patient classification systems* is frequently used, leading to confusion with many other types of patient classification systems such as diagnostic related groups (DRG), case mix groups (CMG), and medical severity of illness systems. Further, many nursing workload measurement systems do not employ the concept of grouping or classification of patients. A common nonclassification approach employs the development of standard times for each nursing task. Staffing calculations are then determined on the basis of the unique set of tasks required for each patient. The terms *nursing severity*, *nursing acuity*, and *patient dependency* systems have also been used to label nursing workload measurement schemes, although these terms suggest a purpose or intent beyond the assessment of nursing care time. Further, the usage of these terms has frequently led to the erroneous assumption that the more acute or serious the patient's condition is, the more nursing care time is required. The preferred and probably most accurate term used in North America appears to be that of nursing workload measurement systems.

A variety of approaches to the measurement of nursing workload has been developed; and although substantial differences exist among the approaches, they all aim to estimate the total hours of nursing care, including both direct and indirect time required to care for patients. Most employ a prospective or predictive approach to the assessment of patients' nursing care needs; however, as the systems are increasingly used for costing out nursing care, retrospective assessments are common. Edwardson and Giovannetti's (1994) integrative review of systems is a comprehensive source for the research base of the systems, whereas Lewis (1989) contains a compendium of many of the systems used in North American hospitals.

The proliferation of systems attests to both the numerous issues that surround the use of nursing workload measurement systems and the complexity of the challenges inherent in determining appropriate nurse staffing levels. The nursing literature is replete with advice on implementation strategies as well as techniques for measuring and monitoring reliability and validity. Recent work by O'Brien-Pallas, Cockerill, and Leatt (1991) and Phillips, Castorr, Prescott, and Soeken (1992) highlighted concerns about the comparability of different systems and thus raised new concerns about their inherent validity. The different systems tested by these investigators revealed a high degree of correlation, yet evidence of comparability was not obtained. This finding has major implications for widespread application of workload and cost comparisons.

In the last decade there has been a surge of research and interest in the area of nurse staffing, resulting in enhanced recognition that the measurement of nursing workload attributed to the nursing needs of patients is only one of the numerous and significant variables to be considered in the provision of safe and competent nurse staffing. Issues related to the mix of nursing staff, educational preparation, evidence-based practice, environmental complexity, nursing work-life conditions, and patient safety, to name a few, have been examined for their impact on both patients and nurses. The reader is directed to several references: O'Brien-Pallas, Irvine, Doran, Peereboom, and Murray (1997); O'Brien-Pallas and colleagues (2001, 2002); Aiken, Clarke, Sloane, Sochalski, and Silber (2002); and Sochalski, (2002).

PHYLLIS B. GIOVANNETTI

Nutrition in Infancy and Childhood

Nutrition in infancy and childhood refers to dietary intake necessary to support optimal growth and developmental processes from birth through the school-age years. Substantial recent research attention has focused on the role of nutrition in health promotion and disease prevention across the life span. Dietary intake has emerged as a major modifiable determinant of numerous chronic diseases including hypertension, osteoporosis, type 2 diabetes, some forms of cancer, and coronary heart disease. Accumulated data suggest that many of these disease processes begin early in life and are influenced over time by patterns of dietary intake. Obesity, the most prevalent nutritional disorder in childhood and adolescence, is linked with many of these chronic conditions. Nutrition has always been a cornerstone of pediatric primary health care; however, these collective diet-disease observations, primarily of adult populations, have placed increasing emphasis on preventive interventions beginning early in life.

Infancy is a time of rapid growth and developmental change in all domains including physical, cognitive, and psychosocial processes. Energy requirements during this period of the life span exceed others and approximate 90 to 100 kilocalories per kilogram (kg) of body weight per day. Recommended (or reference) intakes of most nutrients have now been established and appear to fulfill the unique nutritional needs of infants and young children. The Food and Nutrition Board of the National Academy of Sciences (NAS) has provided Estimated Average Requirement (EAR) and Adequate Intake (AI) reference data for infants (birth to 6 months of age and 7 to 12 months of age), toddlers (1 to 3 years of age), and children of early school-age (4 to 8 years). The currently recommended energy intakes are based on total energy expenditure measured by the doubly labeled water technique plus allowance for growth based on changes in body composition. These are about 15% lower than the previous Recommended Daily Allowance (RDA) established requirements. Sufficient fat for essential fatty acid requirements (0.5–1.0 g/kg/day of linoleic acid plus a smaller amount of alpha-linoleic acid) and sufficient carbohydrate to prevent hypoglycemia and/or ketosis is required (~5.0 g/kg/day). Controversy continues regarding the need for long-chain polyunsaturated fatty acid (LC-PUFA) supplementation (for formula-fed infants). A recent evidence-based report to the Food and Drug Administration reaffirmed selected neurodevelopment benefits associated with this supplementation; however, since results were not consistent across studies, infant formula manufacturers have the option to include LC-PUFA.

The American Academy of Pediatrics Committee on Nutrition (AAP-CON) (1997) recommends human milk as the ideal source of nutrition for the first 4 to 6 months of life. In situations where breast-feeding is not practical or desired, commercial formulas are recommended as the alternative form of infant nutrition. Recent AAP-CON (2004) recommendations reaffirm human milk or commercial formula as the primary milk source throughout the 1st year of life and discourage cow's milk, reduced fat and evaporated milk. In addition, breast-fed infants should receive 400 International Units (IU) of Vitamin D daily and iron supplementation at 4 months of age.

Accumulated data indicate that the age of introduction of supplemental foods should not be rigidly specified; however, 4 to 6 months of age appears to be optimal for the majority of healthy term infants. AAP (2004) emphasizes the introduction of single-ingredient foods, started one at a time at weekly intervals, to allow for the identification of food intolerance. Progression of feeding practices beyond this point may vary as a function of individual, family, cultural, and economic factors. Achievement of individual growth and developmental milestones, however, is universally recommended as a major determinant of nutrition throughout the 1st year of life (AAP).

Although significant advances in the art and science of infant nutrition have been made in the past 2 decades, many challenges remain. A continuing focal point for pediatric health care professionals is increasing the proportion of women who breast-feed in the early postpartum period and throughout the first 6 months of life. Breast-feeding has increased in some segments of the population: however, national goals, as indicated in *Healthy People 2010*, are far from realized. The prevalence of iron-deficiency has decreased in the past several decades; however, data indicate that low income, ethnically diverse infants continue to be a population at-risk.

In addition to supplementation of commercial formulas with LC-PUFA, recent research attention has focused on the relationship of infant nutrient intake and risk factors for adult-onset cardiovascular disease (CVD), the protective role of breast-feeding in prevention of childhood and adolescent overweight, and gene-diet interactions early in life. Answers to questions raised in each of these areas will assist in defining guidelines for preventive interventions relevant to dietary intake in early life.

The epidemic of overweight in children and adolescents in the United States combined with the national emphasis on the role of nutrition in health promotion and disease prevention has prompted several recent surveys of dietary intake in children and youth. Methodological differences make cross-study comparisons difficult to interpret; however, accumulated data indicate that dietary patterns of U.S. children are not consistent with recent recommendations. Data from the National Health and Nutrition Examination Surveys (NHANES) indicate that dietary fat intake has decreased over the past 2 decades from 36.3% to 34% of total food energy intake (EI); however, saturated fat intake (12% to 13% of EI) exceeds current recommendations (≤ 30% of EI). Paralleling the NHANES prevalence and trend data for those who are overweight, minority youth (Black and Mexican-American) have significantly higher fat intakes than their white counterparts. In addition, data from the Youth Risk Behavior Surveillance (YRBS) indicate that almost 80% of schoolchildren do not consume the recommended 5 or more servings of fruits and vegetables per day. Collectively, these observations point to the importance of both high-risk and population-based preventive interventions focused on the determinants of children's patterns of dietary intake.

Numerous agencies have advanced dietary recommendations for children and youth. Recent recommendations reflect the state of knowledge regarding diet-health relationships and place emphasis on prudence and moderation in macronutrient consumption. While specific RDAs vary as a function of age and other individual factors, recent guidelines also emphasize increased consumption of soluble and insoluble fiber and decreased consumption of sucrose and sodium. The American Academy of Pediatrics (2004), and the American Heart Association are consistent in recommending that children's diets should provide calories to support growth and developmental processes, maintenance of desirable body weight, and include a variety of foods. In addition, daily food intake should provide ≤ 30% of total calories from fat, less than 10% from saturated fat, and less than 300 mg of cholesterol.

Pediatric health care professionals are faced with both challenges and opportunities in implementing these guidelines across health care settings. Translating provider-oriented dietary guidelines and recommendations for consumers of varying developmental, educational, and cultural backgrounds is a particular challenge. The revised *Dietary Guidelines for Americans* (forthcoming in 2005) will provide more specific recommendations on implementation. From a pediatric population perspective, numerous factors influence dietary intake including the contexts of family, school, and community. Traditional, individualized approaches to dietary behavior change in children and youth have yielded varying results. Recent data support earlier observations and suggest an ecological approach to improving the nutritional status of U.S. children with efforts that extend beyond the individual level to the school and community environments. By definition, such interventions will be multicomponent, require a multidisciplinary team approach, and involve formulation and implementation of health policies on both local and national levels. With knowledge of nutritional science, human behavior, and experience and expertise across the continuum of health care, nurses and nursing are particularly well-qualified to participate in these efforts.

Programs of nursing and multidisciplinary research focus on feeding practices and dietary intake in infancy and childhood; results to-date have contributed to the existing body of knowledge in these areas of pediatric health care and have influenced clinical practice. Nurse researcher and scholars have also contributed to evidence-based scientific statements and guidelines designed to improve the nutrition of infants, children, and adolescents in clinical and community-based settings As Kennedy (1997) observed, nursing research has contributed substantial information relevant to neonatal and preterm infant feeding. Nurse-initiated research focused on infancy and childhood has been primarily descriptive in design; however, nurses have contributed in various roles in multidisciplinary research that incorporated dietary interventions. Relevant programs of nursing research focused on promotion and determinants of breastfeeding in diverse populations include those conducted by Dr. Linda Brown and colleagues at the University of Pennsylvania and Dr. Paula Meier at the University of Michigan. Drs. Mary and Marguerite Engler at the University of California-San Francisco have implemented a program of research focused on enthothelial function and dyslipidemia in children with emphasis on the effects of antioxidants. Using a gene-diet-environment interaction paradigm, they are currently extending this research with inclusion of additional genetic determinants of CVD. With emphasis on prevention and management of type 2 diabetes in children and youth, Dr. Margaret Grey and colleagues at Yale University include nutritional assessment and management as a major component of this well-established program of research. Finally, in developing programs of research in Thailand, nurse researchers Pulsuk Siripul and Piyanuch Jittanoon are focusing on school-based programs for improving dietary intake in children and youth.

A major challenge for all school-based and other nutrition interventions is maintenance of behavioral change over time. From a health-promotion and disease-prevention perspective, adherence to dietary recommendations continues to be a viable area for nursing and multidisciplinary research.

LAURA HAYMAN

Nutrition in the Elderly

Research on nutrition in the elderly focuses on the older person's (age 65 years and older) balance of nutrient intake, physiological demands, and metabolic rate along a continuum from optimum to poor nutrition (DiMaria-Ghalili, 2002). Older persons are particularly vulnerable to poor nutrition as a result of normal aging, chronic diseases, and social, psychological, and economic factors. In a recent review, prevalence rates for malnutrition in the elderly ranged from 10% to 85% (Chen, C. C., Schilling, & Lyder, 2001). While researchers in other disciplines have significantly contributed to the science of geriatric nutrition, nurse researchers are also making notable additions. As the population continues to age, it is even more imperative for nurses to examine nutrition in the elderly, since assessing the nutritional needs of patients is an important role for the nurse (Nightingale, 1969) in the promotion, prevention, and restoration of health.

Nurse scientists have focused on varied aspects of nutrition in the elderly including feeding the older person with late-stage dementia, examining the relationship between nutritional status and health outcomes in elderly coronary artery bypass graft patients, evaluating the role of arginine on wound healing in the elderly, and identifying predictors of malnutrition in nursing home residents. Amella (1999) examined the interaction that occurs between elderly nursing home residents with dementia and the relationship with nurse aide caregivers on the amount of food consumed. The quality of the reciprocal relationship was found to be related to the proportion of food consumed. Extending this work, the resistance or willingness to accept assistance at meals by persons with dementia was shown to be related to personal interaction and contextual factors. The quality of the interaction between the caregiver and the person being fed is one important determinant in the resistance to feeding persons with dementia. These findings provided a framework for a study evaluating a mealtime intervention that can be used by in-home caregivers to maintain or increase food intake in older persons with dementia. This program of research is significant in that it provided evidence that it is not merely the quantity of nutrients consumed that impacts nutrition in older persons with dementia, but the contextual aspects of feeding and eating are also important.

In a study evaluating the changes in nutritional status and postoperative outcomes in elderly persons undergoing elective coronary artery bypass grafting (CABG) surgery, DiMaria-Ghalili (2002) demonstrated that older persons lose weight from the preoperative (preop) period to the 4–6 weeks postdischarge period. Furthermore, the more weight lost, the lower the older person's self-reported physical health and the higher the likelihood of hospital readmission. The initial weight lost from preop to postdischarge is never fully recovered, since weight at 18 month follow-up is still lower than preop weight. Older persons with depressive symptoms postdischarge also lost more weight than those persons without depressive symptoms postdischarge. While both older and younger persons experience weight loss from preop to postdischarge, older persons never recovered the initial weight lost, even 3 years after surgery. This work is significant because weight loss is an ominous sign in older persons and an indictor of frailty. Future directions include development of an explanatory model of factors contributing to weight loss in the elderly as the basis for a targeted intervention study.

Arginine, a nutrient shown to enhance inflammatory and immunological responses in animal models (Stechmiller, Childress, & Porter, 2004), is being evaluated in a prospective randomized trial as a supplement in older nursing home residents with pressure ulcers. This work is significant because it is targeted at a vulnerable group of elderly at nutritional risk who could benefit from specific nutritional interventions. In order to restore optimal health, additional programs of research in which targeted interventions are developed and tested for a specific group of older people with nutritional risk are needed.

Determining the prevalence of malnutrition in any group of older adults is not a "novel" research topic, but the ability to determine the prevalence from large data sets has important implications for the ease in which the older person at nutritional risk is identified. Crogan, Corbett, and Short (2002) have shown the most significant predictors of protein-calorie malnutrition on admission using the Minimum Data Set to be weight loss, leaving 25% or more of food uneaten at most meals, psychiatric/mental diagnosis, deteriorated ability to participate in activities of daily living, and old age. These findings are significant in that they could lead to development of a set of routine factors identifying older patients at nutritional risk upon nursing home admission without extensive anthropometric and invasive laboratory analysis so that appropriate nutrition interventions can be instituted in a timely fashion, thereby promoting positive health outcomes.

Since nutrition is a complex phenomenon, there is no gold standard in the measurement of nutritional status. A variety of anthropometric data (weight, height, skin-fold thickness, muscle circumference, bio-impedance analysis), visceral protein levels (serum albumin, transferrin, pre-albumin), nutritional screening tools (Determine Your Nutritional Health Checklist, Mini-Nutritional Assessment, Subjective Global Assessment), and dietary intake studies (food recalls, diet diaries, measurement of food consumed) are used in studies on nutrition in the elderly. The ability to quantify nutrition using several measurement tools often detracts from the ability to consistently compare the results of nutrition studies in the elderly. The positive aspect of a variety of measurement tools is that it facilitates the ease by which a researcher can measure components of nutrition status if there is limited access to a specific measurement tool.

For the last 3 decades, the prevalence of poor nutrition in hospitalized and institutionalized older people has been clearly documented. The Nutrition Screening Initiative (NSI), a 5-year multifaceted effort to promote routine nutrition screening and better nutrition care for older Americans communicated the importance of malnutrition in the elderly to professional and lay groups (NSI, 1991). Four major nursing organizations (National League for Nursing, American Nurses' Association, National Gerontological Nurses Association, and National Association of Directors of Nursing Administration in Long-Term Care) served on the Blue Ribbon Advisory Committee for the NSI. The work of the NSI is important in that it was a response to the Department of Health and Human Services' call to increase the proportion of health providers who provide nutrition screening in the *Health People 2000* report. The work of the NSI also validates the important research effort that must be continued to promote, maintain, and restore optimal nutrition in the elderly.

Future studies need to be aimed at identification of the most vulnerable older people who would benefit most from targeted nutritional interventions to promote positive outcomes. It is quite obvious that poor nutrition is not an "all or nothing phenomenon," particularly in this age group. Malnutrition is an indicator for the complex phenomenon of frailty. The major factors related to frailty are sarcopenia, atherosclerosis, cognitive impairment, and malnutrition (Morley, 2003). To promote optimal nutritional health, designing studies that solely focus on dietary interventions may not be sufficient without yconsidering the antecedent or contributing factors to poor nutrition in this age group. A bio-behavioral approach to studying nutrition in the elderly is warranted so that the physiological, psychological, and social factors can also be examined.

Rose Ann DiMaria-Ghalili

O

Obesity as Cardiovascular Risk Factor

With over 60% of the American population classified as overweight or obese, and with the medical costs attributable to obesity ranging upwards from $100 billion per year, the national, indeed global, crisis of obesity stands in the ignominous position of being the one epidemic that nursing research has virtually ignored. In the last few years there has been a slow increase in the number of studies and publications by nurses that focus on obesity. While cardiovascular disease (CVD) and many of its risk factors have been prominent in the nursing literature for quite some time, the intersection of obesity and cardiovascular risk has been virtually unexplored from a nursing perspective. The most common approach of nurses studying obesity and CVD has been to include body weight, either directly measured or self-reported, in descriptive studies of CVD risk factors. This data point subsequently is analyzed as Body Mass Index (BMI), calculated as weight/height (kg/m).

Children. Among 340 elementary school children, 53% had one or more risk factors for CVD (Cowell, Warren, & Montgomery, 1999). Moreover, 25% of the children were obese, and among the children who were obese, 47% had additional risk factors for CVD. Despite a low prevalence of poor fitness, 84% of the low-fitness children also had high blood pressure or were obese. In a study involving 32 third-grade children (Skybo & Ryan-Wenger, 2002), the most prevalent risk factors for heart disease were high body fat percentage and environmental tobacco smoke in the home. Few children had a body fat percentage within the healthy range. Thus, the investigators suggested that the third-grade children possessed some of the known risk factors for CVD, with some of the risk factors being under the control of the child.

Women. A study was conducted to determine whether there was a difference between African-American and Caucasian women in the self-reported CVD risk factors of obesity, physical inactivity, and smoking (Harrell & Gore, 1998). In that study of 1,945 women aged 23–53 years, African-American women of low and middle socioeconomic status (SES) were much more likely than high SES African Americans to be obese, inactive, and smokers. Among Caucasian women, however, only those with low SES had the greatest prevalence of these three risk factors for CVD. After controlling for income and education, African-American women were more than twice as likely as Caucasian women to be obese and inactive. A secondary analysis of the Canadian National Population Health Survey (Cycle I: 1994/95; Cycle II: 1996/97) focused on the CVD risk factors of physical inactivity, hypertension, cigarette smoking, diabetes, obesity, and socioeconomic status (SES) among women aged 20 years and older (Wong & Wong, 2002). Results indicated an increased prevalence of obesity, diabetes, hypertension, and physical activity from Cycle I to Cycle II, and supported previous studies that there is an SES gradient for CVD risk factors. In this study age, physical activity, hypertension, and household income—but not obesity—emerged as significant predictors of heart disease.

Older adults. In a study of patients after coronary artery bypass grafting (CABG), female sex (odds ratio 4.7) and obesity (odds ratio 3.7) significantly predicted hospital readmission (Sabourin & Funk, 1999). Other investigators used a cross-sectional design to assess CVD risk factors in Korean-American elderly, aged 60–89 years, who resided in a large city in the eastern United States (Kim, M. T., Juon, Hill, Post, & Kim, 2001). In these older adults, hypertension was the leading CVD risk factor, followed by high blood cholesterol, overweight, sedentary lifestyle, and smoking.

Intervention studies. Intervention studies of obesity as a CVD risk factor where major dependent variables were physiological, were only found when nurses appeared as members of multidisciplinary investigator teams. One of these teams (McMurray, Ainsworth, Harrell, Griggs, & Williams, 1998) examined cardiovascular fitness (VO_{2max}) and physical activity (PA) rather than obesity per se as CVD risk factors in young adult men and women. A cross-sectional analysis revealed that those in the highest tertile of VO_{2max} had a reduced relative risk for elevated cholesterol, blood pressure, and obesity, while those in the highest tertile of self-reported PA only had a lower relative risk for high systolic blood pressure (BP). After a 9-week exercise program for low-fit young adults, only those who increased VO_{2max} had a reduction in relative risk for high cholesterol and systolic BP, but not for diastolic BP or obesity.

From a research program focusing on obesity and sedentariness as major risk factors for CVD in postmenopausal women, and the corresponding lifestyle modifications of weight loss and physical activity to mediate these risks, Nicklas and colleagues reported the physiological aspects of these phenomena in numerous publications. The sequential effects of a 2-month American Heart Association (AHA) Step I diet and subsequent weight loss through 6 months of hypocaloric AHA diet and low-intensity walking were examined for their effects on lipoprotein lipids in obese, postmenopausal women (Nicklas, Katzel, Bunyard, Dennis, & Goldberg, 1997). The AHA diet alone lowered concentrations of total, low-density lipoprotein (LDL-C) and high-density lipoprotein (HDL-C) cholesterol. Weight loss increased HDL-C concentrations, but brought no additional changes in total cholesterol or LDL-C. Reductions in total cholesterol and LDL-C were significant for participants with hypercholesterolemia, but not for normocholesterolemic women. The investigators conjectured that because the AHA diet alone lowered HDL-C in the total sample of women, a low-fat diet without substantial weight loss may not be beneficial for improving lipoprotein lipid risk factors for CVD in obese, postmenopausal women with normal lipid profiles. In research to determine the specific dietary factors associated with the decrease in HDL-C on an AHA diet alone (Bunyard, Dennis, & Nicklas, 2002), the one significant dietary change was the increase in the percent of energy consumed from simple sugar. There were no relationships between changes in HDL-C and changes in the percentage of energy consumed from total, saturated, polyunsaturated, or monounsaturated fat.

Findings from a study of racial differences in resting metabolic rate (RMR) fat oxidation and VO_{2max} in obese, postmenopausal women showed that RMR, adjusted for differences in lean mass, fat oxidation rate, and VO_{2max}, were significantly higher in white than in black women (Nicklas, Berman, Davis, Dobrovolny, & Dennis, 1999). In a multiple regression model including race, body weight, lean mass, and age, lean mass was the only independent predictor of RMR, while race was the only independent predictor of fat oxidation. The best predictors of VO_{2max} were lean mass and race. The efficacy of a 6-month hypocaloric AHA diet and low-intensity walking in improving CVD risk factors in obese Caucasian and African-American postmenopausal women was evaluated by measurements of body composition (dual-energy x-ray absorptiometry), abdominal fat areas (computed tomography scan), lipoprotein lipids, insulin, glucose tolerance, and blood pressure (Nicklas, Dennis, et al., 2003). Although absolute weight loss was similar in the two races, Caucasian women lost relatively more fat mass. Women across the sample decreased fat in the abdominal region with no differences in magnitude by race. The intervention decreased triglycerides and increased HDL-C in both races, and decreased total and LDL-C in the Caucasian women. Fasting glucose and glucose area during an oral glucose tolerance test decreased in Caucasian women, whereas there were no racial differences in the decreased insulin area. Blood pressure decreased the most in women with higher blood pressures at baseline. Changes in lipids, fasting glucose, and insulin, their responses during the oral glucose tolerance test, and blood pressure were not different between racial groups.

The accumulation of visceral fat, independent of total body obesity, is widely acknowledged for its association with the development of dyslipidemia, hypertension, glucose intolerance, and hyperinsulinemia in women. Examining whether the loss of visceral adipose tissue (VAT) was related to improvements in VO_{2max} during a hypocaloric diet and low-intensity walking intervention, Lynch and colleagues (Lynch, Nicklas, Berman, Dennis, & Goldberg, 2001) found significant declines in visceral as well as subcutaneous adipose tissue areas, with no change in lean body mass. Women with an average 10% increase in VO_{2max} reduced VAT by an average of 20%, significantly more than women who did not increase VO_{2max}, despite comparable reductions in total body fat, fat mass, and subcutaneous adipose tissue area. In a cross-sectional analysis of peri- and postmenopausal women 45–65 years old, who ranged widely in adiposity and fat distribution (Nicklas, Penninx, et al., 2003), women in the lowest quintile for VAT (< 105 cm^2) had significantly higher concentrations of HDL-C, lower LDL-C/HDL-C ratios, triglyceride concentrations, fasting glucose, and insulin concentrations than women in the four remaining quartiles. Women in the two highest VAT quintiles (≥ 163 cm^2) had the highest glucose and insulin concentrations. A VAT greater than 105 cm^2 was associated with a higher risk of having low HDL-C, while a VAT greater than 163 cm^2 also was associated with a higher risk of having a high LDL-C/HDL-C ratio and a higher risk of being glucose intolerant.

Findings from additional studies in overweight and obese postmenopausal women conducted by this same multidisciplinary research team suggested that a reduction in adipose tissue lipoprotein lipase activity (AT-LPL) with weight loss was associated with improvements in lipid metabolic risk factors from weight loss and diminished weight regain. In genetic studies, variations in the lipoprotein lipase gene *PvuII* were associated with AT-LPL activity and lipoprotein lipid and glucose concentrations, which resulted in a more problematic CVD risk factor profile for these women. Women with variation in the peroxisome proliferator-activated receptor (PPAR)-gamma2 gene (Pro12Ala) regained more weight during follow-up than those who were homozygous for the Pro allele.

Obesity is a global epidemic with a complex etiology of physiologic, metabolic, genetic, cognitive, psychological, behavioral, environmental, social, and political factors. Obesity also is a major risk factor for CVD, the leading cause of mortality in women as well as men.

KAREN E. DENNIS

Observational Research Design

Observational designs are nonexperimental, quantitative designs. In contrast to experimental designs in which the investigator manipulates the independent variable and observes its effect, the investigator conducting observational research observes both the independent and the dependent variables. In observational studies, variation in the independent variable is due to genetic endowment, self-selection, or occupational or environmental exposures. Because of the myriad sources of bias that can invalidate naturally occurring events, rigorous designs and methods are required to minimize bias. Observational designs should not be confused with observational methods of data collection.

Observational designs are used when there is not enough knowledge about a phenomenon to manipulate it experimentally. Sometimes research involving human subjects is restricted to observational designs because of the nature of the phenomenon; that is, experimental research is precluded for ethical reasons.

Observational designs include quantitative, descriptive studies as well as analytical studies that are designed to test hypotheses. Descriptive, observational studies provide a basis for further study by describing and exploring relationships between variables, informing the planning of health services, and describing clinical practice for individual clients or groups of clients. In contrast, analytic research is designed to test specific hypotheses in order to draw conclusions about the impact of an independent variable or set of variables on an outcome or dependent variable under scrutiny. Observational designs are classified as longitudinal or cross-sectional. In a cross-sectional study, all the measurements relate to one point in time; in the longitudinal approach, measurements relate to at least two points in time.

A cross-sectional study, sometimes referred to as a correlational study, is conducted to establish that a relationship exists between variables. The term *correlational* refers to a method of analysis rather than a feature of the design itself. Cross-sectional studies are useful if the independent variable is an enduring or invariable personal characteristic, for instance, gender or blood type. Cross-sectional studies are also useful for exploring associations between variables.

Longitudinal comparative designs are usually undertaken to explain the relationship between an independent variable and an outcome. One type of longitudinal, comparative design is referred to as a cohort study. Although the investigator does not manipulate the independent variable, the logic and flow in a cohort study is the same as the logic of an experiment. Subjects are measured or categorized on the basis of the independent variable and are followed over time for observation of the dependent variable. In a cohort study it is established at the outset that subjects have not already exhibited the outcomes of interest (dependent variable). Thus, the time sequencing of events can be established. In other words, it can be demonstrated that the independent variable preceded the occurrence of the dependent variable.

Another type of longitudinal, comparative design is a case-comparison study. In this design the flow is the opposite of a cohort study. Subjects are selected and categorized on the basis of the dependent variable (the outcome of interest). The purpose of the study is to test hypotheses about factors in the past (independent variables) that may explain the outcome. Although case-comparison designs are not prevalent in the nursing research literature, they have great potential for studies of outcomes that occur infrequently. Furthermore, this design is very efficient because it is possible to achieve greater statistical power with fewer subjects than in other types of observational designs.

Longitudinal comparative designs are also classified according to the time perspective of the events under study in relation to the investigator's position in time. A study is retrospective if, relative to when the investigator begins the study, the events under investigation have already taken place. A study is prospective if the outcomes that are being investigated have not yet taken place when the study is initiated. Various hybrid designs are also possible; referred to as ambidirectional studies, they combine features of both designs.

As in experimental research, observational research designs and methods are selected with the aim of minimizing bias. Bias refers to distortion in the result of a study. A biased study threatens internal validity if the distortion is sufficient to lead to an erroneous inference about the relationship between the independent and dependent variable. Potential sources of bias that can threaten the internal validity of observational studies are those related to selection, measurement, and confounding.

Selection bias is a distortion in the estimate of effect resulting from (a) flaws in the choice of groups to be compared; (b) inability to locate or recruit subjects selected into the sample, resulting in differential selection effects on the comparison groups; and (c) subsequent attrition of subjects who had initially agreed to participate, which changes the composition of the comparison groups.

Measurement bias occurs when the independent variable or outcome (dependent variable) is measured in a way that is systematically inaccurate and results in distortion of the estimate of effect. Major sources of measurement bias are (a) a defective measuring instrument, (b) a procedure for ascertaining the outcome that is not sufficiently sensitive and specific, (c) the likelihood of detecting the outcome dependent on the subject's status on the independent variable, (d) selective recall or reporting by subjects, and (e) lack of blind measurements when indicated.

Because of the lack of randomization in a nonexperimental study, uncontrolled confounding variables are a major threat to internal validity. Unless confounding factors are controlled in the design of the study or in its analysis, distortion in the estimate of effect will result. A confounding factor operates through its association with both the independent and the dependent variables. It can distort the results in either direction; that is, it can lead to an overestimation of the relationship between the independent and dependent variables by producing an indirect statistical association, or it can lead to an underestimate of the relationship between the independent and dependent variables by masking the presence of an association between the independent and dependent variables. A distinction between confounding bias and other types of bias is that confounding is correctable at the design or analysis stage of the study, whereas bias due to selection and measurement problems are usually difficult or impossible to correct in the analysis. Confounding can be controlled or minimized at the design stage of the study by restricting the study sample or by matching the comparison groups. At the analysis stage confounding can be controlled or minimized by using a multivariable approach to the statistical analysis to adjust for the confounding factors or by examining the independent-dependent variable relationship within specified levels or categories of the confounding factors (stratified analysis). Confounding variables should not be confused with mediator and moderator variables.

In summary, observational designs are prevalent in nursing research because they are used to describe phenomena in early stages of knowledge development and provide a basis for designing experimental interventions. Additionally, they are the only feasible approach to hypothesis testing when it is unethical to manipulate the independent variable. In the absence of randomization and manipulation, myriad sources of bias can influence observations and conclusions drawn from naturally occurring events, thus, rigorous observational designs and methods are essential.

JANET C. MEININGER

Online Journal of Knowledge Synthesis for Nursing

The Online Journal of Knowledge Synthesis for Nursing (OJKSN) is a full-text peer-reviewed electronic journal published by Sigma Theta Tau International. The journal began publication in January 1994 and was the first peer-reviewed electronic journal in nursing. There is no paper version; it is completely electronic.

The purpose of the journal is to publish timely, synthesized knowledge to guide nursing practice and research. Knowledge synthesis is the gathering of research studies on a topic, assessing the validity of the findings, and asserting implications for practice from the valid findings. The process includes identifying gaps in the knowledge base that would provide direction for future research on the topic. OJKSN provides critical reviews of research pertinent to clinical practice and research situations that nurses can access and use immediately. The journal does not have articles that are reports of a single study, such as you would find in other nursing research journals.

An online electronic journal delivers articles across commercial telecommunications to a computer terminal at a workstation or a personal computer. Transmission is through the Internet. The OJKSN is accessible on the World Wide Web through Sigma Theta Tau International's web site (http://stti-web.iupui.edu). It is available through subscription, which may be either individual or institutional. A combined subscription with the *Registry of Nursing Research* is also available.

All articles include a statement of the practice problem, a summary of the research, annotated critical references, practice implications, directions for future research, search strategies used, and references. Features of the journal include full-text searches, access to graphical displays such as tables and charts, links to referencing in external bibliographical databases such as *Cumulative Index to Nursing and Allied Health Literature* (CINAHL) and MEDLINE.

"Statement of the Practice Problem Issue" is a brief statement explaining the scope of the article. "Summary of the Research" contains the review, analysis and synthesis of the research on the topic. The review is a state of the science for the topic. The extensiveness of the review depends on the depth and breadth of the research on the topic. The summaries differ from a literature review in that there is an assessment of the validity of the information contained in the research reports. It may include a meta-analysis, the statistical manipulation of findings from multiple research studies. The narrative is used to make summary statements about the research as a whole, and tables are used to describe the individual review of studies and the significant variables and findings. "Annotated Critical References" contains an abstract of the most significant research publications on the topic. A maximum of seven are annotated.

In "Practice Implications," the specific implications for practice based on the research are presented and discussed. This section delineates what practitioners can or should do as a result of the research on the topic. The research references are cited for all practice directives so that the clinician can refer to them if desired. "Research Needed" discusses the various directions for future research and the questions that remain unanswered. Knowing about the knowledge that does not exist is often as important as knowing what exists. This section is a good guide for directing master's theses and doctoral dissertations, as well as for clinical research studies. "Search Strategies" describes how the research cited was identified, the citation bases searched, the search terms that were used, and the years that were searched. References cited are listed in the American Psychological Association format. Each reference listed in MEDLINE or CINAHL has a hypertext link so that the entire citation, including abstract, can be accessed.

There are many advantages to an online journal. These include faster publication, immediate access, continuous publication, hypertext links, and instant access. Once a manuscript for a paper journal is accepted and revised, it may be anywhere from 6 to 24 months before it is out in print. With the electronic journal, articles are brought online generally within weeks after final acceptance and editing. The journal is available online 24 hours a day, 7 days a week. Although it may take weeks or months for an international journal to come through the mail, with a computer journal there is instant access.

Unlike a traditional print journal, where there are numerous issues a year with a varying number of articles per issues, an electronic journal has continuous publication. As an article is finalized, it is brought online. Articles are identified by the year and the article number for that year (e.g., 1997, No 11). Uniform standards are being developed for citing electronic publications.

Hypertext links allow direct access to the database of a reference (e.g., MEDLINE) for scanning the abstract of the reference. Once the abstract is read and perhaps printed, the reader is able to click back into the article at the same spot. There is instant access to all previously published articles in the journal; keeping paper copies of back issues is unnecessary.

Subscription information is accessed through the Sigma Theta Tau International web site at http://stti-web.iupui.edu or by requesting subscription information through the international headquarters. Once a subscription is processed, the user is sent a user guide, authorization, and password.

There is a tremendous amount of knowledge available for use in nursing practice. The key is accessing, synthesizing, and having it organized to readily make clinical decisions. The OJKSN greatly increases nursing's opportunities for knowledge-based practice, education, and research.

JANE H. BARNSTEINER

Orem's Self-Care Deficit Nursing Theory

One of nursing's grand theories, Orem's Self-Care Deficit Nursing Theory (SCDNT), is a vital component of nursing's philosophical foundation. The impetus of the theory, to define a curriculum for practical nursing, led Orem to recognize that effort needed to be exerted on the conceptualization of nursing and nursing's relationships to patient needs and patient care. Orem proposed that nurses should be expected to have specialized abilities that qualifies a person to nurse. These abilities she called nursing agency which, together with patient needs and patient abilities, became the structure and focus of the SCDNT (Melnyk, K. A., 1982).

In 1952, working as a hospital consultant nurse with the Indiana State Board of Health, Dorothea Orem was concerned about the state to which nursing was evolving. Nurses were engaging in nursing practice but were not able to articulate what nursing was. "Nursing" of the patient provided a major part of patient care. A person becomes a patient because of a legitimate inability to care for himself or herself when recovering from illness or injury. One of the problems Orem evaluated was how patient care did not truly meet patient needs. The advances in medical and allied research and treatment changed the way nurses evaluated and planned patient care. A broader concept of patient care was necessary. The active participation of patients in their treatment would be required to successfully meet the changing perspectives of patient care. Understanding the care needs of the patient was the obvious starting point for Orem. "The act of nursing is practiced by 'doing for' the person with the disability, by 'helping him to do for himself,' and/or by 'helping him to learn how to do it for himself'" (Orem, 1956, p. 85).

This general nursing theory is accepted as a relationship between self-care agency and therapeutic self-care demands, distinguishing self-care deficit from dependent care. Orem deliberately selected the term "deficit" for this relationship to be interpreted as insufficient, not as a human disorder. The incapacity to meet demands of self-care reflects the fact that a need for nursing exists. Orem recognized an apparent discontinuity between patient care and patient needs. The concept that nurses had of their practice had not evolved at the same pace as had patient needs. The obvious starting point for Orem toward understanding the care needs of the patient was to define, "What is self-care?" "When is nursing needed?" and "How do nurses provide nursing care?" The answers to these questions are derived from three interconnected theories central to the SCNDT: the theory of nursing systems, the theory of self-care, and the theory of self-care deficit. All three theories combined become one general theory of nursing, with self-care deficit as the most comprehensive and at the core of her ideas. The relationship between the three theories is described in the following way. In the theory of self-care, self-care is an activity initiated on one's own behalf in the interest of health and well-being. The theory of self-care deficit is the relationship between therapeutic self-care demand and self-care agency whereas self-care capabilities are not known or able to be met. The theory of nursing systems is the deliberate practice actions of nurses carried out to meet the therapeutic self-care or develop the patients self-care agency. This answers the questions about the nature of care and the nature of nursing.

The central concepts of Orem's theory consist of (a) Self-Care—caring for one's self to maintain life, health, and well-being; (b) Self-Care Demands—varied degrees and kinds of care requirements needed at specific times or over a duration of time for meeting all of an individual's needs; (c) Self-Care Agency—the power and capabilities to engage in self-care, influenced by external and internal factors; (d) Nursing Agency—the broad ability of nurses to perform nursing; (e) Self-Care Deficit—the actions and demands needed for self-care that are greater than the person's current capability for self-care; (f) Conditioning Factors—internal or external factors that affect an individual's ability to engage the kind and degree of self-care required (Orem, 2001). This view distinguishes self-care from dependent care and nursing care, in which the agent acts on behalf of another person. However, the substantive theoretical and practical knowledge of self-care is the foundation for both dependent care and nursing care. From this theoretical view, it is essential that nurses have substantive knowledge about self-care and understand that human beings are both the focus of their actions and the agents of their actions (Orem, 1991). In conclusion, nurses utilize the self-care deficit theory of nursing to aid them in their practice. Many clinical studies have shown that implementing Orem's theory has a positive effect on patients, nurses, and health care organizations. Orem's seminal work, originally published in 1971, *Nursing: Concepts of Practice*, has been revised to its current 6th edition in 2001. Orem's book remains a standard, having been published in seven languages and implemented by nurses in over 19 countries. Beginning in 1989, the World Congress of Self-Care Deficit Nursing Theory, offers a forum for international developments for practitioners, researchers, administrators, and educators (World Congress of Self-Care Deficit Nursing Theory, 2004).

EILEEN VIRGINIA ROMEO
MARY JO DEVEREAUX

Organizational Culture

An organization's culture is understood by shared beliefs, norms, values, policies, work group rules, shared meanings, expectations, and myths. Organizational culture is often used interchangeably with organizational climate (Sleutel, 2000). Reichers and Schneider (1990) traced the development of these two unique concepts. Organizational climate (the older term, traceable to the 1930s) is the group's perceptions about the organization, whereas organizational culture (dating to the 1970s) is determined by the message inherent in the organization which gives shared meaning. Strength of the culture refers to the consistency of the message/meaning found when examining norms, values, etc. For example, strength of the research culture in hospitals was determined by a survey that looked for evidence in mission, goals, policies, and activities (Martin, P., 1993). The organizational culture is an important part of nurses' work environment and has been shown to influence the worker, the work, and the outcomes of the work.

The work of Coeling has done most to show the utility of the concept "organizational culture" in nursing. In her 1988 article with Wilcox, she showed how to not only understand the work group's culture, but how knowing the culture should inform management decision making (Coeling & Wilcox, 1988). How culture can impede or be a catalyst for change has been the primary focus of her work (Coeling & Simms, 1993). This body of research stressed the importance of understanding that culture for both the staff nurses and their leadership when implementing change. The work showed not how one must fit into a prevailing culture, but how understanding organizational culture can assist in innovations and other positive changes needed for the good of the work group. Coeling asserted that organizational culture is important to inform plans for moving the organization both in new directions and more efficiently and effectively along the same path.

Organizational culture is important to assess before a nurse accepts a position or before a nurse manager selects a new employee (Barowsky, 2003; Dowd, Davidhizar, & Giger, 1999). All these authors address "fit" between new employee and the new work group. Employers are looking for indications of shared values and compatible goals; the nurse seeking a position is looking for similar matches. Consistency of message in values and verifying interpretations can lead to the right match from both manager and employee perspectives.

The leader/manager/supervisor has an important responsibility in developing the most appropriate organizational culture (Bruhn, 2001). The leader is in the best position to know the values and group rules necessary for the work important to the organization as a whole. Consistency among workers and in the work toward the organization's mission and goals can be orchestrated through work policies, rewards, and structure. Communication is a critical means of establishing and maintaining the most appropriate culture. A leader may need to change an undesirable work culture, one that contradicts or fights with the organization's mission and goals (Baker, C., Beglinger, King, Salyards, & Thompson, 2000). Crow and Hartman (2002) demonstrated how important it is for the leader to understand, use, and, if necessary, systematically change the culture in order to execute the work and attain the outcomes expected by the organization.

The relevance of organizational culture to outcomes has been a major topic in research, professional, and management journals the last 10 years (Larson, 2002; McDaniel & Stumpf, 1993). Sometimes the concept "organizational culture" is unnamed, but the research demonstrated that policies and practices which could be conceptualized as organizational culture provide a pronounced effect on outcomes. The outcomes identified include worker retention, quality/nature of the work, success in strategic initiatives, productivity, and quality of the outcomes. Some of these outcomes are direct, and others are indirect. What is clear is that organizational culture and the consistency of the message about key values and priorities is an important—and may be the most important—responsibility of the administrative/management team. While culture may be a major factor in dysfunction, it can be revised or revived with dramatic positive results.

The state of research currently is hampered by the limited availability of empirical tools to measure organizational culture that have good psychometric properties. Anthropology, from which the concept of culture was adopted, uses qualitative research approaches. This qualitative tradition has appropriately followed the concept into the discipline of nursing and organizational research; however, the research to a large degree often omits or does not report the accepted qualitative rigor. A quantitative approach may better link the phenomenon of organizational culture to outcomes in a causal way, clarifying the nature of the relationship. Whether organizational culture is a phenomenon that can be appropriately captured quantitatively could be debated. Because of the promise organizational culture shows for guiding both the practicing nurse and nurse managers/administrators in their interface with the work setting, the concept continues to call for more research to explicate how the environment can best be managed to support excellence in practice and quality outcomes.

Supported in part by 1 R01 NR 007738 from the National Institute of Nursing Research, National Institutes of Health

PATRICIA A. MARTIN

Organizational Redesign

Organizational redesign, or restructuring, as some experts refer to the process, is the transformation of an organization's architecture and methods for providing services. It involves a revamping of structures and processes for purposes of achieving efficiency and maximum production outcome. In the case of health care organizations, the redesigned production process is expected to produce improved employee, patient, and organizational outcome. Although the term "organizational redesign" generally implies a fundamental change in the way things are done, the term also is commonly used to describe a variety of changes occurring at the unit, department, or organizational level. This variation in level of focus and measurement has posed difficulties in measuring the true effect of organizational redesign on employee and care delivery outcomes.

Studies of organizational redesign increased dramatically during the 1990s after health care institutions across the U.S. and elsewhere began instituting varying degrees of organizational change. Most of this research was conducted after health care organizations made the decision to redesign. Consequently, most redesign initiatives were implemented without the benefit of supporting evidence to guide the changes made or the effects proposed. As a result, a number of the redesign efforts failed and many institutions have reinstituted some of the processes eliminated during the redesign activities.

Nursing studies of organizational redesign have explored a number of individual and organizational factors that contribute to the outcomes seen. Most investigations have focused on the employee's response to redesign, although a few have included organizational and patient outcome indicators as well. Findings are mixed, with some studies showing improvements in nurse perceptions of work group collaboration, interpersonal relationships, and job satisfaction (Ingersoll et al., 2002) and others reporting increased uncertainty (Blythe, Baumann, & Giovannetti, 2001), worry (Barry-Walker, 2000), emotional stress (Denton, Zeytinoglu, Davies, & Lian, 2002; Greenglass & Burke, 2001), dissatisfaction (Barry-Walker; Denton et al.; Greenglass & Burke), disempowerment (Blythe et al.), anger, despair (Ingersoll, Fisher, Ross, Soja, & Kidd, 2001), anxiety, emotional exhaustion, depression, cynicism (Greenglass & Burke), fragmentation of relationships (Blythe et al.), and mistrust of administration (Ingersoll et al., 2001). When redesign initiatives are targeted at the institution as a whole, redesign impact is felt at all levels of the organization, with midlevel managers also reporting feelings of inadequacy, ambiguity, frustration, and loss of position power as a result of redesign activities (Ingersoll, Cook, Fogel, Applegate, & Frank, 1999). A survey of chief executive officers in one study supported employee beliefs that the overall gains in quality of care are not as substantial as the cost savings to the institution and that the cost savings are overpowered by the serious dissatisfaction of the staff (Urden & Walston, 2001).

Several studies of organizational redesign suggested that individual and organizational characteristics can reduce the negative effects of the organizational change. Employees with higher levels of perceived self-efficacy and positive coping (Greenglass & Burke, 2001) reported less distress in response to organizational redesign. In addition, organizations that promote increased nurse involvement in decision making (Ingersoll, Kirsch, Merck, & Lightfoot, 2000; Laschinger, Finegan, Shamian, & Almost, 2001) and that have a prior history of effective change processes, which has been defined in one study as organizational readiness (Ingersoll et al.) were less likely to report serious negative effects from redesign initiatives.

Regardless of the extent of the redesign underway, staff reaction is strong. Clearly evident in the reports of organizational redesign is a level of employee disruption that is well beyond what was anticipated by the administrators undertaking the redesign initiatives. Even when information was shared, concerns were expressed about what to expect and when the disruption would end. Staff nurse and manager worry about quality of patient care also is a consistent theme across studies.

Investigations of the impact of organizational redesign on patient outcomes are less evident, although a few do exist. In a study by Sovie and Jawad (2001), redesign outcomes were assessed primarily through a comparison of nurse resource variables and their impact on patients and cost. In this study, most hospitals had implemented reductions in RN staff as a component of their redesign initiatives. Findings suggested that hospitals with the greatest reductions in RN staff have the poorest outcomes. An important finding of this study was the increased cost per patient discharge in hospitals with lower rather than higher percentages of RN staff. This cost-outcome finding was supported in a small study by Barry-Walker (2000), in which costs of care per patient-day increased rather than declined following organizational redesign.

Most of the research concerning organizational redesign has been conducted either during the course of or shortly after the redesigns were implemented. Little information is available concerning the long-term effect of these change processes and whether any or all of the redesign components remain intact. Follow-up studies would be useful to clarify which elements have been sustained or refined over time. Moreover, because the studies reflected immediate postimplementation time frames, some of the observed effect may have been the result of the turbulence caused by the change rather than the components of the redesign models themselves.

Evident in the research concerning organizational redesign is the need for better methods for determining cause and effect relationships between redesign components and outcomes seen. Determining the effect of organizational, environmental, and individual factors on redesign outcomes also is important, as preliminary results suggest differences exist across employees and work settings. Attention to the organization's culture and history of (readiness for) change experiences, likewise, appears to be an important aspect of successful organizational redesign. Opportunities for staff nurse involvement in decision making and planning for change also is apparent.

Future investigations of organizational redesign initiatives also should focus on both the processes used to implement the redesigns and the outcomes they are expected to achieve. Without an indication of what was done, which is best identified through the process component of an organizational assessment, no cause/effect determinations can be made about the changes in the outcomes seen. In addition, the consistent use of reliable, valid instruments developed according to some theoretical framework is essential for cross-comparisons of study findings and the development of databased recommendations. The establishment of standards for the collection of organizational performance and patient outcome indicators also would be useful, with national clearinghouses for the development of comparison benchmarks. Some work is currently underway in this regard, but not all institutions can afford to participate in the data analysis processes required and many are unaware of the resources available. Published standards of practice, organizational processes, and benchmarked outcome indicators would help eliminate this concern.

GAIL L. INGERSOLL

Osteoarthritis

Osteoarthritis, the most common of the rheumatic diseases, is characterized by progressive loss of articular cartilage and by reactive changes at the margins of the joints and in subchondral bone. Clinical features can include pain in the involved joint, which is typically worse with activity and relieved by rest; stiffness after periods of immobility; enlargement of the joint; instability; limitation of motion; and functional impairment. Depending on the absence or presence of an identifiable local or systemic etiological factor, osteoarthritis has been classified into idiopathic (primary) and secondary forms. Classification of the disease is based on various combinations of clinical, radiographic, and laboratory parameters.

The prevalence of osteoarthritis is strikingly correlated with age; it is uncommon in adults under 40, but it is the number-one chronic disease in late life, with more than 80% of those over the age of 75 being affected. Osteoarthritis is a major cause of disability in older adults, and knee osteoarthritis is more likely to result in disability than osteoarthritis of any other joint. However, the prevalence of osteoarthritis at all joint sites increases progressively with age, which is the most powerful risk factor for the disease. Women are about twice as likely as men to be affected, and African-American women are twice as likely as Caucasian women to have knee osteoarthritis. The pattern of joint involvement also differs with sex: women have a greater number of joints involved and more frequent complaints of morning stiffness, joint swelling, and nocturnal pain. Factors that appear to be associated with osteoarthritis, based on cross-sectional and longitudinal studies, include obesity, bone density, trauma and repetitive stress, and genetic factors.

The impact of osteoarthritis on function and costs of care are substantial. Patients with osteoarthritis are more likely to be limited in the amount and kind of major activities they can perform, have more restricted bed days, and are more likely to report disability. When disease prevalence figures were applied to estimates of health care utilization and disability for both rheumatoid arthritis and osteoarthritis, an aggregate economic impact some 30-fold greater was found for osteoarthritis than for rheumatoid arthritis. In addition to the functional disability and economic impact of osteoarthritis, older people with this disease experience an inordinate amount of suffering, depression, and diminished quality of life.

Treatment approaches to patients with osteoarthritis have been mainly pharmacological, usually combined with physical therapy and sometimes surgery. Although these interventions are useful, they often fail to control disease progression, and symptoms may be associated with high costs and many toxicities. In addition, they frequently fail to address important issues of patient concern, such as psychological stress, quality of life, and autonomy. Because of the chronicity of the disease, patients must learn to manage and cope with osteoarthritis on a day-to-day basis. The ability to succeed in this task differentiates those who are incapacitated from those who continue to lead full and active lives in the face of equal disease severity. For this reason, health education has a potentially important role.

One of the most common educational interventions used for chronic disease is self-management. Self-management has been described as the day-to-day tasks an individual must undertake to control or reduce the impact of disease on health status; it includes all the tasks for handling clinical aspects of the disease away from the hospital or physician's office. For persons with osteoarthritis this may include using medications, managing acute episodes and emergencies, maintaining adequate exercise and activity, using relaxation and stress-reducing techniques, seeking information, using community services, adapting to work, managing relations with significant others, and managing emotions and psychological responses to the illness.

The "graying of America" and its concomitant increase in the prevalence of osteoarthritis poses problems for an ever spiraling health care budget. Incurable by definition, management of osteoarthritis extends over time, creating continuous costs to both patient and provider. It is important that we examine innovative ways to deliver high-quality care for older adults with osteoarthritis in as efficacious and economical a manner as possible.

CAROL E. BLIXEN

Osteoporosis

Bone mass density (BMD) accounts for 70% of bone strength, is measured as grams of mineral per area, and is reflective of both peak bone mass and the amount of bone loss

(National Institutes of Health [NIH], 2000). Osteoporosis is not only the result of accelerated bone loss during aging, but may also develop because of sub-optimal bone growth in childhood and adolescence. "Osteoporosis is a pediatric disease with geriatric consequences" (Drugay, 1997, as cited in Gueldner, 2000). Bone quality, a poorly understood factor, is thought to result from the bone's micro and macro structure, biochemical composition, distribution and integrity of material components within the bone, turnover, and microdamage accumulation. That a 50 year-old woman with low bone density has a much lower risk of fracture than an 80 year-old woman with the same bone density speaks to changes in bone quality (Kolata, 2003).

Pregnancy-associated osteoporosis is a rare and temporary condition that occurs during the 3rd trimester or postpartum period of a first pregnancy. Symptoms include back pain, loss of height, and vertebral fractures. Lactation is also associated with transient bone loss, with recovery of full bone density within 6 months (National Women's Health Information Center, 2003).

In the United States, using the same criteria of BMD of the hip, prevalence of osteoporosis ranges from 3.9% of Caucasian-American women 50–59 years, to 47.5% for those older than 80 years (World Health Organization [WHO], 2003b). The National Osteoporosis Foundation (NOF, 2002) estimates that 55% of all Americans aged 50 years and older in the year 2002, nearly 44 million people, had either osteoporosis or low bone mass. Based on the 2000 Census, prevalence estimates increase to 52 million women and men for the year 2010, and to 61 million in 2020. Prevalence varies by gender, race, and ethnic group. Both men and women experience a decline in BMD starting in midlife, with women experiencing more rapid bone loss in the immediate years after menopause. Of the 44 million Americans estimated to have osteoporosis and low bone mass in the year 2002, 32% (14 million) of them were men and 68% (30 million) were women (NOF). "These estimates challenge the long-held myth that osteoporosis is a sex-segregated problem" (Wolf, Penrod, & Cauley, 2000, p. 7). Asian and white non-Hispanic women have the lowest bone mineral densities throughout life, and African-American women have the highest. Mexican-American women have bone densities that are intermediate between the two groups. Japanese and Native-American women (limited data) have peak BMD that are lower than white non-Hispanic women (NIH, 2000).

Osteoporosis may be viewed as a silent systemic disease or as a progressive risk factor for fractures. Several factors associated with low bone density and/or risk for fractures have been identified by large prospective studies, including the 35-state National Osteoporosis Risk Assessment (NORA) (Siris et al., 2001). These risk factors are classified as either primary or secondary (Field-Munves, 2000; NIH, 2000; NOF, 2002). Primary causes include:

- Female gender
- Advancing age
- White or Caucasian and Asian races
- Estrogen deficiency as a result of menopause, especially early or surgically induced. This may also be categorized as secondary.
- Low weight and body mass index, having a small frame
- Personal history of fracture after age 50 years
- Family history of osteoporosis
- History of fracture in a first-degree relative
- Cigarette smoking
- Low lifetime calcium and Vitamin D intake
- An inactive lifestyle.

Sometimes listed as a contributing factor, lack of sun exposure, especially in many older adults and during the winter months in higher latitudes, significantly reduces cutaneous production of Vitamin D essential for calcium absorption (Feskanich, Willett, & Colditz, 2003). Other suspected predictors of low bone mass, such as use of alcohol and caffeine-containing beverages, have been proven to be inconsistent in their association (NIH,

2000). In fact, the NORA study of 200,160 postmenopausal women aged 50 years or older found that alcohol consumption significantly decreased the likelihood of osteoporosis (Siris et al., 2001). Other data from this large diverse population found that higher body mass index, African-American heritage, estrogen use, diuretic use, and exercise are BMD protective factors, while age, personal or family history of fracture, Asian or Hispanic heritage, smoking, and cortisone use were significant predictors of osteoporosis. Many diseases and drug therapies are also associated with osteoporosis and increased fracture risk (Field-Munves, 2000; NIH). A comprehensive list is outlined in the National Osteoporosis Foundation Physician's Guide to Prevention and Treatment of Osteoporosis (NOF, 2003).

Osteoporosis causes skeletal changes resulting in chronic morbidity and mortality. It has profound physical, financial and psychosocial consequences for the individual, family, and community (Gueldner, 2000; NIH, 2000). Changes in bone mass or quality, however, occur without symptoms, and are usually not detected until a fracture occurs. Fractures of the proximal femur (hip), vertebrae (spine), and distal forearm (wrist) are the most clinically apparent complications of osteoporosis, and profoundly affect quality of life (Delmas & Fraser, 1999; NIH; NOF, 2003; Wolf, Penrod, & Cauley, 2000). Bone loss associated with the aforementioned risk factors and age-related changes, such as a decrease in proprioception and balance, leads to an increased risk of fracture.

The risk of fracture rises when BMD declines. The use of BMD, therefore, to identify those at risk for fractures is analogous to the use of blood pressure monitoring to identify those at risk for stroke (Wolf et al., 2000). The estimated lifetime risk for wrist, hip, and vertebral fractures is 15%, similar to that for ischemic heart disease (Brundtland, 2000). The majority of these fractures in persons over 50 years of age result from osteoporosis, but attempts to classify fractures have been less than ideal. Use of the hip fracture rate to calculate the osteoporosis fracture burden is promising (WHO, 2003).

Worldwide, the incidence of hip fractures was estimated to be 1.66 million in 1990 (WHO, 2003). Increasing exponentially with age, virtually all occur in persons aged 35 years and older, with 80% of these occurring in women. The highest incidence rates are reported from northern Europe, the northern part of the United States, and among South-East Asian populations, and the lowest are from African countries. The rates, however, differ within racial groups, for example, "rates vary by a factor of about 10 between Sweden and Turkey" (WHO, p. 31). The differences in incidence of hip fractures between countries are greater than those between genders.

Hip fractures are associated with lengthy hospital admissions, difficulty in activities of daily life, nursing home placement, death, and the corresponding economic burden. There is an increase in mortality of 10% to 20% within 1 year of fracture; 30% of fracture patients will fracture the opposite hip; up to 25% require long-term nursing home care; 40% have full recovery to prefracture walking status (NOF, 2003). Mortality is related to comorbid diseases, such as stroke or chronic lung disorders, and to complications arising from immobility and/or treatment of the fracture (Wolf et al., 2000).

Vertebral fractures, often called crushing fractures, result in the characteristic physical changes often associated with osteoporosis, most notably kyphosis or dowager's hump. This collapsing of the vertebral column onto itself impacts other body systems: gastrointestinal, respiratory, genitourinary, and craniofacial, and produces concomitant morbidity: height loss, abdominal protuberance and fullness, inhibited breathing patterns, back pain, back disability, and functional limitations in walking, bending, and reaching (Gueldner, 2000; NIH, 2000; NOF, 2003; Wolf et al., 2000).

The psychosocial ramifications of osteoporosis, though many, are often underaddressed when considering the sequelae of this disorder. Fear, anxiety, anger, depression, and loss of self-esteem threaten the individual's successful adaptation to lifestyle and cosmetic changes, chronic pain, and physical limitations. Often, the decrease in functional abilities leads to social isolation (Gueldner, 2000). The high morbidity and consequent loss of mobility and independence associated with osteoporosis have a ripple effect on the family system, the community, and society. The demands of chronic care, whether formal or informal, strain family, social, health care, and government networks. Global "graying" will further magnify this major public health problem.

The economic burden of osteoporosis to society is formidable. In the United States, the National Osteoporosis Foundation (2003) estimates that the annual cost to the health care system associated with osteoporotic fractures was $17 billion in 2001 dollars. Because these fractures occur in a mainly aged, retired population, costs are associated with direct care services, inpatient and outpatient services, and nursing home care, rather than weighted by a loss of wages (Wolf et al., 2000). Few financial cost estimates are available for the total burden of osteoporosis and all its consequences.

A recent literature search of the CINAHL database entering the keywords *nursing research* and *osteoporosis* for the years 1997–2003 revealed 333 articles. For the year 2003, 43 articles were found, 10 of which were original nursing studies. These studies fell into 5 categories: dealing with patients with hip fractures (3), effect of physical activity on osteoporosis (3), knowledge of osteoporosis (2), attitudes on menopause (1), and development of tools to assess risk factors for osteoporosis (1). The nursing profession, integral to health care from the cradle to the grave, needs to increase osteoporosis awareness, and to research the prevalence, prevention, and adaptation of individuals to this chronic disease.

One ongoing nursing research project is profiling the incidence of osteoporosis in peri- and postmenopausal women in Pennsylvania and the southern tier of New York (Gueldner et al., 2003). Preliminary results of 234 women (mean age, 56.12; median age, 55; range, 32 to 87) found that nearly 24% (23.5%) of these women had heel ultrasound T-scores ≤ -1.0. Data were also analyzed for relationships among demographic variables, risk factors, and T-scores. Age ($p = .012$) and the final score on the Merck Osteoporosis Evaluation SCORE Sheet ($p < .001$) were inversely correlated with T-scores; the older the subject and the higher the score on composite risk factors, the lower the T-scores. Age at menopause was positively correlated with T-scores ($p = .032$); the higher the age at menopause, the higher the T-scores. In addition, women who had taken estrogen had significantly higher T-scores ($p = .038$) than those who had not. Comparison of self-report of height to the measured height on the day of data collection found that self-reported height was significantly lower than measured height ($p < .001$).

These preliminary findings have several implications for clinical practice. That 23.5% of this sample has low bone mass or osteoporosis underscores the importance of early screening in order to develop awareness and provide education on bone health. The high correlation of the SCORE questionnaire with T-scores suggests that this instrument may alone effectively identify "at risk" women for follow-up. This study also supports the unique contribution of estrogen to bone strength, and in light of recent evidence of hormone replacement therapy risks, the need for research on alternative therapies. Lastly, the finding on height discordance mandates the accurate objective measurement of height and weight during health care visits, rather than relying on self-report.

SARAH HALL GUELDNER
GERALDINE BRITTON
SHERI STUCKE

Outcome Measures

Outcomes of nursing and health care encompass changes in both client variables and organizational variables as a consequence of specific processes. Examples of client outcomes include satisfaction and preferences, disease- or problem-specific indicators, functional status, and quality of life. Examples of organizational outcomes include internal customer satisfaction (i.e., nurse or physician satisfaction), personnel safety (i.e., injuries from needles and other "sharps"), and cost-effectiveness. Client-focused variables that cross multiple diseases and conditions, such as mortality, nosocomial infections, falls, skin integrity, and medication errors, have been reported as both client and organizational outcomes.

The national thrust toward outcomes management and research emanates from studies of medical practice variation, which became a priority research agenda in the 1980s. Outcomes management is an ongoing, research-based quest to meet specified quality goals. Outcomes research seeks to determine whether specific interventions or practice models are beneficial in naturalistic environments. It is aimed at broad-based populations and includes service settings other than academic medical centers or large urban environments. In addition to randomized clinical trials, investigators attempt to link information about client outcomes with large administrative and clinical databases. Given an impetus to improve the outcomes of nursing care, investigators must solve various puzzles around appropriate target populations, the right outcome variables, and the associated process and structure variables.

Outcome measures incorporate intermediate clinical variables, such as blood pressure, as well as more extended outcomes, such as return to work. Researchers and managers are challenged to select or design outcome measures and establish their reliability and validity by issues related to sensitivity, specificity, situational contaminants such as severity of illness, and response set and other biases. Variations in definitions, formulas, and data collection procedures frustrate between-group comparisons, particularly for researchers who work with the large databases available from government agencies and organizations within the health care industry. Contextual factors influence client outcomes, including organization ownership (public/private, profit/not for profit), involvement in teaching, case mix, volume of patients treated, organization size, and the extent to which the organization engages in high-tech procedures. Still to be determined is the impact on client outcomes of the integration of health care providers into complex networks.

Projects to develop standardized measures abound. For example, John Ware Jr. and colleagues (Medical Outcomes Trust, 1993) published the *SF-36 Health Survey*, which investigators are using with increasing frequency to assess health status and quality of life from the client's point of view. The SF-36 measures eight concepts: (a) limitations in physical activities because of health problems, (b) limitations in social activities because of physical or emotional problems, (c) limitations in usual role activities because of physical health problems, (d) psychological stress and well-being, (e) limitations in usual role activities because of emotional problems, (f) bodily pain, (g) vitality, and (h) general health perceptions.

Prominent among efforts to standardize measures for outcomes research is the ongoing project conducted by McCloskey and Bulechek (1996), M. Johnson and Maas (1997), and their colleagues at the University of Iowa College of Nursing to develop and maintain taxonomies of nursing interventions and outcomes. In a different arena, the Joint Commission on Accreditation of Healthcare Organizations (1997) has initiated a program that will require organizations seeking accreditation to report patient outcomes. Under that program, *Oryx Outcomes: The Next Evolution in Accreditation*, hospitals choose two clinical performance indicators for reporting from among 60 measurement systems; the selected outcomes must relate to at least 20% of the hospital's patient population. The Agency for Health Care Policy and Research (AHCPR) and the president and fellows of Harvard College have released a computerized compendium of approximately 1,200 clinical performance measures developed by public and private sector organizations to examine the quality of health care. *CONQUEST 1.0* (*CO*mputerized *N*eeds-Oriented *Qu*ality Measurement *E*valuation *System*) can be accessed and downloaded from the AHCPR World Wide Web home page at (http://www.ahcpr.gov/).

ROMA LEE TAUNTON

P

Pain

Pain is "an unpleasant sensory and emotional experience associated with actual or potential damage or described in terms of such damage; pain is always subjective" (International Association for the Study of Pain, 1979, p. 250). People in pain not only suffer considerably but are at risk for long-term adverse effects. Pain is a common component of illness and is the most common reason that people seek medical attention. People experience pain in different ways and only those who have the pain know what it is really like. Communication of that pain to caregivers is dependent on the verbal abilities of the patient, with those who are very young and those who are cognitively impaired being at risk for misunderstanding of its effects.

Pain generally is classified into two types: acute and chronic. However, there are many different types and causes of pain. There is acute pain following surgery and injury, and during labor, sickle cell crisis, and health care procedures. Chronic pain can occur in the musculo-skeletal system, the gastrointestinal system, and the urinary system, and can be recurrent or constant. Cancer pain is from the enlarging tumor, its metastases, or its treatment and is often chronic, increases in intensity and extent; also acute pain can break through the usual pain. Some types of pain are classified by the context in which they occur. These include pain in infants, the critically ill, the cognitively impaired, and at the end of life. Acute pain subsides as healing takes place. Acute pain has a predictable end and is of brief duration, usually less than 3 to 6 months. Chronic pain is said to be that which lasts for longer.

The undertreatment of pain has been well documented for at least the past 30 years (Marks & Sachar, 1973). Barriers to the effective treatment of pain include clinicians' lack of knowledge of pain management principles, clinician and patient attitudes toward pain and drugs, and overly restrictive laws and regulations regarding use of controlled substances. The undermanagement of pain has been particularly pronounced in children, the elderly, and those who cannot speak. Pain relief in palliative care and at the end of life is receiving increased attention in research and practice.

The gate control theory published by Melzack and Wall (1965) provided a theoretical basis for showing how pain, transmitted peripherally to the brain, can be influenced by cognitive and affective as well as physiological factors. Theories of pain have evolved in recent years to the idea of a mind-body unity that Melzack (1996) calls a neuromatrix. An active brain is part of a whole person who has been shaped by genetics and learning to respond to noxious stimuli in individually characteristic patterns. Recent studies of the role of genetics, endorphins, and immune factors, imaging studies of the thalamus, the anterior cingulate, the limbic system, and the cortex, support a holistic theory that goes beyond the mechanics of transmission of noxious messages. An appreciation of the mind-body experience of pain provides a basis for multidisciplinary research and practice, multicultural responses, and multimodal strategies for managing pain.

Within the neuromatrix of a whole and active person, tissue damage causes the release of pain-producing substances, such as serotonin, histamine, bradykinin and substance P, which stimulate nerve endings called nociceptors. Action potentials travel along the peripheral nervous system, are modified in the dorsal horn of the spinal cord, and travel to the brain where sensory, affective, and cognitive responses occur. Nerve fibers descending from the brain to the dorsal horn can inhibit the perception of pain. Opiate receptors in the brain or spinal cord react both to opiates that are externally administered and to enkephalins and endorphins produced by one's own body to modulate pain.

Pain management includes pharmacological, cognitive-behavioral, physical, radiation, anesthetic, neurosurgical, and surgical techniques. Analgesics administered orally or intravenously are needed for moderate to severe pain, and cognitive-behavioral techniques such as relaxation, music, and distraction can increase the relief. More complex pain, such as that experienced by patients with reflex sympathetic dystrophy or by cancer patients who have unrelieved pain from several origins as well as neurogenic and breakthrough pain, may require evaluation and treatment by a multispecialty pain management team. The successful management of pain generally depends on a careful assessment of the pain, patient education for pain management, appropriate pharmacological and nonpharmacological intervention, reassessment to determine the effectiveness of interventions used, and reintervention until satisfactory relief is obtained (Good, 2003).

Pharmacological management of pain usually is treated by three types of drug: (a) aspirin, acetaminophen, and nonsteroidal anti-inflammatory drugs (NSAIDS); (b) opioids; and (c) adjuvant analgesics. NSAIDS decrease the levels of inflammatory mediators generated at the site of tissue injury, thus blocking painful stimuli. They are useful in the management of mild pain and may be used in combination with opioids for moderate to severe pain. Opioids are morphine-like compounds that produce pain relief by binding to opiate receptors. They are used with moderate and severe pain and can be administered orally, subcutaneously, intramuscularly, intravenously, rectally, transdermally, epidurally, nasally, intraspinally, and intraventricularly. Patient-controlled analgesia (PCA) can be accomplished by mouth or by use of equipment set to prescribed parameters to administer a drug intravenously, subcutaneously, or epidurally. Adjuvant drugs are used to increase the analgesic efficacy of opioids, to treat other symptoms that exacerbate pain, or to provide analgesia for specific types of pain.

Physical modalities for pain management include use of heat and cold, counterstimulation such as transcutaneous electrical nerve stimulation (TENS), and acupuncture. Cognitive techniques are focused on perception and thought and are designed to influence interpretation of events and bodily sensations. Providing information about pain and its management, helping patients think differently about pain, and distraction strategies are examples of cognitive techniques. Behavioral techniques are directed at helping patients develop coping skills and modify their reactions to pain. Cognitive-behavioral techniques commonly used by nurses and other clinicians include relaxation, music, imagery, distraction, and reframing. Psychotherapy, support, and hypnosis also have been used successfully in pain management.

When the use of drugs, with or without physical and cognitive behavioral modalities, is not adequate to manage pain, other management techniques may be used. These depend on the cause of the pain and may be temporary or permanent. Radiation therapy is used to relieve metastatic pain and symptoms from local extension of primary disease. Nerve blocks include the injection of a local anesthetic into a spinal space and peripheral nerve destruction. Surgical procedures are used to remove sources of pain, such as debulking a tumor that is pressing on abdominal organs or removing bone spurs that are compressing nerves. Neuroablation techniques include peripheral neurectomy, dorsal rhizotomy, cordotomy, commissural myelotomy, and hypophysectomy.

In recent years, various agencies and organizations have published guidelines for the management of pain. These have included guidelines published by the Agency for Health Care Policy and Research on the management of acute pain, cancer pain, and low-back problems. In addition there are three books from the American Pain Society (APS): on analgesic use, guidelines for pain in arthritis, and pain in sickle-cell disease. In the near future APS will publish two new guidelines for cancer pain and for fibromyalgia. The Joint Commission for Accreditation of Healthcare Agencies has included policies and procedures for pain management in their standards. Pain relief is a patient's right, but there is greater consensus regarding management of acute and cancer pain than for chronic nonmalignant pain.

MARION GOOD
ADA JACOX

Pain Management: A Mid-Range Theory

The theory of a balance between analgesia and side effects proposes that multimodal therapy, attentive care, and patient education contribute to a balance between pain relief and minimal side effects of analgesic medication (Good, 1998, 2004; Good & Moore, 1996). Multimodal therapy consists of a combination of strong analgesics and pharmacological adjuvants (e.g., nonsteroidal antiinflammatory drugs) plus nonpharmacological adjuvants (e.g., relaxation, music, guided imagery). Attentive care means vigilance and consists of regular assessment of pain and side effects, plus identification of inadequate relief, intervention, reassessment, and reintervention. Patient education consists of patient teaching for pain management and mutual goal-setting between the nurse and patient. The three principles are proposed to result in more relief and less side effects than simply giving analgesic medication (Good, 1996, 1998, 2004). The theory is based on the premise that a balance between analgesia and its side effects is the desired goal in acute pain. It is a new conceptualization of acute pain management compared to the previous notion of only giving analgesics (Moore, S. M., 2004).

The theory of a balance between analgesia and side effects is the first integrated, prescriptive nursing theory for acute pain management in adults. Middle-range nursing theories are more useful in practice and research if they have empirical support. Useful sources of mid-range theories are clinical practice guidelines that are based on research and consensus of interdisciplinary experts. Such guidelines can provide a jump-start for empirically based theories and a body of scientific knowledge for practicing nurses. The resulting knowledge then can be taught, used, and developed further. The acute pain management guidelines published by the Agency for Health Care Policy and Research (Acute Pain Management Guideline Panel, 1992) were the source that Good and Moore (1996) used to develop a mid-range pain management theory.

Although analgesic medication is the mainstay of pain therapy after surgery, especially at first, there are large differences in individual response to pain and analgesics. In addition, there may be a mind-body effect from relaxation and soft music. These nonpharmacological modalities have been found to reduce the pain further. Good and colleagues (1999) found that they reduced pain up to 31% more than patient-controlled opioids alone at ambulation and rest. The findings supported the integrated mid-range intervention theory.

The assumptions of the theory are practical. First, the nurse and physician must have current knowledge of pain management and collaborate to achieve relief. Second, the theory is expected to be applied with acute pain in situations in which systemic opioid analgesics or epidural anesthesia are prescribed and medication for side effects is administered as needed. Third, it is applicable to adults who have the ability to learn, set goals, and communicate symptoms (Good, 1998, 2004; Good & Moore, 1996).

This theory has not directly been applied to labor pain, cognitively impaired adults, or patients with special problems such as opioid tolerance, shock, trauma, or burns. However, other theories can be developed from the acute pain management guidelines or from other practice guidelines. For example, Huth and Moore (1998) published an integrated prescriptive theory of acute pain management for infants and children which has been supported by research (Huth, Broome, & Good, 2004). Ruland and Moore (1998) published a mid-range theory of the peaceful end of life based on existing standards of care.

Articles about this theory contain examples of testable research concepts and hypotheses that can be deduced from it. In addition, this literature contains hypothetical cases that ground the theory in reality and illustrate its use with surgical patients and in clinical research (Good, 1998, 2004). It has been republished in part in a textbook of theory development (McEwen, 2002), and practicing nurses taking graduate courses ask about its usefulness for research and practice.

When the theory was created, it was based on empirical support for two of its three propositions and on a consensus of experts for the third one about patient teaching and goal setting (Acute Pain Management Guideline Panel, 1992; Good & Moore, 1996). Since then, there have been research findings that support the effect of nonpharmacological therapies in providing additional pain relief when used with analgesics after surgery (Good & Chin, 1998; Good et al., 2001; Good et al., 1999; Roykulcharoen & Good, in press). These studies took place in the U.S., Taiwan, and Thailand. The largest was a randomized controlled trial of 500 abdominal surgical patients in the U.S., which demonstrated that jaw relaxation, music, and the combination of both had a small to medium effect size compared to analgesics alone. Supported by the National Institute of Nursing Research (NINR), the interventions were effective on postoperative days 1 and 2 and at ambulation and rest (Good et al., 1999). The same music as used in the U.S. study had large effects after gynecological surgery in Kaoshiung, Taiwan (Good & Chin). A test of a longer, whole-body relaxation technique resulted in a large effect size in postoperative abdominal surgical patients in Bangkok, Thailand (Roykulcharoen & Good). A current randomized controlled trial, funded by NINR, is underway to study the effects of nonpharmacological interventions on side effects of opioids after surgery and also the effects of patient teaching for pain management (Good, Anderson, Albert, & Wotman, 2001–2005).

Critical reviews of this theory have noted the clear theoretical and operational definitions given and the clarity and consistency in the use of concepts and prescriptive propositions, making it easy to test in randomized controlled trials (Moore, S. M., 2004; Suppe, 1996). The theory presents a comprehensive approach to clinical management of acute pain, yet with only three propositions it is fairly parsimonious, which is important when teaching it to others. It is reality based, as is evident in the assumptions, concept names, and principles; they are in terms that practicing nurses can easily understand and use. The criteria for a theory in the middle range are met. It is narrow in scope because it is limited to acute pain. It is appropriate for testing because hypotheses can be deduced. Nevertheless it is abstract enough to be useful in practice (Moore, S. M.).

Pain management is important to quality of life. Surgical events are critical stressors in people's lives—a few days when nursing interventions are key factors in preventing ongoing pain and in patients' satisfaction and memory of the event. Pain is a complex phenomenon because human response to pain varies greatly. Pain management is central to good nursing care and relief calls for continual growth of prescriptive knowledge for practitioners. Mid-range theories that clearly and parsimoniously describe this knowledge for nurses can help meet this basic human need in our society. Although more research on the theory is needed and encouraged, what is known thus far can be used to educate the next generation of nurses on management of acute pain.

Marion Good
Shirley M. Moore

Parental Response to the Birth and Hospitalization of a High Risk Infant

Recognizing that parents play an important role in the lives of their infants, nurses have long been concerned about the needs of parents of high-risk infants, that is, preterm and term infants with serious health problems who are hospitalized in neonatal intensive care units (NICUs). The recent thrust on family-centered care in the NICU is a direct result of these concerns about parental needs. Thus, a major focus of research in maternal-child nursing has been on parents of preterm infants hospitalized in an NICU, with a few studies also focusing on parents of term infants with serious health problems. Over the past 2 decades, much of nursing research in this area has focused on two broad areas: (a) describing the sources of stress experienced by parents and identifying factors related to this stress, and (b) examining the emotional responses of parents. Research in this area reflects the works of nurses across the world.

Identification of the stressors experienced by parents related to the hospitalization of their infant in an NICU was greatly facilitated by the development of the Parental Stressor Scale: Neonatal Intensive Care Unit (PSS: NICU) (Miles, Funk, & Carlson, 1993). Worldwide research has been conducted using this scale. In general the findings indicate that aspects of the parental role, such as not being able to protect the baby, feeling helpless, separation, and the appearance and behavior of the sick infant, such as seeing the child experiencing pain or apnea, seeing needles and tubes put into the child, and watching the respirator breath for the child, cause the most distress (Miles, Funk, & Kasper, 1992; Miles & Holditch-Davis, 1997; Shields-Poe & Pinelli, 1997). Limited focus has been placed on parents' perception of their relationship with nursing and medical staff, particularly related to life-and-death decisions, and to the interplay between the nurses and parents as they each assume responsibility for the sick infant.

The emotional distress of parents that results from having a sick infant hospitalized in an NICU has been another direction of research. Studies have focused primarily on depression, anxiety, and general psychological adjustment (Doering, Moser, & Dracup, 2000; Meyer et al., 1995; Miles et al., 1992; Miles, Holditch-Davis, Burchinal, & Nelson, 1999; Shields-Poe & Pinelli, 1997). It has been hypothesized that mothers' responses are similar to those reported for posttraumatic stress (Holditch-Davis, Bartlett, Blickman, & Miles, 2003). While most of this research has focused on negative outcomes, there is a beginning focus on positive outcomes and growth (Miles et al., 1999).

In general, this research suggested that parents of preterm and seriously ill infants experience stress during hospitalization and have intense emotional responses, particularly anxiety and depressive symptoms. Several studies have reported that mothers reported more stress than fathers (Doering et al., 1999; Meyer et al., 1995; Miles et al., 1992; Shields-Poe & Pinelli, 1997). However, most of these studies use small convenience samples of mostly Caucasian, married fathers. More research is needed regarding the experience and needs of single and married fathers and fathers from diverse ethnic backgrounds. Also important is understanding the father's contribution to maternal mental health and parenting and to infant outcomes.

Most of the studies have used quantitative descriptive studies with limited use of conceptual frameworks to explore factors related to parental distress (Miles & Holditch-Davis, 1997). A handful of studies have found that parent and family characteristics and characteristics of the infant's illness are related to stress and emotional distress (Doering et al., 2000; Miles et al., 1999; Shields-Poe & Pinelli, 1997). Few longitudinal studies have been conducted, leaving the findings inconclusive regarding the long-term implications of this distress (Miles & Holditch-Davis). As preterm infants often experience long hospitalizations and the assumption and attainment of the parental role with newborn infants is known to be a process that occurs over time, it is essential that we study parental responses over time to really understand the process and outcomes of this experience. Likewise, we need to link parents and the infants conceptually or methodologically in the design of these studies in order to understand how parental emotional distress and other responses influence parenting behaviors in the critical care period and parenting and the parent-child relationship during childhood. While there is another body of literature related to parent-infant interaction within the NICU, this research is rarely linked to parental emotional responses (Holditch-Davis & Miles, 1997). There are only a limited number of studies using methods of qualitative design that could add more depth to our understanding of parental experiences.

Given the amount of descriptive research on parental stress in the NICU, few researchers have developed and tested interventions aimed at reducing the distress of parents and enhancing their parental role with their infant. Melnyk and colleagues (Melnyk, B. M., et al., 2001) tested a parent-empowerment intervention and reported positive outcomes for low-birthweight infants and their mothers, who reported less stress related to the NICU environment and a better understanding of their preterm infants' behavior.

Future research should be more firmly grounded in developmentally sensitive ecological conceptual models that explore personal and illness-related factors that affect parental responses and link parental responses to parenting and child outcomes. Methods of qualitative and quantitative research should be used and even combined to gain a fuller picture of parental experiences. Longitudinal and repeated measures designs are essential. Research on emotional distress and mental health of parents should include both problematic responses and growth outcomes. Of utmost importance is the need to examine how parents from different ethnic groups respond to birth and hospitalization of a high-risk infant.

In conclusion, nurse researchers internationally have made important contributions to the study of parental responses to birth and hospitalization of a preterm or seriously ill infant. This research has undoubtedly influenced nursing interventions with parents. NICUs generally have open visiting hours, recognize the important role of parents, and work hard to facilitate the development of the parental role even while the infant is critically ill.

MARGARET SHANDOR MILES

Parenting

Parenting is a process that involves a complex set of responsibilities, including being present for the child; caregiving, teaching, protecting, and encouraging the child; and advocating on behalf of the child. These responsibilities evolve over time as the child and parent mature and change in response to environmental contexts and any special needs of the child.

Parenting is a major focus of nursing research. Currently three nursing diagnoses relate to parenting: altered parenting, parental role conflict, and altered parent-infant attachment (Sparks, 1995). The diagnosis of altered parenting involves at-risk or problematic parenting. Parental role conflict involves the changes in parenting that occur when a child is ill, such as providing illness-related care, comforting the child, and stimulating the child's growth and development. Altered parent-infant attachment is an interference with the development of appropriate parental relationship.

An identifiable group of nurse researchers who study parents and parenting has emerged (Beeber & Miles, 2003; Faux, 1998; Holditch-Davis & Miles, 1997; Hoyer, 1998; McBride & Shore, 2001; Mercer, 1995; Miles, 2003). Like parenting researchers from other disciplines, nurse researchers agree that parenting plays a critical role in child development. However, the other side of parenting—its effects on the lives of adults—has received relatively little attention (McBride & Shore). The substantive focus of nursing research on parenting includes parenting during the transition to parenthood, parenting of high-risk infants, parental responses to children's acute and chronic illnesses, parenting of healthy children, and problematic parenting.

Parenting during the transition to parenthood has probably received the most attention from nurse researchers (Mercer, 1995). Areas of research include maternal identity and competence, adjustments to parenting a newborn, parent-infant interactions, and the effects of stressors such as older maternal age, infertility, or a high-risk pregnancy. Fathers are beginning to be studied. Researchers also have studied the development of the parental identity during pregnancy, maternal-fetal attachment, and the emotional tasks of pregnancy.

A related area of research focuses on parenting high-risk infants, including infants who are premature, technologically dependent, prenatally exposed to substances, multiple births, or temperamentally difficult. A number of descriptive studies has explored the emotional distress and sources of stress of parents during the infant's neonatal intensive care hospitalization (Holditch-Davis & Miles, 1997). Of particular concern is the impact of parental distress and parent-infant separation on subsequent parent-child interactions and attachment. Parental influences on development of high-risk infants have also been identified through longitudinal studies. Recently, nurse researchers have tested a number of intervention studies for this population, including support programs in the intensive care unit and home visiting programs (Kearney, York, & Deatrick, 2000).

Another focus of nursing research has been on parents of ill children. Although much of this research has been focused on the family, parents are the most important element of family responses (Faux, 1998). Studies of parents of children with chronic illnesses or developmental disabilities have focused on the impact of the child's diagnosis, stressors associated with treatments and repeated hospitalizations, and parental management of the illness (Miles, 2003). Similarly, researchers have focused on the experiences of parents of acutely ill children, exploring parental emotional responses, participation in care, and stress during hospitalization (Youngblut, 1998). Recently, a few studies have moved beyond physical illnesses and have begun to explore the effect of child psychiatric conditions, such as attention deficit disorder, conduct disorder, and schizophrenia, on parenting. A small but important body of descriptive research about parents' relationships with nurses and other health care providers demonstrates the powerful role nurses have in affecting parental responses and maintaining the parental role, especially during acute illnesses.

Studies of parents of ill children have largely been limited to descriptive, cross-sectional studies done with small convenience samples from one institution. Very few are longitudinal even within the period of hospitalization. More research is needed to explore the nature of the interaction of health care providers and parents and how to strengthen those interactions. More research on the influence of parenting on health and developmental outcomes in ill children is also needed.

Nurse researchers have also studied parenting of normal, healthy children. Preschool children have been studied the most, with less attention to parenting the school-aged, adolescent, and young adult child. Much of this research has looked at parental perceptions of the child or parental effects on child outcomes, such as obesity or substance abuse, rather than parenting per se. However, discipline as an aspect of parenting has received attention. This research has examined the effects of maternal employment, supports for parenting, and issues involved in parenting by grandparents, parenting after divorce, parenting during maternal chronic illness, or parenting after the death of a spouse. In addition, nurse researchers have begun to study ethnic differences in parenting.

Problematic parenting has been another focus of nursing research. Studies have examined the impact of maternal mental health problems or substance abuse on parenting and parents who are abusive to their children. Another important aspect of problematic parenting has focused on parenting by low-income parents (Beeber & Miles, 2003), but the area receiving the most attention from nurse researchers has been adolescent parenting (Hoyer, 1998). Although a number of intervention studies has been conducted to improve parenting in these at-risk groups (Kearney et al., 2000), many of the interventions were atheoretical. More theoretically based intervention studies aimed at improving parenting and removing situational or environmental obstacles to positive parenting are needed.

The theoretical models used as frameworks for nursing research on parenting have been as diverse as the substantive foci. Researchers interested in the transition to parenthood often build on the concepts put forth by Rubin based in role-attainment theory from sociology and adapted by Ramona Mercer and Lorraine Walker. Another commonly used framework is ecological-systems theory, influenced by the work of Uri Bronfenbrenner, Jay Belsky, and Arnold Sameroff, and based in psychology. Within nursing, Kathryn Barnard's theory follows in this tradition.

Other theories used in parenting research by nurses include attachment, cognitive, and stress theories. Attachment theory has its origins in ethology and is influenced by the work of John Bowlby and Mary Ainsworth. This framework is widely used in infancy and preschool parenting research. Cognitively based theories of parenting, such as that developed by Karen Pridham, are used in studies of mothering during the prenatal and postpartal periods. Finally, stress models, influenced by Richard Lazarus and Hans Selye, have been used in studies of the impact of acute illness on parents.

Despite this theoretical diversity, much of the nursing research conducted in the area of parenting remains atheoretical and highly descriptive. Therefore, the findings in this area of research are generally fragmented, and often nurse researchers are not building a coherent science on parenting. The major gaps in the parenting literature in nursing include a need for more information about fathering and about parenting of adolescents and young adults. There is also a need for research that examines parenting from a cultural perspective. Nursing researchers need to go beyond comparing ethnic groups and move toward understanding what is effective and adaptive for parents from varying ethnic backgrounds. Likewise, nurse researchers need to conduct more longitudinal studies that study parenting as a process that unfolds over time.

DIANE HOLDITCH-DAVIS
MARGARET SHANDOR MILES

Parkinson's Disease

Parkinson's Disease (PD) is a progressive, degenerative neurological disorder that manifests severe physical symptoms and also brings emotional issues to the surface. PD is not a new illness; as far back as 1817 an article was written by James Parkinson in which he described a "shaking palsy." The cause, which was a mystery then, remains one today. The symptoms of PD result from a significant degeneration of the neurotransmitter dopamine located in the substantia nigra of the brain. Dopamine is responsible for maintaining the normal function of the extrapyramidal motor system, including control of posture, support, and voluntary motion. The symptoms of PD may vary greatly from individual to individual. However, the "classic" triad of symptoms includes: tremor, rigidity, and bradykinesia. Patients may complain of hand tremors as their first symptom. As the disease progresses, patients become rigid as their muscles lose the ability to relax. The third symptom many people complain about is related to the slowing of movement. Patients can describe feeling "frozen" and they become stuck in one place. It may take them up to several minutes to begin moving again. Due to the degenerative nature of the disease, many patients begin with mild symptoms and over time become significantly debilitated. Pharmacological therapy is the mainstay in treatment for PD. There are several well-known medications in use, the most common being Carbidopa/Levodopa (Sinemet). Sinemet is effective in treating PD by allowing more dopamine to be available for use in the brain. Unfortunately, over time, this and many of the other drugs become less effective, causing a return of symptoms.

Nurses can be pivotal forces in helping patients live with PD. C. Hayes (2002) identified important issues for people living with PD. Her research focused on seven key areas: Anatomy and Physiology/Medical Aspects, Activities of Daily Living, Lifestyle, Mobility, Psychological Issues, Medication, and Advice. The three most important issues identified in the study were available treatments, maintaining independence, and the effects of PD on the brain (Hayes).

Due to the debilitating nature of PD, many spouses often find themselves assuming the caregiver role. Many times relationships drastically change as people assume new roles. Caregiving can be a 24-hour responsibility, and the needs of caregivers as well as the needs of patients must be addressed. Edwards and Scheetz (2002) explored the factors that contribute to the perceived burden of caregivers of PD patients. This study supported the hypothesis that caregivers are affected when their spouse/significant other is diagnosed with PD, and their needs must also be addressed when formulating a plan of care. It was suggested that the nurse prepare and support the family for the progression of the disease. The nurse should assume the role of counselor, educator, and supporter. Nurses should recognize that caregivers have varying abilities, and support groups can be an indispensable avenue for venting feelings and emotions (Edwards & Ruettiger, 2002).

Future research in PD will continue to explore the causes and treatments of this disease. Nursing research will continue to investigate ways in which patients with this disease and their caregivers can obtain the most appropriate treatment, while maintaining the highest possible level of function and quality of life. Lifestyle alterations as well as medications are necessary when treating Parkinson's disease, and the physical as well as emotional needs of patients must remain a top priority in research surrounding this disease.

Andrea Calaluce

Parse's Theory of Nursing: Human Becoming Theory

Human becoming theory (Parse, 1992, 1995) was first entitled *Man-Living-Health: A theory of nursing* (Parse, 1981). In 1998, Parse published *The Human Becoming School of Thought: A Perspective for Nurses and Other Health Professionals* (HBST), a welcome second edition of her original work. This new book gives clear undated explanations of the model, reflecting and elaborating on the research and practice methodologies that were developed after the publication of the first edition. Parse's theory evolved from concern about the use of the medical model applied to the nursing discipline. She was dissatisfied with the mechanistic view of human beings and its lack of congruence with the focus and goals of nursing. The human becoming theory describes a theory of nursing that views the mysteries and uniqueness of humans as unitary beings in mutual process with a multidimensional universe.

Parse (1998) draws from Roger's Science of Unitary Human Beings and the writings on existential phenomenology when she defines the person as being in a process of continuous becoming within the HBST. Humans are described as unitary living beings who are a unity and have more than the sum of their parts. Each person cocreates reality in mutual process with the environment. Quality of life is a central concept within the HBST. According to Parse, any individual capable of the experiences of a living person has a quality of life. She further clarifies that quality of life is subjective and that the nurse should accept quality of life as the patient sees it regardless of the nurse's objective assessment of the patient's quality of life. The goal of nursing is quality of life in Parse's theory

(Parse) thus demonstrating the importance of this concept with the theory.

Within the HBST Parse states that human's health is becoming and is a way of living. She clarifies this by stating that health is nonlinear and therefore one cannot have degrees of health. According to this definition it appears that all one needs to have health is the ability to lead a human life. Human Becoming Theory is guided by nine philosophical assumptions about human beings and becoming that were synthesized from Rogers' Science of Unitary Human Beings and the writings on existential phenomenology. Becoming is "the human's patterns of relating value priorities" (Parse, 1998, p. 20). It is the way one leads one's life. The choices an individual makes identify not only that individual's value priorities but also the type of person he identifies himself as being.

Three principles about human becoming constitute the theoretical structure. Principle 1 states, "structuring meaning multidimensionally is cocreating reality through the languaging of valuing and imaging" (Parse, 1998, p. 35). The major conceptual processes of this principle are imagining, valuing, and languaging (Parse). Principle 2 is that "cocreating rhythmical patterns of relating is living the paradoxical unity of revealing-concealing, enabling-limiting, and connecting-separating" (Parse, p. 42). Principle 3 states, "cotranscending with the possibles is powering unique ways of originating in the process of transforming" (Parse, p. 46). The key conceptual processes for this principle are powering, originating, and transforming (Parse). Parse identifies two types of research within the HBST, basic and applied (Parse, p. 61). Basic research is research that explores the lived experience and human becoming, while applied research evaluates HBST and its application in nursing practice. The basic research focuses on the individual's life experiences. Parse has developed a specific research methodology based on phenomenological hermeneutic methods. It is a qualitative method that focuses on universal human experiences described by research participants. There are three phases involved in this research, dialogical engagement (researcher-participant), extraction-synthesis (dwelling with the data), and heuristic interpretation (Parse). The foci of knowledge development for the discipline within this type of research are the universal lived experiences of individuals, such as hope, joy-sorrow, grieving, and persevering.

In addition, Parse (1998) has delineated a practice method that guides the practice of nurses implementing the theory. She has developed dimensions and processes to guide nurses within the HBST. The goal of nursing is quality of life from the perspective of the patient. The artistic medium employed by the nurse is described as true presence, the basis of nursing practice. True presence is an "intentional reflective love" (Parse, p. 71). The nurse engages with the person by devoting one's attention to the person and trying to immerse oneself in that person's universe. Nurses must understand that both the individual's perspective of his illness and the views of his family about his illness are very important. Within the HBST, nursing provides suitable conditions so that the patient and the family can accept the health concern. Parse does not expect the nurse to change anything apart from providing optimum conditions to facilitate acceptance in the patient and family.

Parse (2004) continues to expand her theoretical perspectives with the introduction of the human becoming teaching-learning processes. The human becoming teaching-learning model is made up of essences, paradoxes, and processes. The essences are semantic coherence, synergistic patterning, and aesthetic innovating (Parse). The paradoxes are rational-intuiting, clarifying-obscuring, waring-woofing, ebbing-flowing, considering-composing, and beholding-refining (Parse). The processes are living with ambiguity, appreciating the mystery, potentiating integrity, weaving multidimensionally, honoring wisdom, and witnessing unfolding (Parse). Parse believes that these essences, paradoxes, and processes provide a model for teaching-learning in which pattern-seeing-see-changing-all-at-once shifts understanding in the never-ending journey of coming-to-know. Nurse educators have incorporated the teaching-learning processes into student's experiences through development of a reflective journaling process to enhance the normally expected journaling experience (Letcher & Yancey, 2004). The teaching-learning processes used by Letcher and Yancer included *living with ambiguity, appreciating the mystery, honoring the wisdom, inventing the possibles*, and *witnessing the unfolding*. Through reflective journaling the students explored the meaning of their teaching-learning experience. An outgrowth of this work was the development of an interactive distance learning experience between two groups of students at different schools of nursing so that they could explore the meaning of this experience with others. Recommendations for future work include linking groups of students earlier in their nursing program and development of distance strategies for such linkage (Letcher & Yancey). The human becoming teaching-learning model provides new approaches to journaling and networking with students while enriching the nursing experience from a theoretical perspective.

Bunkers (2002) has developed a theoretical perspective on lifelong learning through linking Parse's theory of human becoming to seven Da Vincian principles identified by Gelb (1998). The Da Vincian principles reflect all the salient features of Parse's model. This unique link provides a nursing theory perspective on lifelong learning and sets out a framework for the development of new possibilities for lifelong learning. Nurse educators are exploring teaching strategies that address the needs of today's student, such as opportunities to learn theoretical underpinnings of nursing and availability of distance courses. J. R. Norris (2002) explored one-to-one tele-apprenticeship as a teaching and learning strategy for Parse's model. Tele-apprenticeship is defined as a one-to-one learning relationship, developed solely by e-mail, between a mentor and student. This was useful in guiding a student in the theoretical aspects of the Parse model but was unable to provide the depth and skills required to become expert in the practice methodology of the theory. Further research is needed in this area, particularly looking at the synchronized versus nonsynchronized discussions, video conferencing, chat rooms, and other technology that potentially could benefit this teaching-learning strategy.

Diana Lynn Morris
Updated by Mary T. Quinn Griffin

Participant Observation

Participant observation is an approach to data collection that is most often associated with naturalistic or qualitative inquiry, and it involves the researcher as a participant in the scene or observation that is being studied. The primary purpose is to gain an insider's, or emic, view of an event, setting, or general situation. The researcher focuses on the context of the scene along with the ways that individuals are behaving. Examples might include making and participating in observations in a busy emergency room, observing the ways in which people carry out rites of passage, or participating in a special feast or occasion. The researcher attempts to make sense of the situation by interpreting personal experiences and observations and talking with individuals who are present, while simultaneously being fully involved in all of the experiences that occur in that setting. In this way participant observation enables the researcher to gain a view of a society but also serves as a way to validate verbal information that was provided by members of a society or group being studied. Another way in which participant observation may be used in research is with populations in which there is limited communication, such as very small children, the mentally impaired, or elderly stroke survivors. The challenge for the researcher is to combine the activities of observation and participation so that understanding is achieved while maintaining an objective distance.

To carry out participant observation the researcher needs to decide on (a) the role of the observer, (b) the degree to which the role is known to others, (c) the degree to which the purpose is known to others, (d) the amount of time that will be spent in conducting the observation, and (e) the scope of the observational focus. There is a continuum along which the role of the observer may be involved that ranges from involvement of the researcher in all aspects of the observational experience to only partial or minimal involvement. The researcher bases this determination on the research question and the nature of the research. For example, a researcher who assists in a homeless shelter may wish to be involved in all aspects of the daily routine; another researcher may wish only to conduct observations in a busy emergency room for which the routine is more complex. On the other hand, an invitation to participate in a special ceremony or ritual may involve only partial participation.

The degree to which the observer's role and the purpose of the observation are known to others also is related to the intent of the research. In some cases the role of the researcher will be known to all, and in others it may not. If the purpose of the study is to know and understand a particular ritual or religious ceremony, for example, the role of the researcher may be known to all involved in the situation. In other cases the role of the researcher may be minimized, as in situations in which the informants may not fully understand the researcher's participation: observing children on a playground or in a children's unit in a hospital. However, ethical and moral issues arise when the nature and role of the researcher are not made known to all of the individuals being observed. The extent to which individuals are informed varies greatly, from full disclosure to no disclosure, and is often based on the researcher's estimation of how scientific truth can best be obtained.

The amount of time the researcher spends in observation and the scope or focus of the observation also depend on the purpose and intent of the research. In some cases the participant observation experiences are carried out for the length and duration of the research. In other research studies, participant observation may occur at only one point during the study. For example, sometimes a researcher may choose to enter the field and become a participant observer prior to conducting interviews. This gives the researcher time to learn about a community, group of people, or situation and then to use this knowledge to develop questions for subsequent interviews. In addition, the focus and intent of the observations may vary from making general observations of the entire situation, context, or event to very focused observations. For example, a focused observation might include personal interactions or a specific nursing or caring behavior.

One major concern in using participant observation is the degree to which subjects may become sensitized to the researcher's presence and may not behave as they normally would if the researcher were not present. The issue of subject sensitization can be addressed by increasing the duration of time the researcher spends in the observational experience. A longer time spent in observing can also enhance and strengthen the researcher's credibility, as well as any theoretical and empirical generalizations that are made.

In summary, participant observation is a commonly used approach to data collection that is used in naturalistic or qualitative research. It is an approach that allows the researcher to gain an insider's perspective on a social situation or event and can permit the researcher to be totally or minimally involved.

KATHLEEN HUTTLINGER

Patient Classification

Patient classification is a generic term referring to the grouping or categorization of patients according to a predetermined set of characteristics. Until the late 1980s, this term was used almost exclusively to refer to the classification systems for grouping patients according to their requirements for nursing care and nursing resource determination and allocation. The exclusive use of the term to represent nursing systems became inappropriate with the widespread development of other patient classification systems (diagnostic related groups, case mix groups, and medical severity of illness systems) to capture medical resource use and complexity as the basis for hospital case costing.

With some peril, the terms *severity* and *acuity* systems were and continue to be used as equivalent terms. Connotations associated with these terms from the perspective of medical status led to misconceptions, as neither patient severity nor patient acuity correlates uniformly with nursing workload. In contrast, patient dependency and nursing intensity have been offered as more suitable labels to describe the intent of the patient classification systems designed for nursing. During the past decade, however, a shift in the use of terms has occurred. Those patient classification schemes that form the basis for the measurement of patients' requirements for nursing care for the express purpose of nursing resource determination and allocation are now referred to as nursing workload measurement systems.

The process of classifying is defined as the ordering or arranging of objects or concepts into groups or sets based on relationships among the objects or concepts. The relationships can be based on observable or inferred properties. Classification theory also includes the distinction between monothetic and polythetic classifications. Monothetic schemes refer to those in which the classes established differ by at least one property that is uniform among the members of each class. In contrast polythetic schemes refer to those in which the classes share a large proportion of the properties but do not necessarily agree on any one property. Patient classification schemes for nurse staffing are recognized as polythetic, and their development coincides with the principles of this type (Giovannetti, 1978).

Work by Connor, Flagle, Hsieh, Preston, and Singer (1961) at the Johns Hopkins Hospital during the 1960s introduced the concept of classification into the study and measurement of nursing workload. The critical indicators or predictors of nursing care emanating from this work appear in most contemporary nursing patient classification systems.

Two types of patient classification systems, prototype evaluations and factor evaluations, were identified by Abdellah and Levine (1979). Prototype evaluations rely on the creation of several mutually exclusive and exhaustive patient categories. These are graded in terms of an ordinal scale in which the categories represent greater or lesser requirements for nursing care. The patient is classified into the category that most closely matches the profile or prototype description. Factor evaluation systems employ the selection of specific elements or indicators of care, representing either unique care activities or clusters of care activities. Ratings on individual elements are combined on the basis of a predetermined set of decision rules to provide an overall rating that determines the appropriate category.

The end product of the two types of evaluations is essentially the same. The difference lies in the method of rating; in prototype, the patient is rated on a number of characteristics simultaneously, whereas in factor, the characteristics are evaluated one by one. Edwardson and Giovannetti (1994) noted that many systems have been developed by vendors and consequently were not fully described in the published literature. More systems have been developed or modified at the institutional level and also not published.

Transforming classification schemes for their ultimate use as resource determination and allocation methods requires an estimate of the nursing care time required of patients in each category. The literature is replete with techniques for doing so and discussions of the central issues of reliability, validity, and comparability. Similar to nursing workload measurement system research, research on patient classifications systems has much to offer nursing practice, nursing administration, health care administration nursing, and other institutional policy formation. Information on patient classification systems is available in professional, scholarly, management, and policy journals as well as in texts and government reports.

Phyllis B. Giovannetti

Patient Contracting

Patient contracting is an intervention for promoting patient adherence in practice or research settings. Patient contracting provides an opportunity for patients to learn to analyze their behavior relative to their environment and to select behavioral strategies that will promote learning, changing, or maintaining adherence behaviors (Boehm, 1992). Patient contracting is relevant to nursing practice and research because it can assist patients to adhere to treatment regimens, such as medication taking, meal planning, and physical activity.

Research on the effectiveness of patient contracting in nursing has been reported for a variety of behaviors across settings and disorders. For example, patient contracting has been used to control serum potassium levels (Steckel, 1974) and serum phosphorus levels (Laidlaw, Beeken, Whitney, & Reyes, 1999) in patients on dialysis; to increase knowledge and consistency in use of contraceptive methods by sexually active college women from a student gynecology clinic (Van Dover, 1986); to increase knowledge, keep appointments, and reduce diastolic blood pressure in hypertensive outpatients (Steckel & Swain, 1977; Swain & Steckel, 1981); and to keep appointments, lose weight, and reduce blood pressure among outpatients with arthritis, diabetes, and hypertension (Steckel & Funnell, 1981). Patient contracting did not reduce blood glucose and glycosylated hemoglobin in patients with diabetes (Boehm, Schlenk, Raleigh, & Ronis, 1993; Morgan, B. S., & Littell, 1988; Steckel & Funnell).

Patient contracting is the process in which the nurse and patient negotiate an individualized, written, and signed agreement that clearly specifies the behavior and identifies in advance the positive consequences to be given when the patient has successfully performed the behavior (Steckel, 1982). The patient chooses the behavior and reinforcer in the contract with direction by the nurse. Patient contracting is based on the principle of positive reinforcement, which states that when a behavior is followed by a reinforcing consequence, there is an increased likelihood of the behavior being performed again (Boehm, 1992).

The nursing process provides the context within which to develop the patient contract. The nursing process provides the clinical data that can be jointly used by nurses and patients to establish priorities for adherence behaviors (Steckel, 1982). The adherence behavior is the ultimate complex behavior to be learned or changed. The adherence behavior is broken down into successive approximations or small steps. By performing small steps of the behavior, the patient gradually achieves performance of the adherence behavior. Over a series of patient contracts, the patient will specify a variety of behaviors, which include such behavioral strategies as self-monitoring, arranging and rearranging antecedent events, practicing small steps of the adherence behavior, and arranging positive consequences (Boehm, 1992). The first several patient contracts are usually for self-monitoring to identify the successive approximations of the adherence behavior and the antecedents and consequences of the behavior. In later patient contracts, patients specify behavioral strategies related to arranging antecedent events, practicing a small step of the behavior, or arranging positive consequences. Self-monitoring is ongoing throughout the behavior change process to provide data about the effectiveness of the new antecedents, the performance of the small steps of the behavior, and the new positive consequences.

Behavioral analysis is the foundation of the patient contracting intervention. Behavioral analysis is the process by which the patient's behavior is observed, recorded, and analyzed in order to describe the successive approximations of the adherence behavior, the antecedent events that precede the behavior, and the consequences that follow the behavior. The behavioral data used in the analysis are obtained by the patient through self-monitoring (Boehm, 1992). Behavioral analysis begins with the patient self-monitoring the adherence behavior. Self-monitoring provides baseline data that can be used to determine the effectiveness of the behavioral strategies implemented later in the behavior change process. By using the patient's self-monitoring records, the nurse can teach the patient to identify antecedent events that precede the behavior, small steps that comprise the behavior, and consequences that follow the behavior. Based on the behavioral analysis, behavioral strategies are specified that will assist in the behavior change.

Behavioral analysis can identify the multiple small steps that comprise the adherence behavior. When the small steps are identified, the behavioral strategy is to perform a small step of the adherence behavior for a designated period of time. When that small step is being successfully performed, the patient moves onto the next small step. Eventually, patients gradually achieve performance of the adherence behavior (Steckel, 1982). This behavioral strategy is effective because patients are often overwhelmed by expectations of a treatment regimen, which can lead to nonadherence. For example, sedentary patients who are beginning a walking program might start by walking 5 minutes three times per week. Each week the walking goal is gradually increased until they achieve their goal of accumulating 30 minutes of moderate-intensity walking 5 days per week.

Positive reinforcement is the behavioral strategy in which a positive consequence is provided contingent upon performance of the desired behavior, which results in an increase in performance of the behavior. Behavioral analysis can identify positive consequences for behaviors and provide ideas for new consequences (Boehm, 1992). The behavioral strategy is to arrange positive reinforcement to acquire or maintain a desired behavior. For example, adopting a walking program will be strengthened if a positive consequence follows each walking goal that is met. Positive consequences can be pleasurable items and activities; social reinforcement, such as praise; and cognitive reinforcement, such as feelings of pride. Conversely, eliminating positive reinforcement can be used to decrease or extinguish an undesired behavior. For example, eating with selected companions may eliminate positive consequences for inappropriate food item selections.

There are several directions for future research. First, studies are needed to determine the frequency of contact needed with subjects to produce progressive changes in adherence interventions using patient contracting. Second, patient contracting during the maintenance phase of adherence interventions has not been studied. Third, electronic self-monitoring by personal digital assistants or Internet web sites could be utilized during studies. Fourth, studies could include objective measures of adherence behaviors, such as, electronic event monitors to assess medication adherence and accelerometers or pedometers to assess physical activity.

ELIZABETH A. SCHLENK

Patient Education

Patient education is defined as a planned learning experience using a combination of methods such as teaching, counseling, and behavioral strategies that influence the patient's knowledge and behavior (Bartlett, 1985). Since the mid-19th century patient education has been a fundamental cornerstone of health care and today it is an integral component of professional standards of care issued by nursing organizations, such as "A Patient's Bill of Rights" published by the American Hospital Association, and the regulations of the Joint Commission on Accreditation of Healthcare Organizations. Its importance rests on the fact that the well-being of individuals, whether or not they have a diagnosed disease, often is dependent on health-related actions those individuals take on their own behalf. In the managed care environment of today, with its concomitant decrease in the incidence and length of hospitalizations for specific health problems, and the shortening of time allocated to outpatient office visits to a health practitioner, patient's and family's responsibility has increased while the time to provide traditional face-to-face patient education has decreased. Innovative strategies for delivering patient education, such as the use of electronically mediated technologies, need to be explored (e.g., CD-ROM or Internet-based education, or education as a component of telehealth). Strategies to increase effective self-management such as patient empowerment, collaborative goal setting, and problem-solving skills (Wagner, Davis, Schaefer, Von Korff, & Austin, 2002) may need to be added to traditional didactic content.

Research on the effect of patient education began in the early-1960s, and in the late 1980s meta-analyses of this research began to be published. Major researchers in this area and the patient population that was the focus of their review(s) include: A. C. Bernard-Bonnin and associates, and J. P. Guevara and associates (children/adolescents with asthma); S. A. Brown, and Gary and associates (adults with diabetes); E. C. Devine and associates [(1) adults having surgery, (2) adults with hypertension, (3) adults with cancer, (4) adults with chronic obstructive pulmonary disease, and (5) adults with asthma]; E. Monninkhof and associates (adults with chronic obstructive pulmonary disease); W. J. Huestron and associates (women at risk for preterm birth); P. D. Mullen and associates [(1) adults with coronary disease, (2) adults with arthritis, (3) pregnant women who smoke]; and A. M. Peterson (medication adherence).

Many but not all of the meta-analyses of the effect of patient education have found that it is beneficial for the patients receiving it. These beneficial effects have included not only increased patient knowledge, but also positive effects on a wide range of disease-specific outcomes (e.g., blood pressure control among individuals with hypertension [Devine & Reifschneider, 1995]; pain among cancer patients [Devine, 2003]; blood sugar control at 6 months postintervention among adults with diabetes [Brown, S. A., 1992]), and lung function, school absenteeism, and number of visits to the emergency department in children and adolescents (Guevara, Wolf, Grum, & Clark, 2003). However, statistically significant positive effects have not always been found. For example, there was not a consistent beneficial effect of patient education on hospital admissions and lung function among adults with chronic obstructive pulmonary disease, although there was a decrease in the need for rescue medication (Monninkhof et al., 2003). Preterm-birth prevention education did not decrease the preterm delivery or the neonatal death rates among high-risk women (Hueston, Knox, Eilers, Pauwels, & Lonsdorf, 1995). There were short-term but not long-term effects on both blood sugar levels in diabetics (Brown, 1992) and on disability, joint counts, psychological status, and depression in adults with rheumatoid arthritis (Riemsma, Kirwan, Taal, & Rasker, 2003). Clinicians wanting to apply patient education research findings in their practice will need to review the research carefully to find primary research or meta-analyses of research that match both their client group and the outcomes they want to affect.

Critical issues for the profession remain. These include: What combinations of treatment components and modes of treatment delivery are the most effective? To what extent have educational interventions been tested in minority populations? Are culturally-specific interventions needed with minority populations? How do we adapt patient education for nonliterate populations? How do we make the best use of newer computer-based technologies (e.g., the Internet)? How do we educate patients to evaluate and make good use of Internet-based information?

While many of the reviews of patient education research suggested that patient education is beneficial for patients, the research was less clear about which specific types of patient education and which modes of treatment delivery are the most effective for which types of patients. This limitation arises from three problems. First, it is common for patient education researchers to contrast the experimental patient education program with usual health care for the setting, and yet they rarely described the patient education included in usual care. Second, very few studies contrasted different types of patient education or different modes of treatment delivery in the same study. Third, many studies failed to provide detailed descriptions of the subjects included in their sample. Because of these limitations, it is difficult to make causal inferences about which types of content and which modes of treatment delivery are the most effective ones for which types of patients. More research in this area is needed.

Clinicians and researchers interested in patient education will face many new opportunities and challenges as use of the Internet increases. Many patients, from their homes or local libraries, can use the Internet to access an almost limitless amount of health-related information (e.g., from literature searches, professional or consumer organizations, support groups, and disease-specific chat groups). This provides an opportunity for clinicians and researchers to provide patient education in innovative ways that allows the patient to have some control over the topic, timing, and pacing of the education. Some innovative educational programs also allow patients to submit questions using electronic mail and receive a response from their health care provider. The Internet will also provide many challenges to clinicians and researchers. Patients may receive inaccurate information over the Internet and be ill-equipped to judge its trustworthiness. In some situations patients may become aware of the latest research findings (e.g., on treatment options for their health problem) before their nurses and doctors. Clinicians and researchers should determine if their patients are using the Internet to seek health-related information, and be prepared to help their patients make good use of this resource. When appropriate, they also should direct them to authoritative sources of information that are appropriate for health care consumers (e.g., http://www.nlm.nih.gov/medlineplus.html).

Given the research base for patient education and the professional standards that dictate its use, clearly the question is no longer simply: Does research suggest that systematic patient education should be provided? The many remaining researchable questions are at a finer level such as: Is it possibly to improving patient education through the use of technology, or are culturally-specific education programs more effective in underserved groups?

There are ethical and professional mandates to educate patients so that they can make informed decisions about their health. These mandates are undoubtedly over time helping to change the patient education included in usual care. This dynamic nature of care makes it even more important for researchers and clinicians to be aware of the patient education typically provided as part of usual care in their setting.

ELIZABETH C. DEVINE
DEBORAH L. GENTILE

Patient Safety

Past efforts to reduce costs and streamline the delivery of health care have led to significant changes, not always with a positive effect. The Institute of Medicine's (IOM) report, *To Err is Human*, which spotlighted the problem of patient safety, reported that tens of thousands of Americans die each year as a result of human error in the delivery of health care (Institute of Medicine, 2000). The second report in this series described broader quality issues and defined six aims: These included that care should be (1) safe, (2) effective, (3) patient-centered, (4) timely, (5) efficient, and (6) equitable (Institute of Medicine, 2001). The most recent report found that nursing is inseparably linked to patient safety, emphasizing that poor working conditions for nurses and inadequate nurse staffing levels threaten patient safety and increase the risk of errors (Institute of Medicine, 2003).

To improve patient safety, common definitions should be used and it should be understood that not all adverse events are patient safety problems. Essentially, patient safety applies to initiatives designed to prevent adverse outcomes resulting from errors and near misses. Near misses are of interest because of the high probability of the event causing harm to the patient. Unfortunately, many adverse events and near misses are related to low nurse staffing levels or unskilled and inexperienced clinicians.

Health care leaders and managers should strive to create nursing work environments that are conducive to patient safety. To do this, evidence-based management (EBM) strategies are suggested. Most clinicians are now familiar with the notion of evidence-based practice, defined as the conscientious, explicit, and judicious integration of current best evidence to inform clinical decision making. However, EBM is a fairly new term and framework (Sacket et al., 1996). EBM implies that managers, like clinical practitioners, search for, critically appraise, and apply empirical evidence from management research in their practice. Currently, both managers and clinicians have little research-based evidence to apply and are often not experienced in the use of such evidence.

In a seminal study on leadership, *transactional* leaders were differentiated from the more potent *transformational* leaders (Burns, J., 1978). Transactional leadership typifies most leader-follower relationships; it involves a "you scratch my back, I'll scratch yours" exchange. In contrast, transformational leadership occurs when leaders engage with their followers in jointly held goals. This leadership approach is recommended because it transforms all workers—both managers and staff—in the pursuit of the higher collective purpose of patient safety and quality care.

An emerging evidence base is finding a strong correlation between higher staffing levels and lower occurrence of adverse events. In an study of 589 hospitals in 10 states, the registered nurse (RN) staffing level was found to be inversely related to urinary tract infections (UTI) and pneumonia after major surgery ($p < .0001$) (Kovner & Gergen, 1998). In another study of 799 hospitals from 11 states, researchers found UTI and pneumonia to have a consistently strong inverse relationship with nurse staffing ratios (Needleman, Buerhaus, Mattke, Stewart, & Zelevinski, 2001).

A line of research with a broader focus than staffing levels is the investigations involving Magnet hospitals (i.e., hospitals that attract nurses, hence the term Magnet). When Magnet hospitals were matched with control hospitals, controlling for case mix, Aiken and colleagues observed a Medicare mortality rate that was lower by 4.6 per 1,000 discharges (95% confidence interval 0.9 to 9.4) (Aiken, Smith, & Lake, 1994). However, besides the attainment of Magnet status, specifics were not identified. Magnet hospitals are known for higher nurse-to-patient ratios, lower staff turnover rates, and higher rates of nursing satisfaction

Nurses are in the position of being "at the sharp end" of health care interventions by being the patient's advocate, providing care that may result in an error, or witnessing the error(s) of other clinicians. Accidents, errors, and adverse outcomes result from a chain of events involving human decisions and actions associated with active failures and latent failures. Many of these failures are associated with individual performance that is impaired by stress, distractions/interruptions, and fatigue.

Care delivery needs to be redesigned respecting human limitations, particularly the debilitating effects of stress and fatigue on performance (Norman, 2002). Research continues to confirm that clinicians with the appropriate skill, experience, and workload are less likely to make patient safety errors. Yet one of the barriers to improving patient safety, considering the level and types of interactions among clinicians and components within health care, is the ability to recognize and correct errors (Kohn, Corrigan, & Donaldson, 2000).

There is increasing consensus that the organizational culture impacts patient safety and the quality of care (Gershon, Stone, Bakken, & Larson, 2004). Important aspects of safety cultures include communication, nonhierarchical decision making, constrained improvision, training, and rewards and incentives (IOM, 2003a).

Organizational and individual commitment to improving patient safety requires effective leadership and proactive interventions. Patient safety improvements need to draw from qualitative and quantitative research describing work processes and responsibilities, methods to improve performance respecting human limitations, and designs of patient safety supportive communication and team approaches to health care delivery.

PATRICIA W. STONE
RONDA G. HUGHES

Patient Satisfaction

Patient satisfaction has become increasingly popular as a critical component in the measurement of the quality of care. Donabedian (1988) theorized that the quality of medical care could be evaluated from three perspectives: its process (how and what things are done), structure (the setting in which the care is administered), and outcomes (e.g., the effects on health status and patient satisfaction). Few studies of patient satisfaction existed prior to the 1970s. After that time, there was an increase in the research conducted in this area. The number of studies of patient satisfaction parallels the research on consumer satisfaction, which has historically been conducted by industries interested in maintaining and/or increasing their market share. Research on patient satisfaction has continued to gain momentum with the Total Quality Management (TQM) and "outcomes" movements of the 1980s and 1990s, and over the last decade as the health care marketplace has become more competitive.

Patient satisfaction is a complex concept with several dimensions. Ware, Davies-Avery, and Stewart (1978) developed a detailed taxonomy of patient satisfaction from their review of 111 studies published over the 25-year period prior to 1975. The taxonomy initially included the art of care, technical quality of care, accessibility/convenience, finances, physical environment, availability, efficacy, and continuity. After decades of continued research, the dimensions of care were refined to include the following six dimensions: nursing and daily care, hospital environment and ancillary staff, medical care, information, admissions, and discharge and billing (Ware & Berwick, 1990).

Risser (1975) developed an instrument to ascertain patient satisfaction that was specific to nursing care. The Risser Patient Satisfaction Scale (PSS) included 25 questions and three subscales: Technical/Professional Area, Educational Relationship Area, and Trusting Relationship Area. The PSS was originally developed to measure the care of ambulatory patients and was later adapted to the hospital setting through minor rewording and a replication study (Hinshaw, A. S., & Atwood, 1982). La Monica, Oberst, Madea, and Wolf (1986) further developed the PSS to reflect nursing behaviors in the acute care setting and additional items were added and then subjected to psychometric testing to ensure reliability and validity (Munro, Jacobsen, & Brooten, 1994).

Patient satisfaction with nursing care has consistently been found to be correlated with overall satisfaction with care, and has been defined as the "patient's subjective evaluation of the cognitive/emotional response that results from the interaction of the patient's expectations of nursing care and their perception of the actual nurse behaviors/characteristics" (Erikson, 1995, p. 71). Measuring patient satisfaction with care is instrumental to the success of providing patient-centered care and allows consumers to participate in the evaluation process.

The majority of studies on patient satisfaction have been cross-sectional and descriptive in nature. Characteristics of providers or organizations that result in more "personal" care have been associated with higher levels of satisfaction (Cleary & McNeil, 1988). The nurse work environment has been found to be both directly and indirectly (through nurse burnout) related to patient satisfaction (Vahey, Aiken, Sloane, Clarke, & Vargas, 2004). Patients cared for on units which nurses characterized as having adequate staff, good administrative support for nursing care, and good relations between doctors and nurses were more than twice as likely as other patients to report high satisfaction with their care; additionally, their nurses reported significantly lower burnout. Patient satisfaction has also been found to be associated with patient adherence to care provider recommendations and intent to return for or refer services (Hill, M. H., & Doddato, 2002).

It is clear that there are many important implications for assessing and improving patient satisfaction with nursing care. The American Nurses Association (ANA), the Joint Commission on Accreditation of Health Care Organizations (JCAHO), and others have identified patient satisfaction as an important quality indicator (American Nurses Association, 1996, 2000a; Donabedian, 1988; Joint Commission on Accreditation of Healthcare Organizations, 2003a). However, there are several challenges facing researchers in the 21st century.

A major challenge is the need for psychometrically sound, reliable, and valid measures (McDaniel & Nash, 1990). Patient satisfaction with nursing care is a multidimensional phenomenon and therefore a single item will not suffice. However, researchers must consider the burden to patients and limit the number of items to only those that are essential. Additionally, a standardized approach to the measurement of patient satisfaction will allow care providers to benchmark their services and consumers to adequately compare across providers in order to make informed decisions about their care. Currently, the ANA and the Centers for Medicare and Medicaid Services (CMS) are working toward this goal by developing multisite databases. The ANA is sponsoring the National Database for Nursing Quality Indicators (NDNQI), which plans to collect data on patient satisfaction with pain management, educational information, nursing care, and overall care (National Center for Nursing Quality, 2004). The CMS has implemented a three-state pilot project to test and refine a standardized "Patient Experience of Care" (Centers for Medicare & Medicaid Services, 2003).

Another challenge is for health care researchers to refine the methodological strategies so that techniques with greater sensitivity can be achieved. Cross-sectional studies limit the ability to identify causal relationships and generalize findings. Results from mail and telephone surveys, which are the most common methodologies, can be biased because of the timing of these surveys and the rigor in which responses are obtained. Moreover, it is argued that patients tend to report "socially desirable" ratings, which result in data that are skewed and typically reported as high levels of satisfaction. Some researchers therefore have recommended that health care providers focus only on areas of dissatisfaction or patient complaints. Future research should consider other methods for assessing patient satisfaction, which may include focus groups, observation, or qualitative studies. These methods may help isolate "critical moments"—such as specific episodes of care or interactions with care providers, or more clearly identify patient expectations prior to service and whether they are met—which is likely to be a more effective and efficient way to assess important dimensions of care and to make improvements.

Finally, one of the main indications for measuring patient satisfaction with nursing care is to identify areas for improvement; however, few studies have examined the effects of interventions. Recognizing the contributions of nursing to improved patient outcomes and the quality of care will lead to the provision of safe patient-centered care. Designing studies to evaluate interventions that take into consideration increasing patient acuity, shorter lengths of stay, and the cultural diversity of patients will provide for enduring changes resulting in high-quality health care that benefits both patients and providers.

Doris C. Vahey

Pediatric Primary Care

Pediatric primary care has existed for a long time and has been provided by family practice physicians and pediatricians. In the last 25 years, primary care has changed to include pediatric nurse associates who are now called pediatric nurse practitioners (PNPs). PNPs were the first nurse practitioners; they are advanced practice nurses who are educated to provide primary care services to children. Dr. Henry K. Silver and Dr. Loretta Ford started the PNP program in Colorado in 1964. Although the role has remained much the same from its inception, one major change is the level of education required. Originally it was a 4-month continuing education program and now it is a 2-year educational program culminating with a master's degree. National certification is required, in some states to allow PNPs to practice. There are two certifying organizations for PNPs: the American Nurses Credentialing Center (ANCC) and the Pediatric Nursing Certification Board (PNCB).

Currently, there are differences in health care outcomes between minority and majority ethnic groups. Children in minority groups are at much greater risk for poor health care factors, and there is a lack of culturally competent health care providers. In 1998, President Clinton presented the Initiative to Eliminate Racial and Ethnic Disparities in Health. This proposal seeks to eliminate disparities by the year 2010, and focuses on the same goals and outcomes as Health People 2010: infant mortality, child and adult immunizations, HIV/AIDS, diabetes, cardiovascular disease and stroke, and cancer screening and management. Access to health care and quality of health care are also part of the focus (Stinson, 2003)

Childhood immunizations, particularly in children less than 2 years of age, continue to be a major health concern in primary care. Health People 2000 and the President's Childhood Immunization Initiative mandated a goal of 90% immunizations for children younger than 2 years of age by the year 2000. In 1992, only 55% of children under the age of 2 years had received an adequate number of immunizations. By 1994, the rate had risen to 73%, and now it is close to the 90% goal. While these are excellent numbers, there still remain pockets primarily in large cities where immunizations rates are much lower. Data from the CDC National Immunization Survey suggest that minority children, primarily African-American and Hispanic, children living below the poverty level, children of teen mothers, children in large families, children of parents who lack education, families with transportation problems, and children of mothers who lack social support have lower rates of receiving immunizations by age 2 years than the national average.

Obesity is another health issue commonly seen in primary care. It is a complex issue and not fully understood. The number of obese children has increased substantially in the last 20 years, putting them at risk for serious health problems as adults including cardiovascular disease and stroke, diabetes, hypertension, arthritis, and psychological problems. Obesity during infancy and childhood increases the risk of obesity in adolescence and adulthood. Children with a body mass index equal to or more than the 95th percentile are more likely to become obese adults. Obesity is considered to be multifactorial with both genetic and environmental components. Family lifestyle, stress, socioeconomic status, and maternal characteristics are some of the environmental components. Sowan and Stember (2000) studied infants until 15 months of age to identify parental characteristics and to see whether obesity was linked to any of these characteristics. Age of the mother at the time of the infant's birth was predictive of obesity in the infant at 10 months of age. The chances of obesity increased in the infant with every 5 years of age increase in the mother. For every 25 pound increase in the mother's usual weight, the chances of the infant being obese at 7 months of age increased. Maternal smoking increased the chances of infant obesity at 1 and 7 months of age. The usual stressors one might think could cause childhood obesity such as family stresses, socioeconomic status, and family life were found not to be significant predictors.

Faulkner (2002) studied 18 mothers of preschool children enrolled in a nutrition clinic for mothers and children in low-income households. Mothers were questioned in a 1-hour focus group as to how they defined overweight, how they thought their children became overweight, and what barriers existed in preventing and managing obesity. Interestingly, the mothers described their children as strong or solid and did not think that standardized growth charts reflected a healthy weight. As long as children were active the mothers did not consider them overweight but if they were lazy or lay around then they were considered overweight. The mothers thought that heredity and the environment determined the child's weight. In their attempts to manage their children's weight, the mothers had lots of difficulty. Food was used as a reward by some, others did not want to deny their children food, and with others, family members did not want the mother restricting the child's diet. Mothers also thought that their own obesity affected their management of their child's weight.

Prevention of obesity and development of effective programs for those who are overweight are critical to reversing the devastating long term effects. Unfortunately, there are not many effective programs available for children. Dietary management, increasing physical activity, and parental behavior management are critical ingredients in any program (Betz, 2000). Primary care providers need to include appropriate eating patterns, types of foods and amounts when talking with parents during well-child visits. Parents have a crucial role in how children's eating habits develop and how that affects their overall health and psychological well-being.

K. James (2000) introduced a school-based intervention to reduce television and video viewing and then measured body mass index (BMI) at baseline and 7 months later. The children in the intervention group had a significant decrease in BMI when compared to those in the control group. There are few studies which demonstrate significant reduction in children's weight. More innovative low or no cost programs aimed at families and children need to be developed and perhaps schools are the place for implementation.

It is imperative that adequate and appropriate health services are available to children and families to help ensure positive outcomes. A variety of health care providers, including nurse practitioners with knowledge of the needs of children, is essential for changes to occur.

Virginia Richardson

Pender's Health Promotion Model

Pender's Health Promotion Model (HPM) has been classified as a middle-range theory. The model seeks to explain and predict how the complex interaction among perceptual and environmental factors influences the health-related choices that people make. Specifically, Pender intended the focus of the model to be high-level wellness and health promotion, instead of disease prevention. The model has been used internationally as the basis for nursing research, practice, and education (Pender, 2001b, *Most frequently asked questions*).

Pender's representation of healthy behavior is deductive in that it was originally based on concepts from the Health Belief Model, Expectancy Value Theory, and Social Cognitive Theory (Pender, 1982). However, the model is also inductively formulated because over time Pender has made modifications based on research findings. Since her first published model in 1982, Pender has made two major revisions to her model resulting in a 1987 version and a 1996 version. Changes were based on research that supported using fewer variables with more direct and indirect relationships.

The assumptions of the Health Belief Model stress the interactive nature of client and environment. They include:

1. People desire conditions that facilitate the expression of their individual potential.
2. People have the capacity for self-awareness.
3. People value positive growth, and attempt to balance change and stability.
4. There is a natural human desire to control one's own behavior.
5. Humans both change their environment and are changed by it.
6. As part of the environment, health care workers influence others.
7. Lasting behavior modification is based on self-initiated change (Pender, Murdaugh, & Parsons, 2002).

The theoretical propositions of the revised HPM state that characteristics and beliefs of an individual will influence the person's level of commitment and likelihood of demonstrating the health promotion behavior. The HPM consists of nine groups of interrelated variables. Some of the variables that are proposed to indirectly and directly influence one's commitment to a healthy plan of action are past behavior and personal characteristics, positive emotions, perceived self-efficacy, perceived benefits and barriers, expectations of others, environment, and competing demands (Pender et al., 2002).

In Pender's conceptual map (1996) related variables are clustered together and separated into three main categories. The antecedents to action are the Individual Characteristics and Experiences, which include variables that have been determined by past experiences, genetics, or biopsychosocial influence. The majority of the other variables that are based on beliefs and outside influences are fused together under the heading Behavior Specific Cognitions and Affect. Both of these groupings are related to the last cluster of variables termed the "behavioral outcome." The desired outcome is the health promotion behavior, which is influenced by competing demands and making a commitment to changing behavior.

Pender's HPM has been used in research, clinical practice, and nursing education. Dozens of published nursing articles have used the model as a theoretical framework. Research based on the HPM covers a variety of clinical applications such as the use of hearing protection, smoking cessation, exercise, sexual behaviors and contraceptive use, dietary goals and cholesterol levels, use of seat belts, job strain/absenteeism/productivity, and stress reduction. Nursing implications derived from the HPM research offer specific nursing interventions that can be readily used in clinical practice. Information about how to promote healthy choices and lasting behavior modification is valuable to both health care professionals and the public. Pender has also published an article specifically outlining health promotion recommendations for BSN, MSN, and PhD nursing curricula (Pender, Barkauskas, Hayman, Rice, & Anderson, 1992).

The HPM offers a high degree of generalizability to many diverse groups of people. Pender has consulted internationally in such countries as Japan, Korea, Dominican Republic, Jamaica, England, New Zealand, and Mexico (Pender, 2001a, *Biographical sketch*). Currently the HPM is available in English, Spanish, Japanese, and Korean translations (Pender). Research based on the model has tested both males and females at all ages from preschool children to older adults. Research participants have been from a variety of settings including inpatient, outpatient, primary care, and community dwellings. Most importantly, the research based on the HPM has not been limited to healthy subjects. Some populations that have been studied have included people diagnosed with CAD, HIV, asthma, cancer, hypertension, cognitive disorders, and chronic disease.

Past critiques of the model have suggested that Pender needs to further clarify interactions among the variables (Tillett, 1994). In her most recent revision, she has clustered and labeled the variables differently in order to specify relationships. The HPM may also be inappropriate when nurses are interacting with clients who are cognitively impaired or unable to communicate. Examples would include infants or individuals with severe neurological deficits. Overall, the predictive power of the model will always be limited by the inherent uniqueness and variation of each human's behavior.

Strengths of the HPM include its use of concepts that are logical and basic, its generalizability, and its usefulness in research and clinical practice. Pender's model also addresses the barriers to action that are important areas to focus nursing intervention. Lastly, Pender has taken a truly holistic approach, considering sociocultural, psychological, and biological variables. The content of the HPM model is consistent with contemporary beliefs that health promotion is a national and international priority and a cost-effective alternative to sick care.

CARYN A. SHEEHAN

Peplau's Theoretical Model

Hildegard Peplau (1909–1999) formulated her theoretical ideas about the therapeutic process of nursing in the 1940s and published them in the now-classic 1952 book, *Interpersonal Relations in Nursing*, after a lengthy dispute with publishers about the ability of a nurse to author a book. At a time when nurses were "doers" for patients and "followers" of physicians' orders, Peplau's theoretical work and teachings helped catapult nursing from an occupation to a profession. Peplau's ideas provided a foundation for nurses to understand health from a nursing theoretical perspective and to establish interpersonal relationships with patients as the significant context in which nurses facilitate patients' well-being.

Through Peplau's therapeutic relationship, the patient develops inner resources for healthy behaviors by actively participating with the nurse in a developmental process of change. Peplau's interpersonal relationship is also a process through which nursing knowledge is developed and validated (Reed, 1996b). Peplau (1992) purposefully linked her theory to practice and research, as evidenced in her basic assumption that "what goes on between people can be noticed, studied, explained, understood, and, if detrimental, changed" (p. 14).

Peplau's theoretical model derives from the perspective of a critical philosophy that integrates both the science and practice of nursing in theory development. Peplau's theoretical model was based upon her study, observation, and analyses of nurses and patients and was influenced by Harry Stack Sullivan and others' psychodynamic perspectives. Peplau's (1952) classic descriptions of nursing express the nature and goals of the interpersonal process: "Nursing is a human relationship between an individual who is sick or in need of health services, and a nurse especially educated to recognize and to respond to the need for help" (pp. 5–6). Nursing is an "educative instrument, a maturing force, that aims to promote forward movement of personality in the direction of creative, constructive, productive, personal, and community living" (p. 16). Peplau (1988) further described nursing as an "enabling, empowering, or transforming art" (p. 9). Health, according to Peplau (1952), is a "word symbol that implies forward movement of personality and other ongoing human processes in the direction of creative, constructive, productive, personal and community living" (p. 12). Illness forces a "stock-taking by the sick person, which nurses can use to promote learning, growth and improved competencies for living" (Peplau, 1992, p. 13). Health and illness are closely linked to successful management of anxiety, which ranges from pure euphoria to pure anxiety. An optimal level lies between these anxiety extremes, as determined by nurse and patient.

Through the therapeutic relationship, the nurse uses a complex set of strategies to assist the patient in using energy provided by the anxiety to identify and grow from a problematic situation (O'Toole & Welt, 1989; Reed, 2005). The nurse-patient relationship is fundamental to providing nursing care and derives from the human need for connectedness that is still essential in the 21st century (Peplau, 1997). Through this interpersonal relationship, nurses assess and assist people to: (a) achieve healthy levels of anxiety intrapersonally and (b) facilitate healthy pattern integrations interpersonally, with the overall goal of fostering well-being, health, and development. This relationship also provides the context for the nurse to develop, apply, and evaluate theory-based knowledge for nursing care. Nurse interpersonal competencies, investigative skill, and theoretical knowledge as well as patient characteristics and needs are all important dimensions in the process and outcomes of the relationship (Peplau).

The structure of the interpersonal relationship was originally described in terms of four phases: orientation, identification, exploitation, and resolution (Peplau, 1952). Forchuk (1991), with the support of Peplau, clarified the structure as consisting of three main phases: orientation, working (which incorporated identification and exploitation), and termination. In a 1997 publication, Peplau endorsed this three-phase view and explained that the phases were overlapping, each having unique characteristics. Throughout these phases the nurse functions cooperatively with the patient in the nursing roles of stranger, resource person, counselor, leader, surrogate, and teacher. The nurse's range of focus includes the patient in relationship with the family, other health care providers, and community (Peplau, 1952, 1997).

The orientation phase marks a first step in the personal growth of the patient and is initiated when the patient has a "felt need" and seeks professional assistance (Peplau, 1952, p. 18). The nurse focuses on "knowing the patient as a person" and uncovering erroneous preconceptions, as well as gathering information about the patient's mental health problem (Peplau, 1997). The nurse and patient collaborate on a plan, with consideration of the patient's educative needs. Throughout the process, the nurse recognizes that the power to accomplish the tasks at hand resides within the patient and is facilitated through the workings of therapeutic relationship.

The focus of the working phase is on: (a) the patient's efforts to acquire and employ knowledge about the illness, available resources, and personal strengths, and (b) the nurse's enactment of the roles of resource person, counselor, surrogate, and teacher in facilitating the patient's development toward well-being (Peplau, 1952, 1997). The relationship is flexible enough for the patient to function dependently, independently, or interdependently with the nurse, based on the patient's developmental capacity, level of anxiety, self-awareness, and needs.

Termination is the final phase in the process of the therapeutic interpersonal relationship. Patients move beyond the initial identification with the nurse and engage their own strengths to foster health outside the therapeutic relationship (Peplau, 1952, 1988). In addition to addressing closure issues, the nurse and patient engage in planning for discharge and potential needs for transitional care (Peplau, 1997).

Peplau's theoretical model can be categorized as a middle-range theory. It is narrower in scope than a conceptual model or grand theory and addresses a clearly defined number of measurable concepts (e.g., therapeutic relationship, anxiety). The theory has a specific focus on the characteristics and process of the therapeutic relationship as a nursing method to help manage anxiety and foster healthy development. As such, the model is directly applicable to research and practice.

Peplau was explicit in promoting research-based theory. Research based on Peplau's theoretical model has addressed topics related to both nurse behaviors and patient health conditions. Nurse-focused topics include: (a) the practices of psychiatric mental-health nurses, (b) family systems nursing, and (c) the nature of the nurse-patient relationship in reference to roles and role changes over the trajectory of a mental illness, boundary issues in pediatric nursing, and concepts such as therapeutic intimacy. Patient-focused research has addressed health conditions including depression, psychosis, sexual abuse, Alzheimer's disease, and multiple sclerosis. A particularly notable Peplau-based researcher is Forchuk (e.g., Forchuk, 1994; Forchuk et al., 1998; Forchuck, Jewell, Tweedell, & Steinnagel, 2003) who, along with colleagues, has conducted a program of research into applications of the interpersonal relationship process in psychiatric mental-health nursing care.

Peplau's model is historically significant for practice in that it propelled psychiatric nursing from custodial-based care to interpersonal relationship theory-based care. Peplau is considered the founder of professional psychiatric mental-health nursing and was the first to initiate an area of advanced practice nursing. Her theoretical ideas continue to be significant in contemporary nursing for their relevance in not only psychiatric mental-health nursing practice but practice anywhere a nurse-patient relationship exists. Applications of the model are found in individual psychotherapy, reminiscence therapy, terminal illness care, and group and family therapy. Practices based upon Peplau's theory range from hospital to community and home-based.

Peplau's theory has provided an enduring educational foundation for teaching the nurse-patient relationship as a pivotal nursing process in all contexts of practice. A common philosophy underlying all nursing curricula is a belief in the value of a therapeutic nurse-patient relationship that promotes active participation of patients in their health care. Peplau's theoretical work has also promoted a "paradigm of professionalization" and empowerment for educating nurses for the 21st century (Sills, 1998).

Peplau's theoretical model continues to influence nursing research, practice, and education (O'Toole & Welt, 1989), although her original contributions have become knowledge in the public domain and are not always explicitly acknowledged. Internationally, nurses are recognizing Peplau's legacy and the enduring relevance of her theory for nursing in the new millennium (e.g., Barker [2000]). The clinical significance of the therapeutic relationship is likely to increase as health problems shift to those related to stress-related conditions, chronic illness, aging processes, and end of life, where medical-surgical approaches alone have little success in promoting well-being. Peplau's interpersonal relationship theory is expected to withstand the current health care crisis and provide a cost-effective and satisfying resource for patient well-being across a variety of nursing contexts.

The reawakening of nursing by Peplau's ideas in the 1950s continues today through exploration, study, and use of the science-based practice of interpersonal relations theory. Beeber's (1998) research and theory development have extended Peplau's model in important ways, using aesthetic knowing to elaborate on the concept of interpersonal pattern and formalizing Peplau's (1997) idea of transitions in a practice theory of depression. Metatheoretical writings of Peden (1998) and Reed (1996a), inspired by Peplau's practice-based strategy of theory development, portend an emerging philosophy of nursing science that sanctions clinicians as well as traditional researchers as knowledge-builders. Through the creative scholarship of nurses, Peplau's theoretical model can continue to evolve and inspire development of nurse-patient processes that meet contemporary health needs of society.

Pamela G. Reed
Nelma B. Shearer

Pet Therapy

Pet therapy (use of a companion animal to benefit the health of humans) has become a very popular intervention for a variety of clients, and many nurses as well as pet owners have become involved in its delivery. While at the intuitive level pet therapy appears to be beneficial, there are relatively few scientific studies to support its effectiveness. This growing body of research on pet therapy has largely been generated by multidisciplinary scholars, of which nurses have been active participants.

In general, the research on pet therapy generated by nurses falls into three distinct categories: research on the bio-physiological effects of pet therapy; research on the effects of companion animals in alleviating the distress of children undergoing painful procedures; and research on the effectiveness of companion animals for the elderly. This review is divided into these three categories. Studies are included if at least one of the authors is a nurse.

One of the earliest studies that demonstrated the health benefits of companion animals was coauthored by a nurse, Sue Ann Thomas (Friedmann, Katcher, Lynch, & Thomas, 1980). A group of patients who had been admitted to either coronary care or intensive care units with diagnoses of myocardial infarction or angina pectoris were followed for 1 year after discharge. At one year, 28% of the patients who did not own pets had died, but only 6% of the pet owners had died. Caring for the animal was not a factor in the survival rate, and pet ownership was correlated with survival but not with the physiological severity of the disease. Thomas also coauthored a subsequent study that demonstrated that the presence of a friendly animal could modify children's perceptions of an experimental situation and result in lower blood pressures while the children were resting and while they were reading (Friedmann, Katcher, Thomas, Lynch, & Messent, 1983).

The first controlled trial of the effect of interaction with a companion dog on blood pressure was published in *Nursing Research* in 1984 (Baun, Bergstrom, Langston, & Thomas, 1984). Prior to this time, several investigators outside of nursing had released findings from non-experimental observations that seemed to indicate that petting a dog could lower blood pressure, but these studies were never published as scientific journal articles. Thus, the *Nursing Research* article became a landmark study in the fledgling field of the human-animal bond. The study used a within subject, repeated measures design to measure blood pressure (systolic, diastolic, and mean), heart rate, and respiratory rate across three protocols (interacting with a dog to whom the subject was attached, interacting with an unknown [control] dog, and reading quietly). There was a statistically significant difference among the three protocols. Interaction with a known dog resulted in greater decreases in BP than either interacting with the control dog, or reading quietly. This study was the first to suggest that attachment to the animal played an integral role the in the human's physiological responses to that animal. Subsequent nursing studies on hypertensives (Schuelke et al., 1991) and other subjects (Oetting, Baun, Bergstrom, & Langston, 1985) confirmed these findings.

Children and animals seem drawn to each other and several studies have explored the benefits of this relationship in the clinical setting. In a study of the effects of the presence of a companion animal on physiological arousal and behavioral distress exhibited by preschool children during a routine physical examination, a within subject, time series design was used to study healthy children during two physical examinations, with and without a dog present, conducted in a behavioral laboratory (Nagengast, Baun, Megel, & Leibowitz, 1997). Statistically significant differences were found with greater reductions in subjects' systolic and mean arterial pressure, heart rate, and behavioral distress when a dog was present.

A follow-up study was conducted on preschool children attending a pediatric clinic using a two-group, repeated measures design, in which the experimental group had a therapy dog present during their pediatric examination and the control group did not have the dog present (Hansen, Messinger, Baun, & Megel, 1999). Physiological measures of blood pressure and finger temperature were not statistically significantly different between the dog and no-dog groups but were found not to be good measures of physiologic arousal in this age group. Behavioral distress was statistically significantly less in the dog group versus the no-dog group. These findings replicated those of Nagengast and colleagues (1997) and suggested that companion animals may be useful in a variety of health care settings to decrease procedure-induced distress in children.

A third study evaluated the effectiveness of a companion animal on physiologic arousal and behavioral distress among children undergoing a dental procedure (Havener et al., 2001). A two-group, repeated measures experimental design was used to study school age children undergoing procedures in a pediatric dental children. Half the children had the dog present during the procedure and half did not. Children who initially verbalized distress on arrival at the clinic had decreased physiologic arousal during the time the child was on the dental table waiting for the dentist to arrive. Both of these studies demonstrated that a therapy dog could be used in clinical settings to alleviate procedural distress in children.

The majority of studies of the benefits of companion animals have been conducted with the institutionalized elderly, both cognitively intact and cognitively impaired. One of the earliest landmark studies was conducted by nurses in the Veterans Administration system (Robb, Boyd, & Pristash, 1980). At different times a wine bottle, a plant, or a caged dog were placed in the day room of a long-term care division and socially interactive behaviors were measured. Of the three stimulus objects, the caged puppy produced the most dramatic increase in social behavior.

Two early studies addressed the effect of a dog on social interaction among nursing home residents, one on cognitively intact residents (Buelt, Bergstrom, Baun, & Langston, 1985) and the second on cognitively impaired residents (McArthur, Brunmeier, Bergstrom, & Baun, 1986). Within subject, repeated measures designs were used in both studies to measure socially interactive behaviors, which increased in the presence of a dog although the majority of the behaviors were directed at the dog.

Caged birds were placed in the rooms of elderly residents of skilled rehabilitation units, and before and after measures of depression, loneliness, and morale were completed on admission and after 10 days (Jessen, Cardiello, & Baun, 1997). The experimental group (bird) had a significant decrease in depression but not in morale or loneliness compared to the control group (no bird). Results of this study supported the use of companion animals other than dogs to lessen the negative effects of hospitalization in institutionalized elderly.

The use of a therapy dog with persons with Alzheimer's disease (AD) has resulted in increased socialization (Batson, McCabe, Baun, & Wilson, 1998; Churchill, Safaoui, McCabe, & Baun, 1999), improved social behaviors (Kongable, Stolley, & Buckwalter, 1990) and decreased agitation (Churchill et al.). When a resident dog was introduced on an AD special care unit, the number of problem behaviors decreased and remained decreased across the entire 4 weeks of the study (McCabe, Baun, Speich, & Agrawal, 2002). Residents of AD special care units increased nutritional intake, which continued over 6 weeks when aquariums were introduced in the dining rooms. This increased nutritional intake resulted in increased weight gain among the residents (Edwards & Beck, 2002).

From the studies cited above it is clear that quantity of research on the health benefits of companion animals has increased steadily and that nurses have been active investigators in a multidisciplinary field. Published studies on human-animal interactions generally have had significant findings and support the use of animals to benefit the health of humans. Thus, there is some support for pet therapy, although a lot more research on the health benefits of companion animals still needs to be conducted.

MARA M. BAUN

Phenomenology

Phenomenology refers to both a philosophical movement and a research method. The philosophical underpinnings of phenomenology are first summarized to provide a backdrop for what this methodology aims to accomplish. One of the philosophical tenets of phenomenology is intentionality, which refers to the inseparable connectedness of human beings to the world (Husserl, 1962). Subject and object are united in being in the world. One cannot describe either the subjective or objective world but only the world as experienced by the subject (Merleau-Ponty, 1964). The observer is not separate from the observed. One can know what one experiences only by attending to perceptions and meanings that awaken conscious awareness. Phenomenologists hold that human existence is meaningful only in the sense that persons are always conscious of something. Meaning emerges from the relationship between the person and the world as the person gives meaning to experiences. Phenomenology focuses on lived experience, that is, human involvement in the world.

Perception is one's original awareness of the appearance of a phenomenon in experience (Merleau-Ponty, 1962). In phenomenology the process of recovering our original awareness is called reduction. Through phenomenological reduction one refrains from preconceived notions and judgments. Schutz (1973) described reduction as a process that is completed in degrees. Little by little, one's layers of preconceived meaning and interpretation are peeled away, leaving the perceived world. The layers of meaning provided by a researcher's knowledge and interpretation are preserved by being temporarily set aside—that is, bracketing. Through phenomenological reduction the world of everyday experience becomes accessible.

Edmund Husserl is considered the father of phenomenology. His is a descriptive phenomenology. He was interested in the epistemological question, How do we know about man? The goal of his phenomenology is the description of the lived world. Husserl's student, Martin Heidegger, took phenomenology in a different direction. Heidegger (1962) was more interested in the ontological question, What is being? The goal of his phenomenology, called hermeneutic phenomenology, was understanding. This understanding is achieved through interpretation. Heidegger argued that it was not possible to bracket one's being-in-the-world.

The phenomenological philosophies of Husserl and Heidegger have different methodological implications for nurse researchers. Husserlian phenomenology focuses on the analysis of the subject and object as the object appears through consciousness. Bracketing is essential in this descriptive phenomenology. In Heideggerian phenomenology, bracketing is not used because this phenomenology views people as being in the world. This notion of being-in-the-world allows researchers to bring their experiences and understanding of the phenomenon under study to the research.

As a research method, phenomenology is inductive and descriptive. Phenomenology provides a closer fit conceptually with clinical nursing and with the kinds of research questions that emerge from clinical practice than does quantitative research. The goal of phenomenological research is to describe the meaning of human experience (Merleau-Ponty, 1964). In its focus on meaning, phenomenology differs from other types of research, which may, for example, focus on statistical relationships among variables. Phenomenology tries to discover meanings as persons live them in their everyday world. It is the study of essences, that is, the grasp of the very nature of something (Merleau-Ponty, 1962). Essence makes a thing what it is; without it, the thing would not be what it is. The phenomenological approach is most appropriate when little is known about a phenomenon or when a fresh look at a phenomenon is indicated.

As a research method, there are various interpretations of the phenomenological method available, from which nurse researchers may choose. Examples of descriptive phenomenology include Van Kaam's (1966), Colaizzi's (1978), and Giorgi's (1985) approaches. Van Manen's (1990) method is a type of hermeneutic phenomenology. Specific examples of how these different methods were used in nursing research are provided.

Van Kaam's (1966) phenomenological method of analysis was used by C. T. Beck

(1992a) in exploring the meaning of nursing students' caring with physically/mentally handicapped children. The 36 nursing students' written descriptions of their caring experiences yielded 199 descriptive expressions related to the phenomenon under study. The next step in Van Kaam's method focuses on grouping these descriptive expressions into "necessary constituents," which are moments of the experience expressed either implicitly or explicitly in the majority of the participants' descriptions.

The following six necessary constituents of a caring experience between a nursing student and an exceptional child were revealed: authentic presencing, physical connectedness, reciprocal sharing, delightful merriment, bolstered self-esteem, and unanticipated self-transformation. In the final step in Van Kaam's (1966) analysis the necessary constituents are synthesized into one description of the experience being studied. In Beck's (1992a) study this description of caring between a nursing student and an exceptional child was as follows: "an interweaving of authentic presencing with physical connectedness and reciprocal sharing overflowing into delightful merriment, bolstered self-esteem, and an unanticipated self-transformation" (pp. 3–4).

An example of Colaizzi's (1978) phenomenological method is found in Beck's (1992b) study of the lived experience of postpartum depression. After reading and rereading the transcriptions of interviews with seven mothers, 45 significant statements that directly pertained to postpartum depression were extracted. Meanings were then formulated from each of these significant statements. Next in Colaizzi's method is the clustering of these formulated meanings into themes. Eleven themes describing mothers' experiences of postpartum depression emerged. These themes captured the women's unbearable loneliness, uncontrollable anxiety attacks and obsessive thoughts, haunting fear that their lives would never return to normal, consuming guilt, inability to concentrate, loss of control of their emotions, insecurity, lack of positive emotions and previous interests, and contemplating death. Finally, these 11 theme clusters were integrated into an exhaustive description of the experience of postpartum depression.

Bennett (1991) used Giorgi's (1985) method of phenomenological analysis to uncover the meaning of adolescent girls' experience of witnessing marital violence. Interviews with five adolescent girls who had grown up in violent homes were read and reread to identify what Giorgi labeled as "meaning units." These units were segments of the interviews that revealed some aspect of the phenomenon under study. These meaning units were then transformed into statements that expressed implicit or explicit meaning. Next, the transformed meaning units were synthesized into a summary of each adolescent's experience of witnessing physical violence directed toward her mother by her father. Giorgi refers to this synthesis as the "situated level description." The final phase of Giorgi's analysis called for an integration of each of these individual descriptions into one "general level description" that was composed of shared themes and meanings. Bennett's general level description of violence experienced included the following seven themes: (a) remembering, (b) living from day to day, (c) feeling the impact, (d) escaping, (e) understanding, (f) coping, and (g) resolving or settling.

Lauterback (1993) used Van Manen's (1990) method of "doing" phenomenology to study the meaning of mothers' experiences of the perinatal death of wished-for babies. The following four concurrent procedural activities in Van Manen's method were incorporated in this study: turning to the nature of lived experience, existential investigation, phenomenological reflection, and phenomenological writing. Data analysis and interpretation of the data yielded the discovery of the essences in meaning of mothers' experiences. These essential themes included (a) the essence of perinatal loss; (b) reflective pulling back, recovering, reentering; (c) embodiment of mourning loss; (d) the narcissistic inquiry; (e) the finality of death of the body; (f) living through and "with" death; (g) altering worldviews; (h) death overlaid with life; and (i) falling and trying again.

Diverse clinical specialties of nursing such as maternal-child, gerontological, and medical-surgical nursing provide fertile ground for phenomenological research. These studies illustrate the breadth of applicability of this qualitative research method for nursing.

CHERYL TATANO BECK

Philosophy of Nursing

A philosophy of nursing lays the essential foundation for nursing knowledge. Whether explicitly articulated or just implied, all nursing knowledge begins and ends with a philosophy of nursing. A philosophy of nursing is important because it represents the values, visions, and convictions of nurses about what ought to be nursing's central phenomena, that is, those phenomena that are both necessary and sufficient to provide a viable framework for the discipline and practice of nursing (Silva, 1997). Therefore, to generate nursing knowledge, nurses must understand what are considered to be nursing's central phenomena. To better understand the underpinnings of nursing's central phenomena, nurses must turn to the relationship between philosophy and philosophy of nursing.

Philosophy is a specific discipline that deals with ultimate or first-cause questions and phenomena that transcend other disciplines and cannot be answered by science or scientific investigation, for example, what is reality? Like philosophy, nursing is viewed as a specific discipline; thus, a philosophy of nursing should address big or ultimate questions about nursing and its phenomena. Examples follow:

What ought to be the basic phenomena of the discipline of nursing?

What are the metaphysical and ontological claims that underlie the phenomena of the discipline of nursing?

What are the moral claims that underlie the phenomena of the discipline of nursing?

What are the aesthetic claims that underlie the phenomena of the discipline of nursing?

How can the basic phenomena of the discipline of nursing be known?

How should the basic phenomena of the discipline of nursing articulate with basic phenomena of other human, helping-service disciplines?

As health care professionals living in the 21st century, distinct disciplinary boundaries are blurring rapidly and more interdisciplinary fields are emerging. As this trend continues, so too will the questions that constitute the essence of nursing philosophy. In summary, the preceding questions raised about nursing have metaphysical, ontological, moral, and aesthetic claims that emerge from philosophy but manifest themselves in phenomena related to nursing and ultimately to nursing philosophy.

As a philosopher, Rescher (2001) believes that human beings have an innate curiosity "rooted in the need-to-know" (p. 6) answers to life's questions. To get at these answers, Rescher advocates philosophical inquiry as a methodology; this methodology includes a systematic process of "constructing a doctrinal system that answers . . . [life's] questions in a coherent and comprehensive way" (p. 1). But, according to Rescher, there is more: philosophers not only must deal with the estimation of truth that involves errors of omission and/or commission but also must discern what constitutes "the data of philosophy" (p. 15).

Philosophical inquiry in nursing is one approach to advancing nursing knowledge. It follows the same method of philosophizing as described previously by Rescher (2001) but applies the method to substantive philosophical questions in nursing. The goal is coherent and comprehensive answers to nursing's philosophical questions (e.g., Jacobs, B. B., 2001; Jones, T., 2003; Newman, 2002) with the best-fit estimation of truth (e.g., Pilkington & Mitchell, 2003). Like philosophical inquiry in philosophy, nurses who conduct philosophical inquiry in nursing must discern what constitutes the data of nursing.

Philosophy is not science, and nursing philosophy is not nursing science. But philosophy is the foundation of science, and nursing philosophy is the foundation of both nursing science (i.e., the body of nursing's scientific knowledge) and nursing research (e.g., the process of obtaining not only nursing's body of scientific knowledge but also the process of obtaining knowledge derived from scholarly critical analyses).

Implicit in nursing research are assumptions about human beings (i.e., study subjects or participants), about selected phenomena of the discipline (e.g., variables), and about how the selected phenomena can be known (i.e., the research method). In addition, in qualitative research the meaning or artistry of the selected phenomena is often addressed (e.g., hermeneutics, photography). Finally, regardless of whether the research is quantitative, qualitative, and/or scholarly critical analysis, it must be ethical. Thus, all research grounded in nursing contains explicit or implicit philosophies of nursing that determine research approaches.

Future directions about philosophies of nursing and about nurses and nurse researchers include the following: (a) nurses need greater knowledge about and appreciation for the discipline of philosophy; (b) nurse researchers must interact regularly with nurse philosophers to grasp more fully that a philosophy of nursing provides a foundation for nursing science and other nursing knowledge; (c) nurses must commit themselves in greater numbers to philosophical inquiry as a legitimate method of obtaining nursing knowledge; and (d) nurses must prepare themselves for the blurring of distinct disciplinary boundaries as more interdisciplinary fields emerge.

MARY CIPRIANO SILVA

Physical Restraints

A physical restraint is any device or object attached to or adjacent to a person's body that cannot be removed easily and restricts freedom of movement. Bilateral full-length siderails and some types of furniture are also considered restraints when used to limit movement. Although this entry focuses mainly on physical restraints, it is important to keep in mind that these devices are often used in conjunction with psychopharmacologic drugs. When such drugs are given for the purposes of discipline or convenience and are not required to treat specific medical or psychiatric conditions, they are considered chemical restraints.

The prevalence of physical restraints in non-psychiatric settings, estimated in 1989 to affect 500,000 elderly persons daily in hospitals and nursing homes, led many to conclude that a restraint crisis existed. High prevalence in the United States was sharply contrasted with what at the time appeared to be lesser use in several countries in Western Europe. The historical antecedents for these differences appeared related to American beliefs that were embedded by the end of the 19th century: restraint use was therapeutically sound, necessary to control troublesome behavior, and prevented tragic accidents and injuries.

For nearly 100 years those beliefs were largely unchallenged; debate concerning the efficacy of physical restraint was limited, and alternative interventions were rarely considered. The efforts of advocacy groups and committed clinicians, change in nursing home regulation and standards for accreditation of hospitals, warnings from the Food and Drug Administration (FDA), and research demonstrating successful restraint reduction have forced a complete reexamination of their use. Although prevalence has declined in U.S. nursing homes to approximately 8.86%, restraint use and the problems associated with it remain a global concern.

Physical restraints are applied in hospitals and nursing homes primarily for three reasons: fall risk, treatment interference, and behavioral symptoms. To date, no scientific basis of support demonstrates the efficacy of restraints in safeguarding patients from injury, protecting treatment devices, or alleviating such behavioral symptoms as wandering or agitation. Several recent studies, in fact, suggest relationships between physical restraints and falls, serious injuries, or worsened cognitive function (Capezuti, Strumpf, Evans, Grisso, & Maislin, 1998).

Nevertheless, health care professionals and other caregivers see few alternatives to restraint use in some situations. Misplaced fears about legal liability, lack of interdisciplinary discussions about decisions to restrain, and staff perceptions about individual behaviors also influence restraint practices. Insufficient staffing levels and the costs of hiring additional employees have long been regarded as obstacles to minimal use of physical restraints. Hospital studies offer indirect links between staffing levels and restraint use by demonstrating that weekend days and night shifts are the most frequent times when restraints are used (Bourbonniere, Strumpf, Evans, & Maislin, 2001; Whitman, Davidson, Sereika, & Rudy, 2001). Several reports of restraint reduction in nursing homes and one clinical trial show that prevalence of physical restraints can be significantly reduced without increasing serious injuries or hiring more staff (Evans, L. K., et al., 1997). Data show that caring for nursing home residents without restraints is less costly than caring for residents who are restrained (Phillips, C. D., Hawes, & Fries, 1993).

Hospitals and nursing homes often do not have personnel with expertise in aging or with the requisite skills for assessing and treating clinical problems specific to older adults. Studies provide promising evidence that a model of care using advanced practice nurses specializing in geriatrics can reduce restraint use in nursing homes and hospitals through staff education and consultation (Evans, L. K., et al., 1997; Sullivan-Marx, Strumpf, Evans, Capezuti, & Maislin, under review).

Continued use of physical restraints is paradoxical in view of mounting knowledge about their considerable ability to do harm. Physical restraints are known to reduce functional capacity and exert physical and psychological effects (Castle & Mor, 1998; Evans, L. K., & Strumpf, 1989). Furthermore, restraint use can lead to accidental death by asphyxiation (Miles, S. H., & Irvine, 1992). Persons who are likely to be restrained are usually those of advanced age who are physically and mentally frail, prone to injury and confusion, and experiencing invasive treatments. The evidence is compelling that prolonged physical restraint further contributes to frailty and dysfunction.

Restraint-free care can be accomplished through implementation of a range of alternative approaches to assessment, prevention, and response to the behaviors routinely leading to restraint. For such practices, however, changes in fundamental philosophy and attitudes among institutions and caregivers must occur. In settings where restraints have been reduced, there is strong emphasis on individualized, person-centered care; normal risk taking; rehabilitation and choice; interdisciplinary team practice; environmental features that support independent, safe functioning; involvement of family and community; and administrative and caregiver sanction and support for change. The presence of professional expertise, particularly expert nurses and physicians with education and skill in geriatrics, is crucial for sustained cultural change.

Although legislation and other forms of external regulation or control do not in and of themselves change beliefs or entirely alter entrenched practice, the Nursing Home Reform Act, part of the Omnibus Budget Reconciliation Act (OBRA) of 1987 (enacted in 1990), helped to raise standards in nursing homes. The FDA, in response to the known risks of physical restraints and reports of restraint-related deaths, mandates that all devices carry a warning label concerning potential hazards.

Following a decade of emphasis on restraint reduction/elimination in nursing homes, clinicians, researchers, and regulators have recently focused attention on these practices in acute care settings. As with nursing homes, the Joint Commission on Accreditation of Healthcare Organizations and the Centers for Medicare and Medicaid Services define restraint use as both physical and chemical. Standards mandate that restraints be used only to improve well-being in cases where less restrictive measures have failed to protect the patient or others from harm. In addition, continual individualized assessment and reevaluation of the patient by clinicians and consultation with the patient's own provider must occur with restraint use. Direct care staff must also be trained in proper and safe use of restraining devices.

Current approaches to restraint reduction vary along a continuum from promotion of restraint-free care to an attitude of tolerance for restraint use under certain circumstances. To some extent, successful reduction of physical and chemical restraints in nursing homes underscores the need to achieve the same changes in hospitals, where a disproportionately high incidence of iatrogenesis occurs, much of it exacerbated by the use of physical restraints and adverse reactions to psychoactive drugs. The resulting complications—especially delirium, pressure ulcers, infections, and fall-related serious injuries—can add dramatically to the cost of care by contributing to further loss of function.

Although professional organizations in nursing and medicine have endorsed nonuse of physical restraints and appropriate use of psychoactive drugs as the standard of care in all health care settings, the intensity of debate surrounding physical restraint use in hospitals has escalated (Maccioli et al., 2003). Clinicians caring for specialty populations, such as those found in critical care, trauma, neurology and neurosurgery, and hematology/oncology, are confronted with the need to identify, test, and implement interventions that reduce reliance on physical restraints. A standard of least restrictive care will challenge professional caregivers to use comprehensive assessment to make sense of individual behaviors and to employ a range of interventions that enhance physical, psychological, and social function, as well as to acknowledge and affirm the uniqueness and dignity of the older person.

MEG BOURBONNIERE
NEVILLE E. STRUMPF
LOIS K. EVANS

Physiological Monitoring

Physiological monitoring is used by nurse scientists to measure biological functioning in living organisms. Generally, it refers to data collected through an interface of technological instrumentation with a living organism. Technological instrumentation can be relatively simple, such as a thermometer, or as complex as combined hemodynamic and clinical laboratory instrumentation used to measure oxygen utilization in the critically ill patient. Physiological monitoring is used to examine both normative functions (e.g., homeostasis) and disordered responses (e.g., illness and related manifestations). Physiological monitoring occurs in vivo and in vitro, among animal models, in laboratory settings, and in clinical practice areas. Information about physiological parameters promotes understanding about the phenomena with which nurses are concerned: health-supporting and health-restoring human responses.

A variety of physiological variables are measured by nurses: (a) electrical potentials of the brain, heart, laboring uterus, and muscle; (b) pressures in arteries, veins, lungs, mouth, esophagus, bladder, vagina, uterus, and brain; (c) sound (mechanical) waves in the ear and heart; (d) temperature and the concentration of gases in the lungs and blood; (e) physical symptoms such as size and color of bruising, stool, and wounds; and (f) serum levels of hormones, coagulation factors, and molecular proteins that influence local and systemic responses to injury, illness and infection. The most common physiological measures reported in nursing research are blood pressure, heart rate, weight, and temperature. Monitoring of physiological measures can be either direct or indirect, can be utilized continuously or at a particular point in time, and can include physical, electronic, and biochemical devices. Physiological monitoring devices are found in the acute care setting, home health care settings, and outpatient and surgical environments and offer a rich data source for clinical research.

Research by nurses using physiological monitoring has increased steadily since the

1980s (Sechrist & Pravikoff, 2002). Increased numbers of nursing scientists are prepared with a strong theoretical and experiential base for designing physiological studies. One aspect of their work has been to evaluate the accuracy, selectivity, precision, sensitivity, and error of physiological measures so that reliability and validity are supported. Another important focus of physiological monitoring has been to link physiologic responses to patient/client outcomes studies. A third and relatively new area of investigation is the examination of biomarkers, linking physiological monitoring with cellular and molecular responses to illness and interventions. Examination of changes that occur as a consequence of nursing practice has produced a broad range of research, as evidenced by the variety of physiological studies listed by CINAHL and PubMed in the past 10 years.

CHRIS WINKELMAN

Pilot Study

A pilot study is a smaller version of a proposed or planned study that is conducted to refine the methodology for a larger study. A pilot study uses subjects, settings, and methods of data collection and data analysis similar to those of a larger study.

It is recommended that all large-scale studies have either pilot work or other preliminary work as evidence of feasibility of the project and to demonstrate the competence of the investigator with the area of study. Feasibility issues that might be addressed in a pilot study include the availability of subjects and estimating the time required for recruitment of subjects, the conduct of the investigation, and the cost of the study. Particularly when planning studies with populations that may not be easily available or accessible, a pilot study is an opportunity to develop or refine sampling methods and to evaluate the representativeness of a sample.

Preliminary work in the form of a pilot study provides an opportunity to identify problems with many aspects of study design. One important design issue that can be evaluated during the pilot work is determining the number of data collection points and the optimal time between phases of data collection. Pilot work can be used to develop, test, or refine a study protocol, including the treatment or intervention to be used in an experimental or quasi-experimental study. Sufficient pilot work is necessary to support the efficacy of an intervention prior to proposal submission for a large-scale intervention study. During a pilot study extraneous variables that had not been considered in the design may become apparent, and methods to control for them can be introduced when the larger study is designed.

Pilot work also allows the development or refinement of data collection instruments, including questionnaires and equipment. The performance of instruments with a particular sample under specific conditions also can be evaluated in the pilot project. When collecting quantitative data, the reliability and validity of instruments and the ease of operation and administration can be evaluated prior to data collection in a large-scale study. This is an important step whether the data collection instruments are interview schedules, questionnaires, computers databases, or equipment to gather biophysical data. For example, during pilot work, questionnaires can be evaluated for clarity of instructions, wording of questions, reading level, and time required for completion. For qualitative studies, pilot work may be important for gaining experience in interacting with the sample and with aspects of data collection, coding, and analysis.

The results of a pilot study are likely to be significant for the larger proposed study. If the pilot study is of sufficient size, estimates about the relationships between variables and of effect sizes can be made. This is essential not only for statistical power analysis but for a better understanding of the phenomena under study. Pilot studies often provide important insights into the problem being investigated and may lead to reconceptualization of the problem or refinement of the research questions.

Carol M. Musil

Population Health

The term population health is fairly new. Current emphasis on improving health outcomes, eliminating health disparities, and reducing health care costs amplify its importance, but a single accepted definition of population health has yet to emerge. Szreter (2003) traces the origin of the concept of population health back to an historic 18th century debate over the relationship between economic growth and human health. In an article titled *Producing Health, Consuming Health Care,* R. G. Evans and Stoddart (1990) merged concepts and principles from economics and epidemiology to support the idea that health is determined by multiple factors. In 1997 in a book titled *Purchasing Population Health: Paying for Results*, Kindig defined population health as "the aggregate health outcome of health adjusted life expectancy (quantity and quality) of a group of individuals, in an economic framework that balances the relative marginal returns from multiple determinants of health" (p. 47). Kindig's definition proposed a unit of measure for population health and underscored a relationship between economics and health.

In 2001, two models for implementing population health were published, one in Canada and the other in the United States. In July 2001, Health Canada published a draft document titled *The Population Health Template: Key Elements and Actions That Define a Population Health Approach*. The publication consolidated current understandings of population health and outlined procedures and processes for implementing a population health approach. The Health Canada template defined population health as "the health of a population as measured by health status indicators and as influenced by social, economic, and physical environments, personal health practices, individual capacity and coping skills, human biology, early childhood development, and health services" (Health Canada, p. 2). The population health template also identified eight key elements of a population health approach: (1) focusing on the health of populations, (2) addressing the determinants of health and their interactions, (3) basing decisions on evidence, (4) increasing upstream investments, (5) applying multiple strategies, (6) collaborating across sectors and levels, (7) employing mechanisms for public involvement, and (8) demonstrating accountability for health outcomes (Health Canada).

The Department of Defense Tricare Management Activity (DoDTMA) published a *Population Health Improvement Plan and Guide* in December 2001. The guide adopted Kindig's definition of population health and outlined an approach to population health improvement focused on balancing awareness, education, prevention, and intervention activities to improve the health of a specified population (DoDTMA, 2001). Much like the Health Canada template, the DoDTMA guide identified several process steps for population health improvement: (a) identifying the population, (b) forecasting demand, (c) managing demand, (d) managing capacity, (e) implementing evidence-based primary, secondary, and tertiary prevention, (f) community outreach, and (g) analyzing performance and health status.

In 2003, McAlearney published a model for population health in a book titled *Population Health Management: Strategies to Improve Outcomes*. The author used the term "population health management" to describe a variety of approaches developed to foster health and quality-of-care improvements while managing costs. McAlearney outlined several major steps for implementing population health management programs: targeting the program, selecting the strategies, implementing and managing the program, and integrating critical factors.

In March of 2003, in an article titled *What is Population Health?*, Kindig and Stoddart attempted to distinguish population health from public health, health promotion, and social epidemiology. The authors also set out to determine if population health was a field of study of health determinants or a concept of health. Following a critique of existing definitions and understandings of population health dating back to the early 1990s, the authors concluded that population health is concerned with both the definition and measurement of health outcomes and the roles of determinants. Kindig and Stoddart defined population health as the health outcomes of a group, including the distribution of the outcomes within the group, and argued that the field of population health included health outcomes, patterns of determinants of health, and interventions and policies that link outcomes with determinants.

Current understandings and definitions of population health emphasize the link between multiple determinants of health and health outcomes. Population health is focused on improving the health status of populations, enhancing health care quality and access, and decreasing costs. A population health approach targets entire populations; intervenes with families, communities, systems, and individuals; recognizes and emphasizes multiple determinants of health; incorporates primary, secondary, and tertiary prevention; and includes ongoing assessment, monitoring, and improvement.

Sandra C. Garmon Bibb

Populations and Aggregates

In a very broad sense the term *population* refers to a collection of entities that have one or more characteristics in common. According to Kendall and Buckland (1960), "in statistical usage the term 'population' is applied to any infinite collection of individuals. It has displaced the older term 'universe' . . . it is practically synonymous with 'aggregate' and does not necessarily refer to a collection of living organisms" (p. 223). The conception of population is basic to an understanding of inductive or inferential statistics. Stated succinctly by Blalock (1960), "the purpose of statistical generalizations is to say something about various characteristics of the populations studied on the basis of known facts about a sample drawn from that population or universe" (p. 89). In statistics, population characteristics are called parameters and are denoted by Greek letters; sample characteristics, called statistics, are denoted by Roman letters. According to Blalock, in inductive statistics "it is the population, rather than any particular sample, in which we are really interested." As a matter of convenience, a sample is selected but the goal is "practically always to make inferences about various population parameters on the basis of known, but intrinsically unimportant sample statistics" (p. 90). The underlying foundation for making inferences from samples to the population is the mathematical theory of probability.

Within the health field, particularly in public health, the disciplines of epidemiology and biostatistics, and the nursing specialization of public health nursing, the term *population* usually refers to biological entities such as people, animals, or microorganisms that hold characteristics in common. Population has a very prominent position in epidemiology. In discussing the classical understanding of epidemiology, J. N. Morris (1964) referred to it as "the study of the health and disease of populations" (p. 4). More recently, Mausner and Kramer (1985) defined epidemiology as "the study of the distribution and determinants of diseases and injuries in human populations" (p. 1).

Historically, public health specialists such as health officers focused on populations and subpopulations as the target for planning, service programming, and evaluation efforts. Although public health nurses provided clinical services in public health programs directed to target populations such as children under 6 years or prenatal clients, predominant focus was clinical, at the level of the patient or the family. The concept of using a population or aggregate approach to the practice of public health nursing first began to be seriously discussed in the literature in the 1970s (Williams, C. A., 1977). The conceptual shift from a focus on individual patients, the thrust in the clinical preparation of nurses, to a focus on populations, which is the concern of public health, can be difficult. However, it is necessary to understand public health and the specialization of public health nursing.

Taking a population approach to decision making in health care, that is, defining problems and proposing solutions for a population or aggregate, may facilitate health services and care delivery research and the utilization of research in practice for two reasons. First, such an approach involves obtaining data on each member of the population and summarizing it in meaningful ways. Adopting strategies and methods used by nurse researchers, epidemiologists, and others who study community-based or clinical populations may be used. This process may be sufficiently systematic and rigorous to make a contribution to the research literature. Second, a population approach to decision making is highly compatible with the empirical thinking of researchers.

Researchers study samples of populations with specific characteristics. The extent to which a finding in a sample from a particular population can be predicted in another can be assessed primarily by determining the comparability between the populations. If the individuals in a clinical or community-based program were identified as a population or subpopulation, with key characteristics in common, rather than unique individuals, the program population could be compared with another studied population.

Although a population-focused approach has traditionally been central to public health practice, the spread of capitated managed care has precipitated a growing interest in the concept of populations and decision making at the population level throughout the health care industry. The population emphasis has many positive implications for health services and care delivery research and for a more systematic, rational, and data-based approach to decision making in the health care system.

CAROLYN A. WILLIAMS

Postpartum Depression

Postpartum depression (PPD) is an important women's mental health problem because of its timing, prevalence, and associated risks. PPD is believed to affect approximately 13% of women following delivery; however, when self-report depression measures are used to identify women with milder symptom levels, higher percentages are reported. According to the *Diagnostic and Statistical Manual of Mental Disorders* (DSM-IV-TR) (American Psychiatric Association, 2000), diagnostic criteria specify onset within 4 weeks postpartum. The most frequent symptoms are feelings of inadequacy, sadness, fatigue, anxiety, worry, compulsive thoughts, and diminished functioning that can occur from within 2 weeks postpartum to beyond 1 year. Women experiencing PPD can experience symptoms severe enough to require a combination of pharmacological interventions and either short- or long-term counseling and therapy and even hospitalization. Nonetheless, after a comprehensive review of PPD treatment literature, Boath and Henshaw (2001) concluded that treatment efficacy has not been clearly established, with recovery varying from 2–3 months to as long as 2 or more years.

PPD is distinguished from commonly experienced "postpartum or maternity blues" and postpartum psychosis. Postpartum blues is characterized by onset during the first 2 weeks after delivery, presence of mild depressed symptoms with typically rapid resolution, and prevalence as high as 80% in the United States. In addition, postpartum blues wane without need for intervention. Postpartum psychosis, in contrast, is a rare (1–2/1,000) and severe disorder. Symptoms may emerge as early as 1 month before delivery, and rapid postpartum onset within 4 weeks postpartum is characteristic. Hallucinations, delusions, and paranoia are hallmarks and can be associated with suicidal and homicidal ideation. Therefore, risk of harm to the infant is a major concern with psychosis and with severe PPD when cognitive distortions are present (American Psychiatric Association, 2000). A more recently identified disorder, postpartum obsessive-compulsive disorder (OCD) (Sichel & Driscoll, 1999), is not specified within the diagnostic nomenclature as a recognized postpartum syndrome. However, expert practitioners have described heightened vigilance about the possibility of harm to the baby as characteristic of postpartum OCD.

A range of risk factors have been identified with the development of PPD, including a history of depression, difficult infant temperament, marital or partner relationship problems, child care stress, low self-esteem and poor social support. Researchers have extended examination of PPD to include samples from various cultures and countries around the world. For example, a multisite study involving 892 women from nine countries was designed to compare differences in postpartum depressive symptomatology across samples at 4–6 weeks and 10–12 weeks postpartum (Affonso, De, Horowitz, Andrews, & Mayberry, 2000). Average depression scores for women from countries in which postpartum cultural traditions are practiced were significantly higher than depression scores for women from Europe, Australia, and the United States—"western" industrialized countries without such widespread rituals. In focus groups conducted in each of the countries, similar patterns of symptoms were described (Horowitz, J. A., Chang, Das, & Hayes, 2001). Fatigue and pain were common physical symptoms, with irritability, anxiety, loneliness, worrying, indecisiveness, and poor concentration being emotional and cognitive symptoms. Role and relationship conflicts were described within the context of cultural variations. These findings demonstrate that additional research is needed to explore postpartum cross-cultural adjustment problems and to test strategies for relieving distressing symptoms. Furthermore, a growing body of literature indicates that PPD affects women around the world and challenges earlier assumptions that PPD is a culturally based syndrome primarily associated with westernized countries without widespread postpartum traditions (Affonso et al., 2000; Posmontier & Horowitz, 2004).

PPD disrupts maternal-infant interactions and children's cognitive and emotional development. Withdrawn, disengaged, and intrusive maternal behavior patterns may result in fussy, aggressive, less affectionate, and less responsive infants. Reduced vocalization and slower neurological growth and motor skill development have been documented among infants of depressed mothers (Abrams, Field, Scafidi, & Prodromidis, 1995; Field, T., 1995; Tronick & Weinberg, 1997). In response to growing evidence of PPD's negative effects on infant development, investigators have begun to focus on evaluating interventions to promote improved mother-infant relationships. One clinical trial designed to test the efficacy of an interactive coaching approach delivered by a trained home visiting nurse produced promising findings (Horowitz, J. A., Bell, et al., 2001). The intervention had a positive effect on maternal-infant responsiveness among mothers. According to the nurse investigators, subsequent research is needed with diverse samples to test additional interventions to reduce negative effects of maternal depression on child development. Inclusion of partners or other family members to examine family processes related to maternal depression was also recommended (Horowitz, J. A., Bell, et al.).

Nurse investigators are also involved in testing better tools for early detection of PPD. The Postpartum Depression Screening Scale (PDSS) (Beck & Gable, 2001) is a promising, 35-item self-report instrument to identify women who are at high risk for postpartum depression. Given the importance of PPD as a clinical problem, mental health evaluation of all postpartum women should be standard care.

Recommendations for future research directions are: (a) a screening feasibility project to demonstrate ways to implement cost-effective early PPD identification; (b) clinical trials to test non-pharmacologic treatments for PPD and interventions to enhance the quality of mother-child interaction; (c) longitudinal studies to examine the course of maternal depression over time; (d) family research to explore consequences of PPD on family health and test family-oriented interventions; and (e) cross-cultural studies and inclusion of diverse samples within the United States to document prevalence rates, discern risk and protective factors, and test culturally relevant interventions.

LINDA J. MAYBERRY
JUNE ANDREWS HOROWITZ

Pregnancy

Nurses continue to conduct research in various areas related to pregnancy. Predominant areas of inquiry include nutrition/obesity/gestational weight gain, physical activity and exercise during pregnancy, the experience and symptoms of pregnancy, HIV prevention and care, preventing negative consequences of adolescent pregnancy, care during labor and birth, and health promotion.

Nutrition, obesity, and gestational weight gain can impact birth outcomes and how well a woman feels during pregnancy. Nutrition research has focused on identifying optimal nutrition during pregnancy to promote fetal growth and development while preventing excessive maternal weight gain (Bechtel-Blackwell, 2002; Wiles, 1998). Excessive weight gain during pregnancy can contribute to postpartum weight retention and long-term weight gain and later obesity (Walker, 1996). Adequate nutrition during pregnancy influences maternal weight gain. Pattern of weight gain during pregnancy is significant. Nurses have been instrumental in researching patterns of gestational weight gain associated with optimal birth outcomes.

Obesity results from an imbalance of energy. Over time, when more nutrients are consumed than burned, weight gain occurs. Over time excessive nutrient intake results in weight gain and obesity. Excessive weight gain during pregnancy, particularly over multiple pregnancies, contributes to overweight and obesity in women. Women who begin pregnancy overweight are at higher risk for increased gestational weight gain, postpartum weight retention, and complications of pregnancy, including malpresentation, arrested labor, and instrumental delivery.

Physical activity and exercise have been another predominant theme of nurse researchers who study pregnancy. While it has been known for quite some time that exercise and physical activity have benefits at every life stage, exercise research during pregnancy has expanded in recent years. This expansion is partly due to the problem of obesity and excessive weight gain during pregnancy, but also because exercise has been a useful modality in health promotion and disease prevention efforts. For example, pregnant women who exercise on a regular basis have improved birth outcomes and more energy. Recent investigations have focused on the use of exercise during pregnancy to prevent and treat hypertensive disorders and to keep weight gain within normal limits, as recommended by the Institute of Medicine (IOM) based on prepregnancy body mass index (BMI).

Symptoms of pregnancy and their relief are another focus for nurse researchers. Maloni and others have extensively investigated the symptoms of women placed on bed-rest during pregnancy (Maloni, Kane, Suen, & Wang, 2002; Maloni & Schneider, 2002; Maloni, Brezinski-Tomasi, & Johnson, 2001). Nausea and vomiting during pregnancy have also been investigated (Steele, N. M., French, Gatherer-Boyles, Newman, & Leclaire, 2001; O'Brien, Evans, & White-McDonald, 2002; Zhou, O'Brien, & Soeken, 2001). F. H. Chou, Lin, Cooney, Walker, and Riggs (2003) found that depressive symptoms were correlated with nausea and vomiting and that social support was negatively related to nausea and vomiting. Depressive symptoms were also found to be correlated with fatigue; however, the investigators did not examine which symptom appeared first. Other investigators have examined the pregnancy experience among various groups, including adolescents with a planned pregnancy (Montgomery, 2000, 2001, 2002), adolescent mothers, women with a high-risk pregnancy, women with pregnancies conceived via in vitro fertilization, women pregnant with multiples, pregnancy after previous loss, and the experiences of new fathers (Finnbogadottir, Svalenius, & Persson, 2003). In addition, pregnancy and childbirth experiences of women of various cultures have been investigated.

HIV prevention and care during pregnancy have also been investigated by nurse researchers. HIV-positive pregnant women are a diverse group. Many women discover their HIV status following conception. However, with increasing frequency women who are HIV-positive are planning to become pregnant. Nurse investigators have examined HIV-positive women's desire for pregnancy despite their HIV disease and found that women do not wish to give up the experience of motherhood and that they have a healthy focus on living life and not limiting themselves based solely on their HIV diagnosis (Sowell & Misener, 1997). Women also noted that with current medical advances their chances of having a healthy pregnancy and uninfected infant are better than ever before. HIV-positive women need a tremendous amount of support and care during pregnancy and beyond. Nurses have taken the lead in identifying the specific needs and care for this group of women.

While the rates of adolescent pregnancy have decreased in recent years and continue to decline, there are still nearly 1 million adolescents who become pregnant each year. Nurses have investigated various support and education programs to assist these young women with pregnancy and the transition to motherhood (Nuguyen, Carson, Parris, & Place, 2003). Successful programs begin during pregnancy and continue through the child's early years. The focus of these programs is health promotion and teaching, illness prevention, social support, accessing services, and networking (Koniak-Griffin et al., 2003). Nurse researchers have also examined HIV prevention among pregnant adolescents who are often at risk because they lack resources, social status, and knowledge to protect themselves (Lesser, Oakes, & Koniak-Griffin, 2003).

Nurse researchers have investigated various aspects of care during labor and birth, including labor and pushing management among women with epidural anesthesia (Mayberry, Strange, Suplee, & Gennaro, 2003), use of birth plans (Lundgren, Berg, & Lindmark, 2003), labor support by nurses and others, cultural variations in the labor and birth experience (Callister, 2004), childbirth education strategies, and pain reduction with interventions such as ice (Waters & Raisler, 2003). M. R. Sleutel (2002) developed and tested the Labor Support Scale with positive results.

Additional areas related to labor and birth that need to be examined include excessive rates of labor inductions present in many hospitals throughout the U.S., Cesarean sections on demand, implications of increased physician malpractice insurance leading to few physicians attending deliveries and how this affects nursing care, birth outcomes, and the practice of certified nurse midwives (CNMs). Complementary and alternative therapies to relieve labor pain also warrant additional research by nurses.

Pregnancy is one of the few instances in which health promotion efforts can have a direct and immediate impact. Various nurse researchers have investigated health promotion during pregnancy in both a general sense of health promotion behaviors and specific behaviors, such as nutrition in pregnant adolescents (Symon & Wrieden, 2003), physical activity, smoking cessation (Maloni, Albrecht, Thomas, Halleran, & Jones, 2003), and drug and alcohol avoidance. Considerable research effort has also focused on prevention of abuse and violence during pregnancy (Denham, 2003).

The vast majority of research with pregnant women has been focused on birth outcomes, including rates of live birth, prematurity, low birth-weight, congenital malformations, and other complications of pregnancy, labor, and/or birth.

KRISTEN S. MONTGOMERY

Premenstrual Syndrome

Until the 1970s, misogynist views of menstrually-related experiences prevailed. Notably, an article written by a Johns Hopkins University physician, Erle Henrikson, in 1948 described premenstrual tension as the "Bitch Syndrome." After "carefully observing" many nurses and other "perfectionistic" women, Henrikson declared in his study that women who were both high achievers and "not satisfied" with their work or roles had more severe symptoms (Speroff, 1988). With the advent of the 1970s, critique and counterpoint arguments to negative classification of perimenstrual experiences were beginning to be published. Feminist scholars recommended the use of the word "change" over "symptom," as in "premenstrual changes" (Delaney, Lupton, & Toth, 1976; Parlee, 1973). In 1979, feminist epidemiologist and nurse researcher Nancy Woods first used the term "premenstrual symptoms or experiences" (Woods & Hulka, 1979). In the mid-1980s, professional medical organizations in the United States and United Kingdom met to define premenstrual syndrome (PMS) for clinical trials and scientific research. The published proceedings established the medical basis for the presentation and clinical existence of PMS as a disease classification (Dawood, McGuire, & Demers, 1985; Halbreich, 1997). From this point forward, misogynist labeling shifted to medical diagnosis. Notably, psychiatry and the Biological Psychiatry Branch of the National Institute of Mental Health provided the leadership in biomedical research (Rubinow & Schmidt, 1995).

In 1986, the Board of Trustees of the American Psychiatric Association (APA) voted to include a PMS label as a diagnosis in the research appendix of the *Diagnostic and Statistical Manual,* 3rd edition (DSM-IIIR) (American Psychiatric Association, 1986). Although the diagnostic term, Late Luteal Phase Dysphoric Disorder (LLPDD), was included in the 1987 DSM-IIIR in the "category requiring further study" (or research appendix), it was given a diagnostic code, title, list of symptoms, and cutoff points exactly like diagnostic categories in the main text of the DSM that is supported by scientific evidence. In spite of the recommendation of its own subcommittee that there was little substantive science to support a diagnosis of premenstrual mental illness, the APA included a revised label of premenstrual dysphoric disorder (PMDD) in the DSM-IV research appendix and in main text under Depressive Disorders. While symptom assessment requires one of four mood symptoms and four physical or somatic symptoms to qualify for the PMDD diagnosis, only antidepressant drugs were recommended for psychiatric treatment.

It has been argued that the controversy over the labeling and treatment of PMS and its symptoms was not restricted to conflict between feminists and the APA, nor was it a natural result of scientific progress. Rather, using terms such as PMS or PMDD gives a diagnostic (dysfunctional) label to premenstrual experiences and ignores the underlying social causes, allowing the status quo to be maintained. Subsequently, women internalize patriarchal beliefs about femininity and pathology and blame their individual biology for their feelings of dissatisfaction, rather than challenge the cultural traditions by looking for a political or social solution.

So what's all of the fuss about a label? More than an issue of semantics, the terminology we use to describe women's experiences influences social, political, and medical institutions. Classification of health-related signs and symptoms generally leads to the identification of diagnostic criteria but is ultimately a social process, and as such it is influenced by multiple social forces. Unfortunately, biomedical language has predominated with little attention paid to alternative perspectives from other disciplines and, more importantly, from a woman's perspective.

Nursing research has independently and collectively, with colleagues in the Society for Menstrual Cycle Research (SMCR), been at the forefront of a woman-centered agenda for understanding menstrual cycle experiences as both normative and illness processes. One early example of an outcome of the cross-disciplinary SMCR conferences was the 1981 Guidelines for Non-Sexist Research (Psychology of Women Division). These guidelines, sponsored by the SMCR, were a result of 2 years of effort by a national task force of psychologists appointed by Division 35 (Psychology of Women Division of the American Psychological Association, 1981) of the American Psychological Association and endorsed by them in 1981.

A long history of funded research programs also demonstrates the scope, sophistication, and scientific rigor of nursing research in these areas. Since 1986, the National Institute for Nursing Research has been actively supportive of research addressing the cause and consequences of menstrual cycle and menopause-related health conditions (Reame, 2001). Nurse researchers have focused on comorbidities related to menstruation or menstrual cycle phase, such as sleep function and disturbance, fatigue, fibromyalgia, gastrointestinal function and irritable bowel syndrome, brain function and neurocognition, depression, mood states, stress responsivity, circadian rhythms, pain and analgesic responses, bone biomarkers and osteoporosis, HIV and AIDS, violence and posttraumatic stress syndrome, as well as chronic diseases such as heart disease variability, diabetes, epilepsy, cancer, and arthritis (Golding, Taylor, Menard, & King, 2000; Taylor, D., 1999; Woods, Lentz, Mitchell, & Kogan, 1994; Shaver, Giblin, Lentz, & Lee, 1988; Heitkemper et al., 1995; Reame, 2001; Williams, 2003).

Attention to the context in which menstruation occurs has been an important part of nursing research into the menstrual cycle. Studies have documented the importance of stressful life circumstances in association with symptoms, as well as the importance of socialization for menstruation. Nurse researchers have made clear the consequences for women of a social context in which menstrual symptoms such as PMS are invalidated or used to invalidate women's complaints and abilities. Nancy Woods with her team, first at the University of North Carolina and later at the University of Washington, developed and tested multivariate models of "perimenstrual symptoms and experiences" that included sex role orientation, socialization, social context, stress, well-being, health status, health practices, and health seeking (Brown, M. A., & Woods, 1986; Brown, M. A., & Zimmer, 1987a, 1987b; Macdougall, 2000; Mitchell, E., Woods, Lentz, & Taylor, 1991; Mitchell, 1999; Mitchell, E. S., Woods, & Lentz, 1987, 1993; Mitchell, E. S., Woods, Lentz, Taylor, & Lee, 1992; Mitchell, E. S., Woods, & Mariella, 2003; Oleson & Woods, 1986; Taylor, D. T., & Woods, 1991; Taylor, D., Woods, Mitchell, & Lentz, 1987; Woods, 1985). Other nurse investigators have looked beyond negative mood and personal variables to consider positive feelings and experiences, generational differences of mood and physical experiences across social, monthly and seasonal cycles, and development of biopsychosocial conceptual models that clarify the limitations of the biomedical model and provide a basis for hypothesis testing (Cahill, 1998; Costos & Gleason, 1995; Lee, S., 2001; Taylor, D., 1990; Taylor, D., & Woods, 1991).

As a normative experience, nurses have carefully described the experience of women across menstrual cycle phases and transitions. Patterns of perimenstrual symptoms, including Premenstrual Syndrome (PMS), Premenstrual Magnification (PMM), and dysmenorrhea symptoms, have been described carefully as the basis for treatment. The existence of a symptom pattern consistent with definitions of PMS has been described, and the possibility for its idiosyncratic experience has been theoretically developed and tested. Definitions and criteria for clinical assessment based on daily recordings as well as retrospective assessment have been established.

One of the first epidemiologic studies of premenstrual mood change in a healthy, community-based sample was conducted by Woods in which women's daily experience of feelings, cognitions, and physical changes were assessed across three menstrual cycles using prospective daily diaries in multiple, non-clinical samples of regularly menstruating women (Woods, Most, & Dery, 1982; Woods & Hulka, 1979; Woods, Mitchell, Lentz, Taylor, & Lee, 1987). An important contribution by Nancy Woods to understanding what is and is not PMS is the redesign of the epidemiologic approach to estimating the prevalence of PMS. Instead of assuming a set of a priori symptoms or signs attributed to the label of PMS, she turned the epidemiologic model on its head by asking women about their daily experiences across multiple menstrual cycles. Factor and cluster analysis methods allowed classification of these data based on women's lives across all menstrual cycle phases rather than only the premenstrual or menstrual phase.

The measurement of perimenstrual experiences has become increasingly sophisticated as well as reflecting its complex, nonlinear nature. Ellen Mitchell and colleagues (Mitchell, E. S., et al., 1991; Mitchell, E. S., et al., 1987, 1993; Mitchell, E. S., et al., 1992) have made important contributions to advancing the definition of PMS through their data-based models of perimenstrual experience classification (perception, evaluation, response patterns). Research methods that go beyond the traditional quantitative approaches are now better able to capture the women's subjectivity (lived experience) and diversity, such as the interview method, cross-cultural research, ethnography, and feminist experimental methods. A number of studies have compared views and experiences of menstrual cyclicity, including PMS, of women from other cultures (Berg, J., 1999; Beyene, Taylor, & Lee, 2001; Brown, M., & Zimmer, 1986; Dan & Al-Gasseer, 1991). Social and physical environmental effects on the menstrual cycle and PMS experience have been explored, examining the effects of perimenstrual symptoms on work, marital relationships, mother-daughter relationships, and family functioning (Brown, M., & Zimmer, 1986; Roberts, S. J., & Garling, 1980; Robinson, K., 1997).

Nursing research has been influential in expanding therapeutic studies beyond the context-free clinical drug trials while maintaining the "gold-standard" experimental methods—placebo controlled, randomized clinical trial designs. The earliest studies included nonrandomized trials of the effectiveness of biofeedback and autogenic training for menstrual pain, feminist self-help groups, community education strategies, combined self-help and professional support groups, and behavioral (transpersonal approach, relaxation training, telephone counseling, and exercise) therapies (Amato, 1987; Heczey, 1980; Heinz, 1986; Miota, Yahle, & Bartz, 1991; C. Morse, Dennerstein, Farrell, & Varnavides, 1991; Morse, G., 1999; Taylor, D., & Bledsoe, 1986). In the 1990s, well-designed, controlled clinical trials of complementary therapies and cognitive-behavioral therapies were reported (Cohen, S. M., 1989; Groer, 1993; Morse, G., 1999). The first NIH-funded, randomized clinical trial of a pilot-tested, non-pharmacologic treatment included personal symptom management strategies as well as strategies for controlling social stress (Taylor, D., 1996, 1999, 2000). This clinical trial demonstrated how environmental stress management was as important as personal stress management strategies for coping with mood and physical symptoms.

Putting the science back into self-care has been a major contribution of menstrual cycle research by nurse scientists, resulting in research dissemination to consumers. In 2002, Diana Taylor published one of the first science-based self-help books for women that described effective, non-drug remedies for relieving PMS (Taylor, D., & Colino, 2002). Progress has also been made within professional and clinical communities to translate research into practice, using both empirical research as well as women's experiences as an important aspect of the base of evidence. One national organization of women's health nurses has implemented a model of clinical guideline development—the Association of Women's Health, Obstetric and Neonatal Nursing (2003). This professional organization of women's health care providers developed an innovative clinical practice guideline (Association of Women's Health, Obstetrical & Neonatal Nursing) based on a broad range of clinical, empirical, and theoretical evidence and subsequently evaluated the guideline in nursing practice through a research-based practice project (Collins-Sharp, Taylor, Kelly-Thomas, Killeen, & Dawood, 2002). In this guideline, they recommend the term Cyclic Perimenstrual Pain and Discomfort (CPPD) to differentiate normal cyclic changes associated with menstruation from the severe, debilitating menstrual and premenstrual symptom experiences that require professional or pharmacologic intervention. Albeit the label references the negative end of the perimenstrual experience spectrum, it is based on a range of empirical studies using quantitative and qualitative methods of women's experiences, not just hypothetical pigeonholing.

As more nurses assume roles as primary care providers for women, the need for these evidence-based therapeutic models is critically important. Clinical trials of treatment models, coupled with interventions to promote the understanding of menstruation, symptoms, and self-care options, should be aggressively pursued.

DIANA L. TAYLOR

Preoperative Psychological Preparation for Surgery

Study of methods for preparing adult patients for the experiences associated with having surgery comprises one of the largest bodies of research important to the practice of nursing. The first experimental study of preparation for surgery was published in the early 1960s by a nurse, Rhetaugh Dumas (Dumas, R. G., & Leonard, 1963). Since then more than 190 investigations of preparation for surgery were conducted by nurses, physicians, or psychologists.

Concerns about the prevention of pulmonary, gastrointestinal, or circulatory complications of surgery guided much of the early research. Many investigators examined various strategies to help patients deal with the discomfort and anxiety caused by getting out of bed, walking, and coughing, and deep breathing exercises were designed to aid recovery and prevent surgical complications. These studies were often guided by pragmatic concerns, such as whether structured or unstructured teaching, group versus individual teaching, or different methods of information delivery produced less anxiety and aided patients in performing these preventive activities. Other early studies examined the effects of provider-patient interaction. These interventions were highly individualized to identify and meet patient needs. Another approach to preparation for surgery included descriptions of routines of care such as skin preparation, preoperative medication, and transport to surgery and to the recovery room following surgery. This type of orienting information was derived from content found in textbooks or hospital procedure manuals and was often called procedural information.

Although theories about stress and coping began to appear in the literature in the 1950s and 1960s, the research about preparing patients for the stressful experience of having surgery generally remained atheoretical through much of the 1970s. Beginning in the mid 1970s some investigators began to test more theoretically derived interventions to help patients cope with the experience of having surgery. One of these interventions was preparatory sensory information, later called concrete objective information. Based on self-regulation theory (Johnson, J. E., 1999), this intervention describes in concrete and objective terms the typical physical sensations associated with the experience of having surgery; that is, what patients would see, feel, hear, or taste. These sensory experiences are linked to their cause. Examples include description of the sensations associated with preoperative medication (e.g., drowsiness), incisional sensations (e.g., burning, stinging) and how these sensations may change with activity and over time, being in the recovery room with frequent checks of vital signs, and the timing of expected changes in physical activity following surgery. Other interventions related to stress and coping that have been studied include a variety of relaxation methods, hypnosis, and positive thinking. Relaxation strategies have been more frequently studied in persons having surgery than have the latter two interventions.

Because many studies were atheoretical, most outcome indicators used to assess intervention effects were based on expectations drawn from clinical experience and inferences made about how the intervention was expected to improve specific patient outcomes. Outcomes most frequently used included length of stay, medications, pain, and emotions. Most studies assessed outcomes only during hospitalization; however, a few investigators assessed intervention effects on continued recovery and return to usual activities following hospital discharge.

The authors of a series of meta-analyses of studies testing preparatory interventions in patients having surgery (Devine & Cook, 1986; Hathaway, 1986; Devine, 1992) and at least one narrative review (Johnson, J. E., 1984) have drawn similar conclusions: patients who received any of the experimental preoperative preparatory interventions experienced more positive outcomes than patients not receiving such intervention, and these effects are substantive. There also was some evidence that combining intervention strategies produced greater positive effects than did single interventions. Cost savings derived from intervention effects on length of stay and medical complications also were demonstrated in the meta-analysis of studies published between 1961 and 1983 (Devine & Cook), although the magnitude of the effect was less, particularly for length of hospital stay, in the later years. Cost savings also were demonstrated in one study of psychoeducational care delivered by staff nurses after implementation of the diagnosis-related groups prospective payment system (Devine, O'Connor, Cook, Wenk, & Curtin, 1988). The ability to replicate similar cost savings in today's clinical environment is less likely because of even more changes in the delivery of surgical care that reduce the length of hospitalization for many patients.

Research concerning the preparation of patients for surgery has a long history, and it is clear that patients benefit from these interventions. The research findings were published in numerous journals over these years and they are also now included in nursing textbooks. The use of preparatory interventions for surgical patients is a common nursing practice. Because interventions frequently were combined in many studies, it is difficult to determine the specific contribution of each intervention to these positive effects. Such information would enhance clinical decision-making in selecting an intervention(s) to include in the preoperative care of surgical patients. Increased use of theories in the study of preoperative care, such as was done with self-regulation theory, will aid clinician decisions in selecting interventions for preoperative care and the appropriate outcomes for evaluation.

The nature of surgical care has changed dramatically in recent years. The shift to "same day" or ambulatory surgery with admission the day of surgery, discharge upon recovery from anesthesia, or very short post-operative hospital stays created the need for changes in the delivery of preoperative care. It also shifted much of the responsibility for ensuring that preoperative procedures were followed and that postoperative assistance and monitoring of recovery were provided to patients and their families. Even when patients are hospitalized following surgery, the postoperative stays are shorter and patients frequently return home with need for continuing assistance from their families. The practice of minimally invasive surgery also has become prevalent. These changes in surgical practices not only require changes in how preoperative nursing care is provided, but also suggest that new or different care for patients and families may be needed. At the same time there were fewer studies of preoperative preparation for surgery.

Because of these changes in surgical practices and postoperative care, there is need for new research about psychological preparation for surgery. This research should draw on prior research about preparation for surgery and theories relevant to coping with health care experiences. In an environment of cost containment, new research must consider assessing cost outcomes. While preoperative preparation most likely will not decrease hospital stays, using theory may suggest new ways to assess intervention cost effects. For example, in a study of cardiac surgical patients (Kim, Garvin, & Moser, 1999), one group received routine preoperative information consistent with procedural information. Another group received concrete objective information about mechanical ventilation and communication during ventilation plus procedural information. Patients receiving concrete objective information reported less negative mood and communication difficulty, as expected. They also were intubated for less time than the comparison group. The latter effect was unexpected but interpreted within self-regulation theory. Considering intubation time as a recovery indicator for intervention effects suggests using intubation-related costs as an outcome. Social costs of care, such as family member loss of income, out-of-pocket costs, or other costs related to recovery and care in the home, might also be considered when relevant to theoretical expectations.

Lastly, it is acknowledged that many of the insightful, important ideas expressed by Johnson in the first edition of *The Encyclopedia of Nursing Research* are retained in the above paragraphs—although possibly in less detail or in different ways.

NORMA J. CHRISTMAN

Pressure Ulcers

Pressure ulcers remain a common health problem throughout the health care system. It has been conservatively estimated that annually 1 million adults develop pressure ulcers. The incidence rates vary greatly depending on the health care sector. However, pressure ulcer incidence rates for hospitals range from 0.4% to 38%, for skilled nursing facilities from 2.2% to 23.9%, and for home health agencies from 0% to 17% (Cuddigan, Ayello, Sussman, & Baranoski, 2001). The annual cost to treat pressure ulcers has been estimated at $1,335 billion, with an average cost range of $1,190 to $10,185 or more (Kerstein et al., 2001).

The development of pressure ulcers occurs when there is sufficient pressure over time to cause capillary destruction, resulting in tissue necrosis. Although the amount of time and pressure needed to obstruct normal capillary closure vary (acuity of patient), research has found that capillary pressure ranges from 20 mm Hg to 40 mm Hg, with 32 mm Hg considered the average. However, this goal standard is being revisited, since it is possible to develop pressure ulcers at much lower pressures.

The development of a pressure ulcer and/or failure to prevent the ulcer from progressing to a more severe stage can result in negative consequences for the health care system. Litigation has significantly increased related to pressure ulcer development. Moreover, the U.S. Centers of Medicare and Medicaid Services (formerly, Health Care Financing Administration) consider the development of pressure ulcers as a failure in delivery of quality services, since the prevention of these ulcers depends on the cooperation from the entire health care team.

Nursing research has remained at the forefront in building the knowledge base related to pressure ulcer prevention. The first step in effective pressure ulcer prevention is identifying those patients at risk for ulcers. Conservatively, there are over 100 health factors associated with pressure ulcer development. The development of pressure ulcer prediction tools has made a significant difference in identifying those vulnerable adults and children at risk for ulcer development. Nursing research has lead to the development of pressure ulcer prediction tools. Some of the most common prediction tools are the Braden Scale for Predicting Pressure Ulcer Risk and the Norton Scale (U.S. Agency for Health Care Policy and Research, 1992). The Braden and Norton Scales have good sensitivity (83%–100% and 73%–92% respectively) and good specificity (64%–77% and 61%–94% respectively), but have low positive predictive value (approximately 40% and 20% respectively) (Bergstrom, Braden, Laguzza, & Holzman, 1987; Norton, D., McLaren, & Exton-Smith, 1975). Thus, there are patients who are receiving preventive interventions that are truly not at risk. Moreover, optimal cut-off scores may be different depending on patient population; thus continued research in this area is greatly needed.

The use of pressure ulcer prediction tools in non-White populations has been questioned, since many of the prediction tools being used have not been validated in non-White populations.

Several nursing research studies examining the predictive validity of these pressure ulcer prediction tools have emerged in the nursing research literature. Lyder and others (1999) examined the predictive validity of the Braden Scale in Blacks and Hispanics. The scale was found to be highly predictive ($p = .01$) when an optimal cut-off score of 18 or below was used. Conversely, Pang and Wong (1998) investigated the predictive validity of the Braden Scale, the Norton Scale, and the Waterlow Scale (primarily used in the United Kingdom) in a Chinese population. These researchers found that the Braden Scale had the best sensitivity (91%) and specificity (62%). It appears that the Braden Scale may provide an overall better sensitivity and specificity in non-White populations; however there remains a paucity of nursing research examining both risk factors and validation of prediction scales in non-White populations.

The development of the Agency for Health Care Policy and Research (now the Agency for Health Care Research and Quality) guidelines for pressure ulcer prevention was a milestone for both distilling and disseminating current research knowledge on the most effective methods for preventing these ulcers. Led by nurse researcher Dr. Bergstrom, these guidelines provided key areas for clinicians to consider for pressure ulcer prevention (risk assessment, repositioning, use of support surfaces, etc.). Because pressure ulcer development is a multivariate problem, no studies could be found that successfully implemented the guidelines in its entirety. Gunningberg, Lindholm, Carlsson, and Sjoden, (2001), investigating the incidence of pressure ulcers in 1997 and 1999 among patients with hip fractures, found significant reduction in rates (55% in 1997 to 29% in 1999). They attributed these reductions in pressure ulcer incidence rates to performance of systematic risk assessment upon admission, accurately staging pressure ulcers, using pressure-reducing mattresses, and continuing education of staff. Similar results have been noted in other studies when they implement similar pressure ulcer prevention program (Xakellis, Frantz, Lewis, & Harvey, 1998; Lyder, Shannon, Empleo-Frazier, McGehee, & White, 2002). Although nursing research studies have identified the principles of pressure ulcer prevention, additional studies are needed to determine optimal titration levels for preventive strategies based on the patient pressure ulcer risk levels and cost of interventions to the health care system (resources, staff burden, etc.).

In 1994, the Agency for Health Care Policy and Research (led by Dr. Nancy Bergstrom) published guidelines on the treatment of pressure ulcers. Nurse researchers have been quite active in leading the knowledge development in specific areas of pressure ulcer treatment, in particular, tools to objectively monitor pressure ulcer healing. Bates-Jensen, Vredevoe, and Brecht (1992) developed the Pressure Sore Status Tool (PSST) to assessing the healing of pressure ulcers. The content validity of the PSST was established by a panel of 20 experts. Interrater-reliability was established, $r = .91$ for first observation and $r = .92$ for second observation (Bates-Jensen et al., 1992). Another area in which nurse researchers have made an impact has been the evaluation of dressings to assist in the healing of pressure ulcers. Studies have found that, compared to traditional gauze, modern wound dressings heal pressure ulcers faster, are more economical, and save on caregiver time (Bolton, van Rijswick, & Shaffer, 1997).

Much research is still needed on examining the outcome (healing rates, costs, etc.) of standardized protocols for pressure ulcer treatment. Nursing studies are needed on developing and implementing alternative therapies for healing pressure ulcers. Qualitative studies are needed to understand the "lived experience" of patients with pressure ulcers. Finally, nursing researchers can take the lead on developing and evaluating appropriate levels of pressure ulcer care for patients receiving palliative care.

COURTNEY H. LYDER

Prevention of Preterm and Low-Birthweight Births

The prevention of preterm and low-birthweight (LBW) births continues to be a major health care challenge in the United States. Preterm or premature births are defined as those occurring before 37 completed weeks of gestation, with very preterm births considered to be those occurring before 32 completed weeks of gestation. Low-birthweight is defined as a weight of less than 2,500 grams (5 lbs 8 oz), while very-low-birthweight (VLBW) indicates a weight of less than 1,500 grams (3 lbs 4 oz). In spite of major advances in prenatal and perinatal health care, the incidence of preterm birth in the United States increased by 27% between 1981 and 2001, now representing 11.9% of all births. In 2001, preterm birth with low-birthweight was the leading cause of death in the 1st first month of life, accounting for 23% of all neonatal deaths, and further, is a leading contributor to infant morbidity including: mental retardation, cerebral palsy, vision and hearing deficits, and chronic lung disease. Demographically, there is an increasing disparity in rates of preterm and low-birthweight births by African-American mothers (17.5% in 2002) and those by white mothers (11.1% in 2002) (Centers for Disease Control and Prevention, National Center for Health Statistics, 2003). This growing disparity is not explained by known risk factors for preterm births.

The occurrence of preterm births and low-birthweight births are a distinct but highly related phenomena, with 98% of VLBW births and 66% of LBW births associated with prematurity. Additionally, 20%–30% of low-birthweight births are associated with maternal smoking. The specific causes of preterm birth remain unclear at this time despite intensive research. However, risk factors associated with preterm birth include: maternal use of alcohol, tobacco or other drugs during pregnancy; low maternal weight pre-pregnancy or low weight-gain during pregnancy; short interpregnancy interval; maternal infections including periodontal disease; social stress; maternal age; and domestic violence. Reflecting the continuing concern regarding preterm and LBW births in the United States, two of the objectives of Healthy People 2010 are the reduction in the incidence of low-birthweight and very-low-birthweight births, and the reduction of preterm births.

Research related to preterm and LBW births includes descriptive, correlational, and historical studies exploring the relationships among possible risk factors and birth outcomes; the evaluation of common interventions (traditionally designed prenatal care and bedrest for prevention of preterm labor) designed to reduce the incidence of preterm and low-birthweight births; and testing interventions directed at modifiable risk factors.

One of the areas intensively studied is the role of prenatal care in reducing the incidence of LBW births. In 1985 the Institute of Medicine (IOM) published a report concluding that, based on available research, early and comprehensive prenatal care was effective in reducing the incidence of LBW (Institute of Medicine, 1985). This conclusion promoted a national policy advocating universal and early prenatal care. However, in a recent meta-analysis of original research, systematic reviews, other meta-analyses, and commentaries evaluating the content, timing, and context of prenatal care, Lu, Tache, Alexander, Kotelchuk, and Halton (2003) conclude that there is little evidence that prenatal care as currently practiced is effective in preventing preterm or LBW births. In a critical review of current science related to preterm and LBW births, Lu and colleagues propose that the content of prenatal care be redesigned to include risk assessments for neuro-endocrine, immune-inflammatory, and vascular mechanisms now thought to have a causative role in preterm and LBW births. Further, they challenge the timing of prenatal care, suggesting that many of the antecedents to preterm and LBW births occur early in the life of the mother, before the initiation of prenatal care or pregnancy. Factors including maternal nutritional status, early exposure to infectious or inflammatory disease, and early chronic maternal stress may be related to later negative birth outcomes. Thus, the timing of "prenatal care" needs to be reconceptualized to include early and comprehensive health care rather than limited to the period of the pregnancy. Finally, they propose that prenatal care that does not address the social and environmental context of the mother is likely to be ineffective. The experience of racial discrimination, air and water pollution, neighborhood safety concerns, and the lack of a socially supportive environment have all been linked to an increased incidence of preterm and LBW births.

The effectiveness of a second common intervention, prolonged bedrest to prevent preterm labor, has been challenged by nurse researchers. Maloni (1996) describes the common side effects of prolonged bedrest during pregnancy, including depression, anxiety, and muscle weakness. In a sample of 141 women treated with prolonged antepartum bedrest, maternal weekly weight-gain was lower than the IOM recommendations ($p < 0.001$) and infant birthweights were lower than the national mean when matched with the national average for each infant's race, gender, and gestational age ($p < 0.001$) (Maloni, Alexander, Schluchter, Shah, & Park, 2004). In addition, while the prescription of bedrest continues to be a common intervention to prevent preterm labor, no controlled studies have been reported to support its effectiveness.

Two interventions evaluated in controlled studies are the effectiveness of smoking cessation programs and community-based nursing telephone follow-up. Maternal smoking during pregnancy accounts for 20%–30% of all LBW births in the United States (Healthy People 2010, 2000) and is one of the most important modifiable causes of poor pregnancy outcomes. Smoking cessation programs as part of prenatal care have been studied to determine their impact on maternal smoking behaviors. A nurse-managed smoking cessation program consisting of a 15-minute individualized intervention combined with telephone follow-up after 7–10 days was evaluated with 178 pregnant women (Gebauer, Kwo, Haynes, & Wewers, 1998). At 6–12 weeks after the intervention, the intervention group had a 19% self-reported abstinence and a 15.5% abstinence confirmed by saliva cotinine, compared with 0% in the control group. In related work, the 6th Research Based Practice program developed by the Association of Women's Health, Obstetrical and Neonatal Nurses (AWHONN) focused on the development of an evidence-based protocol to address smoking in pregnancy (Maloni, Albrecht, Thomas, Halleran, & Jones, 2003). The AWHONN program uses translational research to create protocols for integration directly into clinical practice. The protocol to address smoking cessation during pregnancy includes screening strategies and counseling during prenatal care.

In a prospective, randomized trial with a sample of 1,554 women receiving prenatal care, the effectiveness of a nursing telephone intervention was tested. Women in the intervention group received telephone calls from a registered nurse one-two times per week during the 3rd trimester of their pregnancies. In a cohort of African-American women 19 years of age or older, the incidence of LBW births was reduced from 15.3% in the control group to 11.3% in the intervention group (Muender, Moore, Chen, & Sevick, 2000).

In summary, the mechanisms leading to preterm and LBW births are not clearly understood. Therefore, much of current research is focused on the elucidation of causation and on the evaluation of interventions to reduce known risk factors. Interventions reported to be effective include smoking cessation classes and telephone follow-up and support by nurse clinical specialists. Controversies continue regarding the effectiveness of prenatal care as it is commonly provided and the use of bedrest for the prevention of preterm labor.

MARILYN J. LOTAS

Primary Care

Primary care is prevention-oriented general wellness and illness care of individuals and families. Primary care is characterized as being accessible, affordable, continuing, comprehensive, and coordinated. This form of personal health care delivery evolved to its contemporary state in the 1960s from earlier public health nursing and general medicine practices. Later, primary care became the foundation and entryway to secondary and tertiary care, especially in managed care systems. The Institute of Medicine (IOM) defined primary care as "the provision of integrated, accessible health care services by clinicians who are accountable for addressing a large majority of personal health care needs, developing a sustained partnership with patients, and practicing within the context of family and community" (Donaldson, Yordy, Lohr, & Vaneslow, 1996, p. 33). Primary care can be defined according to the type of provider, actual service, level of acuity of the illness, delivery setting, and client-provider relationship (Marion, 1996; Starfield, 1998).

Primary care is facing major challenges to its value in the United States. Primary care delivery is unequal in access and quality according to race, income, type of employment, and other factors (IOM, 2003). Also, primary care medicine is reported to be in crisis (Moore, G., & Showstack, 2003) due to consumer preference for specialists and emergency departments, less use of primary care physicians as managed care gatekeepers, slipping salaries and unfilled residencies, and increased access to alternative health care providers. Cooper, Getzen, McKee, and Laud (2002) predicted a shortage of primary care physicians in the near future.

In the face of change and challenges inherent in the U.S. health care system without coverage for many of its residents, advanced practice nurses (APNs) have entered the field of primary care delivery in increasing numbers. Teams of APNs have influenced traditional primary care and created innovative models through basic health and health care knowledge transfer. Nurse researchers, with funding by the National Institutes of Health (NIH) and other funding sources, have investigated health phenomena and have conducted "translational" research by evaluating utilization of basic science and applied science. In addition to the traditional nursing research doctorate (PhD) for generating new knowledge, there has been a resurgence of the practice doctorate to support evidence-based practice and new delivery model development (Marion et al., 2003).

The nursing perspective is largely congruent with that of the 1996 Institute of Medicine, except that the family as well as the individual is considered to be a primary care client. Also, nurses place primary care in the context of primary health care, a set of beliefs and principles concerning rights and responsibilities of individuals, communities, and providers as partners (World Health Organization, 1978). Finally, nurses emphasize their teaching/coaching, case management, and caring competencies in providing primary care (National Organization of Nurse Practitioner Faculties [NONPF], 2002).

The ideal primary care team is multidisciplinary, with nursing, medical, and other types of professionals collaborating in a mutually respectful way to capitalize on each member's individual strengths. Outcomes of this arrangement have shown potential for reducing utilization while maintaining health status (Sommers, Marton, Barbaccia, & Randolph, 2000). Nurses who deliver primary care include advanced practice nurses (APNs), such as nurse practitioners, certified nurse midwives, nurse specialists, and generalist nurses with basic nursing preparation. Primary care physicians are prepared in family and internal medicine, obstetrics and gynecology, and pediatrics. Health care specialists often provide primary care services to their clientele, and these specialists may or may not ensure that a full range of primary care services are delivered within the specialty system.

Primary care research can generally be categorized into health services delivery, effectiveness of diagnostic methods and care regimens for specific health needs, and client-provider interaction research. Primary care as a method of health service delivery includes health services access and utilization: cost; process and outcomes according to type of provider, health care system, setting, geographic region, and payment mechanism; client satisfaction; barriers to care; and continuity-of-care models. Defining primary care, determining essential (diagnosis and treatment) and cutting edge (technology and genomics) primary care competencies, and identifying preferred providers for specific activities are topics for further research. Distance care, such as telehealth to support self-care, is a health services delivery modality that is receiving much attention from researchers. Targeting care to groups of individuals with common needs and tailoring care to the actual individual are foci of health promotion and chronic disease management. To understand commonalities appropriate for group interventions, researchers are analyzing large data sets to identify what individuals fit into groups, such as for cost effective disease management (Bodenheimer, 2003). To tailor interventions to the individual, qualitative and mixed methods help to plan intervention protocols for testing. Related to health services delivery is health care policy research. The effects of policy on primary care and the effects of primary care trends in policy are explored and described in this field of research.

Effectiveness among diagnostic methods and care regimens for client-specific health needs has been a main focus of primary care research. Primary care client needs span most of the health continuum from health promotion to palliative care. Various forms of effectiveness research encompass the development and evaluation of (a) screening protocols based on the epidemiology of the problem and the community; (b) diagnostic procedures; (c) pharmocotherapeutics; (d) exercise, nutrition, and other health promotion prescriptions; (e) alternative therapies; (f) comfort measures; and (g) others. Effectiveness measures include benefits such as health/illness and functional status, quality of life, costs, and client (individual and family) satisfaction. Translating new knowledge to care delivery through evidence-based guidelines is a priority for the NIH Roadmap (NIH, 2003).

Client-provider interaction is of great interest to primary care researchers. Interaction is a vehicle to gain and deliver information, demonstrate caring and support, and plan health care on a mutual basis. Besides the development of a trusting relationship, interaction is largely directed at improving client health behaviors and supporting adherence to recommended regimens for specific health problems. Because the client is ultimately responsible for these activities, client-provider interaction is crucial to the health outcome. Increasingly, providers are using methods such as computerized-based tailored interventions to extend their reach to more people and to get better outcomes. Reaching the right balance of face-to-face and other methods of behavior change and support is a focus in primary care research today.

Research on nursing within a primary care context has mostly centered on APN processes and outcomes in comparison of those of physicians and physician assistants using medical care models (Marion, 1996). Also, primary care APN data are often buried and unidentifiable within physician and insurance data sets. The numerous small studies with limitations provided a convincing picture of competence and cost effectiveness. More recently, Mundinger and others (2000) conducted a randomized trial comparing primary care patient outcomes between physicians and nurse practitioners with the same authority, responsibilities, productivity, and administrative requirements, and the same patient populations. The investigators concluded that the patient outcomes of health status, health service utilization, and satisfaction were comparable.

In 1996, The American Academy of Nursing, with initial funding from the Agency for Health Care Policy and Research (now Agency for Healthcare Research and Quality [AHRQ]), Department of Health and Human Services, began to explore the possibility of a practice-based research network (PBRN) to study primary care among primary care APNs to describe their clientele, practices, and health delivery systems. Since that time, two APN primary care PBRNs have been established with funding by AHRQ: one in the Northeast and another in the Midwest. The Michigan Academic Consortium of nurse-managed academic centers has undergone comparative financial analyses among the four centers (Vonderheid, Pohl, Barkauskas, Gift, & Hughes-Cromwick, 2003).

The potential for future APN primary care PBRNs exists in evolving networks in national organizations. In 2004, the National Organization of Nurse Practitioner Faculties has approximately 1,200 faculty members, with over three quarters in clinical practice. These members represented over 100 graduate nursing programs with academic nursing centers, and many of these programs had several primary care delivery sites. These sites include school and college-based clinics, occupational health settings, mental health facilities, churches, homeless shelters, public housing, and other community agencies. At the same time, the National Nursing Center Consortium is increasing numbers of nursing centers throughout the nation and has adopted a minimum data set for data collection.

In summary, primary care research has a broad base, covering health phenomena of individuals, families, and communities and the delivery of health services, with the goal of improving the health of the nation.

LUCY N. MARION

Primary Health Care

The interdependence and complimentary nature of health with social and economic development is a basic premise of primary health care. A PHC approach emphasizes full development of human potential, community mobilization, and collaborative decision-making between health professionals and community members.

The World Health Organization (WHO) and the United Nations Children's Fund (UNICEF) sponsored the International Conference on Primary Health Care held in Alma-Ata, USSR, in 1978. The Declaration of Alma-Ata, endorsed by member governments of the United Nations at the 32nd World Health Assembly in 1979, provided foundational explication and a definition for Primary Health Care. The basic components of PHC were derived from case studies (Djukanovic & Mach, 1975; Newell, 1975) that examined diverse international health care programs, functioning with limited human, technological, and financial resources, to identify the common structures and strategies across cases.

Primary Health Care is essential health care based on practical, scientifically sound, and socially acceptable methods and technology. It is made universally accessible to individuals and families in the community through their full participation and at a cost that the community and country can afford to maintain at every stage of their development in the spirit of self-reliance and self-determination. It forms an integral part both of the country's health system, of which it is the central function and main focus, and of the overall social and economic development of the community. It is the first level of contact of individuals, family, and community with the national health system, bringing health care as close as possible to where people live and work, and it constitutes the first element of a continuing health care process (World Health Organization, 1978).

Five basic principles for implementation of PHC are: (a) equitable distribution ensuring accessibility of health services to all of the population, (b) maximum community involvement in the planning and operation of health care services, (c) a focus on health services that prevent disease and promote health rather than cure disease, (d) the use of appropriate technology and local resources that are socially acceptable and sustainable, and (e) a multisectoral approach that integrates health programs with social and economic development (WHO, 1985).

Implementation of Primary Health Care is contextually grounded. The development of PHC policies and services are based on the predominant health concerns of communities, and adapted to the cultural, political, and economic conditions of each country or community. Decentralization enables local community involvement in planning and implementation. Through collaboration, community members and health professionals shape programs and services to the particular socio-cultural circumstances of the community. A system of PHC services requires political commitment and appropriate economic policies locally, nationally, and internationally. Community development, multisectoral collaboration, and multilevel coordination facilitate implementation of services in keeping with the PHC standards of what is acceptable, affordable, appropriate, effective, and sustainable.

Primary Health Care teams interact to coordinate community health activities. The composition of a Primary Health Care team is determined by program needs, availability of health professionals, and local practices. Lay community health workers (CHWs) and traditional practitioners are often provided with basic health education. CHWs serve on health teams with nurses, midwives, social workers, physicians, or other appropriate multisectoral personnel.

While disease prevention and health promotion activities are given priority by a PHC team, curative and rehabilitative services are provided within a referral network. A predominant function of the health team is provision of education for communities and clients. Health education includes relevant information about common health concerns, and strategies that enable community mobilization for full participation in community-based health programs. PHC team members facilitate community involvement in an assessment process that identifies local resources and capabilities for community health and development. The Primary Health Care process promotes health through self-learning, self-determination, self-care, and self-reliance.

The terms "Primary Health Care" and "Primary Care" have frequently been used interchangeably. However, they each have distinctive characteristics. Primary Care, as a level of care focused on individuals, is one component of a comprehensive Primary Health Care framework that addresses population-based issues at community and country levels.

The essence of Primary Health Care is community participation in defining and addressing problems; practical understanding of the integral relationships among social, economic, and health conditions of a community; commitment to essential health services; and collaboration between community residents, health professionals, and a multisectoral network of other professionals. Therefore, PHC is an interactive approach to health care where community residents are expected to be knowledgeable in health matters, and to actively engage in their health care management. Moreover, PHC addresses self-care practices for physical and mental aspects of community health, as well as community social and environmental conditions. The basic goal of Primary Health Care is the attainment of optimum health, expressed in the internationally recognized slogan "Health for All."

Primary Health Care programs and literature are frequently integrated with other conceptual frameworks. Adult and popular education concepts, primarily based on Friere's work, and concepts of community assets and capacities have guided PHC implementation with strategies that engage communities in identifying their issues and resources. Community development concepts have been merged with PHC approaches from the time of Alma-Ata. In more recent years, social capital and social cohesion have emerged as concepts incorporated to facilitate PHC discourse and the growth and development of PHC programs.

Over the years, various international and national nursing organizations have promoted PHC as a means for meeting the health needs of the public, with special attention to vulnerable and underserved populations. To this end, Dr. Halfdan Mahler (WHO, 1986), the Director-General of the World Health Organization until 1988, recognized the potential for nurses to be a powerhouse for change if they mobilized around advancement of PHC ideas and convictions. Nursing leadership in PHC is illustrated in the National Institute of Nursing Research (NINR) Agenda for Community-Based Health Care (NINR, 1995). The document presents an NIH priority expert panel's adoption of Primary Health Care as a key concept for community-based health care, providing a basis to identify strategies for developing nursing knowledge for practice in urban and rural settings. Within the region of the Americas, nurses have engaged in PHC through the Florence Nightingale tradition of combining political activism and scholarly work, development of community programs, and educating community health workers as change agents for community health (McElmurry, Marks, & Cianelli, 2002). Nurses' contribution to the development and continuation of PHC is also evident in PHC literature. An integrative literature review of curricular applications of PHC found ongoing commitment to PHC, with 184 nurse authors from a global sample presenting PHC concepts consistent with the Alma-Ata definition (MacIntosh & McCormack, 2000). A multisectoral literature review, with predominant sampling from nursing publications, identified five categories within the PHC literature: concepts, social discourse, human resources, implementation, and participatory evaluation (McElmurry & Keeney, 1999). This review highlighted the participation of nursing in international PHC arenas and provided direction for nursing leadership in present and future development of PHC policy, services, and research. Overall, PHC concepts offer a framework for constructing future directions for nursing within a rapidly changing health care environment.

Since the ratification of the Alma-Ata Declaration, health policies and systems have shifted, beginning with major international initiatives and funding for PHC implementation, then moving to include health policy discourse that has questioned the effectiveness of PHC. With the 2004 celebration of the twenty-fifth anniversary of the declaration, international leaders have named lack of attention, misinterpretation, and oversimplification of PHC principles as basic critiques for not achieving PHC goals and assert that it is essential for the global community to reclaim the comprehensive approach for PHC as delineated at the Alma-Ata Conference (Tejada de Rivero, 2003). The World Health Organization has continued to refer to PHC as a cornerstone for international health initiatives, with the Pan American Health Organization (PAHO, the WHO Americas Regional Office) passing a resolution in 2004 reaffirming commitment to Primary Health Care as a strategy for continuing to work towards the goal of equity and "Health for All" (PAHO, 2004).

BEVERLY J. MCELMURRY
GWEN BRUMBAUGH KEENEY

Primary Nursing

Primary nursing is a nursing care delivery system that places the nurse-patient relationship at its center. One nurse is accountable and responsible for planning, management, delivery, and evaluation of a patient and his or her family's nursing care. Primary nurses practice with a small group of associate nurses who care for the patient in their absence. Continuity between nurse and patient is essential. Primary nursing flourishes best in an environment that recognizes the unique contributions of the professional nurse and supports the various components of professional practice. Typically, a decentralized approach to nursing management featuring a clinical nurse manager, participation in professional committees, and strong systems of accountability are present. Autonomy and authority over nursing practice are emphasized.

Primary nursing was initially conceived in the early 1970s by Manthey, Ciske, Robertson, and Harris (1970). Giovannetti (1980) extended this work, and Clifford (Clifford & Horvath, 1990) is widely recognized for expanding a nursing care delivery system into a professional practice model. Historically, primary nursing has been anecdotally identified as a strong predictor of patient and nurse satisfaction. Research on primary nursing has been fraught with conceptual and methodological challenges. Many studies lack conceptual and operational definitions, theoretical frameworks are not explicitly stated, instrumentation is frequently flawed, and research design less than rigorous.

Despite this lack of research rigor, primary nursing was widely implemented. Many of the original magnet hospitals, for instance, used a primary nursing model. Lack of cost-benefit analyses and measures of efficacy contributed to a building sense in many hospitals that primary nursing was no longer affordable, and many of the myths associated with primary nursing were promulgated. Many believed, for example, that a 100% RN skill mix was necessary for primary nursing.

Recent pressures to decrease the cost of inpatient hospital care and wide spread adoption of reengineering principles have resulted in new patient care delivery models. Many of the patient-focused care models herald a return to the team or functional nursing care delivery models of the past. Concepts such as the nurse-patient relationship, professional nursing practice, and continuity between nurse and patient are conspicuously absent in many of the new patient-focused care models. Rather than recognizing primary nursing as one of the earliest process redesigns in health care, elaborate new systems are being promoted that actually create numerous handoffs between team members. Clinical nurses are in jeopardy of being pulled further from patients to coordinate an increased volume of support tasks. Interestingly, many of the methodological flaws present in the initial evaluation of primary nursing have returned to the evaluation of patient-focused care models. Instruments lacking validity and reliability, inappropriate sampling methods, and lack of operational definitions prevail. Once again, major decisions are being made about nursing care delivery without rigorous evaluation.

Those institutions that have reaffirmed a commitment to primary nursing and professional practice models offer another opportunity to scientifically assess the outcomes of this nursing care delivery system. Rigorous qualitative and quantitative methods are required in this important area of investigation.

MAUREEN P. MCCAUSLAND

Prostate Cancer

Prostate cancer is the most prevalent visceral cancer in men in the United States; some 1.3 million men now live with it (American Cancer Society, 2003b). It has been estimated that 70% of men who survive to 80 years of age have evidence of histologic or latent prostate cancer (Pienta & Esper, 1993). Some researchers, and a great many clinicians and their patients, believe histologic prostate cancer eventually leads to clinically evident cancer (Pienta, Goodson, & Esper, 1996). Thus, in an effort to influence the natural history of prostate cancer, intensive screening efforts dominated by the use of prostate-specific antigens (PSA) in the past 2 decades have led to the diagnosis of scores of asymptomatic, latent cancers. These efforts have resulted in reports of both increased incidence and prevalence of prostate cancer (Newschaffer, 1997), accounting for a doubling of incidence of prostate cancer in the U.S. in the 10-year period from 1984 to 1994 (Parkin, Pisani, & Ferlay, 1999).

Approximately 80% of the 220,900 men diagnosed with prostate cancer in 2003 will learn that they have locally confined disease—early stage prostate cancer (Jemal et al., 2002). Therapeutic alternatives for early stage prostate cancer include radical prostatectomy, external beam radiotherapy, brachytherapy, cryosurgery, and observation ("watchful waiting"). Although approximately one third of patients with early stage prostate cancer elect radical prostatectomy, none of the active treatments has been shown to offer a survival advantage over observation, although an interim analysis of one trial suggests a small reduction in prostate cancer specific efficacy but not overall mortality (Harris & Lohr, 2002; Holmberg et al, 2002). Moreover, each of the active treatments, including radical prostatectomy, is associated with physical side effects, including urinary, bowel, and sexual dysfunction, which may have substantial effects on quality of life.

Most research on "quality of life" outcomes in early prostate cancer has focused on the often-problematic side effects of active treatment, including urinary, bowel, and sexual dysfunction (Talcott et al., 1998). Recent prospective studies have shown that after brief declines, generic measures of quality of life return to baseline levels by 12 months after primary prostate cancer treatment. However, for some, urinary and sexual dysfunction may persist indefinitely, accounting for varying levels of psychological distress related to changes in masculine identity, stigmatization, or demoralization (Powel, 2002; Clark, Rieker, Propert, & Talcott, 1999; Pirl & Mello, 2002).

Prior to the PSA era prostate cancer was a malignancy often detected only in late stages, and associated with imminent death (Litwin, 1994). In the past 20 years the proportion of late to early stage disease has shifted dramatically. Recent findings indicated that there has been a significant reduction in the incidence of metastatic stage disease at diagnosis, and men are being diagnosed at an earlier age. These findings have supported the emphasis on local treatment (i.e., radical prostatectomy and external beam radiotherapy), for which the 5-year survival rate approximates 100%. However, the survival curve declines with longer follow-up, with 54% of those determined to be at low risk of recurrence (risk derived from initial PSA, Gleason score, and clinical stage) recurring by 15 years (D'Amico et al., 1998). The mean onset of clinical metastasis (e.g., symptomatic skeletal metastasis) corresponds to Gleason score; those men with Gleason scores of less than 8 having a 27% chance of disease progression at 5 years after biochemical recurrence, whereas men with Gleason scores of 8 to 10 have a 60% chance of clinical metastasis at 5 years (Pound et al., 1999; Kupelian, Elshaikh, Reddy, Zippe, & Klein, 2002). Thus, while intensive screening has led to the diagnosis of earlier stage disease and improved local therapy, many are left with lifelong physical consequences of primary treatment, and recurrence is increasingly common within 5 years. Thus, prostate cancer represents a significant health problem.

Medical research is addressing many of the clinical challenges endemic to prostate cancer management. Research that is underway relates to the genetic predisposition of prostate cancer and mechanisms of carcinogenesis, updates in the screening of prostate cancer, improved imaging techniques, recent advances in the technical aspects of local therapies, the use of nomograms to predict outcome probabilities, advances in hormonal treatment for prostate cancer, including mechanisms potentially useful in reducing the risk of prostate cancer, the role of dietary and complementary therapies in prostate cancer, the role of chemotherapy in the treatment of hormone-refractory prostate cancer, and the integration of bisphosphonates, radioisotopes, and radiation therapy in the treatment of bone metastasis. While these studies represent impressive strides, other clinical concerns are not well studied. With an estimated 380,000 new cases of prostate cancer expected by 2025, research conducted by nurses over the next few decades is warranted.

In an *Index Medicus* search of manuscripts on prostate cancer written by nurses, 170 articles were found from 1974–2003. Of these, 45 were reports of original research on 16 different topics, including: cancer-related fatigue (2), complementary/alternative care (1), coping (2), couples (6), culturally-sensitive care (1), decision making (3), spirituality (2), men's concerns (2), quality of care (2), quality of life (7), screening (6), sexuality (1), survivors (1), treatment outcomes (5), uncertainty (1), and watchful waiting (2).

In essence, nursing research on prostate cancer has focused on screening of high-risk individuals and effects of local therapy, including feelings of uncertainty, impact on quality of life, and impact of prostate cancer on couples. Two themes were common to many of these reports: (1) patients do not receive sufficient information to make informed decisions about treatment, and (2) patients are infrequently asked about their experiences related to prostate cancer and its treatment.

Several studies found that men have a poor understanding of prostate cancer and its treatment, what conditions to expect after treatment, and how to manage postoperative symptoms and the emotional consequences of primary treatment. Investigators addressed this issue at various time points in the treatment experience—just after diagnosis, while waiting for surgery or radiotherapy, and immediately postoperatively. While several studies interviewed only men, others included a spouse or partner in the interview either individually, as a dyad, or both. The studies that interviewed men typically focused on the impact of physical changes men experienced after local therapy, whereas those that included couples addressed concerns that were slightly different. For example, in one study couples expressed the need to readdress their marital relationship after the illness as well as a cohesive message from the couple about how much information they would share with others about the cancer (Gray, Fitch, Phillips, Labrecque, & Klotz, 1999). In another study, couples were concerned with how to cope with the changes and the uncertainty of their future (Harden et al., 2002). Three intervention studies used psychological distress as an outcome of insufficient information to increase information-sharing that was consistent with the subject's interest and decision-making style. All showed decreased psychological distress as a result of information-related interventions (Davidson, Goldenberg, Gleave, & Degner, 2003; Johnson, J., Fieler, Wlasowicz, Mitchell, & Jones, 1997; Johnson, J., 1996).

When an investigator takes the time to ask about patients' experiences, patients tell them. The problem is that they are not being asked very often. When they are asked, they do not often feel as if their concerns are legitimized. Indeed several papers articulated the value of in-depth interviewing as a method of ascertaining sensitive information from men regarding feelings about changes in physical function following primary treatment and the impact it has had on their relationships and lifestyle. This concern was also apparent in two studies focusing on measuring cancer-related fatigue, a particularly distressing problem for men with recurrent disease. They found that dimensions of fatigue, particularly as it related to patients with metastatic cancer, had not been well articulated. The investigators recommended that more time be spent on extrapolating meaning from people's experiences rather than being so quick to measure them with instruments that assess cancer-related fatigue and therefore may not include all of the attributes that patients experience.

In addition to the papers that related to these themes, Weinrich and colleagues' (2004) impressive program of research in prostate cancer screening warrants mention. These investigators have focused on screening in African-American men, in whom prostate cancer is disproportionately present, as well as rural low- and middle-income men. They have crafted population-specific interventions that have improved screening by attempting to understand barriers as well as what motivates individuals to participate in screening.

The nature of the concerns that men with prostate cancer describe warrants attention by nurse researchers. Given the recent evidence on prostate cancer screening, researchers will be challenged to help interpret these findings in a way that informs men's choices. Treatment choices are incredibly complex and thus studies that address the information gap that men have articulated must be addressed. The physical consequences of primary treatment, such as urinary incontinence and erectile dysfunction, often invoke difficult behavioral, emotional, and interpersonal changes that are poorly understood and therefore require attention. A clearer understanding of the emotional and physical issues related to cancer recurrence is necessary in order to provide appropriate care to men who face recurrent prostate cancer. To date much of the research conducted by nurses has been descriptive or exploratory; additional research is needed.

LORRIE L. POWEL
MARY H. PALMER

Psychosocial Interventions (PSI)

According to Rössler and Haker (2003) in their review of the literature on the topic of psychosocial interventions, there is a paucity of research in this area. The authors noted that in their search of the databases Medline and PsycINFO (2002/2003) (search date June 20, 2003), only 3% and 1.2%, respectively, of the psychiatric articles addressed psychosocial interventions. A further concern was noted by authors Saks, Jeete, Granholm, and others (2002) and by L. L. Street and Luoma (2002) about the ethics of psychosocial intervention research, especially in regard to the issue of having control groups.

Psychosocial intervention (PSI) is often an inadequately defined concept. According to Gazzola and Muskin (2003): "The goals of all psychosocial interventions are determined by the stress on the individual and the coping skills available to that individual" (p. 373). An intervention can be considered to be in the psychosocial category if the intervention is designed to give people the opportunity to participate more fully in their interactions with their community and with society at large.

Psychosocial interventions are those used by people to deal with stressors in their lives. There are many types of interventions, and the ones used are often determined by what techniques are available and/or fit the unique needs of the individual/family. Most authors on this subject agree that it is essential that trust and a therapeutic alliance be established in order for PSI to be successful (Rössler & Haker, 2003; Gamble & Hart, 2003; Schein, Bernard, Spitz, & Muekin, 2003). Relapse is often seen with PSI, such as the return to addictive behaviors (i.e., smoking and illicit drug use) after treatment is finished (Schein et al.).

The objective of all psychosocial interventions is to integrate affected people into the community, and as such, increase their sense of autonomy. The importance of a person's right to self-determination regarding which PSI meets their unique needs cannot be overstressed.

Gamble and Hart (2003) explained how PSI can be implemented in an acute psychiatric inpatient unit. They listed the following as psychosocial interventions: engagement and outcome-oriented assessment, the family's assessment of the patient's needs, psychological management of psychosis-cognitive behavioral therapies, coping strategy enhancement, self-monitoring approaches and training in problem solving, and medication management via motivational interviewing techniques. They stated, however, that there is a great deal of resistance by staff in acute care settings to implement PSI. Some of this is related to staffing levels, its time-consuming nature, and inexperience either in the techniques or in general. Using a case example, they demonstrated that both patients and their families can benefit greatly from the use of psychosocial interventions in the acute care setting.

In their article, J. A. Baker, O'Higgins, Parkinson, and Tracey (2002) indicated that the Department of Health, United Kingdom (UK), identified the provision of psychosocial interventions as a priority in the treatment of the severely mentally ill, PSI being seen as the only training that improved clinical skills (United Kingdom Central Council, 1999). They also confirmed what other researchers have indicated—that there is often difficulty with the implementation of psychosocial interventions, partially related, they believe, to lack of organizational support for such measures (Tarrier, Barrowclough, Haddock, & McGovern, 1999). In response to this identified problem, Baker and colleagues designed a care pathway specific for the implementation of these types of interventions on an acute inpatient care unit in the UK. The model was based on research and evidence-based practice and was one of the first systematic approaches to deal with this issue. All members on the health delivery team participated in the implementation of this approach from its exploration phase through implementation and final evaluation phase. The outcomes were positive and received a certificate of excellence Lilly award. The authors do, however, indicate that the model needs further testing and implementation (J. A. Baker et al.).

Often in today's high-tech world of medical care, the use of psychosocial interventions by health care providers is sorely limited. Schein and colleagues (2003) stated that they believe that health care providers, specifically physicians, often find it hard to keep up with the rapidly increasing onslaught of technology, and therefore focus on the specific illness they are treating rather than the individual as whole. Although much evidence has been collected on the power of the mind over body, the referral of the medically ill patient to clinicians trained in the area of psychosocial interventions is frequently forgotten and therefore not done.

The impact of the use of psychosomatic interventions in coping with physical illness has been documented. Dreher (1998) reviewed the literature of preop preparation on postop outcomes, including a meta-analysis of over 200 prior studies, and found that there were significant outcomes related to things like decrease in need for pain medication and faster wound healing.

Rössler and Haker (2003) also mentioned that there is an emerging trend for online self-help groups to increase interactions and therapeutic alliances between clients and practitioners via the Internet. This will continue to be a growing trend as the use of technology increases in the 21st century.

Huibers, Buerskens, Bleijenberg, and van Schayck (2004) conducted a literature review to determine the effectiveness of PSI when used by general practitioners (GPs). Studies were eligible for inclusion if they were published before January 2002 and were in the categories of controlled clinical studies, controlled patient preference trials, and randomized control trials. A total of eight studies met the criteria and addressed different psychosocial interventions. The results indicated that depression was effectively impacted by GP problem-solving behaviors, but that the data was limited or conflicting on other interventions included in the review, such as counseling to help patients stop smoking or cognitive-behavioral group therapy. The authors indicated that further research is needed on the use of PSI by general practitioners.

Overall, the subject of psychosocial interventions has received little research attention. It will be crucial that these important treatment techniques be a focus for future study and nurses are uniquely qualified to conduct and publish research in this area.

Doris Troth Lippman

Pulmonary Changes in Elders

Most of the pulmonary changes associated with aging are gradual, giving elders the opportunity to adapt (Stanley & Beare, 1999). Normal lung aging is a benign process with relatively few clinical implications. A decline in physiologic reserve is the only consistent finding in healthy adults. This does not affect usual activities of daily living and only has a minor effect on exercise capabilities (Braunwald et al., 2001). However, the physiologic and functional consequences of age-related anatomic changes, altered gas exchange, ventilatory changes, and altered pulmonary-protective mechanisms are important considerations in the comprehensive assessment of the older adult.

Smoking accelerates the age-related decline in pulmonary function. Smoking, unlike other risk factors, can be eliminated. Smoking cessation, even after the age of 60, has been found to halt the progressive decline in pulmonary function (Higgins et al., 1993). Smoking cessation strategies for elders should encompass appropriate modalities, including the use of nicotine patches, oral medications, and behavioral interventions. Smoking-cessation interventions must be planned, should consider any medications being taken concurrently, and should be sensitive to the difficulties associated with a long-standing nicotine addiction.

Dyspnea or shortness of breath is a frequently reported symptom associated with illnesses such as chronic obstructive pulmonary disease (COPD), asthma, lung cancer, and heart failure. Dyspnea is the most common reason for emergency department visits and increases the likelihood for hospital admission (Parshall, 1999). Studies have shown that self-report of dyspnea does not always correlate with pulmonary function testing. In a longitudinal study of elders with COPD, individual ratings of dyspnea were not directly linked to changes in lung impairment (Lareau, Meek, Press, Ansholm, & Roos, 1999). This blunted perception is thought to be caused by physiologic adaptation over time. Assessment of dyspnea can be accomplished using several available scales. The use of a visual analogue scale (VAS) to measure dyspnea in elderly persons with COPD has been validated by Gift (1989). This type of measure provides a quick and reliable measure of dyspnea. The Pulmonary Functional Status and Dyspnea Questionnaire (PFSDQ) designed by Lareau, Carrieri-Kohlman, Janson-Bjerklie, and Roos (1994) is another reliable scale which has been used to measure dyspnea intensity and changes in functional ability in elderly persons with pulmonary disease.

Elders who present with a pulmonary infection often do so atypically. Often this is due to poor patient perception of their symptoms. Initial symptoms of pulmonary infection can be misdiagnosed as a pulmonary embolism or as heart failure (Blair, 1990). The classic triad of cough, elevated temperature, and pleuritic pain may not be present, or it may be blunted in elders. Instead, such subtle changes as increased respiration, increased sputum production, confusion, loss of appetite, and hypotension can be clues to possible pulmonary infection. Signs of sepsis may already be evident when elders present with a pulmonary infection (Stanley & Beare, 1999). Elders who have neurological illnesses such as Alzheimer's disease or Parkinson's disease, or who have sustained a cerebrovascular accident (CVA), are at risk for aspiration pneumonia and should be closely monitored for dysphagia. Interventions aimed at diminishing the risk for aspiration are critical.

Altered pulmonary-protective mechanisms have implications for elders undergoing surgery. In any given year, about 25% of the 600,000 elders who undergo major abdominal or thoracic surgical procedures in the United States experience postoperative pulmonary complications. Common interventions aimed at preventing such complications include cessation of smoking, bronchial hygiene, and incentive spirometry. Prevention of venous thrombosis with possible pulmonary embolization is critical in the elder population undergoing abdominal, thoracic, or orthopedic surgery. This is best accomplished with low-dose heparin, administered subcutaneously every 12 hours, and with the use of pneumatic stockings. For elders at high risk for pulmonary embolism, more frequent subcutaneous dosing of heparin may be used, or coumadin may be ordered.

ELIZABETH MCGANN

Q

Qualitative Research

Taken literally, qualitative research includes all modes of inquiry that do not rely on numbers or statistical methods. However, the terms *qualitative* and *quantitative* research are misnomers, albeit commonly used. The terms *qualitative* and *quantitative* actually refer to the forms of the data, not to specific research designs. It is more accurate to discuss naturalistic and positivistic designs during which qualitative or quantitative data may be collected. For this reason, the subject usually considered under the topic of qualitative research will be called naturalistic inquiry here.

Naturalistic approaches comprise a wide array of research traditions, most often in the categories of ethnography, grounded theory, and phenomenology but also including ethnology, ethnomethodology, hermeneutics, oral/life histories, discourse analysis, case study methods, and critical, philosophical, and historical approaches to inquiry. Each tradition has a distinct set of undergirding philosophical or theoretical orientations, strategies for data collection and analysis, and forms of research products.

The ultimate purpose of all research is the generation of new knowledge. However, different modes of inquiry produce different kinds of knowledge. Knowledge developed from naturalistic methods is at the level of rich description or in-depth understanding. Naturalistic inquiry tends to be exploratory in nature and is particularly useful in identifying important contextual features of the phenomenon. Naturalistic approaches are called for when the purpose of the research is to obtain in-depth information about a phenomenon, when little is known about a topic, or when new perspectives are needed. Secondary purposes for naturalistic approaches include hypothesis generation, obtaining the range of possible items for instrument development, providing illustrative examples or cases, and delineating the context from which other data may be better interpreted.

There are several features that are common to most naturalistic studies. A basic tenet is that reality is socially constructed; as such, there are multiple realities for any phenomenon, given the multiple lenses through which different individuals perceive and experience a situation. Naturalistic approaches favor conducting research in the field setting (vs. an artificial laboratory) in order to observe phenomena as they are lived and to preserve the contextual elements of the phenomena. In contrast to positivist approaches, which use established instruments, in naturalistic inquiry the investigator is the instrument. However, investigators are aware that their own experiences, biases, and perceptual sets particularize both the data that they elicit from informants and ultimately the data analysis/interpretation. There are generally accepted standards for rigor in naturalistic approaches. These include the degree of intimacy of the investigator to the informants, the auditing of interviews and coding structures, trustworthiness, dependability, conformability, meaning-in-context, and saturation/redundancy.

Naturalistic approaches (also known as constructivist or inductive inquiry, Paradigm II, or field approaches) are often contrasted with positivist approaches (also called empiricism, Paradigm I, or experimental approaches). Naturalistic and positivistic modes of inquiry provide different types of data. However, these data sets are most fruitfully viewed as complementary rather than in opposition. Together they provide a more complete understanding than can be obtained by using either approach singly. Sometimes the methods can be employed simultaneously (methodological triangulation); at other times the methods must be applied sequentially in order to satisfy the requirements of each. The reciprocal interweaving of naturalistic and positivist research builds nursing knowledge as each contributes different but important information.

Specific approaches to naturalistic inquiry were developed primarily in the social sciences and philosophy. For example, phenomenology as a method derived from phenomenological and existentialist philosophy, ethnography from anthropologists' study of culture, grounded theory, and ethnomethodology from sociology (specifically the school of symbolic interactionism).

In the discipline of nursing, there were several early reports of qualitative data without a specified naturalistic approach. In 1952 the first issues of the first volume of *Nursing Research*, articles report the qualitative results of unstructured interviews. Orlando (1961) used data from participant observation to describe case examples and advocated the use of open-ended interview techniques followed by validation to determine each patient's individual needs. Although not giving a formal name to this approach, she used data grounded in clinical nursing observations to inductively derive her theory concerning deliberative nursing practice.

In 1962 nurse scientist graduate training programs were initiated through the Division of Nursing for the purpose of increasing the number of nurse research scientists with doctorates in basic physiological or social sciences. As a result, many nurses completed programs that trained them in the qualitative methods developed in the social sciences. Many nurse anthropologists were trained during this period. Similarly, from 1962 to 1967, Benoliel served as a member of the three-person team (with Glaser and Strauss) studying dying and developing what was to be called grounded theory.

Over the decade of the 1960s the number and methodological specificity of naturalistic inquiry increased. By the end of the 1960s, *Nursing Research* had published articles specifically using grounded theory methods, ethnographic methods, and other naturalistic approaches. *Image: the Journal of Nursing Scholarship* was initiated in 1966 and also published research using naturalistic methods (although positivist approaches predominated in both journals). With the advent of the *Western Journal of Nursing Research* in 1978, edited by Brink, there emerged an outlet with a balanced representation of qualitative research. In 1976, Paterson and Zderad published a book based on phenomenological observations and Brink's (1976) book contained a series of methodological articles on conducting qualitative (largely ethnographic) research. Nearly a decade later two broad-based books on qualitative research were published (Field & Morse, 1985; Leininger, 1985b). With the advent of the journal *Qualitative Health Research* in 1991, also edited by a nurse-anthropologist, Morse, an entire journal was fully dedicated to reporting naturalistic research.

Research conferences and societies also have been influential in fostering the development of naturalistic inquiry. The series Communicating Nursing Research, co-sponsored by the Western Interstate Commission for Higher Education and the Division of Nursing, and The Transcultural Nursing Care series organized by Leininger from 1977 to the present offered an opportunity for the presentation of naturalistic research. More recently, regional research societies such as the Midwest Nursing Research Society have added qualitative research sections that meet annually, sponsor symposia, and disseminate newsletters.

The selection of a particular naturalistic approach depends on the purpose of the research. For example, phenomenology is the method of choice when the purpose is to understand the meaning of the lived experience of a given phenomenon for informants; grounded theory is selected to uncover or understand basic social processes; and ethnography is selected to understand patterns and/or processes grounded in culture.

Although most qualitative approaches do not employ formal theoretical frameworks, they do rest on established philosophical assumptions. However, some naturalistic inquiry (particularly ethnography) is conducted in the context of theoretical orientations that reflect the training of the investigator and may focus attention on particular phenomena, relationships, data collection techniques, or research products.

In most forms of naturalistic inquiry, investigators typically use participant observation, informant interviews, and document analysis. However, the extent to which the investigator relies on any one strategy will vary. For example, phenomenology relies primarily on informant interviews, ethnography, and grounded theory and generally has a more even reliance on participant observation and interviewing, whereas ethnology relies primarily on observations.

Methods for data manipulation include strategies for taking notes, making memos, and coding and indexing systems. More recently, computerized software programs such as ETHNOGRAPH, NUD*IST, and MARTIN have been fruitfully employed to aid in the management of data. Methods used in data analysis are inductive and include matrix, thematic, and domain analysis. Finally, the form of the final product may vary. In grounded theory, a substantive theory with a process model is common; in ethnoscience (a form of ethnography) a taxonomic structure is the product.

In summary, naturalistic inquiry most commonly occurs in field settings, with investigators collecting data through participant observation and unstructured interviews and analyzing data through thematic content analysis. It developed initially in the social sciences and began to be incorporated in nursing research in the 1960s and 1970s. Today it is an accepted scientific approach that complements knowledge derived from positivist inquiry.

TONI TRIPP-REIMER
LISA SKEMP KELLEY

Quality of Care

Interest in measuring the quality of health care is a recurring theme in the U.S. health care system. Attempts to measure this concept date back to the 1970s and have more recently taken center stage, with the emphasis on reducing costs of care becoming a key focus of the 1980s and 1990s. Care providers today are expected to provide high-quality care at a reasonable cost while attending to the increasing demand by consumers for more information about care choices and the outcomes of specific providers, whether they be hospitals or other providers of care. Gallagher and Rowell (2003) suggested that the provision of outcome-oriented, cost-effective health care is no longer a goal but a mandate. Part of the issue in health care today, according to these authors, is that the costs, processes, and outcomes of care are so interrelated and reciprocal that changes in one of these areas may have significant effects on the other components.

A recent report by the Institute of Medicine (IOM) stated that "Health care today harms too frequently and routinely fails to deliver its potential benefits" (IOM, 2001, p.1). This report further states that all health care should be "safe, effective, patient-centered, timely, efficient, and equitable" (p. 6). In this report four key aspects of the current health care environment have been identified as the underlying reasons for inadequacy of the health care provided in the U.S. These are the increasing complexity of the fields of science and technology, the increasing issues of chronic health conditions, a poorly structured health delivery system, and constraints on capitalizing on the revolution in information technology today.

The Institute of Medicine adopted a definition that states that "quality is the degree to which health services for individuals and populations increase the likelihood of desired outcomes and are consistent with current professional knowledge" (IOM, 2001, p. 244). Patients receive quality care when the services provided are technically competent, provide good communication, share decision-making with the patient and family, and are culturally sensitive. Donabedian's model (1980) of quality measurement based on structure, process, and outcome has become the foundation of most current strategies to measure quality of care in health care systems. Using Donabedian's model, quality can be evaluated based on the three components of structure, process, and outcomes (IOM). Using this framework, *structural quality* evaluates the capacity of the health care structure to provide high-quality care. In nursing this requires nurses to evaluate how the unit's structure and that of the larger organization affect quality of care for the patients under their care. Measures of structure have primarily included cost and financial resources required to provide care as well as human resources such as skill mix, staff characteristics, patient severity of illness factors, and environmental factors of the hospital or care agency. During the 1970s and 1980s, patient classification systems were developed but never were extensively implemented. More recently, Diagnosis Related Groups and Nursing Diagnoses are frequently used separately or together to describe patient characteristics in research and care effectiveness evaluations.

A second component of quality is *process quality* that focuses on the interactions of nurses with their clients. In nursing, a very process-focused discipline, we see the historical contribution of care plans as an important process tool, and more recently, critical paths and care maps have added to this process focus. The best process measures are based on research evidence that the process leads to better outcomes for patients. In today's health care system, most attempts to measure quality focus on process evaluation by assessing the appropriateness of care and the adherence to professional standards. Discharge Planning and Case Management are nursing interventions included in the Nursing Interventions Classification (NIC) that focus on achieving quality care through a process format (Dochterman & Bulechek, 2004).

A third component of quality is *outcomes* that provide evidence of the effectiveness of the interventions nurses provide for the health problems and concerns of patients. The IOM report states that the best measures of outcomes are those tied to the process of care. Attempts by nurses to enhance quality strategies, such as *critical paths* and *care maps*, have challenged the sacred "care plan" in nursing and have shifted nurses thinking from goals to outcomes. Some of these paths and maps have included standardized nursing languages as content areas for nursing. The Nursing Outcomes Classification (NOC) (Moorhead, Johnson, & Maas, 2004) was developed to measure the effectiveness of nursing interventions. Used with the Nursing Interventions Classification and diagnoses from the North American Nursing Diagnosis Association (NANDA) international, the outcomes are designed to measure the effectiveness of the nursing process. Linkage of these three classifications through a recent publication assists nurses and students to use these languages more effectively (Johnson, M., et al., 2001). The NOC has 330 outcomes that measure along a continuum an individual, family, or community state, behavior, or perception in response to a nursing intervention. Each outcome has an associated set of indicators that are measured to determine the patient, family, or community status in relation to the outcome. Examples of some of the outcomes relevant to a discussion of quality are Pain Control, Symptom Control, Quality of Life, Participation in Health Care Decisions, Asthma Self-Management, Cardiac Disease Self-Management, Risk Control, and Knowledge Disease Process. Use of this classification in practice settings with an evaluation of the outcomes achieved provides needed knowledge to nurses related to the effectiveness of the interventions provided and the care planning process. This evaluation of real patient data on outcomes allows for a continual review of the structure, process, and outcomes of nursing care.

The current environment also is challenged to meet patient expectations. Because of this, NOC has added 14 client satisfaction outcomes to measure patient perceptions of their care. While many would argue that the patients can not usually judge quality as well as health providers can, their impression of quality is very relevant to the discussion. Private nonprofit organizations such as the National Committee for Quality Assurance have been created to improve health care. This organization evaluates health plans in the areas of patient safety, confidentiality, consumer protection, access, and continuous improvements. They have both accreditation and performance measurement programs that provide information to consumers.

The challenges to measure quality are not new issues in the health care system, but we are facing intensive pressure to provide safe, cost-effective, patient-focused quality health care. Attention must remain on these key factors as nurses and other health care providers develop better structures, processes, and outcome measures to evaluate the effectiveness of the care we provide. This desire for providing quality of care is central to nursing practice.

SUE MOORHEAD

Quality of Life

Quality of life (QOL) is a multifaceted construct without a single definition. QOL is used by many disciplines concerned with conditions of human life, including social, environmental, political, economic, and health (Anderson, K. L., & Burckhardt, 1999). Nursing and health care researchers are interested in determining how disease or injury, or the treatment of disease or injury, affects QOL. Health promotion researchers may use QOL measures to ascertain the effectiveness of measures taken to enhance or improve mental, physical, social, or spiritual health. Despite a lack of consensus on what quality of life is, three broad approaches for defining QOL have been suggested (Haas, 1999; Carr, Gibson, & Robinson, 2001; Dijkers, 2003). One category characterizes QOL as evaluations or reactions such as well-being, happiness, satisfaction, morale, or positive and negative affect. Another category describes QOL in terms of normality, meeting societal standards, and status or achievements. Ability to function and fulfill basic needs are examples of this QOL domain. A third approach suggests QOL is a matter of perception regarding the differences between expectations, what is valued or considered important in life, and current life experiences. Many QOL instruments are multi-dimensional, combining the conceptual dimensions of evaluation, normality, and/or perception.

The importance of quality-of-life research is evident through federal funding of health research. One of the five future research priorities identified in September 2003 by the National Institute of Nursing Research includes quality-of-life research in chronic illness (www.nih.gov/ninr/research/themes.doc).The Centers for Disease Control also has a division for health-related quality of life that provides measures and data for tracking various aspects of population health (www.cdc.gov/hrqol/index.htm). The prevalence of QOL as a variable in nursing studies is demonstrated through a CINAHL search, using the phrase "quality of life" and limited to research and nursing journals. The search yielded 1,744 articles published between 1982 and November 2003, with 824 or 47% entered since the year 2000.

QOL measurements are classified into five types (Garratt, Schmidt, Mackintosh, & Fitzpatrick, 2002). *Generic* measures, such as the Medical Outcomes Study SF-36, can be used with any patient population, or any disease or health condition. *Disease or population specific* instruments have been found to be more sensitive to changes in QOL since these tools are designed to measure more specifically how a disease or illness affects life dimensions. The European Organisation for

Research into the Treatment of Cancer quality-of-life questionnaire (EORTC QLQ-C30) is an example of a population-specific tool. *Dimension-specific* measurements focus on specific aspects of health, such as well-being or depression. *Utility measures*, exemplified by the Health Utilities Index, are beneficial in evaluating economic aspects of health treatments and require respondents to choose between alternative health states, with economic or other costs associated with the choices. *Individualized* QOL tools, such as the Patient Generated Index or the Schedule for the Evaluation of Individual Quality of Life, ask respondents to identify and weigh what they deem important in their lives. The individualized approach is considered by some to be the most appropriate way to measure quality of life, because the research participants are the only ones who can say what matters most in their lives (Joyce, Hickey, McGee, & O'Boyle, 2003; Macduff, 2000).

Because QOL is defined in a variety of ways, many methods and tools are available to measure QOL as a research variable. The MAPI Research Institute (Lyon, France) offers a free catalog describing over 1,000 QOL instruments and provide access to these instruments for a subscription fee (http://www.qolid.org). Considerations for selecting or developing a QOL instrument include: deciding who is evaluating QOL, what aspects or dimensions of QOL are to be evaluated, whether the measurement needs to be able to detect changes over time, and how the information gained from the measurement will be used. The research participant's age, communication ability, severity of illness, and cognitive ability will determine whether QOL is scored by an outside observer or proxy, such as a parent, spouse, or health care provider (Addington-Hall & Kalra, 2001). The Scientific Advisory Committee of the Medical Outcomes Trust (2002) suggests the following criteria for evaluating QOL instruments: the conceptual and measurement model underlying the instrument, psychometric properties of reliability and validity, sensitivity or responsiveness to change over time, ease of interpreting and understanding scores, respondent or administrative burden, alternative modes of administration, and cultural and language adaptations of the instrument for use in other populations.

Whether a study is cross-sectional or longitudinal will also influence the instrument choice. Tools used in longitudinal studies need to be sensitive to change, without floor or ceiling effects associated with items in the tool (Hyland, 2003). Hyland also suggests that tools in longitudinal studies be relatively short, have multiple-response items such as Likert scales, and include items that describe problems common and relevant to the population being studied. QOL questionnaires used in cross-sectional studies need to be able to discriminate among respondents who will have varying differences in QOL (Hyland). QOL tools for cross-sectional studies may have more items with two or three response choices, may include items that have floor and ceiling effects, and may not be relevant to all respondents.

Because of the variety of definitions and tools, QOL may be difficult to compare across studies (Garratt et al., 2002). Thorough knowledge of conceptual and psychometric aspects of a QOL measure is essential for selecting the right tool for a research study. Using the same instrument as other researchers may not be appropriate if the instrument does not adequately capture the researcher's conceptualization of quality of life, or if the tool is not sensitive to change over time and the study is a longitudinal design. Thus, definitional and measurement issues may hamper building a body of knowledge about quality of life.

The dynamic nature of life also presents challenges for measuring QOL (Carr et al., 2001). People adapt to illness and their expectations about interventions may change over time, so what effects QOL at one time may not at another. Priorities in life also change, so what a person considers important at one time may be less important at another. Aggregation of QOL data within a population may be difficult because people's expectations regarding the effects of a disease or intervention may differ. Despite these difficulties in measuring QOL, it is an important concept for nursing, and will continue to be an outcome variable in nursing studies.

Carol D. Gaskamp
Carol E. Smith

Quantitative Research

Quantitative research consists of the collection, tabulation, summarization, and analysis of numerical data for the purpose of answering research questions or hypotheses. The term *quantitative research* is of recent origin and is distinguished from qualitative research in design, process, and the use of quantification techniques to measure and analyze the data. The vast majority of all nursing studies can be classified as quantitative.

Quantitative research uses statistical methodology at every stage in the research process. At the inception of a research project, when the research questions are formulated, thought must be given to how the research variables are to be quantified, defined, measured, and analyzed. Study subjects are often selected for a research project through the statistical method of random sampling, which promotes an unbiased representation of the target population among the sample from whom generalizations will be made. Statistical methods are used to summarize study data, to determine sampling error, and in studies in which hypotheses are tested, to analyze whether results obtained exceed those that could be attributed to sampling error (chance) alone. The important role of statistical methodology in quantitative research should not obscure the fact that other methodologies and scientific disciplines play important roles in nursing research. These methods are used in the delineation of research questions and hypotheses, exposition of conceptual frameworks and hypotheses, design of data collection instruments and tools, and interpretation of study data, particularly determination of the clinical significance of the data and dissemination of findings.

Much of the history of nursing research involves quantitative research. Florence Nightingale, who was a skilled statistician, used quantitative measures to describe and evaluate hospital performance (Nightingale, 1858). Studies of nursing in the United States, beginning in the 1940s, used quantitative techniques to survey and analyze nursing education and supply and distribution of nurses. In the 1960s, with support from the federal government, research in nursing began to use advanced research designs, such as controlled experiments, which made extensive use of quantitative tools, techniques, and processes (Hasselmeyer, 1961).

Quantitative data collected in quantitative research are obtained by the use of measurement scales. There are three distinct types of scales: nominal, ordinal, and continuous. Nominal scales consist of two or more ungraded or unranked categories of variables, such as eye color (green, blue, brown) or political affiliation (Republican, Democrat). Ordinal scales possess categories that are ranked or graded, from high to low, small to large, near to far. Graded scales, such as the Likert and Guttman scales, are commonly used in nursing research to measure intensity of opinions, attitudes, and other psychological variables. When nominal and ordinal scales are used, quantitative summaries of the data collected consist of aggregating the number of responses in each scale category, converting them to relative frequencies such as percentages, and if hypotheses are being tested in the research, applying one of many nonparametric techniques available to test the statistical significance of the data.

Continuous scales have continuous quantitative values rather than verbal categories, as in nominal and ordinal scales. These include the scientific measuring instruments widely used in nursing to measure variables such as temperature, weight, height, blood pressure. Continuous measurement scales have certain advantages over other scales because they yield more precise and sensitive data. Also, the statistical significance of continuous data can be analyzed by the more powerful parametric techniques.

Quantitative research is concerned with making generalizations from a study sample to a target population, a process called statistical inference. There are two categories of generalizations in quantitative research: (a) estimates of the quantitative value of selected characteristics of a target population, and (b) results of tests of statistical hypotheses concerning relationships among variables in the target population. Studies in the first category are called descriptive studies; those in the second category are called analytical or explanatory studies. The focus of many early nursing studies was to describe nurses and nursing practice using questionnaire or interview techniques to collect data from large samples of respondents. Recent studies using conceptual frameworks from emerging nursing theories and models have tested hypotheses in controlled or semicontrolled settings.

Statistical techniques are used extensively in descriptive studies to compute summary measures, such as means, standard deviations, and coefficients of correlation, and to determine the sampling error of the measures. In explanatory studies, statistical techniques are used to test whether there are significant relationships among study variables that are delineated in the hypotheses, meaning relationships that cannot be explained by random sampling error (chance). Widely used statistical techniques to test hypotheses include parametric tests such as the *t* test and analysis of variance and nonparametric tests such as chi-square and rank-order correlation.

Quantification in nursing research has helped advance nursing as a scientific discipline. Quantification offers many advantages to nursing research. There is a rich set of statistical tools available for data analysis that can be applied to practically every research question to assist in summarizing the data and evaluating their statistical significance. The internal and external validity of the data of quantitative research can be readily verified by other researchers. Results of similar quantitative studies can be synthesized and analyzed by the meta-analysis technique to shed new light on the research questions. Dissemination of the results of quantitative research is facilitated by the clarity and objectivity possessed by quantitative data.

Some studies in nursing tend to overquantify. Reports of these studies are dominated by statistical data and tests, with a minimum of narrative discussion, providing little interpretation of the clinical significance of results. Sometimes too little time is spent on evaluation of the quality of data used or on the appropriateness of the statistical tests. Qualitative research, with its focus on meaning and interpretation of data, can help to enrich the results of quantitative studies in nursing. The approach called triangulation, which utilizes and integrates methodology from quantitative and qualitative research in a single study, can help achieve the best of both worlds of research methodology.

The history of nursing research reveals a trend from purely descriptive studies of nurses and nursing to the evaluation of the effects of nursing care. Properly applied quantitative research can advance the scientific basis of nursing as well as provide a potent tool for defining and evaluating the outcomes of nursing care. In the future, quantitative research will play an increasingly valuable role in nursing effectiveness studies. The randomized clinical trial (RCT) method, perhaps the most quantitative of all research methods, will find increasing application in nursing as attempts are made to determine the efficacy of nursing interventions. Clinically oriented research using methods such as randomized clinical trials requires development of quantitative outcome measures of variables such as quality of care and quality of life. This will stimulate quantitative research to provide the needed measures and indicators. As more replications of quantitative nursing research become available, the research synthesis techniques of meta-analysis will be increasingly applied to expand nursing's knowledge base.

EUGENE LEVINE

Quantitative Research Methodology

Research methodology is the term commonly used for the procedures employed to accomplish the specific aims of a research project.

In other words, research methodology is the means by which we collect data to answer research questions or to test hypotheses.

The methods are derived from the research design and generally include sample, interventions (if applicable), instruments, data collection procedures, and plans for data analysis. A research design, according to Kerlinger (1986), "expresses both the structure of the research problem and the plan of investigation used to obtain empirical evidence on the relations of the problem" (p. 279).

There is no "best" design. The appropriate design is the one that fits the theoretical formulation underlying the research questions or hypotheses. Theory generation often requires qualitative approaches, whereas relation, association, and theory testing often require quantitative data.

Quantitative designs are often divided into experimental, quasi-experimental, or nonexperimental. We often think of experiments as having been around for a long time, but actually it was only in the 1930s that the first experiments were conducted. Sir Ronald Fisher's (1935) book *The Design of Experiments* provided the first details of experimental techniques. The purpose of experimental design was to gain greater control and thus improve validity. The aim is to associate a treatment with its outcome by minimizing the effect of other variables on the outcome and reducing error introduced by extraneous or confounding variables. Random assignment to groups, manipulation of the independent variable, and control of extraneous variation are the key elements in experimental design.

Originally, experiments were conducted in laboratories; then the social sciences adopted the techniques, and other designs emerged, such as quasiexperimental designs. In quasi-experimental designs there is an experimental intervention, but one or more of the other elements of experimental design are missing. There may be no random assignment to groups. In such cases, the investigator should address the issue of group equivalence by comparing the groups on relevant variables. There may be no control group, as when a group of subjects is measured over time or under different conditions. This is usually referred to as a within-subjects design.

In nonexperimental designs there is no investigator-controlled intervention. Because the investigator does no control the independent variable, it is more difficult to test the direct effects of one variable on another. What is usually tested is the relationship between and among variables. This includes the testing of models through techniques such as path analysis and structural equation modeling.

One type of experimental design that is of special interest to health care professionals is the randomized clinical trial. In such an experimental design the intervention is tested in practice rather than in a controlled laboratory experiment. In the United States the first randomized clinical trial was reported in 1951 by Yale researcher Cadman (1994). He studied the effectiveness of penicillin in treating pneumococcal pneumonia. Another Yale researcher, Dumas (Dumas, R. G., & Leonard, 1963), published the first report of the use of experimental design in nursing research. In 1963 she reported on nursing interventions to reduce postoperative vomiting.

In all designs, sample selection is crucial. Whether the sample consists of an N of 1, or of thousands, the sample must represent the population of interest. Additionally, the size of the sample must be adequate for subsequent analyses.

Sample designs are often divided into probability and nonprobability designs. Some form of random sampling is used in probability sampling. This enables the researcher to make use of probability theory to determine the accuracy of results through the computation of standard errors. The notion is that all potential subjects have an equal possibility of being included in the sample.

Nonprobability sampling includes several techniques, including selecting subjects based on some criteria (purposive or judgmental), taking those subjects that are available when the study is conducted (convenience or accidental), accruing a set number of subjects in various categories (quota), and advertising for volunteers.

The procedures for implementation of the study and for data collection are designed to maintain the integrity of the study. In experimental designs, methods for assignment to groups and implementation of the experimental conditions must be determined. Careful attention should be paid to ensuring that there is no contamination of experimental intervention across study groups.

D. T. Campbell and Stanley (1963) coined the phrases "internal" and "external" validity. Internal validity refers to the integrity of the study through which we can infer the relationships among the variables under study. External validity refers to how generalizable the results of the study are to other samples, settings, and so forth.

All variables included in the design must be defined and measured. Selection of psychometrically sound instruments and establishment of controlled methods for data collection are necessary for the integrity of the data. Data analysis is based on the questions being answered, the characteristics of the data collected, the size of the sample, and the assumptions underlying the statistical techniques.

Quantitative research methods from design through data collection and analysis must be carefully explicated prior to embarking on a study. Careful attention to all aspects of the methodology is necessary to produce valid results.

BARBARA MUNRO

Quasi-Experimental Research

Under "Experimental Research" in this encyclopedia, T. Cook and Campell's (1979) definition that experiments are characterized by manipulation, control, and randomization was cited. However, when conducting research in field settings, it is not always possible to implement design that meets these three criteria. Quasi-experimental research is similar to experimental research in that there is manipulation of an independent variable. It differs from experimental research because either there is no control group, no random selection, no random assignment, and/or no active manipulation.

Quasi-experimental research is a useful way to test causality in settings when it is impossible or unethical to randomly assign subjects to treatment and control groups or to withhold treatment from some subjects. The main disadvantage of quasi-experimental research is the increased threat to internal validity (see "Experimental Research" for a review of types of design validity). Within quasi-experimental designs, a distinction is made between preexperimental, nonequivalent control group designs, and interrupted time series designs. Note also that the boundaries between experimental and quasi-experimental research have blurred. Often investigators like to define their study as experimental when in fact it is quasi-experimental.

Preexperimental designs are the weakest of the quasi-experimental designs. They may lack a control/comparison group, observation before the intervention (commonly known as pretests), or both. Their use is strongly discouraged because they do not permit even remote inferences about the direction and dynamics of change and causality.

Nonequivalent control group designs refer to situations in which naturally occurring groups of subjects are used as control/comparison group or those in which it is impossible or unethical to withhold treatment from a given group. In spite of the absence of randomization, nonequivalent control group designs can be considered relatively strong designs. The use of a control group and a pretest significantly increase the strength of nonequivalent control group designs. Good pretest data will enable the researcher to improve the level of analysis. When subjects from different settings are used, a nonequivalent control group design may control some threats to internal validity, such as compensatory rivalry and demoralization of controls. When subjects in each group are naturally kept separate, it is less likely that they will have contact with each other, and it is often useful to minimize contact between treatment and control groups.

In time series designs the researcher does not always use a control group and does not use randomization. An interrupted time series study uses several observations of subjects over time with a treatment given at a specified point (or longitudinally over time, with start and end time points). A time series study can be designed to study the same individuals at specified intervals or to study different individuals at some common point in time. When the researcher studies one group of subjects, the subjects act as their own controls, which provides the researcher with equivalent control groups. Time series designs are used when a control group population is not available. When only one group is available to the researcher, the time series design significantly increases the strength of the research.

Ivo L. Abraham
Lynn I. Wasserbauer

R

Reliability

Reliability refers to the consistency of responses on self-report, norm-referenced measures of attitudes and behavior. Reliability arises from classical measurement theory, which holds that any score obtained from an instrument will be a composite of the individual's true pattern and error variability. The error is made up of random and systematic components. Maximizing the instrument's reliability helps to reduce the random error associated with the scores, although the validity of the instrument helps to minimize systematic error (see "Validity"). The "true" score or variance in measurement relies on the consistency of the instrument as reflected by form and content, the stability of the responses over time, and the freedom from response bias or differences that could contribute to error. Error related to content results from the way questions are asked and the mode of instrument administration. Time can contribute to error by the frequency of measurement and the time frame imposed by the questions asked. Error due to response differences results from the state or mood of the respondent, wording of questions that may lead to a response bias, and the testing or conceptual experience of the subject.

There are generally two forms of reliability assessment designed to deal with random error: stability and equivalence. Stability is the reproducibility of responses over time. Equivalence is the consistency of responses across a set of items so that there is evidence of a systematic pattern. Both of these forms apply to self-report as well as to observations made by a rater. For self-report measures, stability is examined through test-retest procedures; equivalence is assessed through alternative forms and internal consistency techniques. For observational measurement intra- and interrater techniques assess the two forms of reliability respectively.

Stability reliability is considered by some to be the only true way to measure the consistency of responses on an instrument. In fact, stability was the primary manner in which early instruments were examined for reliability. Stability is measured primarily through test-retest procedures in which the same instrument is given to the same subjects at two different points in time, commonly 2 weeks apart. The scores are then correlated, or compared for consistency, using some form of agreement score that depends on the level of measurement. Typically, data are continuous; thus, correlation coefficients and difference between mean scores are usually assessed. A correlation tells the investigator whether individuals who scored high on the first administration also scored high on the second. It does not provide information on whether the scores are the same. Only a test that looks at the difference in mean scores will give that information.

The problem with stability is that it is not always reasonable to assume that the concept will remain unchanged over time. If the person's true score on a concept changes within 2 weeks, instability and high random error will be assumed—when, in effect, it is possible that the instrument is consistently measuring change across time. Reliance on a 2-week interval for measuring stability may be faulty.

The time interval chosen must directly relate to the theoretical understanding of the concept being measured.

A special case of stability occurs with instruments that are completed by raters on the basis of their observations. Intrarater reliability refers to the need for ratings to remain stable across the course of data collection and not change due to increased familiarity and practice with the instrument. The same assessment procedures are used for intrarater reliability as for test-retest reliability.

Equivalence is evaluated in two major ways. The first of these predated the availability of high-speed computers and easily accessed statistical packages. This set of techniques deals with the comparison of scores on alternate or parallel forms of the instrument to which the subject responds at the same point in time. Parallelism means an item on one form has a comparable item on the second form, indexing the same aspect of the concept, and that the means and variances of these items are equal. These scores are compared through correlation or mean differences in a similar manner to stability. Consistency is assumed if the scores are equivalent. Assessment with alternative/parallel forms is not comparison with two different measures of the concept. It is comparison of two essentially identical tests that were developed at the same time through the same procedures. Therefore, a difficulty with this approach to equivalent reliability is obtaining a true parallel or alternative form of an instrument.

A more common way to look at equivalence is through internal consistency procedures. The assumption underlying internal consistency is that the response to a set of scale items should be equivalent. All internal consistency approaches are based in correlational procedures. An earlier form of internal consistency is split-half reliability, in which responses to half the items on a scale are randomly selected and compared to responses on the other half.

Currently Cronbach's (1951) alpha reliability coefficient is the most prevalent technique for assessing internal consistency. Developed in the 1950s, the formula basically computes the ratio of variability between individual responses to the total variability in responses, with total variability being a composite of the individual variability and the measurement error. As a ratio, the values obtained can range from 0 to 1, with 1 indicating perfect reliability and no measurement error. The ratio then reflects the proportion of the total variance in the response that is due to real differences between subjects. A general guideline for use of Cronbach's alpha to assess an instrument is that well-established instruments must demonstrate a coefficient value above .80, whereas newly developed instruments should reach values of .70 or greater. This should not be taken to indicate that the higher the coefficient, the better the instrument. Excessively high coefficients indicate redundancy and unnecessary items. A special case of alpha is the Kuder-Richardson 20, which is essentially alpha for dichotomous data.

Cronbach's alpha is based on correlational analysis, which is highly influenced by the number of items and sample size. It is possible to increase the reliability coefficient of a scale by increasing the number of items. A small sample size can result in a reduced reliability coefficient that is a biased estimate. A limitation of alpha is that items are considered to be parallel, which means they have identical true scores. When this is not the case, alpha is a lower bound to reliability; and other coefficients for internal consistency, based within models of principal components and common factor analysis (e.g., Theta and Omega), are more appropriate. Obtaining an adequate alpha does not mean that examination of internal consistency is complete. Item analysis must be accomplished and focused on the fit of individual items with the other items and the total instrument.

Again, observational measures are a special case and require different formulas for the determination of equivalence. Interrater reliability refers to the need for ratings to be essentially equivalent across data collectors and not to differ due to individual rater variability. The most common assessment procedure, kappa, is based on percent agreement and controlling for chance.

Any discussion of reliability as approached through classical test theory should note more recent proposals for test consistency. Of these proposals, generalizability theory (G theory) has received the most attention. Unlike classical test theory reliability, G theory can estimate several sources of random error in one analysis; in the process a generalizability coefficient is computed. Proponents of G theory believe that its concentration on dependability rather than reliability offers a more global and flexible approach to estimating measurement error.

PAULA M. MEEK
JOYCE A. VERRAN

Reminiscence and Life Review

The words reminiscence and life review are often used interchangeably. They are however two different methodologies of recall; their one commonality is that they both use memory to operationalize themselves as concept and intervention. Reminiscence is a multifaceted, multipurpose, naturally occurring mental phenomenon manifested across the life span in a variety of forms and contexts. Life review is one of those forms of reminiscence, but it differs in that it is more intense and has more depth. The life review covers the life span, is more structured, and has an evaluative component in which people review, revise, and reintegrate both good and bad memories into a newly organized picture of their lives as they were lived. Often life review is performed on a one-to-one basis rather than in groups.

Presently other types of recall that have many similarities to life review and reminiscence are popular and may be confused with life review modalities. One of these is oral history, where the fact and the content are sought rather than the effect on the person recalling the memories. Reminiscence, life review, and oral history differ in their origin, in that oral history arises from a historical/sociological base and life review/reminiscence arises from a psychological base. Narrative therapy is still another form of recall and arises from psychiatry. In narrative therapy the individual tells the story surrounding a particular problem, a problem for which he has sought help from a psychiatrist. While retelling the story, new insights are gained by both the patient and the psychiatrist, and in the process, the story tends to mend the problem. Story is becoming a term with common use in psychology as scholars and researchers begin to report stories in the narrative and analyze them qualitatively.

In the last 10 years alone, there have been 150 new publications with increased rigor and a more scholarly approach. One of the most important advances in this field of research has been that researchers and practitioners alike now define their process so that others can easily understand it, making outcomes more comparable. Two books with integrated reviews on the work done in the past 10 years, by Haight and Webster (1995) and Webster and Haight (2002), will be especially helpful for additional information on reminiscence and life review.

Reminiscence and life review research use both quantitative and qualitative paradigms. In the last decade researchers have begun to use the whole life story and larger sample sizes while employing diverse ways to look at functions, processes, and outcomes.

A variety of theories have been used in reminiscence research. The most common one is the Eight Ages of Man. Erickson described the last stage of life as integrity and further stated that people who do not reach integrity will be in a continual state of despair. He defined integrity as accepting one's life as it has been lived. For many researchers the life review is seen as the process for reaching integrity. As people review their lives and begin to accept and reintegrate their life events, they also accept their lives as they were lived, thus reaching integrity.

Tornstam (1999) argued that the theory of gerotranscendence is a better way of studying reminiscence, because gerotranscendence and reminiscence functions are intertwined. Tornstam suggested that reminiscence contributes to the reconstruction of identity and the understanding of reality as a process of reorganization and reconstruction. Webster (2003) took still another approach, trying to marry the fields of autobiographical memory and reminiscence with a circumplex model that would serve as a bridging technique within and between reminiscence and autobiography.

Haight, Michel, and Hendrix (2000) conducted a longitudinal study with 256 newly admitted nursing home residents. They not only discovered a positive effect on depression; they found that the therapeutic outcomes increased over time for at least 2 years in those receiving a life review. This is the only longitudinal study published to date that looks at the effect of life review over time and the information can be very important to practice, showing that in 2 years the client may be ready for another dose of life review to reinforce the positive response.

Another very interesting study by a nurse used life review psychotherapy with depressed homebound older adults. McDougall, Blixen, and Lee-Jen (1997) conducted a retrospective analysis of notes from 80 patients over 65 years of age who were discharged from a psychiatric hospital with a primary diagnosis of depression. Home health nurses then used life review as an intervention and facilitated the ability of these patients to live at home and remain independent. Most importantly, McDougal and colleagues showed that these nurses were able to bill for the intervention as a part of their services.

A critical review and synthesis of literature on reminiscing in older adults was recently published in the *Canadian Journal of Nursing Research*. In this analysis and synthesis the authors reported that despite the many publications on the topic only a few were research-based. However, they did conclude that the analysis resulted in clarity regarding the operational definitions of reminiscence and life review and provides guidance for the design of imaginative programs (Buchanan et al., 2002).

Qualitative analysis is an excellent way to study people's experiences to determine what makes them what they are. The life story is a rich resource and can contribute an enormous amount to the study of people.

Heliker (1997) used a narrative approach similar to a modified life review to gather data on volunteers over the age of 75 years living in a nursing home. She used a seven-step hermeneutical method to analyze the data. Her results indicated that the revelation of personal and shared meaning could guide the development of new, innovative patient care interventions.

Melia (1999) collected life stories from sisters of three religious orders to examine the question of whether the old-old undergo additional developmental stages after reaching ego integrity in their younger old age. She used a narrative approach to collect the stories and then used grounded theory to analyze 35 interviews. She found continuity and continued growth in the lives of the religious women.

Much of the new research in 2000 looks at the functions of reminiscence, how it works, and on whom it works best. Continuing this work is necessary to understand the process. Additionally, reminiscence as intervention has been effective particularly with depression and partially with Alzheimer's disease and should be explored more fully in future work.

BARBARA K. HAIGHT

Replication Studies

Replication involves repeating or reproducing a research study to investigate whether similar findings will be obtained in different settings and with different samples. Replication is needed not only to establish the credibility of research findings but also to extend generalizability. Blomquist (1986) listed five reasons why replication studies should be encouraged in nursing: (a) scientific merit is established, (b) Type I and Type II errors are decreased, (c) construct validity is increased,

(d) support for theory development is provided, and (e) acceptance of erroneous results is prevented. Replication studies are essential for developing a scientific knowledge base in nursing. Incorporating research findings into nursing practice has been seriously hampered by the limited number of replication studies. Clarification of replication terminology can assist in advancing replication research. Three of the most often cited classifications of replication research have been developed by Finifter (1975), LaSorte (1972), and Lykken (1968).

Lykken (1968) identified three methods of replication: literal, operational, and constructive. Literal replication is an exact duplication of the original researcher's sampling, procedure, experimental treatment, data collection techniques, and data analysis. Operational replication involves an exact duplication of only the sampling and experimental procedures in the original research to check whether the original design when used by another leads to the same results. In constructive replication duplicate methods are purposely avoided.

Finifter (1975) listed four replication strategies: identical, virtual, systematic, and pseudo. Identical replication involves a one-to-one duplication of the original study's procedures and conditions. In virtual replication the methods of the original study are re-created in varying degrees. In systematic replication neither the methods nor the substance of the original study are duplicated. Pseudoreplication is similar to identical and virtual replication; however, data for pseudoreplication are collected at the same time as those for the original study. The simultaneous confirmation of the study is built into the original design.

LaSorte (1972) described retest, internal, independent, and theoretical replication. Retest replication involves repeating an original study with few, if any, significant changes in the research design. Internal replication is incorporated into the original study. Data for both the original study and its replicated study are collected simultaneously to provide a cross-check for the reliability of the original results. In independent replication, significant modifications in the design of the original study are made to verify the empirical generalization. In theoretical replication the inductive process is used to examine the feasibility of fitting the empirical findings into a general theoretical framework.

A comparison of these three replication classifications reveals that Finifter's (1975) identical replication is similar to Lykken's (1968) literal replication. The three classifications include strategies to approximate the original research design. Finifter calls this virtual replication, Lykken labels it operational, and LaSorte (1972) describes it as retest replication. The purpose of choosing this type of replication is to determine if the original findings can be confirmed when modest changes in the research conditions have been made. When original findings are replicated, confidence in the reliability of these results is enhanced.

All three classifications include an approach to increase empirical generalization by significantly modifying the original design. Finifter (1975) labels this systematic replication, Lykken (1968) describes it as constructive replication, and LaSorte (1972) calls it independent replication. This type of replication strategy is used when the researcher not only wants to validate earlier work but also wants to extend the results and determine the degree of generalizability.

Both Finifter (1975) and LaSorte (1972) specifically identify types of replication where data for both the original and replication studies are collected at the same time. According to Finifter, this is pseudoreplication, and to LaSorte it is internal replication. This type of replication provides additional data, which is used as a cross-check of the data's reliability. LaSorte's classification is the only one that includes a replication strategy to develop and verify theory.

Replication studies conducted in nursing have addressed topics such as nursing education, nurses' characteristics, perioperative nursing, body image during pregnancy, cardiac care, fetal monitoring, and time perception.

When publishing replicated studies nurse researchers should include the following information: (a) identification of the specific type of replication that is conducted, (b) provision of specific information on how a replicated study is the same as and different from the original study, and (c) explanation of what is replicated and how. This information will help readers to more clearly understand how the researchers methodically revised previous studies in a progressive manner. When publishing original studies, researchers also should explicitly detail the important points of their sampling and data collection techniques and their research design to aid replication of their work. Authors must be more diligent in identifying the minimum essential conditions and controls necessary for producing findings because replication is crucial for the further development of nursing knowledge.

CHERYL TATANO BECK

Representation of Knowledge for Computational Modeling in Nursing: The Arcs© Program

There are a number of computational approaches to management and application of knowledge to clinical situations in medicine, and to a small degree, nursing. Computers can apply domain knowledge to data to diagnose and suggest treatment of diseases. Computers can also discover new knowledge. Much of this discovery research uses databases of observations of scientific phenomena and falls into two categories: empirical laws and formation of theories. In contrast, *arcs©* uses the scientific findings reported in the research literature as data with which to propose theoretical models.

Historically, discovery of new knowledge in nursing has been more likely to start with theory than with clinical data. Many nursing observations (data) were discarded from the care record and thus not systematically available for inducing hypotheses. Thus, nurse researchers and theorists have traditionally used the scientific literature to develop theoretical models of a process or event, then empirically test the hypotheses suggested by these models.

Knowledge is found in experts, in the books and journals of a domain, and one might say, in clinical databases if one knows how to acquire it. The process of searching the literature to find knowledge needed to build a testable theoretical model is an appalling task. Scientists want to know what variables were studied together with what result. For them to obtain this knowledge, they must sort through bibliographic databases and/or specific journals and/or work with their "invisible college." The "invisible college" is a term that refers generally to a self-selected group of researchers (or theorists) working in the same field who stay in touch to keep up with one another's work instead of waiting for publications to come out. Bibliographic searches are generally designed so that the searcher either finds too much that is not relevant and not enough that is. Upon finding the desired literature set, one must wade through pages that represent the knowledge in numeric relationship displays and text. An alternative would be to index research by variable names and findings. The scientist can then go directly to the literature that reports on the knowledge established between those variables.

Although *arcs* does not help the user directly with the literature search, *arcs* does demonstrate a methodology for indexing the research literature by variables studied so that all users could go directly to the studies that are of interest to them with 100% sensitivity and 100% specificity. Although *arcs* does not currently eliminate the work of wading through pages of prose to identify the knowledge contained within the research article, it does demonstrate an alternative methodology for reporting and storing research knowledge that immediately makes the knowledge and the salient characteristics obvious and a basis for computational modeling of nursing knowledge. These methods are now enjoying practical application at the Virginia Henderson International Nursing Library of Sigma Theta Tau International (STTI).

The *arcs* program was developed initially as a knowledge engineering project. Knowledge engineering takes knowledge in one form (in this case the scientific literature) and processes it into a more easily used form (in this case textual and graphic relational maps, also called causal/associational maps or concept maps). Knowledge must be represented in the computer so that the computer can process it predictably.

The first step of the *arcs* project was to identify and formalize a definition of knowledge by examining the way it is structured in the scientific literature. A further decision was made to delimit the project to knowledge expressed relationally and generated from empiricist designs, published in English-language journals, and involving only reports of research with humans. Numerous research articles from nursing, psychology, and sociology journals were used. For each article, the expression of the finding(s) was recorded. The overall structure of these knowledge expressions was virtually the same across disciplines. All contained names of variables, stated the relationship studied, and the results. On the basis of these investigations, a structure of scientific knowledge was defined grossly as *the result or finding about the (statistical) relationship between two or more variables, given the design, methods and conditions, and source* (Graves, 1990).

The second step of the project was to devise a knowledge-base structure that would store a unit of knowledge as defined above. In order to retain the original research language, variables are named as designated by the researcher at their operational (measured) level. To collect the potentially numerous variable names into manageable models, a higher level abstraction term may be assigned by the researcher or by the knowledge base builder. In addition to names, other attributes of variables (measurement, dependency [and thus directionality]) were added. Numerical relationships were largely statistical and were categorized as descriptive, associational, directional, difference, and structural. Together, these categories incorporated all types of statistical tests. A number of attributes were added to further describe the conditions of the study and the certainty associated with the finding, including direction and magnitude.

Next, this structure was implemented by using relational database software. Instead of calling the resulting product a database, it is called a knowledge base because it stores the entire unit of knowledge. Before it could be tested by anyone other than the author, however, a menu system had to be added to allow users to interact with the software without learning a database query language. The first program produced a text-based model of a focal variable with three levels of relationships. One had to draw one's own relational map, using the text model.

It was next necessary to test the generalizability of the knowledge structure. This was done by having selected doctoral students use the program in their dissertation literature reviews. It was found that they could use the program to store units of knowledge from very different domains, including research from multiple disciplines.

When it was established that there was sufficient generalizability between research domains, the software was then ported to a machine that could more easily be programmed to build graphical knowledge models. The name was changed from Arks© to *arcs* to denote the mathematical concept of *arc* as a relationship (directional or nondirectional) between two entities in the world—a natural model for representing relational knowledge.

Testing of this version consisted of entering subsets of knowledge in different domains to test the functionality of the program, the accuracy of the models, and the value of the graphics to a user. The program was modified to incorporate suggestions from users as appropriate. The *arcs* program was next converted to a Microsoft Windows™ environment and can be used on a Macintosh with Soft Windows™. It is in active use for building knowledge bases at Sigma Theta Tau.

The *arcs* computer program uses the concept of a knowledge base that contains linked data about all essential elements of a unit of knowledge as defined above. Data must be entered into the program by the user, who must obtain the data from research studies published in a domain of knowledge. The *arcs* program builds the models of knowledge from the data entered by the user about *pairs of variables*, the *relationship* studied between then, *direction*, *sign*, and effect size of the finding. Each statistical relationship is represented by a different type of line that includes the directionality of each relationship, if any. Indirect relationships can be modeled to two more levels. Discovery is supported only passively now; the user must examine models to identify gaps and conflicts in the modeled domain. However, the later version of *arcs* will use a mathematical approach to identifying gaps and conflicts. Work is also in progress to design and test an algorithm to provide an estimate of belief in models, depending on such things as research design and conflicting findings.

There are many more attributes of a unit of knowledge that can be stored in *arcs*. It is up to the user to decide how much detail will be of value in modeling. This, in turn, will depend on the characteristics of the domain being modeled. Virtually all of the attributes can be used to *condition* (restrict or specify) the model. For example, one can elect to model only studies that have certain validity scores or effect sizes or studies of a single sample type, such as children. By conditioning the model to address time of publication, *arcs* models will illustrate changes in what is being studied in a domain over time, changes in level of testing, and methodologies, even variable names. The amount of replication will be visible in the models. Because new findings can be added as they are published, the model stays up-to-date.

The *arcs Tracker* is a menu-guided interface for building queries. The results are reported as text and can be used to build text models as well as to summarize (count) various attributes in the knowledge base. The *arcs* program provides a guided validity review and produces a graph of validity distributions for the user who wishes to describe validities in a domain. Heuristic, internal, and external validities are graphed separately. In addition, *arcs* provides a metastructure map that graphs the frequency with which pairs of variables are studied, using the metastructure categories of person, environment (health or nursing) focus, intervention, and intervention outcome. The *arcs* program is labor-intensive in the data input phase. Some research articles require up to an hour for extraction of all the relevant data about the knowledge, especially when the knowledge is embedded in text and not represented in numeric relationship displays. This limits usefulness.

The broader modeling concepts of *arcs*, however, are implemented in the STTI *Registry for Nursing Research*. In this case, the researchers themselves register their work and enter the details of their studies, so the data does not have to be extracted from published articles. This provides a new paradigm for publishing nursing knowledge and allows researchers access to unpublished as well as published nursing knowledge. Over time, the STTI *Registry for Nursing Research*, not a traditional library of documents, will be the knowledge base with which computational modeling of nursing knowledge will take place.

Judith R. Graves

Research Careers

Research expands the body of knowledge of a discipline and profession. To ensure that students have an opportunity to learn about the importance of nursing research to the profession, the National League for Nursing Accrediting Commission currently mandates that baccalaureate nursing programs teach nursing research methods and incorporate the utilization and evaluation of nursing research into their curricula. For baccalaureate nursing graduates, the expectations are to evaluate and utilize research in their practice. The expectation of master's program graduates is to participate in nursing research and to facilitate research utilization; the expectation of doctorally prepared graduates is that they conduct and disseminate their research. Every nurse has a professional obligation to use research findings to inform his or her practice. Some nurses choose a career in which the conduct of research is one expectation, and others, nurse researchers, choose a career in which the primary expectation is the conduct of research, including the facilitation of research by others.

As a result of their educational and practice experiences, nurses may decide to pursue research careers in a broad continuum of clinical and/or practice areas. Research careers in nursing, as in other disciplines, follow a developmental course, from novice to experienced to senior researcher, with each stage posing different demands and expectations and offering different satisfactions.

The educational preparation for a nursing research career is an earned doctorate with specialized courses in statistics and research methodology. Generally, a nurse formally begins his or her research career with doctoral work. With the doctoral committee members, a research area of interest, a research problem, and senior research advisor are identified. In doctoral work the student has the opportunity to be actively involved in each step of the research process, to develop research skills, and to be formally socialized and mentored in the research environment.

Nurses at this beginning stage of a research career are intimately involved in building a sound foundation in research design, completing data collection and analysis, and starting to develop a scholarly identity through publication. The demands at this stage of a research career revolve around obtaining initial funding, prioritizing time for completing the research data collection and analysis, and working with peers to develop a network of research colleagues. The satisfaction of the novice researcher is in making a contribution to the body of knowledge in a specific area, acquiring a scholarly identity, and presenting and publishing the results of research studies that build the scientific base.

Experienced nurses with evolving nursing research careers are challenged to maintain continued funding, serve as role models for students and other nurses, further develop their research trajectory, and extend their research network. Nurses at this level of their research careers find satisfaction in their growing reputation as researchers, the ability to extend their study to addressing new questions, and working with colleagues on multisite studies.

The challenges facing the senior researcher are to continue and extend their own scholarly research, with interdisciplinary colleagues as appropriate, finding funding sources to support large studies and mentoring novice researchers and students. Senior researchers find career satisfaction in serving as consultants to other nurse researchers and interdisciplinary research teams, mentoring novice researchers, developing as nursing scholars, and making significant contributions to the body of nursing knowledge.

For the nursing profession to remain viable in a changing world, the continuous development of nurse researchers is necessary. To promote this development, the National Institute of Nursing Research (NINR), the institute for nursing research within the National Institutes of Health, has funded core centers for research at universities across the nation. Examples of those funded are University of Pittsburgh, University of California at San Francisco, University of North Carolina, University of Iowa, University of Pennsylvania, and University of Washington. The specific areas of research identified for each university center are chronic disorders, symptom management, chronic illness in vulnerable people, gerontological nursing interventions, advancing care in serious illness, and women's health, respectively.

These core centers support the creation of interdisciplinary collaborative nursing research programs in specific areas of basic and/or clinical nursing research and offer opportunities for nurses to consult with nursing experts in these areas, train with mentors, and develop professional networks with other interdisciplinary researchers. Other schools of nursing have research centers (funded through other sources), and these also provide the infrastructure necessary to support the research careers of faculty.

Financial support for individuals seeking a research career is also available from NINR. There are funding mechanisms to support nurses at various stages of research career development: (a) predoctoral fellowships for researchers beginning their research careers, (b) postdoctoral fellowships for nurses who want to expand the knowledge gained in their doctoral study, and (c) senior fellowships for investigators who have already been successful in a research arena and want to acquire new research capabilities or pursue new directions of research. For information about this funding source, contact National Institute for Nursing Research, 31 Center Drive, MSC 2178 Building 31, Bethesda MD 20892-2178. Professional nursing organizations are additional sources of research funding. Examples of these funding sources include Sigma Theta Tau International, Oncology Nursing Foundation, and American Association of Critical Care Nurses.

Research career development in nursing historically was confined to faculty in a university setting. With recent changes in the health care delivery systems, opportunities for research careers in industry, at clinical centers, and in outpatient care facilities are increasing. Hospitals and integrated systems of health care delivery are increasingly employing nurse researchers to study practice improvements, care quality, and health outcomes. Nurse researchers also assist in the development of the informatics systems used in these settings to support studies of comparison of practices, outcomes, and the benchmarking efforts required.

A research career offers nurses the opportunity to engage in a lifelong process of building a research program that attempts to find answers to the questions that are central to the discipline and professional practice. To pursue this career pathway requires a strong educational foundation, mentoring in the research environment, and available funding. Research centers established by the NINR and other sources serve as resources for beginning, experienced, and seasoned nurse researchers to extend their research trajectories. The future holds many opportunities for nursing research careers in integrated health systems, industry, and academe.

MARY J. MCNAMEE
ADA M. LINDSEY

Research Dissemination

Research dissemination is the purposeful communication of research, particularly the findings and implications of those findings to members of society who can utilize them. Dissemination is initiated by those who "know" and extend to those who "do not know" but might apply the findings if they knew (Rogers, E., 1995). As a practice profession, nursing cannot be satisfied with just awareness but is always interested in the application prospects of the research.

Dissemination is sometimes differentiated from diffusion when the latter term is reserved for spontaneous spread and use of research. Most writers on dissemination and diffusion talk about a purposeful process aimed at spread and use of research. Utilization is another related term. Utilization is specifically focused on application and is more likely to be initiated at the user end, whereas dissemination is focused on knowledge acquisition and more likely is initiated at the researcher end. The two are obviously linked with overlapping phases in their processes.

A principal writer/researcher whose work has directed research dissemination is Rogers, who writes on the "diffusion of innovations." E. Rogers (1995) noted that in 1962, at the time of his first book, 405 publications were found on innovation diffusion, whereas by 1995 the number approached 4,000. Recently, dissemination/diffusion is seen as a less linear process where the potential users of research have a responsibility to contribute to the dialogue so that the movement from innovation to application can occur (Rogers, E.).

E. Rogers's (1995) innovation-decision process has five stages: knowledge, persuasion, decision, implementation, and confirmation. In the knowledge stage, whether the need for the innovation or the innovation occurs first is ambiguous. Three types of knowledge about innovations are essential: awareness, how-to, and principles. Each type represents a more thorough understanding of the innovation. In the persuasion stage a positive or negative impression of the innovation is formed. Here the potential user clearly engages in more active innovation information seeking, the outcome of this stage being formation of an attitude toward the innovation. Although knowledge and attitudes are important factors in the use of the innovation in practice, practice is clearly based on more. Major factors contributing to the knowledge-attitude-practice (KAP) gap include (a) whether the practice of the innovation is outside individual control; (b) whether the individual has interpersonal communication from a near-peer supporting the adoption; (c) individual characteristics toward being an early or late adopter, perhaps based on a sense of efficacy; and (d) whether the nature of the innovation is preventive. Adoption of prevention-focused innovations occurs more slowly.

The ultimate focus of this diffusion process is on the application of the innovation (Rogers, E., 1995) as evidenced by the last three stages. The adoption decision is made in the decision stage. At this stage the process begins to have more relevance for research utilization than for research dissemination. In the implementation stage the innovation is put to use. The final stage, confirmation, is where individuals seed reinforcement for their decision to adopt. In confirmation the innovation is evaluated, an outcome being continuation or discontinuation. The first two stages can guide dissemination; the latter stages, utilization.

Explicit dissemination occurs as researchers present their findings, implications, and recommendations in articles, papers, and posters. Usually, these communications include details of the research process that facilitates a scholarly critique. The criticism is that too often these communications occur between researchers and that the nurse caregiver is not linked into the research communication networks. Fortunately, some practitioners do attend research conferences and some practice-focused conferences devote programming to research.

A model for dissemination reported by S. Funk, Tournquist, and Champagne (1989) included practice-oriented research conferences, edited (specifically for practice) monographs of presentations, and an information center. The evaluation of the conference found the general responses extremely positive, but still major communication problems existed in both oral and written reporting. These problems persisted even with a great deal of support to the research communicators. This communication deficit leaves a practitioner, who is unsure, responsible for deciding about practice utility (persuasion). Because the "old way" is usually comfortable, the innovation may not move from knowledge awareness to the more advanced how-to or principles knowledge. Consequently, the nurse prepared at the graduate level has an important role in dissemination in a clinical agency. This nurse is usually the reader of research, can interpret the findings, and sees the application possibilities. Through means like continuing education and journal clubs, the nurse from a graduate program can assist in filtering the research literature to match closely the practicing nurses' concerns and interests.

Implicit dissemination also occurs. This dissemination occurs when educators (academe, staff development, and continuing education) incorporate relevant research into their offerings. Audiences frequently trust that presenters have carefully critiqued the research they cite. Although this assumption usually is well founded, the scholarly practitioner will seek references and do a personal review.

As more nurses are university educated, including nurse administrators, familiarity with the relevant research has become a standard of practice in some organizations. Although this practice is not yet the norm, practice policies, standards, and procedures should be written, with a literature review that includes applicable research from nursing and other relevant disciplines. With a policy or procedure focusing on the "need to know" for the practitioner, the review of relevant research can be productive in practical dissemination by providing a context for considering whether to move into the application/utilization phases of knowledge diffusion.

An additional means of dissemination is currently evolving, and that is via the Internet. Universities, professional organizations, and individuals have home pages that more and more are including research information. Online journals also are available. Some of the home pages include only researcher names and topics; others include abstracts and findings. The additional caveat needed is that few of the sites have any type of peer review for quality and should be read with that in mind. Sigma Theta Tau's *Online Journal of Knowledge Synthesis for Nursing* is an example of a site with peer-reviewed content.

With the pressure on health care providers to be effective and efficient, the responsibility to break the "knowledge creep and decision accretion" situation (Weiss, C., 1980) is incumbent upon providers. To speed the dissemination process and facilitate utilization, the outcomes of any research project must be communicated with clarity, especially for the practice implications and for future research. One approach is to "market" research findings. This is a persuasive approach and would require more than not speaking solely in "researcher terms" but also addressing the four factors in Rogers's KAP gap. Marketing also addresses who is the persuader; witness the number of nurses selling pharmaceuticals and medical supplies. Clinician partners, especially clinical nurse specialists, are appropriate disseminators of research. A larger proportion of research funds should be spent on dissemination, not just for the "telling" but also for the necessary dialogue for quality research (Backer & Koon, 1995). Although graduate education makes a substantial contribution to dissemination, students must know how to do more than tell. They should learn also to persuade and dialogue. Educators, administrators, and clinicians must all take responsibility with researchers for strengthening the dissemination process so that research can guide nursing practice.

PATRICIA A. MARTIN

Research in Nursing Ethics

Recent developments in technology have created increased awareness on the part of society and health professionals about the ethical dimensions of high-tech care. It is now recognized that our ability to deal with human and ethical issues has not kept pace with the rapid advancements made possible through various technologies being applied in health care.

Nursing ethics has evolved from the use of etiquette or rules of conduct to the philosophical or empirical analysis of (1) the moral phenomena found in nursing practice, (2) the moral language and ethical foundations of nursing practice, and (3) the ethical judgments made by nurses (Fry, 1995).

It is a salutary development of the past two decades that nurse investigators in increasing numbers have engaged in ethical inquiry. Earlier studies on ethical inquiry were mainly philosophical and normative. In more recent years empirical and descriptive studies have predominated, utilizing both qualitative and quantitative methods. The aim of these studies, collectively, has been to understand nurses' ethical decision making and actions under a variety of conditions of ethical ambiguity and conflict, along with the factors that affect these actions and decisions (ethical practice, moral behavior). In addition, there has been interest in understanding how nurses reason about moral choice (moral reasoning) and what conditions promote high-quality reasoning.

Moral reasoning is defined as a cognitive and developmental process involving a sequential transformation in the way social arrangements and ethical problems are interpreted. Each successive stage (of six stages) is more complex, comprehensive, and differentiated than the preceding stage. It has been theorized that certain conditions stimulate moral development. These include cognitive development and the nature of the educational and social climates, such as when opportunities are provided for assumption of responsibility or when cognitive disequilibrium is created to show inadequacies in one's mode of thinking (Kohlberg, 1978).

This conception of morality is ostensibly based on notions of rights, obligations, and justice and is said to reflect a male-oriented perspective. Gilligan (1982) challenged this perspective by proposing the ethic of care or care-based reasoning, reflecting the way women reason about moral choice. This mode of reasoning does not involve the application of abstract ethical principles; rather, moral conflict and possible choices of action are constructed and defined by the context of the situation and the relationship of self to others who are involved in the conflict. Research to date does not support the polarization of and gender identifications with care (as feminine) and justice (as masculine).

Further, Gilligan (1982) contended that moral problems can be viewed from both justice and care perspectives by the same person, and both perspectives contain important moral injunctions; they entail different (but not opposite) ways of approaching moral judgments. Several instruments have been developed to measure care orientation in women. In a few studies using the Ethic of Care Interview, significant relationships have emerged between age, ego identity, and use of care orientation among women.

In an integrative review published in 1989, Ketefian reported on empirical studies conducted in ethical practice and moral reasoning and updated this information by a literature search conducted in 1996. Nurse investigators have studied moral reasoning as a dependent variable, trying to predict its development from various educational, cognitive, environmental, and personal demographic variables. Recently, a number of studies have focused on qualitative descriptions of nurses' reasoning and whether they used the care or the justice conceptions of morality. No clear direction emerged.

Ethical practice refers to nursing decisions and actions that reflect high ethical standards, such as those set forth by the nursing profession. Various indices of ethical behavior have been proposed, which makes comparisons across studies difficult. The measures vary as well. The most frequently used tool is Judgments about Nursing Decisions (Ketefian, 1989), but many investigators have developed their own measures. Ethical practice, moral behavior, and ethical decision making are terms utilized interchangeably and have been studied as dependent variables. Educational variables, moral reasoning, and organizational and personal variables have been used as predictors of ethical practice with inconsistent and mixed results.

Caring behaviors originate from a strong interest in something or someone that contributes to the good, worth, dignity, or comfort of others. A number of descriptive studies on nurses' caring behaviors have been conducted. In samples composed of patients or others, several aspects of nurses' caring behaviors have been identified—empathic communication, competence, providing continuity, meeting needs, and being respectful, nonjudgmental, and solicitous. These aspects of nurses' behaviors provide a starting point for further research on the effects of nurse behaviors on patient satisfaction and patient outcomes.

A few studies have identified the attitudes and values of nurses concerning ethical issues, the extent to which nurses understand the concept of ethical dilemmas, physicians' and nurses' perceptions of ethical problems, how nurses address ethical concerns in their practice, nurses' perceptions of powerlessness in influencing ethical decisions, ethical conflicts related to pain management, and ethical issues in caring for patients receiving long-term tube feedings. Other studies have examined nurses' role in end-of-life treatment decisions, practices concerning assisted suicide and euthanasia, and differences among nurses and physicians in their ethical decision making.

In addition, studies have identified and compared the ethical decision making of nurses in various practice settings. Only a few studies have included variables such as the frequency with which nurses encounter specific ethical issues in their practice, how disturbed they are by them, the relationship of demographic and work-related variables to frequency and disturbance, the resources that nurses use to clarify ethical issues, and nurses' knowledge of patient care ethics committees.

A promising area of research relates to the way in which organizational variables impinge on the quality of nurses' reasoning, behavior, and judgments. There is a need for clearer definition and measurement. Typically, studies in nursing ethics tend to be isolated, individual projects; many are conducted as dissertations, and few are published. There is a need to move toward a programmatic and cumulative approach, along with a need for replications, so that a meaningful body of science can emerge, one in which we can have a degree of confidence.

SHAKÉ KETEFIAN
SARA T. FRY

Research Interviews (Qualitative)

The interview is a major data collection strategy in qualitative research that aims to obtain textual, qualitative data reflecting the personal perspective of the interviewee. The interview creates an interactional situation in a face-to-face encounter between researchers and participants. In the study the interviewer acts as the instrument and through carefully designed questions, attempts to elicit the other person's opinions, attitudes, or knowledge about a given topic. Research interviews have historically provided the foundation for sociological and anthropological studies that attempted to understand other societies and cultures. As nurse scientists were trained in these methods in the late 1960s and the 1970s, they began using research interviews in nursing studies. Some researchers who seek quantitative data from questionnaires may refer to the structured, standardized survey that is administered face-to-face to large groups of people. The present definition, however, refers to the in-depth and generally less structured interview used in qualitative research.

The research method (e.g., grounded theory, phenomenology, ethnography) suggests the style and purpose of the interview questions. The research objectives are fundamental to the interview questions to maintain the integrity of the research. Grounded theory research intended to discover contexts, phases, and processes of a given phenomenon requires questions designed to acquire knowledge, such as, what is the context of death in a nursing home or at home or what are the phases of dying? Phenomenological research that aims to capture what is referred to as "the lived experience" may use only one general question: Please tell me all that you can about dying. Ethnographic research that is focused on culture may ask about which family members are involved in decisions concerning death and what their roles are.

Interviews are structured in phases—the introduction, the working phase, and termination. In the introduction the researcher gives a personal introduction, states the anticipated length of time of the interview, and makes some initial comments to relax the participant and to assist with the transition from social conversation to research interview. In the working phase the themes of the research are introduced, and the researcher and participant work toward generating a shared understanding. In the termination phase the interview draws to a close, and often brief social conversation occurs again.

The interview demands careful thought about the nature, wording, and sequence of questions. Generally, questions move from general to specific, becoming more focused as themes emerge and as data from other participants suggest additional leads. Questions should be unambiguous, meaningful, and successful in involving the interviewee in the process. The participants in the research are often helpful in critiquing the usefulness and appropriateness of the questions and suggesting others that may be more relevant or successful in obtaining the desired data.

Interviews are of two types: formal and informal. Formal interviews are scheduled as to time and place and generally occur over a period of 1 to 2 hours. Informal interviews are those used in participant observation, when the interviewer spends time in a specific environment and interviews participants as they appear on the scene or around a significant event. Although effective interviews, especially informal ones, may appear simple and comfortable, an expert interviewer is always both in and out of the interview. The interviewer listens carefully to the interviewee and anticipates how to direct the interview to accomplish the aims of the research.

Interviews are characterized as structured and focused when all questions are given in the same order to participants. Interviews in qualitative research studies are generally semifocused ones in which information about a certain subject is desired from all participants, but the phrasing and sequence of the questions may be varied to reflect the characteristics of the participants in the context. Time is permitted to encourage participants to introduce other subjects they believe are relevant and to elaborate, often with the help of interviewer's probes, on earlier comments. Participants' interpretations of meanings and definitions are valued. Such information is obtained only through open-ended questions and free-flowing conversation that follow the thinking of the interviewee. In a sense, the interviewee teaches the researcher about a particular experience or event.

Interviews are generally tape-recorded, and the researcher takes handwritten notes that jog his or her memory during the interview to return to a topic, to ask a hypothetical question, or to request new, related information. These taped interviews are transcribed as soon as possible by the researcher or a transcriptionist and cross-checked against the audiotape for accuracy.

Interviewing establishes the foundation for data analysis. The researcher's interview questions and responses to the interviewee must be analyzed in a reflexive manner to ascertain the quality of the interview. Is the interviewer cutting off the interviewee? Is the interviewer asking closed instead of open-ended questions? Is the interviewer asking relevant questions in a sensitive way? Is the interviewer giving the interviewee time to reflect and to complete his or her comments? Unfocused, insensitive interviewing yields poor data. Quality data result from the expression of affective responses and detailed personal information.

The complexity of interviewing becomes apparent in varied contexts. Interviewing individuals from a culture different from that of the interviewer presents other issues; likewise interviewing the extremely poor or the extremely rich has it own sets of problems. In the past, nurses have relied on sociological and anthropological researchers for guidance. Nurse methodologists agree that it is now time to identify and address issues in interviewing that are especially relevant to nursing topics and populations.

Good interviews provide access to the heart. Such personal information, essential to qualitative research that aims to access human meaning, is a gift. The researcher reciprocates by listening carefully and attempting to render or interpret the experience of the other as accurately as possible. An insensitive interviewer can harm the interviewee, leaving the person psychologically depleted or even wounded. Good interviewers leave interviewees feeling that they gained from the interview.

Sally A. Hutchinson
Holly Skodol Wilson

Research on Interactive Video

Interactive video (IAV) is defined as a technology in which a video program is under the control of a computer, with user choices affecting program branching. The video source for IAV was videotape in early days of development, but current applications use the videodisk.

Development of IAV programs for nursing education began in the early 1980s, and commercially produced programs appeared in 1989. However, the body of research in this area is relatively small, and many studies were dissertations. Studies generally fall into six categories: cost-effectiveness, expert and usage surveys, effectiveness, learning in groups, learner attributes, and strategies to facilitate learning.

Parker examined a large-scale IAV project initiated in 1981 to provide continuing education for nurses scattered across 30 different locations in Florida. She reported significant savings in time and money when IAV was compared with traditional workshops.

In 1987, Rizzolo solicited experts to participate in a three-round Delphi study. Twelve significant factors that were impeding the development of new programs in nursing were identified. Participants were able to identify clearly the content they wanted in IAV programs, especially applications for simulations. They agreed on the benefits of IAV for students but were less certain about how it might affect faculty roles. Conservative predictions were made about how technology might change nursing education in the future.

Two surveys examined the status of interactive video in nursing education. In 1989, Clark surveyed 504 BSN programs. Of the 369 respondents, 66 reported that they were using IAV. One year later Cambre and Castner conducted a study funded by FITNE, Inc. Of the 1,120 schools that responded, 207 were using IAV. Visits and phone interviews revealed positive attitudes about IAV but limited integration into the curriculum.

Several early studies compared IAV to another form of instruction, usually a linear videotape or lecture. Most found no significant differences in achievement. A few reported other positive findings attributable to IAV programs such as higher scores on retention, more positive attitudes toward content, or savings in time required to accomplish objectives.

Weiner et al. found that students who completed an IAV on labor and delivery, along with clinical experience, had significantly greater clinical confidence and learning than those who had only clinical experience. Wittstadt found no difference in confidence levels of nurses who used an interactive video program on infusion pumps as compared to those who learned the material in lecture. Froman et al. found that the sequence of lecture followed by IAV produced the largest gains in self-efficacy by students learning IV procedures.

Middlemiss evaluated IAV as a teaching strategy to help students develop ethical decision-making skills. Students wrote about and analyzed an ethical dilemma, then completed an IAV program and analyzed the event again. She found that students focused more on emotions in their first analysis and used a rational approach after completing the IAV program.

Conflicting results were reported in studies of students using IAV in groups. Rizzolo (1994) compared the pre- and posttest scores of students who worked though case study simulations in a large classroom situation to those who worked independently. Although both achieved significant increases in scores, the classroom group scored significantly higher on the posttest. Garcia's study used one case from the same IAV program and found no significant differences among students working individually, in groups of 2 or 3, and in groups of 10 to 12.

Battista-Calderone studied three groups who worked through an IAV tutorial. Some worked individually, some in groups of 2 or 3, the rest in groups of 7 to 10. Results revealed no significant differences in learning and attitude. Moyer (1996) audiotaped students in groups of two and four as they worked through six IAV programs and also had every student write journal entries. Content analysis revealed more problem-solving behaviors in the tetrad groups. Most felt the group experience was not as beneficial for those who learned more slowly nor for content like ethical decision making, particularly when a group member was very opinionated.

Several studies examined the interaction between learner attributes and achievement or attitudes. Glavin-Spiehs examined field dependence, and Hasset studied psychological type. Neither found significant differences.

Billings and Cobb evaluated the effects of learning style preferences, attitude, and GPA on learner achievement. The strongest predictor was attitude toward computer-based instruction. In a later study, Billings assessed student learning style and attitude toward IAV instruction, then students worked through an IAV program either in a group or alone, as they wished. Students who studied in a group reported greater comfort, but there was no significant difference in learning outcomes.

Yoder's (1994) study measured preferred learning style, then randomly assigned students to IAV or linear videotape instruction. Students who preferred to learn through active experimenting learned better with IAV; those who preferred to learn by reflective observing scored higher after learning with linear videotape.

Most of the research on interactive video has implications for newer multimedia formats such as CD-ROM and interactive offerings on the World Wide Web. It seems clear that well-designed programs can teach content just as well if not better than traditional strategies. Some researchers are even using IAV programs as a tool for research. Predko tracked decisions made by cardiac care nurses as they worked through case study simulations to examine the effect of clinical experience and education on clinical decision-making skills.

Nurse researchers can look to instructional design and educational technology researchers for models and suggestions for future investigation. Their studies include approaches based on cognitive psychology, systems modeling, and instructional events and have suggested researchable propositions to test the validity of underlying assumptions about the technology to discover the conditions of effective use.

Although much additional research is needed on how people learn, nursing students are a diverse group, and qualitative studies might produce more useful data. Studies that identify ways to help students effectively choose and use technology-based applications to learn offer an important area of exploration.

Because studies found little integration of IAV into the curriculum and revealed that most faculty use IAV only for supplementary assignments, research on faculty use of technology is an important area of inquiry. Faculty can easily evaluate program content, but can they evaluate program design to determine if appropriate strategies and media are employed to match content and objectives? Can they decide if the degree of fidelity is appropriate for intended learners? These important questions must be answered so that faculty can select and use technology appropriately and design curricula that free the teacher to provide those experiences than only human interaction can accomplish.

MARY ANNE RIZZOLO

Research Utilization

S. Rodgers (1994) defined research utilization as a "process directed toward the transfer of research-based knowledge into nursing practice" (p. 907) with the ultimate goals of improving patient care and advancing the discipline of nursing. The importance of using research findings in clinical practice has been discussed for at least 45 years; however, there are relatively few initiatives actually taking place in clinical or nursing education settings.

The first research utilization models were developed in the 1970s, beginning with the Western Interstate Commission for Higher Education in Nursing (WCHEN) Regional Program for Nursing Research Development (Krueger, 1978). Other models included the Conduct and Utilization of Research in Nursing (CURN) project (Horseley, Crane, Crabtree, & Wood, 1983), the Stetler/Marram model (Stetler, 1994), the Iowa model of research in practice (Titler et al., 1994), and the retrieval and application of research in nursing (RARIN) model (Bostrom & Wise, 1994). This list is not exhaustive; rather it is a representation of several well-known and referenced models found in the literature.

The WCHEN model was focused on cross-organizational planning and enhancing the value for research utilization. Nurses from a variety of clinical agencies were provided with 3 days of research training. Each clinician would identify a clinical problem, review the research in that area, and develop a plan for implementing and evaluating the outcomes of the practice change. The annual Communicating Nursing Research conferences also resulted from the initial WCHEN work group, with emphasis on dissemination of research results across academic and nursing service settings. There have been 30 conferences prior to 1997.

The CURN project was a federally funded initiative that focused on the use of a team approach for reviewing research results related to specific patient care problems, developing clinical protocols, and then testing the protocol in an acute care clinical setting. A key component of research utilization in this model was replication of previous studies. The focus of the Iowa model was similar to that of the CURN project, with particular attention to developing support for research utilization strategies at the organizational level. Both models were developed specifically to bridge the gap between research and practice. Both recommended that organizational resources such as personnel, equipment, time, and money be available to support the nursing staff. Policy, procedures, committee structures, and role expectations must exist in relation to staff involvement in research utilization activities. Both models also supported a fundamental belief that research can and must be applied to practice if patient care is to improve.

The Stetler/Marram model was developed primarily for use at the individual level and specifically outlined the role clinical specialists have in facilitating the application of research findings to clinical practice. The model includes specific steps related to the need for a sound foundation in the conduct of research, and what is more important, it demonstrates how to interpret and validate findings that can be used to change practice.

The RARIN model, funded by a National Library of Medicine grant, was developed at Stanford University Hospital in Palo Alto, California. Distinct from the other models, which focused on providing nurse education, skill building, and organization support strategies, the RARIN model focused on improving staff access to research findings through the use of computerized linkages to established research databases. Training a small set of nurses from each unit on the use of the computer network and the basics of the research critique was the other major component. The computer technology provided direct access to the MEDLINE citation system (including CINAHL) as well as databases of research abstracts that were written by experts. Hence, nurses could access almost any database, via use of the developed tools and technologies, while working in a patient care unit. The model assumption was based on a belief that if access to research findings was improved and the findings were represented in an easily understood yet clinically sound framework, then practicing nurses would be able to improve patient care.

Outcome results from these and other models have been limited. Numerous barriers to transferring research-based knowledge into nursing practice persist. Staff nurses reported the following as barriers to research utilization: (a) insufficient skills and knowledge about evaluating research, (b) lack of awareness or access to research, (c) minimal value of research for practice, (d) insufficient authority to actually change practice, (e) insufficient time to read research and to learn research skills and how to implement changes when necessary, (f) lack of cooperation and support from administration and other staff, (g) little personal benefit, (h) unclear and unhelpful statistical representation of results, (i) few replication studies to determine if sufficient evidence exists to change practice, and (j) lack of access to databases and research literature. Nurse administrators also reported barriers, such as (a) isolation from research colleagues, (b) lack of time because of heavy workloads, (c) difficulty in reading and interpreting research findings and statistics, (d) insufficient skills in research critique, (e) lack of replication studies to determine if practice requires change, and (f) lack of access to databases and research literature.

Facilitators for the research utilization process have also been identified. They include (a) creating practice environments that require research-based clinical standards, (b) providing expert consultation and activities such as research committees to increase adequacy of research skills, (c) improving access to computerized databases and research literature, (d) allotting time and money to support conference attendance and participation, (e) developing performance standards that include behavioral expectations to support research-based practice, and (f) obtaining grants to support research projects.

The literature related to research utilization is almost exclusively focused on nursing practice environments, with little attention to how research utilization is introduced into the nursing curricula at all levels. Research utilization is a critical professional accountability issue to resolve if the discipline of nursing is to advance. Therefore, it is essential for nursing educators to socialize students at all levels to the value of research utilization and to model the required skills. For example, most teaching about the research process at the baccalaureate level is isolated from discussions about actual caregiving and how that care might be improved by applying research findings. Graduate students are not adequately prepared for the integration of research into the care of specific patient populations and have little preparation in areas of quality improvement and outcomes-evaluation methodologies. Doctoral education continues to be focused on the conduct of research, with minimal emphasis on how to report results in ways that are understandable to practicing clinicians. Although learning a thesis format of writing is important, it is equally important to learn how to convert research jargon into useful, specific, and direct reports for clinicians. In addition, more value and attention should be given to replication research that would advance results that are more generalizable and easily applied to clinical practice.

The health care environment is changing rapidly, with increased attention to outcomes-based practice, evaluating patient outcomes, and demonstrating cost efficiency and effectiveness. Research utilization must become a matter of professional accountability for each nurse and every health care organization. Nurses must be better prepared to actively participate in and facilitate research utilization. More attention should be given to implementing strategies that remove the barriers identified in previous research. Technology is now available to provide much access to research and relevant databases; however, there is still need for timely and readable reports of completed research.

The critical challenge is how students, practitioners, educators, executives, and researchers can create learning environments in which research utilization will become an integral part of nursing practice. When nurse colleagues share a common vision related to improving the health of our communities, then research utilization becomes one method to ensure research-based care delivery models, with all nurses accountable for achieving optimal outcomes.

CAROL A. ASHTON

Resourcefulness

Resourcefulness is a collection of cognitive and behavioral skills that are used to attain, maintain, or regain health. Resourcefulness involves the ability to maintain independence in daily tasks despite potentially adverse situations (i.e., personal resourcefulness or self-help) (Rosenbaum, 1990) and to seek help from others when unable to function independently (i.e., social resourcefulness or help-seeking) (Nadler, 1990). Thus, two forms of resourcefulness exist, and the skills comprising the two are complementary and equally important for health promotion. Both the self-help skills constituting personal resourcefulness and the help-seeking skills constituting social resourcefulness are believed to be learned through either formal or informal instruction. Since resourcefulness is thought to be learned (Rosenbaum), the self-help and help-seeking skills that comprise it can be taught. Numerous studies since the early 1980s have suggested that teaching personal and social resourcefulness skills is beneficial in promoting and maintaining healthy physical, psychological, and social functioning across the life span.

Contextual factors affecting personal and social resourcefulness are both intrinsic and extrinsic. Intrinsic factors that have been identified from empirical research are demographic characteristics (e.g., age, gender, race/ethnicity), number of chronic conditions, presence of illness symptoms, and perceived stress (Fingerman, Gallagher-Thompson, Lovett, & Rose, 1996; LeFort, Gray-Donald, Rowat, & Jeans, 1998; Zauszniewski, & Chung, 2001; Zauszniewski, Chung, & Krafcik, 2001). Extrinsic factors include social network size, social support, and health care orientation (Dirksen, 2000; Rapp, S. R., Schumaker, Schmidt, Naughton, & Anderson, 1998).

Zauszniewski (1996) reported significant associations between depressive cognitions and lower self-help (personal resourcefulness) and help-seeking (social resourcefulness) behaviors in healthy, community-dwelling elders. Self-esteem, an affective regulator, has also been reported to be significantly associated with personal resourcefulness and well-being in women survivors of breast cancer (Dirksen, 2000). Health self-determinism, a motivational regulator, was found to be a significant predictor of self-help (personal resourcefulness) and informal help-seeking (social resourcefulness) in chronically ill elders (Zauszniewski et al., 2001). Although studies have identified uncertainty as an antecedent of personal resourcefulness (Dirksen; LeFort et al., 1998), uncertainty may also function as a motivational process regulator, which intervenes between contextual variables and resourcefulness. To date, no published studies have examined the effects of energy as a process regulator. Yet studies of concepts related to resourcefulness and quality of life suggest that energy level may play a mediating or moderating role in the relationships between contextual variables and resourcefulness or quality of life. The specific roles played by various process regulators in affecting personal and social resourcefulness need more systematic examination.

Positive health outcomes of personal and social resourcefulness have been well-documented through empirical research. These outcomes, including adaptive functioning in depressed adults (Zauszniewski, 1995, 1996), life satisfaction in persons with chronic pain and in healthy elders (LeFort et al., 1998; Zauszniewski, 1996), perceived health in caregivers and in diabetic women (Rapp et al., 1998; Zauszniewski et al., 2001), psychological well-being in women survivors of breast cancer and in elders (Dirksen, 2000; Zauszniewski et al., 2001), and health practices in women with type 2 diabetes (Zauszniewski & Chung, 2001), fall under the "umbrella" concept called quality of life. Self-rated health and caregiver well-being, which are also indicators of quality of life, have been reported as outcomes of social resourcefulness in primary caregivers of persons with dementia (Rapp et al.). However, while significant associations between both personal and social resourcefulness and indicators of quality of life have been consistently reported in the literature, few studies have examined personal and social resourcefulness simultaneously in relation to quality-of-life indicators. In one of the few studies, Zauszniewski (1996) found that in healthy elders life satisfaction was a significant outcome of both forms of resourcefulness. However, both forms of resourcefulness in a study of chronically ill elders found that only personal resourcefulness significantly predicted physical functioning and psychosocial well-being (Zauszniewski, Chung, & Krafcik, 2001).

There are reliable and valid measures of both personal and social resourcefulness. Personal resourcefulness, also termed learned resourcefulness, has been measured using Rosenbaum's (1990) Self-Control Schedule. The Self-Control Schedule (SCS) consists of 36 Likert-type items using a six-point scale. Subjects indicate the degree to which each item describes their behavior, ranging from extremely descriptive to extremely nondescriptive; a higher composite score indicates greater personal resourcefulness. Internal consistency estimates have ranged from .78 to .85 in adults, including elders (Rosenbaum). As would be expected, the SCS is moderately related to locus of control, religious orientation, anxiety, and depressive symptoms, supporting its construct validity (Rosenbaum). The Social Resourcefulness Scale (SRS) developed by Rapp and colleagues (1998) consists of 20 Likert-type items using a five-point scale. Subjects indicate the frequency of use of behaviors to obtain and maintain help from others, ranging from never to always. Higher composite scores indicate greater social resourcefulness. An internal consistency estimate was found with elders (Rapp et al.), and construct validity was supported by significant correlations with social support and self-control (Rapp et al.).

Fostering the development and maintenance of both personal and social resourcefulness is well within the purview of nursing interventions. Clinical trials are currently examining various methods for teaching personal and social resourcefulness skills to elders with chronic conditions. Additional research with children, adolescents, and ethnically diverse populations is needed.

JACLENE A. ZAUSZNIEWSKI

Retirement

The increased birth rate of the mid-1900s and longer life expectancies have resulted in an increase in the number of persons who are, or are soon going to be, retired (Anderson & Weber, 1993). In addition, the concept of retirement has changed. While retirement may simply mean the cessation of employment at a given age, the term is generally considered to be much more complex. In preindustrial times, people did not retire; they simply continued to work until their physical capabilities would no longer allow them to continue (Mulley, 1995). Many current older workers want to continue to work, or have "bridge employment" (Kim, S., & Feldman, 2000), but they often want a new career or to work on different terms (AARP, 2003). As a result, determining what retirement is and who is "retired" can be difficult, and the numbers can be equally misleading. The Social Security Administration (2003) provided an estimate of 29.4 million retirees in June 2003, based on the number of people receiving retired-worker benefits. This is indeed a substantial population. Another indicator of the number of retirees is the number of people in the civilian workforce by age group. In 2000, of the 281,421,906 U.S. population, the Administration on Aging (2000) estimates that 34,991,753 people were 65 years of age or older. In a trend analysis for years 1950–2005, workforce "participation rates of men aged 50 and older have been falling for all ages, and the rates for women have been rising sharply for those aged 50 to 54 and 55 to 59" (Bureau of Labor Statistics, 1992), but little change was noted for women over 65. The labor force of workers who are 55 and older is expected to grow by about 8.5 million by 2010, and the 55–64 year old group is expected to increase by 7.2 million (Fullerton & Toossi, 2001). The retirement age is declining, with or without social security benefits (Bureau of Labor Statistics, 2001).

This is particularly important when examining the overall characteristics of older citizens as well as the changes that have occurred over the last several decades. In *A Profile of Older Americans: 2002* (Administration on Aging, 2002), it was reported that in 2000 there were 35.0 million Americans who were 65 years or older, and they represented 12.4% of the U.S. population. In the same year, the 65–74 age group (18.4 million) was eight times larger than it was in 1900, and the 75–84 group (12.4 million) was 16 times larger. Nearly one-half (46%) of all older women in 2001 were widows and there were four times as many widows as widowers. The American Association of Retired Persons (AARP, 1999a) reports, "Outliving men by an average of seven years, women typically have to finance those longer lives with lower wages, fewer benefits, and no pensions. The result? Three quarters of the older Americans living in poverty are women." In 1997 approximately 1 in 7 (14.2%) households that had an elderly head of the family had an income of less than $15,000, and in 1995 older citizens accounted for approximately 40% of all hospital stays (Administration on Aging, 1998). These data have major implications not only for retirees and their families and friends, but also for the health care delivery system and the rising costs of health care. For those who are mobile, states are actively recruiting retirees with sufficient incomes to positively impact on the state's economy (Duncombe, Robbins, & Wolf, 2003).

Several theories of aging have been used to better understand retirement and as frameworks for retirement research. The major ones include continuity theory, activity theory, role theory, disengagement theory, and political-economy theory. Each has it own set of criticisms—as well as contributions—to the overall understanding of the retirement phenomenon. Continuity theory suggests that people develop habits and preferences that become an integral part of them and that persist into their retirement years (Atchley, 1977). According to activity theory, people adjust most effectively in older age when they maintain previously established activities (Friedman, E., & Havighurst, 1954). Role theories suggest that society is structured around various roles that provide both norms and expectations regarding a person's attitudes and behavior (Richardson, 1993). Disengagement theory is based on the premise that people tend to withdraw from some of the roles and activities as they age and enter retirement (Cumming & Henry, 1961). Political-economy theory (Estes, C., Linkins, & Binney, 1996) posits that retirement is the result of decisions on the part of business and industry to reduce the workforce; as a result, retirement adjustment would depend on the personal resources of the individual.

Retirement marks a transition into the later stages of life (Floyd et al., 1992), and as a part of the Normative Aging Study, researchers suggest that retirement is now a normative event, not the unplanned occurrence it used to be (Bossé, Aldwin, Levenson, Spiro, & Mroczek, 1993). Increased longevity and a greater number of healthy older adults have changed expectations for retirement. Retirement may be a time for new recreational pursuits, such as travel, and presents an opportunity to develop new routines (Watts, 1987); however, economic constraints may place limits on these activities, and changes in the health of the retiree or significant other may interfere with previous plans.

Upon retirement, relationships with coworkers are terminated (van Tilburg, 1992), and this has an impact on the life of the retiree. As noted earlier, some retirees continue working after their initial retirement. In fact, eight out of ten "baby boomers" reported that they plan to work at least part-time after retirement (AARP, 1999b). M. Carter and Cook (1995) noted that retirement is a time of redefining roles. Retirement can also have an impact on marital relationships. The retirement of one partner in a marriage suggested a reorganization of roles as the couple begins the transition to full-time retirement (Henretta, O'Rand, & Chan, 1993), and differences have been found in the division of household tasks among retirees and nonretirees (Szinovacz & Harpster, 1994). During retirement, spouses have been found to become increasingly aware of their partners' faults (Johnston, T., 1990), and women may have problems of infringement when husbands spend more time at home (Vinick & Ekerdt, 1989). Lee and Shehan (1989) found no beneficial effects of retirement on marital satisfaction among husbands and wives. T. Gall, Evans, and Howard (1997) found that while interpersonal satisfaction and psychological health peaked 1 year after retirement, it declined significantly by the 6th or 7th years. Yet, they never fell below preretirement levels.

In recent years there have been a number of studies on retirement among women (Slevin & Wingrove, 1995). "Because of the prevailing 'myth' among women that they will be cared for in old age and women's fear of growing old, women often do not aggressively plan for their retirement" (Perkins, K., 1992, p. 526). Some studies suggest that women who have had recent employment are healthier in their later years than women who have not been employed (Hibbard, 1995). Keddy and Singleton (1991) found that among the women they studied, the primary concerns related to finances, the use of leisure time, and keeping a positive attitude in retirement. Women's adaptation to retirement may be more affected by life events than men's (Szinovacz & Washo, 1992).

Retirement is frequently treated as a point in time rather than a complex process (Siegel & Rees, 1992); yet planning for retirement was the second strongest predictor of retirement satisfaction among male respondents in a study by Dorfman (1989). Preretirement planning tends to focus primarily on financial planning without taking into account all of the psychosocial adjustment factors (Rosenkoetter, Garris, & Engdahl, 2001). Among the elderly, a leisure repertoire is of concern due to the abundance of free time that accompanies retirement (Mobily, Lemke, & Gisin, 1991). Differences have been noted across race. K. Allen and Chin-Sang (1990) used a qualitative research approach to study older black women and found that they continued their history of self-reliance in the context of leisure experiences and service to others in old age.

Numerous psychosocial changes have been found to occur with retirement (Rosenkoetter & Garris, 1998), and depression is a factor for at least some retirees (Rosenkoetter, Garris, & Hendricksen, 1997). The effect of retirement on mental health and health behaviors was investigated in the Kaiser Permanente Retirement Study (Midanik, Soghikian, Ransom, & Tekawa, 1995). Atkinson (1990) found that problem drinking in the elderly is a public-health problem of moderate proportion, and that many geriatric cases are not properly identified.

Retirement is an important concept for both nursing practice and nursing research; yet it receives little emphasis in the nursing literature as a significant life event, transition, stressor, or component of routine nursing assessments and interventions. While marriage, divorce, childbearing, and the like have received much attention not only as events but as transitions, considerably less attention has been directed toward retirement. Greater emphasis is needed on the impact of retirement on health and health care and its implications for nursing. Nurses need to be attending to the issues of retirement when working with retirees and their significant others, as well as with those who are in the preretirement phase. Assuming that retirement is a positive experience may not be appropriate or in the best interests of clients and their families or friends.

MARLENE M. ROSENKOETTER

Rights of Human Subjects

Rights are just claims that are due to someone. Legal rights are valid claims recognized by a legal system. Moral rights are valid claims derived from customs, traditions, or ideals which may be upheld or protected by the law. Human rights are valid claims that are due to members of the human species and may be legal, moral, or both.

The rights of human subjects in research include the right to informed consent, the right to privacy, the right to refuse to participate in research, and the right to withdraw from a research study, without penalty, at any time. These four rights are all derived from a general right to liberty and are both moral and legal. They are supported by moral principles of the social community, professional codes of research ethics, and by legal protections. They become relevant in nursing research because all nurses have a responsibility to protect, and sometimes defend, the basic rights of patients within the health care system. When the nurse is also a researcher, the nurse has the added responsibility to make sure that these particular rights are not violated by the research process.

Informed consent is a process that protects research subjects' autonomy, protects research subjects from harm, and assists the researcher to avoid fraud and coercion in the role of researcher. It is also a process that encourages researcher responsibility for how information is communicated in research, promotes rational decision making by human subjects, and involves the public in promoting self-determination as a social value. Informed consent has information elements and consent elements.

Information Elements. For adequate disclosure of information, the research subject must be informed on the procedures to be used throughout the study. Information about available alternative treatment procedures, a discussion of risks and benefits of these procedures, and the opportunity for questions about or withdrawal from the project after treatment has begun, should all be provided to the research subject.

For adequate comprehension of information, the research subject must have time to consider the information and to ask questions. This means that when the ability to comprehend information is limited (such as when a subject's mental competence is limited), the researcher must allow the research subject additional opportunity to consider whether or not to participate in the study.

Consent Elements. Voluntary consent to participate in research means that the research subject has exercised choice, free of coercion and other forms of controlling influence by other persons. A research subject's consent is valid only if it is voluntarily given. Voluntariness protects the patient's right to choose goals and to choose among several goals when offered options. But consent cannot be given unless the research subject is "competent," or can make decisions based on rational reasons. Both competence and voluntariness are required for a subject's consent to be truly informed.

Nursing research on the informed consent of human subjects has focused on the comprehension of information by research subjects, subjects' competency for informed consent (i.e., adolescents, mentally retarded minors), and the factors that influence the informed consent of adolescents and adults. The study designs have been exploratory and quasi-experimental and have included relatively small sample sizes.

Right to Privacy. The right to privacy includes the right to keep personal information about oneself private, undisclosed, and away from public scrutiny. It also includes the right to bodily integrity, or freedom from unwanted intrusions on body parts. One way that the research subject's right to privacy is protected is by following rules of confidentiality. For example, information about the research subject may not be disclosed without the subject's permission and then only under certain conditions. In a like manner, research data is not publicly connected to the research subject, thereby assuring subject privacy.

Another way that the research subject's right to privacy is protected is by obtaining an informed consent and signed permission for invasive procedures used during the research process. For example, informed consent must be obtained before passing a Levine tube to obtain gastric contents for analysis. Nursing research on the privacy of human subjects is not yet documented. Potential areas for nursing research are identifying how research studies protect or do not protect the privacy of human subjects, describing research subjects' perceptions of how their privacy was protected or not protected during a study, identifying researchers' attitudes toward rules of confidentiality under different research conditions, and identifying institutional review board (IRB) members' knowledge of and attitudes toward protection of human subject privacy in research studies.

Right to Refuse to Participate in Research. The right to refuse to participate in research protects the subject from being coerced to participate in research and assures that research subjects are truly voluntary. Nursing research on the right to refuse to participate in research is not yet documented. Potential areas for nursing research are identifying the conditions under which research subjects refuse to participate in a study and describing why subjects have refused to participate in particular types of research studies.

Right to Withdraw from a Research Study. Human subjects have the right to withdraw from a research study without any untoward treatment of them. Even though they had previously consented to participate in a research study, subjects have the right to change their minds and withdraw from the study at any time.

Nursing research on the right to withdraw from a research study is not yet documented. Potential areas for nursing research are identifying the conditions under which research subjects withdraw from a study and describing the course of treatment of subjects who do and do not withdraw from studies involving particular diseases.

The protection of human rights in research studies is important to the moral integrity of nursing research. International and professional codes of research ethics strongly support the morality of research, and the American Nurses Association's *Ethical Guidelines in the Conduct, Dissemination, and Implementation of Nursing Research* (Silva, 1995) supports the morality of nursing research. However, nursing research on the protection of human rights in research is at an early stage of development. As the 21st century approaches, nursing research should include studies of how human rights are protected in research and the factors that inhibit or promote their protection in various kinds of research designs.

SARA T. FRY

(Martha E.) Rogers Science of Unitary Persons

Since 1970, when Martha Rogers initially published *The Science of Irreducible Unitary Human Beings* (1990), the response to the conceptual model has varied. The work has been described as too abstract to be useful in practice; yet its influence on practice, research, and education continue to grow internationally.

The model is derived from many disciplines and results in an integrated whole, unique to nursing. It does not set out to define practice, but is considered a means of stimulating the development of a body of knowledge. It is simple and elegant in design, although it did not seem so initially.

It is important to understand that when she first wrote her book, we had just come out of a one of the most tumultuous decades in American history: the 1960s. We were still grappling with an event that had stunned the nation—the assassination of a vibrant young president—shown repeatedly and graphically, for the first time in our history, on television. To understand the mood, one can compare it to the relentless replay of 9/11/01—the fall of the World Trade Center towers and the devastating and prolonged after-effects of this experience for people in this country. We were in the grip of the war in Vietnam, which divided the country in ways similar to the war in Iraq today. We had just landed a man on the moon and Woodstock and the Beatles were to become national icons.

The majority of nurses were graduates of diploma schools. The mode was to follow the doctor's orders and the oral tradition of previous generations of nurses. Few thought of a career in nursing as being more than just a job. We thought that "we"—the medical experts, led by the physician, knew what was best, and that patient's needed to learn to be compliant with what we prescribed and advised. Nursing theory did not exist.

Within this cultural framework, Rogers writes about the natural process of change, the *inherent* quality of human beings' right to choose, and the *infinite* nature of the relationship between man and the universe. Her description of nursing as a *learned profession*, resulting from a strong academic preparation and based in knowledge unique to nursing, was equally stunning and controversial.

Through 1994, she revised and refined her theory. She makes several assumptions to be tested so that further nursing knowledge can be formulated: *the human being is greater than the sum of his parts; there is constant, progressive interaction between the human being and environment; the environment is infinite—it extends to the universe and beyond; reality is as it appears—it is constructed; energy is matter is energy; the human being can choose to engage in change.*

Rogers defines four postulates as the basis of her theory:

Energy fields—in Rogers' world we *are* energy fields, as is everything around us. She uses the term "unitary" to describe the indivisible and irreducible nature of the human being-environment interaction.

Openness—an attribute of all energy fields—a constant mutual interaction and flow, as *opposed* to a cause and effect relationship.

Pattern—the manifestation of energy fields and exchange which is experienced and known by all senses, including intuition.

Pandimensionality—the boundlessness of the universe, without spatial or linear limits.

In unison with these assumptions and postulates she proposed three principles of homeodynamics:

Helicy—continuous, nonrepetitive and innovative patterning (moving forward/ diversifying).

Resonancy—patterning which changes from lower to higher frequency (responsiveness—increasing vibration).

Integrality—the continuous mutual process between person and environment (feeling "at one" with the universe).

Rogers, whatever one's opinion of her theory, has to be credited with thinking "outside of the box" (another unfamiliar concept in 1970).

Her accomplishments were remarkable for the nursing profession. She established that professional nursing required knowledge gleaned from the arts and science and self-understanding on the part of the individual nurse. She provided the basis for the formulation of nursing theory. She understood that ongoing change, which is inherent in her theory, applied to her own work and she revised it accordingly until her death on March 13, 1994. She studied and understood information from all she read and experienced and synthesized it into a body of knowledge unique to nursing.

Martha Rogers epitomized her theory: open, constantly changing, diverse, thinking without boundaries, and resonating to her world, her profession, and the future.

JOHN PHILLIPS
UPDATED BY ELAINE K. SHIMONO

Roy Adaptation Model

The Roy adaptation model for nursing defines person as a holistic adaptive system that is in constant interaction with the environment (Roy & Andrews, 1999). As a holistic adaptive system the person can be described as a set of interrelated arts with inputs, control and feedback processes, and outputs functioning as a whole for some purpose. Inputs for the system are stimuli received externally from the environment (external stimuli) and internally from within the self (internal stimuli). These stimuli are classified as focal, contextual, or residual. The stimuli immediately confronting the person are called focal stimuli. All other stimuli in the situation that contribute to the effect of the focal stimuli are called contextual stimuli. Stimuli whose effects on the given situation are unclear are called residual stimuli. Thus the environment comprises all the possible inputs for the human adaptive systems (Roy & Andrews).

The control processes of the system are two coping mechanisms, the regulator and cognator subsystems, to adapt or cope with a changing environment. The process of perception links the regulator and cognator subsystems. Outputs of the system are responses, called behaviors, that result from regulator and cognator activity. Behaviors are manifested in four adaptive modes physiological, self-concept, role function, and interdependence. Behavior can be observed, measured, or subjectively reported, and in collaboration with the person, judged as adaptive or ineffective. Adaptive responses maintain or promote integrity or health, whereas ineffective responses disrupt integrity. Through feedback processes, behaviors (responses) provide further input for the person as a system.

The goal of nursing is "the promotion of adaptation in each of the four modes, thereby contributing to the person's health, quality of life, and dying with dignity" (Roy & Andrews, 1999, p. 55). Roy defines health as "a state and a process of being and becoming an integrated and whole person" (Roy & Andrews, p. 54). In essence, health reflects adaptation of the individual's adaptative systems in an ever-changing environment. The role of the nurse is to promote health through promotion of adaptation and enhancing the person-environment interaction through the use of the nursing process. Within the Roy adaptation model, nursing interventions are conceptualized as the management or manipulation of stimuli. Assumptions of the Roy adaptation model are both scientific and philosophical. The scientific assumptions are derived from systems theory and adaptation level theory, whereas the philosophical assumptions are related to humanism (Roy & Andrews).

The elements and assumptions of the Roy adaptation model provide a perspective for nursing research by suggesting what phenomena to study, identifying the research questions, and identifying appropriate methods of inquiry. The phenomena of study are persons as individuals or in groups. The distinctive nature of the research questions is related to basic life processes and patterns, coping with health and illness, and enhancing adaptive coping. Multiple methods are appropriate when conducting research based on the Roy adaptation model (Roy & Andrews, 1999).

A search of the literature revealed numerous studies that used the Roy adaptation model as the conceptual framework for the research, with considerable variability in the clarity and specificity of the links between the Roy adaptation model and the research. Some studies used the model in the development of data collection instruments within the four adaptive models, while other studies used the four adaptive modes as a framework for data analysis. Chiou (2000) conducted a meta-analysis of nine empirical studies based on Roy's adaptation model to determine the magnitude of the interrelationships of the four modes. The results indicated that more research is needed to determine the credibility of Roy's adaptation model (Chiou). Additional studies identified specific concepts from the model, such as interdependence mode or physical self, and used them as the basis for the research.

A number of studies identified specific links, conceptually and operationally, between the Roy adaptation model and the research variables. In these studies specific concepts were linked to the various aspects of the model, including focal, contextual, and residual stimuli control processes and adaptive modes. Yeh (2003) used this approach in research examining the relationships among social support, parenting stress, coping style, and psychological distress in parents caring for children with cancer. Zhan (2000) examined the relationship between cognitive adaptation processes and self-consistency in hearing-impaired elderly. These concepts were then operationalized by identifying specific measurement tools. Several studies identified nursing interventions as the management or manipulation of stimuli, and some specifically tested propositions derived from the model. A urine control theory of the middle range substructed from Roy's adaptation model was studied to explain the phenomenon of urine control in memory-impaired incontinent elders at home (Jirovec, Jenkins, Isenberg, & Baiardi, 1999). This intervention study found that Roy's adaptation model was a useful model to explain the phenomenon of urine control (Jirovec et al.).

Among the studies there were differences in methodologies, designs, data collection procedures, and data analysis techniques. A review of the research designs used in the studies revealed both cross-sectional and longitudinal designs, as well as prospective and ex-post-facto designs. Case study, single group, and comparison group designs were all represented in the studies reviewed. Additionally, designs ranged from exploratory, including descriptive-correlational and descriptive-comparative, to experimental and quasiexperimental.

Similarly, variety was found in the approaches used for data collection. Data were collected by record reviews, observation, interviews, researcher-developed questionnaires, and standardized questionnaires such as the Norbeck Social Support Questionnaire and the State-Trait Anxiety Inventory. Methods of data analysis were both quantitative and qualitative. Several studies used qualitative data analysis procedures such as content analysis and the constant comparative method for grounded theory. Shyu (2000) illustrated the role function mode in Roy's adaptation model using constant comparison to analyze the data. Yeh (2001) used a qualitative approach to establish a framework for the adaptation process of Taiwanese children with cancer. The studies reviewed revealed that the Roy adaptation model was appropriate for guiding research in a variety of settings and populations. Shyu's study was conducted in Taiwan with families whereas Zhan (2000) recruited older hearing-impaired individuals from the northeastern part of the United States. Villareal (2003) demonstrated the use of Roy's adaptation model in young women contemplating smoking cessation. Roy's adaptation model has also guided research related to menopausal women (Cunningham, 2002).

Among those who have built a program of research using the Roy adaptation model are J. Fawcett, S. E. Pollock, and L. Tulman. Fawcett and Tulman (1990) conducted methodological instrument development and substantive research related to childbearing families. Retrospective and longitudinal studies examined factors associated with functional status during the postpartum period, and one study (Fawcett, 1990) tested an intervention derived from the Roy adaptation model. Pollock (1993) and colleagues conducted a series of five longitudinal studies to examine human responses to chronic illness by identifying predictors of adaptation to chronic illness and determining whether adaptive responses differed by diagnostic group. These studies by Fawcett, Pollock, and Tulman demonstrate the usefulness of the Roy adaptation model as a guide for nursing research and support the credibility of the model. Using the Roy adaptation model to guide nursing research has contributed to both the basic and the clinical science of nursing. Increased understanding of the factors influencing adaptive responses are examples. Studies have provided some confirmation for the model, demonstrated its ability to generate new information, and contributed to clinical practice.

Research that continues to test the model and the relationships among its components is needed. One area that has been identified as a research concern is the overlap between the four adaptive modes. Further research may clarify this issue. Additional research should test nursing interventions to promote adaptive responses. Overall, the Roy adaptation model is a very useful model in practice and as a guide to research. The Roy adaptation model continues to make a significant contribution to nursing science as it continues to evolve.

MARY E. TIEDEMAN
UPDATED BY MARY T. QUINN GRIFFIN

Rural Health

Capturing the parameters of *rural* may appear quite simple, as each individual has a personal view of rural life. For some it is the place where, for generations, they have engaged in farming, ranching, mining, or logging, and for others it is an escape from urban tensions—a place to recreate and to relax. For those providing health care, there are unique challenges and opportunities in the rural setting.

Rural health requires an understanding of the clients being served. While rural America is still the site of our food production, it is also evolving into a new place with a new demographic profile and new opportunities. The economic base is marked by increasing diversification, with consumer services accounting for 23% of rural earnings in 1999, along with manufacturing (21%), public sector (20%), recreational services (4%), and only 5% from agriculture (Economic Research Services, 2000). The increasing variety in occupations and rapid advances in technology are quickly blurring differences within rural populations and between urban and rural residents.

Sketching a rural health profile is complicated by the increasing diversity of the population, disparities in definition, inadequate measurement, and lack of adequate health statistics. Yet, from observation and statistical reports, it is clear that significant health disparities are present in certain segments of rural America.

Rural dwellers often have limited access to health care, high rates of poverty, high rates of uninsured and underinsured, transportation problems, and high risks for chronic illness and accidental death. Among rural men, the suicide rate is 54% higher than in urban areas (Dotinga, 2002). Rural women tend to have less access to health education, lower rates of cancer screening, fewer choices in insurance plans, fewer options for cancer treatment, and less access to oncologists than urban women (Hoekstra, 2001). The rural homeless need particular attention in terms of research and policy development (Bushy, 2000). Among Native Americans and migrant workers, homelessness is largely a rural phenomenon (National Coalition for the Homeless, 1999). Rural residents have a greater likelihood of working in hazardous occupations, with exposure to chemicals, hearing loss from farm machinery noise, and serious farm equipment injuries. Other health concerns are domestic violence, smokeless tobacco use, heavy drinking and smoking, unintentional firearms injuries, and suicide.

For small towns in the rural plains, loss is a defining characteristic. There has been a slow demographic collapse with the young moving out, businesses closing, factories emptying, and poverty increasing. Most alarmingly, polls show a "quiet crisis of confidence." Rural people feel powerless to control their lives and are pessimistic about the future (Egan, 2003).

The intention is not to create an exhaustive list of rural health problems. This sample of health disparities serves as an indicator of the complexity of social and health issues in rural areas and the challenges to those engaged in evidence-based rural nursing practice. As noted in *Rural Healthy People 2010*, this type of discussion should not diminish the advantages and attractions that many rural areas already offer to residents and visitors, and to the successes in many communities that are a reflection of the hard work and commitment of rural people unwilling to accept existing conditions (Gamm, Hutchison, Dabney, & Dorsey, 2003).

Optimal nursing care is provided when nurses and health care decision-makers have access to a synthesis of the latest research and a consensus of expert opinion as a basis for their judgment in planning and providing care. There are persisting deficits along with areas of optimism in rural nursing research that guide evidence-based care. There continues to be a limited number of databased articles in the rural nursing literature. Continuing shortfalls in the literature include small sample sizes, lack of random sampling, cross-sectional designs, problems with operationalization and measurement of rurality, and small specific populations. Studies lack clear descriptions of comparison groups and often fail to adequately account for key variables.

Positive signs of the growth of rural nursing science are appearing. Among these are a new online rural nursing journal, programs of rural nursing research including multisite projects, a National Institute of Nursing Research-funded exploratory research center focused on rural health, interest in doctoral preparation in rural health, and use of new technology for education and in nursing research (Weinert, 2002).

The *Online Journal of Rural Nursing and Health Care*, which focuses on dissemination of rural nursing research and health care information, is a sign of progress. There are now a cluster of projects addressing some of the pressing health issues such as women's health, children and adolescents, the elderly, caregiving, and issues associated with managing cancer, stroke, Alzheimer's disease, and end-of-life care in the rural setting. Programs of rural nursing research are developing: Fahs and associates, at Binghamton University, on cardiovascular disease and rural women; Magilvy and colleagues, at the University of Colorado, on community health needs of elderly rural populations; and Weinert and colleagues, at Montana State University-Bozeman, using computer-based technology to provide support and health information to isolated rural women living with a chronic health condition. Cross-state studies are being designed to tease out which characteristics are somewhat universal across rural populations and which may be specific to a certain rural population. One example is the work of Shreffler-Grant, at Montana State University-Bozeman and her colleagues at the University of North Dakota, who are exploring the use of complementary therapy by rural older adults. The launching of a nursing doctoral program at Binghamton University will increase the number of individuals prepared to conduct necessary rural research. The Center for Research on Chronic Health Conditions in Rural Dwellers at Montana State University-Bozeman, funded through the NINR Exploratory Centers Program, provides an opportunity to strengthen rural research and is forging research linkages between Montana nurse scientists and rural nurse investigators in Oregon, Iowa, Wyoming, North Dakota, and Nebraska. The explosion of activity in the arena of telecommunications has been a boon to rural nursing education, brought current practice and research knowledge to the finger tips of nurses in the remotest of areas, extended the reach of the community health nurse through telehealth, and enhanced computer-based research designs. There is progress in the development of the body of knowledge about rural health, with the crafting of more sophisticated and methodologically sound studies and an increase in the number of programs of nursing research. A foundation has been laid for expanding the field of rural nursing through a journal, doctoral program, and research center. These advances in nursing science, along with better understanding of historical factors, changing demographics, health disparities, strengths, and resources of rural communities/individuals, enhance the delivery of evidence-based nursing care in the rural setting.

CLARANN WEINERT

S

Sampling

Sampling is a process or way in which one selects a representative part of the population of interest to make valid inferences and generalizations. A sample is not only more feasible, economical, and practical than using the whole population; it is often more accurate. A sample, in contrast to the greater number of cases in an entire population, decreases the likelihood of nonsampling errors such as measurement errors, nonresponse biases, and recording and coding errors. Most researchers think of sampling as important for accurately representing the population in descriptive terms, that is, external validity or generalization. Sampling, however, also is concerned with the relationships found. Therefore, sampling errors or biases may threaten internal validity as well. Also, strictly speaking, samples are not "representative," "unbiased," or "fair" (Stuart, 1968). Because the researcher never knows the true population values, one cannot determine if any given sample is truly representative of the population. It is the sampling *process* that is representative, unbiased, or fair.

There are several types of sampling. Simple random sampling is a procedure that may involve the use of a table of random numbers or the flip of a coin to determine who or what will be included in the sample. This approach, however, is often impractical and tedious and is infrequently used. Systematic random sampling involves the use of a random start and then the selection of every *k*th case or incidence. This approach is more convenient than simple random sampling, but it can have variance estimation problems (Kish, 1965).

A minimum of two systematic random samples with independent random starts is needed to estimate variance, unless one can assume a random distribution of the cases on the list used for sampling. Also, when using systematic random sampling, one must be careful that the list does not have some systematic order or periodicity. If so, systematic random sampling may lead to a seriously misrepresented sample or pattern. For example, one might inadvertently select all head nurses if the sampling interval mimicked the sequencing of head nurses on the list. Or one might obtain blood samples only when certain hormones are at their peaks if the sampling time interval mimicked when the hormone peaked.

Stratified sampling is another method of random sampling. It involves identifying one or more classification variables for sampling purposes. With stratified sampling, one randomly samples within each nonoverlapping stratum of the classification variables. For example, if sex is the classification variable, one randomly samples men and women separately. Stratified sampling is intended to decrease sampling variability by increasing the homogeneity of the strata. For research purposes, it is best to select classification variables on the basis of their assumed association with the dependent variable, choosing those that are uncorrelated with each other. Stratified sampling facilitates obtaining subgroup parameter estimates, may increase the statistical efficiency of estimates if proportional allocation is used, and may be more convenient if sampling lists are organized according to the selected strata. However, stratified sampling also may be more costly and complex and generally is applied to some, but not all, variables of interest.

Cluster sampling is a fourth type of random sampling. Here the elements of interest for the study and the sampling units are not the same. The sampling unit or cluster is a convenient, practical, and economical grouping, such as practice sites, whereas the elements of interest for the study may be the individual patients obtained at the practice sites. Thus, one randomly samples the clusters and takes all elements (or a relevant, random subset) within each cluster. In contrast to stratified sampling, where one samples from all strata of the classification variable, one samples only some clusters in cluster sampling. In contrast to desiring homogeneous strata, clusters should be as heterogeneous as possible. To the extent that the clusters are not heterogeneous, one loses some precision, and the cluster sample is less efficient than a simple random sample of the same size. At the extreme, if the cluster is completely homogeneous, one achieves no gain from more than one case per cluster.

Finally, convenience samples, or nonprobability samples, are frequently used in nursing research. However, it is not possible to estimate sampling errors with such samples. Therefore, the validity of inferences drawn from nonprobability samples to the population remains unknown. Moreover, whenever nonrandom selection is used, the potential for serious sample selection biases exists. It is well-known that sample selection bias may threaten internal as well as external validity. For this reason, sampling on one's dependent variable should never be done.

LAUREN S. AARONSON

Schizophrenia

Schizophrenia, the most serious and persistent of the brain diseases in psychiatry, strikes at least one in every hundred people. About 1.3% of the population worldwide develops the disease regardless of race, ethnic group, gender, or country of origin. Between two and three million people in the United States suffer from schizophrenia and the accompanying stigma. In three out of four cases the illness begins between the ages of 17 and 25, robbing its victims of their most productive young adult years. The average life span of a person with schizophrenia is 20% shorter than that of the general population.

Schizophrenia is a chronic illness that is five times more common than multiple sclerosis, six times more common than insulin-dependent diabetes, 60 times more common than muscular dystrophy, and 80 times more common than Huntington's disease. To date schizophrenia is unpreventable, its exact cause is unknown, and it is not reliably curable. The word schizophrenia is a combination of two Greek words, *schizein* meaning to split and phren meaning mind. The word refers to a split from reality, not split personality.

The criteria for diagnosis in the American Psychiatric Association's (2000) *Diagnostic and Statistical Manual* (4th edition text revision) requires that at least two of the following be present for a significant portion of time during a 1-month period: delusions; hallucinations; disorganized speech; grossly disorganized or catatonic behavior; and, negative symptoms which refer to cognitive deficits such as alogia, poverty of speech, avolition, and flattening of affect. For a significant portion of the time since the onset of the disturbance, one or more major areas of functioning, such as work, interpersonal relations, or self-care, is markedly below the level achieved prior to the onset. Continuous signs of the disturbance must persist for at least 6 months.

Approximately 400,000 acute episodes occur annually in the U.S. and three million occur worldwide. Schizophrenia is ranked fourth of the top ten of all diseases worldwide in terms of burden of illness. The top three are unipolar disorder, alcohol use, and bipolar disorder. Schizophrenia ranks second in women age 14–44 years of all diseases worldwide in terms of burden of illness. It is projected that by 2020 neurobiological illnesses will account for almost 15% of all illnesses worldwide.

Schizophrenia accounts for 40% of all long-term-care days. $104 billion, 3% of the total United States health care expenditure, is spent annually on schizophrenia-related costs not including loss of productivity. Twenty-five percent of all United States hospital beds are occupied with someone diagnosed with schizophrenia. Twenty to fifty percent of patients with schizophrenia attempt suicide, while 10% succeed.

Recent research aided by new technological advances has redefined schizophrenia as a major neurobiological disease, a concept in psychiatry that now replaces outdated psychological theories of causation. There is now indisputable evidence of anatomical, neurophysiological, biochemical, and electrical abnormalities, including loss of gray matter in the frontal and prefrontal lobes and enlarged ventricles. Further biological evidence for the brain disease model of schizophrenia has come out of studies of genetics, epidemiology, neuroimmunology, and neuroradiography. Understanding of this disease is rapidly increasing with recently developed advanced brain-imaging technologies.

A CINAHL search of nursing research in schizophrenia since 1998 returned 117 citations. The majority of these were descriptive reports of program development and/or nursing interventions. Ongoing nursing research has been focused on 14 major categories. These categories are: (1) symptom management and relapse prevention; (2) caregiver and family burden; (3) treatment adherence and medication side effects; (4) management of hallucinations and delusions: (5) wellness, lifestyle, and medical comorbidity; (6) psychoeducation; (7) psychosocial rehabilitation; (8) outcomes measures and assessment tools; (9) inpatient treatment; (10) empathy and hope; (11) suicide and depression; (12) children and adolescents; (13) psychotherapies; and (14) women's issues. All 117 citations will be described.

Qualitative and quantitative research related to symptom management and relapse prevention is ongoing at the University of Washington in Seattle (Kennedy, Schepp, & O'Connor, 2000). Additional relapse prevention research is being conducted in the Netherlands by van Meijel, van der Gaag, Kahn, and Grypdonck (2002a, 2002b, 2003a, 2003b) and in South Africa by Mwaba and Molamu (1998).

A large corpus of literature is evolving in the area of family and caregiver burden. Tool development for sibling burden is being conducted at the University of Iowa by Friedrich, Lively, Rubenstein, and Buckwalter (1999, 2002), and Friedrich, Lively, and Buckwalter (1999). Researchers in Great Britain (Gall, Elliot, Atkinson, & Johansen, 2001, 2003) have developed a training program to support caregivers of relatives with schizophrenia. Also in Great Britain, Macinnes (1998) reported on differences between health professionals in assessment of caregiver burden. Saunders (1999, 2003; Saunders & Byrne, 2002) at the University of Texas has ongoing studies on overall family functioning. Hope in relationship to family caregivers is documented in Bland and Darlington (2002). Wuerker (2000) has ongoing family research at the University of California in Los Angeles. Canadian researchers at the University of British Columbia is studying the family illness experience (Teschinsky, 2000) while the Ryerson Polytechnic University in Toronto is focusing on parents of individuals experiencing a first episode of schizophrenia. Milliken (2001), Milliken and Northcott (2003), and Milliken and Rodney (2003) are studying the burden of families caring for adult children with schizophrenia at the University of Victoria in British Columbia. German researchers at the University of Leipzig are also looking at subjective burden of parents of patients with schizophrenia (Jungbauer, Wittmund, Dietrich, & Angermeyer, 2003) as are Korean researchers, Y. M. Lim and Ahn (2003) and Jung (2000). Researchers at Khon Kaen University in Thailand are studying psychological morbidity of rural families as well as religious practices used as interventions (Rungreangkulkij, Chafetz, Chesla, & Gilliss, 2002; Rungreangkulkij & Chesla, 2001). The effects of support groups on caregivers in China is reported by K. Chou, Liu, and Chu (2003). Attitudes and beliefs in families is researched in South Africa (Mbanaga et al., 2002). The reliability and validity of the concept as expressed in families and nurses in Hong Kong is articulated by Arthur (2002).

Another growing body of research is in the area of adherence with the treatment regimen. Australian researchers Pinikahana, Happell, Taylor, and Keks (2002) provided a comprehensive review of the complex issues involved with compliance. In Great Britain, Gray, Wykes, and Gournay (2002) are addressing compliance with antipsychotic medications while N. R. Harris, Lovell, and Day are studying consent. L. Jennings and colleagues (2002) are evaluating effects of knowledge of illness, insight, and attitudes toward taking medications. In Atlanta, Jarboe and Schwarz (1999) and Jarboe (2002) are also researching compliance with antipsychotics. Kozuki and Froelicher (2003) reported on lack of awareness as a factor in nonadherence. The evidence base for compliance is being studied in Scotland by Marland (1999) and by Marland and Sharkey (1999). Marland and Cash (2001) are also studying why patients decide not to take prescribed medications. In Israel, Navon and Ozer (2003) are exploring the patient's reasoning regarding compliance. Managing medication side effects to effect compliance is ongoing in Berkshire, England (Sin & Gamble, 2003). Scandinavian researchers are studying the morality of using depot neuroleptics (Svedberg, Hallstrom, & Lutzen, 2000). The role of the community mental health nurse in doing more than just giving injections is reported by Muir-Cochrane in 1998.

The management of hallucinations has been of concern to nurses throughout the history of psychiatric nursing. Ongoing research at the University of California at San Francisco involves randomized controlled trials of a specific psychoeducational intervention (Buccheri et al., 2004; Trygstad et al., 2002). Similar research is ongoing in Great Britain (Wykes, Parr, & Landau, 1999). Also in Britain and Holland, Baguley and Davies (1999a, 1999b) are studying the complications added to managing hallucinations and delusions when the patient is abusing substances. Sayer, Ritter, and Gournay (2000) are researching patient beliefs about their voices and the effects on coping.

Wellness, medical comorbidity, and lifestyle in relationship to management of schizophrenia is also a prominent focus of current research. The effects of antipsychotic medication on quality of life, including weight management and metabolism, is intensely researched by the ProMedica Research group in Georgia (Littrell, Hilligoss, Kirshner, Petty, & Johnson, 2003; Littrell & Littrell, 1999). Health promotion is being addressed by Beebe (2003) while Chafetz and Ricard (1999) are addressing biopsychosocial approaches. Health outcomes related to satisfaction with social functioning and general health are reported by Badger and colleagues in 2003. The association of cigarette smoking to schizophrenia is reviewed by McCloughen (2003) and by Forchuk and colleagues (2002). A 2 1/2 year follow-up study on smoking, body mass index, and risk of heart disease following the first episode of schizophrenia is reported by Luty, Kelly, and McCreadie (2002). Risk of HIV infection in the schizophrenic population is being studied by Gray, Brewin, Noak, and colleagues (2002). The primary care needs of people with schizophrenia is reported by J. Rodgers, Black, Stobbart, and Foster (2003).

Psychoeducation was studied intensely in the 1980s and 1990s, primarily by the allied health disciplines. Current nursing research is being conducted in Hong Kong (Chien, W. T., & Norman, 2003; Chien, W. T., & Lee, 2002; Chien, W. T., Kam, & Lee, 2001) and in Australia (Fung & Fry, 1999).

The topic of psychosocial rehabilitation, overall quality of life, and community-based care is appearing in the general nursing literature as well as in specific psychiatric nursing journals. Antai-Otong (2003) provided a comprehensive review of psychiatric rehabilitation while C. C. Williams and Collins (2002) are looking at the social construct of disability. Social function and quality of life for persons with schizophrenia is described by J. McDonald and Badger (2002) and by Walton (2000). A comparison between psychiatric nurses, psychiatrists, and the public regarding beliefs about interventions is presented by Caldwell and Jorm (2000). The cognitive aspects of activities of daily living is a focus at the University of Kansas (Rempfer, Hamera, Brown, & Cromwell, 2003). Functioning in the community is being studied in the United States by Hampton and Chafeftz (2002), B. Johnson and Montgomery (1999), and Beebe (2001, 2002). Australian researchers are studying grounded research in the willingness to access community mental health services (McCann, T. V., & Clark, 2003) while Pinikahana, Happell, Hope, and Keks (2002) are looking at overall quality of life. In Sweden the focus is the effect of living in a homelike setting (Pejlert, Asplund, & Norberg, 1999). In Taiwan work is ongoing in the area of social skills training (Chien, H. C., et al., 2003). In Hong Kong, Chan, S., Mackenzie, and Jacobs (2000), Tin-Fu, Chan, and Jacobs (2000), and Chan, S., MacKenzie, A., Tin-Fu, and Leung (2000) are studying cost effectiveness of case management versus routine community care, as are Lin, Yin, Kuo, and colleagues in Taiwin. Japanese researchers are studying client empowerment by public health nurses (Kayama, Zerwekh, Thornton, & Murashima, 2001). Anger management is also being studied in Hong Kong (Chan, H., Lu, Tseng, & Chou, 2003). Needs assessment and quality of life in Scandinavia is described in a 5-year follow-up study by Foldemo and Bogren (2002).

An increasing number of studies are focusing on tool development for various measures. In 1999 nursing students developed a tool for assessing safety (Blanchard et al., 1999). In Manchester, England, Lockwood and Marshall (1999) have been studying the importance of standardized and reliable assessment tools in schizophrenia research. Sherrell, Buckwalter, Bode, and Strozdas (1999) are evaluating cognitive abilities screening tools in the assessment of elderly schizophrenics. Beebe (2003b) is emphasizing the importance of the vulnerability model to guide research in schizophrenia. Menzies and Farrell (2002) remind psychiatric nurses of the importance of the traditional Abnormal Involuntary Movement Scale in evaluating patients for side effects related to antipsychotic medications. McCay and Seeman (1998) developed a scale to measure impact of schizophrenia on self-concept.

The use of critical pathways to guide inpatient care at the Chinese University in Hong Kong is emphasized by S. W. Chan and Wong in 1999 and also in London by A. Jones (2000, 2001). At the University of Hawaii, Anders, Kawano, Mori, Kokusha, and Tokunaga (2001) are studying inpatient treatment in Japan, Thailand (Anders, Thapinta, Wiwatkunupakan, Kitsumban, & Vadtanapong, 2003) and the U.S. (Anders, 2000). From the patient perspective, Finnish researchers Koivisto, Janhonen, and Vaisanen (2003) are studying the patient's experience of psychosis using phenomenological methodology. In India, Mahato (2000) studied the relationship between the length of hospitalization and the ability to resume self-care.

Depression and suicide is being studied in Australia by Pinikahana, Happell, and Keks (2003) and in Italy by Pompili, Mancinelli, Girardi, and Tatarelli (2003). In the United States, Menzies (2000) at the University of Virginia is studying the neglected aspect of postpsychotic depression. The concept of hope is being studied by Kirkpatrick, Landeen, Woodside, and Byrne (2001), T. V. McCann (2002), and Salerno (2002).

The use of psychotherapeutic techniques include cognitive behavioral therapy (Siddle & Kingdon, 2000), transactional analysis (Paley & Shapiro, 2001), sense of coherence (Bengtsson-Tops & Hansson, 2001), general psychosocial interventions (McCann, E., 2001), insight (Baier et al., 2000; Baier & Murray, 1999), the nurse-patient relationship (Forchuk, Westwell, et al., 2000), and Newman's theory (Yamashita, 1999).

Women's issues (Clarke, Chernomas, & Chisholm, 2001) and sexuality (McCann, E., 2000) are beginning to appear in the literature; however there was only one study documented related to children and adolescents with schizophrenia (Lambert, L. T., 2001).

In the past 5 years, the quality and quantity of nursing research in schizophrenia has expanded around the globe. Psychiatric nurse researchers are contributing significantly to the improvement of care for individuals with schizophrenia and their families. The corpus of research is maturing with the appearance of randomized controlled trials involving nursing interventions. Research that has been presented in poster format at major research conferences but has yet to be published in refereed journals is demonstrating increased sophistication in methodology in each of the 14 major areas.

MARY MOLLER

Scientific Development

Scientific development is a term defining the process of producing and making available new knowledge through systematically testing theories against empirical reality in order to solve problems. The term *scientific* is used as an attribute of the human knowledge interpreting natural, social, economic, historical, and psychological systems as parts of the empirical world. Scientific knowledge consists of systems of theories able to explain and solve scientific problems. Its essence is testability (Popper, 1969); it requires agreement among individuals about the nature of the problem and the validity of the explanation.

Controversies exist about what scientific knowledge is. For instance, the traditional empirical rationalism perspective holds the position that knowledge is scientific only when it has passed certain rigorous standards of method. Thus, only when reality has been defined in a measurable way and tested under sufficiently controlled conditions as an "objective" phenomenon (well protected from the investigators' subjective biases) can the generated knowledge be defined as scientific and therefore valid and reliable. Deductive reasoning facilitates objectivity by encouraging examination of a phenomenon in light of findings from previous research, conceptualizations contributed by other scholars, and testing of more than one prediction. In this perspective, scientific knowledge progresses by a process of formulating bold conjectures and then subjecting them to equally bold criticism and test.

The main criticism against empirical rationalism comes from the phenomenological perspective originated by preeminent philosophers such as Husserl, Heidegger, and Merleau-Ponty. From the phenomenological point of view it does not make sense to objectify our knowledge because reality consists of the meanings one assigns throughout experiences. Therefore, to the phenomenologist there is no reality separated from the interaction of a person as a perceiving, meaning-giving being. Reality cannot be known independently of a person's experience with all its meanings: "My knowledge of the world, even my scientific knowledge, is gained from my own particular point of view, or from some experience of the world without which the symbols of science would be meaningless" (Merleau-Ponty, 1962, p. vii).

The development of modern science can be defined from different theoretical perspectives; each one provides a rational framework (or methodology) for understanding the historical development of human science. Each framework provides a set of rules for the validation of testable theories; those rules also can be used as criteria for demarcation between common and scientific knowledge. At least four different frameworks can be identified, each one characterized by a specific set of rules finalized to accept or reject theories or research programs.

Inductivism dictates that only those propositions describing hard facts or true generalizations of those facts (or very probable generalizations in the neoinductivist version) can be accepted as scientific. Inductivism's basic assumption is that primitive propositions can be directly derived from facts, and it has been widely criticized. An inductivist accepts a scientific proposition when proved true; otherwise it will be rejected. This approach has a very strict scientific rigor: a proposition has to be demonstrated by facts or inductively-deductively derived from propositions proved to be true. However, inductivism does not offer any explanation about directions of the scientific development, nor can it rationally explain the reasons for the main scientific progress of humankind.

Conventionalism defines science development as the building of systems organizing facts into a consistent whole. When inconsistencies arise, a conventionalist changes or modifies the system, assuming that it can be considered true or false by convention. According to this approach, science develops by accumulation on the level of facts and progresses through simplifications or better conventional explanations. For example, Einstein's theory was progressive because it provided a simpler explanation than former theories. For a conventionalist, false assumptions can lead to true conclusions; therefore, false theories may have great predictive power (this is a solid philosophical position, not to be confused with instrumentalism). Under conventionalism any idea can be acceptable and used for scientific inquiry; what cannot be used is not considered nonscientific, as in the inductivist approach.

Falsificationism admits that the basic assumptions about facts can be accepted by agreement, but this does not apply to the theories. According to this approach, a theory is scientific only if it can be tested against a basic assumption or if it can be experimentally falsified. Thus, a theory must be rejected if it conflicts with accepted assumptions. Popper (1969) stated that, in order to be considered scientific, a theory has to predict new facts (new because they are not considered by other rival theories), has to be empirically testable, and must not be adjustable with ad hoc hypotheses. In the latter, more conventionalist version of this approach, some inductive principles are accepted.

Falsificationists define the development of science as a process of falsifying the dominant theories: behind each important discovery there is a theory proved false. Scientific development is related to the importance of the falsified theories; the more important they are, the more progress that has been made.

Research programs have been proposed by Lakatos (1968) as methods of analysis for scientific development. Research programs are identified as testable results in terms of progressive and regressive "problem shifts." Scientific revolutions consist in substitution of a research program with a more advanced one. According to this approach, a positive heuristic has to dictate the choice of problems for research instead of anomalies or incoherences, as in the falsificationism and inductivism methodologies. Therefore, the development of scientific theories is characterized by high degrees of freedom and is not influenced by the dominant paradigms. Thus, a research program progresses because its theoretical development anticipates the empirical one. It is regressing when it can provide only post hoc explanations because the empirical development is predominant over the theoretical one.

Each one of the four frameworks defines scientific development in a specific way. However, each perspective has to be integrated by external empirical theories able to explain the nonrational factors involved in scientific development, such as the social context and the historical period, because these are powerful forces driving or opposing any scientific development.

A method of analysis that can define how knowledge evolves is essential for understanding scientific development in general as well as in a particular disciplinary field. Three approaches can be proposed to understand nursing's scientific development: (a) revolution, (b) evolution, and (c) integration.

Development by Revolution. The concept of revolution was first used by Kant (1781/1991) to explain his idea that from an initial revolution a discipline will find a secure path for its scientific development. Kuhn (1970) introduced the idea that, under particular circumstances, the whole traditional paradigm (all theories, methods, applications, and instruments made available throughout a consistent tradition of research) is subject to change, not just a theory or a research program. Important progress in scientific development is possible through a series of transitions, from crisis or revolutions to normal science, when members of the field accept in a unified way a common, dominant paradigm (later defined as disciplinary matrix). Using a revolutionary perspective, nursing is in a preparadigmatic stage. Because there may not be periods of normal science (even if nursing knowledge is progressing), it is possible that the nursing scientific revolution may never come (Meleis, 1997).

Development by Evolution. In this approach, knowledge progress is a gradual process of change and differentiation toward a higher level of complexity. It is a process of generating new ideas in continuity with the old ones and therefore systematically accumulating knowledge following a well-defined course. Propositions of one theory are used as premises for another; they are tested against practice, and vice versa. As in the Darwinian process, environment continuously challenges the existent theories, and only the ones that interpret and meet its demands can temporarily survive. Using this approach to nursing, environmental demands for scientific development come from its practice and the scientific community. However, to date in nursing there are no recognizable trends of systematic development by accumulation.

Development by Integration. According to this approach, new ideas and theories are generated simultaneously without following any specific path. Thus, it is more than a process of testing, accepting, and rejecting theories; it is a process of developing agreement or disagreement about phenomena and methodologies that are most congruent with the subject matter of nursing. It follows, from this perspective, that nursing is greatly affected by external factors; nurse scientists gain insights mostly from the ongoing scientific developments in other fields. Therefore, nursing scientific development proceeds through a process of borrowing and repatterning ideas and theories across disciplines, as well as developing new ideas and differentiating them from the traditional ones; all are competing and coexisting.

From an evolutionist perspective, nursing has not accumulated enough knowledge to deserve the status of discipline; from an integrationist perspective, nursing is a discipline because it is able to provide new questions and answers, including repatterning, inventing, and testing knowledge through research and practice.

RENZO ZANOTTI

Secondary Data Analysis

Secondary data analysis uses the analysis of data that the analyst was not responsible for collecting or data that was collected for a different problem from the one currently under analysis. The data that are already collected and archived in some fashion are referred to as secondary information (Stewart, D. W., & Kamins, 1993). Statistical meta-analysis might be considered a special case of secondary analysis (see Meta-analysis).

Secondary information is an inexpensive data source that facilitates the research process in several ways. It is also useful for generating hypotheses for further research. It is useful in comparing findings from different studies and examining trends. Steward and Kamins (1993) point out that population data sets, such as Bureau of the Census data, may be used to compare sample to population characteristics in order to examine the representativeness of the study sample.

The analysis of secondary information is a useful strategy for learning the research process. The secondary data sets that have used optimum sampling techniques provide an optimum resource for students by virtue of the quality of sampling and the time and expense involved in data collection. Given that students are expected to understand, explain, and defend the data set in terms of purpose, sample selection, methods, and instruments, only the real-life collection and recording of data remain unexperienced by the student. A further virtue of using the analysis from secondary information while learning to do research is that it protects the pool of potential research participants and agencies for participation in studies conducted by qualified researchers.

Every research study is conducted with a specific purpose in mind. Delimitations are specific to the original study and introduce specific types of sampling and other bias into the original study. Operational definitions may not be replicable in a second study. For learning purposes, differences in the original study and data set can be handled through careful critique processes by students. However, the biases and differences that exist may be too extreme to permit a valid secondary analysis outside the practice situation.

Archived data sets are rarely held in the form of raw data because the data is usually summarized. The summarization may or may not be appropriate for the research question under consideration for secondary analysis. To analyze such data further confounds results beyond acceptable limits.

The question of using clinical nursing data sets for secondary analysis comes with the advent of clinical nursing information systems. The use of clinical databases as research data sets must be examined carefully. One difficulty is that restricted data resources force clinicians to choose carefully which data to collect. These data are usually not identical with what the researcher needs.

Beyond data restrictions another major difficulty is that the sample biases of clinical databases and research data sets for randomized control studies are different. This difference in bias of the data from clinical databases and randomized controlled trial research data sets can be exploited as a strategy for doing cross-design synthesis. However, this special case aside, the issue is that of sample representativeness. The research sample is selected for a specific reason, with specific delimitations in mind, to be representative of the general population. In contrast, the clinical population from which the clinical data set is drawn is representative only of that type of patient or client on whom data is being collected in that location and rarely, if ever, typical of the general population or even all persons with that clinical problem. For example, patients with congestive heart failure in Alabama are not necessarily representative of patients with congestive heart failure in New England or California. The same is true of patients with congestive heart failure in a community hospital versus those in a teaching hospital in the same county.

These caveats necessitate close evaluation of data sets to be used for secondary analysis. The information needed for such evaluation must be archived along with the data set. Such information includes study purpose; data collection details, such as who collected the data, when, and where; sampling criteria and delimitations; known biases; operational definitions; and methods of data collection.

Traditionally, nursing has not archived research data sets of its own for use in teaching or secondary analysis. Nursing students and nurse researchers do use large government databases, but none are collected specifically by nurse researchers to answer nursing research questions. This is a problem to the extent that learning takes place best when examples and experiences relate closely to daily (nursing) experience. Certainly, problems peculiar to but not exclusive to nursing research are more easily taught with examples from real life. This is a problem also to the extent that nursing research data sets can, in fact, generate new knowledge, whether by reanalysis or by stimulation of further investigation and hypothesis generation.

Sigma Theta Tau International has begun a program to archive selected research data sets of nurse researchers. The project is still in its infancy, with acquisition and dissemination policy still under study (see Data Stewardship). Descriptions of the research study will be required to fulfill criteria for data set evaluation mentioned above.

JUDITH R. GRAVES

Self-Concept Disturbances and Eating Disorders

Dating from early psychodynamic theories to the more contemporary cognitive approaches, the eating disorders have been characterized as disorders of the self. Research that has focused on the self-concept as a determinant of eating disorder symptomatology has addressed three aspects of the self-concept: body image, self-esteem, and structure of the self-concept. Although the majority of empirical work on the self-concept in the eating disorders has focused on body image and self-esteem disturbances, studies related to structure of the self-concept are distinguished in that they build on early clinical theories that focus on disturbances in the development of the total collection of beliefs about the self as the *core vulnerability* contributing to formation of the disorders. An overview of studies that suggest that disturbances in the structure of the self-concept serve as a cognitive vulnerability that contributes to internalization of unrealistic cultural norms regarding body-weight and the formation of eating disorder symptoms is presented.

Two eating disorders are recognized by the American Psychiatric Association, anorexia nervosa (AN) and bulimia nervosa (BN). Diagnostic criteria for AN include: (a) body weight less than 85% of ideal, (b) amenorrhea for 3 consecutive months, and (c) disordered attitudes toward body-weight. Diagnostic criteria for BN include: (a) going on binges (ingesting large quantities of food within 2 hours while feeling out of control), (b) compensatory weight control behaviors (vomiting, laxative or diuretic use, fasting, or excessive exercise) in response to the binge with the cycle occurring at least twice weekly for 3 months, and (c) disordered attitudes toward body-weight. While important differences between the disorders have been identified, theories of etiology of the two disorders often converge.

Although clinical theories converge to suggest that disturbances in identity and self-concept are the core vulnerability that contributes to development of eating disorders, the lack of clarity in theoretical and operational definitions of these constructs has limited empirical testing of the proposition. The first study to address identity and self-concept disturbances in women with BN utilized no theoretical framework for the self constructs. In this study of 26 women with BN, identity confusion was defined as the subjective experience of inconsistency in beliefs about the self, and enmeshment was defined as high reliance on others to define the self (Schupak-Neuberg & Nemeroff, 1993). Both concepts were measured using scales developed for the study. Identity stability was measured by determining the degree of consistency in self-description over 2 weeks. Despite the limitations, results support the identity disturbance hypothesis showing that women with BN had higher levels of confusion, instability, and enmeshment compared to controls.

More recently, studies that have focused on self-concept disturbances in eating disorders have utilized the cognitive model as the theoretical framework. In this model, the self-concept is conceptualized as a well-developed set of memory structures that are formed through interaction with the social environment and have been shown to play a primary role in information processing and behavioral regulation (Kendzierski & Whitaker, 1997). The total set of memory structures about the self is referred to as the self-concept, which in turn is composed of units of self-knowledge, referred to as self-schemas. Each self-schema is itself an organized collection of memory structures that reflect knowledge of oneself within one specific domain. Self-schemas have been shown to be functional memory structures that influence attention and encoding and recall of stimuli, and motivate and regulate goal-directed behavior. Hence, individual differences in the number, valence, content, and organization of the self-schemas have important implications for emotional and behavioral self-regulation.

Two studies using the cognitive model have focused on the valence and organization of self-schemas. Using a card-sort instrument with 31 women with subclinical BN, Showers and Larson (1999) found that women with BN differed from controls in the following configuration of self-schemas: (a) more negative and fewer positive self-schemas, (b) a negative physical appearance self-schema, and (c) more linkages between the negative physical appearance self-schema and other schemas. Similarly, in a study that examined valence and organization of self-schemas in a sample of women with clinically diagnosed BN, Stein, K. F., Corte, and Nyquist (2004) found that women with BN had fewer positive and more negative self-schemas compared to controls. Furthermore, the number of positive self-schemas positively predicted the availability of a fat self-schema which in turn was highly predictive of eating-disordered attitudes and behaviors.

Finally, another study focused on discrepancies between the content of the current self-schemas and self-guides, which are defined as knowledge structures that reflect the self one would ideally like to be (ideal self-guide), and the self one believes that she is obligated to be (ought self-guide) (Strauman, Vookle, Berenstein, Chaiken, & Higgins, 1991). Previous studies have shown that discrepancies between the way the self is currently defined and 'ideal' and 'ought' self-guides have important affective and motivational consequences (Higgins, 1987). In two studies using nonclinical samples of college students, Strauman found that women with extreme discrepancies between their current and ideal self schemas had high levels of body dissatisfaction and bulimic symptoms, whereas women with extreme discrepancies between their current and ought self-schemas had high dieting and anorexic symptoms.

These studies provided evidence to support the hypothesis that characteristics of the self-concept, including the relative absence of positive self-schemas, the presence of many negative self-schemas, high interconnectedness among the self-schemas, and discrepancies between the content of the current self-schemas and self-guides contribute to formation of a negative body weight/appearance self-schema, which in turn is predictive of disordered eating attitudes and behaviors. These findings are consistent with clinical eating disorder theories that suggest that disturbances in the structure of the self-concept are a *core vulnerability* that contribute to eating disorder symptoms. Furthermore, these findings challenge current eating disorder treatment approaches that focus on modifying weight-related cognitions, and point to the importance of interventions designed to modify the overall structure of the self-concept by building new and separate positive self-schemas and modifying the content of negative self-schemas and self-guides to promote long-term recovery from the eating disorders.

KAREN FARCHAUS STEIN
COLLEEN CORTE

Self-Efficacy

Self-efficacy is one component of social cognitive theory, along with outcome expectations, goals, and impediments (Bandura, 1997). An individual becomes efficacious in a particular domain of function through four mechanisms: enactive mastery experience, vicarious experience, verbal persuasion, and physiological and affective states. Bandura differentiates efficacy beliefs and *outcome expectancies*. An efficacy belief is the conviction that one can successfully execute the behavior required to produce the outcomes. Self-efficacy instruments determine the level, strength, and generality of efficacy beliefs. Outcome expectancy is defined as a person's estimate that a given behavior will lead to certain outcomes. These expectancies are physical, social, and self-evaluative. Bandura included the studies of eight nurse scientists conducting self-efficacy research; however, studies from Gortner, Harvey, Jensen, Laschinger, Lin, and Ruiz were not available. In this review, nursing research in cardiac recovery and/or rehabilitation, chronic disease self-management, memory function, and parent and behavior training are presented as examples of self-efficacy derived programs of nursing research. For a comprehensive review on self-efficacy research and Albert Bandura, see the Information on Self-Efficacy maintained by Professor Frank Pajares at http://www.emory.edu/EDUCATION/mfp/effpage and Bandura's (1997) book on human agency. Two examples of memory self-efficacy research using qualitative designs are provided for future development of self-efficacy theory.

Self-efficacy for activity and exercise following cardiac events has been found to predict better health outcomes, not only in hospitalized patients but also in community residing adults. Investigators have evaluated the contribution of efficacy expectations for coronary bypass surgery, valve replacement, implantable cardioverter/defribillator (ICD), and participation in cardiac rehabilitation (Jenkins & Gortner, 1998; Moore, S. M., Dolansky, Ruland, Pashkow, & Blackburn, 2003). Removing barriers and increasing social support clearly build self-efficacy in these individuals who must sustain their efforts for long periods of time.

Lorig and colleagues (2001) have developed a program of efficacy-based interventions aimed at empowering individuals to self manage their chronic disease. The Chronic Disease Self-Management Program (CDSMP) incorporates three self-management tasks—medical management, role management, and emotional management—and six self-management skills—problem solving, decision making, resource utilization, the formation of a patient-provider partnership, action planning, and self-tailoring. Over 800 participants with heart disease, lung disease, stroke, or arthritis have participated in the CDSMP. The longitudinal outcomes include reduced emergency room visits, times hospitalized, and health distress. In addition, this low-cost program significantly improved self-efficacy in these diverse populations.

Adults begin to lose confidence in their memory after age 40 years, and this is particularly strong in adults older than 60 years of age, regardless of their functional ability and living arrangement. Within the psychometric tradition of intelligence and aging, researchers are moving from a decremental model of cognitive function to a health promotion orientation that values an individuals' ability to improve their cognitive abilities through training or mental discipline. In the short term, memory performance may be improved. However, the ability to sustain these gains may be moderated by an individual's memory self-efficacy. McDougall (2004) found that in community-dwelling older adults greater than 70 years of age, memory self-efficacy predicted everyday memory performance in both black and white elders. The participants in this study had lowered correlates of perceived inefficacy and this negatively influenced their everyday memory performance. Continued investigation of the subjective aspects of memory function are necessary since memory self-efficacy, or one type of subjective evaluation, is associated with actual memory performance.

Problematic behaviors in young children may lead to decreased confidence in the parenting role when the parents believe they cannot successfully master these outbursts with their concomitant untoward outcomes in the emotional and intellectual development of the child. Using self-efficacy-derived psychosocial interventions, Gross and her colleagues (2003) have developed behavioral parent-training interventions for families with toddlers in various settings, most recently in day care and low-income urban communities. The boosting of parents' self-efficacy through behavioral parent-training promotes longitudinal health outcomes in high-risk preschool-age children.

However, research emphasizing outcome expectations may need to include qualitative methodologies (Bandura, 2001). Two examples of qualitative research evaluating memory function with adults are used to elaborate the methodology. In the Seattle Midlife Women's Health Study (SMWHS), 230 women averaging 47 years of age were asked to describe types of memory changes, their attributions about the memory changes, and how these changes affected their life roles and stress (Sullivan, Mitchell, & Woods, 2001). Five categories of memory changes and problems were identified: recalling words or numbers, forgetting related to everyday behaviors, events, concentration problems, and need for memory aids. In addition, the participants identified role burden and stress, getting older, health, menstrual cycle changes/hormones, inadequate concentration, and emotional factors. Memory change was attributed to stress, physical health, and aging, not to the menstrual cycle or use of hormones.

In another study of subjective memory evaluation with 169 healthy older adults averaging 68 years of age, McDougall and colleagues (2003) evaluated unsolicited comments about memory from 26 participants. Fifty individuals were between the ages of 50 and 64, 90 between 65 and 74, and 29 were at least 75 and older. In addition to the qualitative themes, this investigation included two quantitative measures of memory self-efficacy, a subjective evaluation of memory function. One measure consisted of 4 items and the other measure contained 50 items. Content analyses of the qualitative data yielded five themes: memory management, rationalization, information seeking, reflection, and correlation establishment. The majority of the themes related to memory management, and all four questions on the memory self-efficacy questionnaire emphasized maintenance skills to prevent decline and strategies for memory management. The qualitative and quantitative data provided an unusual finding: there were no age-group differences on memory self-efficacy with the 4-item measure, but there were significant age-group differences on the 50-item measure. This study and the previous study provide a glimpse of what adults experience regarding memory function and what they believe is important for health care professionals to know.

Examples of memory phenomena captured through qualitative methods were presented to provide examples of multimethod research to quantify a domain-specific measure of self-efficacy. Both of the examples, including the McDougall and the Mitchell and Woods studies, are a beginning effort to measure outcome expectancies in the domain of cognitive function, specifically memory performance. However, neither study developed a quantitative measure of outcome expectancies in the memory function domain as an outcome of the qualitative analyses. Nevertheless, both studies provided evidence supporting the theoretical distinction between efficacy beliefs and outcome expectancies that enforce the belief that a goal is achievable.

GRAHAM J. MCDOUGALL, JR.

Serious Mental Illness

Serious mental illness (SMI) is a term used to define those disorders that persist over time and result in extensive functional impairment in daily living skills and abilities that involve social interaction, interpersonal relations, and work skills (Johnson, 1997). These disorders include but are not limited to schizophrenia, schizoaffective disorder, recurrent major depression, and bipolar disorder (Lyon, 2001). It has been estimated that about 2.8% of the adult population in the United States experience one of these disorders in a 1-year period (National Institutes of Mental Health [NIMH], 1994). Many of these disorders are considered lifelong and involve some level of disability, rendering the individual vulnerable to poor health outcomes and decreased quality of life. Symptoms of severe mental illness are manifested in cognitive dysfunction, social skills deficits, disruption in emotional and behavioral responses, impaired communication, and self-care deficits.

Cognitive impairment in individuals with chronic mental illness includes impairment in conceptualization, information processing, attention, executive functioning, and memory. The more severe impairments involve the ability to problem solve and process complex information. Insight and judgment are severely limited. This is manifested as the inability to recognize the existence of illness and need for treatment, self-knowledge deficits, and poor decision-making abilities. Cognitive impairments are associated with poor functional outcomes and variances in adaptive functioning. Individuals with serious mental illness have difficulty making decisions, as the ability to process and respond to information is often impaired. Often individuals with serious mental illness are unable to meet their basic needs for food, shelter, and money, resulting in increased risk-taking behaviors. It is not an uncommon practice to barter sexual favors for these items and engage in unsafe sexual practices. Carey, Carey, Weinhardt, and Gordon (1997) measured the behaviors associated with risk of transmission of HIV in a population of 60 adults with serious mental illness. The findings indicated that 48% of men and 37% of women engaged in at least one high-risk behavior.

Social skills deficits result in self-concept changes, decreased stress response, and underassessment of personal resources. Social skills deficits include deficits in conversational capacity and impairments in processing interpersonal stimuli, such as eye contact or assertiveness. Individuals with SMI may look eccentric or disheveled, have poor hygiene and bizarre dress. Other behaviors such as aggression, psychomotor retardation, and regression are often present and misinterpreted by others. Results are decreased financial status secondary to inability to gain employment, stigma, social isolation, financial disparities, and homelessness. Coping skills deficits result in self-concept changes, decreased stress response, and underassessment of personal resources. Many individuals with SMI have suffered the loss of family support and relationships. As the symptoms of SMI progress, an individual becomes increasingly isolated. According to Borge, Martinsen, Ruud, Wante, and Frilis (1999), the degree of loneliness, meaningful leisure time activities, and satisfaction with living environment were identified as the most important factors influencing perceived quality of life in a population of clients with SMI. As social support and factors related to perceived quality of life wane, the individual becomes increasingly susceptible to negative health outcomes.

Examining historical trends in psychiatric care reveals a shift from institutionalization to community-based care for individuals with serious mental illness. In the 1960s, deinstitutionalization became a national objective as deplorable conditions in state facilities were recognized, yet few communities were prepared to care for individuals with serious mental illness. Nonetheless, inpatient populations began to decline as patients were discharged into the community. Often the communities were ill-prepared to care for the large number of individuals with serious mental illness, resulting in increased homelessness and increased numbers of incarcerated individuals with serious mental illness. Fortunately, community programs have emerged providing a range of treatment and rehabilitation services, including case management and residential services. In addition, many advocacy groups have emerged such as the National Alliance for the Mentally Ill. These groups advocate for the rights of those with serious mental illness on both the local, state, and national level. Although there have been advances in understanding and treating serious mental illness and the development of more efficacious medications and community-based treatment services, the likelihood of nurses encountering clients with untreated serious mental illness in a variety of health care and community settings is high. Nurses must be in a position to assess, intervene, and evaluate individuals with serious mental illness in order to provide holistic nursing care.

Rebecca J. Bonugli

Sex and Gender

Sex and gender research has exploded over the course of the past half century and consequently traditional ideas have been challenged and in many cases radically modified. Two factors seemed to be the driving forces behind modern sex research: the need to explain the existence of sexual variation, e.g., prostitution, homosexuality, transvestism, and bisexuality on the one hand, and the desire to find some scientific means of family planning or control of reproduction and disseminating information about this on the other hand. Germany was the home of early researchers such as Magnus Hirschfeld and Richard von Krafft Ebing, who explored what Krafft-Ebing called sexual pathology. Both authors are still read today although the key writings of Hirschfeld on homosexuality and transvestism were not translated into English until the 1990s. In England, the leading figure was Havelock Ellis, who used historical and sociological data to challenge many of the sexual beliefs of his generation. All three were data collectors about human sexual variation but were not able to explain why there was so much variation in human behavior (Bullough, 1994).

In the 20th century two Americans, John D. Rockefeller II and Margaret Sanger, a nurse, were extremely influential in establishing the United States as a center for sexual research. Rockefeller originally was concerned with understanding why prostitution and prostitutes existed, while Margaret Sanger was concerned with family planning. Rockefeller in the 1920s established and financially supported the Committee for Research in the Problems of Sex, which concentrated on research about the biological and psychological sources of human sexuality. Sanger in her campaign for effective birth control realized the importance of changing public attitudes about sexuality, since actual dissemination of any kind of information about birth control or many other kinds of sex information across state lines was illegal in the United States. For her, educating the public about what science knew was all important, while Rockefeller felt finding out about what people did sexually as well as the reasons for doing it was the key. One result of Rockefeller's efforts were the books by Kinsey and colleagues (1948, 1953), which revolutionized the understanding of human sexuality, and the ultimate result of Margaret Sanger's work was the development of the pill for contraception which contributed immeasurably to a changing role and status for women in the United States. Some sexual topics are more controversial than others. For example, concern over the effects of pornography has led to many studies on the topic, with the majority of them concluding that it seems to have little correlation with the actual conduct of the viewer or reader. It is a sort of a fantasy literature, an adult Superman comic, which almost all research indicates is not particularly harmful to the adult reader (Elias et al., 1999).

One of the more intensely studied topics in childhood is that of gender identity. Usually by the time children begin to talk they can apply the appropriate gender identity to themselves, although they do not necessarily understand the concept of gender constancy. A little boy may believe, for example, that at some later point in life he will be a girl or vice versa. Gradually as their gender identity becomes stronger, they also learn gender roles, what is expected of females or males in the culture, and begin to acquire a gender role identification (Money & Ehrhardt, 1972). Not all children accept or adopt the norms expected of them. One study of this nonconformity was by Richard Green (1987). He recruited 66 families in which there was a boy (age 4 to 10 years) who was regarded as extremely feminine and in a longitudinal study over a period of 15 years he compared them with a sample of other boys. He started with the assumption that socialization and parental treatment were the main determinants of gender but found that this was not the case. Most of the feminine boys in his study later identified as homosexuals, a development which did not take place in his control study. This study and similar studies tended to give growing credibility to biological factors in the development of homosexuality, bisexuality, and transgender behaviors, resulting in a deemphasis on psychodynamic theories. There is still a lot that remains unknown. The Bulloughs (1993) in their studies of transvestites and transsexuals argued that there were variations in gender and sexual behavior which had some biological basis and that, instead of one standard of definition of what was male and what was female, individuals appeared on different levels of two bell-shaped curves which had considerable overlap. There were in essence females who had a strong masculine component and males with a strong feminine one. These differences were not due to genetic factors per se (although this might have entered in) but more to developmental factors in the fetal period. Studies have shown that adults who as children witnessed parents engaging in sex were not harmed by so doing (Okami, Olmstead, Abramson, & Pendleton, 1998; Lewis, R. J., & Janda, 1988).

Interestingly, boys and girls who engage in consensual same-sex experiences in boarding schools or other sex-segregated institutions do not seem to become homosexual and lesbian as adults in any greater proportion than those who do not. There are also gender differences. Women as a group seem to have their sexual feelings more strongly influenced by considerations of love and intimacy than men do, and this might result in greater fluidity in their sexual orientation than that of men (Peplau, L. A., & Garnets, 2000; Peplau, L. A., Spaulding, Conley, & Veniegas, 1999). Girls seem to be more traumatized by child sexual abuse than are boys, but the reason why is still not clear.

One of the more difficult problems for researchers to study is that of adult-child sexual interaction. One reason for the difficulty is the intense emotions involved by the public in general to such behavior. Perhaps the easiest way to do so is to survey adult recollections of such experience. Even here results are contradictory. One major study found about 15% of women and 7% of men had at least one childhood sexual experience involving physical contact with an adult (Gorey & Leslie, 1997). But the definition of what physical contact was is unclear. Other contemporary estimates based on random samples of adults indicate different rates, ranging from 12% to 55% for females and from 3% to 6% for males. Figures vary to some extent as a function of the population being sampled, the definition of sexual abuse, and the cut-off age employed (e.g., before 14, 16, or 18). In the national sample by Finkelhor (1990), 9% of the males and 22% of the females who reported being victims of attempted or completed sexual relations during childhood had experienced them with relatives—aunts or uncles, siblings, parents or step-parents, or cousins. In general it appears that children in disrupted, isolated, and economically poor families are at higher risk of sexual abuse than youngsters in more stable and high-income families. The effect of such relationships is not clear. Although most people vehemently condemn them and claim that associations have dire effects on the child that last into adulthood, the data did not necessarily support such a view (Rind, Tromo, Viten, & Bauserman, 1998). This finding, which was a summary of numerous studies, went contrary to popular beliefs and was quickly denounced by the U.S. Congress.

One of the areas in which current research is focused is sexual function in physically compromised, the blind, the deaf, the severely physically handicapped; it is only in the past few years that the sexual problems have begun to be understood (Knuth & Smith, 1984; Rubin, E., 1997). Research into sexuality has revealed a wide variety of sexual behaviors and society is adjusting its attitudes toward the people involved. There are, however, many question that sex research has not yet answered, particularly in how some of these paraphilias develop and what is the prognosis of many of them.

Vern L. Bullough

Shivering

Shivering is defined as involuntary shaking of the body and is the adult human's primary defense against the cold. Characterized by a protracted generalized course of involuntary contractions of skeletal muscles that are usually under voluntary control, thermoregulatory shivering differs from transient tremors or "shivers" associated with fear, delight, or other forms of sympathetic arousal. Shivering occurs when heat loss stimulates specific heat-loss sensors in the skin, spinal cord, and brain. Sensory impulses are received and integrated at the preoptic area of the hypothalamus. Shivering is stimulated when integrated thermosensory information indicates body temperature is falling below optimal "set point" range (see Thermal Balance). The shivering center in the posterior hypothalamus is stimulated, sending impulses via anterior spinal routes of the gamma efferent system.

Heat is generated by oscillation and friction of the fibrous muscle spindles of the fusimotor system. Shivering occurs in fever despite rising temperatures because the set point level is raised to higher levels by circulating cytokines and other pyrogens.

The consequences of shivering for seriously ill or vulnerable patients are sometimes overlooked because they seem to be harmless compensatory warming responses. However, the aerobic activity generated by vigorous shivering activity raises oxygen consumption 3–5 fold, approximately that of shoveling snow or riding a bicycle. The resulting oxidative phosphorylation of glucose and fatty acids raises metabolic demands, but it is only about 11% efficient in raising body temperature. The energy expenditure of shivering may be tolerated by healthy persons who shiver for short periods, but it puts specific patient groups at risk for cardiorespiratory, metabolic, and thermal instability. Uncontrollable shivering is distressful to patients, yet it occurs frequently in situations where ambient temperatures are cool, patients are exposed, or therapies induce fever. Shivering is often recalled by patients as a negative aspect of postoperative recovery, childbirth, antifungal drug administration, blood transfusions, or other hospital experience. Nursing research has documented correlates and sequelae of shivering in an effort to determine adverse consequences in postoperative care, febrile illness, and during induced hypothermia. Intervention studies have tested efficacy of nursing measures to prevent shivering during surface cooling and febrile chills. Important to these studies has been the effort to standardize the measurement of shivering by use of a shivering severity scale, originated by Abbey and colleagues (1973).

Although shivering had been studied extensively by physiologists in healthy humans and animals, little clinical interest was evident until the 1970s. Abbey and Close (1979) used wraps of ordinary terry-cloth towels as insulation to protect thermosensitive regions of the skin during use of cooling blankets. Shivering during surface cooling was a significant problem treated at that time with chlorpromazine, a drug with undesirable side effects. The wrapping intervention was based on existing physiological research demonstrating dominance of the heat loss sensors on hands and feet in stimulating shivering. This landmark pilot study demonstrated that insulation of extremities controls shivering and improves comfort without drugs, even when surface cooling induces hypothermic temperatures.

Major studies by nurse investigators (Abbey & Close, 1979; Holtzclaw, 1998) using more extensive temperature and electromyographic measurements further supported the usefulness of "wrapping" extremities, with theoretical perspective based on Abbey's original work. Stated briefly, insulation blunts the neurosensory stimulus of heat loss from dominant sensors, while larger but less thermosensitive regions of the trunk allow heat exchange without inducing shivering.

Historically, interest in postoperative shivering grew in the mid-1980s with the rise in hypothermic cardiac surgery. Research findings show the hazardous increase in oxygen consumption, carbon dioxide production, and cardiovascular exertion during postoperative rewarming from hypothermic cardiac bypass (Holtzclaw & Geer, 1986; Phillips, 1997). Clinical predictors of shivering became of interest as early prevention was indicated. The *mandibular hum* was detected by palpation of referred masseter vibrations over the ridge of the jaw (Holtzclaw & Geer, 1994). Widening of skin to core-temperature gradients was found to predict shivering in this population, presumed to reflect the discrepancy between hypothalamic set point and peripheral temperatures that initiates shivering. Sund-Levander and Wahren (2000) found that tympanic-to-toe temperature gradients predicted shivering in neurologically injured patients during hypothermic surface cooling and that patients were more likely to shiver if cooled too quickly. This study supported Abbey's (1973) earlier contention that shivering during surface cooling could be reduced by modifying the *rate* of body heat loss. Studies confirm that little difference is found between pharmacologic suppressants, warmed blankets, or reflective wraps in preventing shivering during perioperative rewarming (Hershey, Valenciano, & Bookbinder, 1997); however, newer forced-air warming units (e.g., Bair Hugger) and radiant lamps have been found in medical studies to maintain normothermia more effectively. Extremity wraps were found to effectively reduce febrile shivering severity and duration (See Fever/Febrile Response) in immunosuppressed cancer patients and persons with HIV/AIDS (Holtzclaw, 1990, 1998).

As scientific evidence grows about neuroregulatory and immunological factors influencing shivering, new avenues of study emerge. Little is known about how shivering can be controlled in emergency situations during rescue and evacuation. Few studies have examined outcomes of shivering among children. Surgery, trauma, circulatory bypass, and hypothermia have all been linked in preliminary studies to acute phase reactions that stimulate febrile shivering (Phillips, R. A., 1999). While shivering is common during the last stage of labor, little attention has been paid to its origin and management. Future directions in the study of shivering by nursing will likely address the biobehavioral interface of environmental stimuli, biochemical and neurotransmitter activity, energy expenditure, physics of heat exchange, and thermal comfort.

BARBARA J. HOLTZCLAW

Sigma Theta Tau International Nursing Research Classification System

The first nursing research classification system was developed during the project Survey and Assessment of Areas and Methods of Research in Nursing. It was conducted at Yale University under the direction of Leo W. Simmons, a sociologist. Two other sociologists and Virginia Henderson comprised the survey group (Cowan, M. C., 1956). This system formed the basis for the annotation of English language nursing studies in the *Nursing Studies Index* between the years 1900 and 1959 (Henderson & Yale University). The term *study* was broadly defined as "a structured effort to solve a problem" and included historical and biographical articles and monographs in addition to what Henderson called analytical (research) articles (Henderson & Yale University, 1959, p. vii). This classification system categorized the types of nursing research according to fields on which nurse researchers focused their work.

This research classification system was abandoned because there was a desire to index all the nursing literature, not just the research literature. To facilitate indexing and retrieval of this broad literature, it was decided to switch to a subject headings system. Subject headings permit articles to be located according to what the various articles are about. The headings describe important topics in a field and are usually organized into a tree structure to illustrate relationships between the various topics and subtopics. A subject heading system in and of itself does not enable comparison of studies according to aspects such as research design and methods and the myriad of other comparisons of interest in the body of nursing research.

The idea of a classification system for nursing research was not lost, however. Sigma Theta Tau, the International Honor Society of Nursing (STTI), began work on the *Nursing Research Classification System* (NRCS) in the early 1980s. In addition to categorizing the fields in which nurse researchers did studies and the research subjects and methods in which they had experience, an early purpose was to facilitate identification and location of the nurse researchers. Now in its third edition, the system includes description of studies, variables, and findings. The NRCS serves as the structure for the databases that were combined and came to be known as the (electronic) *Registry of Nursing Research* (Graves, 1994).

In this version it is a representation of the language and the structure of clinical nursing research knowledge as well as the language and structure of research knowledge in related domains in which nurses do research such as education, administration, management, and so forth. In this usage, the term *language* refers to the names of research concepts and of variables studied together. The term *structure* refers to the descriptive details of the research describing any study: (a) the demographics (investigators, dissemination, funding, title, conceptual framework); (b) the sample, methodology and design, and analysis and results; and (c) the relationships (hierarchical arrangement) between these descriptors. Multiple knowledge (generation) theories are accommodated.

The STTI *Nursing Research Classification System* (NRCS) is a detailed description of the structured inquiry process used in individual nursing research studies. It identifies and logically relates salient characteristics of research studies in nursing. Salience is defined by whether a descriptive term (a) permits a comparison of studies according to the details of the research process, such as the design, the subjects, and the findings; (b) enables researchers and other users of research to make a preliminary judgment about the quality of a registered study, given the design; (c) enables direct indexing of the knowledge generated by each study (variable names and results); and (d) permits a comparison between studies that is of interest to the nursing profession, such as funding sources and amounts or domains of research that nurses investigate (education, administration, philosophy, culture, etc.).

In keeping with the original purpose of locating researchers, the category *Researcher* is the primary hierarchical element. The basic organization is described here:

- Each *researcher* may have many *research studies*. The single research study is the basic unit of analysis. A study may or may not be a part of a larger *research project*.
- Each *research study* is classified according to title, theoretical/conceptual framework, research domain, funding, keywords (subject headings), dissemination record, participants/sample, sampling plan, scope of sampling, data collection site, design type, extraneous variables.
- Each *study* may ask many *research questions*.
- Each *research question* may have many *analyses*.
- Each *analysis* is classified according to nature of the inquiry (knowledge theory), procedures, type of analysis, method of data analysis, research concept or names of variables studied together, relationship studied (if applicable), and findings.

The NRCS category *Domain of Research* is analogous to the first 9 of 10 categories of the Henderson nursing research classification system. Although not absolutely identical in detail, the categories are remarkably similar. Henderson's 10th category "Conducting Research," incorporates "Research methods and types including devices and techniques," whereas these characteristics form the primary corpus of the STTI NRCS, with domains being a secondary characteristic.

The NRCS provides a structure for a new archetype for storing and retrieving research knowledge in all disciplines. Of all the health science disciplines, only that of nursing has developed a research classification system. The classification system serves as the logical model for the database that organizes the Virginia Henderson Library's *Registry of Nursing Research©*. The Virginia Henderson International Nursing Library is the only known library to store research studies according to a research classification system and to index that research by the names of the variables or research concept studied.

The NRCS plays an active role in contributing the nursing subject headings maintained by the *Cumulative Index for Nursing and Allied Health Literature* (CINAHL). STTI has permission to use the subject headings from the CINAHL subject heading list in selected NRCS categories (i.e., funding sources, nursing theoretical framework, indexing terms, data collection sites). This prevents the development of still another subject heading system to describe the same topics, thus facilitating searching of both the CI-

NAHL bibliographic database and the STTI *Registry of Nursing Research*. As the NRCS becomes more widely used, new terms in use by researchers will provide real data to influence updates of the CINAHL subject heading list. In turn, the CINAHL subject heading list will be used to maintain the descriptors in selected NRCS categories.

The NRCS identifies the data elements necessary for generating an index to the studies in the *Registry of Nursing Research*©, organized by variable name so that the index lists all studies in which a particular variable is studied.

JUDITH R. GRAVES

Sleep

Sleep is a behavior represented by a series of distinguishing brain and somatic state changes oscillating with waking on a regular basis in synchrony with the environmental light/dark cycle (circadian = every 24 hours). Poor sleep has numerous health-related consequences, including impaired attention, memory, and problem solving as well as physical performance, altered immune system function, and tissue healing; in some cases it may herald early onset of psychiatric impairment, particularly major depression. It has been associated with more injury accidents, absences from work, medical problems, provider visits, and hospitalizations.

In research, sleep can be measured physiologically by using somnography (electroencephalogram [EEG], electromyogram, and electrooculogram) to reveal a series of stages, or by activity monitors that distinguish sleep from waking. Sleep also can be assessed behaviorally (by direct observation) or by self-reported perceptions (retrospective recall or global impressions as histories or concurrent reporting in diaries or logs). Using somnography, sleep begins with transitional signs, progresses into a light stage, and then into deep (slow wave) sleep, followed by a period of rapid-eye-movement (REM) sleep to complete one sleep cycle, taking about 60–90 minutes. Consequently, a full night of sleep consists of 3–6 cycles, depending on total sleep duration. Limitations of sleep measures include that physiological measures are time-consuming, require expensive technology, and can interfere with natural sleep. Behavioral observations are tedious, time-consuming, and potentially inaccurate. Self-report methods are subject to preferred answers and the propensity to report negative impressions indiscriminately. Peoples' impressions of their sleep do not always match physiological documentation.

Biological scientists seek to understand the regulation of sleep/wake states. Behavioral scientists seek to understand the function of sleep, normative patterns across age groups or species, the need for sleep, and insight into features predictive of poor sleep. Abnormal behaviors during sleep (e.g., apneas or large muscle movements) and abnormal bouts or timing of sleep (e.g., narcolepsy) claim the interests of clinical scientists. Nursing scientists most often seek to understand how sleep, or more precisely sleeplessness, is related to health and illness, what can be done to promote sleep, and how sleep is affected by environments and life contexts, which often include care environments, e.g., critical or long-term care, or contexts, e.g., enduring pain, injury, diseases, or major transitions.

Sleep science generated to date by nursing scientists is built on the premise that personal stress impacts sleep/wake quality. The notions that illness/disease and hospitalization are sources of stress that interfere with usual sleep/wake behavior are prominent. The vast majority of work is descriptive and only a few interventions, either individual or environmental, have been tested. K. C. Richards (1998) tested massage and found it tended to improve the sleep of critically ill older men. Other studies done several years ago used ocean sounds with evidence of better perceived sleep in post-coronary-artery-bypass-graft surgery, and progressive muscle relaxation in seniors with evidence of better perceived and somnographic sleep variables. In one review, it has been noted that sleeplessness is very common in infants and children, and clinicians frequently are asked for treatment advice in a review of cognitive-behavioral treatments (Owens, France, & Wiggs, 1999). Studies were reviewed that used behavior extinction and modification of parental behavior believed to reinforce waking behaviors as a theoretical basis, including the use of minimal checks, parental presence, stimulus control, and scheduled awakenings. While these interventions are relevant to nursing practice, only one study appeared to involve nursing scientists: a parent sleep education program showing that a significantly smaller percentage of babies in the intervention groups had settling and night-waking difficulties than in the control group (Kerr, Jowett, & Smith, 1996). Earlier, the use of recorded bedtime stories for effect on the time to fall asleep in hospitalized children was tested with implications that the use of parental voice might prolong time needed to fall asleep. Redeker (2000) in an integrative review of sleep in acute care settings revealed that sleep disturbances are common but highly variable, due to multiple personal, health status, and environmental factors. She advocated systematic research to determine correlates of sleep disturbance to identify those most at risk and to derive theoretical and conceptual bases for sleep-promoting interventions.

K. A. Lee (2001) and colleagues have looked at sleep and fatigue in times of transition in women—during the menstrual cycle, in pregnancy and postpartum, and in nurses working shifts. In the menstrual cycle luteal phase, time to REM sleep was shorter when compared to follicular phase, and women with premenstrual negative affect symptoms had less deep sleep during both menstrual cycle phases. Women transitioning through pregnancy report sleep problems, both prenatal and postpartum and primigravidae more than multigravidae. In a descriptive study of registered nurses working and not working outside of day shifts, shiftwork was associated with more sleep disturbances and sleepiness, but age and family factors, more than alcohol and caffeine intake, contributed to the differences in types of sleep disturbances. This group has also looked at fatigue issues in women with HIV/AIDS.

Two groups of investigators have developed research programs focused on individuals with sleep problems. Roger's group has a program of research investigating subjects with narcolepsy. They have found that those with narcolepsy have disturbed sleep and nap more, that memory is not measurably affected although concentration is, and that timed naps can improve time to fall asleep for certain patients (Rogers & Dreher, 2002). Shaver (2002) and her colleagues have ongoing work describing sleep in midlife (perimenopausal) women and particularly those with insomnia. They have found that menopausal status is not profoundly linked to somnographic sleep except if hot flashes are manifested. One group of midlife women reporting insomnia had high life strain, expressed high psychological distress, but exhibited little abnormality in somnographic sleep patterns and few classical symptoms of menopause such as hot flashes. Another group with insomnia reported hot flash activity but had less overall distress and life strain than the other group. Implications are that intervention to manage hot flash and menopausal symptoms are more warranted in the latter, and that life and stress management skills might be more efficacious in the former group.

Research programs are developing related to sleep and major illness. This includes, for example, in renal dialysis groups (Parker, K. A., 2003); in women with chronic fatigue and fibromyalgia (Landis et al., 2003); related to sleep apnea (Chasens & Umlauf, 2003) and Parkinson's disease; but also with postabdominal surgery, after CABG; with cancer, and in hospitalized adults and children.

In synchrony with a central focus for nursing practice, studies by nursing scientists mainly represent understanding sleep related to illness/disease. The majority of studies incorporate descriptive methodology limited to self-reports of sleep. It is imperative for the development of nursing sleep science that more sustained study is done to predict those at high risk for negative consequences with vulnerable populations, particularly older adults and the chronically ill, those suffering from sleep disorders for which behavioral treatments are prominent (e.g., insomnia, narcolepsy), and those in high-risk environments (e.g., hospitals, high-stress factors). Since sleep is a behavior responsive to behavioral interventions, behavioral intervention tests, including dose response, titration, timing, individualized response types, and the factors affecting behavioral choice and adherence especially are needed. Furthermore, the application of biobehavioral methods that combine physiological and perceptual measures will do much to develop our future knowledge, which is important to symptom management, illness/disease prevention, and health promotion.

JOAN L. SHAVER

Smoking Cessation

Twenty-three percent of all American adults continue to smoke, despite evidence that tobacco is responsible for 430,000 deaths in the United States each year and remains the number one avoidable cause of death and disease in this country (Centers for Disease Control, 2003b). Direct medical costs associated with smoking or smoking-attributable diseases have been estimated by the Centers for Disease Control (CDC) to exceed $50 billion annually. Of concern is the increase in smoking prevalence in adolescents since 1990, with 3,000 children and adolescents becoming regular users of tobacco every day. Seventy percent of the approximately 50 million smokers in the United States have made at least one prior quit attempt, with about 46% percent trying each year (CDC). However, the annual quit rate in the U.S. is only 1.0% approximately, with 4.7% having quit for between 3–12 months in the past year.

Smoking cessation, or smoking abstinence, differs from a quit episode, which is considered as 24 hours of continuous abstinence (Ossip-Klein et al., 1986). Smoking cessation is defined as the discontinuation of a smoking behavior. The behavior is characterized as dynamic and is often accompanied by periods of slips and relapses. Smoking cessation and tobacco use are important areas of research for nurses since, as clinicians, nurses represent key smoking cessation interventionists, capable of implementing effective cessation programs (Fiore et al., 2000).

Sarna and Lillington (2002) conducted a review of databased articles that included the keywords "tobacco use" in *Nursing Research* during the years 1952–2000. Their findings indicated that 40 databased articles included this term in either the sample description or as an independent or mediating variable. Fifty-three percent of these articles had been published since 1990, with 71% of the outcome studies being published within the past 5 years. While the authors recognized that nurses with a program of research in tobacco control have published in other interdisciplinary journals, they concluded that tobacco use and cessation are emerging topics for nursing research (Sarna & Lillington).

According to the *Treating Tobacco Use and Dependence Clinical Practice Guideline*, published by the U.S. Public Health Service Agency for Healthcare Research and Quality (AHRQ), a brief intervention should be provided to all tobacco users at each clinical visit (Fiore et al., 2000). The intervention includes five major steps (the "5 As") to managing tobacco dependence: *ask* the patient about tobacco use, *advise* tobacco cessation, assess *willingness to quit, assist* with the quit attempt, and *arrange* for follow-up to prevent relapse. All tobacco users attempting to quit should receive one of the five AHRQ-recommended first-line pharmacotherapies for smoking cessation.

Katz, D. A., Muehlenbruch, Brown, Fiore, and Baker (2002) conducted a pre- and post-test design study of the AHRQ intervention utilizing usual care as the control group. Participants in the intervention group were willing to set a quit date within 30 days. Those smoking at least 10 cigarettes a day were offered an 8-week supply of transdermal nicotine patches. Self-help material, as well as proactive telephone counseling by a trained cessation counselor, was also provided. The 6-month self-reported quit rate was 21% for the intervention group versus 13% in the control group. Continuous abstinence was reported in 10% of the intervention participants versus 3% of the control participants. It was also concluded that the implementation of a guideline-driven smoking cessation intervention was associated with increased abstinence at two-month follow-up (p = 0.0004) among primary care patients interested in making a quit attempt as compared to abstinence rates at baseline (21% vs. 4%) (Katz et al., 2002).

P. M. Smith, Reilly, Miller, DeBusk, and Taylor (2002) examined the application of a nurse-managed inpatient smoking cessation program. The program included physician advice, bedside education including take-home materials (videotape, workbook, and relaxation audiotape), counseling from a smoking cessation trained nurse, nicotine replacement therapy if requested, and four nurse-initiated postdischarge telephone counseling calls. Patients from Stanford University Hospital were recruited to participate in the program. Of 2,091 patients identified as smokers, 1,077 or 52% enrolled in the program, with only 720 patients eligible for 12-month follow-up. Seventy one percent (n = 509) were reached for the 12-month follow-up and of these 509 participants, 49% reported that they were not smoking. However, a limitation noted by the authors included potential underreporting of smoking by the participant at the time of the 12-month follow-up. The investigators acknowledged that misclassification of smoking status by self-report can be especially problematic in cessation studies of hospitalized patients, due to the "demand" characteristic of wanting to please the provider (Smith, P. M., et al., 2002).

The lack of biochemical verification to confirm smoking status does represent a limitation in smoking cessation intervention research. Cotinine, the major metabolite of nicotine, can be measured in plasma, saliva, and urine, with excellent specificity for tobacco use except in persons utilizing nicotine replacement therapy. Carbon monoxide (CO), a byproduct of cigarette smoke, can be measured in expired air. Unfortunately, CO has a shorter half-life of 2–4 hours and is rapidly eliminated, whereas cotinine may be detected for several days after cessation. However, CO assessments are often used to confirm abstinence in studies where nicotine replacement therapy is ongoing. It is recommended that biochemical verification be used in most or all studies of smoking cessation among special populations, including adolescents, pregnant women, and medical patients with smoking-attributable disease (SRNT, 2002).

Smoking is pronounced in the less educated and poor (CDC, 2003b). Efforts to promote cessation and abstinence in these individuals have, to date, been relatively unsuccessful. Their lack of engagement in preventive health care services may, in part, be due to barriers to access and lack of information about prevention (U.S. Department of Health and Human Services, 2000). While the evidence-based AHRQ clinical practice cessation guideline has been developed (Fiore et al., 2000), its testing among vulnerable populations is limited. As an example, the guideline deserves examination among minority groups, pregnant and postpartum women, HIV+ persons, and smokers who are poor and often experiencing a comorbid condition, such as cancer or chronic obstructive pulmonary disease (COPD).

GRETCHEN HARWOOD
MARY ELLEN WEWERS

Smoking/Tobacco as a Cardiovascular Risk Factor

Smoking is the single most preventable cause of death and disability in the United States today. The death toll associated with smoking approaches 440,000 annually, with more than 4.8 million deaths occurring globally. Moreover, by 2030 the World Health Organization projects that tobacco will kill 10 million individuals annually (Schroeder, 2004).

Smoking is a highly addictive disorder that causes both physiological and psychological dependence. Nicotine, which has both stimulating and tranquilizing effects, is the drug that leads to addiction. Addictive disorders such as smoking are characterized by: (a) predictable withdrawal symptoms, (b) physical dependence and tolerance for the drug, (c) use of the drug despite social and medical disapproval, or harm to physical, social, psychological, or economic well-being, (d) use of the drug to cope with stress, (e) an immediate sense of gratification, and (f) use of the drug to restore physical and psychological comfort. Smoking is also an "over-learned" habit. Smoking is associated with many aspects of daily life such as driving in a car, eating a meal, talking on the telephone, or drinking coffee. Finally, smoking is also used as a coping mechanism. Individuals use smoking to deal with stress, boredom, anger, anxiety, and other emotions. The success of interventions to help smokers must focus on the complexity of the behavior including nicotine addiction, psychosocial influences, and the habit itself.

Since 1965, the prevalence of smoking has declined by 40% among those 18 years of age and older. However, the rate of smoking has plateaued since 1990. In those 18–24 years of age, the prevalence actually rose from 23% to 27% between 1991 and 2000. The prevalence of smoking in the United States in 2001 was 48.1 million (1 in 4 adults), which includes 25.2% of males and 20.7% of females. All such individuals are at risk of a myocardial infarction and stroke, with cardiovascular deaths accounting for at least one third of all smoking-related deaths annually (American Heart Association, 2003).

Smoking prevalence varies considerably from state to state, is highly dependant on the success of tobacco-related legislation and changes in policies within a state, and is most often highest in states where tobacco is grown, such as Kentucky. A strong relationship exists between smoking and level of education, with the prevalence being several times higher among those with less than 12 years of education compared to those with more than 16 years of education. Smoking prevalence is higher (33.3%) among those living below the poverty line than in those with higher income levels (American Heart Association, 2003).

Approximately 80% of people who smoke began to use tobacco before the age of 18 years. The most frequent age of initiation is at 14 to 15 years. In 1998, 1.7 million Americans began to smoke cigarettes daily, which translates to more than 4,000 new smokers per day (American Heart Association, 2003). To slow the rate of cardiovascular disease, prevention strategies must be incorporated into education efforts within schools. It is also known that, for those who use tobacco, it is never too late to quit smoking. According to the World Health Organization, the risk of coronary heart disease (CHD) decreases by 50% within 1 year of quitting. Within 15 years of quitting, the relative risk of dying from CHD approximates that of a nonsmoker. In those with established CHD, smoking cessation reduces both morbidity and mortality to a similar degree in both younger individuals and in those over 70 years of age (Williams, M. A., et al., 2002).

Smoking affects almost every tissue and organ in the body. The deleterious effects on the cardiovascular system include an increase in blood pressure, heart rate, and peripheral vascular resistance; an increase in catecholamines; an impairment in flow-mediated dilation of coronary arteries; increased susceptibility to clotting; and reduction in high-density lipoprotein (HDL) cholesterol. These deleterious effects are often associated with angina pectoris, myocardial infarction, stroke, and death. Smoking significantly compounds the risk of other cardiovascular risk factors such as dyslipidemia, hypertension, and obesity.

Tobacco smoke also increases cardiovascular risk among nonsmokers. The 4,000 chemicals and carcinogens found in tobacco smoke increase the risk of death from cardiovascular disease by as much as 30% in nonsmokers (American Heart Association 2003).

Finally, smoking imposes a significant social burden due to the high costs of tobacco-related illness. Health-related costs to Americans now exceed $157 billion annually. These figures are due to loss of productivity and increased medical expenditures among smoking adults, and increased smoking-attributable neonatal medical expenditures. Many strategies for both prevention and intervention are needed in order to combat the aggressive tobacco industry, which spent $11.2 billion on advertising and promotion in the United States alone in 2001 (Schroeder, 2004).

Several theories and models have been effectively incorporated into smoking interventions. These include the *transtheoretical model* (Prochaska & DiClemente, 1983), classifying individuals into stages based on their desire to quit smoking; *social learning theory*, specifically self-efficacy (Bandura, 1997); and the *cognitive-behavioral model* of relapse which focuses on relapse prevention training (Marlatt & Gordon, 1985).

In 2000, the United States Department of Health and Human Services published the Clinical Practice Guideline entitled *Treating Tobacco Use and Dependence* (Fiore et al., 2000). This guideline reviewed more than 6,000 smoking-related studies conducted from 1975–1999. Strength of evidence, primarily from randomized controlled trials, indicates that tobacco dependence must be considered a chronic disease. This is due to the high rates of relapse that persist for weeks, months, or even years after quitting. Intervention strategies must incorporate persuasive advice, behavioral interventions that anticipate and respond to periods of relapse and remission, and the use of appropriate pharmacotherapies and support to help individuals to remain tobacco-free. Further, more than 70% of smokers state their desire to quit, yet only 5% succeed without assistance.

Evidence from randomized clinical trials cited in the Clinical Practice Guideline, indicated that smoking cessation is fostered by: (a) three-minute messages about the importance of cessation, provided by multiple health care professionals, (b) high-intensity counseling (longer than 10 minutes per session with a total duration of 30 minutes or more), (c) four or more follow-up sessions, and (d) provision of multicomponent interventions such as self-help materials, telephone follow-up, pharmacotherapies, and behavioral counseling. Treatments lasting 8 or more weeks will more than double cessation rates. Pharmacologic therapies including nicotine replacement therapies (NRT) and buproprion chloride (Zyban, Wellbutrin) facilitate quitting. Nicotine replacement therapies including the gum and patch are available over the counter. Newer agents such as the nicotine spray and inhaler are offered only by prescription. Research suggests that unless carefully prescribed and combined with follow-up education, nicotine replacement therapies are often ineffective (Pierce & Gilpin, 2002). Thus, nurses may have a significant role in providing education and ensuring follow-up for patients who elect to use pharmacologic agents.

Nurse investigators have played a key role in developing and testing efficacious interventions in various treatment settings such as hospitals and clinics. Interventions that link identification of smokers, strong physician advice, and nurse-mediated behavioral counseling at the bedside with follow-up telephone contacts have been shown to improve outcomes for both cardiovascular patients and those with various medical and surgical diagnoses (Miller, N. H., Smith, DeBusk, Sobel, & Taylor, 1997; Taylor, Houston Miller, Killen, & DeBusk, 1990). This research has been replicated in cardiovascular patients in Canada, and more recently, in clinical practice settings (Smith, Reilly, Miller, DeBusk, & Taylor, 2002). Research by Froelicher and colleagues (Froelicher et al., 2004) suggests that women with cardiovascular disease may represent a refractory group requiring more intensive intervention, including a systematic plan for follow-up and greater use of pharmacotherapies in conjunction with behavioral interventions.

Cardiovascular disease remains the number one cause of death and disability worldwide. The great strides that have occurred to reduce smoking rates in the U.S. over the past 3 decades offer hope that this addictive behavior may someday be a distant memory. Strong support by the nursing, medical, and public health communities is needed to achieve this goal. Thus, all health care professionals must take an advocacy role in clinical practice and other community settings.

NANCY HOUSTON MILLER

SNOMED International

SNOMED International is a compilation of nomenclatures organized into 11 modules or axes: (a) topography; (b) morphology; (c) living organisms; (d) chemicals, drugs, and biological products; (e) function; (f) occupation; (g) diagnosis; (h) procedure; (i) physical agents, forces, and attributes; (j) social context; and (k) general (Coté, Rothwell, Palotay, & Beckett, 1993). North American Nursing Diagnosis Association (NANDA) diagnoses are included in the functional axis of SNOMED, and a limited number of nursing procedures are included in the procedure module. In contrast to taxonomic vocabulary systems with the primary purpose of disjunctive classification (e.g., *International Classification of Diseases* or *Current Procedural Terminology Codes*), SNOMED terms can be combined for the purposes of concept representation for computer-based systems. For instance, the term "pain" from the function axis can be joined with a severity modifier from the general axis to represent the clinical expression "severe pain" or with an anatomic term from the topography axis to represent "back pain." This multiaxial approach is similar to the proposed architecture of the international classification of nursing practice.

Many investigations have demonstrated the usefulness of SNOMED for physician documentation, and a few have addressed the utility of SNOMED for nursing. Nurses use both NANDA diagnoses and other terms (i.e. symptoms, signs, medical diagnoses) to describe patient problems and that SNOMED terms other than those of NANDA diagnoses were exact matches for terms used by nurses in their clinical documentation. Lange (1996) found that SNOMED terms were useful for representing terms used by nurses in intershift reports. J. Campbell and others (1997) compared SNOMED International with the Read Codes and the Unified Medical Language System (UMLS) on the attributes of completeness, clinical taxonomy, administrative mapping, term definitions, and clarity. Of the 1,929 records in the data set, 390 were nursing documents. Although no separate nursing analyses were reported, SNOMED was judged superior to Read and UMLS on the four categories of information (findings, diagnoses, interventions, and plans of care) that comprised greater than 97% of the nursing text sources and overall on the attributes of completeness, taxonomy, and compositional nature. It received lower ratings than Read and UMLS on administrative mappings. If the analyses related to nursing interventions and plans of care had been reported separately from other health care interventions and plans of care, the findings might have differed on the attribute of completeness because the UMLS includes nursing intervention schema from the *Omaha System*, the *Georgetown Home Health Care Classification*, and the *Nursing Interventions Classification*, although SNOMED does not.

Some utility has been demonstrated, but further work is needed to increase the usefulness of SNOMED for nursing. Two areas relate specifically to SNOMED itself, and the third is a more generic requirement for representing nursing concepts in computer-based systems. First, additional terms for nursing interventions must be added to SNOMED. Second, rules (grammars) for combining terms must be developed, using knowledge formalisms such as conceptual graphs. Third, data models that describe the attribute of nursing data must be developed.

SUZANNE BAKKEN

Social Support

The concept of social support is a complex one that has many dimensions or constructs. Dimensions of social support include the *function* (e.g., emotional support, tangible aid), *source of support* (e.g., coworker, supervisor, spouse), and *structure of support* (e.g., network, frequency of social interactions) (Hobfoll & Vaux, 1993). S. Cohen and Wills (1985) described the function of social support as emotional, instrumental, informational, and social companionship. Emotional support is to provide one with love and care. On the other hand, instrumental support is to provide one with financial aid, material resources, and services, whereas informational support (appraisal support) is to assist one to understand and deal with problematic situations, and social companionship is to spend good time (recreational activities) with others (Cohen & Wills). The bulk of social support studies were conducted during the 1980s and early 1990s. This might be attributed to the increased interest of researchers in occupational stress and its management in the late 1970s. Social support was among the approaches that were investigated in relation to dealing with stress.

Research indicates that nursing is a stressful profession. Occupational stressors, if not managed successfully or effectively, could affect the psychological as well as physiological capacities of the individual. However, some employers might consider the stress of their employees as a personal psychological state and ignore its consequences on the organizations and the physiological and behavioral functions of the employees. Lawrence and Lawrence (1987/88) described some of the behavioral changes occurring as a result of work-related stress as low productivity, low morale, and absenteeism. Moreover, occupational stress also has been associated with problems in physical and mental health such as stomach disorders, high blood pressures, headaches, depression, and emotional outbursts. Such consequences of occupational stress are associated with alienation among staff members (lack of emotional support) more than any other factor (Maslach & Pines, 1978). In short, the direct and indirect effects of stress in terms of job dissatisfaction, low job performance, turnover, and absenteeism motivate researchers to investigate variables such as social support that might offset or reduce the impact of occupational stress and enhance the morale and satisfaction of the staff.

The two models of social support, the direct-effect and the stress-buffering, have been widely discussed (Cohen & Wills, 1985). The direct-effect model indicates the effect of social support on certain variables such as job performance and job satisfaction regardless of the level of stress, whereas the stress-buffering model indicates the effect of social support on certain outcomes through decreasing the level of stress. Selected literature of the direct and buffering effects of social support on organizational outcomes among nurses is discussed below.

The literature revealed the consistency for the direct effect of social support on outcomes such as burnout, job performance, job satisfaction, and intention to stay. Emotional social support has been found to associate negatively with burnout despite the different instruments used to measure social support. Such finding was supported by Hare, Pratt, and Anderaw (1988). Both measurements have adequate reliability and validity. AbuAl-Rub (2004) found that as social support increased, job performance increased. McCloskey (1990) found that social integration (social support from coworkers) was correlated positively with job satisfaction, work motivation, commitment to the organization, and intention to stay. Social integration also was found to buffer the bad effects of low autonomy. The autonomy-integration interactions for intent to stay and organizational commitment at 6 months and job satisfaction at 12 months were statistically significant.

On the other hand, the literature showed inconsistent results for the buffering effect of social support. For example, LaRocco, House, and French (1980) tested the buffering effect of social support on the relationships among stress-strain, strain-health, and stress-health, The results indicated that social support (a) did not buffer the impact of job stress on job strain, (b) did buffer the effect of job stress on overall mental health, and (c) did buffer the impact of job strain on mental health. AbuAlRub (2004) found that social support did not buffer the relationship between job stress and job performance; that is, as perceived job stress increased, nurses with high social support in the workplace did not perform better than nurses with less support.

The results of W. Stewart and Barling (1996), who examined the effect of social support on the stress-performance relationship, indicated that only informational social support moderated or buffered the subjective stress-performance relationship. That is, increased informational social support reduces the negative impact of stress on job performance. Fong (1990) examined the stress-support-burnout relation among nursing faculty. The results showed that support from supervisors and work peers was positively correlated with all dimensions of burnout. On the other hand, the results revealed that support from supervisors and coworkers did not moderate or buffer the stress-burnout relation: that is, as stress increased, the individuals with high support did not experience less burnout than those with less support.

Based on the literature, further research using different designs and methodologies is needed to test the buffering effect of social support. In testing such an effect, control is needed not only for individual differences, but also for other job variables that may mask the buffering or moderating effect of social support. Since hospitals spend a great deal of money in the recruitment and orientation processes of new staff, it becomes more important to keep them. Based on the research studies that provide evidence for the direct effect of social support on the organizational outcomes such as job stress, job performance, and job satisfaction, peer and superior support programs are paramount in order to enhance the well-being and satisfaction of the staff and the quality of care they provide for patients.

Raeda Fawzi AbuAlRub

Spirituality

Spirituality represents the human propensity to reach beyond immediate boundaries of the self to experience a greater reality and meaning. In nursing, spirituality is defined in terms of a variety of human experiences that provide a sense of transcendence or awareness of a connection to something greater than the self without devaluing the self, through intrapersonal, interpersonal, and transpersonal dimensions (Reed, P. G., 1992).

The intrapersonal dimension focuses on looking inward to find personal meaning; concepts within this dimension address purpose in life, inner strength, inner peace, courage, and serenity. The interpersonal dimension focuses on relationships with other people and other living systems, as well as with the broader environment and nature; concepts within this dimension include trust, sense of connectedness, forgiveness, interconnectedness, and love. The transpersonal dimension focuses on one's relationship to the unknown or unseen, mystery, God, a higher being or power, and other supernatural entities or expressions of a reality that exist beyond ordinary experiences. Concepts within this dimension include faith, hope, self-transcendence, acceptance, mystical experiences, awareness of a divine presence, experienced grace, specific religious beliefs and practices, and nonreligious, nontheistic, or existential expressions of transcendence.

Despite the often-cited description of spirituality as ineffable, a unifying force, the essence of human beings, and other immeasurable terms, spirituality is regarded by nursing theorists and researchers as a multidimensional concept that can be studied systematically through various empirical indicators and research methods, as suggested in Reed's (1992) paradigm for investigating spirituality.

Spirituality is considered to be an important area for research and practice in nursing as a human experience or process relevant in everyday life and during health-related events, particularly in times of increased awareness of mortality. Dimensions of spirituality have been addressed by eminent nursing theorists including Florence Nightingale, Martha Rogers, Jean Watson, Betty Neuman, Madeline Leininger, Callista Roy, and Rosemarie Parse, as well as by an increasing number of researchers who are developing middle-range theories. Spirituality is regarded as integral to human wholeness, development, and well-being, and increasingly is considered a fundamental concern of nursing practice.

The turn of the 21st century evidenced fairly active inquiry into spirituality. However, research on spirituality was not considered a legitimate area of nursing science until the mid-1980s when nurse researchers published the first reports of studies on spirituality. Research activity was accompanied if not preceded by the expansion of clinical knowledge about spirituality. Noted examples are two books that addressed spiritual and religious dimensions of nursing practice: Fish & Shelly's 1978 book, *Spiritual Care: The Nurse's Role* and subsequent editions, and Verna Carson's 1989 *Spiritual Dimensions of Nursing Practice.*

Several factors converged to stimulate and nurture the growth of spirituality research in nursing: (a) publications in the social sciences that linked spirituality to various indicators of well-being and mental health, as found in sociologist Moberg's research on religion, therapies based on the transpersonal movement in psychology, and life span developmental theories about the spiritual dimensions of aging; (b) development of instruments that measure spiritually-related concepts such as Ellison's (1983) Spiritual Well-Being (SWB) Scale and Reed's (1987) Spiritual Perspective Scale; (c) maturity of nursing as a discipline that defined itself a science with theories whose focus extended beyond the biomedical to include the breadth of human health experiences and patients' perspectives; (d) scientists' increased attention to the voice of the clinicians (e.g., Highfield & Cason, 1983), whose patients attested to the positive influences of spirituality in health care; and (e) efforts to establish a more holistic approach to nursing diagnosis and assessment that included the spiritual dimension, as found in Ruth Stoll's 1979 "Guidelines for Spiritual Assessment," published in the widely read *American Journal of Nursing.* The number of nurses who currently include spiritually related questions and variables in their research has grown considerably since the mid-1980s.

Research findings, as well as a fund of practice knowledge in nursing, support the relevance of spirituality. Spiritually related variables such as hope, courage, and self-transcendence consistently have been found to be significant and at times critical factors in processes of healing and during health-related events associated with particular life phases such as pregnancy, childhood, aging, and end of life.

Dominant areas of research include: terminal illness and dying, chronic illness, cancer, life-threatening and acute illness, mental health in aging, alcoholism and substance abuse, critical losses and life events, and nurses' and other caregivers' health. The majority of spiritually related research efforts have focused on enhancing well-being during terminal illness. Important examples include Beverly Hall's (1998) work with patients who have HIV/AIDS and research on women with breast cancer at diagnosis and end-stage (Coward, 1991, 1998; Mickley, Soeken, & Belcher, 1992). Research findings from these and many other studies overall support the significance of spiritual factors in patient well-being.

Another area of research is represented in the work of several British nurses (Draper, McSherry, Narayanasamy, Owens, Ross) as well as American nurses (such as Tuck and

Emblen), who focused attention on the nurse's spirituality and approaches to spiritual care as important elements in practice. Ethical questions about the congruence between patient and nurse perspectives, and between the nurse's values and actions relative to spirituality, are especially important to study as nurses assume a more active role in spiritual care.

Researchers predominantly have used quantitative designs that incorporate one or more instruments to measure spirituality and its correlates. One caveat in quantitative study results is that statistically significant correlation coefficients between spiritual variables and well-being variables not infrequently are of small to moderate magnitude. This is attributed to small sample size, measurement error, or the influence of other intervening factors that relate to health and well-being, and has not discouraged continued study of spirituality as a relevant human experience. Increasingly, scientists are employing mixed methods and qualitative methods, notably phenomenology and grounded theory, to better understand spirituality as experienced during significant health experiences or life events.

Methods to study spirituality across time and cultures are expanding the terrain of knowledge. Researchers are just beginning to address questions about potential changes in spirituality over the trajectory of illness or across the life span. Their inquiry employs both qualitative and quantitative longitudinal designs that provide insights into spiritual experiences, practices, and strategies over time. Another trend is the increasing number of researchers who are examining spirituality from a cultural perspective (e.g., Pincharoen & Congdon, 2003).

A final method to be recognized is conceptual or philosophic inquiry. The resulting publications of conceptual articles that integrate clinical knowledge, provide ethical analysis, and clarify the complex concept of spirituality have added substantially to the research literature on spirituality.

There are several pathways to knowledge about spirituality that nurses are likely to choose in the future. A major direction is the intervention-based study. Several potential nursing interventions or patient strategies regarding spirituality have already been identified in the literature: spiritual autobiography, life review, therapeutic relationship, prayer in all its forms, meditation, spiritual counseling, guided imagery, existential therapy, personal writing and reflection, and engagement in altruistic activities.

Nurse scientists also are likely to study spirituality as related to not only psychosocial indicators of well-being, but to biobehavioral indicators as well, including those derived from the psychoneuroimmunological perspective. In contrast, a less likely direction for future nursing research is the study of a purely neurobiological basis for spiritual religious beliefs, as is already occurring among some scientists outside of nursing.

Nurses will continue to publish on the clinical as well as empirical significance of spirituality for patient care, as illustrated, for example, in the extensive writings by Margaret Burkhardt and her colleagues. Understanding the role of spirituality in nursing practice will burgeon as more researchers and clinicians work together to build knowledge about spirituality to generate nursing-theory-based strategies that facilitate well-being (e.g., Coward, 1998; Relf, 1997).

PAMELA G. REED
CHERYL A. LARSON

Statistical Techniques

Analysis of covariance (ANCOVA) is a statistical technique that combines analysis of variance (ANOVA) with regression to measure the differences among group means. The advantages of ANCOVA include the ability to reduce the error variance in the outcome measure and the ability to measure group differences after allowing for other differences between subjects. The error variance is reduced by controlling for variation in the dependent measure that comes from variables measured at the interval or ratio level (called covariates) that influence all the groups being compared. The covariate contributes to the variation and reduces the magnitude of the differences among groups. In ANCOVA the variation from this variable is measured and extracted from the within (or error) variation. The effect is the reduction of error variance and therefore an increase in the power of the analysis.

ANCOVA also has been used in both experimental and nonexperimental studies to "equate" the groups statistically. When the groups differ on some variable, ANCOVA is used to reduce the impact of that difference. Although ANCOVA has been widely used for such statistical "equalization" of groups, there is controversy about such efforts, and careful consideration should be given to the appropriateness of the manipulation.

As with ANOVA there are one or more categorical variables as independent variables; the dependent variable is continuous and meets the requirements of normal distribution and equality of variance across groups. The covariate is an interval- or ratio-level measure.

There are additional assumptions to be met in ANCOVA, and these are very important to the valid interpretation of results. There must be a linear relationship between the covariate and the dependent variable, and ANCOVA is most effective when the correlation is equal to or greater than .30. The direction and strength of the relationship between the covariate and dependent variable must be similar in each group. This assumption is called homogeneity of regression across groups.

ANCOVA is an extension of the ANOVA model that reduces the error term by removing additional sources of variation. It is a means of controlling extraneous variation. As with other types of analysis of variance, post hoc tests are used for pairwise comparison of group means.

Analysis of variance (ANOVA) is a parametric statistical test that measures differences between two or more mutually exclusive groups by calculating the ratio of between- to within-group variance, called the *F* ratio. It is an extension of the *t* test, which compares two groups. The independent variable(s) are categorical (measured at the nominal level). The dependent variable must meet the assumptions of normal distribution and equal variance across the groups. A one-way ANOVA means that there is only one independent variable (often called factor), a two-way ANOVA indicates two independent variables, and an *n*-way ANOVA indicates that the number of independent variables is defined by *n*.

The null hypothesis in ANOVA is that all groups are equal and drawn from the same population. To test this assumption, three measures of variation are calculated. The total variation is a measure of the variability of all subjects around the grand mean and is composed of within-group variation and between-group variation. Within-group variation is a measure of how much the scores of subjects within a group vary around the group mean. Between-group variation is a measure of how much each group's mean varies from the grand mean or of how much difference exists between the groups. Quantifying total between- and within-group variation is accomplished by calculating a sum of squares (the sum of the squared deviations of each of the scores around the respective mean) for each component of the variation.

When the null hypothesis is true, the groups' scores overlap to a large extent, and the within-group variation is greater than the between-group variation. When the null hypothesis is false, the groups' scores show little overlapping, and the between-groups variation is greater.

When the ratio of between- to within-group variation (*F* ratio) is significant, the null hypothesis is rejected, indicating a difference among the groups. When more than two groups are being compared, however, it cannot be determined from the *F* test alone which groups differ from the others. In other words, a significant *F* test does not mean that every group in the analysis is different from every other group.

To determine where the significant differences lie, further analysis is required. Two types of comparisons can be made among group means. They include post hoc (after the fact) comparisons and a priori (planned) comparisons based on hypotheses stated prior to the analysis.

A variety of post hoc techniques exist. The purpose of all is to decrease the likelihood of making a Type I error when making multiple comparisons. The Scheffé test is reported frequently. The formula is based on the usual formula for the calculation of a *t*-test or *F* ratio, but the critical value for determining statistical significance is changed according to the number of comparisons to be made. A Bonferroni correction involves dividing the desired alpha (say .05) by the number of comparisons.

The least significant difference (LSD) test is equivalent to multiple *t* tests. The modification is that a pooled estimate of variance is used rather than variance common to groups being compared. Tukey's honestly significant difference (HSD) is the most conservative comparison test and as such is the least powerful. The critical values for Tukey remain the same for each comparison, regardless of the total number of means to be compared. Student Newman-Keuls is similar to Tukey's HSD, but the critical values do not stay the same. They reflect the variables being compared. Tukey's wholly significant difference (WSD) uses critical values that are the average of those used in Tukey's HSD and Newman-Keuls. It is therefore intermediate in conservatism between those two measures.

Planned comparisons, or a priori contrasts, are based on hypotheses stated before data are collected. Prespecified contrasts that are orthogonal (statistically unrelated) to each other may be developed and tested. Such comparisons are more powerful than post hoc contrasts.

With two or more independent variables in an analysis, interactions between the independent variables can be tested. Testing for an interaction addresses the question of whether or not the results of a given treatment vary depending on the groups or conditions in which it is applied.

An ANOVA may include more than one dependent variable. Such an analysis usually is referred to as multivariate analysis of variance (MANOVA) and allows the researcher to look for relationships among dependent as well as independent variables. When conducting a MANOVA, the assumptions underlying the univariate model still apply, and in addition the dependent variable should have a "multivariate normal distribution with the same variance covariance matrix in each group" (Norusis, 1994, p. 58). The requirement that each group will have the same variance covariance matrix means that the homogeneity of variance assumption is met for each dependent variable and that the correlation between any two dependent variables must be the same in all groups. Box's *M* is a measure of the multivariate test for homogeneity of variance.

In the univariate model, the *F* value is tested for significance. In the multivariate model there are four outcome measures. They include Wilks's lambda, which represents the error variance; Pillai-Bartlett trace, which represents the sum of the explained variances; Roy's greatest characteristic root, which is based on the first discriminant variate; and Hotelling-Lawley trace, which is the sum of the between and within sums of squares for each of the discriminant variates. Wilks's lambda is the most widely used. Analysis of variance is commonly used to test for group differences. Multivariate analysis of variance includes more than one dependent variable.

Repeated measures analysis of variance is an extension of analysis of variance (ANOVA) that reduces the error term by partitioning out individual differences that can be estimated from the repeated measurement of the same subjects. There are two main types of repeated measures designs (also called within-subjects designs). One involves taking repeated measures of the same variable(s) over time on a group or groups of subjects. The other involves exposing the same subjects to all levels of the treatment. This is often referred to as using subjects as their own controls.

Because the observations are not independent of each other, there is correlation among the outcome measures. This necessitates an assumption called compound symmetry. To meet this assumption, the correlations across the measurements (time points) must be the same, and the variances should be equal across measurements. This is important because the general robustness of the ANOVA model does not withstand much violation of this assumption.

Repeated measures ANOVA is a particularly interesting technique because health care providers tend to take repeated measures on clients, and it often makes sense to do so with research subjects as well. There are stringent requirements for this analysis, however. The most important is meeting the criteria for compound symmetry. This assumption is often violated, leading to improper interpretation of results. Most computer programs provide a test of this assumption. If the assumption is not met, several alternatives are available.

First, rather than the univariate approach, in which the repeated measures are treated as within-subjects factors, one might use a multivariate approach (MANOVA). In MANOVA, the repeated measures would be treated as multiple dependent variables. Another approach is to use an epsilon correction. The degrees of freedom are multiplied by the value of epsilon, and the new degrees of freedom, which are more conservative, are used to test the *F* value for significance.

The problems with repeated measures analyses may be seen as "the carry-over effect, the latent effect, and the order or learning effect" (pp. 107–108). When subjects are exposed to more than one treatment, previous treatments may still be having an effect, that is, may be carried over. An interaction with a previous treatment is referred to as a latency effect. This would occur if exposure to one treatment had an enhancing or depressing effect on a subsequent treatment. Randomization of the order of treatment is used to control the order of learning effect.

Repeated measures ANOVA is a very useful technique for research by health professionals. There are fairly stringent requirements for the analysis, however.

Correlation is a procedure for quantifying the linear relationship between two or more variables. It measures the strength and indicates the direction of the relationship. The Pearson product-moment correlation coefficient (r) is the usual method by which the relation between two variables is quantified. There must be at least two variables measured on each subject; and although interval- or ratio-level data are most commonly used, it is also possible in many cases to obtain valid results with ordinal data. Categorical variables may be coded for use in calculating correlations and regression equations.

Although correlations can be calculated with data at all levels of measurement, certain assumptions must be made to generalize beyond the sample statistic. The sample must be representative of the population to which the inference will be made. The variables that are being correlated must each have a normal distribution. The relationship between the two variables must be linear. For every value of one variable, the distribution of the other variable must have approximately equal variability. This is called the assumption of homoscedasticity.

The correlation coefficient is a mathematical representation of the relationship that exists between two variables. The correlation coefficient may range from +1.00 through 0.00 to −1.00. A +1.00 indicates a perfect positive relationship, 0.00 indicates no relationship, and −1.00 indicates a perfect negative relationship. In a positive relationship, as one variable increases, the other increases. In a negative relationship, as one variable increases, the other decreases.

The strength of correlation coefficients has been described as follows:

.00–.25—little if any
.26–.49—low
.50–.69—moderate
.70–.89—high
.90–1.00—very high
(Munro, 1997, p. 235).

The coefficient of determination, r^2, often is used as a measure of the "meaningfulness" of r. This is a measure of the amount of variance the two variables share. It is obtained by squaring the correlation coefficient.

Correlational techniques may be used for control of extraneous variation. Partial correlation measures the relationship between two variables after statistically controlling for the influence of a confounding variable on both of the variables being correlated. It is usually expressed as $r_{12.3}$, which indicates the correlation between variables 1 and 2, with the effect of variable 3 removed from both 1 and 2. Semipartial correlation is the correlation of two variables with the effect of a third variable removed from only one of the variables being correlated. It is usually expressed as $r_{1(2.3)}$, which indicates the correlation between variables 1 and 2, with the effect of 3 removed only from variable 2.

Multiple correlation is a technique for measuring the relationship between a dependent variable and a weighted combination of independent variables. The multiple correlation is expressed as R. R^2 indicates the amount of variance explained in the dependent variable by the independent variables. Canonical correlation measures the relationship between two sets of variables and is expressed as R_c.

There are measures other than the Pearson r for measuring relationships. Before the advent of computers, "shortcut" methods of calculation were developed for certain circumstances. Three such measures are phi, point-biserial, and Spearman rho. These measures usually give the same result as r; their only advantage is for doing hand calculations. Phi is used with two dichotomous variables and is often reported in conjunction with chi-square. Point-biserial can be used to calculate the relationship between one dichotomous and one continuous variable. Spearman rho can be used to measure the relationship between two rank-ordered variables.

There are also nonparametric measures of relationship. These are considered "distribution-free," that is, the assumption of normal distribution of the two variables does not have to be met. Kendall's tau is a nonparametric technique for measuring the relation between two ranked (ordinal) variables. The contingency coefficient can be used to measure the relationship between two nominal variables. It is based on the chi square statistic.

There are also formulas that can be used to estimate the correlation coefficient, r. Biserial can be used when one variable is dichotomized and the other is continuous. Dichotomized means that the variable has been made dichotomous—cut into two levels from a variable that would have been naturally continuous. Biserial estimates what r would be if you changed the dichotomized variable into a continuous variable. The tetrachoric coefficient is an estimate of r based on the relationship between two dichotomized variables.

Eta, sometimes called the correlation ratio, is referred to as the universal measure of the relationship between two variables. The values for eta range from 0 to 1. It can be used to measure nonlinear as well as linear relationships. When it is used with two continuous variables that have a linear relationship, it reduces to r.

Correlational techniques are used to explore and test relationships among variables. They serve as the basis for developing prediction equations through regression techniques.

Logistic regression is used to determine which variables affect the probability of the occurrence of an event. In logistic regression the independent variables may be at any level of measurement from nominal to ratio. The dependent variable is categorical, usually a dichotomous variable.

Although it is possible to code the dichotomous variable as 1/0 and run a multiple regression or use discriminant function analysis for categorical outcome measures (two or more categories), this is generally not recommended. Multiple regression and discriminant function are based on the method of least squares, whereas the maximum-likelihood method is used in logistic regression. Because the logistic model is nonlinear, the iterative approach provided by the maximum-likelihood method is more appropriate.

In addition to providing a better fit with the data, logistic regression results include odds ratios that lend interpretability to the data. The odds of an outcome being present as a measure of association has found wide use, especially in epidemiology, because the odds ratio approximates how much more likely (or unlikely) it is for the outcome to be present given certain conditions. An odds ratio is defined as the probability of occurrence over the probability of nonoccurrence.

The probability of the observed results, given the parameter estimates, is known as the likelihood. "Since the likelihood measure is a small number, less than 1, it is customary to use minus 2 times the log of the likelihood as a measure of how well the estimated model fits the data" (Norusis, 1994, p. 10). In logistic regression, comparison of observed to predicted values is based on the log likelihood (LL) function. A good model is one that results in a high likelihood of the observed results. A nonsignificant –2 LL indicates that the data fit the model.

The goodness of fit statistic compares the observed probabilities to those predicted by the model. Assessment of this is also provided in a classification table where percentages of correct predictions are provided. This statistic has a chi-square distribution. A nonsignificant statistic indicates that the data fit the model.

The model chi-square tests the null hypothesis that the coefficients for all the independent variables equal 0. It is equivalent to the *F* test in regression. A significant result indicates that the independent variables are contributing significantly. As in regression, one must assess the significance of each predictor. In multiple regression the b-weights are used in the calculation of the prediction equation. In logistic regression the b-weights are used to determine the probability of the occurrence of an event.

As with all methods of regression it is of utmost importance to select variables for inclusion in the model on the basis of clear scientific rationale. Following the fit of the model, the importance of each variable included in the model should be verified (Norusis, 1994). This includes examination of the Wald statistic, which provides a measure of the significance (p) value for each variable. Additionally, one can test the model by systematically including and excluding the predictors. Variables that do not contribute to the model on the basis of these criteria should be eliminated and a new model fit. Once a model has been developed that contains the essential variables, the addition of interaction terms should be considered.

Logistic regression has been reported in the medical literature for some time, particularly in epidemiological studies. Recently, it has become more common in nursing research. This is the result of a new appreciation of the technique and the availability of software to manage the complex analysis. This multivariate technique for assessing the probability of the occurrence of an event requires fewer assumptions than does regression or discriminant function analysis and provides estimates in terms of odds ratios that add to the understanding of the results.

Nonparametric statistics are techniques that are not based on assumptions about normality of data. When parametric tests of significance are used, at least one population parameter is being estimated from sample statistics. To arrive at such an estimation, certain assumptions must be made; the most important one is that the variable measured in the sample is normally distributed in the population to which a generalization will be made. With nonparametric tests there is no assumption about the distribution of the variable in the population. For that reason nonparametric tests often are called distribution-free.

At one time, level of measurement was considered a very important determinant in the decision to use parametric or nonparametric tests. Some authors said that parametric tests should be reserved for use with interval- and ratio-level data. More recent studies, however, have shown that the use of parametric techniques with ordinal data rarely distorts the results.

The calculations involved in nonparametric techniques are much easier than those associated with parametric techniques, but the use of computers makes that of little concern. Nonparametric techniques are valuable when using small samples and when there are distortions of the data that seriously violate the assumptions underlying the parametric technique.

Chi-square is the most frequently reported nonparametric technique. It is used to compare the actual number (or frequency) in each group with the "expected" number. The expected number can be based on theory, previous experience, or comparison groups. Chi-square tests whether or not the expected number differs significantly from the actual number. Chi-square is the appropriate technique when variables are measured at the nominal level. It may be used with two or more mutually exclusive groups.

When the groups are not mutually exclusive, as when the same subjects are measured twice, an adaptation of chi-square, the McNemar test, may be appropriate. The McNemar test can be used to measure change when there are two dichotomous measures on the subjects.

When comparing groups of subjects on ordinal data, two commonly used techniques are the Mann-Whitney *U*, which is used to compare two groups and is thus analogous to the *t* test, and Kruskal-Wallis *H*, which is used to compare two or more groups and is thus analogous to the parametric technique analysis of variance.

When one has repeated measures on two or more groups and the outcome measure is not appropriate for parametric techniques, two nonparametric techniques that may be appropriate are the Wilcoxon matched-pairs signed rank test and the Friedman matched samples. The Wilcoxon matched-pairs is analogous to the parametric paired *t* test, and the Friedman matched samples is analogous to a repeated-measures analysis of variance.

In addition to nonparametric techniques for making group comparisons, there are nonparametric techniques for measuring relationships. There is some confusion about these techniques. For example, point-biserial and Spearman rho are often considered nonparametric techniques but are actually shortcut formulas for the Pearson product-moment correlation (*r*). Biserial and tetrachoric coefficients are estimates of *r*, given certain conditions.

True nonparametric measures of relationship include Kendall's tau and the contingency coefficient. Kendall's tau was developed as an alternative procedure for Spearman rho. It may be used when measuring the relation between two ranked (ordinal) variables. The contingency coefficient can be used to measure the relationship between two nominal-level variables. The calculation of this coefficient is based on the chi-square statistic.

Nonparametric techniques should be considered if assumptions about the normal distribution of variables cannot be met. These techniques, although less powerful, provide a more accurate appraisal of group differences and relationships among variables when the assumptions underlying the parametric techniques have been violated.

Regression is a statistical method that makes use of the correlation between two variables and the notion of a straight line to develop an equation that can be used to predict the score of one of the variables, given the score of the other. In the case of a multiple correlation, regression is used to establish a prediction equation in which the independent variables are each assigned a weight based on their relationship to the dependent variable, while controlling for the other independent variables.

Regression is useful as a flexible technique that allows prediction and explanation of the interrelationships among variables and the use of categorical as well as continuous variables. Regression literally means a falling back toward the mean. With perfect correlations there is no falling back; using standardized scores, the predicted score is the same as the predictor. With less than perfect correlations there is some error in the measurement; the more error, the more regression toward the mean.

The regression equation consists of an intercept constant (a) and the b's associated with each independent variable. Given those elements and an individual's score on the independent variables, one can predict the individual's score on the dependent variable. The intercept constant (a) is the value of the dependent variable when the independent variable equals zero. It is the point at which the regression line intercepts the *Y* axis.

The letter *b* is called the regression coefficient or regression weight; it is the rate of change in the dependent variable with a unit change in the independent variable. It is a measure of the slope of the regression line, which is the "line of best fit" and passes through the exact center of the data in a scatter diagram. Beta is the standardized regression coefficient.

In multiple regression the multiple correlation (*R*) and each of the b-weights are tested for significance. In most reports the squared multiple correlation, R^2, is reported, as that is a measure of the amount of variance accounted for in the dependent variable. A significant R^2 indicates that a significant amount of the variance in the dependent variable has been accounted for. Testing the b-weight tells us whether the independent variable associated with it is contributing significantly to the variance accounted for in the dependent variable.

Although variables at all levels of measurement may be entered into the regression equation, nominal-level variables must be specially coded prior to entry. Three main types of coding are used: dummy, effect, and orthogonal. Regardless of the method of coding used, the overall *R* is the same, as is its significance. The differences lie in the meaning attached to testing the b-weights for significance. With dummy coding the b-weight represents the difference between the mean of the group represented by that b and the group assigned 0s throughout. In effect coding the b's represent the difference between the mean of the group associated with that b-weight and the grand mean. With orthogonal coding the b-weight measures the difference between two means specified in a hypothesized contrast. Interactions among variables also may be coded and entered into the regression equation.

When using regression, it is of utmost importance to select variables for inclusion in the model on the basis of clear scientific rationale. The method for entering variables into the equation is important, as it affects the interpretation of the results. Variables may be entered all at once, one at a time, or in subsets. Decisions about method of entry may be statistical, as in stepwise entry (where the variable with the highest correlation with the dependent variable is entered first), or theoretical. Stepwise methods have been criticized for capitalizing on chance related to imperfect measurement of the variables being correlated. It is generally recommended that decisions about the order of entry of variables into the regression equation should be made on the basis of the research questions being addressed.

Problems with multiple regression include a high degree of interrelatedness among the independent variables, referred to as multicollinearity. Selection of variables based on theoretical considerations, followed by careful screening of variables and testing of assumptions prior to analysis, can reduce potential problems. If multicollinearity is a problem, decisions must be made about which variables to eliminate. Residual analysis, conducted as part of the regression procedure, can contribute an additional check on whether or not the assumptions underlying the analysis have been met.

Multiple regression is the most commonly reported statistical technique in health care research. It can be used for both explanation and prediction but is more commonly reported as a method for explaining the variability in an outcome measure.

The *t* test involves an evaluation of means and distributions of two groups. The *t* test, or Student's *t* test, is named after its inventor, William Gosset, who published under the pseudonym Student. Gosset invented the *t* test as a more precise method of comparing groups. The *t* distributions are a set of means of randomly drawn samples from a normally distributed population. They are based on the sample size and vary according to the degrees of freedom.

The *t* test reflects the probability of getting a difference of a given magnitude in groups of a particular size with a certain variability if random samples drawn from the same population were compared. Three factors are included in the analysis: difference between the group means, size of each group, and variability of scores within the groups.

Given the same mean difference, an increase in group size increases the likelihood of a significant difference between two groups, and an increase in group variability decreases the likelihood of significant difference. Increased variability increases the error term and the likelihood of overlap between the scores of the two groups, thereby diminishing the difference between them.

There are three *t* tests. The first is used to compare two mutually exclusive groups when the dependent variable is normally distributed and the variances of the two groups are equal. The equal variance assumption is called homogeneity of variance and indicates that the groups are drawn from the same population. This version of the *t* test is referred to as the pooled or equal-variance *t* test because the denominator contains the variance for all the subjects.

If the assumption of homogeneity of variance is not met, a second formula, called the separate or unequal variance *t* test, can be used. In that case the variance is not pooled for all subjects; instead, the separate variances for each group are contained in the denominator.

When the two sets of scores are not independent, as when two measures are taken on the same subjects or matched pairs are used, a paired or correlated *t* test formula can be used. The formula incorporates the correlation between the two sets of scores.

The *t* tests are very useful when two groups or two correlated measures are being compared. Although analysis of variance can accomplish the same results, the *t* test continues to be used when appropriate as it is easy to present and to understand.

BARBARA MUNRO

Stress

The term "stress" first appeared in the *Cumulative Index to Nursing and Allied Health Literature* (CINAHL) in 1956. Nursing's interest in stress as a focus of research has mushroomed since 1970. Although the word "stress" is familiar to many and has become part of our everyday vocabulary, the term conveys divergent meanings, and multiple theories have been proposed to explain it. Most of the theories attempting to describe and explain stress as a human phenomenon can be categorized under one of three very different orientations to the concept: response-based, stimulus-based, and transaction-based. The response-based orientation was developed by Selye (1976), who defined stress as a nonspecific response of the body to any demand. That is, regardless of the cause, situational context, or psychological interpretation of the demand, the stress response is characterized by the same chain of events or same pattern of physiological correlates.

Defined as a response, stress indicators become the dependent variables in research studies. Nurse researchers who have used the response-based orientation measure catecholoamines, cortisol, urinary Na/K ratio, vital signs, brain waves, electrodermal skin responses, and cardiovascular complaints as indicators of stress. The demand component of Selye's definition is treated as an independent variable, whereas hospitalization surgery or critical care unit transfer were commonly the assumed stressor in much of the nursing research using this orientation. The response-based model of stress is not consistent with nursing's philosophical presuppositions that each individual is unique and that individuals respond holistically and often differently to similar situations (Lyon & Werner, 1987).

The stimulus-based theoretical explanation treats stress as a stimulus that causes disrupted responses. As a stimulus, stress is viewed as an external force similar to the engineering use of the term to represent dynamics of strain in metals or an external force directed at a physical object. Defined in this way stress becomes the independent variable in research studies. The most frequently cited example of a stimulus-based theory is the life event theory proposed by T. H. Holmes and Rahe (1967). Stress is operationalized as a stable additive phenomenon that is measurable by researcher-selected life events or life changes that typically have preassigned normative weights. The primary theoretical proposition of the stimulus-based orientation is that too many life events or changes increase vulnerability to illness. Results of studies (Lyon & Werner, 1983) using the life event perspective have failed to explain illness, accounting for only 2% to 4% of the incidence of illness. Noting the limitations of the stimulus-based orientation yet recognizing the need to attend the "initiator" of a stress experience, Werner (1993) proposed a useful classification of stressors that includes dimensions of locus, duration, temporality, forecasting, tone, and impact.

The third way to conceptualize stress is a transaction between person and environment. In this context stress refers to uncomfortable tension-related emotions that arise when demanding situations tax available resources, and some kind of harm, loss, or negative consequence is anticipated (Lazarus, 1966; Lazarus & Folkman, 1984). As a special note, the Lazarus (1966) reference represents a class work in demonstrating how theory informs research and then how research in turn shapes and reshapes theory. In the transactional orientation, stress represents a composite of experiences, including threatening appraisals, stress emotions (anxiety, fear, anger, guilt, depression), and coping responses. As such, the term "stress" has heuristic value but is a difficult construct to study. Use of a transactional theoretical orientation requires that the researcher clearly delineate which aspects of the person-environment transaction are to be studied (Lazarus; Lazarus & Folkman). Commonly, the independent variables in experimental and quasiexperimental studies based on the transactional orientation are personal resources such as self-esteem, perceived control, uncertainty, social support, and hardiness. Appraisal of threat versus appraisal of challenge is commonly studied as a mediating factor between resource strength and coping responses. Dependent variables often include somatic outcomes such as pain, emotional disturbances such as anxiety and depression, and well-being. The transactional model was deemed by Lyon and Werner (1987) to be compatible with nursing's philosophical suppositions.

Lyon and Werner (1987) published a critical review of 82 studies conducted by nurses from 1974 to 1984. The studies reviewed fell evenly across the three different theoretical orientations, and approximately 25% of the studies were atheoretical in nature. In 1993, Barnfather and Lyon edited a monograph of the proceedings of a synthesis conference on stress and coping held in conjunction with the Midwest Nursing Research Society. This critical review of the research covered 296 studies published from 1980 to 1990. Both the 1987 and 1993 critical reviews noted a disturbing absence of programs of research, making it difficult to identify what we have learned from the discipline's research efforts. A compilation of critical reviews of the nursing research literature from 1991–1995 focused on stressors and health outcomes, stressors and chronic conditions, coping, resources, and appraisal and perception; the influence of nursing interventions on the stress-health outcome linkage consistently noted the increase in well-designed studies (Werner & Frost, 2000). Each of these critical reviews noted knowledge gained and gaps in knowledge to guide future research.

In the landmark *Handbook of Stress, Coping, and Health: Implications for Nursing Research, Theory and Practice* (Rice, 2000), the evolution of the efforts of nurse researchers to test various theoretical models of stress, coping, and health is critically reviewed. Importantly the handbook includes critical reviews of developing programs of nursing research.

It is clear from all of the aforementioned critical reviews that our knowledge of how stress affects health is evolving. The significance of nursing research in the area of stress grows even more important in the era of escalating costs for health care services. It is widely recognized that as many as 65% of visits to physician offices are for illnesses that have no discernible medical cause, and many of those illnesses are thought to be stress-related. Furthermore, productivity in the workplace is thought to be greatly affected by the deleterious effects of stress. Future directions for nursing research in the area of stress will focus on (a) effects of psychological stress on the somatic sense of self, functional ability, the experience of illness, and aberrant behaviors such as abuse and use of alcohol and drugs; (b) the identification of patterns of variables that predict vulnerability or at-risk status for stress-related illness experiences and aberrant behaviors; and (c) intervention studies to evaluate the effects of various stress prevention and stress management strategies including cognitive restructuring, guided imagery, desensitization, meditation on stress-related illnesses, and aberrant behaviors.

BRENDA L. LYON

Stress Management

Stress management is a broad term that encompasses a wide range of methods intended to prevent stress or effectively manage it as evidenced by low levels of stress emotions and improved coping abilities. "Stress management interventions are deliberate actions taught to patients to help achieve outcomes" (Synder, 2000, p. 179). Coping strategies are actions self-initiated by a person to manage stress. Coping strategies are typically categorized as direct action/problem-focused aimed at alleviating or decreasing the intensity of perceived threat, or palliative/emotion-focused aimed at decreasing or keeping in check the intensity of stress emotions experienced (Lazarus & Fokman, 1984).

Nurse researchers have studied stress management interventions and coping strategies in various groups of people including nurses, student nurses, and patients. It is interesting to note that the majority of these studies have been conducted by nurse researchers in European and Asian countries. Some of the coping strategies frequently used by nurses to manage stress include taking action, drawing on past experiences, using problem-solving techniques, using humor, talking over problems with coworkers, accepting the situation, taking breaks (escaping from the situation), using diversions, using relaxation, and exercise (Lewis, D. J., & Robinson, 1986; Petermann, Springer, & Farnsworth, 1995). Coping strategies taken to prevent stress involve balancing demands and resources, focusing on the positive in difficult situations, maintaining perceived choice and sense of personal control, building social support, and viewing difficult situations as challenges that can bring gain or benefit through learning (Dionne-Proulz & Pepin, 1993; Lyon, 1996).

Nursing research studies on the effects of stress management interventions with various patient population groups have yielded equivocal results. M. Snyder (1993) critically reviewed all 54 stress-related intervention studies appearing in the nursing literature from 1980 through 1990. The types of stress management interventions used included relaxation strategies (e.g., progressive muscle relaxation, imagery, meditation, breathing techniques, massage, music), educational strategies, and use of social support groups. A major flaw of most of the intervention studies was an inadequate description of the intervention used, and there was a lack of attempts to explain the theoretical link between the intervention and outcome measures. Manipulation checks as a way to assure that subjects mastered the intervention also were lacking in the intervention studies. Studies using sensation information (e.g., Johnson, J. E., Rice, Fuller, & Endress, 1978) and studies using progressive relaxation techniques (e.g.,

Pender, 1985) have demonstrated positive effects on health-related outcomes such as less anxiety and an increased sense of well-being.

Since 1995 there has been little theoretical knowledge gained through nursing research about the effectiveness of stress management interventions or coping strategies. Two common findings, consistent with Lazarus (1966) and Lazarus and Folkman (1984), are that: (a) direct action or problem-focused coping strategies and cognitive restructuring strategies are related to decreased stress-related outcomes such as anxiety, other negative mood states, and an increased sense of well-being; and (b) palliative or emotion-focused strategies are related to increased anxiety, other negative mood states, and distress. The most common theme is that stress is a subjective phenomenon that is experienced differently by each person. The most common outcomes measured as dependent variables have been stress emotions such as anxiety, other negatively toned mood states, and depression.

Future directions for nursing research should focus on identifying patterns of appraisal, emotions, and coping that result in health-related outcomes. Additionally, for the discipline's research efforts to meaningfully contribute to knowledge generation, it is imperative that nurse researchers clearly define and delineate stress management interventions and offer testable theoretical formulations that explain how the interventions affect outcome variables within specified person and environment contexts. It is also essential that the researcher incorporate manipulation checks into the methodology to verify that the intervention "took." For example, when using a progressive muscle relaxation or autogenic relaxation strategy it is important to verify that the participant experienced a sense of "relaxation." Likewise it is equally important for the researcher to verify that participants implement coping strategies correctly following a psychoeducational intervention. Results must be able to demonstrate that the intervention actually altered the target variable as proposed in the theoretical formulation. Furthermore, research designed to contribute to knowledge generation offers little meaning if the researcher does not reflect on the meaning of the findings in relation to proposed theoretical formulations.

Current developments in testing "ABC" codes (Alternative Link, 2004) representing nonpharmacological interventions and complementary and alternative therapies offer nursing the opportunity to demonstrate effectiveness of stress management interventions in assisting patients to achieve desired health-related outcomes (Lyon, 2000). The latter half of this decade will offer unprecedented opportunities for nurse scientists to demonstrate the cost-effectiveness of stress management interventions in nursing practice.

BRENDA L. LYON

Stroke

Stroke, also known as cerebrovascular accident or apoplexy, is a sudden loss of consciousness due to either a loss of blood flow to the brain or a sudden rupture of a blood vessel in or near the brain. There are two main types of strokes. An *ischemic stroke* is caused by thrombus formation due to narrowing of the arteries from arteriosclerosis, an embolus that has dislodged and traveled to the brain, or a lack of blood flow to the brain due to circulatory failure (American Heart Association, 2004). A *hemorrhagic stroke* results from the rupture of a blood vessel either in the space between the brain and the skull (subarachnoid hemorrhage) or deep within the brain tissue (intracerebral hemorrhage) (American Heart Association). A *transient ischemic attack* (TIA) is a brief disruption of blood flow to the brain causing warning signs to occur. Such warning signs of stroke include (a) sudden numbness or weakness of the face, arm, or leg; (b) sudden confusion, trouble speaking or understanding; (c) sudden trouble seeing in one or both eyes; (d) sudden trouble walking, dizziness, loss of balance or coordination; or (e) a sudden severe headache (American Heart Association). Common disabilities from stroke include hemiparesis (50%), inability to walk without assistance (30%), activities of daily living dependency (26%), aphasia (19%), depressive symptoms (35%), and institutionalization in a nursing home (26%) (American Heart Association, 2003).

Stroke is the third leading cause of death in the United States and about a quarter of first-time stroke survivors die within 1 year of having a stroke (American Heart Association, 2003). Approximately 500,000 people each year experience a stroke for the first time, and another 200,000 suffer a recurrent stroke (American Heart Association). Stroke is also the number one cause of serious, long-term disability in the U.S. (American Heart Association). There are currently about 4,800,000 stroke survivors alive today in the U.S., 1,100,000 of whom report functional limitations or deficits in activities of daily living (American Heart Association). In 2004, stroke was estimated to cost $53.6 billion, with a mean lifetime cost for ischemic stroke estimated at $140,048 per person including inpatient care, rehabilitation, and follow-up care (American Heart Association).

Carotid endarterectomy is the most common surgical procedure and anticoagulants and antiplatelet agents are the most common medications used to prevent stroke (American Heart Association, 2003, 2004). It has only been within the past 10 years that an effective treatment for acute ischemic stroke has been made available to the public. Tissue-type plasminogen activator (tPA) is a drug that must be given intravenously to patients with ischemic stroke within 3 hours of the first warning sign to prevent disability from stroke. Unfortunately, few stroke survivors are able to make it to a physician who can administer tPA within the 3-hour time window. This dilemma has prompted the development of primary stroke centers (Alberts et al., 2000). Recommendations for primary stroke centers include an integrated emergency response system, acute stroke team, inpatient stroke unit, and written care protocols. The acute stroke team must include a physician and a nurse who are available 24 hours a day for rapid evaluation of patients experiencing the warning signs of stroke (Alberts et al.). Once stroke survivors are stabilized, they enter the rehabilitation phase of treatment where they learn how to live with their disabilities from stroke. Multidisciplinary rehabilitation teams consist of physicians, physiatrists, nurses, psychologists or psychiatrists, counselors, and physical, occupational, recreational, and speech therapists (American Heart Association, 2004).

Learning how to live with disabilities resulting from stroke is challenging for not only stroke survivors, but also for their family caregivers. Poststroke depression is a major complication of stroke and can greatly impede recovery (American Heart Association, 2004). Other quality-of-life issues for stroke survivors include disruption of personality and moods, diminished self-care, changes in social and family roles, loss of work or productivity, among others (Williams, L. S., Weinberger, Harris, Clark, & Biller, 1999). Family caregivers often experience negative changes in social functioning, subjective well-being, and perceived health as a result of providing care (Bakas & Champion, 1999). Caregiver tasks perceived as most difficult include managing behaviors and emotions of the stroke survivor, as well as providing household tasks and managing finances after stroke (Bakas, Austin, Jessup, Williams, & Oberst, 2004).

Nurses are involved with the care of stroke survivors throughout the continuum of care. E. T. Miller and Spilker (2003) found that their educational intervention was effective in reducing stroke risk factors and increasing stroke knowledge in a local family practice. Judith Spilker and colleagues (1997) integrated the use of the National Institutes of Health Stroke Scale into current nursing practice as a clinical stroke assessment tool. It is now widely used in stroke centers across the nation. Nursing research is greatly needed in the area of demonstrating best practices in the care of stroke survivors, particularly as new protocols are written and evaluated.

There are few published nursing research articles in the area of stroke survivor quality of life. Perhaps the development of outcome measures, such as the Stroke-Specific Quality of Life Scale (Williams, L. S., et al., 1999), will stimulate more research in this area. A recent search of the Computer Retrieval of Information on Scientific Projects (CRISP) —a database of biomedical research funded by the National Institutes of Health (n.d.)—revealed two studies of interest funded by the National Institute for Nursing Research (NINR). Pamela Mitchell has been funded to evaluate a nurse-delivered psychosocial/behavioral intervention for poststroke depression. Sharon Ostwald has been funded to evaluate her intervention for stroke survivors and spousal caregivers. It is hopeful that these intervention programs will provide promise for the future care of stroke survivors.

Published nursing research focusing on family caregivers of stroke survivors is growing. Brief research instruments that show promise for clinical assessment in practice include the Oberst Caregiving Burden Scale (Bakas et al., 2004) and the Bakas Caregiving Outcomes Scale (Bakas & Champion, 1999). J. S. Grant, Elliott, Weaver, Bartolucci, and Giger (2002) documented the effectiveness of a problem-solving intervention in reducing stroke-caregiver depression and improving caregiver perceived health. A search of the CRISP database (2004) revealed even more studies funded by NINR focused on family caregivers of stroke survivors. Patricia Clark has been funded to explore family function, stroke recovery, and caregiver outcomes. Judith Matthews has been funded to determine the use of technology with stroke caregivers. Rosemarie King was recently funded to evaluate the effectiveness of her problem-solving intervention for stroke caregivers, and Bakas has received funding to develop and pilot test the "Caregiver Telephone Assessment and Skill-Building Kit." Linda Pierce has been funded to test her intervention entitled, "The Caring Web" for stroke caregivers. All of these studies show great potential toward improving the care and well-being of families of stroke survivors. Now is a very fruitful time for nurses to conduct research in the area of stroke and stroke caregivers. With stroke being the number one cause of serious, long-term disability in the U.S., it is imperative that nurses take the lead in developing programs that improve the care of stroke survivors and their family members.

Tamilyn Bakas

Structural Equation Modeling

Structural equation modeling (SEM) is used to describe theoretical and analytic techniques for examining cause-and-effect relationships. It is used interchangeably with the terms causal modeling, covariance structure modeling, and LISREL modeling. The theoretical issues are discussed in "Causal Modeling." A description of the analytic issues when programs such as LISREL or EQS are used will ensue.

Structural equation modeling techniques are extremely flexible. Most models of cause can be estimated. In some models the causal flow is specified only between the latent variable and its empirical indicators, such as in a factor analysis model. This is known as confirmatory factor analysis. In other models, causal paths among the latent variables also are included.

Conducting a confirmatory factor analysis with SEM has many advantages. With SEM, the analyst can specify exactly which indicators will load on which latent variables (the factors), and the amount of variance in the indicators not explained by the latent variable (due to error in either measurement or model specification) is estimated. Correlations between latent variables and among errors associated with the indicators can be estimated and examined. Statistics that describe the fit of the model with the data allow the analyst to evaluate the adequacy of the factor structure, make theoretically appropriate modifications to the structure based on empirical evidence, and test the change in fit caused by these modifications. Thus, confirmatory factor analysis provides a direct test of the hypothesized structure of an instrument's scales.

An advantage of using SEM to estimate models containing causal paths among the latent variables is that many of the regression assumptions can be relaxed or estimated. For example, with multiple regression, the analyst must assume perfect measurement (no measurement error); however, with SEM, measurement error can be specified and the amount estimated. In addition, constraints can be introduced based on theoretical expectations. For example, equality constraints, setting two or more paths to have equal values, are useful when the model contains cross-lagged paths from three or more time points. The path from latent variable A at Time 1 to latent variable B at Time 2 can be set to equal the path from latent variable A at Time 2 to latent variable B at Time 3. Equality constrains also are used to compare models for two or more different groups. For example, to compare the models of effects of maternal employment on preterm and full-term child outcomes, paths in the preterm model can be constrained to be equal to the corresponding paths in the full-term model.

Data requirements for SEM are similar to those for factor analysis and multiple regression in level of measurement but not sample size. Exogenous variables can have indicators that are measured as interval, near-interval, or categorical (dummy-, effect-, or orthogonally coded) levels, but endogenous variables must have indicators that are measured at the interval or near-interval level. The rule of thumb regarding the number of cases needed for SEM, 5 to 10 cases per parameter to be estimated, suggests considerably larger samples than usually needed for multiple regression; thus, samples of 100 for a very modest model to 500 or more for more complex models are often required. Despite the advantages of SEM, these larger samples can result in complex and costly studies.

Structural equation modeling is generally a multistage procedure. First, the SEM implied by the theoretical model is tested and the fit of the model to the observed data is evaluated. A nonsignificant χ^2 indicates acceptable fit, but this is difficult to obtain because the χ^2 value is heavily influenced (increased) by larger sample sizes. Thus, most analytic programs provide other measures of fit. A well-fitting model is necessary before the parameter estimates can be evaluated and interpreted.

In most cases, the original theoretical model does not fit the data well, and modifications must be made to the model in order to obtain a well-fitting model. Although deletion of nonsignificant paths (based on t values) is possible, modifications generally focus on the inclusion of omitted paths (causal or correlational). Any path that is omitted specifies that there is no relationship, implying a parameter of zero; thus, analysis programs constrain these paths to be zero. After estimating the specified model, most programs provide a numerical estimate of the "strain" experienced by fixing parameters to zero or improvement in fit that would result from freeing the parameters (allowing them to vary). Suggested paths must be theoretically defensible before adding them to the respecified model.

Because model respecification is based on the data at hand in light of theoretical evidence and those data are repeatedly tested, the significance level of the χ^2 is actually higher than what the program indicates. Thus, other criteria are necessary to evaluate the adequacy of the final model. First is the theoretical appropriateness of the final model. Comparison of the original model with the final model will indicate how much "trimming" has taken place. In addition, the values and signs of the parameters are evaluated. The signs (positive or negative) of the parameters should be in the expected direction. Parameters on the paths between the latent variable and its indicators should be $\geq .50$ but ≤ 1.0 in a standardized solution. The lower the unexplained variance of the endogenous variables, the better the model performed in explaining those endogenous variables (similar to the $1\text{-}R^2$ value in multiple regression). Results that are consistent with a priori expectations and findings from previous research increase one's confidence in the model.

In summary, SEM is a powerful and flexible analysis technique for testing models of cause, investigating specific cause-and-effect relationships, and exploring the hypothesized process by which specific outcomes are produced. With SEM programs, the researcher has greater control over the analyses than with other factor analysis and multiple regression programs. Model respecification is usually necessary, but the role of theory in selecting appropriate modifications is crucial.

JoAnne M. Youngblut

Substance Abuse and Addiction Among Registered Nurses

Drug use by health professionals has a long history but became the focus of public health concerns in the 1980s. Illicit drug use peaked in the 1970s and alcohol use by more than half of Americans resulted in significant prevalence of alcohol and drug-related problems. These were paralleled in physicians, nurses, pharmacists, and others, causing concern based on the public trust vested in these professionals. Research on substance use/abuse among registered nurses emerged in response to a dearth of accurate data on nurses' drug using and addiction problems, which compromised the development of policy and educational initiatives in this area. The climate of social concern and the visibility of substance-related problems within the profession prompted the American Nurses Association (ANA) and several specialty nursing associations to support research and develop positions on the issue. The American Nurses Association House of Delegates in 1982 passed a resolution on impaired practice, defined as "nursing practice which does not meet the professional ethical code and standards of nursing practice because cognitive, interpersonal, and/or motor skills of the practitioner are impaired by psychiatric illness or excessive use of alcohol and/or other drugs." A policy statement, *Addictions and Psychological Dysfunctions: The Profession's Response to the Problem,* followed (ANA, 1984). Research related to the origins of impaired practice by registered nurses dates from the 1980s, and focuses on patterns of drug and alcohol use; nurse and nursing student attitudes (Engs, 1982; Haack & Harford, 1984); the course, recovery, and relapse of illnesses linked with alcohol and/or other drug problems among registered nurses (Hutchinson, 1986; Sullivan, E., 1987); and more recently, potential contributing factors to the development of addiction (Trinkoff & Storr, 1998a, 1998b).

An estimate of alcoholism at 2% among nurses was first extrapolated from a small descriptive survey by Bissell and Haberman ($N = 407$) of nurses in Alcoholics Anonymous (AA). Although these findings were limited by the size of a small, primarily Caucasian, convenience sample of survivors of addiction, they quickly became normative. Nurses in AA and recovery reported that 55%–63% had used narcotics and between 20% and 64% had used marijuana (Sullivan, E., Bissell, & Leffler, 1990). The estimate of drug and alcohol-related problems first adopted by ANA was 6%–9%, based on estimates from the National Household Drug Survey on alcohol and illicit drug use rates in the female population at large. The first findings of alcohol or drug use and abuse, the primary predispositions to addiction in registered nurses, were those of Trinkoff, Eaton, and Anthony (1991). The Epidemiologic Catchment Area Study (ECA) sponsored by the National Institute of Mental Health (NIMH) was a multisite probability sample, which included 142 nurses working full or part-time. These researchers found that nurses in the study and control group members had similar rates of illicit drug use: nurses 32.9% and nonnurses 31.5% (marijuana, cocaine, heroin, other opiates, psychedelics, tranquilizers, and amphetamines). Nonnurses had a much higher prevalence of alcohol abuse, with 3.8% reporting heavy use and 8.8% reporting pathological use. Nurses' parallel rates were 0.7% heavy use and 4.9% pathological use (Trinkoff, Eaton, & Anthony).

Despite the self-report and retrospective nature of data collection, these findings moved forward efforts to delineate the scope of the use/abuse problem.

Blazer and Mansfield's (1995) randomized descriptive survey (*N* = 1,525), measuring substance abuse in relation to stress and job outcomes, compared 920 nurses with other female employees. They found low levels of use of illicit drugs and alcohol for all subjects, with the lowest prevalence of smoking among nurse subjects and about 79% reporting moderate alcohol use. The same factors which predispose members of the general population to addiction also predispose nurses. These include family history of substance abuse, stress in various life realms, or sexual and/or emotional abuse. Workplace/occupational factors, inasmuch as they increase risk for personal stress, have been recently studied in an effort to understand the likelihood that nurses will develop addiction. One factor, access to controlled substances through prescribing and/or dispensing, such as hypnotics and analgesics, have been linked, for nurses and other health professionals. Findings of The Nurses' Worklife and Health Study, an anonymous, national survey of a stratified sample (4,438 registered nurses with a 78% response rate), indicated alcohol and illicit drug use similar to those of the general population, but higher prescription drug use rates for nurses. Smoking and cocaine/marijuana use was lower than in the general population and binge-drinking rates were comparable (Trinkoff & Storr, 1998a, 1998b). The prevalence of past-year substance use for all substances was 32%; for marijuana/cocaine, 4%; prescription drugs, 7%; cigarette smoking, 14%; and binge drinking, 16%. Males nurses were more likely to misuse prescription drugs, and of drugs misused, opiates were used most frequently (60.3%), and tranquilizers (44.6%) next. This research confirmed the link between easier workplace access and higher rates of substance use and provided direction for further analyses of substance use by nursing specialty.

On further analyses, nurses in certain specialties were found to have much greater likelihood of substance use. Critical care and emergency nurses were more likely to report marijuana or cocaine use, oncology nurses were more like to report binge drinking, and smoking rates were highest among psychiatric, gerontology, and emergency nurses. Trinkoff and Storr (1998) further examined workplace issues in relation to the potential demands and stressor of schedule variations (rotating shifts and overtime). This analysis of the Nurses' Worklife and Health Study revealed that work schedule characteristics were associated with the prevalence and odds of substance use. Working a few days overtime, working shifts longer than 8 hours, and working one or two weekends per month all increased the likelihood of using alcohol. In addition, smoking was more prevalent among night-shift workers and those working several weekends per month, a factor that was also associated with increased drug use. While the survey data used in the foregoing analyses were self-reports of drug use, such data have been found to be valid, although use may be somewhat underestimated.

The trend to correlated workplace factors such as job demands and access to substances represents a new direction from original efforts to estimate prevalence of actual illness by profession. On the whole, health professional groups have been unable to verify the prevalence of addiction to drugs and/or alcohol by profession. Indirect data have been obtained by the review of reasons for disciplinary action, or through the study of nurses participating in peer assistance monitoring programs (Finke, Williams, & Stanley, 1996). Research is just beginning to emerge on the patterns and progress of recovery in programs with various characteristics. A recent survey of nurses returning to work (*N* = 622) describes the challenges and obstacles confronted by these professionals (Brown, J., Trinkoff, & Smith, 2003). These current trends suggest a research emphasis on prevention by deterring contributing workplace conditions, such as easy access, and assisting nurses with addiction to return to health and optimal professional performance.

MADELINE A. NAEGLE

Substruction

Substruction is a heuristic technique, designed to be helpful in planning research and critiquing published research. It was first introduced to the nursing research literature by Hinshaw (1979). She outlined four steps in the process of substruction: (1) identify and isolate major concepts, (2) specify relationships among the concepts, (3) hierarchically order concepts by level of abstraction, and (4) pictorially present relationships among the variables. She provided guidelines for conducting theoretical substruction.

Substruction now comprises two components. The theoretical system explicates the relationship between constructs and concepts through articulating postulates or statements of relationships. For example, the construct of quality of life might postulate that it is composed of three dimensions or concepts, including physical, social, and spiritual. Thus, there is an implicit level of abstraction in substruction, moving vertically down from the most abstract (constructs) to less abstract notions (concepts). It is true that in the English language some authors will consider the words *constructs* and *concepts* to be interchangeable, and this must be recognized as a potential source of confusion when discussing substruction. The labels are less important than the idea of levels of abstraction.

In addition to examining vertical, conceptual relationships, the theoretical system examines across constructs through articulating axioms and propositions. Axioms are statements linking constructs; propositions are statements of relationships between or among concepts. For example, an investigator may hypothesize the relationship between the concepts of severity of illness and quality of life. The study might state as an axiom that there is an inverse, predictable relationship between severity of illness and quality of life. An author might hypothesize that as illness becomes more severe, quality of life diminishes.

The authors may conceptualize severity of illness to have related concepts, just as the construct quality of life had three concepts. Perhaps severity of illness is conceptualized to have two concepts, including physiological status and severity of symptoms.

If one is reading or planning an intervention study, the construct may be the intervention itself, such as patient teaching. There also may be concepts related to the intervention, such as type of delivery technique (group vs. individual) or time spent on teaching activity as a measure of dose of the treatment. Each of these concepts may be operationalized in the operational system as strategies to assess the take of the treatment, even though the treatment may have as its empirical indicator Yes or No or "received treatment" or "did not receive treatment."

The operational system was added by Dulock and Holzemer (1991) in their article on the process of substruction. The operational system requires the investigator to link each concept identified in the theoretical substruction with an empirical indicator or measure. The process of identifying the measures for each concept (or subconcept) highlights for the reader how the investigator operationalized the constructs. Sometimes this process reveals that, although an investigator included a construct or concept, the variable was never actually measured in the study.

This process of identifying the empirical indicators or measures also helps the investigator to give attention to the validity and reliability of each measure selected to ensure confidence in the results of the measurement. Finally, a review of the empirical indicators assists with an analysis of the level of scaling of the measures so that the reader can have confidence that an appropriate statistical analysis was conducted. Labeling the obtained scores from empirical indicators or measures as continuous or discrete leads one directly to the discussion of parametric or nonparametric analyses and which approach might be appropriate.

Dulock and Holzemer (1991) outlined a series of questions that can be generated related to the process of substruction when either planning or critiquing research studies. These questions have been modified and included the following:

1. What is the evidence that supports the relationships between constructs and concepts in the study?
2. What is the evidence that supports the relationships between constructs and concepts?
3. How does the study propose to measure each of the identified concepts?
4. Is there evidence of the validity and reliability of the measures?
5. What level of measurement will result from these instruments?
6. Are the data analysis techniques appropriate for these measures?
7. Is there a logical consistency between the theoretical system and the operational system?

They wrote: "These questions are designed to guide the exploration of the relationships between the theoretical and operational aspects of a study. The analytical process of substructing helps one to focus upon the study as a Gestalt of interrelationships" (p. 86). Substruction has proved to be an extremely useful tool when developing a new research project as well as for analyzing published studies. As a heuristic technique, substruction helps the researcher to understand how to think about the relationships among the selected variables or to understand how the author conceptualized these relationships.

WILLIAM L. HOLZEMER

Suicide

Suicide is defined as a death that is the result of an intentional self-destructive act. Nurses have demonstrated a great deal of clinical and theoretical interest in suicide, suicide attempts, attitudes toward suicide, and assisted suicide but have conducted very little research on these topics. A related topic that has been studied fairly extensively by nurses is suicide survivors, those family members and significant others who are bereaved by a suicide.

Few nursing studies have addressed suicide specifically. Using a qualitative methodology, messages of psychiatric patients who attempted or committed suicide were compared by Valente (1994). She found that clear suicidal messages were sent by most of these psychiatric patients and that the messages of suicide completers and suicide attempters could be differentiated. Demi, Bakeman, Sowell, Moneyham, and Seals (1996) studied suicidality in HIV-infected women and found that suicidal thoughts were common among the women and that family cohesion moderated the effect of HIV-related symptoms on emotional distress. They also found that there were clear differences between women who neither thought about nor attempted suicide and those who thought about or attempted suicide, but there were no significant differences between those who thought about suicide and those who attempted it. Grabbe, Demi, Camann, and Potter (1997) used a national database to assess suicidal risk factors among the elderly during their last year of life; using logistic regression, they confirmed the traditional risk factors of age, race, gender, alcohol use, and mental illness and provided preliminary evidence that cancer is also a risk factor among the elderly.

Several studies addressed adolescent suicide. Burge, Felts, Chenier, and Parrillo (1995), using a national database, studied suicidal behaviors among U.S. high school students and found a significant positive relationship between cocaine use and severity of outcomes of suicide attempts. They also found a significant but less strong relationship between marijuana use, alcohol use, sexual activity, and suicide attempts. Rew, Taylor-Seehafer, and Fitzgerald (2001) found that among homeless youths 35.1% had seriously considered suicide during the past 12 months and 12.3% had actually attempted suicide; they also found that participants with a history of sexual abuse were more likely to have considered suicide in the past 12 months. In another study Rew, Thomas, Horner, Resnick, and Beuhring (2001) found that among a group of triethnic adolescents Hispanic Latina girls had significantly higher suicide attempts than any other ethnic-gender group.

Several studies by nurses have investigated nurses' attitudes toward suicide in diverse groups. Oncology nurses' knowledge and misconceptions about suicide were explored through use of a vignette depicting a suicidal cancer patient. Although the nurses correctly identified a number of risk factors, few knew that race, age, and gender were risk factors. Further, few nurses assessed whether patients had a specific suicide plan, and less than one third identified appropriate interventions to prevent suicide in an at-risk patient. Another study compared nurses' attitudes toward suicide based on their clinical specialty, age, and highest degrees; they found no significant differences on any of the subscales based on clinical specialty, although age and degrees were significant on only the right-to-die subscale. A comparison of doctors' and nurses' attitudes toward the suicide of young people revealed few differences (Anderson, M., Standen, Nazir, & Noon, 2000). Another study explored patients' and psychiatric nurses' opinions regarding care for in-patients; nurses and patients believed that communicating with patients is the most important skill in psychiatric nursing (McLaughlin, 1999).

The only study of nonnurses explored attitudes toward suicide among low-income, elderly, inner city residents and compared attitudes toward suicide of men and women, African Americans and Whites, finding no significant differences. The researchers suggested that social class and place of residence may be better predictors of attitudes toward suicide in the elderly than race and gender (Parker, Cantrell, & Demi, 1997).

Several studies explored the effectiveness of "no-suicide contracts" with conflicting findings. Some found that there is no support for the effectiveness of no-suicide contracts; however, others note that no-suicide contracts are negotiated when there is a high risk of suicide. There is general consensus that there should be national standards for observation of patients identified as at risk for suicide.

Many studies have been conducted on suicide survivors, including parents, spouses, children, siblings, and therapists. Most of the studies of suicide survivors have been descriptive and have found that a death by suicide produces extreme distress in the survivors, with evidence of increased guilt, stigma, and resentment and a continuing questioning of "why" the suicide occurred. Several studies have compared those bereaved by suicide with those bereaved by other modes of death and have reported conflicting findings.

The suicide rates for the elderly are rising. At the same time, there is increased interest in euthanasia and assisted suicide. Nurses are intimately involved with elderly and terminally ill patients who are contemplating suicide and assisted suicide. Matzo and Emanuel (1997) found that nurses were more likely to have performed patient-assisted euthanasia than physicians; however the number who admitted to hastening a patient's death was very small. Much more research attention should be directed to this topic. Researchers should move beyond describing attitudes toward suicide and effects of suicide on survivors and toward studying interventions to prevent suicide, to help nurses cope with requests for assisted euthanasia, and to assist those coping with a death by suicide.

ALICE S. DEMI

Surgery

The preparation of patients for their experience with surgery is one of the largest bodies of clinical investigation relevant to the practice of nursing. The first report of an experimental study was published by a nurse, Rhetaugh Dumas (Dumas & Leonard, 1963), and the topic continued to attract researchers representing nursing, medicine, and psychology for over 20 years. The interest in psychological preparation for the surgical experience started with the discovery that when patients ambulated within hours after the operation, instead of being in bed for 7 to 10 days, morbidity and mortality decreased. This change in practice was anxiety-provoking for both patients and the people who cared for them. Preparing patients for the experience of getting out of bed soon after surgery was a way to deal with the anxiety. Much of the research stemmed from pragmatic concerns about how to help these anxious patients ambulate and perform behaviors believed to reduce postoperative complications. Psychological theories about *coping* with stressful events began to emerge in the late 1950s and 1960s, but most of the research on preparing patients for the stressful experience of undergoing surgery was atheoretical. Connections between the clinical research and theory, when attempted, were often vague.

Research on the effects of various approaches to preparing patients for surgery has been reviewed by a number of people, using meta-analysis and narrative review. It was difficult to conduct a tightly controlled study in the clinical settings, and there were methodological flaws in the studies. Nevertheless, there was consensus among the reviewers for the overall conclusion that preoperative interventions aimed at helping patients deal with their experiences postoperatively had a substantial positive effect on patients' welfare.

The interventions varied in content and focus. The most frequently tested intervention was instruction in the exercises and behaviors that patients were expected to engage in postoperatively to reduce complications. For abdominal and chest surgery patients, the intervention usually consisted of instruction in methods of deep breathing to effectively inflate the lungs, effective coughing techniques, leg exercises to increase circulation, and methods of getting out of bed to minimize incisional pain. The next most frequent intervention consisted of information that oriented patients to the routines of care. These descriptions were based on content in textbooks, manuals used by care providers, and providers' experiences. Patients were told, for example, that their skin would be prepared, that they would receive preoperative medication, and that they would go to the recovery room. The specifics of patients' experiences during those procedures were not included. This type of information has been referred to as procedural information.

In another type of informational intervention, the patient's perspective of the experience of undergoing surgery was emphasized. These descriptions focused on physical sensations associated with the events, when events would occur, and how long they would last. For example, the interventions included statements about how long patients could expect to be in the recovery room and about vital signs being checked frequently, descriptions of the sensations caused by preoperative medication (e.g., dry mouth and drowsiness), descriptions of sensations that abdominal surgery patients experienced when they coughed, and the expected progression of physical activities. This type of information was originally called sensory information and later called concrete objective information because that phrase more accurately described the content. Highly individualized nurse-patient interactions, hypnosis, relaxation, and positive thinking also have been used as interventions in a few studies of surgical patients. The impact of these studies on practice was decreased because of inconsistent findings and the special training required to deliver the intervention.

Clinical experience influenced the aspects of patient response, behaviors, and recovery selected as outcome measures in the research on preparing patients for surgery. Length of postoperative stay, pain medication use, complications, and ambulating behavior are representative of measures derived from clinical experience. Some researchers included patients' psychological responses, such as mood or emotions, pain reports, satisfaction with care, and well-being. Most researchers limited their measurement of outcomes to the time the patient was hospitalized. However, a few researchers were interested in the influence of the interventions on patients' long-term recovery and measured patients return to usual activities and psychological response after discharge from the hospital.

Although as many as 102 studies have been included in reviews, confident conclusions about relationships between content of interventions and specific outcomes cannot be drawn. The practice of combining content in interventions, instead of studying the effects of each type of content separately, contributes to the inability to sort out the content that was associated with specific outcomes. However, reviewers agree that combined interventions have the most consistent effects on outcomes. A frequently used combined content intervention consisted of instruction in postoperative exercises and behaviors and informing patients about routines of care (procedural information). This combined intervention appeared to have a positive effect on outcomes measured during hospitalization. A combination of descriptions of experiences from the patient's perspective (concrete objective information) and instruction in postoperative exercises and behavior also had a positive effect on outcomes measured during hospitalization. An additional benefit of the concrete objective information intervention was that it was associated with patients returning earlier to their usual activities after discharge.

The practice of preparing patients for surgery has been widely disseminated and is included in textbooks of nursing. It has become a part of care in most health care settings. The economic impact has been accepted as self-evident because of the reduction in complications and length of hospitalization and the early return to productive activities. In addition, the interventions had a positive effect on patients' subjective reports of well-being, such as mood and satisfaction with care. The combination of a practice activity having positive effects on cost and quality of care makes it an ideal practice to be widely adopted.

The recent practice of ambulatory surgery with discharge after patients awaken from anesthesia and that of admitting patients the day of surgery with brief hospital stays have changed the nature of patients' experiences when undergoing surgery. Patients and their families have to provide postoperative care. This includes assessing for complications, making decisions about the patient's status, progression of physical activities, and care of the incision. There has been little research on preparing patients for surgery since this change in practice.

Because the needs of surgical patients and their families have changed, new research on preparation for surgery is necessary. That research should draw on the prior research on preparing patients for surgery and advances in theory about coping with health care experiences. Relying on informational processing explanations of behavior, self-regulation theory provides explanations for why specific types of information about an experience, combined with instruction in self-care and coping activities, can help patients and families to cope with the surgical experience.

In the current climate of containment of health care costs, insurance coverage decisions are informed primarily by data about cost of care. There is much less data about how coverage regulations affect patient welfare. Research on preparing surgical patients for their experience at this time has the potential of influencing policies about services covered by health insurance.

JEAN E. JOHNSON

T

Taxonomy

A taxonomy is an organizing structure for a set of concepts/terms that helps identify relationships among the concepts and facilitates use of the concepts. Taxonomy is defined by Fleishman and Quaintance (1984) as "the theoretical study of systematic classifications including their bases, principles, procedures, and rules; the science of how to classify and identify" (p. 22). In recent years the word taxonomy is heard more often in nursing as the use of nursing knowledge classifications (e.g., classifications of nursing diagnoses, interventions, and outcomes). It is helpful to distinguish the term "taxonomy" from other related terms:

Standardized language: agreed-upon terms for specific objects/conditions/actions, with definitions; also called common language.

Classification: a set of concepts/terms that brings sense and some structure to some part of reality; sometimes used interchangeably with taxonomy although it is preferable to think of the taxonomy as the organizing structure for a classification's terms.

Aristotelian Classification: has binary characteristics—present or not present; used in biology, geology, and physics; two types: a monethetic classification has a single set of conditions whereas a polythetic classification has a number of shared characteristics (Bowker & Star, 1999).

Prototype Classification: a broad picture is created and this picture is extended by metaphor and analogy; a best example is called up to see if there is a reasonable resemblance (Bowker & Star, 1999); used more in sociolinguistics, anthropology, and nursing.

Standards: a set of agreed-upon rules for the production of objects; help to make things work together over distance; have significant inertia and can be difficult and expensive to change (Bowker & Star, 1999).

Terminology: words for concepts, the vocabulary; can be the same as standardized language if the terms are agreed upon and have standardized definitions; sometimes used interchangeably with *classification* although it is preferable to think of the terms as the vocabulary within a classification.

Naming and classifying are necessary for communication and for creating order in our lives. Look around your home or office and notice the ad hoc, often unnoticeable classifications; for example, dirty and clean dishes, important mail separated from junk mail, books in a bookshelf organized by topics. The nursing classifications identify and organize nursing knowledge; they make visible the work of nurses. The standardized nursing language in these classifications allows nursing to fit into existing health care memory systems, such as Systematized Nomenclature of Medicine (SNOMED) or the information systems in health care agencies. An excellent reference about classification is the book by Bowker and Star (1999), *Sorting Things Out: Classification and its Consequences.* Chapters in this book include information and analysis of the International Classification of Disease (ICD), the race classification under apartheid in South Africa, the classification of viruses and tuberculosis, and the Nursing Interventions Classification (NIC).

There is considerable confusion and misuse of the terms defined above. The term "taxonomy" is being used here to mean an organizing structure for a classification. In nursing in the United States, there are three comprehensive (across all settings and specialties), clinically useable (have terms that clinicians can plan and document care with), and current (have an ongoing submission and review system in place) clinical nursing classifications: NANDA, NIC, and NOC. Each of these classifications is organized in its own taxonomy as well as a common taxonomy, the Taxonomy of Nursing Practice. Each has a similar structure composed of Domains (the top, most abstract level) and Classes (the second level of the taxonomy, less abstract than the top domain level, in which the concepts of diagnoses, interventions, or outcomes are grouped). Each of the four taxonomies is overviewed briefly below.

North American Nursing Diagnosis Association (NANDA)—Taxonomy 2

Diagnoses are clinical judgments about individual, family, and community responses to problems or life processes that provide the basis for selection of nursing interventions to achieve outcomes for which the nurse is accountable. The NANDA Taxonomy 2 (NANDA, 2003) was approved for adoption by the NANDA members at their conference in April 2000. It consists of 13 domains (e.g., Health Promotion, Nutrition) and 46 classes (e.g., Health Awareness, Ingestion). Each domain and class has a definition and a total of 155 diagnoses are included at the third level of the taxonomy.

Nursing Interventions Classification (NIC)

Interventions are treatments performed based upon clinical judgment and knowledge to enhance patient outcomes. The NIC taxonomy (McCloskey & Bulechek, 2004) consists of seven domains (e.g., Physiological: Basic, Behavioral) and 30 classes (e.g., Activity and Exercise Management, Coping Assistance). Each domain and class has a definition. The 514 interventions are placed in the classes at the third level of the taxonomy.

Nursing Outcomes Classification (NOC)

Outcomes are measurable individual, family, or community states, behaviors, or perceptions influenced by and responsive to nursing interventions. The NOC taxonomy (Moorhead, Johnson, & Maas, 2004) consists of seven domains (e.g., Functional Health, Physiologic Health) and 31 classes (e.g., Energy Maintenance, Growth & Development). Each domain and class has a definition. The 260 outcomes are placed in the classes at the third level of the taxonomy.

Taxonomy of Nursing Practice

The Taxonomy of Nursing Practice (Dochterman & Jones, 2003) consists of four domains and 28 classes. The structure resulted from an invitational conference effort in 2001 to provide an organizing structure useful for all nursing classifications to promote linkages among diagnoses, interventions, and outcomes. It is a structure that is different from the existing structures of NANDA, NIC, and NOC, yet is not a radical departure from any. It is also placed in the public domain, available for use by any group or individual. The 2004 editions of NIC and NOC include placements of interventions and outcomes in this structure as well as their own structures. The NNN Alliance Conference in March 2004 includes sessions to further the ongoing effort to refine and use this common taxonomy.

A taxonomy that classifies nursing knowledge is useful to assist the clinician in identifying related concepts, and assists in the designing of nursing information systems and in organizing nursing curricula. The organization of nursing knowledge helps to identify what is known and can be used to support clinical decision making, and what is not known and needs more research. Multiple other benefits of taxonomy are also mentioned in the literature.

JOANNE MCCLOSKEY DOCHTERMAN

Telehealth

Telehealth is defined as the use of interactive technology for the provision of clinical health care, patient and professional education, and health care administration over small and large distances (American Nurses Association, 1999; Chaffee, 1999). The defining aspect of telehealth is the use of electronic signals to transfer various types of information from one site to another. Information ranges from clinical records to health promotion instructions to still-images of wounds and motion-images demonstrating exercise routines. Throughout the published literatures relevant to the health sciences, telehealth is used interchangeably with telemedicine, and every so often the term telenursing will surface. The term telehealth is embraced as the more encompassing concept, descriptive of the state of technology used in the provision of health care; telemedicine and telenursing are subsets of telehealth.

Telehealth has tremendous potential for nursing, both as a means of communication between nurses, patients, and their caregivers, and as a way to deliver tailored nursing services. Telehealth can serve in nearly every area of nursing care, from emergency response systems to hospital, home, and community care. Telehealth has the potential of expanding health care services beyond traditional geographic boundaries and enabling access to a broader range of care options in previously underserved areas and at times where health care providers commonly are not accessible. It can be used for bedside nursing care, patient education, or to assist nursing care at distant sites. This broad definition includes several means of transmission, including telephone and fax transmissions, interactive video and audio, store and forward technology, patient monitoring equipment, electronic patient records, electronic libraries and databases, the Internet and intranet, World Wide Web (WWW), electronic mail systems, decision and care planning support systems, and electronic documentation systems. When used optimally, telehealth can be used to leverage limited health care resources to better meet the needs of patients (Darkins, Fisk, et al., 1996; Wakefield, Flanagan, et al., 2001).

Most nurses have already been involved in telehealth without realizing it. Examples include telephoning or faxing a patient status report, telephone triage, home health visits via telecommunication for monitoring, and designing websites for educating patients. While much attention has been paid to technology and innovative equipment as a potential to enhance the access and availability of health care services for patients regardless of where they live, very little work has been accomplished in the area of systematically reviewing the efficiency and effectiveness of its applications. An exception is the use of the telephone for consultations. Randomized clinical trials have established the efficacy of telephone consultation to improve patients' outcomes across a broad spectrum of patient populations (Balas, Jaffrey, et al., 1997). Studies of interactive "teleconsultations" have been performed all over the world and most suggest that health care delivery via these technologies is acceptable to patients in a wide variety of circumstances.

Telenursing provides other potentials for nursing practice. A small but persuasive set of research projects (Whitten, Mair, et al., 1997; Hayes, Duffey, et al., 1998; Wootton, Loane, et al., 1998; Hagan, Morin, et al., 2000; Hanson, E. J., & Clarke, 2000; Hanson, E. J., Tetley, et al., 2000; Johnson-Mekota, Maas, et al., 2001; Jerant, Azari, et al., 2003) identified the important components of home care that could be delivered via telecommunications applications, demonstrated the equivalence of technology-mediated assessment with face-to-face approaches and illustrated the feasibility and potential health benefits of information technology designed to intervene in significant health problems.

Research examining telehealth in support of clinical nursing is in its infancy, with most projects, save Brennan's ComputerLink work (Brennan, Moore et al., 1991), occurring since the mid-1990s. This relative youth is a consequence both of the state of Telehealth applications and the expectations of nurses regarding the nature of appropriate interventions. The World Wide Web is but 10 years old and the penetration of computer technology into daily life, while accelerating, has yet to touch the lives of greater than 80% of the American public. Additionally, the nursing discipline has concentrated its professional and scientific attention on the face-to-face encounter with patients (Darkins, Fisk, et al., 1996; Whitten, Cook, et al., 1998; Gardner, Frantz, et al., 2001; Johnson-Mekota, Maas, et al., 2001; Wakefield, Flanagan, et al., 2001; Dansky, Yant, et al., 2003). Preliminary investigations into the use of telehealth for delivery of professional nursing interventions (Brennan & Ripich, 1994; Brennan, S. M., et al., 1995; Brennan, Moore, et al., 2001; Heyn Billipp, 2001) demonstrated the feasibility of the approach and the potential for not only social benefits but also improved health outcomes. However, across all of the studies a persistent theme emerges: the telehealth innovations that work the best are those that complement the existing nursing approaches. Importantly, then, this finding calls for the initiation of studies in which the telehealth innovation is examined as a component of, not apart from, the nursing intervention.

JOSETTE JONES

Terminal Illness

The trajectory of terminal illness may be relatively brief or may transpire over a period of years. The term is generally applied to a person with a degenerative process rather than an episode engendered by trauma sustained as a result of some external force. "A person may be regarded as having a terminal illness when broad agreement has been reached among health professional that there is no longer the possibility of cure and that life-expectancy is limited" (Hughes, N., & Neal, 2000, p. 4). Research in the area of terminal illness has focused on the individual (patient needs, symptom management, and holistic care), family needs (meaning-making, empowerment, anticipatory grief, managing time, and the impact of terminal illness on the family), and system issues (adequacy of care, ethical issues, impact of ethnicity on care, terminally ill patients and research, transfer to hospice, and incarcerated terminally ill persons).

The effects of terminal illness on the patient were studied by B. D. Davis, Cowley, and Ryland (1996), who did so in order to assess whether the services currently available in their region were adequate to meeting these needs. Partially replicating prior studies, the researchers met with the relatives of people dying within the health district but excluded those who died in long-stay geriatric hospitals or nursing homes. It was observed that the symptoms from the cause of death predominated in the last 3 months of life, while symptoms related to a host of other causes were more significant during the last year of life but prior to the last 3 months of life. Of the various terminal illness diagnoses, those diagnosed with cancer obtained better symptom relief that those suffering from other diseases. This may well be because of the attention given to symptom management in oncology and because people with cancer were the patients who received attention from hospice providers, resulting in a body of practice knowledge and research findings.

A continuing question in the care of those with a terminal illness is the role of food and hydration. For relatives and significant others, food has a symbolic value connoting nurturing and life and the hope that death will be forestalled. For patients, food tastes and the desire for food may change due to disease and its treatment. And for health care providers, and particularly nurses, feeding and hydration of patients including subcutaneous fluids was deemed appropriate if it would make the family members more comfortable. The ten nurse respondents in this study of health care providers felt that the decision regarding hydration was to be made by the physician (McAulay, 2001). It would be interesting to see whether this finding would be upheld were the study conducted with a larger number of nurses and if those nurses represented a variety of countries.

The needs of families of those who are terminally ill has also been of interest to researchers. The prevalence of pathologies and decreasing health in the informal caregivers as well as their efforts, often unsuccessful, in getting physicians to give serious attention to symptoms in their terminally ill family members adds to the stress of both patient and caregivers (Davis, B. D., Cowley, & Ryland, 1996). Interestingly, Tang, Aaronson, and Forbes (2004) found that terminally ill persons who did not live with their caregivers had more social support, less pain intensity, higher spirituality, and a significantly better quality of life.

The needs of caregivers of terminally ill children present other issues. Factors that influence how families navigate this terrain include the relationship with health care providers, the availability of information, and the effectiveness of communication between parents (Steele, R. G., 2002). In a grounded theory investigation of a nurse-facilitated empowering intervention of 24 family caregivers of terminally ill patients, it was found that information, education, encouragement, and support were required by these caregivers (Mok, Chan, Chan, & Yeung, 2002). The importance of a trusting relationship with caregivers and the confidence that the caregiver will not be abandoned was also found to be crucial, reinforcing previous findings. The need for information and support was underscored in another study examining the adequacy of primary care and the deployment of visiting nurses in Great Britain (Beaver, Luker, & Woods, 2000).

Examining the management of time in caring for a terminally ill person in the home, K. E. Rose (1998) observed that in addition to the practical and emotional tasks as well as outside demands facing caregivers, there was also the uncertainty that was the context in which these activities transpired. With regard to time this uncertainty means not knowing how many hours, days, weeks, or months are left prior to the patient's demise. Time and uncertainty also interact in the question of what will happen prior to death and how that time until death will be experienced. Finally there is also the uncertainty as to what will happen in the time after the patient's death. Nonetheless, other studies have found that the meaning that is found in caregiving enabled caregivers to develop a new view of life and reach out to help others.

In another qualitative study, Duke (1998) investigated the lived experience of being with a terminally ill spouse and then being bereaved. The themes that emerged during the illness phase were related to sharing the illness experience, being a caregiver and providing comfort, being in limbo, and knowing that this time was a period of creating memories that would be treasured as well as those memories of experiences that were emblematic of the transition along the illness trajectory.

Repeatedly in the research on caregivers of terminally ill persons, the need for information has been stressed. In Norway and Sweden, using 45 forced choice open-ended questions, researchers found that respondents supported ongoing disclosure of information to terminally ill patients (Lorensen, Davis, Konishi, & Bunch, 2003). This contrasts sharply with parts of Europe and Japan where it is the custom to speak with the family rather than the patient. Interestingly this is also the view of many Korean Americans and Mexican Americans in the survey of 800 elderly residents at 31 senior citizen centers in Los Angeles County conducted by Blackhall, Murphy, and Frank (1995). Younger and more affluent Korean Americans and Mexican Americans were more likely to share the views of other Americans and expect to be given information as patients.

Finally caregivers often serve as the source of information about the end-of-life experience of the terminally ill person. Quality of care and satisfaction with care are measured by the reports of family members of the patient's experience. Hinton's (1996) reinterview of 71 relatives showed that there is variable agreement with earlier statements made by these same individuals. This raises a question about the validity and reliability of such measurements when used to indicate the satisfaction with care of the terminally ill person. At the same time, there is no easy answer as to how satisfaction with care of terminally ill persons is to be measured given the fragile condition of persons nearing the end of their lives.

Research with the terminally ill as with other patients demands the calculation of a risk/benefit ratio. In this case, the research may not benefit the individual participant but it may be of benefit to future terminally ill persons. Given the condition of terminally ill persons, qualitative research has been favored as a method of inquiry. That leaves the question of the generalizability of the results; quantitative methods are important for future studies. As the research results accumulate, the translation of the research findings into practice will enhance the care of the terminally ill.

INGE B. CORLESS

Theoretical Framework

A theoretical framework is a group of statements composed of concepts related in some way to form an overall view of a phenomenon. As constructions of our mind, theoretical frameworks provide explanations about our experiences of phenomena in the world. The explanations provided by theoretical frameworks are of two types: descriptive (understanding the interaction among a set of variables) or prescriptive (anticipating a particular set of outcomes) (Dubin, 1978). The term *theoretical framework* often is used interchangeably with the terms *theory*, *theoretical model*, and *theoretical system*. Conceptual frameworks and conceptual models are related to but different from theoretical frameworks in that conceptual frameworks and models are more abstract and more comprehensive than theoretical frameworks and usually are not able to be tested empirically.

Theoretical frameworks consist of the following components: (a) concepts that are identified and defined, (b) assumptions that clarify the basic underlying truths from which and within which theoretical reasoning proceeds, (c) the context within which the theory is placed, and (d) relationships between and among the concepts that are identified. Theoretical frameworks serve as guides for practitioners and researchers in that they organize existing knowledge and aid in making new discoveries to advance nursing practice.

It is important to distinguish an empirical system from a theoretical one. An empirical system is what we apprehend, through senses, in the environment. A theoretical system is what we construct in our mind's eye to model the empirical system (Dubin, 1978). The scientist focuses on making the empirical world and the theoretical world (represented by theoretical frameworks) as congruent as possible. Linkages between the theoretical world and the empirical world to which it applies are made through the formulation and testing of hypotheses. As long as the abstraction of the theoretical framework can be represented with empirical indicators, hypotheses can be generated and empirically tested. Theoretical frameworks are developed and tested through theory-linked research. Theory-generating research is designed to discover and describe concepts and relationships for the construction of theory. Once theory is constructed, theory-testing research is used to validate how accurately the theory depicts empirical phenomena and their relationships.

Generation of theoretical frameworks in nursing has followed an evolutionary process. Initially, nursing grappled with defining theory for a developing discipline. In the

1960s and 1970s early nurse theorists attempted to answer questions such as:

1. Around what phenomena do nurses develop theory?
2. What are the things nurses think about and take action on?
3. What are the boundaries of the discipline?

In response to these questions, a proliferation of conceptual models and philosophies of practice of nursing were developed. These nursing conceptual models are considered at the grand theory level, examples of which are the theories of Johnson, Roy, Neuman, Rogers, and Watson.

The discipline also addressed the question of how to develop theory for nursing and proposed definitions emphasizing the structure, purpose, and use of theory. Nurse scientists and theorists debated methods of developing theory, including reformulation of borrowed theories and development of unique nursing theories based on quantitative and qualitative research. These discussions have led to the acceptance of multiple approaches to theory development in nursing, including both inductive and deductive methods. Recent attention has focused on the need to develop knowledge about the substance of nursing. In response to this call, theoretical frameworks that address specific nursing phenomena and that focus on the clinical processes in nursing are being developed. This knowledge is referred to as middle- and micro-range theory.

The notion of different levels of theory has been a useful way to develop knowledge in nursing. Each level of theory has characteristics and purposes that are specific to that level. The scope or breadth of the concepts and goals of a theoretical framework determine its usefulness for research and practice. As the goal of a theory narrows in scope, it moves from grand to middle range to micro range. Grand theories provide global perspectives of the discipline and offer ways of looking at nursing phenomena based on these perspectives. However, because of the broad scope and abstract concepts of grand theories, they are not testable and therefore are limited in their usefulness to researchers.

Unlike grand theories, the scope of middle-range theories is not as broad as the full range of phenomena of concern to the discipline but involves more concepts than micro-range theories. Middle-range theories are sufficiently abstract to generalize yet specific enough to be empirically tested. In contrast to grand theories, middle-range theories contain concepts close to observed data, from which hypotheses may be logically derived and empirical tested. Examples of middle-range theoretical frameworks are Mishel's theory of uncertainty in illness, Pender's theory of health promotion, and Lenz and colleagues' theory of unpleasant symptoms.

Micro-range theory (also called practice theory) is more specific than middle-range theory and refers to precise goals and actions to achieve goals in a particular nursing practice situation. Although micro-range theory offers specific guidelines for practitioners, it is often situation-specific and thus limited in generalizability. It is generally agreed that the development of theoretical frameworks at all three levels—grand, middle range, and micro-range—are needed and will enhance the knowledge base of nursing.

The process of developing theoretical frameworks that inform nursing practice and drive nursing research is ongoing. Several challenges prevail in the development of nursing theoretical frameworks. One challenge is how to integrate related theoretical frameworks that have arisen from the multiple ways of developing knowledge in nursing. For example, how does the theory about stages of behavior change, developed from grounded theory methods, relate to theories of self-efficacy for health behaviors that were developed using empirical methods? Additionally, what mechanisms are needed to enhance communication between practitioners and researchers about the knowledge produced by both using divergent methods? Also, how do different levels of theory relate to each other? How can one level of theory be used to develop related theories at another level? Another challenge is the need to build programs of research that are substantially large enough to accrue sufficient knowledge around a particular set of phenomena. Such programs of research will require greater use of collaborative approaches to knowledge development than those previously used within the discipline. The efficient development of nursing theoretical frameworks will require extensive collaboration among institutions, disciplines, researchers, and practitioners.

SHIRLEY M. MOORE

Thermal Balance

Thermal balance is defined as a thermal "steady state" in which the loss of body heat is equal to the heat gain. In health, this balance produces a thermoneutral state, optimal for cellular function. In humans, this state averages about 37° C ± .05 for internal temperatures and 33.5° C ± .05 for skin. Variations in body temperature respond to both homeostatic and circadian influences. Circadian rhythm of core temperature is regulated by a remarkably stable endogenous "clock" which has helped to make it the most widely used circadian indicator. Hypothalamic thermoregulatory controls keep internal temperatures fairly stable, despite environmental changes and the propensity of heat to escape to cooler regions. Metabolic and physical activity continually generates heat, even as it is constantly lost to the cooler environment. Current theory is that elaborate thermoregulatory control systems maintain temperatures within the optimal *set point* range. Compensatory cooling or warming mechanisms respond to deviations above or below this range. Temperatures rising above this range evoke vasodilation and sweating, while falling temperatures cause vasoconstriction, shivering, and increased metabolic activity. Each physiological response augments or inhibits the transfer of heat by affecting the *thermodynamics* of conduction, convection, radiation, and evaporation. Vasodilation warms the skin where heat is more easily lost to air, contact surfaces, or liquids. Vasoconstriction creates a poorly perfused insulative layer of tissue that conserves heat. In infants, cold exposure causes metabolic breakdown of *brown fat* to generate heat. In older children and adults, the primary means of heat generation is shivering.

Nurses have recognized the importance of assessing thermal balance as a vital health indicator for as long as the profession has existed. Body temperature provides an important *vital sign* of metabolic, neurological, and infectious activity. Circadian rhythms, monthly cycles, and daily body temperature ranges are assurances of healthy variations. The pregnant mother provides heat exchange both for herself and the fetus; therefore high maternal body temperatures, from fever, hyperthermia, or prolonged "hot tub" use, put the unborn infant at risk for neurological damage. Temperature elevations in the acutely ill and injured may indicate either fever or hyperthermia. Each has its own dynamics and treatment. Fevers are usually self-limiting. Thermoregulatory control is lost during hyperthermia and requires aggressive cooling treatment. Temperatures above 42° C can cause irreversible neural cellular damage. Conductive cooling blankets, ice packs, and cooling fans are used to lower core temperatures. In immunosuppression associated with cancer treatment, fevers may indicate fulminating systemic infection. However, the immunosuppressed HIV-infected patient may become febrile from high cytokine levels, without obvious secondary infection. In both groups, constant assessment of other indicators is necessary to rule out infection.

Situations that promote heat loss or interfere with heat generations put patients at risk for hypothermia. The neonatal nurse must be extremely sensitive to the low-birthweight infant's need for external heat source. Unable to shiver, the neonate expends oxygen to metabolize brown fat and can easily become hypoxic from cold exposure. Declining metabolic and vasomotor activity makes elders particularly susceptible to heat loss during surgery, trauma, or outdoor exposure. Hypothermic states can destabilize thermoregulatory function further, leading eventually to death.

Fever patterns were used to detect the onset and progress of infections since early times. It was recognized that high temperatures could lead to brain damage, so nurses routinely cooled patients with fever or heat stroke with ice packs, cooling sponge baths, or circulating fans. In the 1970s, nurses used conductive cooling blankets, with refrigerated circulating coolant, to treat refractory hyperthermia. Sharp gradients between skin and core temperatures stimulated vigorous and distressful shivering. Interventions to prevent shivering were among the earliest to be tested by nurses. Interest in and awareness of temperature variations became more acute among nurse researchers when advanced technology in thermometry was introduced to clinical settings. In the 1970s, thermistor probes in hemodynamic monitoring systems made pulmonary artery temperatures possible in some critical care settings. As probes became available for bladder, tympanic membrane, and skin temperatures, studies of gradients between body regions and measurement sites were common. Variation in quality and precision of instruments made studies of reliability and accuracy important. Recognition of *malignant hyperthermia*, a rare but lethal genetically-linked disorder occurring when susceptible persons receive anesthetic agents, led to closer surveillance of perioperative body temperature. This precaution reduced mortality from hyperthermia in this uncommon condition, but also brought to awareness the high incidence of *low* body temperatures in most surgical patients. Increased survival of preterm infants in the 1970s created increased concern for thermal balance of vulnerable infants. Studies of environmental influences, warming devices, and skin-to-skin contact were made possible by sophisticated continuous skin temperature monitors.

Temperature measurement issues continue to dominate clinical nursing research, stimulated by commercial development of new technology in thermometers. There is an ongoing program of research in body temperature measurement by Erickson and colleagues (Erickson, R. S., 1999; McKenzie & Erickson, 1996), who have compared oral, skin, rectal, and tympanic membrane measurement sites in children and adults. Findings reassure nurses that oral measurement provided reliable intermittent thermal assessment in afebrile patients. While placement site and method of insertion yield statistically significant differences, they are of less importance clinically. Erickson's work was set apart from other contemporary studies by her appropriate statistical treatment beyond simple correlations and by meaningful interpretation of device reliability, accuracy, and linearity. In the past decade, nurse researchers began drawing inferences from observed relationships between thermal changes and other variables. Gradients between skin and core temperatures initiate thermoregulatory responses (see Shivering). Studies have shown the importance of thermal gradients and rate of cooling in initiating shivering in a comparison of cooling blanket temperatures (Caruso, Hadley, Shukla, Frame, & Khoury, 1992; Sund-Levander & Wahren, 2000). Nursing research has also tested methods to alleviate adverse effects of warming and cooling in patients of all ages. Particularly vulnerable are the preterm infant, the elderly, and patients recovering from surgery, cardiopulmonary bypass, or traumatic injury. Anderson (Anderson, Chiu, et al., 2003) pioneered "kangaroo care" as a method of maintaining thermal balance in preterm and term infants. Drawn from perinatal practices of Western Europe, this method uses skin-to-skin care for infants held against the skin under the mother or father's clothing. Self-demand breast-feeding and lactation were promoted by close constant maternal contact. More recently, the relationships between the infant's body temperature and environment, circadian rhythm, and parental cosleeping have been investigated (Thomas & Burr, 2002). Several studies have compared cooling interventions in febrile adults with similar findings (Caruso et al., 1992; Henker et al., 2001). Most concluded that antipyretic drugs are as effective as cooling without inducing distressful shivering. In a controlled trial with febrile patients with HIV disease, insulating skin against heat loss actually kept peak febrile temperatures lower (Holtzclaw, 1998). While numerous small studies in nursing have tested various products that cool febrile patients or restore heat loss in perioperative patients, they are often empirical in nature. By contrast, the investigations mentioned above are theoretically based on principles of thermodynamics and physiological responses. They seek to explain mechanisms, predict consequences, and alleviate hazards of altered thermal balance.

Some of the newer areas of investigation conducted by nurse scientists related to thermal balance are studies using animal models to demonstrate effects of exercise on thermoregulatory responses (Rowsey, Metzger, & Gordon, 2001) and circadian influences on thermoregulation in obesity (Jarosz, Lennie, Rowsey, & Metzger, 2001). As more nurses enter fields of genetics, immunology, and molecular biology, they will play important roles in seeking origins and mechanism of thermoregulatory responses. New avenues for nursing research in thermal balance emerge as new situations of vulnerability develop and measurement techniques are advanced. At particular risk is the rapidly growing population of the frail elderly. Declining metabolic rate, lower vasomotor sensitivity, and diminishing insulation from body fat make this group vulnerable to extremes in heat or cold. The existence and treatment of thermoregulatory failure in home-bound patients is an area that nursing has not yet systematically studied. Improved survival of individuals with neurological, vasomotor, and endocrine impairments and with extensive burns creates new situations where thermal balance is altered. Only recently have nurses begun to investigate relationships between the circadianicity of body temperature and the effectiveness of other therapies. Study and intervention are needed in addressing thermal balance, thermal perception, and thermal comfort during a variety of life events and health alterations.

BARBARA J. HOLTZCLAW

Time Series Analysis

Time series analysis and statistical time series models are basic to describing and studying change in human responses and behavior. They are appropriate to cyclical patterns as well as periodic or systematic variance across time. Many of the phenomena of interest to nursing are intimately related to time. Thus, time series statistical models are an appropriate and powerful methodology for longitudinal nursing studies of intraindividual differences in rate and patterns of change.

In contrast to inferential statistical models, where aggregate data are generalized to describe changes in human behavior, time series analysis uses individual patterns of change to predict future behavior. Thus, the subject is a unitary entity or system whose behavioral state can be isolated within a given point and measured through a specified window of time. For the purpose of time series analysis, the singular system can be defined at many different levels of complexity and inclusiveness. Examples of individual systems that are legitimate subjects for time series nursing research include cardiovascular response to a cardiac stressor, individuals, families, communities, health care systems, even political institutions.

The characteristic feature of time series analysis is that the phenomenon to be studied has a distinctive temporal component—the behavioral state will vary predictably with the passage of time. Obviously, the passage of time can not be manipulated, thus, differences in patterns of change are not a direct function of time. Time is not the independent variable; it is, instead, a necessary temporal frame or marker in any time series analysis study.

Time series studies can be either univariate or multivariate. However, a time series variable always consists, by definition, of a series of observations that occur in temporal order. Thus, multivariate time series analysis is accomplished by identifying the relationship between or among two or more pairs of univariate time series.

Unlike inferential statistical models, time series data points are not intended to be independent of one another. Each value is highly correlated with every successive value. Thus, any observation in a time series has significantly less individual predictive significance than its inferential counterpart. In time series analysis, predictive power is not a direct function of sample size. Instead, predictive power depends on an accurate hypothesis of the internal temporal structure of the phenomenon, selection of a sampling time window of sufficient length to capture multiple expressions of the change being studied, and identification of a sampling frequency that will adequately capture all critical phases of the evolving pattern.

Although change in behavior is an essential characteristic of many of the phenomena of interest to nursing science, the use of statistical time series models is not always appropriate or feasible. However, although time series analyses are complex and costly, they permit nurse scientists to more completely examine and evaluate trends, cycles, and patterns of change that are framed within predictable spaces of time.

BONNIE L. METZGER

Transitional Care

Transitional care refers to care and services required in the safe and timely transfer of patients from one level of care to another or from one type of health care setting to another (Brooten, 1993). Transitional environments include the hospital, home, nursing home, rehabilitation center, and hospice. Some authors differentiate subacute care from transitional care; others use the terms interchangeably. Those who make the distinction view subacute care as a unit or component of inpatient care in an acute care facility, skilled nursing facility, or freestanding medical or rehabilitation center. Transitional care ideally ends with normal functioning and recovery, functional independence, or stabilization of the patient's condition (Brooten). In the case of many frail children or adults, transitional services end in long-term care.

Key features of transitional care include comprehensive discharge planning from one site of care to another, coordination of post-discharge services, provision of in-home services on a short-term basis, and continued health care follow-up. The most important components of transitional care services are continuity of care across sites of care, communication of the plan of care among the differing providers, and matching patient needs and knowledge with skills of the care providers.

Transitional care services have increased significantly over the past 10 to 15 years in response to changes in health care delivery, especially earlier hospital discharge of patients.

Research issues in transitional care include determining the nature and needed length of the service, risk profiles of patients who need the service, type and level of providers needed, and cost-effectiveness of the service compared to alternative services. The length of transitional services should vary with the specific needs of the patients or group of patients rather than being dictated by the reimbursement plan. However, data are not available demonstrating the most effective and cost-efficient endpoint for services to achieve optimal patient outcomes in specific patient groups or subgroups.

It is generally agreed that vulnerable groups such as the elderly, the technologically dependent, the disabled, and some high-risk infants and children should receive transitional services. Decisions regarding which patients should receive these services are currently based on the patient's functional ability, available caretakers at home, ethnicity, age, previous hospitalization, and technology dependence.

Currently, there is wide variation in the type and level of transitional care provider, and there is disagreement about who should provide the care. Whether APNs are needed for transitional services to all patient groups has not yet been tested. Home care provided by professional nurses (RNs) has been reported to decrease the negative psychosocial impact on parents caring for medically fragile children at home. Improved patient outcomes using home care provided by RNs also has been reported with ventilator-dependent children, with oncology patients, and with elders.

Data also are needed on the cost-effectiveness of transitional care compared to alternative approaches to care. Although the direct costs for transitional care have been calculated in some studies, costs such as prevention of rehospitalization, acute care visits, decreased employment, and burden on family caregivers are less well documented. These data are important in examining the overall cost benefit or cost-effectiveness of transitional services.

Transitional care services are provided through public agencies; private, not-for-profit agencies; freestanding and privately operated proprietary agencies; freestanding and operated for profit, hospital-based agencies; and dedicated units or departments operated by a hospital. Transitional services are provided by community nursing services, hospital home care services, health maintenance organization (HMO) follow-up services, and subacute care units established within hospitals or skilled nursing facilities or as freestanding subacute care hospitals.

Community or public health nurses have historically provided home follow-up to high-risk patients with complex health needs. Their services are well-known and accepted by the general public and health care providers. Unfortunately, over the past 10 to 15 years, budget reductions for community nursing services have virtually eliminated home follow-up services to many patient groups. Current challenges for community nursing services include updating the specialty knowledge and skills of agency nurses with a generalist preparation, maintaining continuity of patient care from the hospital to the home, providing sufficient services to maintain continuity of patient care from the hospital to the home, and providing sufficient services to maintain good patient outcomes as insurers reimburse for fewer services.

As reimbursed length of stay for even high-risk patients decreases, the hospitals' need for improved discharge planning and postdischarge home care services for these groups increases. Documented discharge planning is mandatory for hospitals, and many have hired discharge planners to facilitate earlier discharge. Some hospitals contract with community nursing services or independent home care agencies to provide home care services for their high-risk patients. An increasing number of hospitals are establishing their own home care services.

HMOs have a clear financial incentive for discharging patients early and for preventing costly rehospitalizations. They have used case managers and nurses with specialty knowledge and skills to review patients' discharge and home care needs. Because realizing a profit is essential in the for-profit HMOs, their approach has been one of minimal hospital length of stay and postdischarge services. Home follow-up services vary in number of visits provided, type of nurse provider (nurse generalist or specialist), and length of follow-up. More than the routine allowable for home visits may be reimbursable for a patient, but this must be negotiated between provider and insurer.

Research is needed to determine: the nature, intensity, and length of transitional services required to optimize patient and family outcomes; the profile of patients who would benefit most from these services; the type and level of providers needed to deliver these services; and the costs of such services. Continued study of existing and emerging models of transitional care also is necessary to determine which of these models achieves the highest quality and most cost-effective outcomes.

Study findings suggest that, for selected patient groups or subgroups, discharge planning and home care protocols designed to meet their unique needs are more effective than the general protocols designed for all patients that is currently used by many hospitals and home care agencies. Targeted protocols should be derived from empirical data regarding the unique needs of specific patient groups and their caregivers after hospital discharge. Transitional care protocols should be based on an empirical understanding of the nature of the patients' and caregivers' needs (e.g., lack of knowledge, complexity of therapeutic regimen), strengths (e.g., supportive family) or barriers (e.g., language) to meeting needs, timing of needs (e.g., 24 hours after discharge), most cost-effective strategy to meet needs (e.g., telephone contact vs. home visit), and length of follow-up needed. Unfortunately, for many patient groups, this research base is limited. For these patient groups, research efforts should be targeted first at identifying patients' and caregivers' needs and subsequently at the design and testing of interventions to meet their unique needs.

There is a need for studies that compare and contrast existing and emerging models of transitional care, focusing on differences in both processes and outcomes of care. Knowledge generated from studies of these models would contribute to the ongoing discussion and debate about which providers are most effective and efficient in coordinating transitional care services and providing continuity of care for patients and their caregivers. Study findings also would advance our understanding about effective ways to engage a multidisciplinary team of providers in transitional services. Finally, the knowledge generated from this research would determine the processes of care that available data suggest are important to positive patient outcomes: assessing, communicating, clinical decision making, teaching, collaborating, referring, monitoring, and evaluating.

Dorothy Brooten
Mary Duffin Naylor

Transitions and Health

Nurses provide care to patients and families who are experiencing many kinds of transitions. Developmental transitions (pregnancy, birth, parenthood), situational transitions (immigration, widowhood, relocation), and health/illness transitions (diagnosis of a chronic disease, recovery from surgery, rehabilitation) are examples of the many types of transitions encountered in clinical practice. Transitions also occur in the work setting of nurses and can be classified as organizational transitions. Examples include changes in leadership, new staffing patterns, implementation of new models for nursing care, and structural reorganization. A focus on transitions is so central to nursing practice that it has been argued that the mission of nursing is to facilitate transitions (Meleis & Trangenstein, 1994).

Transition is defined as a passage between two relatively stable periods of time. In this passage the individual moves from one life phase, situation, or status to another. Transitions often are conceptualized in terms of stages in order to capture their movement and direction as they evolve over time. A classic description of transition stages is found in Bridge's (1991) work. He identified three stages: (a) a period of ending or disconnectedness from what had been before, (b) a neutral period characterized by a sense of disruption and disorientation as well as discovery, and (c) a period of new beginnings in which the individual finds new meanings and a sense of control and challenge. Transitions also can be conceptualized in terms of critical points. Critical points are turning points that can lead to either healthy or unhealthy outcomes. The identification of stages, critical points, and strategies for coping during the transition experience provides the basis for nursing therapeutics to support healthy transitions processes and outcomes and to prevent unhealthy transitions.

When using a transition framework in clinical practice or research, several universal properties of transitions must be taken into account. First, transitions are precipitated by significant marker events or turning points that require new patterns of response. These markers prompt the recognition that new strategies are needed to handle familiar daily life experiences. Second, transitions are processes that occur over time. Transition processes encompass the period of time from the first anticipation of a transition until a new identity is formed at the completion of the transition. During this process the context, history, and future of the person are important. A sense of disconnectedness from one's familiar world is another universal property of transition. There is often a sense of loss or alienation from what had been familiar and valued. Another property is that transitions involve fundamental changes in one's view of oneself and the world. During transitions, changes in identity, roles, and patterns of behavior occur. New skills, new relationships, and new coping strategies must be developed.

Persons in transition experience a wide range of responses. They may experience losses or gains, suffer from physical debilitation, have lower or higher immune responses, feel an emergence or loss of spirituality, discover new meanings, or experience traumatic stress symptoms. Indicators of a healthy transition include a sense of well-being, the development of a new identity, mastery of new roles, well-being in relationships, harmony with the environment, renewed energy, and positive quality of life. Indicators of unhealthy transitions may be protracted transitional periods or the continuation of responses, such as role insufficiency or isolation, during the transition period. Previous life patterns may be maintained that are incongruent with the demand for new identities and life patterns.

Goals for knowledge development about transitions include increased understanding of the following: (a) the processes and experiences of human beings who are in transition; (b) the nature of life patterns and new identities that emerge during transitions; (c) the processes or conditions that promote healthy transition outcomes; (d) environments that constrain, support, or promote healthy transitions; and (e) the structure and components of nursing therapeutics that deal with transitions (Meleis, 1993). Numerous theories of family, ecology, problem solving, and self-care can be used to facilitate such knowledge development.

Research has begun to contribute to development of knowledge about transitions. Transition frameworks have been used in research to uncover the experiences of persons living with chronic illness, new mothers, patients recovering from surgery, and persons taking on the caregiving role. Nursing therapeutics tested in research include debriefing, transition services, and role supplementation. Further research is needed to identify the types and dimensions of transitions and the consequences of transition for individuals, families, and communities. Because transitions are processes, appropriate research methods include qualitative and longitudinal approaches.

As a discipline, nursing is concerned with the process and the experiences of human beings undergoing transitions where health and perceived well-being are the outcomes (Meleis & Trangenstein, 1994). The concept of transition was developed as a framework particularly appropriate for viewing nursing phenomena from the perspective of a human science and a practice-oriented discipline. A transition framework provides a way of understanding human responses to events that affect growth and development, health, and person/environment interaction. A transition framework also provides a focus for understanding the content and timing of nursing interventions. From a transition perspective, both the timing and the duration of nursing interventions are of utmost importance. Further, a transition perspective is focused on clients and nurses as dynamic, changing beings evolving within the context of an environment that may be healthy or unhealthy. During the process of transition, clients experience losses and gains. They need new skills to develop new lifestyles or modify lifestyles, prevent illness or live with illness, and enhance or maintain well-being. Nurses and nurses' actions are instrumental in the process of developing these skills.

In summary, the use of transition as a framework facilitates the development of knowledge related to changes in persons, health, and environment. Within this framework, scholarship should focus on uncovering and explaining patterns of responses and critical points in transitions that require nursing interventions.

AFAF IBRAHIM MELEIS
KAREN L. SCHUMACHER

Triangulation

Triangulation, as it is most commonly used in nursing research, refers to the combination of qualitative and quantitative research methods within a single study. There are a number of approaches to triangulation, and it can serve a number of purposes. According to Duffy (1987), triangulation is "the use of multiple methods, theories, data and/or investigators in the study of a common phenomenon" (p. 130). The term *triangulation* has its roots in surveying and navigation and describes the idea of using known points and angles in a triangular fashion to locate an unknown point. D. Campbell and Fiske (1959) are credited as the first to apply this approach in their use of the multitrait-multimethod matrix to establish convergent validity.

Denzin (1989) identified four different approaches to triangulation: methodological, data, theoretical, and investigator. Methodological triangulation, currently the most commonly used triangulation approach in nursing research, involves the use of two or more different methods within a single study. Denzin points out that this approach can involve within-method or between-method triangulation. E. S. Mitchell (1986) emphasized the need for complementarity in the methods used with this approach. Within-method triangulation refers to the use of several different instruments to measure a construct, for example, the use of the Peabody Picture Vocabulary Test—Revised (PPVT-R) as well as the Kaufman Assessment Battery for Children (KABC) to measure different dimensions of child development. Between-method (also known as across-method) triangulation refers to the use of more than one research method to study a phenomenon, for example, the use of a qualitative approach such as phenomenology in concert with a quantitative approach such as a descriptive survey. Between-method triangulation can be accomplished simultaneously or sequentially.

A second type of triangulation, theoretical triangulation, involves analysis of data using several related yet perhaps contradictory theories or hypotheses. The hypothesis supported by the data can be strongly supported because other theories and hypotheses have been discounted (Mitchell, E. S., 1986). This type of triangulation can be utilized within a quantitative or a qualitative methodology; it seeks to avoid a narrow, specialized interpretation of the data (Denzin, 1989). Denzin described this approach, explaining that theoretical triangulation encourages an awareness of the multiple ways data can be interpreted.

A third type, data triangulation, involves data collected from different sources. A fourth type of triangulation is investigator triangulation. Denzin (1989) suggested that the use of more than one data collector helps to ensure the reliability of the data and the uses of multiple analysts to interpret the data guards against the risk of bias associated with only one point of view. E. S. Mitchell (1986) added a fifth variety of triangulation, multiple triangulation, or the combining of two or more types of triangulation, for example, the use of methodological, data and investigator triangulation within a single study.

Originally, triangulation was carried out mainly for purposes of confirmation. Confirmation is analogous to convergent validity and refers to the idea that through the use of multiple methods, data sources, or investigators, a single, obvious conclusion or representation of reality can be researched. Recently, triangulation has been conducted to achieve completeness. This approach can illuminate many of the individual facets of a multidimensional construct. These researchers used qualitative and quantitative methods as they sought both confirmation and completeness in their study of families with a critically ill child. However, not all scholars agree with the notion of triangulation for completeness.

E. S. Mitchell (1986) identified a number of concerns with multiple triangulation that also apply to other triangulation approaches. First, Mitchell noted that a common unit of analysis is essential in any form of triangulation. Second, some forms of triangulation, especially data and investigator triangulation, can be especially costly in terms of time and money. In addition, triangulation places special demands on the investigator because combining methods requires, as Mitchell noted, "a broad knowledge base in research methodology including both qualitative and quantitative methods" (p. 24). Perhaps the greatest challenge of triangulation, however, is found in the area of analysis. Mitchell noted that analysis in a triangulated study presents special challenges, such as the difficulties of combining numerical and textual data. Problems can also arise in interpreting divergent results from these types of data and in weighing data collected from different sources and from different methods.

In spite of these challenges, triangulation of method, data, theories, or investigators can be an important tool in developing nursing science. The concepts of interest to nursing are generally complex, multidimensional human constructs and are difficult to examine by means of a singular research approach. Triangulation is a means to a deeper understanding of these constructs.

THERESA STANDING

U

Uncertainty in Illness

Uncertainty in illness has been defined by Mishel (1988) as the inability to determine the meaning of illness-related events; this occurs in situations where the decision maker is unable to assign definite value to objects and events or is unable to accurately predict outcomes due to lack of sufficient cues. The uncertainty theory by Mishel explains how uncertainty develops in patients with an acute illness and how it is proposed that patients deal with uncertainty. Mishel further defined the original theory to refer to chronic illness in 1990.

Uncertainty regarding an illness has been identified as the greatest single psychological stressor for the patient with a life-threatening illness (Koocher, 1984). Uncertainty is not the total experience in acute and chronic illness, yet it is a constant occurrence from diagnosis through living with a long-term illness or condition. Study of uncertainty dates back to some of the early work by Davis (1960), where he detailed the difference between clinical and functional uncertainty and tied the experience to the delivery of care and the agenda of health care providers. From 1960 through 1974, other classic pieces on uncertainty emerged, which included the work by McIntosh (1974, 1976) on the desire for information among patients with cancer. This work provided some of the first ideas about the ambiguity surrounding diagnosis and prognosis and the impact of this ambiguity upon the patient's psychological state. Work by Wiener in 1975 explored the topic of uncertainty in chronic illness. This classic work on living with uncertainty brought home the invasion of uncertainty into multiple aspects of life and the strategies to tolerate the uncertainty.

Since the publication of the Mishel Uncertainty in Illness Scale (MUIS) (Mishel, 1981), the Parents Perception of Uncertainty Scale (PPUS) (Mishel, 1983b), the exploration of uncertainty scales for specific populations (Mishel, 1983a), along with early conceptualization of the variable within illness (Mishel, 1981), the study of uncertainty has expanded considerably. Both qualitative and quantitative work in nursing and in other fields added to the knowledge on uncertainty in illness. The research has spread to practice through clinical publications (Hilton, 1992; Righter, 1995; Wurzbach, 1992). A second instrument on uncertainty in illness has been developed by Hilton (1994). This instrument is based on the stress and coping framework by Lazarus and Folkman (1984) and is not derived from a nursing theory of uncertainty in illness.

A number of reviews of the research on uncertainty in illness have been published. The first review by Mast (1995) used the uncertainty in illness theory as the framework for the review of research on uncertainty. Similarly the two reviews by Mishel (1997 and 1999) also used the Uncertainty in Illness theory published in 1988 as the framework for review although Mishel (1999) also included the uncertainty theory published in 1990 to evaluate the qualitative work done on uncertainty in chronic illness. Stewart and Mishel (2000) reviewed the research on parent and child uncertainty. Other recent reviews of the research and theory on uncertainty include the review by Neville (2003) with a focus on application to orthopedic conditions and the chapter by Barron (2000) on stress, uncertainty, and health. Further work on the concept of uncertainty, has been published by McCormick (2002) and by Babrow (2001) from the field of health communication. Discussion of the theory of uncertainty has appeared in two sources on nursing theory (Aligood & Tomey, 2002; Mishel & Clayton, 2003).

As noted by Barron (2000) and Mishel (1997), there has been a strong interest in the study of uncertainty; however, most of it has been atheoretical. Most of the quantitative studies of uncertainty in illness have used one of Mishel's uncertainty scales, but the selection of variables had not been tied to the theory of uncertainty in illness. Most of the research has been on uncertainty in specific clinical populations, with the predominance of the quantitative research on acute illness and with more qualitative work on chronic illness. This may be due to the focus of the uncertainty scales on acute illness and hospitalization, with less accurate measurement available for the study of chronic illness.

In the study of uncertainty, most of the studies are cross-sectional and the findings are associative, although the analyses in many studies are often considered predictive when causal modeling is used. At this time, some consistent findings have emerged. Across all illnesses studied to date, uncertainty decreases over time and returns on illness recurrence or exacerbation, and uncertainty is highest or most distressing while awaiting a diagnosis. Current evidence is strong for the role of social support in reducing uncertainty among those with an acute illness. Due to consensus of the findings, if further research is done in this area, it should be focused on building on what is known instead of repeating similar findings.

Concerning the role of personality dispositions as antecedents of or modifiers of uncertainty, the evidence is not solid. In acute illness, there is some support for mastery in a mediating role, but the study of personality dispositions related to uncertainty has been limited to a small number of studies, all with cancer patients receiving treatment. Other acute illnesses require study in order to see which personality dispositions are associated with uncertainty and at which phase in the illness experience. Further research is necessary to determine if the acuity of illness immobilizes personality variables and whether they come into play during the recovery phase or during the management of continual uncertainty in chronic illness.

In chronic illness, interesting findings are emerging from quantitative studies of perceived personal control as a personality disposition for influencing uncertainty and the relationship between uncertainty and mood state. Likewise, spirituality is also being studied for its potential in modifying the impact of uncertainty in mood. Both of these avenues of study are important and point out that in a long-term illness, personality dimensions may come into play for their ability to reduce uncertainty or to reduce the negative impact of uncertainty.

Studies of coping with uncertainty in persons with acute illness have resulted in consistent findings for the relationship between uncertainty and emotion-focused coping. In order to determine if a broader range of coping strategies exists, attention needs to be given to developing instruments that are related to the problem under study. If coping strategies were derived from the setting and population, results may differ from those consistently accrued from global measures of coping.

There is sufficient evidence that uncertainty has a negative impact on quality of life and psychosocial adjustment in acute illness populations. Uncertainty has consistently been found to be related to depression, anxiety, poorer quality of life, less optimism, and negative mood states. Since the evidence is consistent and strong it provides direction for interventions to target outcome variables. There is some evidence for the effectiveness of supportive educational interventions in modifying the adverse outcomes from uncertainty. Recently, interventions for managing uncertainty in breast and prostate cancer have been published reporting strong intervention effect (Braden, Mishel, Longman, & Burns, 1998; Mishel et al., 2002). Repeated testing of these interventions and the development of other theory and research-based interventions that build on the body of existing descriptive research should be the direction of future research.

In chronic illness, the work on management of uncertainty has been enriched by the qualitative investigations where a variety of management methods have been found across a number of chronic illnesses. In contrast to the limited and ineffective coping strategies reported from the use of standardized scales, the findings from qualitative studies indicate that people are very resourceful in finding approaches for living with enduring uncertainty. More research is needed in this area with an attempt to replicate findings across studies so that support for particular strategies can emerge. At the present time, the findings are scattered with no attempt to relate findings from one study to another.

In conclusion, the research on the concept of uncertainty continues to spread across disciplines and countries. Today the uncertainty in illness scales have been translated into more languages and the research continues across all continents.

MERLE H. MISHEL

Unified Language Systems

A unified language system is a network of linked terms that allows integration of existing sets of machine-readable terms, such as thesauri, classification systems, and nomenclatures for the purposes of information retrieval. Whereas a *uniform* language system would necessitate that a common set of terms is utilized for multiple purposes, a *unified* language system builds on the strengths of existing systems that have been designed from a variety of perspectives and for a broad range of purposes. The primary unified language systems of relevance to nursing are the Unified Medical Language System (UMLS) and the Unified Nursing Language System (UNLS).

In 1986 the National Library of Medicine began a long-term research and development project to build the UMLS, utilizing the strategy of successive approximations of the capabilities ultimately desired. The UMLS currently comprises four knowledge sources: the *Metathesaurus*, the *Semantic Network*, the *SPECIALIST Lexicon*, and the *Information Sources Map*. All sources are available via the Internet through the Knowledge Source Server.

The *Metathesaurus* is a database of information on concepts that appear in at least one of a set of controlled source vocabularies. Thirty source vocabularies provide the 252,892 concepts and 542,723 concept names in the 1996 *Metathesaurus* (http://wwwlst.nlm.nih.gov:8000/Docs). These include Medical Subject Headings (MeSH), *International Classification of Diseases: Clinical Modification*, and SNOMED International. Four systems specifically designed for use by nurses are source vocabularies in the Metathesaurus: the North American Nursing Diagnosis Association (NANDA) *Taxonomy 1*, the *Omaha System*, the *Georgetown Home Health Care Classification*, and the *Nursing Intervention Classification* (NIC). The *Metathesaurus* is organized by concept, with entries connecting alternative names for the same concept (e.g., synonyms, lexical variants, translations) from different vocabularies. Thus, shortness of breath, breathlessness, and dyspnea share a common concept identifier but different lexical identifiers in the *Metathesaurus*.

The UMLS *Semantic Network* provides a consistent categorization of concepts represented in the *Metathesaurus* and a set of relationships between the concepts. The 1996 version includes 135 semantic types (http://wwwlst.nlm.nih.gov:8000/Docs). Concepts are broadly categorized into the semantic types of entity or event. Examples of semantic types of relevance to nursing are "Finding," "Individual Behavior," "Therapeutic or Preventive Procedure," and "Disease or Syndrome." The primary relationship among concepts is "IS_A," for example, "Pain Management IS_A Therapeutic or Preventive Procedure." Other relationships include temporal—for example, "Diabetes Mellitus PRECEDES Diabetic Retinopathy"—and causal, for example, "CMV Retinitis is CAUSED_BY cytomegalovirus."

The *SPECIALIST Lexicon* comprises a set of commonly used English and biomedical terms. Entries include the base form of the term and its lexical variants, for example, *assess*, *assesses*, and *assessed*. The *Information Sources Map* describes the publicly available databases of the National Library of Medicine and selected expert systems and databases from outside the National Library of Medicine.

The American Nurses Association Steering Committee on Databases to Support Nursing Practice has endorsed the concept of a unified nursing language system within the structure of the UMLS. The nursing care elements of the nursing minimum data set (NMDS) define the data elements of a UNLS: nursing diagnosis, nursing intervention, nursing outcome, and nursing care intensity (see Table 1). The current UNLS comprises the four nursing systems in the UMLS: NANDA *Taxonomy 1*, the *Omaha System*, the *Georgetown Home Health Care Classification*, and NIC. Extensive research is underway to enhance and refine the existing UNLS, for example, the *Nursing Intervention Lexicon and Taxonomy*, the *Patient Care Data Set*, the *Nursing Outcomes Classification*, and the *International Classification of Nursing Practice*.

SUZANNE BAKKEN

Unlicensed Assistive Personnel

Unlicensed assistive personnel (UAP) is an "unlicensed individual who is trained to function in an assistive role to the licensed nurse" (American Nurses Association, 1992). UAPs provide direct and indirect patient care that has been delegated and is supervised by a registered nurse. Known by a variety of names and practicing in distinctly different sites—Patient Care Assistant (PCA), Nurse Extender (NE), or nurse partner in acute care; Certified Nurse Assistant (CNA) in nursing homes; Resident Assistant (RA) in assisted living residences; Personal Care Attendant (PCA) or Home Care Aide (HCA) in home care; aide, orderly, etc.—job qualifications, training, and nursing activities vary widely. The purpose of this entry is to describe recent studies about UAPs conducted by nurse researchers.

There is a dearth of published information about the content, duration, and effectiveness of UAP-training in acute and home care (including assisted living). In the nursing home (NH) sector, mandatory education and training curricula are set by the federal government and can be no less than 75 hours. Topics include personal care of the elderly person (i.e., activities of daily living [ADLs]), com-

TABLE 1 Elements of NMDS in Systems Comprising the Current UNLS

System	Diagnosis	Intervention	Outcome
NANDA	x		
Omaha	x	x	x
Georgetown	x	x	x
NIC		x	

munication and culture, age-related changes, resident rights, and death and dying. R. A. Burns (1995) reported that this curriculum was sufficient for standard care, but additional hours were needed for CNA-delivered care in subacute special care units. In assisted living (AL) and home care, each state regulates training and curricula. In acute care, it is institution-directed and ranges from 1.5 to 6 weeks, including on unit orientation (Barczak & Spunt, 1999). There is considerable variation in level of required education; only some hospitals require that UAPs have a high school diploma (Bernreuter & Cardona, 1997). A medication administration training program for aides in Maryland AL facilities attributed the successful completion rate and scores on the final examination to high school education (Spellbring & Ryan, 2003). A study of the relationship between literacy skills and job performance found that NH aide literacy was between 5th and 6th grade level (Benjamin, 1995). It is unknown whether or how this might affect reading and comprehension of a written nursing plan of care in any setting.

In their review of studies of UAP implementation in acute care, Bernreuter and Cardona (1997) noted that nurse managers and staff nurses feel that UAPs lack ADL and supportive skills, but had been adequately trained in technical skills. Yet, some nurses feel that training is inadequate, inconsistent, relies too heavily on on-unit training, and fails to teach UAPs how to recognize patient problems.

In most NHs, CNAs constitute 70% of the nursing staff. This has been standard practice for decades although some states regulate the CNA-to-resident ratio. Primary nursing was never a delivery model. The workload for NH CNAs has increased due to staffing cutbacks associated with reimbursement, the nursing shortage, and higher acuity residents. However, quality of care is compromised and turnover increases when CNAs lack time to deliver care, are unsure how to prioritize, and "cut corners" (Bowers & Becker, 1992; Foner, 1994). Nurses and CNAs disagree about the likelihood of implementing individualized care plans (a goal of care), but both groups agree that barriers include inadequate staffing and poor communication (Walker, T., Porter, Gruman, & Michalski, 1999). Hartig (1998) reported that CNAs' and RNs' assessments of residents' functional status were highly correlated but also found that institutionally ascribed "expert" CNAs were performing nursing tasks that exceeded their training and education.

Hospital restructuring, job redesign, and adding UAPS to the skill mix in acute care are attributed to cost containment, managed care, and more recently the shortage of licensed professional nurses. Proponents argue that UAPs free nurses to meet "higher-level" patient care needs. As such, UAPs are assuming more of the bedside, task-based care. In some settings, UAPs draw bloods, take and interpret EKGs, suction and administer respiratory treatments, and perform catheterization. More commonly in acute care than in nursing homes, and most probably in home care, UAPs take blood pressures, perform catheterization, nasopharanygeal and tracheostomy suctioning and trach care, phlebotomy, and enteral tube feeding (Barzak & Spunt, 1999).

An American Nurses Association (ANA) statement to the IOM (Institute of Medicine, 1996) held that reducing RNs and adding UAPs increased costs in many cases related to training UAPs and training RNs for delegation and supervisory roles. The anticipated cost-savings by using UAPs in the delivery of nursing care is equivocal; some studies report reduced costs, others report increased costs, and others are budget neutral (Huston, 1997; McClung, 2000). Most studies fail to incorporate or calculate UAP turnover and training costs, off-unit time for RNs to learn delegation and management skills, and cost reductions (or increases) among ancillary services if UAPs assume, for example, responsibilities for blood specimen collection or food tray distribution (Bernreuter & Cardona, 1997; Zimmerman, 2000). The absence of an accepted methodology to calculate productivity and the failure to recognize variables that could have an impact on costs, productivity, and quality weaken the validity of findings of virtually all studies of cost-effectiveness of UAPs in acute care.

Not surprisingly, UAPs want to be treated with respect, thanked for doing a good job or going the extra mile, and not be thought of as interested only in their paycheck (Burke, Summers, & Thompson, 2001). Responding to an investigator-designed survey (validity and reliability not reported), CNAs felt that poor team communication and negative staff attitudes were barriers to improved care (Curry, Porter, Michalski, & Gruman, 2000). They also felt that they were not respected by other team members and that their suggestions about individualized care were not valued or given a try. These findings were similar to those reported in a study to implement a prompted voiding program in a nursing home in which CNAs were directly responsible (Lekan-Rutledge, Palmer, & Belyea, 1998). Nursing home CNAs feel that communication within the health care team and decisions about care should include the CNAs who, after all, spend more time with the resident than the licensed nurses (Harrington, Carillo, & Wellin, 2001).

Nurses feel they are not prepared to delegate or supervise and are concerned about their legal liability and loss of protection under the collective bargaining provisions of the National Labor Relations Act once they are designated as a supervisor (Huston, 2001). Most, but not all, Boards of Nursing of the 50 states have guidelines for UAP supervision by RNs, but few boards use the ANA or National Council of State Board's (NCSBN) definitions of delegation or assignment (Thomas, S. A., Barter, & McLaughlin, 2000). Most state boards created their own definitions and parameters for delegation and had no plans to standardize UAP training curriculum.

The single largest concern of RNs in institutional settings is the relationship between staff mix and quality of care; this is echoed by consumers as well (Zimmerman, 2000). Notwithstanding that UAPs are responsible for accurate observation, reporting, and documentation of patient status, and are accountable for the nursing tasks delegated to them, several studies found that as the number of RNs in hospital staffing decreased and were replaced by UAPs, adverse clinical outcomes increased (Blegen, Goode, & Reede, 1998; Eastwood & Schechtman, 1999; Huston, 2001; IOM, 1996; Kovner & Gergen, 1998; Zimmerman, 2000). Among the negative outcomes were medication errors, inappropriate use of physical restraints, pressure ulcers, increased mortality rates, patient falls, and postsurgical complications (e.g., pneumonia, UTI). Huston suggested that her finding of less effective pain relief for hospitalized patients with diagnostic related grouping (DRG) 209 (joint and limb reattachment) who were receiving nurse-administered analgesia might be attributed to changes in the staffing mix. On the other hand, M. J. Ventura (1999) reported that hospital RNs felt that UAPs contributed to quality of care.

Sophisticated research designs are needed to look at the complex relationships and factors with a multilevel nursing staff, the most prominent being delegation, achievement needs, communication and interpersonal relations, competency and performance evaluation, and cost-effectiveness. Virtually nothing is known about the number of UAPs who choose to study professional nursing (RN and LPN) and the barriers and facilitators to that movement. Studies of delegation must account for the variables embedded in resources and systems that can affect outcomes.

ETHEL L. MITTY
MIA KOBAYASHI

Urban Health Research: Nursing Research in Urban Neighborhoods

Urban communities are home to heterogeneous ethnic, age, and socioeconomic groups, populations that make up a large share of the underserved in this county. These underserved populations face daunting hurdles that challenge their ability to maintain healthy lifestyles. Moreover, urban environments may provide limited or inaccessible support for individuals seeking health-promotion and disease-prevention information and services. Many urban environments are marred by poverty, strained school systems, crowded housing, unemployment, a pervasive drug culture, periodic street violence, and high levels of stress. Some health issues resulting from the urban environment include high rates of HIV infections and AIDS, increased morbidity and mortality due to violence, increased morbidity and mortality secondary to substance abuse, the resurgence of infectious diseases (tuberculosis and hepatitis B), chronic illness, and maternal/child health problems.

Many of the health problems experienced by residents in urban neighborhoods are preventable, at least in part, through lifestyle changes. Steps also can be taken to reduce health disparities through early identification and treatment. Unfortunately, statistics demonstrate that urban populations do not routinely receive early screening and preventive health care.

When thinking about what *urban* means, nurses are confronted with a number of images, ranging from shining tall buildings, greater opportunities for employment, upscale housing, and community parks to dilapidated buildings, vacant lots sewn with rubble, high rates of unemployment, congested expressways, youth gangs, drug dealers and drug addicts, and, most of all, people. Perhaps the images include the stark difference between cultures—African, Asian, Caribbean, European, Hispanic, Middle Eastern—expressing the diversity and cosmopolitan atmosphere of everyday life in big cities. In some cases the images are those of opportunity; in others, of despair. Historically, urban images in the United States have tended to oscillate between the positive (cities as innovative, progressive, and modern) and the negative (cities as alienated, pathological, and decadent). Today, popularly depicted urban images include culture, arts, and music; recreation and leisure; and the hustle and bustle of commerce, as well as violent crime, rampant drug abuse, crumbling infrastructure, transportation gridlock, and pollution. These images not only depict sharp contrasts between rich and poor but suggest that the worst states of health are found among urban dwellers exposed to substandard housing, poverty, unemployment, and drug abuse.

The process of attaching meaning to these images is multifaceted. However, there is no consensus on a common definition of *urban*. Most definitions include an interrelationship between people (demography) and space: political and administrative boundaries, social and cultural arrangements, economic and technological restructuring. The process of urbanization in the United States has resulted in political, social, economic, environmental, and health changes; at the same time, political, social, economic, environmental, and health changes have influenced the process of urbanization. Urbanization is a dynamic process, and its effects on health are seen and felt in different ways within particular cities and across the nation.

Striking disparities in health outcomes among urban populations provide compelling evidence of the significant health risk these groups experience. The health outcomes described below are observed in nonurban populations but are disproportionally seen in urban populations.

Chronic Illnesses

Hypertension and heart disease: Thirty-eight percent of Blacks suffer from hypertension; of those, only 25% are managing their disease.

Obesity: Forty-four percent of Black and Latino women ages 20 and older are obese, compared to 27% for all women and 37% for low-income women.

Diabetes: The disease is 33% more common among Blacks than among the general population. Latino and Native American populations report elevated morbidity rates from diabetes, often exacerbated by poor nutrition and exercise habits.

Cancer: Major disparity in cancer rates exist among Blacks, Latinos, Native Americans, the elderly, and poor Americans. Failure to screen is often due to fatalism, lack of knowledge, or limited access.

General health habits: Poor nutrition, smoking, alcohol and drug abuse, minimal exercise and stress management, along with other risk factors, appear to be more common among persons with low incomes, who tend to be urban residents.

Violence

Men, young adults, and teenagers within minority populations, particularly Blacks and Latinos, are most likely to be murder victims.

Domestic violence accounts for one of six homicides, particularly among young adults and Blacks.

Child abuse cases make up a significant portion of urban violence, affecting mostly poor families.

Maternal and Child Health

Black, Native American, and Latino infants have the highest morbidity and mortality rates in the United States. Low-birthweight Black babies account for most of these deaths, but even normal-weight Black babies have a greater risk of death.

Asthma risk is increased for poor, minority urban residents, both initial attacks and exacerbations. Environmental factors such as air pollution and cockroach allergens have been correlated with emergency room visits for asthma.

Teen pregnancy has risen for all girls, particularly among poor and ethnic minority groups, with significant social, economic, and health consequences.

HIV and AIDS

The rates of AIDS among Blacks and Latinos are more than triple that of the general population.

Women and their children are one of the largest groups infected.

Sexually active teens are a fast-growing population at risk for HIV infection.

Urban Health Research focuses on the following processes, which form a circular link:

Identifying methodologies and models for developing culturally sensitive research approaches, data collection instruments, and program evaluation instruments.

Building partnerships with community members, nurses, and other health professionals who have community-based practices and with transdisciplinary researchers to identify and prioritize urban health issues that need investigating.

Determining the most effective, culturally sensitive health-promotion and disease-prevention intervention strategies and best-practice models for the targeted urban setting.

Implementing the most effective health-promotion and disease-prevention intervention strategies and best-practice models within the targeted urban community while simultaneously collecting evaluation data that will be used to modify the implementation process as needed.

As nurses we must be concerned about how the issues of urbanization affect the health of urban communities. Residents of such communities are the most reliable sources for this information. However, they are not likely to volunteer this information either because of distrust of researchers or the perception that their opinions or facts are not valued by nurses or researchers. Hence, one of the early steps in the urban health research process is to empower and recruit urban community members, especially minorities, to become active research partners, not just participants, in research programs.

The overall goal of urban-related nursing research is to integrate scientific knowledge, professional skill, community input and support, and political advocacy of health promotion and disease prevention in an effort to create and maintain healthy urban communities. To achieve this goal, nurse researchers in urban settings, with community input, must seek to develop, test, and disseminate health care interventions, tailored to address the major urban health care issues, that are found to be scientifically sound, culturally relevant, and effective. Once identified, the urban-related nursing research process continues with the implementation of effective interventions and best practices within the community while maintaining overall health care costs. When logistically feasible, it is advisable to take the programs or practices to the target populations because this approach tends to foster participant.

Nurses can meet the challenges of addressing the needs of urban community residents by using a multidimensional approach that focuses on their social, psychological, biological, and environmental needs. Historically, nurses have viewed the recipients of their care in a holistic manner, taking into account all domains that have an impact on their lives. This approach is particularly useful with urban minority populations, who tend to experience many different stressors and who also tend to value the interpersonal process.

Through innovative research projects, innovative educational programs, and new strategies for providing services, we can meet their needs. For today, urban health is a priority. With the recent economic trend that is moving health care from hospitals to the community, current nursing students are being prepared to shift their work setting to the community and to interact with clients in their "home environment." This educational preparation should result in better health care as well as stronger client advocacy, another important aspect in the process. Nurses in the future will increasingly work in community-based settings such as homeless shelters, community clinics, small independent practices, schools, and church clinics.

To summarize, for programs of nursing research to be effective in urban communities the researcher must do the following:

- Design programs that are based on a comprehensive needs assessment, including an identification of the target population.
- Make programs accessible and affordable to the target population.
- Ensure that the programs are culturally competent and relevant to the target population (i.e., consistent with norms, attitudes, beliefs, and attitudes). Members of the target populations should be included in program design, implications, and evaluation.
- Ensure that the programs are consistent with the social and community norms of the target population so that program participants will receive consistent messages and reinforcement for the prescribed health behavior plan.
- Address the linguistic needs of the target population (i.e., with translators and health and education reading materials in the community's native language and at the appropriate reading levels).
- When applicable, ensure that programs meet the needs of the deaf and hearing-impaired members of the target population, as well as those with developmental disabilities.

Residents of urban communities have numerous health care challenges. Fortunately, nurses with the proper education and training can emerge to provide excellent compassionate and innovative care and to design culturally competent and theory-driven intervention that will produce positive healthy outcomes. One advantage of meeting this need is the fact that most schools of nursing are located in urban communities, which enhances the interaction between and among nurses, community members, and researchers. Nurse researchers are not the only ones who benefit from such interaction; students and the people in the community also benefit. Nursing research projects designed and implemented by building bridges with the community can provide the most efficacious and cost-effective community-based health care.

LORETTA SWEET JEMMOTT
EMMA J. BROWN

Urinary Incontinence

Urinary Incontinence (UI) is the involuntary loss of urine that creates a social or hygienic problem. It is a common health concern for women (Sampselle et al., 1997). More than 20 million adults are estimated to have UI or Overactive Bladder (OAB). Between 15% and 30% of adult women experience UI, and the prevalence is even greater in the elderly population. UI is present in half the older residents at nursing homes, and in 13% to 56% of home-bound elders (Anonymous, 2003). The Agency for Healthcare Policy and Research (AHCPR) believes that UI was underreported, underdiagnosed, and undertreated in the 1990s. Although Urinary Incontinence is common, it is not a part of the normal aging process and is therefore considered abnormal despite the large numbers of people whose lives are affected by it.

Stress Incontinence is most common in older women. Stress incontinence occurs when urine leaks during lifting, exercise, coughing, sneezing, or laughing. Weakness of the pelvic floor allows the proximal urethra and bladder base to be pushed out of the pelvis during these periods of increased abdominal pressure, resulting in leakage. This type of UI may also be caused by decreased estrogen levels after menopause. Overflow Incontinence is more common among older men, especially those with enlarged prostate glands, which creates constriction of the tube through which urine drains from the bladder. This results in a constant dripping of urine and strained urination.

Urge Incontinence, common in elderly people, occurs when, having had the urge to urinate, the ability to do so is lost, or the need to urinate comes before arriving at the bathroom. An overactive bladder causes involuntary bladder muscle contractions. Some medical conditions, such as stroke, multiple sclerosis, and Parkinson's disease, can cause urge incontinence.

Functional Incontinence occurs when bladder function is normal, but the physical act of getting to a bathroom is hampered, either by cognitive impairment or physical disability. Such conditions impair an individual's ability to appropriately respond to their cues to void. Severe arthritis and severe dementia are examples of hindrances which cause functional incontinence.

Mixed Incontinence is a combination of bladder and urethral dysfunction which causes stress and urge incontinence to occur together.

With a greater understanding among the general population that UI is a treatable medical condition, an increasing number of women are reporting incontinence and seeking treatment. Screening for UI is appropriate at any age but is especially so for older adults due to its increased prevalence in this population. In fact, the at-risk population includes those with immobility, impaired cognition, medications, morbid obesity, environmental barriers, high-impact physical activities, diabetes, stroke, estrogen depletion, and/or pelvic muscle weakness (Dowling-Castronova, 2001).

The economic costs of urinary incontinence in America have been estimated at more than $15 billion annually. There are costs other than economic as well: skin breakdown and infection resulting from rashes and pressure ulcers, urinary tract infections, anxiety, depression, low self-esteem, and social isolation (Johnson, S., 2000). In the nursing home, the economic costs have been estimated to be close to $5 billion annually, including costs associated with staff, laundry, and supplies. UI may also lead to falls among residents with nocturia, urge incontinence, and impaired balance or gait (Ouslander & Schnelle, 1995).

Nursing has traditionally supported behavioral approaches to incontinence management. They include inhibition training (wherein the goal is to eliminate unwanted bladder contractions by decreasing the use of bladder irritants such as caffeine, alcohol, artificial sweeteners, pepper, spicy foods, etc), active bladder relaxation (wherein movement is avoided), general relaxation, and contracting of the pelvic muscles until the urgency sensation goes away and it becomes "safe" to go to the bathroom. The key to success is to not move when the urgency sensation occurs. With the bladder training technique, the patients are to keep a record and show some ability to control urgency. There are three components to bladder training—comprehensive patient education, timed but progressively lengthened voiding intervals, and positive reinforcement (Krissovich & Safran, 1997). Pengelly and Booth (1980) reported, in a prospective trial that included 12 weeks of bladder training, that more than half of the 25 participants who completed the program were completely cured or improved, and that none got worse.

Pelvic Muscle rehabilitation (Kegel exercises) involves using the pelvic floor muscles to regain control over lower urinary tract function. Pelvic muscle strengthening and active use of the pelvic muscles to prevent urge or stress incontinence are key components of this approach. Programs of pelvic muscle exercise have proven to increase muscle strength and reduce incontinent urine loss. Dougherty and colleagues (1993), in a study of 65 women aged 35–75 years, found significant improvement in force (25%) and duration (40%) of muscle contraction, as well as significant reduction (62%) in the amount of urine leakage and reported episodes of incontinence, after a 16-week course of pelvic muscle exercise. Biofeedback Training, which involves electronic and mechanical instruments to relay messages to patients about their physiologic conditions, is known as the most effective method of achieving pelvic muscle rehabilitation. Other methods for augmenting pelvic muscle training include electrical stimulation and vaginal weights. Two randomized controlled trials using 6-week treatment periods reported 70% and 87% cure or significant improvement rates with behavioral therapies (Krissovich & Safran, 1997).

The importance of treating incontinence cannot be overlooked because incontinence impacts psychologically as well as physiologically. Researchers have shown a direct relationship between incontinence and depression as patients become less involved in social activities. Ultimately, this could lead to sadness and overwhelming despair. UI may be associated with depression, social isolation, loss of self-esteem, and altered relationships (Castina, Boyington, & Dougherty, 2002). This negative impact may also be felt by the nursing staff and family members. Caregivers often feel overwhelmed and frustrated as a result of the amount of time and staff required by an incontinent patient. Additionally, but often overlooked, is the economic impact resulting from early retirement or an inability to work. Thus, urinary incontinence can be a devastating experience, with serious psychosocial consequences for both the affected individual and the caregiver (Yu, 1987).

ELLA BLOT

V

Validity

Validity refers to the accuracy of responses on self-report, norm-referenced measures of attitudes and behavior. Validity arises from classical measurement theory, which holds that any score obtained from an instrument will be a composite of the individual's true pattern and error variability. The error is made up of random and systematic components. Maximizing the instrument's reliability helps to reduce the random error associated with the scores (see "Reliability"), although the validity of the instrument helps to minimize systematic error. Reliability is necessary but not a sufficient requirement for validity.

Validity and theoretical specification are inseparable, and the conceptual clarification (see "Instrumentation") performed in instrument development is the foundation for accurate measurement of the concept. Broadly stated, validity estimates how well the instrument measures what it purports to measure. Underlying all assessment of validity is the relationship of the data to the concept of interest. This affects the instrument's ability to differentiate between groups, predict intervention effects, and describe characteristics of the target group.

Literature usually describes three forms of validity: content, criterion, and construct. These forms vary in their value to nursing measurement, and unlike reliability, singular procedures are not established that lead to one coefficient that gives evidence of instrument validity. Instead, validity assessment is a creative process of building evidence to support the accuracy of measurement.

Content validity determines whether the items sampled for inclusion adequately represent the domain of content addressed by the instrument. The assessment of content validity spans the development and testing phases of instrumentation and supersedes formal reliability testing. Examination of the content focuses on linking the item to the purposes or objective of the instrument, assessing the relevance of each item, and determining if the item pool adequately represents the content. This process is typically done by a panel of experts, which may include professional experts or members of the target population. Lynn (1986) has provided an excellent overview of the judgment-quantification process of having judges assert that each item and the scale itself is content-valid. The results of the process produce a content validity index (CVI), which is the most widely used single measure for supporting content validity. Content validity should not be confused with the term *face validity*, which is an unscientific way of saying the instrument looks as if it measures what it says it measures. Although content validity is often considered a minor component for instrument validation, researchers have repeatedly found that precise attention to this early step has dramatic implications for further testing.

Criterion validity is the extent to which an instrument may be used to measure an individual's present or future standing on a concept through comparison of responses to an established standard. Examination of the individual's current standing is usually expressed as concurrent criterion validity, although predictive criterion validity refers to the individual's future standing. It is important to note that rarely can another instrument be used as a criterion. A true criterion is usually a widely accepted standard of the concept of interest. Few of these exist within the areas of interest to nursing.

Construct validity has become the central type of validity assessment. It is now thought that construct validity really subsumes all other forms. In essence, construct validation is a creative process that rarely achieves completion. Instead, each piece of evidence adds to or detracts from the support of construct validity, which builds with time and use. Nunnally (1978) proposes three major aspects of construct validity: (a) specification of the domain of observables; (b) extent to which the observables tend to measure the same concept, which provides a bridge between internal consistency, reliability, and validity; and (c) evidence of theoretically proposed relationships between the measure and predicted patterns. The first aspect is similar to content validity and is essentially handled through formalized concept clarification in instrument development. The inclusion of this specification of the domain under construct validity supports the contention that construct validity is the primary form, with other types forming subsets within its boundaries.

The other two aspects of construct validity are examined formally through a series of steps. These steps form a hypothesis-testing procedure in which the hypotheses are based on the theoretical underpinnings of the instrument. Hypotheses can relate to the internal structure of the items on the instrument. Hypotheses can also refer to the instrument's anticipated relationship with other concepts, based on a theoretical formulation. The first set of hypotheses fall into the second aspect of construct validity testing; the latter relate to the third aspect.

Although there are no formalized ways to examine the hypothesis proposed for construct validity testing, some typical approaches have been identified in nursing research. Primarily, the internal structure of an instrument is tested through factor analysis and related factor analytic procedures, such as latent variable modeling. Factor analysis has become one of the major ways in which nursing researchers examine the construct validity of an instrument. It is important to note that this approach addresses only the second aspect of construct validity testing and in itself is insufficient to support the validity of an instrument. Factor analysis simply provides evidence that the underlying factor structure of the instrument is in line with the theoretically determined structure of the construct.

The third aspect of construct validation provides an opportunity for more creative approaches to testing. Hypotheses proposed have to do with the relationship of the concept being measured with other concepts that have established methods of measurement. These hypotheses deal with convergent and discriminate construct validity, subtypes that examine the relationship of the concept under study with similar and dissimilar concepts. If data evidence a strong relationship with similar concepts and no relationship with dissimilar concepts, evidence is built for the construct validity of the instrument. Should data not support similarities and differences, several options are possible: (a) the instrument under construction may not be accurately measuring the concept, (b) the instruments for the other concepts may be faulty, or (c) the theory on which the testing was based may be inaccurate. The multitrait-multimethod (MTMM) matrix has been proposed as a way to formally test convergent and discriminate construct validity.

Another approach to examining the relationship among concepts involves a known group technique. In this method, the researcher hypothesizes that the instrument will provide a certain level of data from groups with known levels on the concept the instrument has been designed to measure.

The above approaches to testing construct validity are only samples of techniques that can be used. As mentioned, construct validity testing is creative. Researchers can design unique ways to support the validity of their instruments. The important point is that whatever is designed must be based in theory and must be intuitively and logically supported by the investigator.

JOYCE A. VERRAN
PAULA M. MEEK

Violence

Violence is a public health problem in the United States that impacts individuals, families, and communities. The U.S. has experienced a downward trend in violence to 23 million violent and property crimes during 2002, but it remains one the most violent countries in the industrialized world (U.S. Department of Justice, Office of Justice Programs, 2003). The violent crime rate decreased from 25 per 100,000 persons aged 12 years and older in 2001 to 23 per 100,000 aged 12 years and older in 2002. The rate of every major violent and property crime declined from 1993 to 2002. Rape/sexual assault decreased 56%, robbery 63%, aggravated assault 64%, simple assault 47%, household burglary 52%, motor vehicle theft 53%, and property theft 49% (U.S. Department of Justice, Office of Justice Programs).

Victims of violence are violated physically, emotionally, psychologically, spiritually, and socially. Nurses are engaged in providing care to victims and perpetrators of violence in a variety of health care settings. Nursing scholarship related to violence recognizes the complex interaction of community factors (inequality, marginalization, disparity, residential mobility, poverty, lack of education, lack of career opportunities, housing, social and cultural norms, stigmatization and bias, and population density) in addition to individual and familial risk factors that require evidence and research-based preventive measures.

Violence and abuse against women (VAAW) have been recognized globally as a public health problem affecting women regardless of age, culture, or socioeconomic status. Types of VAAW consist of physical, psychological, and sexual; various controlling behaviors by perpetrators; stalking; and workplace violence.

Nursing research has grown out of concern for the victim of abuse and has been focused on risk factors, battering syndrome, intimate partner violence, children of battered women, consequences of abuse, relationships of HIV infections and violence, and abuse during pregnancy. A published review of violence research by Campbell, Harris, and Lee (1995) highlighted significant findings in the area of VAAW. Manfrin-Ledet and Porche (2003) published a meta-analysis of the state of the science in the intersections of violence and HIV infection.

Ethical conduct and safety issues in VAAW research are critical. Future research should focus on interventions for preventing and combating VAAW, lifetime health consequences of violence, and long-term effects of VAAW programs using various methodologies in different cultural settings.

Contributions by nurse researchers related to the study of child abuse have focused on shaken baby syndrome, the battered child, health and sociological consequences of child abuse, risk factors, child sexual assault, and neglect. Clements and Burgess (2002) conducted research to understand children's responses to family member homicide and associations with complicated bereavement, including childhood posttraumatic stress disorder. Future research in the area of child abuse must take into account standards and expectations in differing cultures for parenting behavior, the inclusion of cultural issues, and the long-term effects of child abuse, interventions for prevention and treatment, and empowerment strategies for victims of abuse.

Elder abuse and neglect are significantly underdiagnosed and underreported. The National Center on Elder Abuse (n.d.) defines seven different types of elder abuse: physical, sexual, and emotional abuse; financial exploitation; neglect; abandonment; and self-neglect. Elder abuse is largely hidden under a shroud of family secrecy, in addition to the problem of not being recognized by health care providers.

Researchers have developed valid and reliable instruments to identify elders at risk of abuse. Instruments include screening tools for elder abuse or tools whose purpose is to assess existing cases of elder abuse for future risk. Two elder abuse screening tools are the Hwalek-Sengstock Elder Abuse Screening Test (H-S/EAST) and the Indicators of Abuse Screen. Risk assessment tools for future abuse generally contain a list of indicators or conditions which are rated with regard to the elder's risk for future victimization. Typical indicators include client characteristics, environmental risk factors, support services, historical abuse factors and patterns, and abuse factors (Wolf, 2003).

Nursing scholarship by Fulmer and Gurland (1996) has addressed elder mistreatment and elder abuse assessment. Phillips and Rempusheski (1985) studied diagnostic and intervention decisions in elder abuse and neglect.

The epidemic of adolescent violence forces millions, including youth, families, and communities, to cope with injury, disability, and fatality. Homicide is a leading cause of death for adolescents. Two general trajectories have been proposed to explain the development of adolescent violence. One is the development of violence before puberty and another is violence beginning in adolescence. Earlier development, before age 13 years, is generally associated with more violence and more serious crimes over a longer period of time, continuing into adulthood (U.S. Department of Health and Human Services, 2001a).

Risk factors for adolescent violence include involvement in serious criminal activities, substance use before age 13 years, male gender, hostility, low socioeconomic status, antisocial parents, drug selling, weak social bonds to traditional peers, ties to delinquent peers, and gang membership (U.S. Department of Health and Human Services, 2001a).

Adolescent violence is preventable behavior that needs to be understood and treated. However, nursing research related to adolescent violence has been rather limited. Vessey, Duffy, O'Sullivan, and Swanson (2003) have studied teasing, a precursor to bullying, and developed the Physical Appearance Related Teasing Scale-Revised (PARTS-R) instrument to assess teasing in school-age children. Future research in nursing should take into account risk and protective factors among the biological, psychological, and social-contextual aspects of adolescent violence.

Nursing research, practice, health policy, and political activism have all been instrumental in addressing violence as a health phenomenon. Nursing research on violence has advanced the science of violence prevention and treatment. However, more research remains that builds on the body of scholarship available. A variety of methodological approaches, including quantitative and qualitative designs, is called for in future violence research in nursing. Research data about human responses to violence should provide direction for improved health care, nursing care outcomes, and policy.

DANNY G. WILLIS
LINDA MANFRIN-LEDET
DEMETRIUS J. PORCHE

Virginia Henderson International Nursing Library

The Virginia Henderson International Nursing Library is an electronic library whose resources are digital, not physical. It is supported by Sigma Theta Tau International (STTI), the international honor society of nursing, and is housed at the Center for Nursing Scholarship, international headquarters of STTI in Indianapolis, Indiana. The holdings are distributed worldwide via the Internet and the World Wide Web (WWW).

The goal for the Virginia Henderson Library is encompassed in the mission statement of STTI: "to improve the health of people worldwide by improving nursing scholarship." Three of four objectives for achieving this mission speak directly to nursing knowledge: knowledge development, knowledge dissemination, and knowledge utilization. Of all the nursing organizations in the United States, only the International Nursing Library and Sigma Theta Tau together have the unique mission of nursing scholarship.

The Virginia Henderson Library began early in the 1980s under the sponsorship of STTI in response to continuing dissatisfaction with the limitations of extant bibliographic services to locate nursing literature, particularly nursing research and theory. Bibliographic services distribute information about where knowledge might be found, not the knowledge itself (see Bibliographic Retrieval Systems). Addressing this identified need, the library was envisioned as a repository of nursing research, and collection of biographical data and summary information about nurse researchers began almost immediately, forming the core resource of the library. The first *Directory of Nurse Researchers* was printed in 1983.

In 1989 the library was named for one of the most respected nurse leaders, Virginia Henderson, who developed the first nursing research classification system (see Nursing Research Classification Systems). In that same year, the library became a computer-based electronic resource. Over the next decade, the *Directory of Nurse Researchers* evolved into the *Registry of Nursing Research*, changing in intent from the networking and location of other nurse researchers to the intent of registering all nurse researchers and nursing research, including findings.

The Virginia Henderson Library now has many resources, including data, information, and knowledge, which are designed to serve the scholarship and knowledge mission of STTI. Data services include archived nursing research data sets contributed by various researchers. Although these research data sets may be used for teaching research, their primary purpose is for generating knowledge via secondary analysis by qualified students and researchers. Information services include the STTI *International Book Service*, which provides peer reviews of newly published nursing books in partnership with Doody Publishing, Inc., a leading independent reviewer of health science books. Knowledge services include the *Registry of Nursing Research©* and the *Online Journal of Knowledge Synthesis for Nursing©* (OJKSN).

The *Registry of Nursing Research©* is the premier resource of the Virginia Henderson Library to such an extent that library and Registry are sometimes used synonymously, though incorrectly. Both published and fugitive research are sought for the Registry. Rather than the narrative reporting of knowledge as in published scientific journals, the Registry presents research knowledge as data describing researchers, their studies, and the findings generated by the studies. The data base of the Registry is organized by the STTI *Nursing Research Classification System*, third edition. The knowledge (findings) is indexed directly by variable name. Data for the Registry is submitted by researchers with a special registration form on the WWW or on disks for Macintosh and Windows. Minimum information required is biographical data about the researcher and a structured abstract of each study. More data about the study and findings are required of registrants whose work is funded by STTI. In addition, detailed data are requested of researchers who work in a domain that has been identified as a primary focus area by the STTI research and library committees.

The *Online Journal of Knowledge Synthesis for Nursing* provides critical reviews (i.e., narrative meta-analysis, integrative review, qualitative knowledge synthesis) of research pertinent to clinical nursing practice problems. Author teams composed of a clinical specialist and a clinical researcher provide the reviews in an area of expertise and are expected to update the review when required by new knowledge in the area. A traditional peer review process is used. A major difference in the electronic publication format is that distribution takes place within hours of acceptance, rather than the months required to bring a print version of a publication to subscribers. Articles can be printed at the user's local printer or ordered from a document delivery service. In addition to being able to browse the articles, a user can search for a keyword of interest. Such a search produces all articles that contain the keyword. It is anticipated that the *Online Journal of Knowledge Synthesis for Nursing* is only the first of many electronic publications that will be offered by the Virginia Henderson Library.

Communication services offer an electronic conferencing/bulletin board service for networking, group publishing, group bibliographic citation management, and conducting multisite research. These services are all in the support of knowledge development, dissemination, and utilization goals of STTI.

The Henderson International Library is not the only major nursing library in the world; however, it is the only major nursing library that is completely electronic. It is the only library to register details of nursing research and findings. The Registry can be searched by researcher name, keywords, and research variable or concept names. It is the only known library in the world to index research knowledge by variables studied together.

JUDITH R. GRAVES

Vulnerable Populations

Vulnerable human populations have been identified as being at risk for health problems (Aday, 2001). The combined term, VPs, yields an amalgamated description in reference to generalizing all people who are members of a defined class; who are worthy of being hurt, ignored or helped; and, who are connected by action or process. Aday referred to VPs as societal subgroups in the position of being hurt, ignored, and/or helped by others. She claimed all members of human communities are potentially-vulnerable. Flaskerud and Nyamanthi (2002) summarized typical VPs as women, children, ethnic people of color, immigrants, homosexuals, the HIV-infected, chemically-addicted, mentally-impaired, homeless, and elderly. She contended that these groups have increased susceptibility to health adversities due to discrimination and marginalization (Flaskerud & Nyamanthi).

The legal definition of VPs is "those . . . susceptible to coercive or undue influence; including children, prisoners, pregnant women, mentally disabled, and the economically or educationally disadvantaged" (Stone, T. H., 2003). Economically or educationally disadvantaged are considered *invisible* VPs (Stone, T. H.). When coupled to subgroups, the appellation is *doubly* VPs (Moore, L. W., & Miller, 1999).

WHO *Health for All* highlights health data of subgroups; poverty and limited access to care (ATC) are primary contributors to poor health (Hegavary, 2000). HP 2010 Goals to increase quality-of-health years and eliminate health disparities (HD) distinguishes improved ATC as one measure of goal attainment (http://www.health.gov/healthypeople/table of contents/html.vol#1). The NIH Mission focuses on the study of disease prevention and health promotion among diverse populations to reduce HD and improve ATC. The NINR Mission directs: eliminating substantial HD among different segments of the population, inclusive of certain ethnic groups; ATC; incidence of disease; length of life; and mortality rates (http://www.nih.gov/ninr/about/sepmin02.pdf). The American Nurse Association presents key areas for promoting health for all people. These include: policy development, influence public expectation, increase consumer demand for preventative health, and equitable ATC (http://www.nursingworld.org/about/stratpln.htm). These directives defend the relevance of VPs for nursing research (Edelman & Mandle, 2002).

The relevance of VPs to nursing research is critical (Hinshaw, 2000). NIH has targeted studies that recognize certain ethnic groups' risk for disease, tensions mired in HD, lack of ATC, effects of environmental toxins, and increased risk for obesity. In-depth and comparative studies which determine biological and behavioral factors impacting health are required to better understand VPs. Additionally, NIH seeks longitudinal research which evaluates effects of interventions of healthy behavioral change over time (http://www.nih.gov/ninr/about/sepmin02.pdf).

Two researchers have been instrumental in developing frameworks for vulnerable population research. In 1994, Aday (2001) developed a framework that identified VPs as significant contributors in ATC. Unique to the ATC Model are predictors for populations at risk. Predictors include demographics. In 1998, Flaskerud (2002) developed VPs Conceptual Model that postulates interrelationships among resource availability, relative risk, and health status. The Flaskerud Model is unique because empirical indicators predict health status of populations.

In 1999, NINR funded University of California, Los Angeles (UCLA) School of Nursing (SON), Center for Vulnerable Populations Research (CVPR), to unite scholars focused on HD among VPs. Primary investigators include: Deborah Koniak-Griffin, RN, EdD, Director of CVPR, Professor at UCLASON. Her area of expertise is community-based nursing to reduce risk and promote health of VPs, teens, young parents, and families. Adeline Nyamathi, PhD, ANP, is Associate Director of the CVPR and Associate Dean for Academic Programs at UCLASON. Her areas of interests are homeless adults at risk for HIV, TB, and hepatitis; and VPs at risk for HIV in international settings. Jacquelyn Flaskerud, RN, PhD, is Professor Emeritus at UCLASON. Her research interests are cultural beliefs and practices on prevention/treatment of AIDS and mental illness, utilization of health services by VPs, participatory research (PR) methods, and methodological issues in working with culturally diverse populations. Nancy Anderson, PhD, RN, is Professor Emeritus at UCLASON. Her areas of expertise are qualitative research methods, applications of PR methods, and development of culturally proficient research measures and interventions. For additional faculty participating in this project see http://www.ucla.edu/cvpr.

Fundamental to VPs research are issues of ethics involving human subjects (Mann, 2003). Three cautionary accounts were consistent in the literature. First, consent from participants must be obtained postlocal ethics review boards because many members of VPs are minors, have cognitive problems, or are in custody of government. Second, inclusion by self-selection and/or referral may impact sample purity. Self-selected participants may use the study as an opportunity to be less victimized by circumstance. Referrals might be made for the same reasons (Mann; Stone, T. H., 2003). Watchirs (2002) provided an extensive review of methodologies measuring human rights which includes a review of current law for using VPs in PR. Third, and an important ethical concern, is the prospect of direct health-related benefits. If a health problem is identified, an intervention toward positive outcome must be offered (Stone, T. H.).

VPs are social groups with increased risk of altered health. Researchers and law define these groups differently. Data are lacking to substantiate which groups are at most risks. Financial deprivation and limited ATC are related. Vulnerability is evidenced in worldwide trends of lower life expectancy, reduced ATC, and diminished quality of life. The UCLACVPR follows NIH directives to investigate VPs in terms of HD of minorities and those living in poverty. CVPR investigators aim to advance knowledge about VPs, which includes methods of PR which are subject to ethical scrutiny. In designing research with respect to law and ethics, the substantive study of VPs by nursing has the potential to influence world health and improve ATC for all.

Ann M. Stalter

W

Wandering

In 1980, Irene expressed dismay at the lack of a suitable definition of wandering as well as the lack of nursing articles or research on the topic. She cited only five articles on wandering published between 1941 and 1978. Clearly, many nurses have studied this behavior since that time. A CINAHL search for articles published in English under "dementia wandering" located 14,629 citations for 2003 alone. Among the subtopics identified were risk management, staff development, and observational tools.

As might be expected with such a multifaceted topic, definitions are numerous. Aimless locomotion and cognitive impairment were two elements common to most definitions in the 1970s and 1980s. For example, an early definition of wandering was "a tendency to move about, either in a seemingly aimless or disoriented fashion, or in pursuit of an indefinable or unobtainable goal" (Snyder, L. H., Rupprecht, Pyrek, Brekhus, & Moss, 1978, p. 272).

The increased study of wandering has illuminated its complexity. Algase's (1999b) review of 108 wandering studies revealed four dimensions that characterize wandering in dementia patients. To be classified as wandering, the ambulating had to (1) occur often; (2) seem to be aimless, lapping, or random; (3) exceed environmental limits, possibly into hazardous territory; and (4) reflect spatial disorientation or navigational deficits. Some studies differentiate pacing from wandering whereas others treat them as the same or overlapping phenomena (Algase).

The etiology of wandering remains a topic of debate. Proposed explanations range from physical discomfort and unmet needs to right parietal lobe dysfunction. Positive correlations have been found between wandering and cognitive impairment, spatial disorientation, stress, unmet needs, reduced higher order cognitive and planning abilities, and circadian rhythm disturbances.

Wandering can be viewed as meaningless or as an effort to fulfill felt needs that the patient may or may not be able to communicate. Cohen-Mansfield and Werner (1998) asserted that wandering could be both adaptive and appropriate for the cognitively impaired elder. Wandering probably has physical and psychosocial benefits; however, positive outcomes have received less attention that negative consequences. Algase (1999a) used the need-driven behavior model to explain wandering as the result of the interplay of background (relatively fixed variable such as general health status and neurocognitive status) and proximal factors (dynamic individual or environmental variables such as physiological needs).

Studies of personal characteristics of wanderers have produced variable results. Algase's (1999b) review reported no consistent relationships between wandering and gender, education, or race. Factors that correlated positively with wandering included general health, appetite, fewer medications and medical diagnoses, and other "agitated" behaviors. Factors that correlated negatively with wandering were pain and eating impairment. Studies of the impact of premorbid personality, activity level, and stress-coping strategies on wandering have yielded conflicting results.

A limited number of studies on the effects of environmental conditions on wandering have found that wandering increased in the presence of a low noise level, and with normal lighting and temperature (Cohen-Mansfield, Werner, Marx, & Freedman, 1991; Cohen-Mansfield & Werner, 1995).

During the 1980s wandering research primarily addressed the characteristics and behaviors of wanderers and measures to prevent wandering. Physical and chemical restraints commonly were used to control all types of disturbing behaviors. The passage of the Omnibus Budget Reconciliation Act (OBRA) in 1987 that mandated the use of least restrictive interventions for behavioral problems shifted emphasis from preventing wandering to making it safer. The focus of intervention studies has broadened to include environmental adaptations and caregiver approaches, as well as pharmacologic management.

The simplest suggested adaptations create visual illusions. For example, strips of dark tape placed across the floor in front of exit points may appear as gaps that patients are reluctant to cross. A shower curtain over a door and cloths over doorknobs may disguise the exit. Limited research on visual illusions shows that they work with some, but not all, patients (Price, Hermans, & Grimley, 2003). Differences in patient responses to specific adaptations could be attributed to differences in cognitive skills that characterize each stage of dementia among study subjects.

Increased tolerance of wandering, measures to create safer wandering environments, and caregiver education have made drug therapy a last resort in most cases. When wandering is accompanied by agitation, neuroleptics sometimes are used. A major adverse effect with neuroleptics is orthostatic hypotension. The atypical antipsychotics such as risperidone and olanzapine are preferred for older adults because they have fewer side effects than most older neuroleptics (American Geriatric Society Clinical Practice Committee, 2003). One comparative study found slightly fewer side effects with risperidone than with olanzapine in a sample of 730 adults with dementia (Martin, Slyk, Deymann, & Cornacchione, 2003). Cholinesterase inhibitors generally have been found to improve function, especially in the early stage of dementia, and may also reduce behavioral disturbances (Daly, Falk, & Brown, 2001).

In summary, research on wandering continues to elucidate variables and characteristics associated with wandering. However, emphasis on interventions to maintain safety without undue restrictions is receiving increased attention. Continued efforts to identify and meet underlying needs are warranted. Other suggested topics for future studies might focus on (a) assessment and management in various settings including acute care, transitional settings, assisted living, and private residences, and (b) strategies for locating lost wanderers.

ADRIANNE D. LINTON

Watson's Theory of Human Caring

Watson's Theory of Human Caring can be called a treatise, a conceptual model, a framework, or a middle-range theory, which seeks to provide a moral and philosophical basis for nursing. The Theory of Human Caring (Watson, 2001) was developed between 1975 and 1979 as an "attempt to bring meaning and focus to nursing as an emerging discipline and distinct health profession with its own unique values, knowledge, and practices, with its own ethic and mission to society" (p. 344). Many varied, philosophical views held by Nightingale, Henderson, Krueter, Hall, Leininger, Gadow, Peplau, Maslow, Heidegger, Erickson, Lazarus, deChardin and Sarte influenced the development of the Theory of Human Caring. Perennial philosophy, wisdom traditions, quantum physics, and feminist theory also guided the philosophical and intellectual development of the theory (Fawcett, 2000b). These humanities and sciences provided a phenomenological, existential, and spiritual orientation upon which Watson developed the framework for her theory. Watson (1996) states that, both retrospectively and prospectively, her work "can be read as philosophy, ethic, or even paradigm or worldview" (p. 142). The concepts Watson defined in the Theory of Human Caring were "derived from clinically inducted, empirical experiences [and combined with] philosophical, intellectual and experiential [past experiences, with her early work emerging from her own] values, beliefs, and perceptions about personhood, life, health and healing" (Watson, 1996, p. 143).

The traditional health-illness phenomena defined within nursing and medicine is replaced with the deeply human experiences of life itself. Watson's theory focuses on "the centrality of human caring and on the caring-to-caring transpersonal relationship and its healing potential for both the one who is caring and the one who is being cared for" (Watson, 1996, p. 141).

Watson's Theory of Human Caring includes the following major assumptions as stated in her first book *Nursing: The Philosophy and Science of Caring* (1979):

1. Caring can only be effectively demonstrated and practiced interpersonally.
2. Caring consists of carative factors that result in the satisfaction of certain human needs.
3. Effective caring promotes health and individual or family growth.
4. Caring responses accept a person not only as he/she is now but as what he/she may become.
5. A caring environment offers the development of potential by allowing the person to choose the best action for himself/herself at a given time.
6. Caring is more "healthogenic" than is curing. The practice of caring integrates biophysical knowledge with the knowledge of human behavior to generate or promote health and to provide ministrations to those who are ill. A science of caring is therefore complimentary to the science of curing.
7. The practice of caring is central to nursing.

As Watson (1979/1985a, 1985b) continued in the development of the philosophy and science of her model, she proposed 11 caring paradigm assumptions which further defined nursing's social and ethical responsibilities based upon human values and altruism which are paraphrased below:

1. Care and love are primal, universal forces.
2. Nourishment of care and love, cornerstones of humanness, fulfills humanity.
3. Sustaining the caring ideology of nursing will affect civilization's development and nursing's contribution to society.
4. You must care for yourself before you can care for others.
5. Nursing has always valued caring in regard to people's health.
6. Caring is the essence of nursing.
7. In the health care delivery system, caring has been increasingly deemphasized.
8. Modern technological advances have sublimated nursing's caring framework.
9. Preservation and advancement of human care are significant concerns for nursing now and in the future.
10. Only through interpersonal relationships can human care be effectively demonstrated.
11. Nursing's social, moral, and scientific contributions to mankind and society lie in its commitments to human care ideals in theory, practice, and research (Watson, 1996, pp. 149–151).

The following seven premises based upon the interpersonal-transpersonal-spiritual aspects of Watson's (1985) work provide the foundation for further development of her theory:

1. A person's mind and emotions are windows to the soul.

2. A person's mind and soul are not confined to the physical universe but transcend time and space.
3. Inseparable spheres of the human being, the mind, body, or soul can be accessed by the nurse.
4. The soul or a person exists in and for itself.
5. People need the love and care of each other in order to nourish humanity, advance civilization, and love together.
6. Finding meanings in the context of the human predicament provides solutions.
7. The totality of human experience at any given moment constitutes a phenomenal field.

Key components of the Theory of Human Caring include human care and transpersonal relationships. Reverence and sacredness of life are fundamental. Art and science are converged into a redefined concept of humanistic care in which both the nurse and the individual receiving the care are affected, resulting in a more humanistic, holistic self-transcendence (Watson, 1997). The 10 hierarchical carative factors are aspects of nursing that "actually potentiate therapeutic healing processes for both the one caring and the one being cared for" (Watson, 1996, pp. 154–155) and include:

1. Formation of a humanistic-altruistic system of values
2. Enabling and sustaining faith-hope
3. Cultivation of sensitivity to self and to others
4. Development of a helping-trusting, caring relationship
5. Promotion and acceptance of the expression of positive and negative feelings and emotions
6. Engaging in creative, individualized problem-solving caring processes
7. Promotion of transpersonal-interpersonal teaching-learning
8. Provision for a supportive, protective, and corrective mental, physical, sociocultural, and spiritual environment
9. Assistance with gratification of human needs while preserving human dignity and wholeness
10. Allowance for existential-phenomenological-spiritual dimensions of caring and healing that cannot be fully explained scientifically through modern Western medicine.

According to Watson (2002) the processes of caring and healing occur when transpersonal caring seeks to embrace the soul of the other. This transpersonal caring creates a caring moment, in which the nurse has the ability to center consciousness and intentionality on caring, healing, and wholeness rather than on the pathological processes. This framework provides holistic and complete caring in a caring moment. The spiritual nature of human beings, striving for inner harmony, is the key to understanding the fundamental key of transpersonal caring of humans.

Watson's Theory of Human Caring is used in many published research studies, articles, and book chapters, and has served as a guide for master's and doctoral student research. This theory also serves as the foundation for doctoral educational programs, hospital units, and outpatient services. Human science nursing "allows for the questioning of ultimate meanings and ethical values of human's health and nursing" (Watson, 1985/1999a, p. 16). Watson's theory incorporates the sacredness of the relationship between humans, impacting the caring, healing environment through the art and science of nursing. This theory of transpersonal caring has made and will continue to make a significant and lasting impact on nursing science.

Diana Lynn Morris
Updated by Kristen S. Montgomery

Weight Management

Weight management, defined as deliberate actions to reduce and maintain healthy body weight, is classified as formal and informal. Formal weight management consists of paying for organized services to assist individuals with weight reduction. Informal weight management includes personal weight-loss methods without professional assistance. Weight management usually is targeted at reducing weight (versus gaining) because of societal pressures to be thin and current epidemic incidences of overweight, obesity, and their comorbidities. Overweight is defined as 25 to 29.9 body mass index (BMI) and obesity is defined as BMI ≥ 30 (National Heart Lung and Blood Institute [NHLBI], 1998).

In the United States, the incidence of being overweight increased from 25% to 33% between 1980 to 1991. In 1995, costs related to obesity were $99 billion and escalated to $117 billion in 2000 (NHLBI, 1998). Currently, the Centers for Disease Control reported that almost two thirds of adult Americans and 15% of their children are overweight or obese. Obesity has remained more prevalent among women (33%) compared to men (28%). The Third National Health and Nutrition Examination Survey (NHANES III) showed about half of minority women populations to be overweight or obese, namely African-American (50%), Mexican-American (40%), and non-Hispanic whites (30%). Overweight and obesity increase risk for mortality and morbidity from cardiovascular disease, which remains the number one killer of women in the U.S.

Experts agree that environmental influences, rather than biological reasons, explain the obesity epidemic over the past 3 decades. Four factors explain the environmental stimulus–response nature of the rise in obesity in the U.S.: (1) a fast-paced eating style consisting of fatty, glycemic "fast foods" and super sizing, (2) excessive calorie intake, (3) reduced physical activity and technological dependency, and (4) heightened responsiveness to food as a stimulant (Hill, Wyatt, Reed, & Peters, 2003). To date, few studies focused on psychological, sociocultural, and spiritual aspects of weight management (Timmerman & Gregg, 2003).

Long-term habits of overeating without hunger and with little or no physical exercise in a fast-paced society must be examined as contributors to the growing weight problem among U.S. citizens. Most weight-loss treatments in the U.S. have not helped reduce weight over the long term and have even contributed to the overweight problem (Hill, J. O., Wyatt, Reed, & Peters, 2003). As obesity increased, so did many associated comorbid conditions, including heart disease and hypertension, stroke, gallbladder disease, osteoarthritis, sleep apnea, respiratory problems, cancers, and type 2 diabetes. Insulin resistance syndrome (metabolic syndrome) is estimated to affect about 25% of American adults. The safest, most effective way to reverse insulin resistance, as most of the obesity comorbidities, is through physical activity, dietary intake (less glycemic, more fiber), and weight loss (Tuomilehto et al., 2001).

Failure rates for weight loss treatments in the U.S. are estimated to be as high as 90% to 95%. Even people listed in the National Weight Control Registry, those who reported maintaining an average weight loss of about 30% for 5.5 years, reported 91% failure rate before eventually succeeding. Treatments that fail to promote long-term weight management: (a) are restrictive in calories, choices, and when to eat; (b) are uni-dimensional using one major means to achieve weight loss and do not include regular exercise; and (c) do not permit individuals to tailor weight management to their preferences and lifestyles.

Treatments that restrict calories, choices, and when to eat offer a temporary modification that is unrealistic for the long term. Diets can lead to weight loss but rebound weight gain and psychological consequences remain a concern. Medical treatments (surgery and drugs) can yield short-term weight loss, but fail in the long term. Poston, Haddock, Dill, Thayer, and Foreyt (2001), in a meta-analysis of randomized clinical trials using lifestyle changes with pharmacotherapy, found that most trials used low-calorie diets with pharmacotherapy (41%), low-calorie diets alone

(25%), and only 17% included any form of exercise with pharmacotherapy.

Most behavioral weight-management programs that emphasize stimulus control of intake and output by dieting and behavior modification are usually unidimensional and focus mainly on calorie reduction. Few weight management programs take a holistic, multidimensional approach to lifestyle changes using strategies to correct underlying overeating, lack of exercise, and poor self-esteem. Most weight-management programs place greater emphasis on eating, exercise, *or* psychosocial aspects, rather than *holistic* emphasis on *all three* dimensions.

Treatments that do not permit individuals to tailor weight management to their preferences and lifestyles cannot be lasting. Weight loss treatments fail when program directives are too stringent for individuals to feel ownership and acceptance of weight management strategies as a way of life (Hill et al., 2003). The 1997 American Dietetic Association position statement stated that for adults to successfully achieve long-term weight management, daily physical activity and eating should be *sustainable* and *enjoyable.*

Strategies that concentrate on modifying behavior by differentiating stimuli before, during, and after eating are a healthy *start* toward lasting weight management (i.e., identifying stimuli other than hunger that trigger eating, monitoring amounts and conditions during eating, and rewarding appropriate actions). One reason why behavioral techniques have limited success is because they seek to control the diet and environment without considering eating as a coping mechanism to manage unpleasant feelings (Popkess-Vawter, Brandau, & Straub, 1998). Few current weight-management behavioral approaches, cognitive restructuring, or combinations thereof, directly address how negative beliefs about self and irrational perceptions of the world can trigger negative self-talk with resultant overeating and no exercise responses.

There is growing evidence that 5% of maximum weight lost contributes to positive changes in obesity comorbidities (Yanovski & Yanovski, 2002). The NHLBI weight-management treatment and programs like "America on the Move" are national initiatives that have accommodated people's busy lives by suggesting "real world, do-able" eating and exercise goals for arresting the obesity epidemic; more stringent recommendations of the past have only fueled the epidemic (Hill et al., 2003). Studies are lacking that test the efficacy of holistic approaches that accompany busy lifestyles. A few computer applications related to weight management have emerged, including treatments for smoking cessation, exercise, and food shopping, but Internet obesity studies are rare (Tate, Wing, & Winett, 2001).

The ultimate goal of weight management is to prevent obesity and its comorbidities (Serdula, Khan, & Dietz, 2003). Primary care clinics are frontline settings to approach people about weight management, but structured and practical treatments are still lacking. Many reasons have been reported to account for ineffective weight management—lack of time, inadequate training, labor intensity, and pessimism that intervention is useless. Patients were not satisfied with primary care physicians' weight-loss recommendations (Wadden et al., 2000). Less than half (43%) of surveyed obese patients reported that providers actually advised them about weight loss, and almost 30% reported that they received *no* weight management counseling. Providers may not be aware of their powerful influence in helping patients with weight management. To promote healthy weight among Americans, long-term, lifestyle-change intervention studies are vital, using qualitative and quantitative measurements of physical *and psychosocial* weight-management strategies.

SUE A. POPKESS-VAWTER

Wellness

Wellness is an integrated method of functioning directed toward maximizing the potential of which an individual is capable within the environment where functioning occurs. Wellness is both a process and a goal that can be self-selected by anyone of any age, in any setting, and with any condition of health, illness, or disability. Wellness as a process is a movement toward greater individual awareness of activities that promote health, active engagement in those activities, and the personal satisfaction that results from active engagement. Activities that promote health include physical fitness, positive nutrition, positive relationships, stress management, clear life purpose, consistent belief systems, commitment to self-care, and environmental comfort. The goal of wellness is self-actualization.

Nursing is concerned with the phenomena of human responses to illness and health. Progress has been made to move nursing taxonomic language to descriptors of wellness and its maintenance and promotion. Quality of life is increasingly a focus of health status for clients, family members, health care providers, and other decision-makers. The wellness model focuses on what is "right" with the person and the quality of life an individual enjoys. Most theoretical thinking in nursing includes the integration of body, mind, and spirit; the wellness orientation is consistent with most of this thinking although less well-defined. Nurses in all arenas of practice, education, research, and administration are influential in assisting clients in making personal lifestyle changes directed toward wellness.

Nursing pioneers in the wellness movement adopted a holistic approach and promoted wellness through self-care and self-responsibility. Dimensions of a health-promoting lifestyle encompassing behaviors that serve to maintain or enhance the wellness or self-fulfillment of an individual were identified and scientifically validated by nurse scientists. Those dimensions include health responsibility, nutrition, exercise, stress management, interpersonal support, and self-actualization. Later, wellness practitioners developed these themes into wellness practices. Promotion of health is an appropriate comparison for the wellness model because it emphasizes improving one's general state of health. Further, the construct of health promotion contains concepts that are more readily measurable yielding a stronger conceptual basis for the abstract notion of wellness.

Dunn (1961) was the first to use the term *wellness* nearly 2 decades before the concept of high-level wellness and holistic health were popularized by Ardell, Travis, and others in the late 1970s and early 1980s. Dunn's writings reflect and acknowledge the ideas of thinkers such as Eric Fromm, Carl Rogers, Abraham Maslow, and Hans Selye, who were also concerned about how individuals might achieve their full potential within their world. Dunn equated health with the integration of person-mind-body-spirit and maintained that what people feel, believe, and think affects their physical capabilities and vice versa.

The wellness and holistic health movement of the 1970s evolved outside the traditional health professions. Major threads throughout the movement today continue to reflect the integration of body, mind, and spirit; the ethic of self-responsibility and choice; and the interdependence of individual, social, and environmental wellness originally conceptualized. In fact, these ideas have become increasingly relevant in the scientific community as advances in biological sciences have evolved to support the relationships among these threads.

The terms as well have become popularized and used by lay persons and health professionals alike, often without clear conceptual understanding of what the concepts really mean. Today thousands of web sites and articles in the professional and lay literature use the term wellness without a clear understanding of what it means. Further, the dichotomy between the characteristics of the medical model and the wellness model creates dissonance and makes the use of wellness language inaccurate and confusing in the context of a medically driven system of illness care.

Smith (1983) described distinctive models of health, which include a clinical orientation, a role-performance or functional definition of health, an eudaemonistic definition of health as exuberant well-being, and an adaptive definition of health. The Laffrey Health Conception Scale (Laffrey, 1986) based on Smith's work was developed to measure the perception of health held by individuals. The original Health Promoting Lifestyle Profile, the work of Walker, Sechrist, and Pender (1987), provided a seminal work in this area.

MARION HEMSTROM-KRAINESS

Widows and Widowers

The recent research about widows and widowers addresses younger widowed persons rather than focusing principally upon older widows. However, researchers have continued to concentrate upon the relatively short period of bereavement rather than the longer-term circumstances of living alone. Common concepts surrounding bereavement include: grief, stress, adaptation, coping, and social support. The work reflects four perspectives on bereavement: (a) as loss, (b) as a process of phases and stages, (c) as a stressor, and (d) as a series of tasks.

Loss. Bacon, Condon, and Fernsler (2000) considered support and coping as key factors enabling adjustment to loss of a spouse. They explained why young widowed mothers might find it difficult to participate in a traditional support group. In a descriptive study, they detailed the perceptions of 21 widows (age 31–50 years) about taking part in an electronic self-help group. Responses to closed questions were reported using descriptive statistics; responses to an open question soliciting feelings about participation were submitted to content analysis. Most of the women had not taken part in an internet self-help group previously. They rated the experience positively in reducing the sense of isolation and coping with loss.

An intervention of four support group sessions was tested to determine its influence upon the affect and loneliness of widows over age 55 years (Stewart, Craig, MacPherson, & Alexander, 2001). With repeated measures, within-subjects design standardized tools tapped outcomes related to social support, affect, and loneliness. Perceptions of the intervention's impact were analyzed qualitatively. The intervention diminished the need for other support, enhanced positive affect, and increased satisfaction with support.

Process of phases and stages. Hegge and Fischer (2000) differentiated grief responses of 22 senior widows (age 60–74 years) and 17 older widows (age 75–90 years). Concept analysis was used to detail frequent and troubling problems, coping strategies, support systems, and goal adjustments. There were no major differences by age groups. Grieving had four overlapping phases (numb shock, emotional turmoil, disorganization, and acceptance), which were briefer and less intense for older widows. Loneliness was the most common problem for both groups.

Steeves (2002) did a hermeneutic analysis of field notes and interviews with 29 older bereaved spouses in the rural South to capture data about the duration of grieving. The interviews began before a spouse's death and continued for up to 30 months. The rhythm of grief had three fluid stages: numbness, grief attacks or waves, and loneliness.

Stressor. Referring to a spouse's death as a very stressful life event, Constantino, Sekula, and Rubinstein (2001) studied the effectiveness of the Bereavement Group Postvention (BGP) and the Social Group Postvention (SGP) on bereavement outcomes for 60 widowed survivors of the spouse's suicide. Participants were randomized into the BGP or the SGP, taking part in a weekly 90-minute session for 8 weeks. There were no significant differences between groups on depression, psychological distress, grief, or social adjustment at any time point (pretest, immediate, 6-month, and 12-month postvention). For both groups, there was a significant reduction in depression, distress, and grief over time, and a significant increase in social adjustment. There was no evidence of a confounding effect due to duration of widowhood, but Constantino and colleagues did not rule it out. Because there was no evidence of a differential effect for the two interventions, they suggested that participation in any social group might be beneficial.

In a descriptive, mixed-methods study, sources and nature of social support perceived by 218 Finnish widows and widowers, aged 30 to 87 years, were discerned (Kaunonen, Tarkka, Paunonen, & Laippala, 1999). A standardized tool was used to appraise dimensions of grief, and qualitative data about coping sources were submitted to content analysis. The most common support sources were friends and family, and their time was the most precious resource offered.

Daggett (2002) referred to spousal bereavement as a stressor requiring coping. Daggett used a phenomenological method to describe the grief experience of 8 middle-aged men who had been widowed from 6 months to 6 years. Under a major theme of *irreconcilable loss*, the two categories *responding to the loss* and *living through the loss* were simultaneous occurrences, moving over time to *reclamation and reconstruction of a life*. Daggett described the categories in terms of time-based parameters, much like stages, although she had stated that stage-based theories of bereavement did not capture individual differences in grief experiences.

Series of interwoven tasks. Zonnebelt-Smeenge and DeVries (2003) explained that stage-based theories had given way to task theories of bereavement (Rando, 1993; Worden, 1991) involving spiraling or interwoven behaviors over time (Bowlby, 1981). Zonnebelt-Smeenge and DeVries highlighted the dual-process model (Stroebe, M., & Schut, 1999) of simultaneous grief-work relative to loss and to restoration. (Thus, the idea of living through loss while responding to loss was not original to Daggett [2000].) Viewing the model as consistent with task-related theory, they cited five bereavement tasks (Rando; Worden) and created a tool to determine the frequency and effectiveness of widowed persons' task-related interventions. They reported preliminary findings with 115 widowed persons (age 24 to 90 years, *MD* = 54). Women found it more important to engage in activities leading to acceptance of the reality of the death, whereas more men than women undertook activities to experience all death-related emotions. Persons under age 45 years felt more positive about the future; more persons older than 65 years had taken part in support groups. Variables of resolution were positively correlated with duration of widowhood. Relatively few participants engaged in work to summarize and store memories of the spouse, so practitioners were encouraged to suggest activities enabling bereaved persons to directly address this task.

Two interpretive phenomenological studies were done with older rural widows. With five women, Swensen (1998) explored attachment to place, finding that home was the center of self, caring, and reach. D. C. Roberts and Cleveland (2001) studied the experience of living alone for nine widows who lived on islands near Maine. The three essential themes were characterized as nautical metaphors, such as *securely anchored in a safe harbor*. Although the women were actively engaged, resilient, and resourceful, access to health care was a problem.

Porter has used descriptive phenomenology to explore the essence of older widows' health-related experiences. E. J. Porter (1998a) found that 16 older urban and rural widows sought to *keep the generations separate* by continuing to live alone and by trying not to burden the children. The intention of 9 older rural widows to *stay close to shore* for health care resulted in a new interpretation of access to care as familiarity with the care locale (Porter, E. J., 1998b). In a longitudinal study, E. J. Porter (2001) described the transition of an older widow from her home to assisted living, secondary to changes in payment policies affecting the rural home care agency.

Several studies were not focused on widowhood per se; instead, the researchers were interested in health as a variable affecting widowed persons. In the group studied by Wallace, Molavi, Hemphill, and Fields (1999), which consisted of 931 African Americans over the age of 65 years, neither the ability to perform activities of daily living nor the use of health care services was influenced by widowhood. Among other issues, Crane and Warnes (2001) examined the role of widowhood as an influence upon homelessness in 18 persons over the age of 55 years. The authors concluded that although widowhood had a greater impact on men than on women, it can result in dramatic changes in lifestyle and living arrangements. Finally, T. R. Fitzpatrick and Bosse (2000) studied the effects of employment on the health of 510 widowers (aged 39 to 86 years) up to 3 years after the spouse's death. Employment had a positive effect on the physical health of the widowers, but there was no evidence of an effect upon their mental health.

Nurse researchers have tended to focus on older widowed persons (WP), primarily women (Porter, E. J., 2000). Recently, there has been a new and noteworthy interest in younger widows and WP of both genders. However, without regard to age or gender, there has been an overemphasis on the relatively short period of bereavement and a neglect of the long-term issue of life as a WP. In bereavement studies, most researchers have reviewed generic theories of coping or loss and undertaken qualitative studies with vague methods (such as concept analysis) and small samples. The work of Zonnebelt-Smeenge and deVries (2003) is a notable exception.

Duration of widowhood is a critical variable in research on bereavement as well as studies of life alone, although few researchers noted this other than Constantino and colleagues (2001), Fitzpatrick and Bosse (2000), and Zonnebelt-Smeenge and deVries (2003). Most nurse researchers other than Steeves (2002) and E. J. Porter (2001) have used cross-sectional designs; longitudinal designs yield more information about living alone. Nurse researchers must explore the health-related needs of vulnerable subgroups, such as widowers at risk for suicide and widows at risk for breast cancer. Finally, scholars must attend to revealing the variations in the experience of widowhood among groups of WP who share key demographic characteristics.

EILEEN J. PORTER

Women's Health

"Women's health" is a phrase that has come to signal movement away from a focus on gynecology—synonymous historically with reproductive matters—to gynecology, meaning that overall well-being is shaped by the fit between the woman and her environment. This expanded biopsychosocial perspective is not just concerned with women's diseases, but their dis-eases, too, and coincides with nursing's longstanding emphasis on the interface between and among genetic, physiologic, psychosocial, economic, cultural, generational, developmental, and lifestyle factors in determining health.

Women's health research began as a critique of existing practices and their effects on women's well-being. In 1985, the Public Health Service Task Force on Women's Health Issues examined the role of the Department of Health and Human Services in addressing women's health and found that women were often not included as subjects in health research. Women had historically been excluded from the first two stages of drug testing. Even female animals had typically not been used in constructing animal models because of "their hormonal fluctuations." The health problems that women suffered from disproportionately were also not much studied, for example, osteoporosis, breast and ovarian cancer, urinary incontinence, the autoimmune diseases, violence, and poverty.

Health had been construed so that male behavior was regarded as normative, and research conducted exclusively on males was typically generalized to all human beings. When women did not fare as well with the same treatment, they were regarded as atypical. From Freud to Kohlberg, theoretical models had been constructed so that women were regarded as less developed when they did not act in a fashion similar to men. Even when studied, the sociocultural factors shaping health problems in girls and women were ignored, for example, the relationship between learned helplessness and some kinds of depression, and between anorexia and the popular admonition that you can never be too rich nor too thin.

Social/health systems also had been prejudicial in important respects. Insurance policies did not necessarily cover health matters unique to women, for example, breast prostheses post mastectomy. Women were not in research and policy-making positions proportionate to their numbers, responsibilities, and educational preparation. The burden of family caregiving that women largely bear remained invisible, notably in estimates of the Gross National Product (GNP).

The Office of Research on Women's Health (ORWH) was established in 1990 within the Office of the Director of the National Institutes of Health (NIH) to address these lacunae. A decade later, not coincidentally, the majority of human subjects enrolled in all extramural NIH research were women, and they were represented in Phase III clinical trials.

Often led by nurses, women's health research has become relatively mainstream in the ensuing years. S. K. Donaldson (2000) analyzed the achievements of nursing research between 1960 and 1999, and found substantial strengths in the area of women's health. The Center for Women's Health Research at the University of Washington, supported by the National Institute of Nursing Research (NINR), has increased understanding of menstrual cycle change, including the menopausal transition (Mitchell, Woods, & Mariella, 2002). That Center has also played a role in translational research, for example, offering a video presentation to help women in deciding if hormone replacement therapy (HRT) is appropriate for them (Woods, 2002).

One area of common concern to the five Centers of Geriatric Nursing Excellence funded by the Hartford Foundation is the experience of family caregivers, largely women (Archbold & Stewart, 1996). Nurses have also brought new understandings to other developmental transitions, for example, the experience of women as mothers/grandmothers (McBride & Shore, 2001), and how puberty may differentially affect girls in comparison to their male counterparts (Austin, Dunn, & Huster, 2000). The ORWH has collaborated with various NIH institutes to fund Specialized Centers of Research of Sex and Gender Factors Affecting Women's Health. The one based at the University of Michigan is conducting research on the pelvic floor, and nurses have pioneered therapeutic use of pelvic floor muscle training in women (Miller, J. M., 2002).

Because one of its fundamental beliefs is the need to proceed from an understanding of the person-environment fit, nursing has long been concerned about the importance of context in understanding health behavior. Nurse midwives, for example, tend not to talk about "delivering the baby," preferring instead to focus on the mother and how she would prefer her labor and delivery to go. Nurses were among the first to question a preference for the so-called objective view of the researcher, historically male, over the subjective view of the patient (McBride & McBride, 1981). They took the lead in use of the diary/health journal as a way to analyze the complexity of women's reality. The research that has resulted has been informed by how women describe their lived experience. A feminist ethic has emerged that is neither focused on "doing good" nor "doing unto others what one would wish for oneself" but with providing care that builds on the patient's perceptions of what is good for her.

The ORWH has developed an Agenda for Research on Women's Health for the 21st century (Pinn, 2001). Many of its priorities dovetail with the focus of nursing research; for example, interdisciplinary approaches to chronic multi-system diseases with multi-factorial etiology, caregiving, and health-related quality-of-life issues. Indeed, most of the research centers supported by the NINR focus on either healthy living and the prevention of chronic disorders or quality of life in chronic illness. Developing effective ways to manage chronicity, as opposed to serial management of a number of diseases, is of particular concern to nurse researchers.

Women's health research has made major strides in the inclusion of females as research subjects, but the next challenge is to cease treating women as a monolithic group. Women vary significantly according to their circumstances. Thus, it is important that research not just include girls and women, but overselect for heretofore understudied populations, for example, diverse cultures, women of color, the elderly, rural and inner-city women, the poor, lesbians, and women with disabilities. The resulting findings are likely to fuel the burgeoning movement towards an emphasis on the design of tailored interventions.

In an attempt to reject "biology as destiny," women's health research may also have inadvertently minimized the physiologic pathways involved in responses to stressful psychosocial conditions. Future research must, therefore, be concerned with women's experiences that exist on the interface between the behavioral and the biomedical sciences in order to provide additional insights into sex versus gender differences.

ANGELA BARRON MCBRIDE

Workplace Violence

Workplace violence is defined as "violent acts (including physical assaults and threats of assaults) directed toward persons at work or on duty" (National Institute of Occupational Safety and Health [NIOSH], 2002). Most workplace violence falls into one of four categories:

- Type I (Criminal Intent): Results while a criminal activity (e.g., robbery) is being committed and the perpetrator has no legitimate relationship to the workplace.
- Type II (Customer/Client): The perpetrator is a customer or client at the workplace (e.g., health care patient) and becomes violent while being served by the worker.
- Type III (Worker-on-Worker): Employees or past employees of the workplace are the perpetrators in this case.
- Type IV (Personal Relationship): The perpetrator in this case usually has a personal relationship with an employee (e.g., domestic violence in the workplace).

Homicide has remained among the top three causes of death in the workplace since 1990. According to the Bureau of Labor Statistics (BLS), workplace violence is the third leading cause of occupational injury death among all workers and the leading cause among women. Workplace homicides have declined from a high of 1,080 in 1994 to 609 in 2002; on average 846 workers per year have died as a result of homicide since 1992. Notably, 80% of workplace homicides involve the use of a firearm (NIOSH, 1996).

Nonfatal assaults are much more common than fatal assaults. Although both share many of the same risk factors (e.g., contact with the public, working with volatile persons, working in small numbers, and working in community-based settings) health care rather than retail workers represent the majority of victims of nonfatal workplace violence. According to the Department of Justice's National Crime Victimization Survey (NCVS), 1.9 million incidents of workplace violence occurred in the workplace each year from 1992–1996 (Warchol, 1998). Twelve percent of all victims reported physical injuries; 6% of the workplace crimes resulted in injury that required medical treatment, and only 44% of all incidents were reported to the police.

Workplace violence is a documented occupational hazard in the health care and service sectors (NIOSH, 2002; Lipscomb & Love, 1992; Warchol, 1998). The health care sector leads all other industries in nonfatal workplace assaults. In 2000, 48% of all nonfatal injuries resulting in days away from work from violent acts and assaults occurred in the health and social service sector (BLS, 2001). The incidence rate for violent acts and assaults resulting in days away from work was 9.3 per 10,000 full-time workers for health services workers compared to an overall private sector injury rate of 2 per 10,000 full-time workers (BLS). Among victimizations reported in the NCVS, mental health professionals had an incidence rate of 79.5 per 1,000 workers compared with an overall rate of 14.8 per 1,000 workers. Nurses had an incidence rate of 24.8 per 1,000 workers, the highest rate in the "medical" category (Warchol).

Violence in mental health has an extensive history, with the first documented case of a patient fatally assaulting a psychiatrist in 1849 (Bernstein, 1981). Until the 1990s, most studies that examined the risk of violence to psychiatrists and other therapists focused on the victim's role, the assaultive patient's characteristics, and contextual factors surrounding the assault. Only recently have environmental risk factors been a focus of research and nurses and aides the subjects of study.

Bensley and colleagues (1997) compared the number of workers compensation claims from a Washington State psychiatric hospital, formal incident reports, and the number of incidents of assault reported on a survey measuring attitudes and experiences related to assaults. She found that 73% of staff surveyed reported at least a minor injury related to a patient assault in the past year. Only 43% of those reporting moderate, severe, or disabling injuries related to assault filed a workers compensation claim. The survey found an assault incidence rate of 437 per 100 employees per year, a rate that underestimated incident reports of assaults by a factor of more than five (Bensley et al.).

Environmental and organizational factors have been associated with patient assaults, including understaffing (especially during times of increased activity such as meal times), workplace security, time of day, unrestricted access to movement and transporting patients (NIOSH, 2002). S. S. Lee, Gerberich, Waller, Anderson, and McGovern (1999) found that among 105 nurses who had filed a workers compensation claim for work-related assault injuries, the presence of security personnel reduced the rate of assault while the perception that administrators considered assault to be part of the job, having received assault prevention training, a high patient/personnel ratio, working primarily with mental health patients, and working with patients who had a long hospital stay increased the risk of assault.

The one patient characteristic that has been singled out as a strong risk factor for violence is a history of violent behavior. A number of studies have documented that a small number of patients are responsible for the majority of assaults (Hillbrand, Foster, & Spitz, 1996). Drummond, Sparr, and Gordon (1989) examined an intervention designed to identify patients with a history of violence and found that flagging charts of patients with histories of assaultive or disruptive behavior reduced assaults against staff by 91%.

Many psychiatric settings now require that all patient care providers receive annual training in the management of aggressive patients. However, few studies have examined the effectiveness of such training. Those that have generally found improvement in nurses' knowledge, confidence, and safety after taking an aggressive behavior management program (Hurlebaus & Link, 1997). Carmel and Hunter (1990) examined the relationship between participation in training and aggressive behavior by inpatients on 27 inpatient wards in a California State hospital and found that wards with higher staff attendance at the training experienced lower rates of injury. Lehmann et al. (1983) found significantly higher knowledge and confidence in trained staff.

Runyan, Zakocs, and Zwerling (2000) reviewed 137 papers mentioning violence prevention intervention and found that only ten of the papers reflected databased intervention. All interventions took place in health care; five studies evaluated violence prevention training interventions (including Lehmann and colleagues, and Carmel & Hunter), three examined postincident psychological debriefing programs, and two evaluated administrative controls to prevent violence. All were quasiexperimental, without a formal control group and with equivocal findings.

The health care workplace must be made safe for all health care workers through the use of currently available engineering and administrative controls, such as security alarm systems, and adequate staffing and training. The Occupational Safety and Health Administration published "Guidelines for Preventing Workplace Violence for Healthcare and Social Service Workers." These guidelines describe the key elements of any proactive health and safety program including: management commitment and employee involvement, a written violence prevention program, a worksite analysis, hazard prevention and control, medical management and post incident response, training and education, and record keeping and evaluation of the program. These authors are currently evaluating the effectiveness of these guidelines in preventing violence within the mental health and social service work settings. Preliminary findings from the inpatient mental health workplace indicate that a comprehensive violence prevention program is associated with a reduction in risk factors for violence and workplace threats and assaults (Lipscomb, in preparation).

Research evaluating intervention directly at the primary, secondary, and tertiary prevention of violence across health care settings is critically needed to reduce workplace violence and ultimately improve patient care. A secure and healthful work environment is essential to a positive environment of care.

JANE LIPSCOMB
CASSANDRA OKECHUKWU

REFERENCES

Aaronson, L. S., Pallikkathayil, L., & Crighton, F. (2003). A qualitative investigation of fatigue among healthy working adults. *Western Journal of Nursing Research, 25*, 419–433.

Aaronson, L. S., Teel, C., Cassmeyer, V., Neuberger, G. B., Pallikkathayil, L., Pierce, J., et al. (1999). Defining and measuring fatigue. *IMAGE: Journal of Nursing Scholarship, 31*, 45–50.

Aaronson, N. K. (1990). Quality of life assessment in cancer clinical trials. In J. C. Holland & R. Zitbun (Eds.), *Psychosocial aspects of oncology* (pp. 97–111). Berlin: Springer-Verlag.

AARP. (1999a). *Financial planning: A must for midlife and older women*. Retrieved June 28, 1999, from http://www.aarp.org/finance99/older.html

AARP. (1999b). *Baby boomers envision their retirement: An AARP segmentation analysis*. Retrieved June 23, 1999, from http://research.aarp.org/econ/boomer_seg_1.html

Abbey, J. C., Andrews, C., Avigliano, K., Blossom, R., Bunke, B., Engberg, N., et al. (1973). A pilot study: The control of shivering during hypothermia by a clinical nursing measure. *Journal of Neurosurgical Nursing, 5*(2), 78–88.

Abbey, J., & Close, L. (1979, May 2–5). *A study of control of shivering during hypothermia*. Paper presented at the 12th annual Communicating Nursing Research Conference: WICHEN/WSRN, Denver, CO.

Abdellah, F., & Levine, E. (1965). *Better patient care through nursing research*. New York: Macmillan.

Abdellah, F. G., & Levine, E. (1979). *Better patient care through nursing research* (2nd ed.). New York: Macmillan.

Abete, P., Ferrara, N., Cacciatore, F., Sagnelli, E., Manzi, M., Carnovale, V., et al. (2001). High level of physical activity preserves the cardioprotective effect of preinfarction angina in elderly patients. *Journal of the American College of Cardiology, 38*, 1357–1365.

Abraham, I. L., Bottrell, M. M., Dash, K. R., Fulmer, T. T., Mezey, M. D., O'Donnell, L., et al. (1999). Profiling care and benchmarking best practice in care of hospitalized elderly: The geriatric institutional assessment profile. *Nursing Clinics of North America, 34*(2), 239–255.

Abraham, I. L., Chalifoux, Z., & Evers, G. C. M. (1992). Conditions, interventions, and outcomes: A quantitative analysis of nursing research (1981–1990). In P. Moritz (Ed.), *Patient outcomes research: Examining the effectiveness of nursing practice* (NIH Publication No. 93-3411, pp. 7–87). Bethesda, MD: National Institutes of Health.

Abraham, I. L., Currie, L. J., Neese, J. B., Yi, E. S., & Thompson-Heisterman, A. A. (1994). Risk profiles for nursing home placement of rural elderly: A cluster analysis of psychogeriatric indicators. *Archives of Psychiatric Nursing, 8*, 262–271.

Abrams, S. M., Field, T., Scafidi, F., & Prodromidis, M. (1995). Newborns of depressed mothers. *Infant Mental Health Journal, 16*, 233–239.

Abramson, J., & Mizrahi, T. (1996). When social workers and physicians collaborate: Positive and negative interdisciplinary experiences. *Social Work, 41*, 270–281.

AbuAlRub, R. (2004). Job stress, job performance, and social support among hospital nurses. *Journal of Nursing Scholarship, 36*, 73–78.

Acute Pain Management Guideline Panel. (1992). *Acute pain management: Operative or medical procedures and trauma. Clinical practice guideline* (Vol. AHCPR No. 92-0032). Rockville, MD: Agency for Health Care Policy and Research, Public Health Service, U.S. Department of Health and Human Services.

Adams, W. (1996). Alcohol use in retirement communities. *Journal of the American Geriatrics Society, 44*, 1082–1085.

Aday, L. (2001). *At risk in America* [electronic resource]: *The health and health care needs of vulnerable populations in the United States* (2nd ed.). San Francisco: Jossey-Bass Publishers. Retrieved November 22, 2003, from http://www.netlibrary.com/ebook/

Addington-Hall, J., & Kalra, L. (2001). Who should measure quality of life? *British Medical Journal, 322*, 1417–1420. Retrieved September 29, 2003, from http://www.bmj.com

Administration on Aging. (2000). *Statistics. Census 2000 Data on the Aging*. Retrieved October 3, 2003, from http://www.aoa.gov/prof/Statistics/Census 2000/stateprofiles/agepr ofile-states.asp

Administration on Aging. (2002). *Profile of older Americans: 2002*. Retrieved October 27, 2003, from http://www.aoa.gov/prof/Statistics/profile/profiles2002.asp

Administration on Aging. (2003). *Profile of older Americans: 2002*. Retrieved July 23, 2003, from http://www.aoa.dhhs.gov/aoa/STATS/profile/12.html

Adult Treatment Panel III Guidelines of the National Cholesterol Education Program. (2002). NIH publication no. 01-3305. Bethesda, MD: National Institutes of Health.

Affonso, D. D., De, A. K., Andrews Horowitz, J., & Mayberry, L. J. (2000). An international study exploring levels of postpartum depressive symptomatology. *Journal of Psychosomatic Research, 49*, 207–216.

Agency for Health Care Policy and Research. (1998). *Systematic review of the research literature regarding sleep apnea*. Evidence Report/Technology Assessment: Number 1.

Agency for Health Care Policy and Research (AHCPR). Panel for the Prediction and Prevention of Pressure Ulcers in Adults. (1992, May). *Pressure ulcers in adults: Prediction and prevention*. Clinical practice guideline, number 3 (AHCPR Publication No. 92-0047). Rockville, MD: Public Health Service, U.S. Dept of Health and Human Services.

Agency for Health Care Policy and Research. (2003). Retrieved from http://www.ahcpr.gov/new/press/pr2002/strengpr.htm

Agency for Healthcare Research and Quality. (2003a). *National Quality Measures Clearinghouse*. Retrieved November 23, 2003, from http://www.qualitymeasures.ahrq.gov/

Agency for Healthcare Research and Quality. (2003b). *Research in action*. Retrieved November 23, 2003, from http://www.ahrq.gov/news/riaix.htm

Agency for Healthcare Research and Quality. (2004). *Strategic Plan*. Retrieved August 13, 2004, from http://www.ahrq.gov/about/strateix.htm

Aggarwal, N. T., Bennett, D. A., Bienias, J. L., Mendes de Leon, C. F., Morris, M. C., & Evans, D. A. (2000). The prevalence of dizziness and its association with functional disability in a biracial community population. *Journal of Gerontology, Medical Sciences, 55A*(5), M288–M292.

Agran, P. F., Anderson, C., Winn, D., Trent, R., Walton-Haynes, L., & Thayer, S. (2003). Rates of pediatric injuries by 3-month intervals for children 0 to 3 years of age. *Pediatrics, 111*, e683–e692.

Ahluwalia, I. B., Morrow, B., Hsia, J., & Grummer-Strawn, L. M. (2003). Who is breast-feeding? Recent trends from the Pregnancy Risk Assessment and Monitoring System. *Journal of Pediatrics, 141*, 486–491.

Ahrens, T., Pennick, J. C., & Tucker, M. K. (1995). Frequency requirements for zeroing transducers in hemodynamic monitoring. *American Journal of Critical Care, 4*(6), 466–471.

Aiken, L., & Patrician, P. A. (2000). Measuring organizational traits of hospitals: The Revised Nursing Work Index. *Nursing Research, 49*, 146–153.

Aiken, L. H., Clarke, S. P., Cheung, R. B., Sloane, D. M., & Silber, J. H. (2003). Educational levels of hospital nurses and surgical patient mortality. *Journal of the American Medical Association, 290*, 1617–1623.

Aiken, L. H., Clarke, S. P., Sloane, D. M., Sochalski, J., & Silber, J. H. (2002). Hospital nurse staffing and patient mortality, nurse burnout, and job dissatisfaction. *Journal of the American Medical Association, 288*(16), 1987–1993.

Aiken, L. H., Sloane, D. M., Lake, E. T., Sochalski, J., & Weber, A. L. (1999). Organization and outcomes of inpatient AIDS care. *Medical Care, 37*(8), 760–772.

Aiken, L. H., Smith, H. L., & Lake, E. T. (1994). Lower Medicare mortality among a set of hospitals known for good nursing care. *Medical Care, 32*(8), 771–787.

Aitken, L. (2000). Reliability of measurements of pulmonary artery pressure obtained with patients in 60 degree lateral position. *American Journal of Critical Care, 9*(1), 43–51.

Ajzen, I. (1988). *Attitudes, personality and behavior*. Chicago: Dorsey Press.

Ajzen, I. (2001). Nature and operation of attitudes. *Annual Review of Psychology, 52*, 27–58.

Akers, P. (1991). The algorithmic approach to clinical decision making. *Oncology Nursing Forum, 18*, 1159–1163.

Albee, G. W. (1996). Revolutions and counterrevolutions in prevention. *American Psychologist, 51*, 1130–1133.

Alberdi, E., Taylor, P., Lee, R., Fox, J., Sordo, M., & Todd-Pokropek, A. (2000). CADMIUM II: Acquisition and representation of radiological knowledge for computerized decision support in mammography. In J. M. Overhage (Ed.), *Proceedings of the American Medical Informatics Association Symposium* (pp. 7–11). Bethesda, MD: AMIA.

Albert, N. M., Spear, B. T., & Hammel, J. (1999). Agreement and clinical utility of 2 techniques for measuring cardiac output in patients with low cardiac output. *American Journal of Critical Care, 8*, 464–474.

Albertine, J., Oldehinkel, A. J., Ormel, J., & Neeleman, J. (2000). Predictors of time to remission from depression in primary care patients: Do some people benefit more from positive life change than others? *Journal of Abnormal Psychology, 109*(2), 299–307.

Alberts, M. J., Hademenos, G., Latchaw, R. E., Jagoda, A., Marler, J. R., Mayberg, M. R., et al. (2000). Consensus statement: Recommendations for the establishment of primary stroke centers. *Journal of the American Medical Association, 283*, 3102–3109.

Albrecht, S. L., Miller, M. K., & Clarke, L. L. (1994). Assessing the importance of family structure in understanding birth outcomes. *Journal of Marriage and the Family, 56*(4), 987–1003.

Alessi, C. A., Stuck, A. E., Aronow, H. U., Yuhas, K. E., Bula, C. J., Madison, R., et al. (1997). The process of care in preventive in-home comprehensive geriatric assessment. *Journal of the American Geriatric Society, 45*, 1044–1050.

Alexopoulos, G. S. (2001). Interventions for depressed elderly primary care patients. *International Journal of Geriatric Psychiatry, 16*(6), 553–559.

Algase, D. L. (1999a). Wandering: A dementia-compromised behavior. *Journal of Gerontological Nursing, 25*(9), 10–16.

Algase, D. L. (1999b). Wandering in dementia. *Annual Review of Nursing Research*, 185–217.

Algase, D. L., Beattie, E. R. A., Bogue, E., & Yao, L. (2001). The Algase Wandering Scale: Initial psychometrics of a new caregiver reporting tool. *Journal of Alzheimer's Disease and Other Dementias, 16*(3), 141–152.

Algase, D. L., Beck, C., Kolanowski, A., Whall, A., Berent, A., Richards, K., et al. (1996). Need-driven dementia-compromised behavior: An alternative view of disruptive behavior. *American Journal of Alzheimer's Disease, 11*(6), 10–19.

Allen, J., Blumenthal, R. S., Marholis, S., Young, D. R., Miller, E. R., & Kelly, K. (2002). Nurse case management of hypercholesterolemia in patients with coronary heart disease: Results of a randomized clinical trial. *American Heart Journal, 144*(4), 678–686.

Allen, K., & Chin-Sang, V. (1990). A lifetime of work: The context and meanings of leisure for aging Black women. *Gerontologist, 30*, 734–740.

Alliance for Aging Research. (2003). *Ageism: How healthcare fails the elderly*. Retrieved October 16, 2003, from http://www.agingresearch.org/

Alliance for the Mentally Ill. (2005). www.nami.org

Alligood, M. (2001). Research corner. A theory of nursing empathy in King's Interacting Systems. *Tennessee Nurse, 64*(3), 7.

Alligood, M. R. (1995). King's interacting systems and empathy. In M. A. Frey & C. L. Sieloff (Eds.), *Advancing King's systems framework and theory of nursing* (pp. 66–87). Thousand Oaks, CA: Sage.

Alligood, M. R., & Tomey, A. M. (2002). *Nursing theory: Utilization & application*. St. Louis: Mosby.

Als, H. (1991). Neurobehavioral organization of the newborn: Opportunity for assessment and intervention. *NIDA Research Monographs, 114*, 106–116.

Alter, M. J., Mast, E. E., Moyer, L. A., & Margolis, H. S. (1998). Hepatitis C. *Infectious Disease Clinics of North America, 12*, 13–26.

Alternative Link. (2004). *ABC coding manual for integrative healthcare: Codes for research, management and commerce* (6th ed.). Albuquerque, NM: Author.

Alternative Link Systems. (2001). *The CAM and nursing coding manual*. Albany, NY: Delmar.

Alzheimer, A. (1906). Uber einen eigenartigen schweren krankheitsprozess der hirnrinde. *Neurologisches Centralblatt, 25*, 113–114.

Amato, B. C. (1987). PMS support groups: Creating environments for healing. Efficacy of self care [Abstract]. *7th Conference of the Society for Menstrual Cycle Research*, 58–60.

Amato, B. C. (1987). *PMS support groups: Creating environments for healing. Efficacy of self care* [Abstract]. 7th Conference of the Society for Menstrual Cycle Research, 58–60.

Amella, E. J. (1999). Factors influencing the proportion of food consumed by nursing home residents with dementia. *Journal of the American Geriatrics Society, 47*, 879–885.

Amella, E. J. (2003). Decision making for tube feeding in dementia: When evidence becomes paramount. *Journal of Clinical Nursing, 12*, 703–705.

American Academy of Pediatrics. (2004). *Pediatric Nutrition Handbook*. Elk Grove, Illinois: Author.

American Academy of Pediatrics Committee on Practice and Ambulatory Medicine. (1997). Pediatrician's responsibility for infant nutrition. *Pediatrics, 99*(5), 749–751.

American Association of Colleges of Nursing. (1994). Position Statement: *Certification and Regulation of*

Advanced Practice Nurses. American Association of Colleges of Nursing: Washington, DC.

American Association of Critical-Care Nurses. (1993). Evaluation of the effects of heparinized and nonheparinized flush solutions on the patency of arterial pressure monitoring lines: The AACN Thunder Project. *American Journal of Critical Care, 2*, 3–15.

American Association of Critical-Care Nurses. (2002, June 24). *Research priorities*. Retrieved February 7, 2004, from http://www.aacn.org/research

American Cancer Society. (2003a). Colon and rectum cancer: Prevention and risk factors. *Prevention*. Available from http://www.cancer.org

American Cancer Society. (2003b). *Cancer facts & figures. 2003*. Atlanta, GA: Author.

American Diabetes Association. (2003). Report of the expert committee on the diagnosis and classification of diabetes mellitus. *Diabetes Care, 26*(Suppl. 1), S3–S20.

American Gastroenterological Association. (2002). Gastroenterology. *AGA Technical Review on Irritable Bowel Syndrome, 123*, 2108–2131.

American Geriatrics Society. (1997). Measuring the quality of care at the end of life: A statement of principles. *Journal of the American Geriatrics Society, 45*(4), 526–527.

American Geriatrics Society. (2001). Guideline for the prevention of falls in older persons. *Journal of the American Geriatric Society, 49*, 664–672.

American Geriatrics Society Clinical Practice Committee. (2003). Guidelines abstracted from the American Academy of Neurology's dementia guidelines for early detection, diagnosis, and management of dementia. *Journal of the American Geriatrics Society, 51*(6), 869–873.

American Heart Association. (2001a). Open-heart statistics. *Heart and Stroke Encyclopedia*. Retrieved December 5, 2003, from www.americanheart.org

American Heart Association. (2001b). *Heart and stroke facts and statistics*. Dallas, TX: Author.

American Heart Association. (2003). *Heart disease and stroke statistics—2004 update*. Dallas, TX: Author.

American Heart Association. (2004). *Stroke: Patient education tool kit*. Dallas, TX: Author.

American Journal of Nursing, in conjunction with the National Library of Medicine. (1966). *International nursing index*. New York: Author.

American Medical Association. (1992). *Diagnostic and treatment guidelines on elder abuse and neglect*. Chicago, IL: Author.

American Medical Association. (2000). *Physician's current procedural terminology*. Chicago: Author.

American Nurses Association. (1975). *Human rights guidelines for nurses in clinical and other research*. Kansas City, MO: Author.

American Nurses Association. (1980). *Nursing: A social policy statement*. Kansas City, MO: Author.

American Nurses Association. (1982). *A challenge for change: The role of gerontological nursing*. Kansas City, MO: Author.

American Nurses Association. (1984). *Addictions and psychological dysfunctions: The profession's response to the problem*. Kansas City, MO: American Nurses' Publishing.

American Nurses Association. (1985). *Human rights guidelines for nurses in clinical and other research*. Kansas City, MO: Author.

American Nurses Association. (1992). *Position Statement: Registered Nurse Utilization of Unlicensed Assistive Personnel*. Washington, DC: Author.

American Nurses Association. (1995). *Nursing's social policy statement*. Washington, DC: Author.

American Nurses Association. (1996). *Nursing quality indicators: Definitions and implications*. Washington, DC: Author.

American Nurses Association. (1999). *Core principles on telehealth*. Report of the Interdisciplinary Telehealth Standards Working Group. March 25, 1998. Washington, DC: Author.

American Nurses Association. (2000a). *Nursing quality indicators beyond acute care: Literature review*. Washington, DC: Author.

American Nurses Association. (2000b). *Nurse staffing and patient outcomes in the inpatient hospital setting*. Washington, DC: Author.

American Nurses Association. (2001). *Code of ethics for nurses with interpretive statements*. Washington, DC: Author.

American Nurses Association. (2003). *Nursing's social policy statement* (2nd ed.). Washington, DC: Nursesbooks.org (Publishing Program of ANA).

American Nurses Association Center for Nursing Research. (1980). Generating a scientific basis for nursing practice: Research priorities for the 1980's. *Nursing Research, 29*, 219.

American Psychiatric Association. (1986). *Diagnostic and statistical manual of mental disorders (DSMIIIR)*. Washington, DC: American Psychiatric Publishing.

American Psychiatric Association. (1986). *Diagnostic and statistical manual of mental disorders (DSMIIIR)*. Washington, DC: Author.

American Psychiatric Association. (1999). Practice guideline for the treatment of patients with delirium. *American Journal of Psychiatry, 156*(5, Suppl.), 1–20. Also can be retrieved from http://www.psych.org/psych_pract/treatg/pg/pg_delirium.cfm

American Psychiatric Association. (2000). *Diagnostic and statistical manual of mental disorders* (4th ed., text revision.) Washington, DC: Author.

ANA (American Nurses' Association). (2002). The American Nurse (n.d.). *Helping nurses help caregivers*. Retrieved January 8, 2003, from http://nursingworld.org

Anders, R. L. (2000). Assessment of inpatient treatment of person with schizophrenia: Implications for practice. *Archives of Psychiatric Nursing, 14*, 213–221.

Anders, R. L., Kawano, M., Mori, C., Kokusho, H., & Tokunaga, I. (2001). Assessment of inpatient treatment of patients with schizophrenia in Japan: Implications for practice. *Archives of Psychiatric Nursing, 15*, 265–271.

Anders, R. L., Thapinta, D., Wiwatkunupakan, S., Kitsumban, V., & Vadtanapong, S. (2003). Assessment of inpatient treatment of mentally ill patients in Thailand: Implications for practice. *Contemporary Nurse, 15*, 322–332.

Anderson, C., & Weber, J. (1993). Preretirement planning and perceptions of satisfaction among retirees. *Educational Gerontology, 19*, 397–406.

Anderson, G. C. (1977). The mother and her newborn: Mutual caregivers. *Journal of Obstetric, Gynecologic, and Neonatal Nursing, 6*(5), 50–57.

Anderson, G. C. (1989). Risk in mother infant separation postbirth. *IMAGE: Journal of Nursing Scholarship, 21*, 196–199.

Anderson, G. C. (1991). Current knowledge about skin-to-skin (kangaroo) care for preterm infants. *Journal of Perinatology, 11*, 216–226.

Anderson, G. C. (1995). Touch and the kangaroo method. In T. Field (Ed.), *Touch and infancy* (pp. 35–51). Hillsdale, NJ: Erlbaum.

Anderson, G. C. (1999). Kangaroo care of the premature infant. In E. Goldson (Ed.), *Nurturing the premature infant: Developmental interventions in the neonatal intensive care nursery* (pp. 131–160). New York: Oxford University Press.

Anderson, G. C., Chiu, S. H., Dombrowski, M. A., Swinth, J. Y., Albert, J. M., & Wada, N. (2003). Mother-newborn contact in a randomized trial of kangaroo (skin-to-skin) care. *Journal of Obstetric, Gynecologic, & Neonatal Nursing, 32*, 604–611.

Anderson, G. C., Dombrowski, M. A. S., & Swinth, J. Y. (2001). Kangaroo care: Not just for stable premies anymore. *Reflections on Nursing Leadership, 27*, 32–34.

Anderson, G. C., Moore, E. R., Hepworth, J., & Bergman, N. (2003). *Early skin-to-skin contact for mothers and their healthy newborn infants*. (Cochrane Review). In The Cochrane Library, Issue 2, 2003. Oxford, England: Update Software.

Anderson, J. (1991b). Immigrant women speak of chronic illness. The social construction of the devalued self. *Journal of Advanced Nursing, 16*, 710–717.

Anderson, K. L., & Burckhardt, C. S. (1999). Conceptualization and measurement of quality of life as an outcome variable for health care intervention and research. *Journal of Advanced Nursing, 29*, 298–306.

Anderson, M., Standen, P., Nazir, S., & Noon, J. P. (2000). Nurses and doctors attitudes toward suicidal behavior in young people. *International Journal of Nursing Studies, 37*, 1–11.

Anderson, R. (2002). *Deaths: Leading causes for 2000*. (50) 16. Hyattsville, MD: National Center for Health Statistics. Retrieved from http://www.cdc.gov/nchs/data/nvsr/nvsr50/nvsr50_16.pdf

Anderson, R. A., Hsieh, P. C., & Su, H. F. (1998). Resource allocation and resident outcomes in nursing homes: Comparisons between the best and worst. *Research in Nursing & Health, 21*, 297–313.

Andrew, M. J., Baker, R. A., Kneebone, A. C., & Knight, J. L. (2000). Mood state as a predictor of neuropsychological deficits following cardiac surgery. *Journal of Psychosomatic Research, 48*, 537–546.

Andrews, D. A., & Bonta, J. (1995). *LSI-R: The Level of Service Inventory—Revised*. Toronto, Ontario, Canada: MultiHealth Systems, Inc.

Andrist, L., & MacPherson, K. (Eds.). (2001). *Conceptual models for women's health research: Reclaiming menopause as an exemplar of nursing's contributions to feminist scholarship* (Vol. 19, pp. 29–62). New York: Springer.

Androwich, I., Bickford, C., Button, P., Hunter, K., Murphy, J., & Sensmeier, J. (2003). *Clinical Information Systems: A framework for reaching the vision*. Washington, DC: American Nurses Publishing.

Annells, M., & Koch, T. (2002). Older people seeking solutions to constipation: The laxative mire. *Journal of Clinical Nursing, 11*(5), 903.

Anonymous. (2003). The state of the science on urinary incontinence. *American Journal of Nursing, 103*(3), 45–49.

Antai-Otung, D. (2003). Psychosocial rehabilitation. *Nursing Clinics of North America, 38*, 151–160.

Anthony, W. A., Cohen, M., Farkas, M., & Cohen, B. (2000). Clinical update: The chronically mentally ill. *Community Mental Health Journal, 36*(1), 97–106.

Antonovsky, A. (1998). The sense of coherence: An historical and future perspective. In H. I. McCubbin, E. Thompson, A. Thompson, & J. Fromer (Eds.), *Stress, coping, and health in families: Sense of coherence and resiliency*. Thousand Oaks, CA: Sage.

APA, Psychology of Women Division of the American Psychological Association. (1981). *Guidelines for non-sexist research*. Washington, DC: Author.

Aravanis, S. C., Adelman, R. D., Breckman, R., Fulmer, T., Holder, E., Lachs, M. S., et al. (1993). Diagnostic and treatment guidelines on elder abuse and neglect. *Archives of Family Medicine, 2*(4), 371–388.

Arbogast, K. B., Cornejo, R. A., Kallan, M. J., Winston, F. K., & Durbin, D. R. (2002). Injuries to children in forward facing child restraints. *Annual Proceedings of the Association for the Advancement of Automotive Medicine, 46*, 213–230.

Archbold, P. G., & Stewart, B. J. (1996). The nature of the caregiving role and nursing interventions for caregiving families. In E. Swanson & T. Tripp-Reimer (Eds.), *Series on issues in gerontological nursing* (Vol. 1, pp. 133–156). New York: Springer Publishing.

Arean, P. A., & Cook, B. L. (2002). Psychotherapy and combined psychotherapy/pharmacotherapy for late life depression. *Biological Psychiatry, 52*, 293–303.

Argyris, C. (1987). Seeking truth and actionable knowledge: How the scientific method inhibits both. *Philosophica, 40*, 5–21.

Argyris, C., Putnam, R., & Smith, D. M. (1985). *Action science*. San Francisco: Jossey-Bass.

Argyris, C., & Schön, D. (1974). *Theories in practice: Increasing professional effectiveness*. San Francisco: Jossey-Bass.

Arias, E., MacDorman, M. F., Strobino, D. M., & Guyer, B. (2003). Annual summary of vital statistics—2002. *Pediatrics, 112*(6), 1215–1230.

Aroian, K. J. (2001). Immigrant women's health. In N. Woods and D. Taylor (Volume Eds.), & J. Fitzpatrick (Series Ed.), *Annual Review of Nursing Research, 19* (pp. 179–226). New York: Springer Publishing.

Aroian, K. J., Norris, A. E., & Chiang, L. (2003). Gender differences in psychological distress among immigrants from the former Soviet Union. *Journal of Sex Roles Research, 48*(1/2), 39–51.

Aronheim, J. C., Mulvihill, M., Sieger, C., Park, P., & Fries, B. E. (2001). State practice variation in the use of tube feeding for nursing home residents with severe cognitive impairment. *Journal of the American Geriatric Society, 49*, 148–152.

Arras, J. D. (1995). *Bringing the hospital home: Ethical and social implications of high-tech home care*. Baltimore: John Hopkins University Press.

Arthur, D. (2002). The validity and reliability of the measurement of the concept of 'expressed emotion' in the family members and nurses of Hong Kong patients with schizophrenia. *International Journal of Mental Health Nursing, 11*, 192–198.

Ary, D., Cheser Jacobs, L., & Razavieh, A. (2002). *Introduction to research in education* (5th ed.). New York: Holt, Rinehart and Winston.

Ashton, C., Whitworth, G. C., Seldomridge, J. A., Shapiro, P. A., Weinberg, A. D., Michler, R. E., et al. (1997). Self-hypnosis reduces anxiety following coronary artery bypass surgery. *Journal of Cardiovascular Surgery, 38*, 69–75.

Association of Operating Room Nurses (AORN). (1997). *Perioperative Nursing Data Set*. Boulder, CO: Author.

Association of Operating Room Nurses. (1998). Recommended practices for laser safety in practice settings. *Association of Operating Room Nurses Journal, 67*, 263–264, 267–269.

Association of Women's Health, Obstetrical & Neonatal Nursing. (2003). *Evidence-based clinical practice guideline: Nursing management for cyclic perimenstrual pain and discomfort*. Washington, DC: Author.

Astrup, J., Siesjo, B. K., & Symon, L. (1981). Thresholds in cerebral ischemia—the ischemic penumbra. *Stroke, 12*(6), 723–725.

Atchison, J. H. (1998). Perceived job satisfaction among nurse assistants employed in midwest nursing homes. *Geriatric Nursing, 19*(3), 135–138.

Atchley, R. (1977). *Social forces in later life*. Belmont, CA: Wadsworth.

Atkinson, R. (1990). Aging and alcohol use disorders: Diagnostic issues in the elderly. *International Psychogeriatrics, 2*, 55–72.

Atlas of Canada. (2001). *Health indicators*. Retrieved from http://atlas.gc.ca/maptexts/topic_texts/english/health_ind_e.html

Attree, M. (2001). Patients' and relatives' experiences and perspectives of 'good' and 'not so good' quality care. *Journal of Advanced Nursing, 33*(4), 456–466.

Auerbach, J., Wypijewska, C., Brodie, H., & Hammond, K. (1994). *AIDS and behavior: An integrated approach*. Washington, DC: National Academy Press.

Auerbach, K. G. (2000). Evidence-based care and the breastfeeding couple: Key concerns. *Journal of Midwifery & Women's Health, 45*(3), 205–211.

Austin, J. (1996). A model of family adaptation to new onset childhood epilepsy. *Journal of Neuroscience Nursing, 28*(2), 82–92.

Austin, J. K., & Dunn, D. W. (2000). Children with epilepsy: Quality of life and psychosocial needs. *Annual Review of Nursing Research, 18*, 26–47.

Austin, J. K., Dunn, D. W., & Huster, G. A. (2000). Childhood epilepsy and asthma: Changes in behavior problems related to gender and change in condition severity. *Epilepsia, 41*, 615–623.

Austin, J. K., Harezlak, J., Dunn, D. W., Huster, G. A., Rose, D. F., & Ambrosius, W. T. (2001). Behavior problems in children before first recognized seizures. *Pediatrics, 107*(1), 115–122.

Austin, J. L. (1975). *How to do things with words* (2nd ed.). Oxford, England: Oxford University Press.

Avato, J. L., & Lai, K. K. (2002). Impact of postdischarge surveillance on surgical-site infection rates for coronary artery bypass procedures. *Infection Control Hospital Epidemiology, 23*, 364–367.

Aydelotte, M. (1973). *Nurse staffing methodology: A review and critique of selected literature*. Washington, DC: DHEW Publication No. (NIH) 73-433.

Ayoub, J. L., Vanderboom, C., Knight, M., Walsh, K., Briggs, R., & Grekiw, K. (1998). A study of the effectiveness of an interactive computer classroom. *Computers in Nursing, 16*(6), 333–338.

Aziz, N., & Rowland, J. (2002). Cancer survivorship research among ethnic minority and medically underserved groups. *Oncology Nursing Forum, 29*(5), 789–801.

Baar, A., Moores, B., & Rhys-Hearn, C. (1973). A review of the various methods of measuring the dependency of patients on nursing staff. *International Journal of Nursing Studies, 10*, 195–203.

Babrow, A. S. (2001). Uncertainty, value, communication, and problematic integration. *Journal of Communication, 51*(3), 553–573.

Backer, T., & Koon, S. (1995). Sharing the wealth of ideas: Demonstrate, evaluate, disseminate, repeat. *Foundation News and Commentary, 36*(2), 28–34.

Bacon, E., Condon, E., & Fernsler, J. (2000). Young widows' experience with an internet self-help group. *Journal of Psychological Nursing, 38*(7), 24–33.

Badger, T. A. (1996a). Family members' experiences of living with members with depression. *Western Journal of Nursing Research, 18*, 149–171.

Badger, T. A. (1996b). Living with depression: Family members' experiences and treatment needs. *Journal of Psychosocial Nursing and Mental Health Services, 34*, 21–29.

Badger, T. A., McNiece, C., Bonham, E., Jacobson, J., & Gelenberg, A. J. (2003). Health outcomes for people with serious mental illness: A case study. *Perspectives of Psychiatric Care, 39*, 23–32.

Badovinac, C. C., Wilson, S., & Woodhouse, D. (1999). The use of unlicensed assistive personnel and selected outcome indications. *Nursing Economics, 17*(4), 194–200.

Baggens, C. (2001). What they talk about: Conversations between child health center nurses and parents. *Journal of Advanced Nursing, 36*, 659–667.

Baggs, J. G., & Mick, D. J. (2000). Collaboration: A tool addressing ethical issues for elderly patients near the end of life in intensive care units. *Journal of Gerontological Nursing, 26*(9), 41–47.

Baier, M., DeShay, E., Owen, K., Robinson, M., Lasar, K., Peterson, K., et al. (2000). The relationship between insight and clinical factors for persons with schizophrenia. *Archives of Psychiatric Nursing, 14*, 259–265.

Baier, M., & Murray, R. L. E. (1999). A descriptive study of insight into illness reported by persons with schizophrenia. *Journal of Psychosocial Nursing and Mental Health Services, 37*, 14–21.

Bailey, S. L., & Heitkemper, M. M. (2001). Circadian rhythmicity of cortisol and body temperature: Morningness-eveningness effects. *Chronobiology International, 18*(2), 249–261.

Bakas, T., Austin, J. K., Jessup, S. L., Williams, L. S., & Oberst, M. T. (2004). Time and difficulty of tasks provided by family caregivers of stroke survivors. *Journal of Neuroscience Nursing, 36*, 95–106.

Bakas, T., & Champion, V. (1999). Development and psychometric testing of the Bakas Caregiving Outcomes Scale. *Nursing Research, 48*, 250–259.

Baker, C., Beglinger, J., King, S., Salyards, M., & Thompson, A. (2000). Transforming negative work cultures. *Journal of Nursing Administration, 30*, 357–363.

Baker, F. M., & Bell, C. C. (1999). Issues in the psychiatric treatment of African Americans. *Psychiatric Services, 50*, 362–368.

Baker, J. A., O'Higgins, H., Parkinson, J., & Tracey, N. (2002). The construction and implementation of a psychosocial interventions care pathways within a low secure environment: A pilot study. *Journal of Psychiatric Mental Health Nursing, 9*(6), 737–739.

Baker, R., Wu, A. W., Teno, J. M., Kreling, B., Damiano, A. M., Rubin, H. R., et al. (2000). Family satisfaction with end-of-life care in seriously ill hospitalized adults. *Journal of the American Geriatrics Society, 48*(5), 61–69.

Baker, R. A., Andrew, M. J., Schrader, G., & Knight, J. L. (2001). Preoperative depression and mortality in coronary artery bypass surgery: Preliminary findings. *Australia New Zealand Journal of Surgery, 71*, 139–142.

Bakken, S. (2001). An informatics infrastructure is essential for evidence-based practice. *Journal of the American Informatics Association, 8*, 199–201.

Bakken, S., Campbell, K. E., Cimino, J. J., Huff, S. M., & Hammond, W. E. (2000). Toward vocabulary domain specifications for Health Level 7-

coded data elements. *Journal of the American Medical Informatics Association, 7*(4), 333–342.

Bakken, S., Cashen, M. S., Mendonca, E. A., O'Brien, A., & Zieniewicz, J. (2000). Representing nursing activities within a concept-oriented terminological system: Evaluation of a type definition. *Journal of the American Medical Informatics Association, 7*(1), 81–90.

Bakken, S., Cimino, J. J., & Hripcsak, G. (2004). Promoting patient safety and enabling evidence-based practice through informatics. *Medical Care, 42*, II-49–II-56.

Bakken, S., Coenen, A., & Saba, V. (2004). ISO Reference Terminology Model. *Healthcare Informatics, 21*(9), 52.

Bakken, S., Warren, J. J., Lundberg, C., Casey, A., Correia, C., Konicek, D., et al. (2002). An evaluation of the usefulness of two terminology models for integrating nursing diagnosis concepts into SNOMED Clinical Terms. *International Journal of Medical Informatics, 68*(1–3), 71–77.

Balas, E. A., Jaffrey, F., Kuperman, G. J., Boren, S. A., Brown, G. D., Pinciroli, F., et al. (1997). Electronic communication with patients: Evaluation of distance medicine technology. *Journal of American Medical Association, 278*, 152–159.

Baldacchino, D., & Draper, P. (2001). Spiritual coping strategies: A review of the nursing research literature. *Journal of Advanced Nursing, 34*, 833–841.

Baldwin, Jr., D. (1996). Some historical notes on interdisciplinary and interprofessional education and practice in health care in the USA. *Journal of Interprofessional Care, 10*, 173–187.

Ballantyne, G. H. (2002). Robotic surgery, telerobotic surgery, telepresence, and telementoring. Review of early clinical results. *Surgical Endoscopy, 16*(10), 1389–1402.

Ballantyne, G. H., Hourmont, K., & Wasielewski, A. (2003). Telerobotic laparoscopic repair of incisional ventral hernias using intraperitoneal prosthetic mesh. *Journal of the Society of Laparoendoscopic Surgeons, 7*(1), 7–14.

Baltes, P. B., & Danish, S. J. (1980). Intervention in life-span development and aging. In R. R. Turner & H. W. Reese (Eds.), *Life-span developmental psychology* (pp. 49–78). New York: Academic Press.

Baly, M. E. (1988). Florence Nightingale and "her" schools of nursing. *Humane Medicine, 4*(1), 23–45.

Bandura, A. (1977). Self-efficacy: Toward a unifying theory of behavioral change. *Psychological Review, 84*, 191–215.

Bandura, A. (1994). Social cognitive theory and exercise of control over HIV infection. In R. J. DiClemente & J. L. Peterson (Eds.), *Preventing AIDS: Theories and methods of behavioral interventions* (pp. 25–59). New York: Plenum Press.

Bandura, A. (1997). *Self-efficacy: The exercise of control*. New York: W. H. Freeman.

Banerji, D. (2003). Reflections on the twenty-fifth anniversary of the Alma-Ata Declaration. *International Journal of Health Services, 33*, 813–818.

Banever, G. T., Moriarty, K. P., Sachs, B. F., Courtney, R. A., Konefal, S. H., Jr., & Barbeau, L. (2003). Pediatric hand treadmill injuries. *Journal of Craniofacial Surgery, 14*(4), 487–490: discussion 491–492.

Bankert, K., Daughtridge, S., Meehan, M., & Colburn, L. (1996). The application of collaborative benchmarking to the prevention and treatment of pressure ulcers. *Advances in Wound Care: The Journal for Prevention and Healing, 9*(2), 21–29.

Baradell, J. G., & Bordeaux, B. R. (2001). Outcomes and satisfaction of patients of psychiatric clinical nurse specialists. *Journal of the American Psychiatric Nurses Association, 7*, 77–85.

Baranowski, T. (1997). Families and health actions. In D. S. Gochman (Ed.), *Handbook of health behavior research I: Personal and social determinants* (pp. 179–205). New York: Plenum Press.

Barczak, N., & Spunt, D. (1999). Competency-based education: Maximize the performance of your unlicensed assistive personnel. *Journal of Continuing Education in Nursing, 30*(6), 254–259.

Barkauskas, V. H., Pohl, J. M., Breer, L., Benkert, R., & Wells, M. (2005). Measuring quality in nurse-managed centers using HEDIS measures. *Journal for Healthcare Quality, 27*(1), 4–14.

Barkauskas, V. H., Pohl, J. M., Breer, L., Tanner, C., Bostrom, A., Benkert, R., et al. (2003). Academic nurse-managed centers: Approaches to evaluation. *Outcomes Management, 8*(1), 57–66.

Barker, P. (2000). Commentaries and reflections on mental heath nursing in the UK at the dawn of the new millennium: Commentary 1. *Journal of Mental Health, 9*(6), 617–619.

Barlow, J., Coren, E., & Stewart-Brown, S. (2002). Meta-analysis of the effectiveness of parenting programmes in improving maternal psychosocial health. *British Journal of General Practice, 52*(476), 223–233.

Barnard, K. E., & Eyres, S. J. (1979). *Child health assessment, part 2: The first year of life*. Hyattsville, MD: U.S. Department of Health, Education, and Welfare, Public Health Service, HRA, Bureau of Health Manpower.

Barnard, K. E., Hammond, M. A., Booth, C. L., Bee, H. L., Mitchell, S. K., & Spieker, S. (1989). Measurement and meaning of parent child interaction. In F. Morrison, C. Lord, & D. Keating (Eds.), *Applied developmental psychology* (Vol. 3). New York: Academic.

Barnes, S. J., & Adair, B. (2002). The cognition-sensitive approach to dementia parallels with the Science of Unitary Human Beings. *Journal of Psychosocial Nursing and Mental Health Services, 40*(11), 30–37, 44–45.

Barnfather, J. S., & Lyon, B. L. (1993). *Stress and coping: State of the science and implications for nursing theory, research and practice*. Indianapolis, IN: Sigma Theta Tau International.

Barnsteiner, J. H. (1993, Spring). The online journal of knowledge synthesis for nursing. *Reflections, 19*(1), 8.

Baron, R. A., & Byrne, D. (1994). *Social psychology: Understanding human interaction* (7th ed.). Boston: Allyn and Bacon.

Barowsky, D. (2003). Assessing cultural fit during the interview. *Healthcare Executive, Sept/Oct*, 62–63.

Barratt, E. (1989). Community psychiatric nurses: Their self-perceived roles. *Journal of Advanced Nursing, 14*, 42–48.

Barrett, E. A. M. (2000). *The theoretical matrix for a Rogerian nursing practice*. Retrieved September 12, 2004, from http://www.nurses.info/nursing_theory_person_rogers_martha.htm

Barron, C. R. (2000). Stress, uncertainty, and health. In V. H. Rice (Ed.), *Handbook of stress, coping and health implications for nursing research, theory, and practice* (pp. 517–539). Thousand Oaks, CA: Sage Publications.

Barry-Walker, J. (2000). The impact of systems redesign on staff, patient, and financial outcomes. *Journal of Nursing Administration, 30*, 77–89.

Barsky, A. J,. Peekna, H. M., & Borus, J. F. (2001). Somatic symptom reporting in women and men. *General Internal Medicine, 16*, 266–275.

Bartels, S. J., Dums, A. R., Oxman, T. E., Schneider, L. S., Arean, P. A., Alexopoulos, G. S., et al. (2002). Evidence-based practices in geriatric mental health care. *Psychiatric Services, 53*, 1419–1431.

Barter, M., McLaughlin, F. E., & Thomas, S. A. (1997). Registered nurse role changes and satisfaction with unlicensed assistive personnel. *Journal of Nursing Administration, 27*(1), 29–38.

Barthes, R. (1974). *Introduction to the structured analysis of the narratives* (R. Miller, Trans.). New York: Hill & Wang.

Bartlett, E. E. (1985). At last, a definition. *Patient Education and Counseling, 7*, 323.

Bassett, C. C. (1995). Critical care nurses: Ethical dilemmas, a phemonemological perspective. *Care of the Critically Ill, 11*(4), 166, 168–169.

Bassett, K. (1996). Anthropology, clinical pathology and the electronic fetal monitor: Lessons from the heart. *Social Science and Medicine, 42*, 281–292.

Bates-Jensen, B. M. Vredevoe, D. L., & Brecht, M. (1992). Validity and reliability of the pressure sore status tool. *Decubitus, 5*(6), 20–28

Batson, K., McCabe, B., Baun, M. M., & Wilson, C. (1998). The effect of a therapy dog on socialization and physiologic indicators of stress in persons diagnosed with Alzheimer's disease. In C. C. Wilson & D. C. Turner (Eds.), *Companion animals in human health* (pp. 203–215). Thousand Oaks, CA: Sage.

Bauer, H. M., Rodríguez, M. A., & Pérez-Stable, E. J. (2000). Prevalence and determinants of intimate partner abuse among public hospital primary care patients. *Journal of General Internal Medicine, 15*, 811–817.

Baumann, S. L. (1993). The meaning of being homeless. *Scholarly Inquiry for Nursing Practice: An International Journal, 7*(1), 59–73.

Baun, M. M., Bergstrom, N., Langston, N. F., & Thoma, L. (1984). Physiological effects of human/companion animal bonding. *Nursing Research, 33*(3), 126–129.

Bayley, E. W., MacLean, S. L., Desy, P., & McAMahon, M. (2004). ENAs Delphi study on national research priorities for emergency nurses in the U.S. *Journal of Emergency Nursing, 30*, 96–102.

Beach, S., Schultz, R., Yee, J., & Jackson, S. (2000). Negative and positive health effects of caring for a disabled spouse. *Psychology and Aging, 15*(2), 259–271.

Beach, S. R. H., Sandeen, E. E., & O'Leary, K. D. (1990). *Depression in marriage: A model for etiology and treatment*. New York: Guildford.

Bearn, J., & Wessely, S. (1994). Neurobiological aspects of the chronic fatigue syndrome. *European Journal of Clinical Investigation, 24*, 79–90.

Beaton, R. D., & Murphy, S. A. (2002). Psychosocial responses to biological and chemical terrorist threats and events. *American Association of Occupational Health Nursing Journal, 50*(4), 182–189.

Beaver, K., Luker, K. A., & Woods, S. (2000). Primary care services received during terminal illness. *International Journal of Palliative Nursing, 6*, 220–227.

Beavis, D., Simpson, S., & Graham, I. (2002). A literature review of dementia care mapping: Methodological considerations and efficacy. *Journal of Psychiatric and Mental Health Nursing, 9*(6), 725–736.

Bechtel-Blackwell, D. A. (2002). Computer-assisted self-interview and nutrition education in pregnant teens. *Clinical Nursing Research, 11*, 450–462.

Beck, A. T. (1997). The past and future of cognitive therapy. *Journal of Psychotherapy Practice and Research*, 6(4), 276–284.

Beck, C., Heacock, P., Mercer, S. O., Walls, R. C., Rapp, C. G., & Vogelpohl, T. S. (1997). Improving dressing behavior in cognitively impaired nursing home residents. *Nursing Research*, 46(3), 126–132.

Beck, C., Heacock, P., Rapp, C. G., & Mercer, S. O. (1993). Assisting cognitively impaired elders with activities of daily living. *American Journal of Alzheimer's Care and Related Disorders & Research*, 8, 11–20.

Beck, C. T. (1992a). Caring between nursing students and physically/mentally handicapped children: A phenomenological study. *Journal of Nursing Education*, 31, 1–6.

Beck, C. T. (1992b). The lived experience of postpartum depression: A phenomenological study. *Nursing Research*, 41, 166–170.

Beck, C. T. (1996). A meta-analysis of predictors of postpartum depression. *Nursing Research*, 45, 297–303.

Beck, C. T., & Gable, R. K. (2001). *Postpartum Depression Screening Scale*. Los Angeles: Western Psychological Services.

Beckstrand, J., Ellett, M., Welch, J., Dye, J., Games, C., Henrie, S., et al. (1990). The distance to the stomach for feeding tube placement in children predicted from regression on height. *Research in Nursing & Health*, 13(6), 411–420.

Beebe, L. H. (2001). Community nursing support for clients with schizophrenia. *Archives of Psychiatric Nursing*, 15, 214–222.

Beebe, L. H. (2002). Problems in community living identified by people with schizophrenia. *Journal of Psychosocial Nursing and Mental Health Services*, 40 38–45.

Beebe, L. H. (2003a). Health promotion in persons with schizophrenia: Atypical medications. *Journal of the American Psychiatric Nurses Association*, 9, 115–122.

Beebe, L. H. (2003b). Theory-based research in schizophrenia. *Perspectives in Psychiatric Care*, 39, 67–74.

Beeber, L. S. (1998). Treating depression through the therapeutic nurse-client relationship. *Nursing Clinics of North America*, 33, 153–172.

Beeber, L. S., & Miles, M. S. (2003). Maternal mental health and parenting in poverty. In J. J. Fitzpatrick, M. S. Miles, & D. Holditch-Davis (Eds.), *Annual review of nursing research* (Vol. 21, pp. 303–331). New York: Springer.

Beers, M. H., & Berkow, R. (Eds.). (2000). *The Merck manual of geriatrics* (3rd ed.). Whitehouse Station, NJ: Merck Research Laboratories.

Behl, L. E., Conyngham, A., & May, P. F. (2003). Trends in child maltreatment literature.

Bell, R. P., & McGrath, J. (1996). Implementing a research based kangaroo care program in the NICU. In L. Brown (Ed.), *Nursing clinics of North America:* Vol. 31(2). Maternal/fetal nursing (pp. 387–403). Philadelphia: Saunders.

Bem, S. L. (1974). The measurement of psychological androgyny. *Journal of Consulting and Clinical Psychology*, 42, 155–162.

Benever, G. T., Moriarty, R. P., Sachs, B. F., Courtney, R. A., Konefal, S. H., & Barbeau, L. (2003). *Journal of Craniofacial Surgery*, 14, 487–490.

Bengstsson-Tops, A., & Hansson, L. (2001). The validity of Antonovsky's sense of coherence measure in a sample of schizophrenic patients living in the community. *Journal of Advanced Nursing*, 33, 432–438.

Benjamin, B. A. (1995). Relationship between literacy skills and actual and estimated job performance of the nurse aide (Doctoral dissertation, Teachers College, Columbia University).

Benkert, R., Barkauskas, V., Pohl, J., Tanner, C., & Nagelkerk, J. (2002). Patient satisfaction outcomes in nurse managed centers. *Outcomes Management for Nursing Practice*, 6(4), 174–181.

Benner, P. (1984). *From novice to expert: Power and excellence in nursing practice*. Palo Alto, CA: Addison-Wesley.

Benner, P. (Ed.). (1994). *Interpretive phenomenology: Embodiment, caring and ethics in health and illness*. Thousand Oaks, CA: Sage.

Benner, P., Panner, C. A., & Chesla, C. (1996). *Expertise in nursing practice: Caring, clinical judgement, and ethics*. New York: Springer.

Benner, P., & Tanner, C. (1987). Clinical judgment: How expert nurses use intuition. *American Journal of Nursing*, 87(1), 23–31.

Bennett, L. (1991). Adolescent girls' experience of witnessing marital violence: A phenomenological study. *Journal of Advanced Nursing*, 16, 431–438.

Bennetts, C. (2000). The traditional mentor relationship and the well being of creative individuals in school and work. *International Journal of Health Promotion & Education*, 38(1), 22–27.

Benoliel, J. Q. (1983). Nursing research on death, dying, and terminal illness: Development, present state, and prospects. In H. Hurley & J. Fitzpatrick (Eds.), *Annual review of nursing research* (Vol. 1, pp. 101–130). New York: Springer.

Bensing, J., van Dulmen, S., & Tates, K. (2003). Communication in context: New directions in communication research. *Patient Education and Counseling*, 50, 27–32.

Bensley, L., Nelson, N., Kaufman, J., Silverstein, B., Kalat, J., & Walker, J. (1997). Injuries due to assaults on psychiatric hospital employees in Washington State. *American Journal of Industrial Medicine, 31*, 92–99.

Bentley, M. E., Dee, D. L., & Jensen, J. L. (2003). Breastfeeding among low income, African-American women: Power, beliefs, and decision making. *Journal of Nutrition, 133*, 305S–309S.

Berard, A., Bravo, G., & Gauthier, P. (1997). Meta-analysis of the effectiveness of physical activity for the prevention of bone loss in postmenopausal women. *Osteoporosis International, 7*(4), 331–337.

Berenson, R. A. (1984). *Intensive care units: Clinical outcomes, costs, and decision making* (OTA-HCS-28). Washington, DC: U.S. Government Printing Office.

Berg, A. O., & Atkins, D. (2003). Screening for osteoporosis in postmenopausal women: Recommendations and rationale. *American Journal of Nursing, 103*(1), 73–81.

Berg, J. (1999). *Modifying a perimenopausal symptom treatment package for use with Mexican American midlife women* [Abstract]. Abstracts of the 13th Conference of the Society for Menstrual Cycle Research, 1.

Berg, J., & Taylor, D. (1999). The symptom experience of Filipino American midlife women. *Menopause, 6*(2), 105–114.

Berg, J. (1999). Modifying a perimenopausal symptom treatment package for use with Mexican American midlife women [Abstract]. *Abstracts of the 13th Conference of the Society for Menstrual Cycle Research*, 1.

Bergeron, L. R., & Gray, B. (2003). Ethical dilemmas of reporting suspected elder abuse. *Social Work, 48*(1), 96–105.

Bergstrom, N. (1997). Prevention focused interventions skin breakdown: Preventing pressure ulcers—the status of prediction and success of prevention. Vitality throughout the adult lifecycle: *Interventions to Promote Health Seminar Proceedings*. Retrieved December, 2003, from http://www.nursing.uiowa.edu/centers/gnirc/vitality/abstract12.htm

Bergstrom, N., Braden, B., Laguzza, A., & Holzman, V. (1987). The Braden scale for predicting pressure sore risk. *Nursing Research, 38*, 205–210.

Berkman, L. F., Blumenthal, J., Burg, M., Carney, R. M., Catellier, D., Cowan, M. J., et al. (2003). Effects of treating depression and low perceived social support on clinical events after myocardial infarction: The Enhancing Recovery in Coronary Heart Disease Patients (ENRICHD) Randomized Trial. *Journal of the American Medical Association, 289*, 3106–3116.

Berkman, L. F., Leo-Summers, L., & Horowitz, R. (1992). Emotional support and survival after myocardial infarction: A prospective population based study of the elderly. *Annals of Internal Medicine, 117*, 1003–1009.

Bernard-Bonnin, A. C., Stachenko, S., Bonin, D., Charette, C., & Rousseau, E. (1995). Self-management teaching programs and morbidity of pediatric asthma: A meta-analysis. *Journal of Allergy and Clinical Immunology, 1*, 34–41.

Bernert, G., van Siebenthal, K., Seidl, R., Vanhole, C., Devlieger, H., & Casaer, P. (1997). The effect of behavioral states on cerebral oxygenation during endotracheal suctioning of preterm babies. *Neuropediatrics, 28*(2), 111–115.

Bernreuter, M. E., & Cardona, S. (1997). Survey and critique of studies related to unlicensed assistive personnel from 1995 to 1997, Part 2. *Journal of Nursing Administration, 27*(7/8), 49–55.

Bernstein, H. A. (1981). Survey of threats and assaults directed toward psychotherapists. *American Journal of Psychotherapy, 35*(4), 542–549.

Betz, C. (2000). Childhood obesity: Nursing prevention and intervention approaches are needed. *Journal of Pediatric Nursing, 15*(3), 135–136.

Beyene, Y., Taylor, D., & Lee, K. (2001). More than hot flashes: Cross-cultural symptom patterns and responses in midlife women [Abstract]. *Abstracts of the 13th Conference of the Society for Menstrual Cycle Research*, 52.

Biegel, D., Robinson, E., & Kennedy, M. (2000). A review of empirical studies of interventions for families of persons with mental illness. In J. Morrisey (Ed.), *Research in community mental health: Social factors in mental health and illness*. (Vol. 11). Greenwich, CT: JAI Press.

Biegel, D., Sales, E., & Schulz, R. (Eds.). (1991). Family caregiving in chronic illness. In *Family caregiver application series* (pp. 1–45). Newbury Park, CA: Sage.

Biglan, A., Hops, H., Sherman, L., Frediman, L. S., Arthur, J., & Osteen, V. (1985). Problem-solving interactions of depressed women and their spouses. *Behavior Therapy, 16*, 431–451.

Bilhartz, L. E., & Croft, C. L. (2000). *Gastrointestinal disease in primary care*. Philadelphia: Lippincott Williams & Wilkins.

Billings, A. G., & Moos, R. H. (1985). Psychosocial problems in unipolar depression: Comparing patients with matched community controls. *Journal of Counseling & Clinical Psychology, 53*, 314–325.

Birmaher, B., Ryan, N. D., & Williamson, D. E. (1996). Depression in children and adolescents:

Clinical features and pathogenesis. In K. I. Shulman, M. Tohen, & S. P. Kutcher (Eds.), *Mood disorders across the lifespan* (pp. 51–81). New York: Wiley-Liss.

Birnbaum, H. G., Leong, S. A., & Greenberg, P. E. (2003). The economics of women and depression: An employer's perspective. *Journal of Affective Disorders, 74*, 15–22.

Bischoff, W. E., Reynolds, T. M., Sessler, C. N., Edmond, M. B., & Wenzel, R. P. (2000). Handwashing compliance by health care workers: The impact of introducing an accessible, alcohol-based hand antiseptic. *Archives of Internal Medicine, 160*, 1017–1021.

Bishop, S., & Ingersoll, G. (1989). Effects of marital conflict and family structure on the self-concepts of pre- and early adolescents. *Journal of Youth and Adolescence, 18*(1), 25–38.

Bissell, L., & Haberman, P. C. (1984). *Alcoholism in the professions*. New York: Oxford University Press.

Bithoney, W. G., & Newberger, E. H. (1987). Child and family attributes of failure to thrive. *Journal of Developmental and Behavioral Pediatrics, 8*, 32–36.

Bixo, M., Sundström-Poromaa, I., Björn, I., & Åström, M. (2001). Patients with psychiatric disorders in gynecologic practice. *American Journal of Obstetric & Gynecology, 185*, 396–402.

Bjorklund, A., & Lindvall, O. (2000). Self-repair in the brain. *Nature, 405*, 892–895.

Blackhall, L. J., Murphy, S. T., Frank, G., Michel, V., & Azen, S. (1995). Ethnicity and attitudes toward patient autonomy. *Journal of the American Medical Association, 274*, 820–825.

Blair, K. (1990). Aging: Physiological aspects and clinical implications. *Nurse Practitioner, 2*, 14–28.

Blake, G. J., Rifai, N., Buring, J. E., & Ridker, P. M. (2003). Blood pressure, C-reactive protein, and risk of future cardiovascular events. *Circulation, 108*(24), 2993–2999.

Blalock, H. M. (1960). *Social statistics*. New York: McGraw-Hill.

Blanchard, D., Aswell, L., Goghlan, G., Durnin, M., Lomar, R., Sibley, M., et al. (1999). A student-developed tool for assessing safety in schizophrenic patients. *Nursing Connections, 12*, 37–41.

Bland, R., & Darlington, Y. (2002). The nature and sources of hope: Perspectives of family caregivers of people with serious mental illness. *Perspectives in Psychiatric Care, 38*, 61–68.

Blau, P. M. (1964). *Exchange and power in social life*. New York: Wiley.

Blazer, D. G. (2003). Depression in late life: Review and commentary. *Journals of Gerontology: Series A: Biological Science & Medical Science, 58A*(3), 249–265.

Blazer, L. K., & Mansfield, P. K. (1995). A comparison of substance use rates among female nurses, clerical workers and blue-collar workers. *Journal of Advanced Nursing, 21*, 305–313.

Blegan, M. A. (1993). Nurses' job satisfaction: A meta-analysis of related variables. *Nursing Research, 42*, 36–41.

Blegen, M., Vaughn, T., & Goode, C. (2001). Nurse experience and education: Effect on quality of care. *Journal of Nursing Administration, 31*(1), 33–39.

Blegen, M. A., Goode, C. J., & Reede, L. (1998). Nurse staffing and patient outcomes. *Nursing Research, 47*(1), 43–50.

Bleismer, M. M., Smayling, M., Kane, R., & Shannon, I. (1998). The relationship between nursing staffing levels and nursing home outcomes. *Journal of Aging and Health, 10*(3), 351–371.

Blendon, R. J., Scoles, K., DesRoches, C., Young, J. T., Herrmann, M. J., Schmidt, J. L., et al. (2001). Americans' health priorities: Curing cancer and controlling costs. *Health Affairs, 20*(6), 222–232.

Blomquist, K. (1986). Replication of research. *Research in Nursing and Health, 9*, 193–194.

Bloom, B. (2000). *Gender-responsive supervision and programming for women offenders in the community*. In National Institute of Correction (NIC) Annual issue 2000: Responding to women offenders in the community (No. J1CO-110, pp. 11–18). Longmont, CO: NIC Information Center.

BLS. (2001). *Detailed industry by selected events or exposures*. Retrieved February 10, 2004, from http://www.bls.gov/iif/oshwc/osh/os/ostb0992.pdf

Blue, C. L., Wilbur, J., & Marston-Scott, M. V. (2001). Exercise among blue-collar workers: Application of the theory of planned behavior. *Research in Nursing & Health, 24*, 481–493.

Blumenthal, J. A., Lett, H. S., Babyak, M. A., White, W., Smith, P. K., Mark, B. D., et al. (2003). Depression as a risk factor for mortality after coronary artery bypass surgery. *Lancet, 362*, 604–609.

Blustein, J., & Weiss, L. (1998). The use of mammography by women aged 75 and older: Factors related to health, functioning, and age. *Journal of the American Geriatrics Society, 46*, 941–946.

Blythe, J., Baumann, A., & Giovannetti, P. (2001). Nurses' experiences of restructuring in three Ontario hospitals. *Journal of Nursing Scholarship, 33*, 61–68.

Boath, E., & Henshaw, C. (2001). The treatment of postnatal depression: A comprehensive literature review. *Journal of Reproductive and Infant Psychology*, 215–248.

Bodenheimer, T. (2003). Innovations in primary care in the United States. *British Medical Journal, 326*, 796–798.

Boehm, S. (1992). Patient contracting. In G. M. Bulechek & J. C. McCloskey (Eds.), *Nursing interventions: Essential nursing treatments* (2nd ed., pp. 425–433). Philadelphia: W. B. Saunders.

Boehm, S., Schlenk, E. A., Raleigh, E., & Ronis, D. (1993). Behavioral analysis and behavioral strategies to improve self-management of type II diabetes. *Clinical Nursing Research, 2*, 327–344.

Bogardus, S. T., Yueh, B., & Shekelle, P. G. (2003). Screening and management of adult hearing loss in primary care-clinical applications. *Journal of the American Medical Association, 289*(15), 1986–1990.

Bolton, L. L., van Rijswick, L., & Shaffer, F. A. (1997). Quality wound care equals cost-effective wound care: A clinical model. *Advances in Wound Care, 10*, 33–38.

Bonner, B. L., Logue, M. B., Kaufman, K. L., & Niec, L. N. (2001). Child maltreatment. In C. E. Walker & M. C. Roberts (Eds.), *Handbook of clinical child psychology* (3rd ed., pp. 989–1024). New York: John Wiley & Sons.

Bonner, G. (2000). The CMHN and change. *Mental Health Nursing, 20*(6), 8–12.

Boockvar, V., Brodie, H. D., & Lachs, M. (2000). Nursing assistants detect behavior changes in nursing home residents that precede acute illness: Development and validation of an illness warning instrument. *Journal of the American Geriatrics Society, 48*(9), 1086–1091.

Booth, K., Maguire, P. M., Behir, F. R. C., Butterworth, T., & Hillier, V. F. (1996). Perceived professional support and the use of blocking behaviours by hospice nurses. *Journal of Advanced Nursing, 24*, 522–527.

Borge, L., Martinsen, E., Ruud, T., Wante, O., & Frilis, S. (1999). Quality of life, loneliness, and social contact among long term psychiatric patients. *Psychiatric Services, 50*(1), 81–84.

Borgman, C. L. (1990). Editor's introduction. In C. L. Borgman (Ed.), *Scholarly communication and bibliometrics* (pp. 10–27). Newbury Park, CA: Sage Publications.

Borowicz, L., Jr., Royall, R., Grega, M., Selnes, O., Lyketsos, C., & McKhann, G. (2002). Depression and cardiac morbidity 5 years after coronary artery bypass surgery. *Psychosomatics, 43*(6), 464–471.

Borowicz, L. M., Goldsborough, M. A., Selnes, O. A., & McKhann, G. M. (1996). Neuropsychologic change after cardiac surgery: A critical review. *Journal of Cardiothoracic and Vascular Anesthesia, 10*, 105–111.

Borum, M. L. (1998). Does age influence screening for colorectal cancer? *Age Ageing, 27*(4), 509–511.

Bosek, M. S., Lowry, E., Lindeman, D. A., Burck, J. R., & Gwyther, L. P. (2003). Promoting a good death for persons with dementia in nursing facilities: Family caregivers' perspectives. *JONAs Healthcare Law, Ethics, & Regulation, 5*(2), 34–41.

Bossé, R., Aldwin, C., Levenson, M., Spiro, A., & Mroczek, D. (1993). Change in social support after retirement: Longitudinal findings from the normative aging study. *Journal of Gerontology: Psychological Sciences, 48*, P210–P217.

Bostrom, J., & Wise, L. (1994). Closing the gap between research and practice. *Journal of Nursing Administration, 24*(5), 22–27.

Bottorff, J. L., Steele, R., Davies, B., Garossino, C., Porterfield, P., & Shaw, M. (1998). Striving for balance: Palliative care patients' experiences of making everyday choices. *Journal of Palliative Care, 14*(1), 7–17.

Bottrell, M., O'Sullivan, J. F., Robbins, M. A., Mitty, E., & Mezey, M. D. (2001). Transferring dying nursing home residents to the hospital: DON perspectives on the nurse's role in transfer decisions. *Geriatric Nursing, 22*(6), 313–317.

Boufford, J. I., & Lee, P. (2001). *Health policies for the 21st century: Challenges and recommendations for the U.S. Department of Health and Human Services*. Milbank Memorial Fund. Washington, DC.

Boult, C., Boult, L., Morishita, L., Dowd, B., Kane, R., & Urdangarin, C. (2001). A randomized clinical trial of outpatient geriatric evaluation and management. *Journal of the American Geriatrics Society, 49*, 351–363.

Boult, C., Murphy, J., Sloane, P., Mor, V., & Drone, C. (1991). The relation of dizziness to functional decline. *Journal of the American Geriatrics Society, 39*, 858–861.

Bourbonniere, M., Strumpf, N., Evans, L., & Maislin, G. (2001). Organizational characteristics and restraint use for hospitalized nursing home residents. *Journal of the American Geriatrics Society, 51*, 1079–1084.

Bowers, B., & Becker, M. (1992). Nurse's aides in nursing homes: The relationship between organization and quality. *Gerontologist, 32*(3), 360–366.

Bowker, G. C., & Star, S. L. (1999). *Sorting things out: Classification and its consequences*. Cambridge, MA: MIT Press.

Bowlby, J. (1981). Attachment and loss. In *Loss: Sadness and depression* (Vol. 3). London: Hogarth.

Bowles, K. (2003). *Assessing health related quality of life among frail elders*. Retrieved December, 2003, from http://www.nursing.upenn.edu/research/grants/default.asp?pid=233

Boyce, G. C., Smith, T. B., & Casto, G. (1999). Health and educational outcomes of children who experienced severe neonatal medical complications. *Journal of Genetic Psychology, 160*, 261–269.

Boyce, W. T., Frank, E., Jensen, P. S., Kessler, R. C., Nelson, C. A., Steinberg, L., et al. (1998). Social context in developmental psychopathology: Recommendations for future research from the MacArthur Network on Psychopathology and Development. *Development and Psychopathology, 10*, 143–164.

Boyd, N. (1998). *Gently into the night: Aggression in long-term care*. WCB of British Columbia, Research Report.

Boykin, A., Parker, M. E., & Schoenhofer, S. O. (1994). Aesthetic knowing grounded in a explicit conception of nursing. *Nursing Science Quarterly, 7*(4), 158–161.

Boykin, A., & Schoenhofer, S. (1990). Caring in nursing: Analysis of extant theory. *Nursing Science Quarterly, 3*(4), 149–155.

Boykin, A., & Schoenhofer, S. O. (1993). *Nursing as caring: A model for transforming practice*. New York: National League for Nursing Press.

Boykin, A., & Schoenhofer, S. O. (2001a). *Nursing as caring: A model for transforming practice* (rev. ed.). Sudbury, MA: Jones & Bartlett.

Boykin, A., & Schoenhofer, S. (2001b). Anne Boykin and Savina O. Schoenhofer in nursing as caring. In M. Parker (Ed.), *Nursing theories and nursing practice* (pp. 391–402). Philadelphia: F. A. Davis.

Boykin, A., Schoenhofer, S. O., Smith, N., St. Jean, J., & Aleman, D. (2003). Transforming practice using a caring-based nursing model. *Nursing Administration Quarterly, 27*, 223–230.

Braden, C. J., Mishel, M. H., Longman, A. J., & Burns, L. R. (1998). Self-help intervention project: Women receiving treatment for breast cancer. *Cancer Practice, 6*(2), 87–98.

Brandeis, J., Pashos, C. L., Henning, J. M., & Litwin, M. S. (2001). Racial differences in the cost of treating men with early-stage prostate cancer. *Journal of the American Geriatric Society, 49*(3), 297–303.

Branston, N. M., Symon, L., Crockard, H. A., & Pasztor, E. (1974). Relationship between the cortical evoked potential and local cortical blood flow following acute middle cerebral artery occlusion in the baboon. *Experimental Neurology, 45*(2), 195–208.

Braun, K. L., Suzuki, K. M., Cusick, K. E., & Howard-Carhart, K. (1997). Developing and testing training materials on elder abuse and neglect for nurse aides. *Journal of Elder Abuse & Neglect, 9*(1), 1–15.

Braunwald, E., Fauci, A. S., Kasper, D. L., Hauser, S. L., Longo, D. L., & Jameson, J. L. (2001). *Harrison's principles of internal medicine* (15th ed.). New York: McGraw-Hill.

Brayfield, A. H., & Rothe, H. F. (1951). An index of job satisfaction. *Journal of Applied Psychology, 35*, 307–311.

Breitbart, W., McDonald, M. V., Rosenfeld, B., Monkman, N. D., & Passik, S. (1998). Fatigue in ambulatory AIDS patients. *Journal of Pain and Symptom Management, 15*, 159–167.

Brennan, P. F., Moore, S. M., Bjornsdottir, G., Jones, J., Visovsky, C., & Rogers, M. (2001). HeartCare: An internet based information and support system to facilitate patient's home recovery after coronary artery bypass graft (CABG) surgery. *Journal of Advanced Nursing, 35*, 699–708.

Brennan, P. F., Moore, S. M., & Smyth, K. A. (1991). ComputerLink: Electronic support for the home caregiver. *Advances in Nursing Science, 13*(4), 14–27.

Brennan, P. F., Moore, S. M., & Smyth, K. A. (1995). The effects of a special computer network on caregivers of persons with Alzheimer's disease. *Nursing Research, 44*(3), 166–172.

Brennan, P. F., & Ripich, S. (1994). Use of a home-care computer network by persons with AIDS. *International Journal of Technology Assessment in Health Care, 10*(2), 258–272.

Brenneman, S. K., Lacroix, A. Z., Buist, D. S., Chen, Y. T., & Abbott, T. A. (2003). Evaluation of decision rules to identify postmenopausal women for intervention related to osteoporosis [Abstract]. *Disease Management, 6*(3), 159–168.

Bridges, E. J., Woods, S. L., Brengelmann, G. L., Mitchell, P., & Laurent-Bopp, D. (2000). Effect of the 30 degree lateral recumbent position on pulmonary artery and pulmonary artery wedge pressures in critically ill cardiac surgery patients. *American Journal of Critical Care, 9*(4), 262–275.

Brierley, J. B. (1973). Pathology of cerebral ischemia. In F. H. McDowell & R. W. Brennan (Eds.), *Cerebral vascular disease* (pp. 59–75). New York: Grune & Stratton.

Brierley, J. B., Brown, A. W., & Meldrum, B. S. (1971). The nature and time course of the neuronal alterations resulting from oligaemia and hypoglycaemia in the brain of Macaca mulatta. *Brain Research, 25*(3), 483–499.

Brierley, J. B., Meldrum, B. S., & Brown, A. W. (1973). The threshold and neuropathology of cerebral "anoxic-ischemic" cell change. *Archives of Neurology, 29*(6), 367–374.

Brink, P. J. (1976). *Transcultural nursing: A book of readings*. New York: Haworth Press.

British Geriatrics Society. (1999). *Guidelines for the diagnosis and management of delirium in the elderly.*

Retrieved September 9, 2003, from http://www.bgs.org.uk/publication/publication.htm

Britton, C. (1998). Clinical issues. The influence of antenatal information on breastfeeding experiences. *British Journal of Midwifery, 6*, 312–315.

Brod, M., Stewart, A. L., & Sands, L. (1999). Conceptualization of quality of life in dementia. *Journal of Mental Health and Aging, 5*(1), 7–20.

Bromet, E., Parkinson, D., Schulberg, H., & Gondek, P. (1982). Mental health of residents near the Three Mile Island reactor: A comparative study of selected groups. *Journal of Preventive Psychiatry, 1*, 225–276.

Bromley, D. (1986). *The case-study method in psychology and related disciplines*. Chichester, England: Wiley.

Brooker, C., & Butterworth, C. (1991). Working with families caring for a relative with schizophrenia: The evolving role of the community psychiatric nurse. *International Journal of Nursing Studies, 28*, 189–200.

Brooten, D. (1993). Assisting with transitions from hospital to home. In S. Funk, E. Tornquist, M. Champage, & R. Wiese (Eds.), *Key aspects of caring for the chronically ill: Hospital and home* (pp. 30–37). New York: Springer Publishing.

Brooten, D., Kumar, S., Brown, L. P., Butts, P., Finkler, S. A., Bakewell-Sachs, S., et al. (1986). A randomized clinical trial of early hospital discharge and home follow-up of very-low-birth-weight infants. *New England Journal of Medicine, 315*(15), 934–939.

Brooten, D., & Naylor, M. (1995). Nurses' effect on changing patient outcomes. *Image, 27*(2), 95–99.

Brower, H. (1994). Policy implications for life care environments. *Journal of Gerontological Nursing, 20*, 10–17.

Brown, B., & Bzostek, S. (2003). *Violence in the lives of children* (Pub. 2003-15). Cross Currents: Child Trends DataBank. (1) August. Retrieved from http://www.childtrendsdatabank.org/PDF/Violence.pdf

Brown, B. V., Kinkukawa, A., Michelson, E., Moore, A., Moore, K. A., & Sugland, A. (1999, December). *A century of children's health and well-being*. Research brief prepared for the National Child Health Leadership Conference. Retrieved January 8, 2004, from Child Trends web-site http://www.childtrends.org/PDF/disparities.pdf

Brown, C., Schulberg, H. C., Madonia, M. J., Shear, M. K., & Houck, P. R. (1996). Treatment outcomes for primary care patients with major depression and lifetime anxiety disorders. *American Journal of Psychiatry, 153*, 1293–1300.

Brown, D. R., & Boyce-Mathis, A. (2000). Surrogate parenting across generations: African American women caring for a child with special needs. *Journal of Mental Health and Aging, 6*, 339–351.

Brown, E. L. (1948). *Nursing for the future*. New York. Russell Sage Foundation.

Brown, G. W., & Moran, P. M. (1997). Single mothers, poverty, and depression. *Psychological Medicine, 27*, 21–33.

Brown, J., Trinkoff, A. M., & Smith, L. (2003). Nurses in recovery: The burden of life problems and confidence to resist relapse. *Journal of Addictions Nursing, 14*, 133–137.

Brown, K. E. M. (2000). *Nurses' experiences with spirituality and end-of-life issues*. Doctoral dissertation, University of Alabama at Birmingham.

Brown, L. P., Bair, A. H., & Meier, P. (2003). Does federal funding for breastfeeding research target our national health objectives? *Pediatrics, 111*(4), e360–e364.

Brown, M. A., & Woods, N. F. (1986). Sex role orientation, sex typing, occupational traditionalism, and perimenstrual symptoms. *Health Care for Women International, 7*(1–2), 25–37.

Brown, M., & Zimmer, P. (1986). Personal and family impact of premenstrual symptoms. *Journal of Obstetrical, Gynecological and Neonatal Nursing, 15*(1), 31–38.

Brown, M. A., & Zimmer, P. A. (1987a). Marital quality and partner support in women with varying levels of premenstrual symptomology [Abstract]. *Abstracts of the 7th Conference of the Society for Menstrual Cycle Research*, 38.

Brown, M. A., & Zimmer, P. A. (1987b). Premenstrual interference: Men's perceptions of personal and family disruption [Abstract]. *Abstracts of the 7th Conference of the Society for Menstrual Cycle Research*, 39.

Brown, S. (1999). Patient-centered communication. In J. Fitzpatrick (Ed.), *Annual review of nursing research* (pp. 85–104). New York: Springer.

Brown, S. A. (1992). Meta-analysis of diabetes patient education research: Variations in intervention effects across studies. *Research in Nursing and Health, 15*, 409–419.

Brown, S. A., Garcia, A. A., Kouzekanani, K., & Hanis, C. L. (2002). Culturally competent diabetes self-management education for Mexican Americans: The Starr County border health initiative. *Diabetes Care, 25*, 259–268.

Brown, S. A., & Grimes, D. E. (1995). A meta-analysis of nurse practitioners and nurse midwives in primary care. *Nursing Research, 44*(6), 331–339.

Bruce, M. L. (2002). Psychosocial risk factors for depressive disorders in late life. *Biological Psychiatry, 52*(3), 175–184.

Bruch, H. (1979). Developmental deviations in anorexia nervosa. *Israel Annals of Psychiatry and Related Disciplines, 17*, 255–261.

Bruhn, J. (2001). Managing tough and easy organizational cultures. *Health Care Manager, 20*, 1–10.

Brundtland, G. H. (2000, January). *Address to the scientific group meeting on the burden of musculoskeletal disease: The bone and joint decade, 2000–2010*. Retrieved November 16, 2003, from http://who.int/director-general/speeches/2000/english/20000113_bone_joint.html

Buccheri, R., Trygstad, L., Dowling, G., Hopkins, R., White, K., Griffin, J. J., et al. (2004). Long term effects of teaching behavioral strategies for managing persistent auditory hallucinations. *Journal of Psychosocial Nursing and Mental Health Services, 42*, 19–27.

Buchanan, A. (1988). Principle/agent theory and decision making in healthcare. *Bioethics, 2*(4), 317–333.

Buchanan, D., Moorhouse, A., Cabico, L., Krock, M., Campbell, H., & Spevakow, D. (2002). A critical review and synthesis of literature on reminiscing with older adults. *Canadian Journal of Nursing Research, 34*(3), 293–303.

Buckles, D. C., Sarosiek, I., McMillin, C., & McCallum, R. W. (2004). Delayed gastric emptying in gastroesophageal reflux disease: Reassessment with new methods and symptomatic correlations. *American Journal of Medical Science, 327*(1), 1–4.

Buckwalter, K. C. (Ed.). (1999). Overview of NDB Model (Special Issue). *Journal of Gerontological Nursing, 25*(9), 6–39.

Buckwalter, K. C. (Ed.). (2002). NDB Model Interventions (Special Focus Section). *Journal of Gerontological Nursing, 28*(10), 5–23.

Buckwalter, K. C., Gerdner, L., Kohout, F., Hall, G. R., Kelly, A., Richards, B., et al. (1999). A nursing intervention to decrease depression in family caregivers of persons with dementia. *Archives of Psychiatric Nursing, 16*, 156–167.

Buckwalter, K. C., Kerfoot, K. M., & Stolley, J. M. (1988). Children of affectively ill parents. *Journal of Psychosocial Nursing and Mental Health Services, 26*, 8–14.

Buckwalter, K. C., Maas, M., & Reed, D. (1997). Assessing family and staff caregiver outcomes in Alzheimer disease research. *Alzheimer Disease & Associated Disorders, 11*(Suppl. 6), 105–116.

Budin, W. (1998). Psychosocial adjustment to breast cancer in unmarried women. *Research in Nursing and Health, 21*, 155–166.

Budman, S., & Gurman, A. (1988). *Theory and practice of brief therapy*. New York: Guilford Press.

Budzynski, T. H. (1996). Brain brightening: Can neurofeedback improve cognitive process: *Biofeedback*, 14–17.

Budzynski, T. H., & Budzynski, H. K. (1997). Can an old brain change in EEG? *Newsletter of the Society for the Study of Neuronal Regulation*, Clinical Corner.

Budzynski, T. H., & Budzynski, H. K. (2000). Reversing age-related cognitive decline: Use of neurofeedback and audio-visual stimulation. *Biofeedback*, 19–21.

Buelt, M. C., Bergstrom, N., Baun, M. M., & Langston, N. (1985). Facilitating social interaction among institutionalized elderly through use of a companion dog. *Journal of the Delta Society, 2*(1), 62–63.

Bugental, D. B., Olster, D. H., & Martorell, G. A. (2003). A developmental neuroscience perspective on the dynamics of parenting. In L. Kuczynski (Ed.), *Handbook of dynamics in parent-child relations* (pp. 25–48). Thousand Oaks, CA: Sage.

Bull, M., Hansen, H., & Gross, C. (2000). Differences in family caregiver outcomes by their level of involvement in discharge planning. *Applied Nursing Research, 13*(2), 76–82.

Bullough, V. L. (1994). *Science in the bedroom: A history of sex research*. New York: Basic Books.

Bullough, V. L., & Bullough, B. (1993). *Cross dressing, sex, and gender*. Philadelphia: University of Pennsylvania Press.

Bunkers, S. S. (2002). Lifelong learning: A human becoming perspective. *Nursing Science Quarterly, 15*(4), 294–300.

Bunyard, L. B., Dennis, K. E., & Nicklas, B. J. (2002). Dietary intake and changes in lipoprotein lipids in obese, postmenopausal women placed on an American Heart Association Step 1 diet. *Journal of the American Dietetic Association, 102*(1), 52–57.

Bureau of Justice Statistics. (2003). *Intimate Partner Violence, 1993–2001*. (NCJ Publication #197838) Washington, DC: National Institute of Justice.

Bureau of Labor Statistics. (1992). *Trends in retirement age by sex, 1950–2005*. Retrieved June 23, 1999, from http://stats.bls.gov/opub/mlr/1992/07/art3exc.htm

Bureau of Labor Statistics. (1998a). *Incidence rates of nonfatal occupational injuries and illnesses by industry and selected case types*. Washington, DC: Author.

Bureau of Labor Statistics. (1998b). *Number of nonfatal occupational injuries and illnesses by industry and selected case types*. Washington, DC: Author.

Bureau of Labor Statistics. (1999). *Employment projections. Civilian labor force by sex, age, race, and Hispanic origin, 1986, 1996, and projected 2006*. Re-

trieved June 23, 1999, from http://stats.bls.gov/news.release/ecopro.table1.htm
Bureau of Labor Statistics. (2000). Employed persons by detailed industry, sex, race, and Hispanic origin. *Employment and Earnings*, *47*, 191–195.
Bureau of Labor Statistics. (2001). *Retirement age declines again in 1990s*. Retrieved October 23, 2003, from http://stats.bls.gov/opub/mlr/2001/10/art2exc.htm
Bureau of Labor Statistics. (2003). *National Census of Occupational Injuries*. Retrieved December 8, 2003, from http://www.bls.gov/iif/home.htm
Burge, V., Felts, M., Chenier, T., & Parillo, A. V. (1995). Drug use, sexual activity, and suicidal behavior in U.S. high school students. *Journal of School Health*, *65*, 222–227.
Burgener, S., Jirovec, M., Murrell, L., & Barton, D. (1992). Caregiver and environmental variables related to difficult behaviors in institutionalized, demented persons. *Journal of Gerontological Psychosocial Sciences*, *47*(4), 242–249.
Burger, S. G., Kayser-Jones, J., & Bell, J. P. (2000). Malnutrition and dehydration in nursing homes: Key issues in prevention and treatment. National Citizens Coalition for Nursing Home Reform (publication number 386). *The Commonwealth Fund*. Retrieved from http://www.cmwf.org
Burgess, E. (1926). The family as a unity of interacting personalities. *Family*, *7*, 3–9.
Burgess, G. H., Oh, W., Brann, B. S. 4th, Brubakk, A. M., & Stonestreet, B. S. (2001). Effects of Phenobarbital on cerebral blood flow velocity after endotracheal suctioning in premature neonates. *Archives of Pediatric & Adolescent Medicine*, *155*(6), 723–727.
Burgoyne, R. W., & Saunders, D. S. (2001). Quality of life among urban Canadian HIV/AIDS clinic outpatients. *International Journal of STD & AIDS*, *12*, 505–512.
Burke, G., III, Summers, J., & Thompson, T. (2001). Quality in long-term care: What we can learn from certified nursing assistants. *Annals of Long-Term Care*, *9*(2), 29–35.
Burl, J. B., Bonner, A., Rao, M., & Khan, A. M. (1998). Geriatric nurse practitioners in long-term care: Demonstration of effectiveness in managed care. *Journal of the American Geriatric Society*, *46*, 506–510.
Burnette, D. (1998). Grandparents rearing grandchildren: A school-based small group intervention. *Research on Social Work Practice*, *8*, 10–27.
Burns, J. (1978). *Leadership*. New York: Harper and Row.
Burns, P. A. (1995). *A study of the Omnibus Budget Reconciliation Act of 1987 and the amendments of 1989 and 1990. Mandatory education for nursing assistants and their effect on job performance in two counties in Florida*. Unpublished PhD dissertation, University of North Texas.
Burns, R., Nichols, L., & Martindale-Adams, J. (2000). Interdisciplinary geriatric primary care evaluation and management: Two-year outcomes. *Journal of the American Geriatrics Society*, *48*, 8–13.
Burns, S. M., Carpenter, R., & Truitt, J. D. (2001). Report on the development of a procedure to prevent placement of feeding tubes into the lungs using end-tidal CO_2 measurements. *Critical Care Medicine*, *29*(5), 936–939.
Burns-Tisdal, S., & Goff, W. F. (1989). The geriatric nurse practitioner in home care: Challenges, stresses, and rewards. *Nursing Clinics of North America*, *24*(3), 809–817.
Bushy, A. (2000). *Orientation to nursing in the rural community*. Thousand Oaks, CA: Sage.
Bustan, M. N., & Coker, A. L. (1994). Maternal attitude toward pregnancy and the risk of neonatal death. *American Journal of Public Health*, *84*(3), 411–414.
Butler, R. (1975). *Why survive: Being old in America*. New York: Harper and Row.
Butler, S. M., Ashford, J. W., & Snowdon, D. A. (1996). Age, education, and changes in the Mini-Mental State Exam scores of older women: Findings from the Nun Study. *Journal of the American Geriatrics Society*, *44*, 675–681.
Byerly, E. L. (1990). The nurse-researcher as participant-observer in a nursing setting. In P. J. Brink (Ed.), *Transcultural nursing* (pp. 143–162). Prospect Heights, IL: Waveland Press. (Original work published 1969)
Byrne, M. (2002). Building research competence in nursing through mentoring. *Journal of Nursing Scholarship*, *34*(4), 391–396.
Byrne, M. (2003). A mentored experience in maternal-infant research. *Journal of Professional Nursing*, *19*(2), 66–75.
Cadman, E. C. (1994). The academic physician-investigator: A crisis not to be ignored. *Annals of Internal Medicine*, *120*, 401–410.
Caetano, R., Clark, C. L., & Tam, T (1998). Alcohol consumption among racial/ethnic minorities: Theory and research. *Alcohol, Health & Research World*, *22*(4), 233–238.
Cagney, K., & Agree, E. (1999). Racial differences in skilled nursing care and home health use: The mediating effects of family structure and social class. *Journal of Gerontology B Psychological and Social Sciences*, *54*(4), S223–S236.
Cahill, C. A. (1998). Differences in cortisol, a stress hormone, in women with turmoil-type premenstrual symptoms. *Nursing Research*, *47*, 278–284.

Cairns, R. B., Elder, G. H., & Costello, E. J. (1996). *Developmental science*. Cambridge, England: Cambridge University.

Caldwell, T. M., & Jorm, A. F. (2001). Mental health nurses' beliefs about likely outcomes for people with schizophrenia or depression: A comparison with the public and other healthcare professionals. *Australian and New Zealand Journal of Mental Health Nursing, 10*, 42–54.

Caliandro, G., & Hughes, C. (1998). The experience of being a grandmother who is the primary caregiver for her HIV-positive grandchild. *Nursing Research, 47*(2), 107–113.

Callaghan, L., Jones, J., & Leonard, L. (2001). Evaluation of a childbirth and parenting education service. *Birth Issues, 10*(2), 41–49.

Callister, L. C. (2004). Promoting positive birth experiences. *Journal of Obstetric, Gynecologic and Neonatal Nursing, 33*, 484.

Camberg, L., Woods, P., Ooi, W. L., Hurley, A., Volicer, L., Ashley, J., et al. (1999). Evaluation of simulated presence: A personalized approach to enhance well-being in persons with Alzheimer's disease. *Journal of the American Geriatrics Society, 47*, 446–452.

Campbell, D., & Fiske, D. (1959). Convergent and discriminant validation by the multitrait-multimethod matrix. *Psychological Bulletin, 56*, 81–105.

Campbell, D. T., & Stanley, J. C. (1963). Experimental and quasi-experimental designs for research on teaching. In N. L. Gage (Ed.), *Handbook of research on teaching* (pp. 171–246). Chicago: Rand-McNally.

Campbell, J., Carpentar, P., Sneiderman, C., Cohn, S., Chute, C., & Warren, J. (1997). Phase II evaluation of clinical coding schemes. Completeness, taxonomy, mapping, definitions and clarity. *Journal of the American Medical Informatics Association, 4*, 238, 251.

Campbell, J., Harris, M. J., & Lee, R. K. (1995). Violence research: An overview. *Scholarly Inquiry for Nursing Practice: An International Journal,* 9(2), 105–126.

Campbell, J., Jones, A., Dienemann, J., Kub, J., Schollenberger, J., O'Campo, P., et al. (2002). Intimate partner violence and physical health consequences. *Archives of Internal Medicine, 162*, 1157–1163.

Canadian Study of Health and Aging Working Group. (2002). Patterns and health effects of caring for people with dementia: The impact of changing cognitive and residential status. *Gerontologist, 42*(5), 643–652.

Cannon, C. P., Braunwald, E., McCabe, C. H., Rader, D. J., Rouleau, J. L., Joyal, S. V., et al. (2004). Intensive versus moderate lipid lowering with statins after acute coronary syndromes. *New England Journal of Medicine, 350*(15), 1495–1504.

Capaldini, L. (1998). Fatigue and HIV: Interview with Lisa Capaldini, M. D. Interview by John S. James. *AIDS Treatment News, 291*, 1–6.

Capasso, V. A., & Munro, B. H. (2003). The cost and efficacy of two wound treatments. *AORN Online, 77*, 984, 986, 988–992, 995–997, 1000–1004. Retrieved November 1, 2003, from Ovid.

Capezuti, E., Brush, B. L., & Lawson, W. T. (1997). Reporting elder mistreatment. *Journal of Gerontological Nursing, 23*(7), 24–32.

Capezuti, E., Strumpf, N. E., Evans, L. K., Grisso, J. A., & Maislin, G. (1998). The relationship between physical restraint removal and falls and injuries among nursing home residents. *Journal of Gerontology, 53*, M47–M52.

Caplan, G. (1964). *Principles of preventive psychiatry*. New York: Basic Books.

Caplan, N., & Rich, R. F. (1975). *The use of social science knowledge in policy decisions at the national level*. Ann Arbor: University of Michigan Institute of Social Research.

Carey, M., Carey, K., Weinhardt, L., & Gordon, C. (1997). Behavioral risk for HIV infection among adults with a severe and persistent mental illness: Patterns and psychological antecedents. *Community Mental Health Journal, 33*(2), 133–142.

Caris-Verhallen, W., de Gruijter, I. M., Kerkstra, A., & Bensing, J. M. (1999). Factors related to nurse communication with elderly people. *Journal of Advanced Nursing, 30*(5), 1106–1117.

Caris-Verhallen, W., Kerkstra, A., & Bensing, J. (1997). The role of communication in nursing care for elderly people: A review of literature. *Journal of Advanced Nursing, 25*, 915–933.

Caris-Verhallen, W., Kerkstra, A., van der Heijden, P., & Bensing, J. (1998). Nurse-elderly patient communication in home care and institutional care: An explorative study. *International Journal of Nursing Studies, 35*, 95–108.

Carmel, H., & Hunter, M. (1989). Staff injuries from inpatient violence. *Hospital and Community Psychiatry, 40*(1), 41–46.

Carney, R. M., Saunders, R. D., Freedland, K. E., Stein, P., Rich, M. W., & Jaffe, A. S. (1995). Association of depression with reduced heart rate variability in coronary artery disease. *American Journal of Cardiology, 76*, 562–564.

Carper, B. A. (1978). Fundamental patterns of knowing. *Advanced Nursing Science, 1*, 13–23.

Carr, A. J., Gibson, B., & Robinson, P. G. (2001). Is quality of life determined by expectations or experience? *British Medical Journal, 322,* 1240–1243. Retrieved September 29, 2003, from http://www.bmj.com

Carroll-Johnson, R. M. (Ed.). *Classifications of nursing diagnoses: Proceedings of the Ninth conference*. Philadelphia: Lippincott.

Carter, J., Moorhead, S., McCloskey, J., & Bulechek, G. (1995). Using the Nursing Interventions Classification to implement Agency for Health Care Policy and Research guidelines. *Journal of Nursing Care Quality,* 9(2), 76–86.

Carter, M., & Cook, K. (1995). Adaptation to retirement: Role changes and psychological resources. *Career Development Quarterly, 44,* 67. Retrieved from October 23, 2003, from http://proquest.umi.com/pqdweb?index

Carter-Pokras, O., & Baquet, C. (2002). What is a "health disparity"? *Public Health Reports, 17,* 426–434.

Cartwright, J. C. (2002). Nursing homes and assisted living facilities as places for dying. In *Annual review of nursing research* (Vol. 20, pp. 231–264). New York: Springer Publishing.

Caruso, C., Hadley, B., Shukla, R., Frame, P., & Khoury, J. (1992). Cooling effects and comfort of four cooling blanket temperatures in humans with fever. *Nursing Research, 41*(2), 68–72.

Case Management Society of America. (2002). *Standards of practice for case management* (2nd ed.). Little Rock, AR: Author.

Cashion, A. (2002). Genetics in transplantation. *Medical & Surgical Nursing Journal, 11*(2), 91–94.

Cassem, N. H., & Hackett, T. P. (1971). Psychiatric consultation in a coronary care unit. *Annals of Internal Medicine, 75,* 9–14.

Castina, S., Boyington, A., & Dougherty, M. (2002). Urinary incontinence. *American Journal of Nursing, 102*(8), 85–87.

Castle, N. G., & Mor, V. (1998). Physical restraints in nursing homes: A review of the literature since the Nursing Home Reform Act of 1987. *Medical Care Research and Review, 55,* 139–170.

Catolico, O., Navas, C. M., Sommer, C. K., & Collins, M. A. (1996). Quality of decision making by registered nurses. *Journal of Nursing Staff Development, 12*(3), 149–154.

Cattell, R. B. (1966). The scree test for the number of factors. *Multivariate Behavioral Research, 1,* 245–276.

Caygill, C. P., Charlett, A., & Hill, M. J. (1998). Relationship between the intake of high-fibre foods and energy and the risk of cancer of the large bowel and breast. *European Journal of Cancer Prevention, 7*(Suppl. 2), 11–7.

Centers for Disease Control and Prevention. (1989). Guidelines for prevention of transmission of human immunodeficiency virus and hepatitis B virus to healthcare and public safety workers. *Morbidity and Mortality Weekly Report, 38*(5–6), 3–37.

Centers for Disease Control and Prevention. (1992). Public health focus: Surveillance, prevention, and control of nosocomial infections. *Morbidity and Mortality Weekly Report, 41,* 783–787.

Centers for Disease Control and Prevention. (1998). Recommendation for prevention and control of hepatitis C virus (HCV) infection and HCV-related chronic disease. *Morbidity and Mortality Weekly Report, 47*(RR19), 1–58.

Centers for Disease Control and Prevention. (2000a). *HIV/AIDS Surveillance Report, 12,* 24.

Centers for Disease Control and Prevention. (2000b). Monitoring hospital-acquired infections to promote patient safety—United States, 1990–1999. *Morbidity and Mortality Weekly Report, 49,* 149–153.

Centers for Disease Control and Prevention. (2001). *HIV/AIDS Surveillance Report 2001,* 13.

Centers for Disease Control and Prevention. (2002a). *HIV/AIDS Surveillance Report 2002,* 14.

Center for Disease Control and Prevention. (2002b). *The National Nursing Home Survey: 1999 Summary.* Vital and Health Statistics, series 13, number 152. DHHS Publication No. (PHS) 2002-1723. Hyattsville, MD: National Center for Health Statistics.

Centers for Disease Control and Prevention. (2002c). Guideline for hand hygiene in health-care settings. *Morbidity and Mortality Weekly Report, 51*(RR-16), 1–44.

Centers for Disease Control and Prevention. (2003a). *National diabetes fact sheet: General information and national estimates on diabetes in the United States.* Atlanta, GA: U.S. Department of Health and Human Services. Retrieved December 4, 2003, from http://www.cdc.gov/diabetes/pubs/factsheet.htm

Centers for Disease Control and Prevention. (2003b). Prevalence of current cigarette smoking among adults and changes in prevalence of current and some day smoking—United States, 1996–2001. *Morbidity and Mortality Weekly Report, 52,* 303–307.

Centers for Disease Control and Prevention. (2003c). *Data and statistics.* Retrieved November 23, 2003, from http://www.cdc.gov/scientific.htm

Centers for Disease Control and Prevention. (2003d). National Center for Health Statistics. *National Vital Statistics Report, 52*(10), 89.

Centers for Disease Control and Prevention. (2004). Health Resources and Services Administration. *Maternal, infant, and child health*. Retrieved April 25, 2004, from http://www.healthpeople.gov/Document/HTML/Volume2/16MICH.htm

CDC AIDS Community Demonstration Projects Research Group. (1999). Community-level HIV intervention in five cities: Final outcome data from the CDC AIDS Community Demonstration Projects. *American Journal of Public Health*, 89(3), 336–345.

Centers for Medicare and Medicaid Services. (2001). *MDS frequency report: January 15, 2001*. Retrieved March 17, 2004, from http://www.cms.hhs.gov/states/mdsreports/freq3.asp?var=G1hA&date=3

Centers for Medicare & Medicaid Services. (2004). *Hospital quality information initiative*. Retrieved January 10, 2004, from http://cms.hhs.gov/quality/hospital/

Cesta, T., & Tahan, H. (2003). *The case manager's survival guide: Winning strategies for clinical practice* (2nd ed.). St. Louis, MO: Mosby.

Chafetz, L., & Ricard, N. (1999). The biopsychosocial perspective in psychiatric nursing: Myth or future reality? *Canadian Journal of Nursing Research*, *31*, 17–23.

Chaffee, M. (1999). A telehealth odyssey. *American Journal of Nursing*, 99(7), 27–32, quiz 32–33.

Chaisson, C. M. (1980). Life cycle: A social simulation game to improve attitudes and response to the elderly. *Journal of Gerontological Nursing*, 6, 587–592.

Chan, H., Lu, R., Tseng, C., & Chou, K. (2003). Effectiveness of the anger-control program in reducing anger expression in patients with schizophrenia. *Archives of Psychiatric Nursing*, *17*, 88–95.

Chan, S., Mackenzie, A., & Jacobs, P. (2000). Cost-effectiveness analysis of case management versus a routine community care organization for patients with chronic schizophrenia. *Archives of Psychiatric Nursing*, *14*, 98–104.

Chan, S., MacKenzie, A., Tin-Fu, D., & Leung, J. K. (2000). An evaluation of the implementation of case management in the community psychiatric nursing service. *Journal of Advanced Nursing*, *31*, 144–56.

Chan, S. W., & Wong, K. F. (1999). The use of critical pathways in caring for schizophrenic patients in a mental hospital. *Archives of Psychiatric Nursing*, *13*, 145–153.

Charlton, B. G. (1995). Mega-trials: Methodological issues and clinical implications. *Journal of the Royal College of Physicians of London*, 29(2), 96–100.

Chase, S. K. (1988). Knowledge representation in expert systems: Nursing diagnosis applications. *Computers in Nursing*, 6, 58–64.

Chasens, E. R., & Umlauf, M. G. (2003). Nocturia: A problem that disrupts sleep and predicts obstructive sleep apnea. *Geriatric Nursing*, *24*, 76–81, 105.

Chassagne, P., Landrin, I., Neveu, C., Czernichow, P., Bouaniche, M., Doucet, J., et al. (1999). Fecal incontinence in the institutional elderly: Incidence, risk factors, and prognosis. *American Journal of Medicine*, *106*(2), 185–190.

Chen, C. C., Schilling, L. S., & Lyder, C. H. (2001). A concept analysis of malnutrition in the elderly. *Journal of Advanced Nursing*, *36*, 131–142.

Chen, H. T. (1990). *Theory-driven evaluations*. Newbury Park, CA: Sage.

Chen, Y., Dewey, M., & Avery, A. (2001). Analysis Group of the MRCCFA study. Self-reported medication use for older people in England and Wales. *Journal of Clinical Pharmacy & Therapeutics*, *26*, 129–140.

Chernoff, R. (1999). *Geriatric nutrition* (2nd ed.). Gaithersburg, MD: Aspen Publications.

Chesla, C. A., Fisher, L., Skaff, M. M., Mullan, J. T., Gilliss, C. L., & Kanter, R. (2003). Family predictors of disease management over one year in Latin and European American patients with type 2 diabetes. *Family Process*, *42*, 375–390.

Chesla, C. A., & Rungreangkulkij, S. (2001). Nursing research on family processes in chronic illness in ethnically diverse families: A decade review. *Journal of Family Nursing*, *7*(3), 230–243.

Chesney-Lind, M. (2000). Women and the criminal justice system: Gender matters. In National Institute of Correction (NIC) Annual Issue 2000: *Responding to women offenders in the community* (No. J1C0–110, pp. 7–10). Longmont, CO: NIC Information Center.

Chevalier, S., Gougeon, R., Nayar, K., & Morais, J. A. (2003). Frailty amplifies the effects of aging on protein metabolism: Role of protein intake. *American Journal of Clinical Nutrition*, *78*, 422–429.

Chiang, J., Kowada, M., Ames, A. 3rd, Wright, R. L., & Majno, G. (1968). Cerebral ischemia. Vascular changes. *American Journal of Pathology*, *52*(2), 455–476.

Chien, H. C., Ku, C. H., Lu, R. B., Chu, H., Tao, Y. H., & Chou, K. R. (2003). Effects of social skills training on improving social skills of patients with schizophrenia. *Archives of Psychiatric Nursing*, *17*, 228–236.

Chien, W. T., Kam, C. W., & Lee, I. F. (2001). An assessment of the patients' needs in mental health education. *Journal of Advanced Nursing*, *34*, 304–311.

Chien, W. T., & Lee, I. F. (2002). Educational needs of families caring for patients with schizophrenia. *Journal of Clinical Nursing*, *11*, 695–696.

Chien, W. T., & Norman, I. (2003). Educational needs of families caring for Chinese patients with schizophrenia. *Journal of Advanced Nursing, 44*, 490–498.

Child Trends. (2003). *Teen births*. Child Trends Database. Retrieved from http://www.childtrends databank.org/pdf/13_PDF.pdf

Chinn, P. L., & Kramer, M. K. (2004). *Integrated knowledge development in nursing* (6th ed.). St. Louis, MO: Mosby.

Chiou, C. (2000). A meta-analysis of the interrelationships between the modes in Roy's adaptation model. *Nursing Science Quarterly, 13*(3), 252–258.

Chiu, L. (1999). A phenomenological study on searching for meaning-in-life in women living with breast cancer [Abstract]. *Nursing Research, (China), 7*, 119–128.

Cho, S. H., Ketefian, S., Barkauskas, V. H., & Smith, D. G. (2003). The effects of nurse staffing on adverse events, morbidity, mortality and medical costs. *Nursing Research, 52*, 71–79.

Chobanian, A. V., Bakris, G. L., Black, H. R., Cushman, W. C., Green, L. A., Izzo, J. L. Jr., et al. (2003a). Seventh report of the Joint National Committee on Prevention, Detection, Evaluation, and Treatment of High Blood Pressure. *Hypertension, 42*(6), 1206–1252.

Chobanian, A. V., Bakris, G. L., Black, H. R., Cushman, W. C., Green, L. A., Izzo, J. L., et al. (2003b). The seventh report of the Joint National Committee on Prevention, Detection, Evaluation and Treatment of High Blood Pressure. *Journal of American Medical Association, 289*, 1560–1572.

Chodorow, N. (1978). *The reproduction of mothering: Psychoanalysis and the sociology of gender*. Berkeley: University of California Press.

Chou, F. H., Lin, L. L., Cooney, A. T., Walker, L. O., & Riggs, M. W. (2003). Psychosocial factors related to nausea, vomiting, and fatigue in early pregnancy. *Journal of Nursing Scholarship, 35*, 119–125.

Chou, K., Liu, S., & Chu, H. (2002). The effects of support groups on caregivers of patients with schizophrenia. *International Journal of Nursing Studies, 39*, 713–722.

Chou, L. L. Wang, R. H., Chen, S. J., & Pai, L. (2003). Effects of music therapy on oxygen saturation in premature infants receiving endotracheal suctioning. *Journal of Nursing Research, 11*(3), 209–216.

Chrisman, M., Tabar, D., Whall, A., & Booth, D. (1991). Agitated behavior in cognitively impaired elderly. *Journal of Gerontological Nursing, 17*(12), 9–13.

Christman, N. (1990). Uncertainty and adjustment during radiotherapy. *Nursing Research, 39*, 17–20.

Chumbler, N., Grimm, J., Cody, M., & Beck, C. (2003). Gender, kinship and caregiver burden: The case of community-dwelling memory impaired seniors. *International Journal of Geriatric Psychiatry, 18*(8), 722–732.

Chumlea, W. C., & Guo, S. S. (1994). Bioelectric impedance and body composition: Present status and future directions. *Nutrition Reviews, 52*(4), 123–131.

Churchill, M., Safaoui, J., McCabe, B. W., & Baun, M. M. (1999). Effects of a therapy dog in alleviating the agitation behavior of sundown syndrome and in increasing socialization for persons with Alzheimer's disease. *Journal of Psychosocial Nursing and Mental Health Services, 37*(4), 16–22.

Chyun, D. A., Khuwatsamrit, K., Katten, D. M., Price, W. J., Davey, J. A., Inzucchi, S. E., et al. (2003). Self-management of type 2 diabetes (T2DM) in adults screened for coronary artery disease (CAD), Impact on quality of life (QOL). *Diabetes, 52*(Suppl. 2), A410.

Chyun, D. A., Melkus, G., Inzucchi, S. E., Sun, V., Price, W. J., Davey, J. A., et al. (2002). Depressive symptoms, anxiety, and quality of life (QOL) in adults with type 2 diabetes (T2DM) screened for coronary artery disease (CAD). *Diabetes, 51*(Suppl. 2), A444.

Chyun, D. A., Minicucci, D. S., Katten, D. M., Davey, J. A., Grey, N. J., & Melkus, G. D. (2002). Motivational factors and control of type 2 diabetes (T2DM) and coronary heart disease (CHD) risk factors. *Gerontologist, 42*(Special Issue II), 216.

Chyun, D. A., Vaccarino, V., Murillo, J., Young, L., & Krumholz, H. (2002a). Mortality, heart failure and recurrent myocardial infarction in the elderly with diabetes. *American Journal of Critical Care, 9*, 504–519.

Chyun, D. A., Vaccarino, V., Murillo, J., Young, L. H., & Krumholz, H. M. (2002b). Acute myocardial infarction mortality in the elderly with diabetes. *Heart and Lung, 31*, 327–339.

Chyun, D. A., Young, L. H., Wackers, F. J. T., Inzucchi, S. E., Davey, J., Broadbridge, C., et al. (2003). Investigators. Association of measurements of heart rate variability with asymptomatic myocardial ischemia: Results of the Detection of Ischemia in Asymptomatic Diabetics (DIAD) study. *Clinical Autonomic Research, 13*, 379.

Cimino, J. J. (1998). Desiderata for controlled medical vocabularies in the twenty-first century. *Methods of Information in Medicine, 37*(4–5), 394–403.

Cimprich, B. (1995). Symptom management: Loss of concentration. *Seminars in Oncology Nursing, 11*, 279–288.

Cimprich, B., & Ronis, D. L. (2003). An environmental intervention to restore attention in women with newly diagnosed breast cancer. *Cancer Nursing, 26*(4), 284–292.

Clapcich, J., Goldberg, N., & Walsh, E. (2002). *Be independent: A self help guide for people with Parkinson's disease*. New York: American Parkinson's Disease Association.

Clare, M., Sargent, D., Moxley, R., & Forthman, T. (1995). Reducing health care delivery costs using clinical paths: A case study on improving hospital profitability. *Journal of Health Care Finance, 21*(3), 48–58.

Clark, J., Rieker, P., Propert, K., & Talcott, J. (1999). Changes in quality of life following treatment for early prostate cancer. *Urology, 53*(1), 161–168.

Clarke, D. E,, Chernomas, W. M., & Chisholm, F. A. (2001). Addressing the needs of women living with schizophrenia. *Canadian Nurse, 97,* 14–18.

Clauseen, A. H., & Crittenden, P. M. (1991). Physical and psychological maltreatment: Relations among the types of maltreatment. *Child Abuse & Neglect, 15,* 5–18.

Cleary, P. D., & McNeil, B. J. (1988). Patient satisfaction as an indicator of quality care. *Inquiry, 25,* 25–36.

Clements, P. T., & Burgess, A. W. (2002). Children's responses to family member homicide. *Family & Community Health, 25*(1), 32–42.

Clifford, J., & Horvath, K. (1990). *Advancing professional nursing practice at Boston's Beth Israel Hospital*. New York: Springer Publishing.

Cochrane, C. (2001). The National Institute of Nursing Research/National Institute of Mental Health mentorship program: Building the capacity of psychiatric mental health nurse researchers. *Journal of the American Psychiatric Nurses Association, 7,* 171–172.

Cockerill, R., Pallas, L. O., Bolley, H., & Pink, G. (1993). Measuring nursing workload for case costing. *Nursing Economic$, 11,* 342–349.

Cockrell, J. R., & Folstein, M. F. (1988). Mini-Mental State Examination (MMSE). *Psychopharmacology Bulletin, 24,* 689–690.

Coeling, H., & Simms, L. (1993). Facilitating innovation at the unit level through cultural assessment, part 2: Adapting managerial ideas to the unit work group. *Journal of Nursing Administration, 23,* 13–20.

Coeling, H., & Wilcox, J. (1988). Understanding organizational culture: A key to management decision-making. *Journal of Nursing Administration, 18,* 16–24.

Cohen, E., & Cesta, T. (1997). *Nursing case management: From concept to evaluation* (2nd ed.). St. Louis, MO: Mosby Year Book.

Cohen, H., Feussner, J., Weinberger, M., Carnes, M., Hamdy, R., Hsieh, F., et al. (2002). A controlled trial of inpatient and outpatient geriatric evaluation and management. *New England Journal of Medicine, 346,* 874–888.

Cohen, I. B. (1984). Florence Nightingale. *Scientific American, 250,* 128–137.

Cohen, J. (1988). *Statistical power analysis for the behavioral sciences* (2nd ed.). Hillsdale, NJ: Erlbaum.

Cohen, J. (1994). The earth is round (p < .05). *American Psychologist, 49,* 997–1003.

Cohen, M. Z., Kahn, D. L., & Steeves, R. H. (1998). Beyond body image: The experience of breast cancer. *Oncology Nursing Forum, 25,* 835–841.

Cohen, M. Z., & Palos, G. (2001). Culturally competent care. *Seminars in Oncology Nursing, 17*(3), 153–158.

Cohen, M. Z., Phillips, J. M., & Palos, G. (2001). Qualitative research with diverse populations. *Seminars in Oncology Nursing, 17*(3), 190–196.

Cohen S. (2003). *Living with HPN: A caregivers perspective* (p. 313). Caring for the Caregiver Support Implications Panel, ASPEN Scientific Symposium, in San Antonio, TX.

Cohen, S., & Wills, T. (1985). Stress, social support, and the buffering hypothesis. *Psychological Bulletin, 98,* 310–357.

Cohen, S. M. (1989). Effects of natural progesterone on premenstrual syndrome symptoms. In A. Voda & R. Conover (Eds.), *Proceedings of the 8th Conference of the Society for Menstrual Cycle Research* (SMCR) (pp. 581–588). Salt Lake City, UT: SMCR.

Cohen, S. W., Rousseau, M. E., & Carey, B. L. (2003). Can acupuncture ease the symptoms of menopause? *Holistic Nursing Practice, 17*(6), 295–299.

Cohen-Mansfield, J., & Werner, P. (1998). The effects of an enhanced environment on nursing home residents who pace. *Gerontologist, 38*(2), 199–208.

Cohen-Mansfield, J., Werner, P., Marx, M., & Freedman, L. (1991). Two studies of pacing in the nursing home. *Journal of Gerontology: Medical Sciences, 46,* M77–M83.

Cohen-Mansfield, J., Werner, P., Marx, M., & Freedman, L. (1995). Environmental influences on agitation: An integration summary of an observation study. *American Journal of Alzheimer's Care and Related Disorders and Research, 10,* 32–39.

Coie, J. D., Watt, N. F., West, S. G., Hawkins, J. D., Asarnow, J. R., Markman, H. J., et al. (1993). The science of prevention: A conceptual framework and some directions for a national research program. *American Psychologist, 48,* 1013–1022.

Colaizzi, P. (1978). Psychological research as the phenomenologist views it. In R. Valle & M. King (Eds.), *Existential phenomenological alternative for psychology* (pp. 48–71). New York: Oxford University Press.

Cole, M. (1999). Delirium: Effectiveness of systematic interventions. *Dementia and Geriatric Cognitive Disorders, 10,* 406–411.

Coleman, W., & Garfield, C. (2004). Fathers and pediatricians: Enhancing men's roles in the care and development of their children. *Pediatrics, 113*(5), 1406–1411.

Colenda, C. C., Streim, J., Greene, J. A., Meyers, N., Beckwith, E., & Rabins, P. (1999). The impact of OBRA '87 on psychiatric services in nursing homes. *American Journal of Geriatric Psychiatry, 7*(1), 12–17.

Colling, K. B., & Buettner, L. L. (2002). Simple pleasures: Interventions from the need-driven dementia-compromised behavior model. *Journal of Gerontological Nursing, 28*(10), 17–20.

Collins, C., Stommel, M., Wang, S., & Given, C. W. (1994). Caregiving transitions: Changes in depression among family caregivers of relatives with dementia. *Nursing Research, 43,* 220–225.

Collins, J. J., Byrnes, M. E., Dunkel, I. J., Lapin, J., Nadel, T., Thaler, H. T., et al. (2000). The measurement of symptoms in children with cancer. *Journal of Pain Symptom Management, 19*(5), 363–373.

Collins-Sharp, B., Taylor, D., Kelly-Thomas, K., Killeen, M. B., & Dawood, M. Y. (2002). Cyclic perimenstrual pain and discomfort: The scientific basis for practice. *Journal of Obstetric, Gynecological, and Neonatal Nursing, 31,* 637–649.

Computer Retrieval of Information on Scientific Projects. (2004). Retrieved February 6, 2004, from http://crisp.cit.nih.gov/crisp/crisp_query.generate_screen

Computer Retrieval of Information on Scientific Projects (CRISP)—A database of biomedical research funded by the National Institutes of Health. (n.d.). Retrieved September 29, 2004, from http://crisp.cit.nih.gov/

Con, A. H., Linden, W., Thompson, J. M., & Ignaszewski, A. (1999). The psychology of men and women recovering from coronary artery bypass surgery. *Journal of Cardiopulmonary Rehabilitation, 19,* 152–161.

Conn, V., Taylor, S., & Miller, R. (1994). Cognitive impairment and medication adherence. *Journal of Gerontological Nursing, 20,* 41.

Conner, R. (1960). A hospital inpatient classification system. *Dissertation Abstracts International, 21,* 565.

Connerney, I., Shapiro, P. A., McLaughlin, J. S., Bagiella, E., & Sloan, R. P. (2001). Relation between depression after coronary artery bypass surgery and 12-month outcome: A prospective study. *Lancet, 358,* 1766–1771.

Connor, P. D., & Streissguth, A. P. (1996). Life-stage issues. Effects of prenatal exposure to alcohol across the life span. *Alcohol, Health & Research World, 20*(3), 170–174.

Connor, R. J., Flagle, C. D., Hsieh, R. K. C., Preston, R., & Singer, S. (1961). Effective use of nursing resources: A research report. *Hospitals, 35*(9), 30–39.

Constantino, R., Sekula, K., & Rubinstein, E. (2001). Group intervention for widowed survivors of suicide. *Suicide and Life-Threatening Behavior, 3,* 428–439.

Constantinople, A. (1973). Masculinity-femininity: An exception to a famous dictum? *Psychological Bulletin, 80,* 389–407.

Cook, J. A., Ingersoll, G. L., & Spitzer, R. (1999). Managed-care research, part 1. Defining the domain. *Journal of Nursing Administration, 29*(11), 23–30.

Cook, T., & Campbell, D. (1979). *Quasi-experimentation: Design and analysis issues for field studies.* Chicago: Rand McNally.

Cooley, M. E., & Moriarty, H. J. (1997). An analysis of empirical studies examining the impact of the cancer diagnosis and treatment of an adult on family functioning. *Journal of Family Nursing, 3,* 318–347.

Cooper, M. (2000). Towards a model of safety culture. *Safety Science, 36,* 111–136.

Cooper, R. A., Getzen, T. E., McKee, H. J., & Laud, P. (2002). Economic and demographic trends signal an impending physician shortage. *Health Affairs, 21*(1), 140–154.

Coppola, K. M., Ditto, P. H., Danks, J. H., & Smucker, W. D. (2001). Accuracy of primary care and hospital-based physicians' predictions of elderly outpatients' treatment preferences with and without advance directives. *Archives of Internal Medicine, 161,* 431–440.

Corcoran, S. A. (1986). Planning by expert and novice nurses in cases of varying complexity. *Research in Nursing and Health,* 9(2), 155–162.

Coren, E., Barlow, J., & Stewart-Brown, S. (2003). The effectiveness of individual and group based parenting programmes in improving outcomes for teenage mothers and their children: A systematic review. *Journal of Adolescence, 26*(1), 79–103.

Corless, I. B. (1994). Dying well: Symptom control within hospice care. In J. J. Fitzpatrick & J. Stevens

(Eds.), *Annual review of nursing research* (Vol. 12, pp. 125–146). New York: Springer.

Corley, M. C. (1995). Moral distress of critical care nurses. *American Journal of Critical Care, 4*, 280–285.

Costos, D., & Gleason, J. (1995). PMS as a vehicle for dividing women: An analysis of women's attitudes toward PMS and early education regarding menstruation [Abstract]. *Abstracts of the 11th Conference of the Society for Menstrual Cycle Research*, 69.

Coté, R. A., Rothwell, D. J., Palotay, J. L., & Beckett, R. S. (1993). *SNOMED international*. Northfield, IL: College of American Pathologists.

Courtney, R., & Rice, C. (1997). Investigation of nurse practitioner-patient interactions: Using the nurse practitioner rating form. *Nurse Practitioner, 22*(2), 46–65.

Covington, S. (1998). The relational theory of women's psychological development: Implications for the criminal justice system. In R. Zaplin (Ed.), *Female offenders: Critical perspectives and effectiveness interventions* (pp. 42–58). Gaithersburg, MD: Aspen Publishers.

Covinsky, K., Eng, C., Lui, K., Sands, L., Sehgal, A., Walter, L., et al. (2001). Reduced employment in caregivers of frail elders: Impact of ethnicity, patient clinical characteristics, and caregiver characteristics. *Journals of Gerontology Biological Sciences Medical Sciences, 56*(11), M707–M713.

Covinsky, K. E., Eng, C., Lui, L. Y., Sands, L. P., & Yaffe, K. (2003). The last 2 years of life: Functional trajectories of frail older people. *Journal of the American Geriatrics Society, 51*, 492–498.

Cowan, C. (1995). The use of holistic nursing interventions in the treatment of breast cancer: A pilot study [Abstract]. *New Zealand Practice Nurse, 80*, 82.

Cowan, M. C. (Ed.). (1956). *The yearbook of modern nursing*. New York: G. P. Putnam.

Coward, D. (1991). Self-transcendence and emotional well-being in women with advanced breast cancer. *Oncology Nursing Forum, 18*, 857–863.

Coward, D. (1998). Facilitating self-transcendence in a breast cancer support group. *Oncology Nursing Forum, 25*, 75–84.

Cowell, J. M., Warren, J. S., & Montgomery, A. C. (1999). Cardiovascular risk prevalence among diverse school-age children: Implications for schools. *Journal of School Nursing, 15*(2), 8–12.

Cowen, P. S. (1999). Child neglect: Injuries of omission. *Pediatric Nursing, 25*(4), 401–405.

Cox, M. (1994). *Statistical analysis triangulation of infant outcomes of a nurse managed obstetrical clinic*. Paper presented at the Texas Medical Center National Nursing Research, Conference, Houston, TX.

Cox, S. G., & Turnbull, C. J. (1998). Developing effective interactions to improve breastfeeding outcomes. Part 2: Antenatal empowerment of mothers for postnatal success in breastfeeding. *Breastfeeding Review, 6*(2), 17–22.

Coyne, A. C., Reichman, W. E., & Berbig, L. J. (1993). The relationship between dementia and elder abuse. *American Journal of Psychiatry, 150*(4), 643–646.

Coyne, J. C. (1990). The interpersonal processes of depression. In G. I. Keitner (Ed.), *Depression families: Impact and treatment* (pp. 31–54). Washington, DC: American Psychiatric Press.

Coyne, J. C., Kessler, R. C., Tal, M., Turnbull, J., Wortman, C. B., & Greden, J. (1987). Living with a depressed person. *Journal of Clinical & Consulting Psychology, 55*, 347–352.

Cramer, L. D., McCorkle, R., Cherlin, E., Johnson-Hurzeler, R., & Bradley, E. H. (2003). Nurses' attitudes and practice related to hospice care. *Journal of Nursing Scholarship, 35*, 249–255.

Crane, M., & Warnes, A. M. (2001). Older people and homelessness: Prevalence and causes. *Topics in Geriatric Rehabilitation, 16*(4), 1–14.

Cranney, A., Guyett, G., Griffith, L., Wells, G., Tugwell, P., Rosen, C., et al. (2002). IX: Summary of meta-analyses of therapies for postmenopausal osteoporosis. *Endocrine Review, 23*(4), 570–578.

Cranney, A., Tugwell, P., Adachi, J., Weaver, B., Zytaruk, N., Papaioannour, A., et al. (2002). III. Meta-analysis of risedronate for the treatment of postmenopausal osteoporosis. *Endocrine Review, 23*(4), 517–523.

Cranney, A., Tugwell, P., Zytaruk, N., Robinson, V., Weaver, B., Adachi, N., et al. (2002). IV. Meta-analysis of raloxifene for the prevention and treatment of postmenopausal osteoporosis. *Endocrine Review, 23*(4), 524–528.

Cranney, A., Wells, G., Willan, A., Griffith, L., Zytaruk, N., Robinson, V., et al. (2002). III. Meta-analysis of alendronate for the treatment of postmenopausal osteoporosis. *Endocrine Review, 23*(4), 508–516.

Criddle, L. (1993). Healing from surgery: A phenomenological study. *Image: Journal of Nursing Scholarship, 25*, 208–213.

Crogan, N. L., Corbett, C. F., & Short, R. A. (2002). The minimum data set: Predicting malnutrition in newly admitted nursing home residents. *Clinical Nursing Research, 11*, 341–353.

Cronbach, L. J. (1951). Coefficient alpha and the internal structure of tests. *Psychometrika, 16*, 297–334.

Cronin-Stubbs, D., & Rooks, C. A. (1985). The stress, social support, and burnout of critical care nurses: The results of research. *Heart & Lung, 14*, 31–39.

Cross, I. (2003). Music as a biocultural phenomenon. *Annals of the New York Academy of Science, 999*, 106–111.

Crow, S., & Hartman, S. (2002). Organizational culture: Its impact on employee relations and discipline in health care organizations. *Health Care Manager, 21*, 22–28.

Crowley, M. (1996). Exercise restores seniors' strength and spirits. *Health Progress, 6*, 42–44.

Crum, R., Anthony, J., Bassett, S., & Folstein, M. (1993). Population-based norms for the Mini-Mental State Examination by age and educational level. *Journal of the American Medical Association, 269*, 2386–2391.

Cuddigan, J., Ayello, E. A., Sussman, C., & Baranoski, S. (Eds.). (2001). *Pressure ulcers in America: Prevalence, incidence, and implications for the future*. Reston, VA: National Pressure Ulcer Advisory Panel.

Cuddigan, J. E., Logan, E., Evans, D., & Hoesing, H. (1988). Evaluation of an artificial intelligence-based nursing decision support system in a clinical setting. In N. Daly & K. J. Hannah (Eds.), *Nursing and computers: Proceedings of the third international symposium on nursing use of computers and information science* (pp. 629–636). St. Louis, MO: C. V. Mosby.

Cuffe, S. P., Addy, C. L., Garrison, C. Z., Waller, J. L., Jackson, K. L., McKeown, R. E., et al. (1998). Prevalence of PTSD in a community sample of older adolescents. *Journal of the American Academy of Child & Adolescent Psychiatry, 37*(2), 147–154.

Cuijpers, P., & Smit, F. (2002). Excess mortality in depression: A meta-analysis of community studies. *Journal of Affective Disorders, 72*, 227–236.

Cullen, D. J., Sweitzer, B. J., Bates, D. W., Burdick, E., Edmondson, A., & Leape, L. L. (1997). Preventable adverse drug events in hospitalized patients: A comparative study of intensive care and general care units. *Critical Care Medicine, 25*, 1287–1289.

Cumming, E., & Henry, W. (1961). *Growing old: The process of disengagement*. New York: Basic Books.

Cunningham, D. A. (2002). Application of Roy's adaptation model when caring for a group of women coping with menopause. *Journal of Community Health Nursing, 19*(1), 49–60.

Curry, L., & Hogstel, M. O. (2002). Osteoporosis: Education and awareness can make a difference. *American Journal of Nursing, 102*(1), 26–32.

Curry, L., Porter, M., Michalski, M., & Gruman, C. (2000). Individualized care: Perceptions of certified nurse's aides. *Journal of Gerontological Nursing, 26*(7), 45–51.

Cwikel, J. G., Fried, A. V., Biderman, A., & Galinsky, D. (1998). Validation of a fall-risk screening test, the Elderly Fall Screening Test (EFST), for community-dwelling elderly. *Disability and Rehabilitation, 20*, 161–167.

Czarnecki, M. T. (1996). Benchmarking: A data-oriented look at improving health care performance. *Journal of Nursing Care Quality, 10*(3), 1–6.

Czarnik, R. E., Stone, K. S., Everhart, C. C., & Preusser, B. A. (1991). Differential effects of continuous versus intermittent suction on tracheal tissue. *Heart & Lung, 20*, 144–151.

Czuchta, D. M., & McCay, E. (2001). Help-seeking for parents of individuals experiencing a first episode of schizophrenia. *Archives of Psychiatric Nursing, 15*, 159–170.

Daggett, L. M. (2002). Living with loss: Middle-aged men face spousal bereavement. *Qualitative Health Research, 22*, 625–639.

Daly, E. J., Falk, W. E., & Brown, P. (2001). Cholinesterase inhibitors for behavioral disturbances in dementia. *Current Psychiatry Reports, 3*(3), 251–258.

Dalzell, M. D. (2002). *Has capitation weathered the storm?* Managed Care. Fifth Annual Evergreen Managed Care Indicators. Retrieved from http://www.managedcaremag.com/archives/0212/0212

D'Amico, A., Whittington, R. Malkowicz, S., Schultz, D., Blank, K., Broderick, G., et al. (1998). Biochemical outcome after radical prostatectomy, external beam radiation therapy, or interstitial radiation therapy for clinically localized prostate cancer. *Journal of the American Medical Association, 280*(11), 969–974.

Dan, A. J., & Al-Gasseer, N. (1991). Perimenstrual symptoms among Bahraini women [Abstract]. *Proceedings of the 9th Conference of the Society for Menstrual Cycle Research*, 40.

Dansky, K. H., Yant, B., Jenkins, D., & Dellasega, C. (2003). Professional issues. Qualitative analysis of telehomecare nursing activities. *Journal of Nursing Administration, 33*(7/8), 372–375.

Darkins, A., Fisk, N., Garner, P., & Wootton, R. (1996). Point-to-point telemedicine using the isdn. *Journal of Telemedicine & Telecare, 2*(Suppl. 1), 82–83.

Dartmouth Medical School, Center for the Evaluative Clinical Science. (1998). *The Dartmouth atlas of health care*. Retrieved from http://www.dartmouthatlas.org/atlaslinks/98atlas.php

D'Auria, J. P. (1994). A bibliometric analysis of published maternal and child health nursing research from 1976 to 1990. In S. J. Grobe & E. S. P. Pluyter-Wenting (Eds.), *Nursing informatics: An international overview for nursing in a technological era* (pp. 471–475). Amsterdam: Elsevier.

Davidson, B., Goldenberg, S., Gleave, M., & Degner, L. (2003). Provision of individualized information to men and their partners to facilitate treatment decision making in prostate cancer. *Oncology Nursing Forum, 30*(1), 107–114.

Davis, A. J., & Underwood, P. (1976). Educational preparation for community mental health nursing. *Journal of Psychosocial Nursing and Mental Health Services, 14*, 10–15.

Davis, B. D., Cowley, S. A., & Ryland, R. K. (1996). The effects of terminal illness on patients and their careers. *Journal of Advanced Nursing, 23*, 512–520.

Davis, F. (1960). Uncertainty in medical prognosis clinical and functional. *American Journal of Sociology, 66*, 41–47.

Davis, R. E. (2002). Leave-taking experiences in the lives of abused women. *Clinical Nursing Research, 11*(30), 285–305.

Dawood, M. Y., McGuire, J. L., & Demers, L. M. (1985). *Premenstrual syndrome and dysmenorrhea*. Baltimore: Urban & Schwarzenberg.

Dawson-Hughes, B. (1991). Calcium supplementation and bone loss: A review of controlled clinical trials. *American Journal of Clinical Nutrition, 54*(1, Suppl.), 274S–280S.

Day, J. C. (1996). *Population projections of the United States by age, sex, race and hispanic origin: 1995 to 2050* (U. S. Bureau of Census, Current Population Reports, p. 25–1130). Washington, DC: U.S. Government Printing Office: Retrieved from http://www.census.gov/prod/1/pop/p25-1130/p251130.pdf

Day, L., Fildes, B., Gordon, I., Fitzharris, M., Flamer, H., & Lord, S. (2002). Randomised factorial trial of falls prevention among older people living in their own homes. *British Medical Journal, 325*, 128–133.

Dean, H. (2003). *Mental health reform agenda*. Retrieved from www.mhreform.org/news/9–12-03 dean.htm

Deatrick, J., Knafl, K., & Murphy-Moore, C. (1999). Clarifying the concept of normalization. *Image: Journal of Nursing Scholarship, 31*(3), 209–214.

De Chardin, P. T. (1955). *The phenomenon of man*. London: Collins.

Deci, P. A., Santos, A. B., Hiott, D. W., Schoenwald, S., & Dias, J. K. (1995). Dissemination of assertive community treatment programs. *Psychiatric Services, 46*, 676–678.

DeCostanzo, E. T. (1998). Why women offenders? *Corrections Today, 60*(7), 8–9.

De Geest, S., Abraham, I., & Dunbar-Jacob, J. (1996). Measuring transplant patients' compliance with immunosuppressive therapy. *Western Journal of Nursing Research, 18*, 595–605.

De Geest, S., Borgermans, L., Gemoets, H., Abraham, I., Vlaminck, H., Evers, G., et al. (1995). Incidence determinants, and consequences of non-compliance with immunosuppressive therapy in renal transplant patients. *Transplantation, 59*, 340–347.

De Geest, S., Kesteloot, K., Andriaenssen, G., Lenaerts, K., Thelissen, M., Mekers, G., Sergeant, P., & Daenen, W. (1998). Clinical and cost comparison of three preoperative skin preparation protocols in CABG-patients. *Progress in Cardiovascular Nursing, 11*, 4–16.

De Geest, S., Kestleloot, K., Degryse, I., & Vanhaecke, J. (1995). Hospital costs of protective isolation procedures in heart transplant recipients. *Journal of Heart and Lung Transplantation, 14*, 544–552.

De Geest, S., von Renteln-Kruse, W., Steeman, E., Degraeve, S., & Abraham, I. (1998). Adherence issues with the geriatric population. Complexity with aging. In I. Abraham, T. Fulmer, & K. Milisen (Guest Eds.), Geriatric nursing. *Nursing Clinics of North America, 33*, 467–480.

Dejin-Karlsson, E., Hanson, B. S., Östergren, P., Lindgren, A., Sjoberg, N., & Marsal, K. (2000). Association of a lack of psychosocial resources and the risk of giving birth to small for gestational age infants: A stress hypothesis. *British Journal of Obstetrics and Gynaecology, 107*(1), 89–100.

Delaney, J., Lupton, M., & Toth, E. (1976). The storm before the calm: The premenstrual syndrome. In J. Delaney, M. Lupton, & E. Toth (Eds.), *The curse: The cultural history of menstruation* (pp. 83–106). New York: E. P. Dutton.

Delaney, K., Chisholm, M., Clement, J., & Merwin, E. (1999). Trends in psychiatric mental health nursing education. *Archives of Psychiatric Nursing, 13*, 67–73.

Delaney-Black, V., Covington, C., Ondersma, S. J., Nordstrom-Klee, B., Templin, T., Ager, J., et al. (2002). Violence exposure, trauma, and IQ and/or reading deficits among urban children. *Archives of Pediatrics & Adolescent Medicine, 156*(3), 280–285.

Delbecq, A., Van de Ven, A., & Gustafsen, D. (1975). *Group techniques for program planning: A guide to nominal group and Delphi processes*. Glenview, IL: Scott Foresman.

Dellasega, C., & Zerbe, T. (2002). Caregivers of frail rural older adults: Effects of an advanced practice nursing intervention. *Journal of Gerontological Nursing, 28*(10), 40–49.

DeMarco, R., Ford-Gilboe, M., Friedemann, M., McCubbin, H. I., & McCubbin, M. A. (2000). Stress, coping, and family health. In V. H. Rice (Ed.), *Handbook of stress, coping, and health: Implications for nursing research, theory, and practice*. Thousand Oaks, CA: Sage.

Demi, A., Bakeman, R., Sowell, R., Moneyham, L., & Seals, B. (1998). Suicidal thoughts of women with HIV infection: Effect of stressors and moderating effects of family cohesion. *Journal of Family Psychology, 12*, 1–10.

Demi, A. S., Meredith, C. E., & Gray, M. (1996). Research priorities for urological nursing: A Delphi study. *Urological Nursing, 16*, 3–8.

Demi, A. S., & Miles, M. S. (1987). Parameters of normal grief: A Delphi study. *Death Study, 11*, 397–412.

Demitrack, M. A., Dale, J. K., Straus, S. E., Laue, L., Listwak, S. J., Kruesi, M. J. P., et al. (1991). Evidence for impaired activation of the hypothalamic-pituitary-adrenal axis in patients with chronic fatigue syndrome. *Journal of Clinical Endocrinology and Metabolism, 73*, 1224–1234.

Denham, S. A. (2003). Describing abuse of pregnant women and their healthcare workers in rural Appalachia. *American Journal of Maternal Child Nursing, 28*, 264–269.

Dennis, C. L. (2002). Breastfeeding initiation and duration: A 1990–2000 literature review. *Journal of Obstetrical, Gynecological, and Neonatal Nursing, 31*(1), 12–32.

Denton, M., Zeytinoglu, I. U., Davies, S., & Lian, J. (2002). Job stress and job dissatisfaction of home care workers in the context of health care restructuring. *International Journal of Health Services, 32*, 327–357.

Denzin, N. (1989). *The research act: A theoretical introduction to sociological methods*. Englewood Cliffs, NJ: Prentice-Hall.

Department of Defense Tricare Management Activity. (2001). *Population health improvement plan and guide*. Washington, DC: Tricare Management Activity Government Printing Office. Retrieved from http://www.tricare.osd.mil/mhsophsc/DoD_PHI_Plan_Guide.pdf

Derdiarian, A. K. (1990). The relationships among the subsystems of Johnson's behavioral system model. *Image: Journal of Nursing Scholarship, 22*(4), 219–225.

Derogatis, L. (1983). *The Psychosocial Adjustment to Illness Scale*. Towson, MD: Clinical Psychometric Research.

Desai, M., Pratt, L., Lentzner, H., & Robinson, K. (2001). Trends in vision and hearing among older Americans. *Aging Trends, 2*, 1–8.

Deutsch, F. M., Ruble, D. N., Fleming, A., Brooks-Gunn, J., & Stangor, C. (1988). Information-seeking and maternal self-definition during the transition to motherhood. *Journal of Personality and Social Psychology, 55*(3), 420–431.

Devine, E. C. (1992). Effects of psychoeducational care for adult surgical patients: A meta-analysis of 191 studies. *Patient Education and Counseling, 19*, 129–142.

Devine, E. C. (2003). Meta-analysis of the effect of psychoeducational interventions on pain in adults with cancer. *Oncology Nursing Forum, 30*, 75–89.

Devine, E., & Cook, T. (1983). A meta-analytic analysis of effects of psychoeducational interventions on length of post surgical hospital stay. *Nursing Research, 32*, 267–274.

Devine, E. C., & Cook, T. D. (1986). Clinical and cost-saving effects of psychoeducational interventions with surgical patients: A meta-analysis. *Research in Nursing and Health, 9*, 89–105.

Devine, E. C., O'Connor, F. W., Cook, T. D., Wenk, V. A., & Curtin, T. R. (1988). Clinical and financial effects of psychoeducational care provided by staff nurses to adult surgical patients in the post-DRG environment. *American Journal of Public Health, 78*, 1293–1297.

Devine, E. C., & Reifschneider, E. (1995). A meta-analysis of the effects of psychoeducational care in adults with hypertension. *Nursing Research, 44*, 237–245.

DeVoe, J. F., Ruddy, S. A., Miller, A. K., Planty, M., Snyder, T. D., Duhart, D. T., et al. (2002). *Indicators of school crime and safety 2002*. (NCJ 196753). Washington, DC: U.S. Department of Justice Office of Justice Programs Bureau of Justice Statistics. Retrieved from http://www.ojp.usdoj.gov/bjs/pub/ascii/iscs02.txt

Dew, M. A., Becker, J. T., Sanchez, J., Caldararo, R., Lopez, O. L., Wess, J., et al. (1997). Prevalence and predictors of depressive, anxiety, and substance use disorders in HIV-infected and uninfected men: A longitudinal evaluation. *Psychology Medicine, 17*, 395–409.

Dexter, P. R., Wolinsky, F. D., Gramelspacher, G. J., Eckert, G. J., & Tierney, W. M. (2003). Opportunities for advance directives to influence acute medical care. *Journal of Clinical Ethics, 14*, 173–182.

DeYoung, C., & Tower, M. (1971). *The nurse's role in community mental health centers: Out of uniform and into trouble*. St. Louis, MO: Mosby.

Dharmarajan, T. S., & Ugalino, J. T. (2003). Dementia. In T. S. Dharmarajan & R. A. Norman (Eds.), *Clinical geriatrics* (pp. 293–309). New York: Parthenon Publishing Group.

Diabetes Control and Complications Trial Research Group. (1993). The effect of intensive treatment of diabetes on the development and progression of long-term complications in insulin-dependent diabetes mellitus. *New England Journal of Medicine, 329*, 977–986.

Diamond, M. (1965). A critical evaluation of the ontogeny of human sexual behavior. *Quarterly Review of Biology, 40*, 147–175.

Diamond, M. C. (1988). *Enriching heredity: The impact of the environment on the anatomy of the brain* (pp. 79–87). New York: Free Press.

DiCenso, A., Guyatt, G., Willan, A., & Griffith, L. (2002). Interventions to reduce unintended pregnancies among adolescents: Systematic review of randomized controlled trials. *British Medical Journal, 324*(5), 14–26.

Dickenson-Hazard, N. (1999). Collaboration—Are we really ready? *Journal of Professional Nursing, 15*(5), 261.

Dickerson, S., Stone, V., Panchura, C., & Usiak, D. (2002). The meaning of communication: Experiences with augmentative communication devices. *Rehabilitation Nursing, 27*, 215–220.

Dickinson, J. I., Shroyer, J. L., & Elias, J. W. (2002). The influence of commercial-grade carpet on postural sway and balance strategy among older adults. *Gerontologist, 42*, 552–559.

Dickoff, J., James, P., & Wiedenbach, E. (1968). Theory in a practice discipline: Part I. Practice oriented theory. *Nursing Research, 17*, 415–435.

DiClemente, R. J., & Wingwood, G. M. (1995). A randomized controlled trial of an HIV sexual risk-reduction intervention for young African-American women. *Journal of the American Medical Association, 274*(16), 1271–1276.

Diemer, G. A. (1997). Expectant fathers: Influence of perinatal education on stress, coping, and spousal relations. *Research in Nursing & Health, 20*, 281–293.

Dienemann, J., Boyle, E., Baker, D., Resnick, W., Wiederhorn, N., & Campbell, J. (2000). Intimate partner abuse among women diagnosed with depression. *Issues in Mental Health Nursing, 21*(5), 499–513.

Diers, D., Schmidt, R. L., McBride, M. A., & Davis, B. L. (1972). The effect of nursing interaction on patients in pain. *Nursing Research, 21*, 419–428.

DiIorio, C., Duduley, W. N., Kelly, M., Soet, J. E., Wbwara, J., & Potter, J. S. (2000). A social cognitive-based model for condom use among college students. *Nursing Research, 49*(4), 208–214.

DiIorio, C., Shafer, P. O., Letz, R., Henry, T., Schomer, D. L., Yeager, K., et al. (2003). The association of stigma with self-management and perceptions of health care among adults with epilepsy. *Epilepsy & Behavior, 4*, 259–267.

Dijkers, M. P. (2003). Individualization in quality of life measurement: Instruments and approaches. *Archives of Physical Medicine and Rehabilitation, 84*(Suppl. 2), S3–S14.

Dillman, A. (1978). *Mail and telephone surveys: The total design method*. New York: Wiley.

DiMaria-Ghalili, R. A. (2002). Changes in nutritional status and postoperative outcomes in elderly CABG patients. *Biological Research for Nursing, 4*, 73–84.

DiMartini, A., Rovera, G. M., Graham, T. O., Furukawa, H., Todo, S., Funovits, M., et al. (1998). Quality of life after intestinal transplantation and among home parenteral nutrition patients. *Journal of Parenteral and Enternal Nutrition, 22*, 357–362.

Dionne-Proulz, J., & Pepin, R. (1993). Stress management in the nursing profession. *Journal of Nursing Management, 1*(2), 75–81.

DiPalma, J. A. (2001). Management of severe gastroesophageal reflux disease. *Journal of Clinical Gastroenterology, 32*(1), 19–26.

Dirksen, S. R. (2000). Predicting well-being among breast cancer survivors. *Journal of Advanced Nursing, 32*(4), 937–943.

Ditto, P. H., Danks, J. H., Smucker, W. D., Bookwala, K., Coppola, K. M., Dresser, R., et al. (2001). Advance directives as acts of communication: A randomized controlled trial. *Archives of Internal Medicine, 161*, 421–430.

Djukanovic, V., & Mach, E. P. (1975). *Alternative approaches to meeting basic health needs in developing countries: A joint UNICEF/WHO study*. Geneva: World Health Organization.

Docherty, S. L. (2003). Symptom experiences of children and adolescents with cancer. In *Annual review of nursing research* (Vol. 21, pp. 123–149). New York: Springer.

Dochterman, J. M., & Jones, D. A. (2003). *Unifying nursing languages: The harmonization of North American Nursing Diagnosis Association (NANDA), NIC, and Nursing Outcomes Classification (NOC)*. Washington, DC: American Nurses Association.

Dochterman, J., & Bulechek, G. (2004). *Nursing interventions classification (NIC)* (4th ed.). St. Louis, MO: Mosby.

Doering, L. V., Moser, D. K., & Dracup, K. (2000). Correlates of anxiety, hostility, depression, and psychosocial adjustment in parents of NICU infants. *Neonatal Network, 19*, 15–23.

Donabedian, A. (1980). *Explorations in quality assessment and monitoring* (Vol. 1–3). Ann Arbor, MI: Health Administration Press.

Donabedian, A. (1988). Quality assessment and assurance: Unity of purpose, diversity of means. *Inquiry, 25*, 173–192.

Donahue, M. P. (1996). *Nursing: The finest art* (2nd ed.). St. Louis, MO: Mosby-Year Book.

Donaldson, M., Yordy, K., Lohr, K., & Vanselow, N. (Eds.). (1996). *Primary care: America's health in a new era*. Washington, DC: National Academy Press.

Donaldson, S. K. (2000). Breakthroughs in scientific research: The discipline of nursing, 1960–1999. In J. F. Fitzpatrick & J. Goeppinger (Eds.), *Annual review of nursing research* (Vol. 18, pp. 247–311). New York: Springer Publishing.

Donaldson, S. K., & Crowley, D. M. (1978). The discipline of nursing. *Nursing Outlook, 26*, 113–120.

Dong, M., Anda, R. F., Dube, S. R., Giles, W. H., & Felitti, V. J. (2003). The relationship of exposure to childhood sexual abuse to other forms of abuse, neglect, and household dysfunction during childhood. *Child Abuse and Neglect, 27*(6), 625–639.

Donnelly, E. (2001). An assessment of nursing theory as guides to scientific inquiry. In N. Chaska (Ed.), *The nursing profession: Tomorrow and beyond* (pp. 331–346). Thousand Oaks, CA: Sage Publications.

Donovan, J. M., & Syngal, S. (1998). Colorectal cancer in women: An underappreciated but preventable risk. *Journal of Women's Health, 7*(1), 45–48.

Doornbos, M. M. (2000). King's systems framework and family health: The derivation and testing of a theory. *Journal of Theory Construction & Testing, 4*(1), 20–26.

Doornbos, M. (2002). Family caregivers and the mental health care system: Reality and dreams. *Archives of Psychiatric Nursing, 16*(1), 39–46.

Dorfman, L. (1989). Retirement preparation and retirement satisfaction in the rural elderly. *Journal of Applied Gerontology, 8*, 432–450.

Dotinga, R. (2002). *Suicide on the rise in rural America*. Retrieved from http://www.iwon.com/home/health/helath_article/0,11720,507895/06-29-2002::06:00,00.html

Douaihy, A., & Singh, N. (2001). Factors affecting quality of life in patients with HIV infection. *AIDS Reader, 11*(9), 444–449.

Douglas, M. (2000). The time has come for interventional studies in transcultural nursing. *Journal of Transcultural Nursing, 11*, 246.

Douglas, S., Daly, B., Rudy, E., Song, R., Dyer, M. A., & Montenegro, H. (1995). The cost-effectiveness of a special care unit to care for the chronically critically ill. *Journal of Nursing Administration, 25*(11), 47–53.

Doukas, D. J., & McCullough, L. B. (1988). Assessing the values history of the elderly patient regarding critical and chronic care. In J. J. Gallo, W. Reichel, & L. Anderson (Eds.), *Handbook of geriatric assessment*. Rockville, MD: Aspen.

Dow, K. H., Ferrell, B. R., Haberman, M. R., & Eaton, L. (1999). The meaning of quality of life in cancer survivorship. *Oncology Nursing Forum, 26*, 519–528.

Dowd, S., Davidhizar, R., & Giger, J. (1999). Will you fit if you move to a job in another culture? *Health Care Manager, 18*, 20–27.

Dowdell, E. B. (1995). Caregiver burden: Grandmothers raising their high risk grandchildren. *Journal of Psychosocial Nursing 33*(3), 27–30.

Dowling-Castronovo, A., & Bulkwalter, K. C. (2001). Urinary incontinence assessment. *Gerontological Nursing, 27*(5), 6–7.

Doyle, J. B. (1986). How experts scan journals: Implications for expert systems in text retrieval. In R. Salamon, B. Blum, & M. Jorgensen (Eds.), *MEDINFO 86* (pp. 540–544). North-Holland, Netherlands: Elsevier.

Drachman, D. A. (2000). Occam's razor, geriatric syndromes, and the dizzy patient. *Annals of Internal Medicine, 132*(5), 403–405.

Dracup, K., & Bryan-Brown, C. W. (2003). Nursing morbidity and mortality conferences. *American Journal of Critical Care, 12*(6), 492–494.

Dracup, K., & Moser, D. K. (1991). Treatment-seeking behavior among those with signs and symptoms of acute myocardial infarction. *Heart and Lung, 20*, 570–575.

Dreher, H. (1998). Mind-body interventions for surgery: Evidence and exigency. *Advances in Mind-Body Medicine, 14*, 207–222.

Dreifuss, F. E., & Nordli, D. R. (2001). Classification of epilepsies in childhood. In J. M. Pellock, W. E. Dodson, & B. F. D. Bourgeois (Eds.), *Pediatric epilepsy: Diagnosis and therapy* (2nd ed., pp. 69–80). New York: Demos.

Dretske, F. (1988). *Explaining behavior: Reasons in a world of causes*. Cambridge, MA: MIT Press.

Drevdahl, D., Taylor, J. Y., & Phillips, D. A. (2001). Race and ethnicity as variables in nursing research, 1952–2000. *Nursing Research, 50*, 305–313.

Drew, B. J., Krucoff, M. W., for the ST-segment monitoring practice guideline International Working Group. (1999). Multilead ST-segment monitoring in patients with acute coronary syndromes: A consensus statement for healthcare professionals. *American Journal of Critical Care, 8*, 372–386.

Drinka, T., & Clark, P. (2000). *Health care teamwork: Interdisciplinary practice and teaching*. Westport, CT: Auburn House.

Drossman, D. A. (1995). Diagnosing and treating patients with refractory functional gastrointestinal disorders. *Annals of Internal Medicine, 123*(9), 688–697.

Drossman, D. A., Leserman, J., Li, Z., Keefe, F., Hu, Y., & Toomey, T. (2000). Effects of coping on health outcome among women with gastrointestinal disorders. *Psychosomatic Medicine, 62*(3), 309–317.

Droste, C., & Roskamm, H. (1983). Experimental pain measurement in patients with asymptomatic myocardial ischemia. *Journal of the American College of Cardiology, 1*, 940–945.

Drought, T. S., & Koenig, B. A. (2002). "Choice" in end-of-life decision making: Researching fact or fiction? *Gerontologist, 42*(Special Issue III), 114–128.

Drummond, D. J., Sparr, L. F., & Gordon, G. H. (1989). Hospital violence reduction among high risk patients. *Journal of the American Medical Association, 261*(17), 2531–2534.

Drury, T. (1997). Recognizing the potential for violence in the ICU. *Dimensions of Critical Care Nursing, 16*, 314–326.

Druss, B. G., Marcus, S. C., Olfson, M., & Pincus, H. A. (2002). The most expensive medical conditions in America. *Health Affairs, 21*(4), 105–111.

Druss, B. G., Marcus, S. C., Olfson, M., Tanielian, T., Elinson, L., & Pincus, H. A. (2001). Comparing the national economic burden of five chronic conditions. *Health Affairs, 20*(6), 233–241.

Dube, S. R., Anda, R. F., Felitti, V. J., Chapman, D. P., Williamson, D. F., & Giles, W. H. (2001). Childhood abuse, household dysfunction, and the risk of attempted suicide throughout the life span: Findings from the Adverse Childhood Experiences Study. *Journal of the American Medical Association, 286*, 3089–3096.

Dube, S. R., Anda, R. F., Felitti, V. J., Edwards, V. J., & Croft, J. B. (2002). Adverse childhood experiences and personal alcohol abuse as an adult. *Addictive Behaviors, 27*, 713–725.

Dubin, R. (1978). *Theory building* (Rev. ed.). New York: MacMillan.

DuBois, K., & Rizzolo, M. A. (1994). Cruising the "information superhighway." *American Journal of Nursing, 94*(12), 58–60.

Dubos, R. (1965). *Man adapting*. New Haven, CT: Yale University Press.

Duffield, P., & Podzamsky, J. E. (1996). The completion of advance directives in primary care. *Journal of Family Practice, 42*(4), 378–384.

Duffy, M. (1987). Methodological triangulation: A vehicle for merging quantitative and qualitative research methods. *Image: Journal of Nursing Scholarship, 19*, 130–133.

Duits, A. A., Boeke, S., Tamms, M. A., Passchier, J., & Erdman, R. A. (1997). Prediction of quality of life after coronary artery bypass graft surgery: A review and evaluation of multiple, recent studies. *Psychosomatic Medicine 59*, 257–268.

Duits, A. A., Duivenvoorden, H. J., Boeke, S., Taams, M. A., Mochtar, B., Krauss, X. H., et al. (1999). A structural modeling analysis of anxiety and depression in patients undergoing coronary artery bypass graft surgery: A model generating approach. *Journal of Psychosomatic Research, 46*(2), 187–200.

Duke, S. (1998). An exploration of anticipatory grief: The lived experience of people during their spouses' terminal illness and in bereavement. *Journal of Advanced Nursing, 28*, 829–839.

Dulock, H. L., & Holzemer, W. L. (1991). Substruction: Improving the linkage from theory to method. *Nursing Science Quarterly, 4*, 83–87.

Dumas, P. D., & Fraser, M. (1999). Strong bones in later life: Luxury or necessity? *Bulletin of the World Health Organization, 77*(5), 416–422.

Dumas, R. G., & Leonard, R. C. (1963). The effect of nursing on the incidence of postoperative vomiting. *Nursing Research, 12*, 12–15.

Dunbar-Jacob, J., & Schlenk, E. (1996). Treatment adherence and clinical outcome: Can we make a difference? In *Health psychology over the life span* (pp. 323–343). Washington, DC: American Psychological Association.

Duncan, G. J., & Brooks-Gunn, J. (1997). *Consequences of growing up poor*. New York: Russell Sage Foundation.

Duncombe, W., Robbins, M., & Wolf, D. (2003). Place characteristics and residential location choice among the retirement-age population. *Journals of Gerontology: Social Sciences, 58*, S244–S252.

Dunkin, J. J., & Anderson-Hanley, C. (1998). Dementia caregiver burden. A review of the literature and guidelines for assessment and intervention. *Neurology, 51*(Suppl. 1), S53–S60.

Dunn, D. W., Austin, J. K., & Huster, G. A. (1999). Symptoms of depression in adolescents with epilepsy. *Journal of the Academy of Child and Adolescent Psychiatry, 38*, 1132–1138.

Dunn, H. L. (1961). *High level wellness*. Emmaus, PA: Rodale.

Dunn, M. E. (1980). *High-level wellness*. Thorofare, NJ: Charles B. Slack.

Dunphy, L. H. (1998). *The circle of caring: A transformative model of advanced practice nursing*. Paper presented at the 20th Research Conference of the International Association of Human Caring, Philadelphia.

Eagly, A. H. (1992). Uneven progress: Social psychology and the study of attitudes. *Journal of Personality and Social Psychology, 63*, 693–710.

Earle, J. R., Smith, M. H., Harris, C. T., & Longino, C. F. (1998). Women, marital status, and symptoms of depression in a mid-life sample. *Journal of Women and Aging, 10*(1), 41–57.

East, T., Lugo, A., Morris, A., Parmley, L., Hill, T., Gooder, V., et al. (1999). Efficacy of computerized decision support for mechanical ventilation: Results of a prospective multi-center randomized trial. *Proceedings of the American Medical Informatics Association Symposium*, 251–255.

Eastwood, E. A., & Schechtman, J. (1999). Direct observation nursing: Adverse patient behaviors and functional outcomes. *Nursing Economics, 17*(2), 96–102.

Eckberg, E. (1998). The future of robotics can be ours. *AORN Journal, 67*(5), 1018–1023.

Eckhart, J. G. (1993). Costing out nursing services: Examining the research. *Nursing Economic$, 11*, 91–98.

Economic Research Services, U.S. Department of Agriculture. (2000). *Rural industry: What rural industries provide high-paying, private-sector jobs?* Retrieved from http://www.ers.usda.gov/Briefing/Industry/highpaying/salaryearnings.htm

Edell-Gustafsson, U. M., & Hetta, J. E. (1999). Anxiety, depression and sleep in male patients undergoing coronary artery bypass surgery. *Scandinavian Journal of Caring Science, 13*, 137–143.

Edelman, C. L., & Mandle, C. L (2002). *Health promotion throughout the life span* (5th ed.). St. Louis, MO: Mosby.

Edelson, M. (1970). *Sociotherapy and psychotherapy*. Chicago: University of Chicago Press.

Edvinsson, L., MacKenzie, E. T., & McCulloch, J. (1993). *Cerebral blood flow and metabolism*. New York: Raven Press.

Edwards, N. E., & Beck, A. M. (2002). Animal-assisted therapy and nutrition in Alzheimer's disease. *Western Journal of Nursing Research, 24*(6), 697–712.

Edwards, N. E., & Ruettiger, K. M. (2002). The influence of caregiver burden on patients' management of Parkinson's disease: Implications for rehabilitation nursing. *Rehabilitation Nursing, 27*, 182–186.

Edwards, N. E., & Scheetz, P. S. (2002). Predictors of burden for caregivers of patients with Parkinson's disease. *Journal of Neuroscience Nursing, 34*, 184–189.

Edwardson, S., & Giovannetti, P. (1994). Nursing work-load measurement systems. In *Annual review of nursing research* (Vol. 12, pp. 95–123). New York: Springer Publishing.

Egan, T. (2003, December 1). Amid dying towns of rural plains, one makes a stand. *New York Times*, p. A1.

Egbert, A. M. (1996). The Dwindles: Failure to thrive in older patients. *Nutrition Reviews, 54*, S25–S30.

Eisenberg, J. (1998). Health services research in a market-oriented health care system. *Research and Marketplace, 17*(1), 98–108.

Elfenbein, D. S., & Felice, M. E. (2003). Adolescent pregnancy. *Pediatric Clinics of North America, 50*(4), 781–800.

Elias, J., Elias, V. D., Bullough, V. L., Brewer, G., Douglas J., & Jarvis, W. (1999). *Porn 101*. Buffalo, NY: Prometheus Books.

Elkind, D. (1984). Teenage thinking: Implications for health care. *Pediatric Nursing, 10*(6), 383–385.

Eller, L. S. (1999). Guided imagery interventions for symptom management. In *Annual review of nursing research* (Vol. 17, pp. 57–84). New York: Springer Publishing.

Ellett, M. L. C., & Beckstrand, J. (1999). Examination of gavage tube placement in children. *Journal of the Society of Pediatric Nurses, 4*(2), 51–60.

Ellett, M. L. C., Maahs, J., & Forsee, S. (1998). Prevalence of feeding tube placement errors and associated risk factors in children. *The American Journal of Maternal Child Nursing, 23*(5), 234–239.

Ellison, C. (1983). Spiritual well-being: Conceptualization and measurement. *Journal of Psychology and Theology, 11*, 330–340.

Elstein, A. S., Shulman, L., & Sprafka, S. (1978). *Medical problem solving: An analysis of clinical reasoning*. Cambridge, MA: Harvard University Press.

Emergency Nurses Association. (1994). *Prevalence of violence in emergency departments*.

Emick, M., & Hayslip, B. (1999). Custodial grandparenting: Stresses, coping skill, and relationships with grandchildren. *International Journal of Aging & Human Development, 48*(1), 35–61.

Eng, C., Padulla, J., Eleazur, G. P., McCann, R., & Fox, N. (1997). Program of all-inclusive care for the elderly (PACE): An innovative model of integrated geriatric care and financing. *Journal of the American Geriatrics Society, 45*, 223–232.

Engebretson, J., & Wardell, D. W. (1997). The essence of partnership in research. *Journal of Professional Nursing, 13*, 38–47.

Engel, G. L. (1962). *Psychological development in health and disease*. Philadelphia: W. B. Saunders.

Engle, V. F. (1996). Newman's theory of health. In J. Fitzpatrick & A. Whall (Eds.), *Conceptual models of nursing: Analysis and application* (3rd ed., pp. 275–288). Stamford, CT: Appleton and Lange.

Engle, V. F., & Fox-Hill, E. J. (2005). Newman's theory of health. In J. Fitzpatrick & A. Whall

(Eds.), *Conceptual models of nursing: Analysis and application* (4th ed., pp. 273–296). Upper Saddle River, NJ: Pearson Prentice Hall.

Engler, M. M., Engler, M. B., Malloy, M. J., Chiu, E. Y., Schloetter, M. C., Paul, S. M., et al. (2003). Antioxidant vitamins C and E improve endothelial function in children with hyperlipidemia: Endothelial Assessment of Risk from Lipids in Youth (EARLY) Trial. *Circulation, 108,* 1059–1063.

Engs, R. (1982). Drinking patterns and attitudes toward alcoholism of Australian human services students. *Journal of Studies on Alcohol, 43,* 517–531.

Enhancing Recovery in Coronary Heart Disease Patients (ENRICHD) Investigators. (2003). Effects of treating depression and low perceived social support on clinical events after myocardial infarction: The Enhancing Recovery in Coronary Heart Disease Patients (ENRICHD) randomized trial. *Journal of the American Medical Association, 289,* 3106–3116.

Ensign, J., & Gittelsohn, J. (1998). Health access to care: Perspectives of homeless youth in Baltimore City, U.S.A. *Social Science Medicine, 47*(12), 2087–2099.

Epilepsy Foundation. (n.d.). *Treatment through vagus nerve stimulation.* Retrieved January 7, 2004, from http://www.epilepsyfoundation.org/answerplace/quickstart/newlydiagnosed/qstreatment/qstrvns.cfm

Eriksen, L. R. (1995). Patient satisfaction with nursing care: Concept clarification. *Journal of Nursing Measurement, 3,* 59–76.

Erickson, R. S. (1999). The continuing question of how best to measure body temperature [Editorial]. *Critical Care Medicine, 27*(10), 2307–2310.

Erikson, E. H. (1959). Identity and the life cycle. *Psychological Issues, 1,* 18–164.

Erikson, E. H. (1968a). *Childhood and society* (Rev. ed.). New York: Norton.

Erikson, E. H. (1968b). *Identity, youth, and crisis.* New York: Norton.

Eriksson, P. S., Perfilieva, E., Bjork-Erikkson, T., Alborn, A., Nordborg, C., Peterson, D. A., et al. (1998). Neurogenesis in the adult human hippocampus. *Nature Medicine, 4*(11), 1313–1317.

Essex, M. J., Klein, M. H., Cho, E., & Kalin, N. H. (2002). Maternal stress beginning in infancy may sensitize children to later stress exposure: Effects on cortisol and behavior. *Biological Psychiatry, 52,* 776–784.

Essex, M. J., Klein, M. H., Cho, E., & Kraemer, H. C. (2003). Exposure to maternal depression and marital conflict: Gender differences in children's later mental health symptoms. *Journal of the American Academy of Child and Adolescent Psychiatry, 42,* 728–737.

Essex, M. J., Klein, M. H., Miech, R., & Smider, N. A. (2001). Timing of initial exposure to maternal major depression and children's mental health symptoms in kindergarten. *British Journal of Psychiatry, 179,* 151–156.

Estabrooks, C. A. (1999). The conceptual structure of research utilization. *Research in Nursing and Health, 22,* 203–216.

Estes, C., Linkins, K., & Binney, E. (1996). The political economy of aging. In R. H. Binstock & L. K. George (Eds.), *Handbook of aging and the social sciences* (pp. 346–361). San Diego, CA: Academic Press.

Estes, E. H. (2002). Primary care: Building a model for the new medical environment. *North Carolina Medical Journal, 63*(4), 189–194.

Evans, G., Wilt, D., Alligood, M., & O'Neil, M. (1998). Empathy: A study of two types. *Issues in Mental Health Nursing, 19,* 453–461.

Evans, L. K. (1996). Knowing the patient: The route to individualized care. *Journal of Gerontological Nursing, 22*(3), 15–19.

Evans, L. K., & Strumpf, N. E. (1989). Tying down the elderly: A review of the literature on physical restraint. *Journal of the American Geriatrics Society, 37,* 65–74.

Evans, L. K., Strumpf, N. E., Allen-Taylor, S. L., Capezuti, E., Maislin, G., & Jacobsen, B. (1997). A clinical trial to reduce restraints in nursing homes. *Journal of the American Geriatrics Society, 45,* 675–681.

Evans, M. (2004). My baby's father: Unmarried parents and paternal responsibility. *Contemporary Sociology, 33*(1), 32–33.

Evans, R. G., & Stoddart, G. L. (1990). Producing health, consuming health care. *Social Science and Medicine, 31*(12), 1347–1363.

Executive summary of the third report of the National Cholesterol Education Program (NCEP) Expert Panel on Detection, Evaluation, and Treatment of High Blood Cholesterol in Adults (Adult Treatment Panel III). (2001). *Journal of the American Medical Association, 285,* 2486–2497.

Facts at a Glance. (2003). Child Trends: Washington, DC. Retrieved from http://www.childtrendsdatabank.org/

Fagin, C. M. (2001). Revisiting treatment in the home. *Archives of Psychiatric Nursing, 15*(1), 3–9.

Fagot-Campagna, A. (2000). Emergence of type 2 diabetes mellitus in children: Epidemiological evidence. *Journal of Pediatric Endocrinology & Metabolism, 13,* 1395–1402.

Fairtlough, H., & Closs, S. J. (1996). Patient focused menu planning: An ENB project in hospice. *Nursing Standard, 12*, 44–47.

Farran, C., Loukissa, D., Perraud, S., & Paun, O. (2004). Alzheimer's disease caregiving information and skills. Part II: Family caregiver issues and concerns. *Research in Nursing and Health, 27*(1), 40–51.

Farrell, A. D., & Bruce, S. E. (1997). The impact of exposure to community violence on violent behavior and emotional distress among urban adolescents. *Journal of Clinical Child Psychology, 26*, 2–14.

Farrell, M., Schmitt, M., & Heinemann, G. (2001). Informal roles and the stages of interdisciplinary team development. *Journal of Interprofessional Care, 15*, 281–295.

Fass, R., Longstreth, G., Pimentel, M., Fullerton, S., Russak, S., Chiou, C., et al. (2001). Evidence- and consensus-based practice guidelines for the diagnosis of irritable bowel syndrome. *Archives of Internal Medicine, 161*(17), 2081–2088.

Faulkner, M. (2002). Low income mothers of overweight children had personal and environmental challenges in preventing and managing obesity. *EBN, 5*(1), 27–29.

Faulkner, M. S., Hathaway, D. K., Milstead, E. J., & Burghen, G. A. (2001). Heart rate variability in adolescents and adults with type 1 diabetes. *Nursing Research, 50*, 95–104.

Faux, S. A. (1998). Historical overview of responses of children and their families to chronic illness. In M. E. Broome, K. Knafl, K. Pridham, & S. Feethan (Eds.), *Children and families in health and illness* (pp. 179–195). Thousand Oaks, CA: Sage Publications.

Fawcett, J. (1978). The what of theory development. In *Theory development: What, why, how?* (pp. 17–34). New York: National League for Nursing.

Fawcett, J. (1990). Preparation for caesarean childbirth: Derivation of a nursing intervention from the Roy adaptation model. *Journal of Advanced Nursing, 15*, 1418–1425.

Fawcett, J. (2000a). *Analysis and evaluation of contemporary nursing knowledge*. Philadelphia: F. A. Davis.

Fawcett, J. (2000b). Watson's theory of human caring. In J. Fawcett (Ed.), *Analysis of evaluation of contemporary nursing knowledge: Nursing models & theories* (pp. 657–686). Philadelphia: F. A. Davis.

Fawcett, J., & Giangrande, S. K. (2001). The Neuman Systems Model and research: An integrative review. In B. Neuman & J. Fawcett (Eds.), *The NSM* (4th ed.). Upper Saddle River, NJ: Prentice Hall.

Fawcett, J., & Tulman, L. (1990). Building a programme of research from the Roy adaptation model. *Journal of Advanced Nursing, 15*, 720–725.

Fazio, R. H., & Williams, C. J. (1986). Attitude accessibility as a moderator of the attitude-perception and attitude-behavior relations: An investigation of the 1984 presidential election. *Journal of Personality and Social Psychology, 51*, 505–514.

Feder, G., Griffiths, C., Eldridge, S., & Spence, M. (1999). Effect of postal prompts to patients and general practitioners on the quality of primary care after a coronary event (POST): A randomised controlled trial. *British Medical Journal, 318*, 1522–1526.

Federal Bureau of Investigations. (1999). *Crime in the United States 1998*. Washington, DC: U.S. Government Printing Office. Retrieved from http://www.fbi.gov/ucr/Cius_98/98crime/98cius01.pdf

Federal Interagency Forum on Aging. (2000). *Older Americans 2000. Key indicators of well-being*. Retrieved August 5, 2002, from http://www.agingstats.gov/chartbook2000/population.html

Federal Interagency Forum on Child and Family Statistics. (2003). *America's children: Key national indicators of well-being, 2002*. Washington, DC: U.S. Government Printing Office. Retrieved from http://www.childstatsagingstats.gov/chartbook2000/population.html

Federal Interagency Forum on Child and Family Statistics. (n.d.). *America's children: Key national indicators of well-being 2003*. Retrieved January 9, 2004, from http://www.childstats.gov/ac2003/indicators.asp?IID=121&id=4

Feetham, S. L. (1999). Families and the genetic revolution: Implications for primary care, education, research and policy. *Families, Systems and Health, 17*(1), 27–43.

Feetham, S. L. (2000). Editorial genetics and nursing research: Opportunities and challenges. *Research in Nursing and Health, 23*(4), 257–259.

Feetham, S. L. (Ed.). (2004). *Nursing and 21st century genetics: Leadership for global health*. Geneva, Switzerland: International Council of Nurses.

Feetham, S. L., & Thomson, E. (in press). Genomics and health. *Journal of Nursing Scholarship*.

Fehring, R. J. (1987). Methods to validate nursing diagnoses. *Heart & Lung, 16*(6), 625–629.

Feil, N. (2002). *The validation breakthrough: Simple techniques for communicating with people with "Alzheimer's-Type Dementia"* (2nd ed.). Baltimore, MD: Health Professions Press.

Feinstein, N. F. (2000). Fetal heart rate auscultation: Current and future practice. *Journal of Obstetric, Gynecologic, and Neonatal Nursing, 29*(3), 306–315.

Feldman, M. J., Ventura, M. R., & Crosby, F. (1987). Studies of nurse practitioner effectiveness. *Nursing Research, 36*(5), 303–306.

Fenton, M. (1988). Moral distress in clinical practice: Implications for the nurse administrator. *Canadian Journal of Nursing Administration, 1*, 8–11.

Fenton, M. V., & Brykczynski, K. A. (1993). Qualitative distinctions and similarities in the practice of clinical nurse specialists and nurse practitioners. *Journal of Professional Nursing*, 9(6), 313–326.

Ferketich, A. K., Schwartzbaum, J. A., Frid, D. J., & Moeschberger, M. L. (2000). Depression as an antecedent to heart disease among women and men in the NHANES I study. National Health and Nutrition Examination Survey. *Archives of Internal Medicine, 160*, 1261–1268.

Ferketich, S., & Muller, M. (1990). Factor analysis revisited. *Nursing Research, 39*, 59–62.

Ferrando, S., Goggin, K., Sewell, M., Evans, S., Fishman, B., Robkin, J., et al. (1998). Substance use disorders in gay/bisexual men with HIV and AIDS. *American Journal on Addictions, 7*, 51–60.

Ferrari, A. M. (2002). The impact of culture upon child rearing practices and definitions of maltreatment. *Child Abuse & Neglect, 26*(8), 793–813.

Ferrell, B. R., Grant, M., Funk, B., Otis-Green, S. A., & Garcia, N. J. (1998). Quality of life in breast cancer survivors: Implications for developing support services. *Oncology Nursing Forum, 25*, 887–895.

Ferrucci, L., Cavazzini, C., Corsi, A., Bartali, B., Russo, C. R., Lauretani, F., et al. (2002). Biomarkers of frailty in older persons. *Journal of Endocrinology Investigation, 25*, 10–15.

Feskanich, D., Willett, W. C., & Colditz, G. A. (2003). Calcium, vitamin D, milk consumption, and hip fractures: A prospective study among postmenopausal women. *American Journal of Clinical Nutrition, 77*, 504–511.

Fick, A. (1870). Ueber die Messung des Blutquantums in den Herzventrikeln. *Sitz Physik-Med Ges Wurzburg, 2*, 16–28.

Fick, D. M., Agostini, J. V., & Inouye, S. K. (2002). Delirium superimposed on dementia: A systematic review. *Journal of the American Geriatrics Society, 50*, 1723–1732.

Fick, D., & Foreman, M. D. (2000). The consequences of not recognizing delirium superimposed on dementia in hospitalized elders. *Journal of Gerontological Nursing, 26*(1), 30–40.

Field, P. A., & Morse, J. M. (1985). *Nursing research: The application of qualitative approaches*. Rockville, MD: Aspen.

Field, T. (1995). Infants of depressed mothers. *Infant Behavior & Development, 18*, 1–13.

Field, T. (1998). Maternal depression effects on infants and early interventions. *Preventive Medicine, 27*, 200–203.

Field-Munves, E. (2000). Osteoporosis: Patient identification and evaluation. In S. H. Gueldner, M. S. Burke, & H. Smiciklas-Wright (Eds.), *Preventing and managing osteoporosis* (pp. 63–86). New York: Springer.

Field, M., & Cassell, C. (1997). *Approaching death: Improving care at the end of life*. Washington, DC: Academy Press.

Fingerman, K. L., Gallagher-Thompson, D., Lovett, S., & Rose, J. (1996). Internal resourcefulness, task demands, coping, and dysphoric affect among caregivers of the frail elderly. *International Journal of Aging and Human Development, 42*(3), 229–248.

Finifter, B. (1975). Replication and extension of social research through secondary analysis. *Social Science Information, 14*, 119–153.

Finke, L., Williams, J., & Stanley, R. (1996). Nurses referred to peer assistance programs for drug and alcohol problems. *Archives of Psychiatric Nursing, 10*(5), 319–324.

Finkelhor, D. (1990). Is child abuse overreported. *Public Welfare, 4*.

Finkelhor, D., & Hashima, P. (2001). The victimization of children & youth: A comprehensive overview. In S. O. White (Ed.), *Law and social science perspectives on youth and justice* (pp. 49–78). New York: Plenum Publishing.

Finnbogadottir, H., Svalenikus, E., & Persson, E. K. (2003). Expectant first-time fathers' experiences of pregnancy. *Midwifery, 19*, 96–105.

Finucane, T. E., Christmas, C., & Travis, K. (1999). Tube feeding in patients with advanced dementia: A review of the evidence. *Journal of the American Medical Association, 282*, 1365–1370.

Fiore, M. C., Bailey, W. C., Cohen, S. J., Dorfman, S. F., Goldstein, M. G., Gritz, E. R., et al. (2000). *Treating tobacco use and dependence. Clinical practice guideline*. Rockville, MD: U.S. Department of Health and Human Services. Public Health Service.

Fishbein, M., & Ajzen, I. (1975). *Belief, attitude, intention and behavior: An introduction to theory and research*. Reading, MA: Addison-Wesley Publishing.

Fisher, E. A., Van Horn, L., & McGill, H. (1997). Nutrition and children: A statement for healthcare professionals from the nutrition committee, American Heart Association. *Circulation, 95*, 2332–2333.

Fisher, R. A. (1935). *The design of experiments*. London: Oliver & Boyd.

Fisher, S. E., Burgio, L. D., Tjorn, B. E., Allen-Burge, R., Gerstle, J., Roth, D. L., et al. (2002). Pain assessment and management in cognitively impaired nursing home residents: Association of Certified Nurse Assistant report, Minimum Data Set report, and analgesic medication use. *Journal of the American Geriatrics Society, 50*(1), 152–156.

Fitzgerald, K. (2003). *Quality of life of HPN and bowel transplant*. Unpublished doctoral dissertation, University of Illinois, Chicago.

Fitzpatrick, J. J. (1991). The translation of the NANDA taxonomy into ICD code. In R. M. Carroll-Johnson (Ed.), *Classifications of nursing diagnoses: Proceedings of the Ninth conference*. Philadelphia: Lippincott.

Fitzpatrick, J., & Goeppinger, J. (2000). Focus on chronic illness. In *Annual review of nursing research* (Vol. 18). New York: Springer Publishing.

Fitzpatrick, J. J., & Whaal, A. L. (1989). *Conceptual models of nursing: Analysis and application* (2nd ed.). Norwalk, CT: Appleton and Lange.

Fitzpatrick, J. J., & Whall, A. L. (Eds.). (1996). *Conceptual models of nursing: Analysis and application* (3rd ed.). Stanford, CT: Appleton & Lange.

Fitzpatrick, T. R., & Bosse, R. (2000). Employment and health among older bereaved men in the Normative Aging Study: One year and three years following a bereavement event. *Social Work in Health Care, 32*(2), 41–60.

Fitzsimons, D., Parahoo, K., & Stringer, M. (2000). Waiting for coronary artery bypass surgery: A qualitative analysis. *Journal of Advanced Nursing, 32*(5), 1243–1252.

Flaherty, E., Hyer, K., & Fulmer, T. (2003). Using case studies to evaluate students' ability to develop a geriatric interdisciplinary care plan. *Gerontology and Geriatrics Education, 24*(2).

Flaskerud, J. H. (2000). Ethnicity, culture and neuropsychiatry. *Issues in Mental Health Nursing, 21*, 5–29.

Flaskerud, J. H., Lesser, J., Dixon, E., Anderson, N., Conde, F., Kim, S., et al. (2002). Health disparities among vulnerable populations. *Nursing Research, 51*, 74–85.

Flaskerud, J. H., Lesser, J., Dixon, E., Anderson, N., Conde, F., Kim, S., et al. (2002). Health disparities among vulnerable populations: Evolution of knowledge over five decades in Nursing Research, Publications. *Nursing Research, 51*(2), 1–12.

Flaskerud, J. H., & Nyamathi, A. M. (2000). Collaborative inquiry with low-income Latina women. *Journal of Health Care for the Poor and Underserved, 11*, 326–342.

Fleishman, E. A., & Quaintance, M. K. (1984). *Taxonomies of human performance: The description of human tasks*. Orlando, FL: Academic Press.

Fletcher, K. (1996). Use of restraints in the elderly. American Association of Critical-Care Nurses Clinical Issues. *Advanced Practice in Acute Critical Care, 7*, 611–620.

Fleury, J., Kimbrell, L. C., & Kruszewski, M. A. (1995). Life after a cardiac event: Women's experiences in healing. *Heart and Lung: Journal of Critical Care, 24*, 474–482.

Floyd, F., Haynes, S., Doll, E., Winemiller, D., Lemsky, C., Burgy, T., et al. (1992). Assessing retirement satisfaction and perceptions of retirement experiences. *Psychology and Aging, 7*, 609–621.

Flynn, J. P. (Ed.). (1997). *The role of the preceptor: A guide for nurse educators and clinicians*. New York: Springer Publishing.

Fogel, C., & Woods, N. (Eds.). (1995). *Women's health care*. Thousand Oaks, CA: Sage.

Fogg, D. (1990). Using wall suction for evacuating laser plumes. *AORN Journal, 52*, 408, 410.

Foldemo, A., & Bogren, L. (2002). Needs assessment and quality of life in outpatients with schizophrenia: A five year followup study. *Scandinavian Journal of Caring Sciences, 16*, 393–398.

Folstein, M. (1998). Mini-mental and son. *International Journal of Geriatrics, 13*, 290–294.

Folstein, M. F., Folstein, S. E., & McHugh, P. R. (1975). Mini-mental state: A practical method for grading the cognitive state of patients for the clinician. *Journal of Psychiatric Research, 12*, 196–198.

Fonagy, H., Steele, H., & Steele, M. (1991). Maternal representations of attachment during pregnancy predict the organization of infant-mother attachment at one year of age. *Child Development, 62*(5), 891–905.

Foner, N. (1994). Nursing home aides: Saints or monsters? *Gerontologist, 34*(2), 245–250.

Fong, C. (1990). Role overload, social support, and burnout among nursing educators. *Journal of Nursing Education, 29*, 102–108.

Food and Nutrition Board. Institute of Medicine. (1992). *Dietary reference intakes for energy, carbohydrate, fiber, fat, fatty acids, cholesterol, protein, and amino acids. (Macronutrients)*. Washington, DC: National Academies Press.

Force, L. T., Botsford, A., Pisano, P. A., & Holbert, A. (2000). Grandparents raising children with and without a disability: Preliminary comparisons. *Journal of Gerontological Social Work, 33*(4), 5–21.

Forchuk, C. (1991). Peplau's theory: Concepts and their relations. *Nursing Science Quarterly, 4*(2), 54–60.

Forchuk, C. (1994). The orientation phase of the nurse-client relationship: Testing Peplau's theory. *Journal of Advanced Nursing, 20*, 1–6.

Forchuk, C. (1995). Development of nurse-client relationships: What helps? *Journal of the American Psychiatric Nurses Association, 1*(5), 146–151.

Forchuk, C., Beaton, S., Crawford, L., Ide, L., Voorberg, N., & Bethune, J. (1989). Incorporating Peplau's theory and case management. *Journal of Psychosocial Nursing and Mental Health Services, 27*(2), 35–38.

Forchuk, C., & Brown, B. (1989). Establishing a nurse-client relationship. *Journal of Psychosocial Nursing and Mental Health Services, 27*(2), 30–34.

Forchuk, C., Jewell, J., Tweedell, D., & Steinnagel, L. (2003). Role changes experienced by clinical staff in relation to clients' recovery from psychosis. *Journal of Psychiatric and Mental Health Nursing, 10*, 269–276.

Forchuk, C., Norman, R., Malla., A., Martin, M., McLean, T., Cheng, S., et al. (2002). Schizophrenia and the motivation for smoking. *Perspectives in Psychiatric Care, 38*, 41–49.

Forchuk, C., Westwell, J., Martin, M., Azzapardi, W. B., Kosterewa-Tolman, D., & Hux, M. (1998). Factors influencing movement of chronic psychiatric patients from the orientation to the working phase of the nurse-client relationship. *Perspectives in Psychiatric Care, 34*(1), 36–44.

Forchuk, C., Westwell, J., Martin, M., Bamber-Azzapardi, W., Kosterewa-Tolman, D., & Hux, M. (2000). The developing nurse-client relationship; nurses' perspectives. *Journal of the American Psychiatric Nurses Association, 6*, 3–10.

Forchuk, C., Westwell, J., Martin, M., Bamber-Azzapardi, W., Kosterewa-Tolmun, D., & Hux, M. (2000). The developing nurse-client relationship: Nurses' perspectives. *Journal of the American Psychiatric Nurses Association, 6*(2), 56–62.

Ford-Gilboe, M., & Cohen, J. A. (2000). Hardiness: A model of commitment, challenge, and control. In V. H. Rice (Ed.), *Handbook of stress, coping, and health: Implications for nursing research, theory, and practice*. Thousand Oaks, CA: Sage.

Foreman, M. D., & Vermeersch, P. E. H. (2004). Measuring cognitive status. In M. Frank-Stromborg & S. J. Olsen (Eds.), *Instruments for clinical health-care research* (3rd ed., pp. 100–127). Sudbury, MA: Jones and Bartlett.

Forker, J. E., & McDonald, M. E. (1996). Methodologic trends in healthcare professions: Computer adaptive and computer simulation training. *Nurse Educator, 21*(4), 13–14.

Foucault, M. (1972). *The archeology of knowledge*. London: Tavistock.

Foundations for Health Services Research. (1992). *Health outcomes research: A primer*. Washington, DC: Foundations for Health Services Research.

Fox, K., & Cuite, C. (2001). *Preventive care services in New Jersey and the implementation of the Health Wellness Promotion Act: Report of stakeholder perceptions 2001*. New Brunswick, NJ: Center for State Health Policy.

Fox, K. M., Hawkes, W. G., Magaziner, J., Zimmerman, S. I., & Hebel, J. R. (1996). Markers of failure to thrive among older hip fracture patients. *Journal of the American Geriatrics Society, 44*, 371–376.

Fox, S. D., & Wold, J. E. (1996). Baccalaureate gerontological nursing experiences: Raising consciousness levels and affecting attitudes. *Journal of Nursing Education, 35*, 348–355.

Frank, D. A., & Zeisel, S. H. (1988). Failure to thrive. *The Pediatric Clinics of North America, 35*, 1187–1206.

Frankl, V. E. (1984). *Man's search for meaning: An introduction to logotherapy*. Boston: Beacon Press.

Fredriksson, L. (1999). Modes of relating in a caring conversation: A research synthesis on presence, touch and listening. *Journal of Advanced Nursing, 30*, 1167–1176.

Freiman, M. P., & Zuvekas, S. H. (2000). Determinants of ambulatory treatment mode for mental illness. *Health Economics*, 9(5), 423–434.

French, J. R. P., Jr., Rodgers, W., & Cobb, S. (1974). Adjustment as person-environment fit. In G. V. Coelho, D. A. Hamburg, & J. D. Admans (Eds.), *Coping and adaptation* (pp. 316–333). New York: Basic Books.

Frenchman, I. B., Capo, C., & Hass, H. (2000). Effect of treatment with divalproex sodium and lorazepam in residents of long-term-care facilities with dementia-related anxiety or agitation: Retrospective chart review. *Current Therapeutic Research, Clinical & Experimental, 61*(9), 621–619.

Frengley, J. D., & Mion, L. C. (1998). Physical restraints in the acute care setting: Issues and future direction. *Clinics in Geriatric Medicine, 14*(4), 727–743.

Frenn, M., Lundeen, S. P., Martin, K. S., Riesch, S. K., & Wilson, S. A. (1996). Symposium on nursing centers: Past, present, and future. *Journal of Nursing Education, 35*(2), 54–62.

Freud, S. (1975). *Three essays on the theory of sexuality*. New York: Basic Books.

Frey, M. A. (1995). Toward a theory of families, children, and chronic illness. In M. A. Frey & C. L. Sieloff (Eds.), *Advancing King's systems framework and theory of nursing* (pp. 109–125). Thousand Oaks, CA: Sage.

Frey, M. A. (2004). King's conceptual system and theory of goal attainment. In J. Fitzpatrick & A. Whall (Eds.), *Conceptual models of nursing analysis and application* (4th ed., pp. 225–246). Upper Saddle River, NJ: Pearson Prentice Hall.

Frey, M. A., & Sieloff, C. (1995). *Advancing King's framework and theory for nursing*. Thousand Oaks, CA: Sage Publications.

Frich, L. M. H. (2003). Nursing interventions for patients with chronic conditions. *Journal of Advanced Nursing, 44*(2), 137–153.

Friedman, B., De La Mare, J., Andrews, R., & McKenzie, D. H. (2002). Practical options for estimating costs of hospital inpatient stays. *Journal of Healthcare Finance, 29*, 1–13.

Friedman, E., & Havighurst, R. (Eds.). (1954). *The meaning of work and retirement*. Chicago: University of Chicago Press.

Friedmann, E., Katcher, A. H., Lynch, J. J., & Thomas, S. A. (1980). Animal companions and one-year survival of patients after discharge from a coronary care unit. *Public Health Reports, 95*(4), 307–312.

Friedmann, E., Katcher, A. H., Thomas, S. A., Lynch, J. J., & Messent, P. R. (1983). Social interaction and blood pressure. Influence of animal companions. *Journal of Nervous and Mental Disease, 171*(8), 461–465.

Friedrich, R. M., Lively, S., & Buckwalter, K. C. (1999). Well siblings living with schizophrenia. Impact of associated behaviors. *Journal of Psychosocial Nursing and Mental Health Services, 37*, 11–19.

Friedrich, R. M., Lively, S., Rubenstein, L., & Buckwalter, K. (2002). The Friedrich-Lively instrument to assess the impact of schizophrenia on siblings (FLIISS), Part I—instrument construction. *Journal of Nursing Measures, 10*, 219–230.

Froelicher, E. S., Houston Miller, N., Christopherson, D. J., Martin, K., Parker, K., Amonetti, M., et al. (2004). High rates of sustained smoking cessation in women hospitalized with cardiovascular disease. The Woman's Initiative for Nonsmoking (WINS). *Circulation, 109*, 587–593.

Fry, S. T. (1995). Nursing ethics. In W. Reich (Ed.), *Encyclopedia of bioethics* (2nd ed., pp. 1822–1827). New York: MacMillan.

Fukuda, K., Straus, S. E., Hickie, I., Sharpe, M. C., Dobbins, J. G., Komaroff, A., et al. (1994). The chronic fatigue syndrome: A comprehensive approach to its definition and study. *Annals of Internal Medicine, 121*, 953–959.

Fuller-Thomson, E., & Minkler, M. (2000). African American grandparents raising grandchildren: A national profile of demographic and health characteristics. *Health & Social Work 25*(2), 109–119.

Fuller-Thompson, E., & Minkler, M. (2001). American grandparents providing extensive child care to their grandchildren: Prevalence and profile. *Gerontologist, 41*(2), 201–209.

Fuller-Thomson, E., Minkler, M., & Driver, D. (1997). A profile of grandparents raising grandchildren in the United States. *Gerontologist, 37*, 406–411.

Fullerton, J., & Toossi, M. (2001, November). Labor force projections to 2010: Study growth and changing composition. *Monthly Labor Review*, 21–38.

Fulmer, T., & Abraham, I. L. (1998). Rethinking geriatric nursing. *Nursing Clinics of North America, 33*(3), 387–394.

Fulmer, T. T., Feldman, P. H., Kim, T. S., Carty, B., Beers, M., Molina, M., et al. (1999). An intervention study to enhance medication compliance in community-dwelling elderly individuals. *Journal of Gerontological Nursing, 25*(8), 6–14.

Fulmer, T., Firpo, A., Guadagno, L., Easter, T. M., Kahan, F., & Paris, B. (2003). Themes from a grounded theory analysis of elder neglect assessment by experts. *Gerontologist, 43*(5), 745–752.

Fulmer, T., Guadagno, L., Bitondo Dyer, C., & Connolly, M. T. (2004). Progress in elder abuse screening and assessment instruments. *Journal of the American Geriatrics Society, 52*(2), 297–304.

Fulmer, T., & Gurland, G. (1996). Restriction as elder mistreatment: Differences between caregiver and elder perceptions. *Journal of Mental Health and Aging, 2*, 89–98.

Fulmer, T., & Hyer, K. (1998). Evaluating the effects of geriatric interdisciplinary team training. In E. L. Siegler, K. Hyer, T. Fulmer, & M. Mezey (Eds.), *Geriatric interdisciplinary team training* (pp. 115–149). New York: Springer.

Fulmer, T., Hyer, K., Flaherty, E., Mezey, M., Whitelaw, N., Jacobs, M., et al. (2004). *Geriatric interdisciplinary team training program: Evaluation components*. Manuscript submitted for publication.

Fulmer, T., Mezey, M., Bottrell, M., Abraham, I., Sazant, J., Grossman, S., et al. (2002). Nursing improving care to health systems elders (NICHE), Using outcomes and benchmarks for evidenced-based practice. *Geriatric Nursing, 23*(3), 121–127.

Fung, C., & Fry, A. (1999). The role of community mental health nurses in educating clients and families about schizophrenia. *Australian and New Zealand Journal of Mental Health Nursing, 8*, 162–175.

Funk, M., Naum, J. B., Milner, K. A., & Chyun, D. (2001). Presentation and symptom predictors of coronary heart disease in patients with and without diabetes. *American Journal of Emergency Medicine, 19*, 482–487.

Funk, S., Tornquist, E., & Champagne, M. (1989). Application and evaluation of the dissemination model. *Western Journal of Nursing Research, 11*, 486–491.

Futterman, A., Thompson, L. W., Gallagher-Thompson, D., & Ferris, R. (1995). Depression in later life: Epidemiology, assessment, etiology, and treatment. In E. E. Beckham (Ed.), *Handbook of depression* (pp. 494–538). New York: Guilford Press.

Fuzi, B. L. (1995). Realization impact: Nursing assessment and strategies . . . a process through which family members proceed before facing the fact that their family member could die. *Dimensions of Critical Care Nursing, 14*(6), 316–326.

Gadamer, H. (1989). *Truth and method* (Rev. ed.) (J. Weinsheimer & D. G. Marshall, Trans.). New York: Continuum. (Original work published 1960)

Gagnon, J. H., & Simon, W. (1987). The social scripting of oral genital contacts. *Archives of Sexual Behavior, 16*, 1–25.

Galea, S., Ahern, J. R., Resnick, H., Kilpatrick, D., Bucavalas, M., Gold, J., et al., (2002). Psychological sequalae of the September 11 terrorist attacks in New York City. *New England Journal of Medicine, 346*(13), 982–987.

Gall, S. H., Atkinson, J. M., Elliott, L., & Johansen, R. (2003). Supporting carers of people diagnosed with schizophrenia: Evaluating change in nursing practice following training. *Journal of Advanced Nursing, 41*, 295–305.

Gall, S. H., Elliot, L., Atkinson, J. M., & Johansen, R. (2001). Training nurses to support carers of relatives with schizophrenia. *British Journal of Nursing, 10*, 238–241.

Gall, T., Evans, D., & Howard, J. (1997). The retirement adjustment process: Changes in the well-being of male retirees across time. *Journals of Gerontology: Psychological Sciences, 52*, 110–117. Retrieved October 23, 2003, from http://proquest.umi.com/pqdweb?index

Gallagher, R. M., & Rowell, P. A. (2003). Claiming the future of nursing through nursing-sensitive quality indicators. *Nursing Administration Quarterly, 27*(4), 273–284.

Gamble, C., & Hart, C. (2003). The use of psychosocial interventions. *Nursing Times*, 99(9), 46–47.

Gamm, L., Hutchison, L., Dabney, B., & Dorsey, A. (Eds.). (2003). *Rural Healthy People 2010: A companion document to Healthy People 2010* (Vol. 1). College Station: Texas A&M University Health Science Center, School of Public Health, Southwest Rural Health Research Center.

Garand, L., Buckwalter, K. C., Lubaroff, D., Tripp-Reimer, T., Frantz, R. A., & Ansley, T. N. (2002). A pilot study of immune and mood outcomes of a community based intervention for dementia caregivers: The PLST intervention. *Archives of Psychiatric Nursing, 16*, 156–167.

Garcia Coll, C., Lamberty, G., Jenkins, R., McAdoo, H. P., Crnic, K., Wasik, B. H., et al. (1996). An integrative model for the study of developmental competencies in minority children. *Child Development, 67*, 1891–1914.

Gardner, S. E., Frantz, R. A., Specht, J. K. P., Johnson-Mekota, J. L., Buresh, K. A., Wakefield, B., et al. (2001). How accurate are chronic wound assessments using interactive video technology? *Journal of Gerontological Nursing, 27*(1), 15–20.

Garfield, E. (1985). Citation patterns in nursing journals, and their most-cited articles. In E. Garfield, *Essays of an Information Scientist: 1984* (Vol. 7, pp. 336–345). Philadelphia: ISI Press.

Garlinghouse, J., & Sharp, L. J. (1968). The hemophiliac child's self concept and family stress in relation to bleeding episodes. *Nursing Research, 17*, 32–37.

Garratt, A., Schmidt, L., Mackintosh, A., & Fitzpatrick, R. (2002). Quality of life measurement: Bibliographic study of patient assessed health outcome measures. *British Medical Journal, 324*, 1417–1419. Retrieved September 29, 2003, from http://www.bmj.com

Garvey, C., Gross, D., Delaney, K., & Fogg, L. (2000). Discipline across generations. *Nurse Practitioner Forum, 11*, 132–140.

Gaskamp, C. (2004). Changes in family economic resources and quality of life across a decade in patients and family caregivers managing home parenteral nutrition care. *Nursing Economic$, 22*, 135–139.

Gaspar, P. M. (1999). Water intake of nursing home residents. *Journal of Gerontological Nursing, 25*(4), 22–29.

Gastmans, C. (1998). Interpersonal relations in nursing: A philosophical-ethical analysis of the work of Hildegard E. Peplau. *Journal of Advanced Nursing, 28*, 1312–1319.

Gaston, E. T. (1951). Dynamic music factors in mood change. *Music Educators Journal, 3*, 42–44.

Gates, D. M., Fitzwater, E., & Meyer, U. (1999). Violence against caregivers in nursing homes: Expected, tolerated and accepted. *Journal of Gerontological Nursing, 25*(4), 12–22.

Gatsonis, C. A., & Needleman, H. L. (1992). Recent epidemiologic studies of low-level lead exposure and the IQ of children: A meta-analytic review. In H. L. Needleman (Ed.), *Human lead exposure* (pp. 243–255). Boca Raton, FL: CRC Press.

Gazmararian, J. A., Adams, M. M., Saltzman, L. E., Johnson, C. H., Bruce, F. C., Marks, J. S., et al. (1995). The relationship between pregnancy intendedness and physical violence in mothers of newborns. *Obstetrics and Gynecology, 85*(6), 1031–1038.

Gazzola, L. R., & Muskin, P. R. (2003). The impact of stress and the objectives of psychosocial interventions. In H. I. Spitz (Ed.), *Psychosocial treatment for medical conditions: Principles and techniques* (pp. 373–406). New York: Brunner-Routledge.

Gebauer, C., Kwo, C., Haynes, E. F., & Wewers, M. E. (1998). A nurse-managed smoking cessation intervention during pregnancy. *Journal of Obstetric, Gynecologic, and Neonatal Nursing, 27*(1), 47–53.

Gebbie, K. M., & Lavin, M. A. (1975). *Classification of nursing diagnoses: Proceedings of the First National Conference*. St. Louis: C. V. Mosby.

Gee, J. P. (1991). A linguistic approach to narrative. *Journal of Narrative and Life History, 1*, 15–39.

Gegor, C. L., & Paine, L. L. (1992). Antepartum fetal assessment techniques: An update for today's perinatal nurse. *Journal of Perinatal and Neonatal Nursing, 5*(4), 1–15.

Geibart, R. C. (2000). Integrating web-based instruction into a graduate nursing program taught via videoconferencing; challenges and solutions. *Computers in Nursing, 18*(1), 26–34.

Gelazis, R. S., & Coombe-Moore, J. (1993). Developing a therapeutic relationship. In R. P. Rawlings, S. R. Williams, & C. K. Beck (Eds.), *Mental Health-Psychiatric Nursing* (pp. 109–133). St. Louis, MO: Mosby Year Book.

Gelb, M. (1998). *How to think like Leonardo Da Vinci*. New York: Dell.

Gelles, R. J. (2000). *Changing rates of criminal and family violence: No safety for children*. Washington, DC: National Institute of Justice Journal, U.S. Department of Justice, National Institute of Justice.

Gelles, R. J., & Cornell, C. P. (1990). *Intimate violence in families* (2nd ed.). London: Sage.

Genette, G. (1988). *Narrative discourse revisited*. Ithaca, NY: Cornell University Press.

George, J. B. (2001). Theory of culture care diversity and universality. In J. B. George (Ed.), *Nursing theories: The base for professional nursing practice* (5th ed., pp. 489–518). Upper Saddle River, NJ: Prentice Hall.

George, T. (1996). Women in a South Indian fishing village: Role identity, continuity, and the experience of menopause. *Health Care for Women International, 17*, 271–279.

Germino, B. B. (1998). Uncertainty in prostate cancer. *Cancer Practice, 6*, 107–115.

Geronimus, A. T. (2003). Damned if you do: Culture, identity, privilege, and teenage childbearing in the United States. *Social Science and Medicine, 57*, 881–893.

Gershon, R. M., Stone, P. W., Bakken, S., & Larson, E. (2004). Measurement of organizational culture and climate. *Journal of Nursing Administration, 34*, 33–40.

Geuldner, S. H. (2000a). Introduction and overview. In S. H. Gueldner, M. S. Burke, & H. Smiciklas-Wright (Eds.), *Preventing and managing osteoporosis* (pp. 1–4). New York: Springer.

Geuldner, S. H. (2000b). Target groups for prevention and early detection. In S. H. Gueldner, M. S. Burke, & H. Smiciklas-Wright (Eds.), *Preventing and managing osteoporosis* (pp. 157–174). New York: Springer.

Geuldner, S. H., Burke, M. S., & Smiciklas-Wright, H. (2000). (Eds.). *Preventing and managing osteoporosis*. New York: Springer.

Geusens, P., Hochberg, M. C., van der Voort, D. J. M., Pols, H., van der Klift, M. Siris, E., et al. (2002). Performance of risk indices for identifying low bone density in postmenopausal women. *Mayo Clinic Proceedings, 77*(7), 629–637.

Gewolb, I. H., Bosma, J., Reynolds, E., & Vice, F. (2003). Integration of suck swallow rhythms during feeding in preterm infants with and without bronchopulmonary dysplasia. *Developmental and Behavioral Pediatrics, 45*, 344–348.

Giarelli, E. (2003). Bringing threat to the fore: Participating in lifelong surveillance for genetic risk of cancer. *Oncology Nursing Forum, 30*, 945–955.

Gibbons, C., Bachulis, A., & Allen, G. (1999). A comparison of a computer and paper and pencil assignment. *Computers in Nursing, 17*(6), 286–290.

Gibbons, R., Chatterjee, K., Daley, J., Douglas, J. S., Finn, S. D., Garelin, J. M., et al. (1999). ACC/AHA/ACP-ASIM guidelines for the management of patients with chronic stable angina. *Journal of the American College of Cardiology, 33*, 2092–2197.

Gibson, J. L., Love, W., Hardie, D., Bancroft, P., & Turner, A. J. (1892). Notes on lead poisoning as observed among children in Brisbane. In L. Huxtable (Ed.), *Transactions from the third intercolonial medical congress of Australasia* (pp. 76–77). Syndey, Australia: Charles Potter.

Giebel, G. D., Lefering, R., Troild, H., & Blochl, H. (1998). Prevalence of fecal incontinence: What can be expected? *International Journal of Colorectal Disease, 13*(2), 73–77.

Gift, A. (1989). Validation of a vertical visual analogue scale as a measure of clinical dyspnea. *Rehabilitation Nursing, 14*, 323–325.

Gigliotti, E., & Fawcett, J. (2001). The Neuman Systems Model and research instruments. In B.

Neuman & J. Fawcett (Eds.), *The NSM* (4th ed.). Upper Saddle River, NJ: Prentice Hall.

Gill, T. M., Williams, C. S., Mendes de Leon, C. F., & Tinettit, M. E. (1997). The role of change in physical performance in determining risk of dependence in ADLs among nondisabled community-living elderly persons. *Journal of Clinical Epidemiology*, 60, 765–772.

Gilligan, C. (1982). *In a different voice: Psychological theory and women's development*. Cambridge, MA: Harvard University Press.

Gillis, C. L. (1991). Family nursing research, theory and practice. *Image: Journal of Nursing Scholarship*, *23*(1), 19–22.

Giorgi, A. (1985). *Phenomenology and psychological research*. Pittsburgh, PA: Duquesne University Press.

Giovannetti, P. (1978). *Patient classification systems in nursing: A description and analysis* (DHEW Publication No. HRA 78/22). Washington, DC: U.S. Government Printing Office.

Giovannetti, P. (1980). A comparison of team and primary nursing care delivery systems. *Nursing Dimensions*, *7*(4), 96–100.

Giovannetti, P. (1994). Measurement of nursing workload. In J. M. Hibberd & M. E. Kyle (Eds.), *Nursing management in Canada* (pp. 331–349). Toronto: W. B. Saunders.

Girot, E. A. (2000). Graduate nurses: Critical thinkers or better decision makers? *Journal of Advanced Nursing*, *31*(2), 288–297.

Girou, E., Loyeau, S., Legrand, P., Oppein, F., & Brun-Buisson, C. (2002). Efficacy of handrubbing with alcohol based solution versus standard handwashing with antiseptic soap: Randomised clinical trial. *British Medical Journal*, *325*, 362–366.

Given, B., & Given, C. W. (1992). Patient and family caregiver reaction to new and recurrent breast cancer. *Journal of the American Medical Women's Association*, *47*, 201–207.

Given, B. A., & Given, C. W. (1998). Health promotion for family caregivers of chronically ill elders. In *Annual review of nursing research* (Vol. 16, pp. 197–216). New York: Springer Publishing.

Gjelsvik, A., Verhoek-Oftedahl, W., & Perleman, D. N. (2003). Domestic violence incidents with children witnesses: Findings from Rhode Island surveillance data. *Women's Health Issues*, *13*(2), 68–73.

Gladdish, S., & Rajkumar, C. (2001). Prevention of cardiac disease in the elderly. *Journal of Cardiovascular Risk*, 8, 271–277.

Glaser, B. (1978). *Theoretical sensitivity: Advances in the methodology of grounded theory*. Mill Valley, CA: Sociological Press.

Glaser, B., & Strauss, A. (1967). *The discovery of grounded theory: Strategies for qualitative research*. Chicago: Aldine Publishing Company.

Glaser, D. (2002). Emotional abuse and neglect (psychological maltreatment), A conceptual framework. *Child Abuse & Neglect*, *27*(6), 697–714.

Glass, N., Dearwater S., & Campbell, J. (2001). Intimate partner violence screening and intervention: Data from eleven Pennsylvania and California community hospital emergency departments. *Journal of Emergency Nursing*, *27*(2), 141–149, 215–222.

Gleser, G., Green, B., & Winget, C. (1981). *Prolonged psychological effects of disaster: A study of Buffalo Creek*. New York: Academic Press.

Godin, P. (1996). The development of community psychiatric nursing: A professional project? *Journal of Advanced Nursing*, *23*, 925–934.

Godin, P. (2000). A dirty business: Caring for people who are a nuisance or a danger. *Journal of Advanced Nursing*, *32*, 1396–1402.

Golding, J., Taylor, D., Menard, L., & King, M. (2000). Prevalence of sexual assault in women experiencing severe PMS. *Journal of Psychosomatic Obstetrics & Gynecology*, *21*, 69–80.

Goldman, D. (1998). *Working with emotional intelligence*. New York: Bantam Books.

Goldman, D. (2002). DBH and functional taxonomy of major depressive disorder. *Biological Psychiatry*, *51*, 347–348.

Goldmark, J. (1923). *Nursing and nursing education in the United States*. New York: Macmillan.

Goldrick, B. (2003). Surgical-site infections. *American Journal of Nursing*, *103*(4), 64AA.

Good, M. (1996). Effects of relaxation and music on postoperative pain: A review. *Journal of Advanced Nursing*, *24*, 905–914.

Good, M. (1998). A middle range theory of acute pain management; use in research. *Nursing Outlook*, *46*(3), 120–124.

Good, M. (2003). Pain: Theory of a balance between analgesia and side effects. In S. J. Peterson & T. Bredow (Eds.), *Middle range theories: Application to nursing research*. Philadelphia: Lippincott, Williams & Wilkins.

Good, M., Anderson, G. C., Albert, J., & Wotman, S. (2001–2005). *Supplementing relaxation and music for postoperative pain* (Grant # RO1-05 NR3933). Washington, DC: National Institute of Nursing Research.

Good, M., Anderson, G. C., Stanton-Hicks, M., Grass, J. A., & Makii, M. (2002). Relaxation and music reduce pain after gynecologic surgery. *Pain Management Nursing*, *3*(2), 61–70.

Good, M., & Chin, C. (1998). The effects of Western music on postoperative pain in Taiwan. *Kaoshiung Medical Journal, 14*(2), 93–103.

Good, M., & Moore, S. M. (1996). Clinical practice guidelines as a new source of middle-range theory: Focus on acute pain. *Nursing Outlook, 44*(2), 74–79.

Good, M., Picot, B., Salem, S., Picot, S., & Lane, D. (2000). Cultural responses to music for pain relief. *Journal of Holistic Nursing, 18*(3), 245–260.

Good, M., Stanton-Hicks, M., Grass, J. A., Anderson, G. C., Choi, C. C., Schoolmeesters, L., et al. (1999). Relief of postoperative pain with jaw relaxation, music, and their combination. *Pain, 81*(1–2), 163–172.

Good, M., Stanton-Hicks, M., Grass, J. A., Anderson, G. C., Lai, H. L., Roykulcharoen, V., et al. (2001). Relaxation and music reduce postsurgical pain across activities and days. *Journal of Advanced Nursing, 33*(2), 208–215.

Goodnow, J. J., & Collins, W. A. (1990). *Development according to parents: The nature, sources, and consequences of parents' ideas.* Hilldale, NJ: Lawrence Erlbaum.

Goodrich, H. M., Johnston, P., & Thomson, M. (1996). Conflict and aggression as stressors in the work environment of nursing assistants: Implications for institutional elder abuse. *Journal of Elder Abuse & Neglect,* 8(1), 49–67.

Goodwin, Z., Kiehl, E. M., & Peterson, J. Z. (2002). King's theory as foundation for an advance directive decision-making model. *Nursing Science Quarterly, 15*(3), 237–241.

Gordon, J. S., & Moss, D. (2003). Manifesto for a new medicine. *Biofeedback,* 8–11.

Gorey, K. M., & Leslie, D. R. (1997). The prevalence of child sexual abuse: Integrative review adjustment for potential response and measurement biases. *Child Abuse and Neglect, 21,* 391–398.

Gorham, W. (1962). Staff nursing behaviors contributing to patient care and improvement. *Nursing Research, 11,* 68–79.

Gorski, L. A. (1995). Patient education in high-tech homecare. *Caring, 14,* 22–28.

Gorsuch, R. L. (1983). *Factor analysis* (2nd ed.). Hillsdale, NJ: Lawrence Erlbaum.

Gotlib, I. H., Lewinsohn, P. M., & Steeley, J. R. (1998). Consequences of depression during adolescence: Marital status and marital functioning in early adulthood. *Journal of Abnormal Psychology, 107*(4), 686–690.

Grabbe, L., Demi, A., Camann, M., & Potter, L. (1997). The health status of elderly persons in the last year of life: A comparison of deaths by suicide, injury, and natural causes. *American Journal of Public Health, 87,* 434–437.

Grady, K., Dracup, K., Kennedy, G., Moser, D., Paino, M., Stevenson, L. W., et. al. (2000). Team management of patients with heart failure: A statement for healthcare professionals from the cardiovascular nursing council of the American Heart Association. *Circulation, 102,* 2443–2456.

Grahl, C. (1994). Improving compliance: Solving a $100 billion problem. *Managed Health Care,* S11–S13.

Grandin, C. B. (2003). Assessment of brain perfusion with MRI: Methodology and application to acute stroke. *Neuroradiology, 45*(11), 755–766.

Grant, J. S., Elliott, T. R., Weaver, M., Bartolucci, A. A., & Giger, J. N. (2002). Telephone intervention with family caregivers of stroke survivors after rehabilitation. *Stroke, 33,* 2060–2065.

Grant, R., Finnocchio, L., & the California Primary Care Consortium Subcommittee on Interdisciplinary Collaboration. (1995). *Interdisciplinary collaborative teams in primary care: A model curriculum and resource guide.* San Francisco: Pew Health Commission.

Grap, M. J., Glass, C., Corley, M., & Parks, T. (1996). Endotracheal suctioning: Ventilator vs manual delivery of hyperoxygenation breaths. *American Journal of Critical Care, 5,* 192–197.

Graves, J. (1990). A research-knowledge systems (ARKS) for storing, managing, and modeling knowledge from the scientific literature. *Advances in Nursing Science, 13*(2), 34–45.

Graves, J. R. (1993). Data versus information versus knowledge. *Reflections, 19*(1), 4–5.

Graves, J. R. (1994). STTI Library: A registry of nursing research. *Reflections, 20*(2), 9.

Graves, J. R. (1997). The Virginia Henderson International Nursing Library: Resource for nurse administrators. *Nursing Administration Quarterly, 21*(3), 76–83.

Gray, R., Brewin, E., Noak, J., Wyke-Joseph, J., & Sonik, B. (2002). A review of literature on HIV infection and schizophrenia: Implications for research, policy and clinical practice. *Journal of Psychiatric and Mental Health Nuring, 9,* 405–409.

Gray, R., Fitch, M., Phillips, C., Labrecque, M., & Klotz, L. (1999). Presurgery experiences of prostate cancer patients and their spouses. *Cancer Practice, 7*(3), 130–135.

Gray, R., Wykes, T., & Gournay, K. (2002). From compliance to concordance: A review of the literature on interventions to enhance compliance with antipsychotic medication. *Journal of Psychiatric and Mental Health Nursing, 9,* 277–284.

Gray-Toft, P. A., & Anderson, J. G. (1981). Stress among hospital nursing staff: Its causes and effects. *Social Science and Medicine, 15*, 639–647.

Green, R. (1987). *The "Sissy Boy Syndrome" and the development of homosexuality: A 15 year prospective study*. New Haven, CT: Yale University Press.

Green, S. (2001). Grandma's hands: Parental perceptions of the importance of grandparents as secondary caregivers in families of children with disabilities. *International Journal of Aging and Human Development, 53*(1), 11–33.

Greenfield, L., & Snell, T. F. (1999, December). *Women offenders. Bureau of Justice Statistics Special Report*. Washington, DC: U.S. Department of Justice.

Greenglass, E. R., & Burke, R. J. (2001). Stress and the effects of hospital restructuring in nurses. *Canadian Journal of Nursing Research, 33*, 93–108.

Greenhalgh, R., Slade, P., & Spiby, H. (2000). Fathers' coping style, antenatal preparation, and experiences of labor and the postpartum. *Birth, 27*, 177–184.

Greenough, W. T., Black, J. E., & Wallace, C. S. (1987). Experience and brain development. *Child Development, 58*, 539–559.

Grey, M. (2000). Interventions for children with diabetes and their families. In *Annual review of nursing research* (Vol. 18, pp. 149–170). New York: Springer Publishing.

Grey, M., Berry, D., Davidson, M., Galasso, P., Gustafson, E., & Melkus, G. (2004). Preliminary testing of a program to prevent type 2 diabetes among high risk youth. *Journal of School Health, 74*, 10–15.

Grey, M., Boland, E., Davidson, M., Li, J., & Tamborlane, W. (2000). Coping skills training for youth with diabetes mellitus has long-lasting effects on metabolic control and quality of life. *Journal of Pediatrics, 137*, 107–113.

Grey, M., Knafl, K., Gilliss, C., & McCorkle, R. (in press). A framework for the study of self and family management.

Grier, B., & Grier, M. (1978). Contributions of the passionate statistician. *Research in Nursing and Health, 1*, 103–109.

Griffith, H., & Fonteyn, M. (1989). Let's set the payment record straight. *American Journal of Nursing, 89*, 1051–1058.

Griffith, H. M., Dickey, L., & Kamerow, D. B. (1995). Put prevention into practice: A systematic approach. *Journal of Public Health Management and Practice, 1*(3), 9–15.

Griffith, H. M., & Robinson, K. R. (1992). Survey of the degree to which critical care nurses are performing Current Procedural Terminology-coded services. *American Journal of Critical Care, 1*, 91–98.

Griffith, H. M., & Robinson, K. R. (1993). Current Procedural Terminology (CPT) coded services provided by nurse specialists. *Image: Journal of Nursing Scholarship, 25*, 178–186.

Griffith, H. M., Thomas, N., & Griffith, L. (1991). MDs bill for these routine nursing tasks. *American Journal of Nursing, 91*(1), 22–27.

Groer, M. (1993). Menstrual cycle lengthening and reduction in premenstrual distress through guided imagery [Abstract]. *Abstracts of the 10th Conference of the Society for Menstrual Cycle Research*, 52.

Grondin, J. (1995). *Sources of hermeneutics*. Albany: State University of New York Press.

Gross, D. (1996). What is a "good" parent? *American Journal of Maternal Child Nursing, 21*, 178–182.

Gross, D., & Conrad, B. (1995). Temperament in toddlerhood. *Journal of Pediatric Nursing, 10*, 146–151.

Gross, D., Fogg, L., Webster-Stratton, C., Garvey, C., Julion, W., & Grady, J. (2003). Parent training of toddlers in day care in low-income urban communities. *Journal Consulting and Clinical Psychology, 71*(2), 261–278.

Gross, D., Sambrook, A., & Fogg, L. (1999). Behavior problems among young children in low-income urban day care. *Research in Nursing & Health, 22*, 15–25.

Grossman, S., & Valiga, T. (2000). *The new leadership challenge: Creating the future of nursing*. Philadelphia: F. A. Davis.

Grov, E. K. (1999). Death at home—how can the nurse contribute in making death at home possible for people with terminal cancer. *Nursing Science & Research in the Nordic Countries, 19*(4), 4–9.

Grunbaum, J., Kann, L., Kinchen, S., Williams, B., Ross, J., Lowry, R., et al. (2002). Youth risk behavior surveillance—United States, 2001. *Morbidity and Mortality Weekly Report, 51*, 1–62.

Grzeczkowski, A. M., & Knapp, M. (1988). The gerontological nurse practitoners as director of nursing in the long-term facility. *Nursing Management, 19* (4 Long Term Care Ed.), 64B–64D, 64F.

Gueldner, S. H. (2000). *Preventing and managing osteoporosis*. New York: Springer Publishing.

Gueldner, S. H., Britton, G. R., Stucke, S. A., Skorupa, S., Ferrario, J., Grabo, T., et al. (2003, November). *Profiling the incidence and risk of osteoporosis in a Pennsylvania population using ultrasound measurement of bone density and assessment of risk factors*. Poster presented at the Eleventh Annual Clinical Campus Research Poster Session, State University of New York Upstate Medical University, Binghamton.

Guevara, J. P., Wolf, F. M., Grum, C. M., & Clark, N. M. (2003). Effects of educational interventions for self management of asthma in children and adolescents: Systematic review and meta-analysis. *British Medical Journal, 326*, 1308–1313.

Guise, J. M., Palda, V., Westhoff, C., Chan, B. K. S., Helfand, M., & Lieu, T. A. (2003). The effectiveness of primary care-based interventions to promote breastfeeding: Systematic evidence review and meta-analysis for the U.S. Preventive Services Task Force. *Annals of Family Medicine, 1*(2), 70–78.

Gunningberg, L., Lindholm, C., Carlsson, M., & Sjoden, P. O. (2001). Reduced incidence of pressure ulcers in patients with hip fractures: A 2-year follow-up of quality indicators. *International Journal of Quality Health Care, 13*, 399–407.

Gunter, L., & Estes, C. (1979). *Education for gerontic nursing*. New York: Springer Publishing.

Guralnik, J. M., Ferrucci, L., Pieper, C. F., Leveille, S. G., Markides, K. S., Ostir, G. V., et al. (2000). Lower extremity function and subsequent disability: Consistency across studies, predictive models, and value of gait speed alone compared with the short physical performance battery. *Journals of Gerontology: Biological and Medical Sciences, 55*, M221–M231.

Gurney, J. G., & Bondy, M. L. (2002). Epidemiologic research methods and childhood cancer. In P. A. Pizzo & D. G. Poplack (Eds.), *Principles and practice of pediatric oncology* (4th ed.). Philadelphia: J. B. Lippincott.

Gurvich, T., & Cunningham, J. A. (2000). Appropriate use of psychotropic drugs in nursing homes. *American Family Physician, 61*, 1437–1446.

Guttmacher, A. E., & Collins, F. S. (2002). Genomic medicine: A primer. *New England Journal of Medicine, 347*, 1512–1520.

Guttman, L. (1954). Some necessary conditions for factor analysis. *Psychometrika, 19*, 149–161.

Guzzetta, C. E. (1988). Music therapy: Hearing the melody of the soul. In B. M. Dossey, L. Keegan, C. E. Guzzetta, & L. G. Kolkmeier (Eds.), *Holistic nursing: A handbook for practice* (pp. 617–640). Rockville, MD: Aspen.

Guzzetta, C. E. (1997). Music therapy. In B. M. Dossey (Ed.), *American Holistic Nurses' Association: Core curriculum for holistic nursing*. Gaithersburg, MD: Aspen.

Haack, M. R., & Harford, T. C. (1984). Drinking patterns among student nurses. *International Journal of Addictions, 19*, 577–583.

Haas, B. K. (1999). Clarification and integration of similar quality of life concepts. *Image: Journal of Nursing Scholarship, 31*(3), 215–220.

Haber, L. C., Fagan-Pryor, E. C., & Allen, M. (1997). Comparison of registered nurses' and nursing assistants' choices of interventions for aggressive behaviors. *Issues in Mental Health Nursing, 18*(2), 113–124.

Hackett, T. P., & Cassem, N. H. (1974). Development of a quantitative rating scale to assess denial. *Journal of Psychosomatic Research, 18*, 93–100.

Hackett, T. P., & Cassem, N. H. (1982). Coping with cardiac disease. *Advanced Cardiology, 31*, 212–217.

Haddon, W., Jr., & Baker, S. P. (1980). Injury control. In D. Clark & B. MacMahon (Eds.), *Preventive medicine*. Boston: Little, Brown.

Hagan, L., Morin, D., & Lépine, R. (2000). Evaluation of telenursing outcomes: Satisfaction, self-care practices, and cost savings. *Public Health Nursing, 17*(4), 305–313.

Haggerty, L. A. (1999). Continuous electronic fetal monitoring: Contradictions between practice and research. *Journal of Obstetric, Gynecologic, and Neonatal Nursing, 28*(4), 409–416.

Haight, B., Christ, M. A., & Dias, J. (1994). Does nursing education promote ageism? *Journal of Advanced Nursing, 20*, 382–390.

Haight, B. K., Michel, Y., & Hendrix, S. (2000). The extended effects of the life review in nursing home residents. *International Journal of Aging & Human Development, 50*(2), 151–168.

Haight, B. K., & Webster, J. D. (Eds.). (1995). *The art and science of reminiscing: Theory, research, methods, and applications*. Washington, DC: Taylor and Francis.

Hajjar, I., & Kotchen, T. A. (2003). Trends in prevalence, awareness, treatment, and control of hypertension in the United States, 1988–2000. *Journal of the American Medical Association, 290*(2), 199–206.

Halbreich, U. (1997). Menstrually related disorders—towards interdisciplinary international diagnostic criteria. *Cephalalgia, 17*, 1–4.

Haley, R. A., Culver, D. H., White, J., Morgan, W. E., & Emori, E. G. (1985). The nationwide nosocomial infection rate. A new need for vital statistics. *American Journal of Epidemiology, 121*, 159–167.

Hall, B. (1998). Patterns of spirituality in persons with advanced HIV disease. *Research in Nursing & Health, 21*, 143–153.

Hall, G. R., & Buckwalter, K. C. (1987). Progressively lowered stress threshold: A conceptual model for care of adults with Alzheimer's disease. *Archives of Psychiatric Nursing, 1*, 399–406.

Hall, J. M., Stevens, P. E., & Meleis, A. I. (1994). Marginalization: A guiding concept for valuing diversity in nursing knowledge development. *Advances in Nursing Science, 16*(4), 23–41.

Hall, M. J., Norwood, A. E., Ursano, R. J., Fullerton, C. S., & Levinson, C. J. (2002). Psychological and behavioral impacts of bioterrorism. *PTSD Research Quarterly, 14*(3), 1–2.

Halloran, E. (Ed.). (1995). *A Virginia Henderson reader: Excellence in nursing.* New York: Springer.

Halloran, E. (1995). Preserving the essence of nursing in a technological age. In V. Henderson & E. Halloran (Eds.), *A Virginia Henderson reader: Excellence in nursing* (pp. 96–115). New York: Springer.

Halloran, E. J., & Hadley-Vermeersch, P. (1987). Variability in nurse staffing research. *Journal of Nursing Administration, 17,* 26–32.

Halpern, L. F., MacLean, W. E., Jr., & Baumeister, A. A. (1995). Infant sleep-wake characteristics: Relation to neurological status and the prediction of developmental outcome. *Developmental Review, 15,* 255–291.

Hamit, F. (1993). Virtual reality and the exploration of cyberspace. *SAMS Publishing,* 254–256.

Hammen, C. (2003). Interpersonal stress and depression in women. *Journal of Affective Disorders, 74,* 49–57.

Hammond, K. R. (1964). An approach to the study of clinical inference in nursing: Clinical inference in nursing: A methodological approach. *Nursing Research, 13,* 315–319.

Hampton, M. D., & Chafetz, L. (2002). Factors associated with residential placement in an assertive community treatment program. *Issues in Mental Health Nursing, 23,* 677–689.

Hamric, A. B., Spross, J. A., & Hanson, C. M. (1996). *Advanced practice nursing: An integrated approach.* Philadelphia: W. B. Saunders.

Hannigan, B. (1997). A challenge for community psychiatric nursing: Is there a future in primary health care? *Journal of Advanced Nursing, 26,* 751–757.

Hansen, K. M., Messinger, C. J., Baun, M. M., & Megel, M. (1999). Companion animals alleviating distress in children. *Anthrozoös, 12*(3), 142–148.

Hanson, E. J., & Clarke, A. (2000). The role of telematics in assisting family carers and frail older people at home. *Health and Social Care in the Community,* 8(2), 129–137.

Hanson, E. J., Tetley, J., & Shewan, J. (2000). Elderly care. Supporting family carers using interactive multimedia. *British Journal of Nursing,* 9(11), 713–719.

Hanson, R. F., Saunders, B., Kilpatrick, D., Resnick, H., Crouch, J. A., & Duncan, R. (2001). Impact of childhood rape and aggravated assault on adult mental health. *American Journal of Orthopsychiatry, 71*(1), 108–119.

Hanson, R. L. (1979). Predictive criteria for length of nasogastric tube insertion for tube feeding. *Journal of Parenteral & Enteral Nutrition,* 3(3), 160–163.

Happ, M. B., Capezuti, E., Strumpf, N. E., Wagner, L., Cunningham, S., Evans, L., et al. (2002). Advance care planning and end-of-life care for hospitalized nursing home residents. *Journal of the American Geriatrics Society, 50*(5), 829–835.

Happ, M. B., Williams, C. C., Strumpf, N. E., & Burger, S. G. (1996). Individualized care for frail elders: Theory and practice. *Journal of Gerontological Nursing, 22*(3), 7–14.

Harada, N., Chiu, V., Damron-Rodriguez, J., Fowler, E., Siu, A., & Reuben, D. B. (1995). Screening for balance and mobility impairment in elderly individuals living in residential care facilities. *Physical Therapy, 75,* 462–469.

Harden, J., Schafenacker, A., Northhouse, L., Mood, D., Smith, D., Pienta, K., et al. (2002). Couples experiences with prostate cancer: Focus group research. *Oncology Nursing Forum, 30*(1), 107–114.

Hardiker, N. R., & Rector, A. L. (1998). Modeling nursing terminology using the GRAIL representation language. *Journal of the American Medical Informatics Association,* 5(1), 120–128.

Hardiker, N. R., & Rector, A. L. (2001). Structural validation of nursing terminologies. *Journal of the American Medical Informatics Association,* 8, 212–221.

Hare, J., Pratt, C., & Anderaw, D. (1988). Predictors of burnout in professional and paraprofessional nurses working in hospitals and nursing homes. *International Journal of Nursing, 25,* 105–115.

Harmer, B., & Henderson, V. (1939). *Textbook of the principles and practice of nursing* (4th ed.). New York: Macmillan.

Harmer, B., & Henderson, V. (1955). *Textbook of the principles and practice of nursing* (5th ed.). New York: Macmillan.

Harrell, J. S., & Gore, S. (1998). Cardiovascular risk factors and socioeconomic status in African American and Caucasian Women. *Research in Nursing and Health, 21,* 285–295.

Harrell, J. S., McMurray, R. G., Gansky, S. A., Bangdiwala, S. I., & Bradley, C. B. (1999). A public health vs. a risk-based intervention to improve cardiovascular health in elementary school children: The Cardiovascular Health in Children Study. *American Journal of Public Health, 89,* 1529–1535.

Harrell, R., Toronjo, C. H., McLaughlin, J., Pavlik, V. N., Hyman, D. J., & Dyer, C. B. (2002). How geriatricians identify elder abuse and neglect. *American Journal of Medical Science, 323*(1), 34–38.

Harrington, C., Carillo, H., & Wellin, V. (2001). *Nursing facilities, staffing, residents, and facility deficiencies, 1994 through 2000*. San Francisco: University of California, Department of Social and Behavioral Sciences.

Harrington, C., Kovner, C., Mezey, M., Kayser-Jones, J., Burger, S., Mohler, M., et al. (2000). Experts recommend minimum nurse staffing standards for Nursing Facilities in the United States. *Gerontologist, 40*(1), 5–16.

Harrington, C., Zimmerman, D., Karon, S. L., Robinson, J., & Beutel, P. (2000). Nursing home staffing and its relationship to deficiencies. *Journal of Gerontology: Social Sciences, 55B*(5), S278–S287.

Harrington, V., Lackey, N., & Gates, M. (1996). Needs of caregivers of clinic and hospice cancer patients. *Cancer Nursing, 19*(2), 118–125.

Harris, N. R., Lovell, K., & Day, J. C. (2002). Consent and long-term neuroleptic treatment. *Journal of Psychiatric Mental Health Nursing, 9*, 475–482.

Harris, R., & Lohr, J. (2002). Screening for prostate cancer: An update of the evidence for the U.S. Preventative Service Task Force. *Annals of Internal Medicine, 137*, 917–929.

Harris, S. (2002). Nurses' views on withdrawing ECMO: A grounded theory study. *Nursing in Critical Care, 7*(3), 144–151.

Harris, Z. S. (1952). Discourse analysis. *Lg, 28*, 1–30.

Hart, B. (2002). Promoting positive outcomes for elderly persons in the hospital: Prevention and risk factor modification. *Advanced Practice in Acute and Critical Care, 13*(1), 22–33.

Hart, L. B. (2000). Integrating technology and traditional methods to simulate different cognitive styles in a critical care course. *Journal for Nurses in Staff Development, 16*(1), 31–33.

Hartig, M. T. (1998). Expert nursing assistant care activities. *Western Journal of Nursing Research, 20*(5), 584–601.

Hartley, C. C. (2002). The co-occurrence of child maltreatment and domestic violence: Examining both neglect and child physical abuse. *Child Maltreatment, 7*(4), 349–358.

Hartley, S. S., & McKibbin, R. C. (1983). *Hospital payment mechanisms, patient classification systems and nursing: Relationships and implications*. Kansas City, MO: American Nurses Association.

Hasselmeyer, E. G. (1961). *Behavior patterns of premature infants* (USDHS Publication No. 840). Washington, DC: U.S. Government Printing Office.

Hathaway, D. (1986). Effect of preoperative instruction on postoperative outcomes: A meta-analysis. *Nursing Research, 35*, 269–275.

Hatlebakk, J. G. (2003). Gastric acidity—comparison of esomeprazole with other proton pump inhibitors. *Alimentary Pharmacotherapeutics, 17*(suppl.), 10–15.

Hauenstein, E. J. (1996). Testing innovative nursing care: Home intervention with depressed rural women. *Issues in Mental Health Nursing, 17*, 33–50.

Hauenstein, E. J. (2003). No comfort in the rural South: Women living depressed. *Archives of Psychiatric Nursing, 17*(1), 3–11.

Hauenstein, E. J., & Peddada, S. (in revision). Prevalence of major depressive disorder in rural women using primary care. *Journal of Rural Health.*

Hauser, W. A., & Hesdorffer, D. C. (1990). *Epilepsy: Frequency, causes, and consequences*. New York: Demos Publications.

Havener, L., Gentes, L., Thaler, B., Megel, M., Baun, M., Driscoll, E. A., et al. (2001). The effects of a companion animal on distress undergoing dental procedures. *Issues in Comprehensive Pediatric Nursing, 24*(2), 137–152.

Hawkins, J. D., Herrenkohl, T., Farrington, D. P., Catalano, R. F., Harachi, T. W., & Cothern, L. (2000). *Predictors of youth violence*. Washington, DC: U.S. Department of Justice, Office of Justice Programs, Office of Juvenile Justice and Delinquency Prevention. Retrieved from http://www.ncjrs.org/pdffiles1/ojjdp/179065.pdf

Hayes, C. (2002). Identifying important issues for people with Parkinson's disease. *British Journal of Nursing, 11*, 91–97.

Hayes, R. P., Duffey, E. B., Dunbar, J., Wages, J. W., & Holbrook, S. E. (1998). Staff perceptions of emergency and home-care telemedicine. *Journal of Telemedicine & Telecare, 4*(2), 101–107.

Hayman, L. L., Williams, C. L., Daniels, S. R., Steinberger, J., Paridon, S., Dennison, B. A., et al. (2004). Cardiovascular health promotion in the schools. A statement for health and education professionals and child health advocates from the Committee on Atherosclerosis, Hypertension, and Obesity in Youth (AHOY) of the Council on Cardiovascular Disease in the Young, American Heart Association. *Circulation, 110*, 2266–2275.

Haynes, R., McDonald, H., Garg, A., & Montague, P. (2003). *Interventions for helping patients to follow prescriptions for medications*. The Cochrane Database for Systematic Reviews.

Hays, B., Norris, J., Martin, K., & Androwich, I. (1994). Informatics issues for nursing's future. *Advances in Nursing Science, 16*(4), 71–81.

Hayslip, B., Emick, M. A., Henderson, C. E., & Elias, K. (2002). Temporal variations in the experience of custodial grandparenting: A short-term longitudinal study. *Journal of Applied Gerontology, 21*, 139–156.

Hayslip, B., Shore, R. J., Henderson, C. E., & Lambert, P. L. (1998). Custodial grandparenting and the impact of grandchildren with problems on role satisfaction and role meaning. *Journal of Gerontology: Social Sciences, 53*, S164–S173.

Haywood, T. W., Kravitz, H. M., Goldman, L., & Freeman, A. (2000). Characteristics of women in jail and treatment orientations: A review. *Behavior Modification, 24*(3), 307–324.

Hazlett, R. L., Tusa, R. J., & Waranch, H. R. (1996). Development of an inventory for dizziness and related factors. *Journal of Behavioral Medicine, 19*, 75–85.

Health Canada. (2001). *The population health template: Key elements and actions that define a population health approach* [Draft]. Ottawa, Ontario, Canada: Health Canada Population and Public Health Branch, Strategic Policy Directorate. Retrieved from: http://www.hc-sc.gc.ca/hppb/phdd/pdf/discussion_paper.pdf

Health Care Financing Administration and Bureau of Data Management and Strategy. (1990). *HCFA, BDMS, BMAD system procedure file*. Washington, DC: U.S. Department of Health and Human Services.

Healthy People 2010: Understanding and improving health. (2000). In Office of Women's Health, U.S. Department of Health and Human Services (Ed.), *HHS blueprint for action on breastfeeding* (2nd ed.). Washington, DC: U.S. Government Printing Office.

Heath, J. M., Dyer, C. B., Kerzner, L. J., Mosqueda, L., & Murphy, C. (2002). Four models of medical education about elder mistreatment. *Academe, 77*(11), 1101–1106.

Hebda, T., Czar, P., & Mascara, D. (2001). *Handbook of informatics for nurses and health care professionals* (2nd ed.). Upper Saddle River, NJ: Prentice-Hall.

Hebert, L. E., Scherr, P. A., Bienias, J. L., Bennett, D. A., & Evans, D. A. (2003). Alzheimer disease in the US population: Prevalence estimates using the 2000 census. *Archives of Neurology, 60*(8), 1119–1122.

Heczey, M. D. (1980). Effects of biofeedback and autogenic training on dysmenorrhea. In A. Dan, E. Graham, & C. Beecher (Eds.), *The menstrual cycle: A synthesis of interdisciplinary research* (Vol. 1, pp. 283–291). New York: Springer.

Hedström, M., Haglund, K., Skolin, I., & Von Essen, L. (2003). Distressing events for children and adolescents with cancer: Child, parent, and nurse perceptions. *Journal of Pediatric and Oncology Nursing, 20*(3), 120–132.

Hefferman, P., & Heilig, S. (1999). Giving "moral distress" a voice: Ethical concerns among neonatal intensive care unit personnel. *Cambridge Quarterly of Healthcare Ethics, 8*, 173–178.

Hegavary, S. (2000). Scholarship for a new era. *Journal of Nursing Scholarship, 32*(1), 4–5.

Hegge, M., & Fischer, C. (2000). Grief response os senior and elderly widows: Practice applications. *Journal of Gerontological Nursing, 25*(2), 35–43.

Hegleson, V. S., & Heidi, F. (1999). Cognitive adaptation as a predictor of new coronary events after percutaneous transluminal coronary angioplasty. *Psychosomatic Medicine, 61*, 488–495.

Heidegger, M. (1962). *Being and time* (J. Macquarrie & F. Robinson, Trans.). New York: Harper & Row. (Original work published 1927)

Heidegger, M. (1993). In D. Krell (Ed.), *Basic writings* (Rev. ed.). San Francisco: Harper. (Original work published 1927)

Heidegger, M. (1996). *Being and time: A translation of Sein und Zeit* (J. Stambaugh, Trans.). New York: Harper and Row. (Original work published 1927)

Heinemann, G., & Brown, G. (2001). Instruments for health care teams. In G. Heinemann & A. Zeiss (Eds.), *Team performance in health care: Assessment and development*. New York: Kluwer.

Heinemann, G., Schmitt, M., & Farrell, M. (1994). The quality of geriatric team functioning: Model and methodology. In J. R. Snyder (Ed.), *Interdisciplinary health care teams* (pp. 77–91). Proceedings of the Sixteenth Annual Conference in Indianapolis: Indiana University Medical Center.

Heinig, M. J. (2001). Host defense benefits of breastfeeding for the infant. *Pediatric Clinics of North America, 48*(1), 105–123.

Heinz, S. (1986). Premenstrual syndrome: An assessment, education, and treatment model. In V. Oleson & N. F. Woods (Eds.), *Culture, society, and menstruation* (pp. 153–157). New York: Hemisphere, Harper & Row.

Heiss, W. D., & Rosner, G. (1983). Functional recovery of cortical neurons as related to degree and duration of ischemia. *Annals of Neurology, 14*(3), 294–301.

Heitkemper, M. M., & Bond, E. F. (2003). State of nursing science: On the edge. *Biological Research for Nursing, 4*(3), 151–62.

Heitkemper, M., Carter, E., Ameen, V., Olden, K., & Cheng, L. (2002). Women with irritable bowel syndrome: Differences in patients' and physicians' perceptions. *Gastroenterology Nursing, 25*(5), 192–200.

Heitkemper, M. M., Jarrett, M., Caudell, K. A., & Bond, E. (1998). Women with gastrointestinal symptoms: Implications for nursing research and practice. *Gastroenterology Nursing, 21*(2), 52–58.

Heitkemper, M., Jarrett, M., Cain, K. C., Shaver, J., Walker, E., & Lewis, L. (1995). Daily gastrointestinal symptoms in women with and without a diagnosis of IBS. *Digestive Diseases and Sciences*, *40*(7), 1511–1519.

Heliker, D. (1997). A narrative approach to quality care in long-term care facilities. *Journal of Holistic Nursing*, *15*(1), 68–81.

Heller, B. W., Flohr, L. M., & Zegans, L. S. (Eds.). (1989). *Psychosocial interventions with physically disabled persons*. New Brunswick, NJ: Rutgers University Press.

Henderson, A. (2001). Factors influencing nurses' response to abused women: what they say and why they say they do it. *Journal of Interpersonal Violence*, *16*(12), 1284–1306.

Henderson, V. (1939). *Harmer and Henderson's textbook of the principles and practice of nursing* (4th ed.). New York: Macmillan.

Henderson, V. (1955). *Harmer and Henderson's textbook of the principles and practice of nursing* (5th ed.). New York: Macmillan.

Henderson, V. (1978). The concept of nursing. *Journal of Advanced Nursing*, *3*, 113–130.

Henderson, V. (1991) *The nature of nursing: Reflections after 25 years*. New York: National League for Nursing.

Henderson, V. (1997). *ICN basic principles of nursing care*. Geneva, Switzerland: International Council of Nurses. Retrieved from http://nursingworld.org/books

Henderson, V. (2004). *ICN basic principles of nursing care*. Geneva, Switzerland: International Council of Nurses. Published first in 1960 and revised in 1969, 1977, 1997.

Henderson, V., & Nite, G. (1978). *Principles and practice of nursing* (6th ed.). New York: Macmillan.

Henderson, V., & Nite, G. (1997). *Principles and practice of nursing*. Geneva, Switzerland: International Council of Nurses.

Henderson, V., & Yale University School of Nursing Index Staff (1963, 1966, 1970, 1972). Nursing Studies Index, Volumes IV, III, II, I. Philadelphia: J. B. Lippincott. Re-printed in 1984 by Garland Publishing: New York.

Hendrickson, M. H., & Paganelli, B. (1994). Facing the challenges of nurse expert systems in the future. In S. J. Grobe & E. S. P. Pluyter Wenting (Eds.), *Nursing informatics: An international overview for nursing in a technological era* (pp. 336–340). Amsterdam, Netherlands: Elsevier.

Henker, R., Rogers, S., Kramer, D. J., Kelso, L., Kerr, M., & Sereika, S. (2001). Comparison of fever treatments in the critically ill: A pilot study. *American Journal of Critical Care*, *10*(4), 276–280.

Henretta, J., O'Rand, A., & Chan, C. (1993). Gender differences in employment after spouse's retirement. *Research on Aging*, *15*, 148–169.

Henry, S. B. (1991). Effect of level of patient acuity on clinical decision making of critical care nurses with varying levels of knowledge and experience. *Heart & Lung*, *20*(5 Pt. 1), 478–485.

Henry, S. B., Holzemer, W. L., Randell, C., Hsieh, S.-F., & Miller, T. J. (1997). Comparison of Nursing Interventions Classification and Current Procedural Terminology codes for categorizing nursing activities. *Image: Journal of Nursing Scholarship*, *29*(2), 133–138.

Henry, S. B., Holzemer, W. L., Reilly, C. A., & Campbell, K. E. (1994). Terms used by nurses to describe patient problems: Can SNOMED III represent nursing concepts in the patient record? *Journal of the American Medical Informatics Association*, *1*(1), 61–74.

Henry, S. B., & Mead, C. N. (1997). Nursing classification systems: Necessary but not sufficient for representing "what nurses do" for inclusion in computer-based patient record systems. *Journal of the American Medical Informatics Association*, *4*(3), 222–232.

Henry, S. B., Warren, J. J., Lange, L., & Button, P. (1998). A review of major nursing vocabularies and the extent to which they have the characteristics required for implementation in computer-based systems. *Journal of the American Medical Informatics Association*, *5*, 321–328.

Herrenkohl, T. I., Hawkins, J. D., Chung, I. J., Hill, K. G., & Battin-Pearson, S. (2001). School and community risk factors and interventions. In R. Loeber & D. P. Farrington (Eds.), *Child delinquents: Development, intervention, and service needs* (pp. 211–246). Thousand Oaks, CA: Sage Publications.

Herrmann, N. (2001). Recommendations for the management of behavioral and psychological symptoms of dementia. *Canadian Journal of Neurological Sciences*, *28*, 96–107.

Hershey, J., Valenciano, C., & Bookbinder, M. (1997). Comparison of three rewarming methods in a postanesthesia care unit. *Journal of the Association of Operating Room Nurses*, *65*(3), 597–601.

Hervada, A. R., & Hervada-Page, M. (1995). Infant nutrition: The first two years. In F. Lifshitz (Ed.), *Childhood nutrition* (pp. 43–52). Boca Raton, FL: CRC Press.

Hess, D. R., Kallstrom, T. J., Mottram, C. D., Myers, T. R., Sorenson, H. M., & Vines, D. L. (2003). AARC evidence-based clinical practice guidelines. Care of the ventilator circuit and its relation to ventilator-associated pneumonia. *Respiratory Care*, *48*(9), 869–879.

Hess, G. (1969). Perception of nursing role in a developing mental health center. *Journal of Psychiatric Nursing and Mental Health Services, 7*, 77–81.

Hewitt-Taylor, J. (2002). Evidence-based practice. *Nursing Standard, 17*, 47–52.

Heyn Billipp, S. (2001). The psychosocial impact of interactive computer use within a vulnerable elderly population: A report on a randomized prospective trial in a home health care setting. *Public Health Nursing, 18*(2), 138–145.

HHS News. (2001, October). *HHS issues report on community health in rural, urban areas.* Retrieved from http://www.cdc.gov/nchs/releases/01news/hus01.htm

Hibbard, J. (1995). Women's employment history and their post-retirement health and resources. *Journal of Women & Aging, 7*(3), 43–54.

Hicks, C. F., Deloughery, G. L., & Gebbie, K. M. (1971). Progress in community mental health nursing: Is role diffusion ending? *Journal of Psychosocial Nursing and Mental Health Services, 9*, 28–29.

Higgins, E. T. (1987). Self-discrepancy: A theory relating self and affect. *Psychological Review, 94*, 319–340.

Higgins, M., Enright, P., Kronmal, R., Schenker, M., Anton-Culver, H., & Lyles, M. (1993). Smoking and lung function in elderly men and women: The cardiovascular health study. *Journal of the American Medical Association, 269*, 2741–2748.

Highfield, M. F., & Cason, C. (1983). Spiritual needs of patients: Are they recognized? *Cancer Nurse, 6*, 187–192.

Hildebrandt, E. (1994). A model for community involvement in health (CIH) program development. *Social Science Medicine, 39*(2), 247–254.

Hildebrandt, E. (1996). Building community participation in health care: A model and example from South Africa. *Image: Journal of Nursing Scholarship, 28*(2), 155–159.

Hill, C. (2004). Gastroesophageal reflux disease. In S. E. Meiner (Ed.), *Care of gastrointestinal problems in the older adult.* New York: Springer Publishing.

Hill, J. O., Wyatt, H. R., Reed, G. W., & Peters, J. C. (2003). Obesity and the environment: Where do we go from here? *Science, 299*, 853–855.

Hill, M. H., & Doddato, T. (2002). Relationships among patient satisfaction, intent to return, and intent to recommend services provided by an academic nursing center. *Journal of Cultural Diversity, 9*, 108–112.

Hill, N. (2002). Use of quality-of-life scores in care planning in a hospice setting: A comparative study. *International Journal of Palliative Nursing, 8*, 540–547.

Hill, R. (1958). Social stresses on the family. *Social Casework, 39*, 139–150.

Hillbrand, M., Foster, H. G., & Spitz, R. T. (1996). Characteristics and costs of staff injuries in a forensic hospital. *Psychiatric Services, 47*(10), 1123–1125.

Hilton, B. A. (1992). Perceptions of uncertainty: Its relevance to life-threatening and chronic illness. *Critical Care Nurse, 12*(1), 70–73.

Hilton, B. A. (1994). The Uncertainty Stress Scale: Its development and psychometric properties. *Canadian Journal of Nursing Research, 26*(3), 15–30.

Hiltunen, E. F., Medich, C., Chase, S., Peterson, L., & Foroow, L. (1999). Family decision making for end-of-life treatment: The SUPPORT nurse narratives. *Journal of Clinical Ethics, 10*(2), 126–134.

Hinds, P., Hockenberry, M., & Schum, L. (2002). Research. In C. R. Baggott, K. P. Kelly, D. Fochtman, & G. V. Foley (Eds.), *Nursing care of children and adolescents with cancer* (3rd ed.). Philadelphia: W. B. Saunders.

Hinrichs, M., Huseboe, J., Tang, J. H., & Titler, M. G. (2001). Research-based protocol. Management of constipation. *Journal of Gerontological Nursing, 27*(2), 17–28.

Hinshaw, A. S. (1979). Theoretical substruction: An assessment process. *Western Journal of Nursing Research, 1*, 319–324.

Hinshaw, A. (2000). Nursing knowledge for the 21st century: Opportunities and challenges. *Journal of Nursing Scholarship, 2*(32), 117–123.

Hinshaw, A. D., Feetham, S., & Shaver, J. (1999). *Handbook of clinical nursing research.* Thousand Oaks, CA: Sage Publications.

Hinshaw, A. S., & Atwood, J. R. (1981). A patient satisfaction instrument: Precision by replication. *Nursing Research, 31*, 170–175, 191.

Hinton, J. (1996). How reliable are relatives' retrospective reports of terminal illness? Patients' and relatives' accounts compared. *Social Science & Medicine, 43*, 1229–1236.

History of the American Association of Critical-Care Nurses. (2003). Retrieved February 6, 2004, from http://www.aacn.org/AACN/mrkt.nsf/vwdoc/HistoryofAACN

Ho, V. W., Thiel, E. C., Rubin, H. R., & Singer, P. A. (2000). The effect of advance care planning on completion of advance directives and patient satisfaction in people with HIV/AIDS. *AIDS Care, 12*, 97–108.

Hobbs, C. J., Hanks, H. G., & Wynne, J. M. (1999). *Child abuse and neglect: A clinician's handbook* (2nd ed.). London: Churchill Livingstone.

Hobbs, F., & Stoops, N. (2001). *Demographic trends in the 20th century*. Washington, DC: U.S. Government Printing Office.

Hobfoll, S., & Vaux, A. (1993). Social support: Social resources and social context. In L. Goldberger & S. Breznitz (Eds.), *Handbook of stress: Theoretical and clinical aspects* (2nd ed., pp. 685–705). New York: Free Press.

Hoekstra, J. (2001, April). Hard luck in the heartland. MAMM, 3, 36, 57.

Hogan, N., Greenfield, D., & Schmidt, L. (2001). Development and evaluation of the Hogan Grief Reaction Checklist. *Death Studies, 25*, 1–32.

Hogan, N., & Schmidt, L. (2002). Testing the grief to personal growth model using structural equation modeling. *Death Studies, 26*, 615–634.

Hogenmiller, J. (2004). Measures and predictors of pap smear screening participation among inner city sheltered women. (Doctoral dissertation, University of Nebraska Medical Center, 2004) submitted to Dissertation Abstracts International.

Hogstel, M. O. (2001). *Gerontology: Nursing care of the older adult*. Albany, NY: Delamar Publishers.

Holaday, B. (1997). Johnson's behavioral system model in nursing practice. In M. Alligood & A. Marriner-Tomey (Eds.), *Nursing theory: Utilization and application* (pp. 49–70). St. Louis, MO: Mosby Year-Book.

Holder, D., & Anderson, C. (1990). Psychoeducational family interventions for depressed patients and their families. In G. I. Keitner (Ed.), *Depression families: Impact and treatment* (pp. 159–184). Washington, DC: American Psychiatric Press.

Holditch-Davis, D., Bartlett, T. R., Blickman, A. L., & Miles, M. S. (2003). Post-traumatic stress symptoms in mothers of premature infants. *Journal of Obstetric, Gynecologic, and Neonatal Nursing, 32*, 161–171.

Holditch-Davis, D., Blackburn, S., & Vandenberg, K. A. (2003). Newborn and infant neurobehavioral development. In C. Kenner & J. W. Lott (Eds.), *Comprehensive neonatal nursing care: A physiologic perspective* (3rd ed., pp. 236–284). Philadelphia: Saunders.

Holditch-Davis, D., & Miles, M. S. (1997). Parenting the prematurely born child. In J. J. Fitzpatrick & J. Norbeck (Eds.), *Annual review of nursing research* (Vol. 15, pp. 3–34). New York: Springer Publishing.

Holick, M. F. (2003). Vitamin D deficiency: What a pain it is. *Mayo Clinic Proceedings, 78*(12), 1457–1459.

Holland, M., Baguley, I., & Davies, T. (1999a). Hallucinations and delusions. 2: A dual diagnosis case study. *British Journal of Nursing, 8*, 1095–1102.

Holland, M., Baguley, I., & Davies, T. (1999b). Psychological methods of treating hallucinations and delusions: 1. *British Journal of Nursing, 8*, 998–1002.

Holley, J. L., Stackiewicz, L., Dacko, C., & Rault, R. (1997). Factors influencing dialysis patients' completion of advance directives. *American Journal of Kidney Diseases, 30*(3), 356–360.

Holmberg, L., Bill-Axelson, A., Helgesen, F., Salo, J. O., Folmerz, P., Haggman, M., et al. (2002). A randomized trial comparing radical prostatectomy with watchful waiting in early prostate cancer. *The New England Journal of Medicine, 347*, 781–789.

Holmes, G. L. (1987). *Diagnosis and management of seizures in children*. Philadelphia: W. B. Saunders.

Holmes, T. H., & Rahe, R. (1967). The social readjustment rating scale. *Journal of Psychosomatic Research, 12*, 213–218.

Holohan-Bell, J., & Brummel-Smith, K. (1999). Impaired mobility and deconditioning. In J. Stone, J. Wyman, & S. Salisbury (Eds.), *Clinical gerontological nursing: A guide to advanced practice* (pp. 267–287). Philadelphia: W. B. Saunders.

Holt, L. E. (1897). *Diseases of infancy and childhood*. New York: D. Appleton.

Holtzclaw, B. J. (1990). Control of febrile shivering during amphotericin B therapy. *Oncology Nursing Forum, 17*(4), 521–524.

Holtzclaw, B. J. (1998). *Final Report: Febrile symptom management in persons with AIDS* (R01 NR03988). Bethesda, MD: National Institute of Nursing Research, National Institutes of Health.

Holtzclaw, B. J., & Geer, R. T. (1986). Shivering after heart surgery: Assessment of metabolic effects. *Anesthesiology, 65*(Suppl. 3A), A18.

Holtzclaw, B. J., & Geer, R. T. (1994). Clinical predictors and metabolic consequences of postoperative shivering after cardiac surgery. *Key Aspects of Caring for the Acutely Ill: Technological Aspects, Patient Education, and Quality of Life, 5*, 226–233.

Holzemer, W. L., Henry, S. B., Dawson, C., Sousa, K., Bain, C., & Hsieh, S. F. (1997). An evaluation of the utility of the Home Health Care Classification for categorizing patient problems and nursing interventions from the hospital setting. *Studies in Health Technology & Informatics, 46*, 21–26.

Holzemer, W. L., Henry, S. B., Portillo, C. J., & Miramontes, H. (2000). The Client Adherence Profiling-Intervention Tailoring (CAP-IT) intervention for enhancing adherence to HIV/AIDS medications: A pilot study. *Journal of the Association of Nurses in AIDS Care, 11*(1), 36–44.

Holzemer, W. L., & Reilly, C. A. (1994). Variables, variability, and variations research: Implications for medical informatics. In Informatics: The infrastructure for quality assessment and improvement in nursing. *Proceedings of the Fifth International Nursing Informatics Symposium Post-Conference* (pp. 47–51). San Francisco: University of California Nursing Press.

Holzemer, W. L., Spicer, J., Wilson, H., Kemppainen, J., & Coleman, C. (1998). Validation of quality of life scale; living with HIV. *Journal of the Association of Nurses in AIDS Care, 28*, 622–630.

Homans, G. (1961). *Social behavior: Its elementary forms*. New York: Harcourt, Brace and World.

Homes for the Homeless. (1998). *Ten cities: 1997–1998: A snapshot of family homelessness across America*. New York: Homes for the Homeless & Institute for Children and Poverty.

Hong, T. C., Callister, L. C., & Schwartz, R. (2003). First-time mothers' views of breastfeeding support from nurses. *American Journal of Maternal/Child Nursing, 28*(1), 10–15.

Hope-Stone, L., & Mills, B. (2001). Developing empathy to improve patient care: A pilot study of cancer nurses. *International Journal of Palliative Nursing, 7*(3), 146–150.

Horgas, A., & Dunn, K. (2001). Pain in nursing home residents. Comparison of residents' self-report and nursing assistants' perceptions. *Journal of Gerontological Nursing, 27*(3), 44–53.

Horowitz, J. A., Bell, M., Trygulski, J., Munro, B. H., Moser, D., Hartz, S. A., et al. (2001). Promoting responsiveness between mothers with depressive symptoms and their infants. *Journal of Nursing Scholarship, 33*, 323–329.

Horowitz, J. A., Chang, S., Das, S., & Hayes, B. (2001). Women's perceptions of postpartum depressive symptoms from an international perspective. *International Nursing Perspectives, 1*, 5–14.

Horowitz, R. S., & Fuller, S. S. (1982). Concurrence in content descriptions: Author vs. medical subject headings (MESH). *Proceedings of the American Society for Information Science Annual Meeting, 19*, 139–140.

Horsley, J. A., Crane, J., Crabtree, M. K., & Wood, D. J. (1983). *Using research to improve nursing practice: A guide*. New York: Grune & Stratton.

Hoskins, C. N., Baker, S., Bohlander, J., Bookbinder, M., Budin, W., Ekstrom, D. (1996a). Adjustment among spouses of women with breast cancer. *Journal of Psychosocial Oncology, 14*, 41–69.

Hoskins, C. N., Baker, S., Bohlander, J., Bookbinder, M., Budin, W., Ekstrom, D. (1996b). Social support and patterns of adjustment to breast cancer. *Scholarly Inquiry for Nursing Practice: An International Journal, 10*, 99–123.

Hospice and Palliative Nurses Association. (2003). *Hospice and Palliative Care Nurses Association position statement: Artificial nutrition and dehydration*. Retrieved November 10, 2003, from http://www.hpna.org/position_ArtificialNutrition.asp

Howard, L., & Malone, M. (1996). Current status of home parenteral nutrition in the United States. *Transplant Proceedings, 28*(5), 2691–2695.

Howard, L. V., West, D., & Ossip-Klein, D. J. (2000). Chronic constipation management for institutionalized older adults. *Geriatric Nursing, 21*(2), 78–82.

Howland, J., Lachman, M. E., Peterson, E. W., Cote, J., Kasten, L., & Jette, A. (1998). Covariates of fear of falling and associated activity curtailment. *Gerontologist, 38*, 549–555.

Hoyer, P. J. (1998). Prenatal and parenting programs for adolescent mothers. In J. J. Fitzpatrick (Ed.), *Annual review of nursing research* (Vol. 16, pp. 221–249). New York: Springer Publishing.

Hsu, C., Pu, C., & Sewell, K. L. (1996). Systemic lupus erythematosus as a cause of failure to thrive in older people. *Journal of the American Geriatrics Society, 44*, 337–338.

Huang, C. Y., & Menke, E. M. (2001). School-aged homeless sheltered children's stressors and coping behaviors. *Journal of Pediatric Nursing, 16*(2), 102–109.

Hubbard, H., Walker, P., Clancy, C., & Stryer, D. (2002). Outcomes and effectiveness research: Capacity building for nurse researchers at the agency for healthcare research and quality. *Outcomes Management, 6*(4), 46–151.

Hudson, M., Mertens, A., Yasui, Y., Hobbie, W., Chen, H., Gurney, J., et al. (2003). Health status of adult long-term survivors of childhood cancer: A report from the Childhood Cancer Survivor Study. *Journal of the American Medical Association, 290*(12), 1583–1592.

Hueston, W. J., Knox, M. A., Eilers, G., Pauwels, J., & Lonsdorf, D. (1995). The effectiveness of preterm-birth prevention educational programs for high-risk women: A meta-analysis. *Obstetrics and Gynecology, 86*, 705–712.

Hughes, J. R., Keely, K. P., Niaura, R. S., Ossip-Klein, D. J., Richmond, R. L., & Swan, G. E. (2003). Measures of abstinence in clinical trials: Issues and recommendations. *Nicotine & Tobacco Research, 5*, 13–25.

Hughes, N., & Neal, R. D. (2000). Adults with terminal illness: A literature review of their needs and wishes for food. *Journal of Advanced Nursing, 32*, 1101–1107. Retrieved January 26, 2004, from http://gateway1.ovid.com/ovidweb.cgi

Huibers, M. J. H., Buerskens, A,J. H., Bleijenberg, G., & van Schayck, C. P. (2004). *The effectiveness of psychosocial interventions delivered by general practitioners*. Oxford, England: Cochrane Library.

Humphreys, B. L., Lindberg, D. A. B., Schoolman, H. M., & Barnett, G. O. (1998). The Unified Medical Language System: An informatics research collaboration. *Journal of the American Medical Informatics Association, 5*(1), 1–11.

Hunt, M. (1974). *Sexual behavior in the 1970s*. Chicago: Playboy Press.

Hunt, S., Baker, D., Chin, M., Cinquegrani, M. P., Feldman, A. M., Francis, G. S., et al. (2001). ACC/AHA guidelines for the evaluation and management of chronic heart failure in the adult: Executive summary. *Journal of the American College of Cardiology, 38*, 2101–2113.

Hurlebaus, A., & Link, S. (1997). The effects of an aggressive behavior management program on nurses' level of knowledge, confidence, and safety. *Journal of Nursing Staff Development, 36*(12), 1312–1314.

Hurley, R. (1991). The continuing care retirement community executive: A manager for all seasons. *Hospital and Health Services Administration, 36*, 365–381.

Hurley, A., Volicer, B., Hanrahan, P., Houde, S., & Volicer, L. (1992). Assessment of discomfort in advanced Alzheimer patients. *Research in Nursing and Health, 15*, 369–377.

Hurst, N. M., Meier, P. P., Engstrom, J. L., & Myatt, A. (2004). Mothers performing in-home measurement of milk intake during breastfeeding of their preterm infants: Maternal reactions and feeding outcomes. *Journal of Human Lactation, 20*, 178–187.

Hurt, H., Malmud, E., Brodsky, N. L., & Giannetta, J. (2001). Exposure to violence: Psychological and academic correlates in child witnesses. *Archives of Pediatric Adolescent Medicine, 155*, 1351–1356.

Husserl, E. (1962). *Ideas: General introduction to pure phenomenology*. New York: Macmillan.

Huston, C. J. (2001). Contemporary staffing-mix changes: The impact on post-operative pain management. *Pain Management Nursing, 2*(2), 65–72.

Hutchinson, S. (1986). Chemically dependent nurses: The trajectory toward self-annihilation. *Nursing Research, 34*(4), 196–201.

Hutchinson, S. A. (1993). Grounded theory: The method. In P. L. Munhall & C. O. Boyd (Eds.), *Nursing research: A qualitative perspective* (pp. 213–236). New York: National League for Nursing Press.

Huth, M. M., Broome, M. E., & Good, M. (2004). Imagery reduces children's post-operative pain. *Pain, 110*, 439–448.

Huth, M. M., & Moore, S. M. (1998). Prescriptive theory of acute pain management in infants and children. *Journal of the Society of Pediatric Nurses, 3*(1), 23–32.

Huttlinger, K. W. (1985). *Keeping adolescents healthy: Face-care*. Unpublished manuscript, University of Arizona, Tucson.

Hwang, S. S., Chang, V. T., & Kasimis, B. S. (2003). A comparison of three fatigue measures in veterans with cancer. *Cancer Investigation, 21*, 363–373.

Hwu, Y. -J., Coates, V. E., & Boore, J. R. P. (2001). The evolving concept of health in nursing research: 1988–1998. *Patient Education and Counseling, 42*, 105–114.

Hyer, K., Flaherty, E., Fairchild, S., Bottrell, M., Mezey, M., & Fulmer, T. (2001). *Geriatric Interdisciplinary Team Training: The GITT kit*. New York: New York University.

Hyer, K., Heinemann, G., & Fulmer, T. (2002). Teams skills scale. In G. Heinemann & A. Zeiss (Eds.), *Team performance in health care* (pp. 159–161). New York: Klewer.

Hyer, K., Skinner, J., Kane, R., Howe, N., Whitelaw, N., Wilson, N., et al. (2003). Using scripted video to assess interdisciplinary team effectiveness training outcomes. *Gerontology and Geriatrics Education, 24*(2), 75–91.

Hyland, M. E. (2003). A brief guide to the selection of quality of life instrument. *Health and Quality of Life Outcomes, 1*, 24. Retrieved from http://www.hqlo.com/content/1/1/24

Hymes, D. (1964). Introduction toward ethnographies of communication. *American Anthropologist*, 66, 6–56.

Hyun, S., & Park, H. A. (2002). Cross-mapping the ICNP with NANDA, HHCC, Omaha System and NIC for unified nursing language system development. *International Nursing Review, 49*, 99–110.

Iglesias, G. H. (1998). Role evolution of the mental health clinical nurse specialist in home care. *Clinical Nurse Specialist, 12*, 38–44.

Im, E.-O., Meleis, A., & Park, Y. (1999). A feminist critique of research on menopause experience of Korean women. *Research in Nursing & Health, 22*, 410–420.

Im, E., & Chee, W. (2003). Issues in internet research. *Nursing Outlook, 51*, 6–12.

Ingersoll, G. L. (1996). Evaluation research. *Nursing Administration Quarterly, 20*(4), 28–39.

Ingersoll, G. L, Cook, J., Fogel, S., Applegate, M., & Frank, B. (1999). The effect of patient-focused redesign on midlevel nurse managers' role responsibilities and work environment. *Journal of Nursing Administration, 29*(5), 21–27.

Ingersoll, G. L., Fisher, M., Ross, B., Soja, M., & Kidd, N. (2001). Employee response to major organizational redesign. *Applied Nursing Research, 14*, 18–28.

Ingersoll, G. L., Kirsch, J. C., Merck, S. E., & Lightfoot, J. (2000). Relationship of organizational culture and readiness for change to employee commitment to the organization. *Journal of Nursing Administration, 30*, 11–20.

Ingersoll, G. L., & Schmitt, M. (2003). Interdisciplinary collaboration, team functioning, and patient safety. In A. Page (Ed.), *Keeping patients safe. Transforming the work environment of nurses* (pp. 341–383). Washington, DC: National Academy Press.

Ingersoll, G. L., Spitzer, R., & Cook, J. A. (1999). Managed-care research, part 2. Researching the domain. *Journal of Nursing Administration, 29*(12), 10–16.

Ingersoll, G. L., Wagner, L., Merck, S. E., Kirsch, J. C., Hepworth, J. T., & Williams, M. (2002). Patient-focused redesign and employee perception of work environment. *Nursing Economics, 20*, 163–170.

Inouye, S. K., Acampora, D., Miller, R. L., Fulmer, T., Hurst, L. D., & Cooney, L. M., Jr. (1993a). The Yale Geriatric Care Program: A model of care to prevent functional decline in hospitalized elderly patients. *Journal of the American Geriatrics Society, 41*(12), 1345–1352.

Inouye, S. K., Bogardus, S. T., Jr., Charpentier, P. A., Leo-Summers, L., Acampora, D., Holford, T. R., et al. (1999). A multicomponent intervention to prevent delirium in hospitalized older patients. *New England Journal of Medicine, 340*, 669–676.

Inouye, S. K., Foreman, M. D., Mion, L. C., Katz, K. H., & Cooney, L. M., Jr. (2001). Nurses' recognition of delirium and its symptoms: Comparison of nurse and researcher ratings. *Archives of Internal Medicine, 161*, 2467–2473.

Inouye, S. K., Wagner, D. R., Acampora, D., Horwitz, R. I., Cooney, L. M., Jr., & Tinetii, M. E. (1993b). A controlled trial of a nursing-centered intervention in hospitalized elderly medical patients: The Yale Geriatric Care Program. *Journal of the American Geriatric Society, 41*(12), 1353–1360.

Insel, K. C., & Cole, L. (in review). Environmental cuing to improve medication adherence among older adults. *Applied Nursing Research.*

Institute of Medicine. (1985). *Committee to study the prevention of low birth weight. Preventing low birth weight.* Washington, DC: National Academy Press

Institute of Medicine. (1994). *Reducing risks for mental disorders—Frontiers for preventive intervention research.* Washington, DC: National Academy Press.

Institute of Medicine. (1995). *Health services research: Work force and education issues.* Washington, DC: National Academy Press.

Institute of Medicine. (1996). *Nursing staff in hospitals and nursing homes: Is it adequate?* Washington, DC: National Academy Press.

Institute of Medicine. (2000). *To err is human: Building a safer health system.* In L. T. Kohn, J. M. Corrigan, & M. S. Donaldson (Eds.). Washington, DC: National Academy Press.

Institute of Medicine. (2001). *Crossing the quality chasm: A new health system for the 21st century.* Washington, DC: National Academy Press.

Institute of Medicine. (2003a). *Keeping patients safe: Transforming the work environment of nurses.* Washington, DC: National Academy Press.

Institute of Medicine. (2003b). *Unequal treatment: Confronting racial and ethnic disparities in health care.* Washington, DC: National Academy Press.

International Association for the Study of Pain. (1979). Pain terms: A list with definitions and notes on usage. *Pain, 6*, 249.

International Council of Nurses. (1996). *The international classification for nursing practice: A unifying framework.* Geneva, Switzerland: ISO.

International Council of Nurses. (2002). *The international classification for nursing practice: A unifying framework.* Geneva, Switzerland: ICN Press.

Ireton-Jones, C. (1998). Nutrition support in home care. In M. Gottschlich, L. Matarese, & W. B. Saunders (Eds.), *Nutrition support: A clinical guide* (pp. 611–623). Philadelphia: Saunders.

Irvine, D., Brown, B., Crooks, D., Roberts, J., & Browne, G. (1991). Psychosocial adjustment in women with breast cancer. *Cancer, 67*, 1097–1117.

Irvine, D. M., & Evans, M. G. (1995). Job satisfaction and turnover among nurses: Integrating research findings across studies. *Nursing Research, 44*, 246–253.

Irvine, D. M., Vincent, L., Bubela, N., Thompson, L., & Graydon, J. (1991). A critical appraisal of the research literature investigating fatigue in the individual with cancer. *Cancer Nursing, 14*, 188–199.

Irwin, S. (2000). The experiences of the registered nurse caring for the person dying of cancer in a nursing home. *Collegian: Journal of the Royal College of Nursing, Australia, 7*(4), 30–34.

Isaacs, N. E., Kennedy, B., & Graham, J. D. (1995). Who's in the car? Passengers as potential interveners in alcohol-involved fatal crashes. *Accident: Analysis and Prevention, 27*, 159–165.

Iscoe, N. J., Williams, J. P., & Osoba, D. (1991). Prediction of psychosocial distress in patients with cancer. In D. Osoba (Ed.), *Effect of cancer on quality of life* (pp. 41–59). Boston: CRC Press.

Jacelon, C. (2003). Peer mentoring for tenure-track faculty. *Journal of Professional Nursing, 19*(6), 335–338.

Jacob, S. (1996). The grief experience of older women whose husbands had hospice care. *Journal of Advanced Nursing, 24*, 280–286.

Jacobs, B. B. (2001). Respect for human dignity: A central phenomenon to philosophically unite nursing theory and practice through consilience of knowledge. *Advances in Nursing Science, 24*(1), 17–35.

Jacobs, T., & Johnson, S. L. (2001). Sequential interactions in the parent-child communications of depressed father and depressed mothers. *Journal of Family Psychology, 15*, 38–52.

Jacobson, G. P., & Newman, C. W. (1990). The development of the Dizziness Handicap Inventory. *Archives of Otolaryngology and Head and Neck Surgery, 116*, 424–427.

Jacobson, S. P., & McGraw, H. M. (1983). *Nurses under stress*. New York: John Wiley.

James, K. (2000). A school based intervention to reduce television use decreased adiposity in children in grades 3 and 4. *EBN 3*(2), 43–45.

James, N., Burrage, J., & Smith, B. (2003). Commentary on: Scientific integrity: A review of the Institute of Medicine's (IOM) reports. *Nursing Outlook, 51*, 239–241.

Jameton, A. (1984). *Nursing practice: The ethical issues*. Englewood Cliffs, NJ: Prentice-Hall.

Jameton, A. (1993). Dilemmas of moral distress: Moral responsibility and nursing practice. *Clinical Issues in Perinatal and Women's Health Nursing, 4*, 542–551.

Jarboe, K. (2002). Treatment nonadherence: Causes and potential solutions. *Journal of the American Psychiatric Nurses Association, 8*, S18–S25.

Jarboe, K., & Schwartz, S. K. (1999). The relationship between medication noncompliance and cognitive function in patients with schizophrenia. *Journal of the American Psychiatric Nurses Association, 5*, S2–S8.

Jarosz, P. A., Lennie, T. A., Rowsey, P. J., & Metzger, B. L. (2001). Effect of genetic obesity on thermoregulatory activity responses to inversion of the light/dark cycle. *Biological Research for Nursing, 2*(4), 249–256.

Jarr, S., Henderson, M. L., & Henley, C. (1998). The registered nurse: Perceptions about advance directives. *Journal of Nursing Care Quality, 12*(6), 26–36.

Jarrett, N., & Payne, S. (1995). A selective review of the literature on nurse-patient communication: Has the patient's contribution been neglected? *Journal of Advanced Nursing, 22*, 72–78.

Jarrett, N., & Payne, S. (2000). Creating and maintaining 'optimism' in cancer care communication. *International Journal of Nursing Studies, 37*, 81–90.

Jarvis, W. R. (1996). Selected aspects of the socioeconomic impact of nosocomial infections: Morbidity, mortality, cost, and prevention. *Infection Control and Hospital Epidemiology, 17*, 552–557.

Jaycox, L. H., Stein, B. D., Kataoka, S. H., Wong, M., Fink, A., Escudero, P., et al. (2002). Violence exposure, posttraumatic stress disorder, and depressive symptoms among recent immigrant schoolchildren. *Journal of the American Academy of Child & Adolescent Psychiatry, 41*(9), 1104–1110.

Jeffers, B. R. (2001). Human biological materials in research: Ethical issues and the role of stewardship in minimizing research risks. *Advances in Nursing Science, 24*(2), 32–46.

Jemal, A., Thomas, A., Murray, T., & Thun, M. (2002). Cancer statistics. *CA: A Cancer Journal for Clinicians, 52*(1), 23–47, *52*(2), 119.

Jemmott, L. S. (2000). Saving our children: Strategies to empower African-American adolescents to reduce their risk for HIV infection. *Journal of The National Black Nurses Association, 11*(1), 4–14.

Jenkins, L. S., & Gortner, S. R. (1998). Correlates of self-efficacy expectation and prediction of walking behavior in cardiac surgery elders. *Annals of Behavioral Medicine, 20*(2), 99–103.

Jennings, C. P. (2000). Influencing health policy and the impact of health policy on nursing policy in the USA. In D. Hennessey & P. Spurgeon (Eds.), *Health policy and nursing* (pp. 42–47). New York: MacMillan Press.

Jennings, L., Harris, B., Gregoire, J., Merrin, J., Peyton, J., & Bray, L. (2002). The effect of a psychoeducational programme on knowledge of illness, insight and attitudes toward medication. *British Journal of Forensic Practice, 4*, 3–10.

Jerant, A. F., Azari, R., Martinez, C., & Nesbitt, T. S. (2003). A randomized trial of telenursing to reduce hospitalization for heart failure: Patient-centered outcomes and nursing indicators. *Home Health Care Services Quarterly, 22*(1), 1–20.

Jessen, J., Cardiello, F., & Baun, M. M. (1997). Avian companionship in alleviation of depression, loneliness, and low morale of older adults in skilled rehabilitation units. *Humans & Other Species, 8*(2), 16.

Jezewski, M. (1993). Culture brokering as a model for advocacy. *Nursing and Health Care, 14*, 78–85.

Jezewski, M. (1995). Staying connected: The core of facilitating health care for homeless people. *Public Health Nursing, 12*(3), 203–210.

Jezewski, M. A., & Finnel, D. S. (1998). The meaning of DNR status: Oncology nurses' experiences with patients and families. *Cancer Nursing, 21*(3), 212–221.

Jezewski, M. A., Meeker, M. A., & Schrader, M. (2003). Voices of oncology nurses: What is needed to assist patients with advance directives. *Cancer Nursing, 26*(2), 105–112.

Jirovec, M. M., Jenkins, J., Isenberg, M., & Baiardi, J. (1999). Urine control theory derived from Roy's conceptual framework. *Nursing Science Quarterly, 12*(3), 251–255.

Johnson, B., & Montgomery, P. (1999). Chronic mentally ill individuals reentering the community after hospitalization. Phase II: The urban experience. *Journal of Psychiatric Mental Health Nursing, 6*, 445–451.

Johnson, D. (1959). A philosophy of nursing. *Nursing Outlook, 7*, 198–200.

Johnson, D. (1997). Overview of severe mental illness. *Clinical Psychology Review, 17*(3), 247–257.

Johnson, D. A., & Fennerty, M. B. (2004). Heartburn severity underestimates erosive esophagitis severity in elderly patients with gastroesophageal reflux disease. *Gastroenterology, 126*(3), 660–664.

Johnson, D. E. (1961). The significance of nursing care. *American Journal of Nursing, 61*(11), 63–66.

Johnson, D. E. (1980). The behavioral system model for nursing. In J. P. Riehl & S. C. Roy (Eds.), *Conceptual models for nursing practice* (2nd ed.). New York: Appleton-Century-Crofts.

Johnson, J. (1996). The effects of nursing care guided by self-regulation theory on coping with radiation therapy. *Oncology Nursing Forum, 19*(1), 1041–1050.

Johnson, J., Fieler, V., Wlasowicz, G., Mitchell, M., & Jones, L. (1997). The effects of nursing care guided by self-regulation theory on coping with radiation therapy. *Oncology Nursing Forum, 24*(6), 1041–1050.

Johnson, J. A., & King, K. B. (1995). Influence of expectations about symptoms on delay in seeking treatment during a myocardial infarction. *American Journal of Critical Care, 4*, 29–35.

Johnson, J. E. (1984). Coping with elective surgery. In H. H. Werley & J. J. Fitzpatrick (Eds.), *Annual review of nursing research* (Vol. 2, pp. 107–132). New York: Springer Publishing.

Johnson, J. E. (1999). Self-regulation theory and coping with physical illness. *Research in Nursing and Health, 22*, 435–448.

Johnson, J. E., Rice, V. H., Fuller, S. S., & Endress, M. P. (1978). Sensory information, instruction in coping strategy and recovery from surgery. *Research in Nursing and Health, 1*, 4–17.

Johnson, J. G., Williams, J. B., Rabkin, J., Goetz, R. R., & Remien, R. H. (1995). Axis I psychiatric symptoms associated with HIV infection and personality disorder. *American Journal of Psychiatry, 152*, 551–554.

Johnson, M., Bulechek, G., Dochterman, J., Maas, M., & Moorhead, S. (2001). *Nursing diagnoses, outcomes, interventions: NANDA, NOC, and NIC linkages*. St. Louis, MO: Mosby.

Johnson, M. B. (1990). The holistic paradigm in nursing: The diffusion of an innovation. *Research in Nursing and Health, 13*, 129–139.

Johnson, M. R., & Maas, M. (Eds.). (1997). *Nursing outcomes classification (NOC)*. St. Louis, MO: Mosby.

Johnson, M., Maas, M., & Moorhead, S. (2000). *Nursing outcomes classification (NOC)* (2nd ed.). St. Louis, MO: Mosby.

Johnson, R. A. (2002). Commentary. Human-animal interaction research as an area of inquiry in nursing. *Western Journal of Nursing Research, 24*(6), 713–715.

Johnson, R. J., & Wolinsky, F. D. (1993). The structure of health status among older adults: Disease, disability, functional limitations and perceived health. *Journal of Health and Social Behavior, 34*, 105–121.

Johnson, S. (2000). From incontinence to confidence. *American Journal of Nursing, 100*(2), 69–75.

Johnson-Mekota, J., Maas, L. M., Burash, K. A., Gardner, S. E., Frantz, R. A., Specht, J. K. P., et al. (2001). A nursing application of telecommunication: Measurements of satisfaction for patients and providers. *Journal of Gerontological Nursing, 27*(1), 28–33.

Johnston, M., Langton, K., Haynes, B., & Mathieu, A. (1994). A critical appraisal of research on the effects of computer-based decision support systems on clinician performance and patient outcomes. *Annals of Internal Medicine, 120*, 135–142.

Johnston, T. (1990). Retirement: What happens to the marriage. *Issues in Mental Health Nursing, 11*, 347–359.

Joint Commission on Accreditation of Healthcare Organizations. (1997). *Oryx outcomes: The next evolution in accreditation*. Oakbrook Terrace, IL: Author.

Joint Commission on Accreditation of Healthcare Organizations. (2002). *Sentinel event policy and procedures* (revised July 2002). Retrieved from http://www.jcaho.org/accredited+organizations/hospitals/sentinel+events/index.htm

Joint Commission on Accreditation of Healthcare Organizations. (2003a). *The comprehensive accreditation manual for hospitals: The official handbook (CAMH)* (Automated version). Oakbrook Terrace, IL: Author.

Joint Commission on Accreditation of Healthcare Organizations. (2003b). *Performance measurement.* Retrieved November 23, 2003, from http://www.jcaho.org/pms/index.htm

Jones, A. (2000). Implementation of hospital care pathways for patients with schizophrenia. *Journal of Nursing Management*, 8, 215–225.

Jones, A. (2001). Hospital care pathways for patients with schizophrenia. *Journal of Clinical Nursing*, *10*, 58–69.

Jones, J. (2001). Telehealth: Can nursing values be preserved? *Nursing Leadership Forum*, *5*(2), 40, 51.

Jones, S. (1996). Mental illness as a brain disorder. *Archives of Psychiatric Nursing*, *12*, 1–2.

Jones, T. (2003). The virtues of nonreduction, even when reduction is a virtue. *Philosophical Forum*, *34*(2), 121–140.

Jones, T. H., Morawetz, R. B., Crowell, R. M., Marcoux, F. W., FitzGibbon, S. J., DeGirolami, U., et al. (1981). Thresholds of focal cerebral ischemia in awake monkeys. *Journal of Neurosurgery*, *54*(6), 773–782.

Jònsdòttir, H., & Baldursdòttir, L. (1998). The experience of people awaiting coronary artery bypass graft surgery: The Icelandic experience. *Journal of Advanced Nursing*, *27*, 68–74.

Jordan, E. A., Dugan, A. K., & Hardy, J. B. (1993). Injuries in children of adolescent mothers: Home safety education associated with decreased injury risk. *Pediatrics*, *91*, 481–487.

Jordan, S., Tunnicliffe, C., & Sykes, A. (2002). Minimizing side-effects: The clinical impact of nurse-administered 'side-effect' checklists. *Journal of Advanced Nursing*, *37*, 155–165.

Joyce, C. R. B., Hickey, A., McGee, H. M., & O'Boyle, C. A. (2003). A theory-based method for the evaluation of individual quality of life: The SEIQoL. *Quality of Life Research*, *12*, 275–280.

Jung, M. (2000). Lives of two Korean mothers of children with schizophrenia: An interpretive approach. *Journal of the American Psychiatric Nurses Association*, 6, 87–92.

Jungbauer, J., Wittmund, B., Dietrich, S., & Angermeyer, M. C. (2003). Subjective burden over 12 months in parents of patients with schizophrenia. *Archives of Psychiatric Nursing*, *17*, 126–134.

Kaas, M. J., Dahl, D., Dehn, D., & Frank, K. (1998). Barriers to prescriptive practice for psychiatric/mental health clinical nurse specialists. *Clinical Nurse Specialist*, *12*, 200–204.

Kabel, A., & Roberts, D. (2003). Professionals' perceptions of maintaining personhood in hospice care. *International Journal of Palliative Nursing*, *9*, 283–289.

Kane, R. L., Garrard, J., Skay, C. L., Radosevich, D. M., Buchanan, J. L., McDermott, S. M., et al. (1989). Effects of a geriatric nurse practitioner on process and outcome of nursing home care. *American Journal of Public Health*, *79*(9), 1271–1277.

Kannel, W. (1997). Cardiovascular risk factors in the elderly. *Coronary Artery Disease*, *8*, 565–575.

Kannus, P., Parkkari, J., Niemi, S., Pasanen, M., Palvanen, M., Jarvinen, M., et al. (2000). Prevention of hip fracture in elderly people with use of a hip protector. *New England Journal of Medicine*, *343*(21), 1506–1513.

Kant, I. (1991). *Critique of pure reason*. London: Dent. (Original work published 1781)

Kao, A. C., Nanda, A., Williams, C. S., & Tinetti, M. E. (2001). Validation of dizziness as a possible geriatric syndrome. *Journal of the American Geriatrics Society*, *49*(1), 72–75.

Kaplan, N. M. (1994). *Clinical hypertension*. Baltimore: Williams and Wilkins.

Kaplan, P. S., Bachorowski, J. A., & Zarlengo-Strouse, P. C. (1999). Child-directed speech produced by mothers with symptoms of depression fails to promote associative learning in 4-month-old infants. *Child Development*, *70*(3), 560–570.

Kaplun, A. (Ed.). (1992). *Health promotion and chronic illness: Discovering a new quality of life*. Copenhagen: World Health Organization.

Karasek, T., & Theorell, T. (1990). *Healthy work*. New York: Basic Books.

Karel, M. J., & Hinrichsen, G. (2000). Treatment of depression in late life: Psychotherapeutic interventions. *Clinical Psychology Review*, *20*, 707–729.

Karlsson, I., Berglin, E., & Larsson, P. A., (2000). Sense of coherence: Quality of life before and after coronary artery bypass surgery—a longitudinal study. *Journal of Advanced Nursing*, *31*(6), 1383–1392.

Kasper, C. E., Maxwell, L. C., & White, T. P. (1996). Alterations in skeletal muscle related to short-term impaired physical mobility. *Research in Nursing and Health*, *19*, 133–142.

Katon, W., Sullivan, M., & Walker, E. M. (2001). Medical symptoms without identified pathology: Relationship to psychiatric disorders, childhood and adult trauma, and personality traits. *Annals of Internal Medicine*, *134*, 917–925.

Katon, W. J. (2003). Clinical and health services relationships between major depression, depressive symptoms and general medical illness. *Biological Psychiatry*, *54*, 216–226.

Katz, D. A., Muehlenbruch, D. R., Brown, R., Fiore, M. C., & Baker, T. B. (2002). Effectiveness of a clinic-based strategy for implementing the AHRQ

Smoking Cessation Guideline in primary care. *Preventive Medicine, 35*, 293–302.

Katz, S. J., Kessler, R. C., Frank, R. G., Leaf, P., Lin E., & Edlund, M. (1997). The use of outpatient mental health services in the United States and Ontario: The impact of mental morbidity and perceived need for care. *American Journal of Public Health, 87*(7), 1136–1143.

Kaunonen, M., Tarkka, M., Paunonen, M., & Laippala, P. (1999). Grief and social support after the death of a spouse. *Journal of Advanced Nursing, 30*, 1304–1311.

Kavey, R. E., Daniels, S. R., Lauer, R. M., Atkins, D. L., Hayman, L. L., & Taubert, K. (2003). American Heart Association Guidelines for primary prevention of atherosclerotic cardiovascular disease beginning in childhood. *Circulation, 107*, 1562–1566.

Kayama, M., Zerwekh, J., Thornton, K. A., & Murashima, S. (2001). Japanese expert public health nurses empower clients with schizophrenia living in the community. *Journal of Psychosocial Nursing and Mental Health Services, 39*, 40–47.

Kayser-Jones, J. (2002). The experience of dying: An ethnographic nursing home study. *Gerontologist, 42*(Special issue III), 11–19.

Kayser-Jones, J., & Schell, E. (1997). The effect of staffing on the quality of care at mealtimes. *Nursing Outlook, 45*(2), 64–72.

Keane, A., Brennan, A., & Pickett, M. (2000). A typology of residential fire survivors' multidimensional needs. *Western Journal of Nursing Research, 22*, 263–285.

Kearney, M. H., York, R., & Deatrick, J. A. (2000). Effects of home visits to vulnerable young families. *Journal of Nursing Scholarship, 32*, 369–376.

Keddy, B., & Singleton, J. (1991). Women's perceptions of life after retirement. *Activities, Adaptation & Aging, 16*, 57–65.

Keitner, G. I., Archambault, R., Ryan, C. E., & Miller, I. W. (2003). Family therapy and chronic depression. *Journal of Clinical Psychology, 59*, 873–884.

Keitner, G. I., Miller, I. W., Epstein, N. B., Bishop, D. S., & Fruzzetti, A. E. (1987). Family functioning and the course of major depression. *Comprehensive Psychiatry, 1*, 54–64.

Keitner, G. I., Miller, I. W., & Ryan, C. E. (1993). The role of the family in major depressive illness. *Psychiatric Annals, 23*, 500–507.

Kellar, N., Martinez, J., Finis, N., Bolgar, A., & von Gunten, C. F. (1996). Characterization of an acute inpatient hospice unit in a U.S. teaching hospital. *Journal of Nursing Administration, 26*, 16–20.

Kelley, S. J., Whitley, D., Sipe, T. A., & Yorker, B. C. (2000). Psychological distress in grandmother kinship care providers: The role of resources, social support, and physical health. *Child Abuse and Neglect, 24*, 311–321.

Kelley, S. J., Yorker, B. C., Whitley, D., & Sipe, T. A. (2001). A multimodal intervention for grandparents raising grandchildren: Results of an exploratory study. *Child Welfare, 80*, 27–50.

Kelly, J. A., St. Lawrence, J. S., Diaz, Y. E., Stevenson, L. Y., Hauth, A. C., Brasfield, T. L., et al. (1991). HIV risk behavior reduction following intervention with key opinion leaders of population: An experimental analysis. *American Journal of Public Health, 82*(11), 168–171.

Kelly, K. J. (1964). An approach to the study of clinical inference in nursing: Utilization of "lens model" method to study the inferential process of the nurse. *Nursing Research, 1*, 319–322.

Keltner, N. L. (2000). Neuroreceptor function and psychopharmacologic response. *Issues in Mental Health Nursing, 21*, 31–50.

Kempe, A. (1994). *Forming alliances: Toward a grounded theory of the nurse caring for the family caregiver of a schizophrenic member.* Detroit, MI: Wayne State University.

Kempe, C. H., Silverman, F. N., Steele, B. F., Droegemuller, W., & Silver, H. K. (1962). The battered child syndrome. *Journal of the American Medical Association, 181*, 17–24.

Kempermann, G., & Gage, F. H. (1999). New nerve cells for the adult brain. *Scientific American, 265*, 48–53.

Kempermann, G., Kuhn, H. G., & Gage, F. H. (1997). More hippocampal neurons in adult mice living in an enriched environment. *Nature, 386*, 493–495.

Kempf, W. L. (2004). Soothing the burn: Management of gastroesophageal reflux disease. *Advance for Nurse Practitioners, 12*(1), 47–50.

Kemppainen, J. K. (2001). Predictors of quality of life in AIDS patients. *Journal of the Association of Nurses in AIDS Care, 12*(1), 61–70.

Kemppainen, J. K., Holzemer, W. L., Nokes, K., Eller, L. S., Corless, I. B., Bunch, E. H., et al. (2003). Self-care management of anxiety and fear in HIV disease. *Journal of the Association of Nurses in AIDS Care, 14*(2), 21–29.

Kendall, M. G., & Buckland, W. R. (1960). *A dictionary of statistical terms.* New York: Hofner.

Kendzierski, D., & Whitaker, D. (1997). The role of self-schema in linking intentions with behavior. *Personality and Social Psychology Bulletin, 23*, 139–147.

Kennedy, C. (1997). Childhood nutrition. In J. J. Fitzpatrick & J. Norbeck (Eds.), *Annual review of nursing research* (Vol. 16). New York: Springer Publishing.

Kennedy, M., Schepp, K., & O'Connor, F. (2000). Symptom self-management and relapse in schizophrenia. *Archives of Psychiatric Nursing, 14*, 266–275.

Kerem, E., Yatsiv, I., & Goitein, K. J. (1990). Effect of endotracheal suctioning on arterial blood gases in children. *Intensive Care Medicine, 16*(2), 95–99.

Kerlinger, F. N. (1986). *Foundations of behavioral research* (3rd ed.). New York: Holt, Rinehart & Winston.

Kerr, M. E. (1998). Nursing diagnosis. In J. J. Fitzpatrick (Ed.), *Encyclopedia of nursing research*. New York: Springer Publishing.

Kerr, M. E., Rudy, E. B., Brucia, J., & Stone, K. S. (1993). Head-injured adults: Recommendation for endotracheal suctioning. *Journal of Neuroscience Nursing, 25*, 86–91.

Kerr, S. M., Jowett, S. A., & Smith, L. N. (1996). Preventing sleep problems in infants: A randomized controlled trial. *Journal of Advanced Nursing, 24*, 938–942.

Kerstein, M. D., Gemmen, E., van Rijswijk, L., Lyder, C. H., Phillips, T., Xakellis, G., et al. (2001). *Disease Management and Health Outcomes, 9*, 651–663.

Kessler, R. C. (2003). Epidemiology of women and depression. *Journal of Affective Disorders, 74*, 5–13.

Kessler, R. C., Berglund, P., Demler, O., Jin, R., Koretz, D., Merikangas, K. R., et al. (2003). The epidemiology of major depressive disorder: Results from the National Comorbidity Survey Replication (NCS-R). *Journal of the American Medical Association, 289*(23), 3095–3105.

Kessler, R. C., McGonagle, K. A., Zhao, S., Nelson, C. B., Hughes, M., Eshleman, S., et al. (1994). Lifetime and 12 month prevalence of DSM-III-R psychiatric disorders in the United States. *Archives of General Psychiatry, 51*, 8–19.

Kessler, R. C., Walters, E. E., & Forthofer, M. S. (1998). The social consequences of psychiatric disorders, III: Probability of marital stability. *American Journal of Psychiatry, 155*(8), 1092–1096.

Ketefian, S. (1989). Moral reasoning and ethical practice in nursing. In J. J. Fitzpatrick & R. L. Taunton (Eds.), *Annual review of nursing research* (Vol. 7, pp. 173–195). New York: Springer Publishing.

Ketterer, M. W., Huffman, J., Lumley, M. A., Wassef, S., Gray, L., Kenyon, L., et al. (1998). Five-year follow-up for adverse outcomes in males with at least minimally positive angiograms: Importance of "denial" in assessing psychosocial risk factors. *Journal of Psychosomatic Research, 44*, 241–250.

Kety, S. S. (1950). Blood flow and metabolism of the human brain in health and disease. *Transactions & Studies of the College of Physicians of Philadelphia, 18*(3), 103–108.

Kety, S. S., & Schmidt, C. F. (1948). The nitrous oxide method for the quantitative determination of cerebral blood flow in man: Theory, procedure and normal values. *Journal of Clinical Investigation, 27*, 476–483.

Khatri, P., Babyak, M., Clancy, C., Davis, R., Croughwell, N., Newman, M., et al. (1999). Perception of cognitive function in older adults following coronary artery bypass surgery. *Health Psychology, 18*(3), 301–306.

Khatri, P., Babyak, M., Croughwell, N., Davis, R., White, W. D., Newman, M. F., et al. (2001). Temperature during coronary artery bypass surgery affects quality of life. *Annals of Thoracic Surgery, 71*, 110–116.

Kiely, M., Byers, L. A., Greenwood, R., Carroll, E., & Carroll, D. (1998). Thermodilution measurement of cardiac output in patients with low output: Room-temperature versus iced injectate. *American Journal of Critical Care, 7*(6), 436–438.

Kim, H. S. (1994). Action science as an approach to develop knowledge for nursing practice. *Nursing Science Quarterly, 7*, 134–138.

Kim, H., Garvin, B. J., & Moser, D. K. (1999). Stress during mechanical ventilation: Benefit of having concrete objective information before cardiac surgery. *American Journal of Critical Care*, 8, 118–126.

Kim, M. J., McFarland, G. K., & McLane, A. M. (1995). *Pocket guide to nursing diagnoses* (2nd ed.). St. Louis, MO: Mosby.

Kim, M. T., Juon, H. S., Hill, M. N., Post, W., & Kim, K. B. (2001). Cardiovascular disease risk factors in Korean American elderly. *Western Journal of Nursing Research, 23*(3), 269–282.

Kim, S., & Feldman, D. (2000). Working in retirement: The antecedents of bridge employment and its consequences for quality of life in retirement. *Academy of Management Journal, 43*, 1195–1210. Retrieved October 23, 2003, from http://proquest.umi.com/pqdweb?index

Kindig, D. A. (1997). *Purchasing population health: Paying for results*. Ann Arbor: University of Michigan Press.

Kindig, D., & Stoddart, G. (2003). What is population health? [Electronic version]. *American Journal of Public Health, 93*(3), 380–383.

King, I. M. (1981). *A theory for nursing: General concepts of human behavior*. New York: Wiley.

King, I. M. (1992). King's theory of goal attainment. *Nursing Science Quarterly, 5*(1), 19–26.

Kinsey, A. C., Pomeroy, W. B., & Martin, C. E. (1948). *Sexual behavior in the human male.* Philadelphia: Saunders.

Kinsey, A. C., Pomeroy, W. B., Martin, C. E., & Gebhard, P. (1953). *Sexual behavior in the human female.* Philadelphia: Saunders.

Kirby, D. (2002). *Do abstinence-only programs delay the initiation of sex among young people and reduce teen pregnancy.* Retrieved from http://www.teenpregnancy.org/resources/data/pdf/abstinence_eval.pdf

Kirk, R. (1997). *Managing outcomes, process, and cost in a managed care environment.* Gaithersburg, MD: Aspen.

Kirkpatrick, H., Landeen, J., Woodside, H., & Byrne, C. (2001). How people with schizophrenia build their hope. *Journal of Psychosocial Nursing and Mental Health Services, 39,* 46–53.

Kirksey, K., Goodroad, B., Kemppainen, J., Holzemer, W., Bunch, E., Corless, I., et al. (2002). Complementary therapy use in persons with HIV/AIDS. *Journal of Holistic Nursing, 20*(3), 264–278.

Kirmayer, L. J., & Robbins, J. M. (1996). Patients who somatize in primary care: A longitudinal study of cognitive and social characteristics. *Psychological Medicine, 26,* 937–951.

Kish, L. (1965). *Survey sampling.* New York: Wiley.

Kitchen, J., & Rouch, J. (1990). Life-care resident preferences: A survey of the decision-making process to enter a CCRC. In R. D. Chellis & P. J. Grayson (Eds.), *Life care: A long term solution* (pp. 49–60). Lexington, MA: Lexington.

Klauber, J. (1996). Arzneiverordnungsreport. In U. Schwabe & D. Paffrath (Eds.), Gustav Fisher Verlag (pp. 497). Stuttgart.

Klein, D., & White, J. (1996). *Family theories: An introduction.* Thousand Oaks, CA: Sage.

Kleinman, A. (1988). *The illness narratives: Suffering, healing and the human condition.* New York: Basic Books.

Kleinpell, R. M., & Ferrans, C. E. (1998). Factors influencing intensive care unit survival for critically ill elderly patients. *Heart and Lung, 27*(5), 337–343.

Knafl, K. A., Breitmayer, B., Gallo, A., & Zoeller, L. (1996). Family responses to childhood chronic illness: Description of management styles. *Journal of Pediatric Nursing, 11,* 315–326.

Knapp, T. R., & Brown, J. K. (1995). Ten measurement commandments that often should be broken. *Research in Nursing and Health, 18,* 465–469.

Knaus, W., Draper, E., Wagner, D., & Zimmerman, J. (1986). An evaluation of outcomes from intensive care in major medical centers. *Annals of Internal Medicine, 104,* 410–418.

Knight, D. C., & Eden, J. A. (1996). A review of the clinical effects of phytoestrogens. *Obstetrics and Gynecology, 87*(5 Pt. 2), 897–904.

Knowlton, D. (1996). Stages of managed-care evolution. *Endocrine Practice, 2*(6), 425–428.

Knuth, J. L., & Smith, S. E. (1984). Sexuality from the perspective of the visually impaired. *Siecus Report,* 12.

Kockler, M., & Heun, R. (2002). Gender differences of depressive symptoms in depressed and nondepressed elderly persons. *International Journal of Geriatric Psychiatry, 17,* 65–72.

Kohlberg, L. (1978). The cognitive-developmental approach to moral education. In P. Scharf (Ed.), *Readings in moral education* (pp. 36–51). Minneapolis, MN: Winston Press.

Kohn, L. T., Corrigan, J. M., & Donaldson, M. S. (Eds.). (2000). Institute of Medicine Committee on Quality of Health Care in America. *To err is human: Building a safer health system.* Washington, DC: National Academy Press.

Koistinen, P. (1996). How nurses experience a patient's death. *Hototiede* (Finland), 8(1), 11–19.

Koivisto, K., Janhonen, S., & Vaisanen, L. (2003). Patients' experiences of psychosis in an inpatient setting. *Journal of Psychiatric Mental Health Nursing, 10,* 221–229.

Kolata, G. (2003, September 28). Bone diagnosis gives new data but no certain answers. *New York Times,* pp. A1, A28.

Kolb, D. (1982). *Experiential learning.* Englewood Cliffs, NJ: Prentice Hall.

Kolcaba, K. (1991). A taxonomic structure for the concept comfort. *Image: Journal of Nursing Scholarship, 23*(4), 237–239.

Kolcaba, K. (1994). A theory of holistic comfort for nursing. *Journal of Advanced Nursing, 19,* 1178–1184.

Kolcaba, K. (2001). Evolution of the mid range theory of comfort for outcomes research. *Nursing Outlook,* 49(2), 86–92.

Kolcaba, K. (2003). *Comfort theory and practice.* New York: Springer Publishing.

Kolcaba, K. (1997, updated continuously). The comfort line. Retrieved from http://www.uakron.edu/comfort/

Kolcaba, K., & Kolcaba, R. (1991). An analysis of the concept of comfort. *Journal of Advanced Nursing, 16,* 1301–1310.

Kongable, L., Stolley, J., & Buckwalter, K. C. (1990). Pet therapy for Alzheimer's patients: A survey. *Long Term Care Administration, 18*(3), 17–21.

Kongsvedt, P. R. (1995). *Essentials of managed health care*. Rockville, MD: Aspen.

Koniak-Griffin, D., Verzemnieks, I. L., Anderson, N. L., Brecht, M. L., Lesser, J., Kim, S., et al. (2003). Nurse visitation for adolescent mothers: Two-year infant health and maternal outcomes. *Nursing Research, 52*, 127–136.

Koocher, G. P. (1985). Psychosocial care of the child cured of cancer. *Pediatric Nursing, 11*, 91–93.

Koons, B. A., Burrow, J. D., Morash, M., & Bynum. T. (1997, October). Expert offender perceptions of program elements linked to successful outcomes for incarcerated women. *Crime and Delinquency, 43*(4), 512–532.

Kosowski, M. M., & Roberts, V. W. (2003). When protocols are not enough: Intuitive decision making by novice nurse practitioners. *Journal of Holistic Nursing, 21*(1), 52–72.

Kotechi, C. (2002). Baccalaureate nursing students' communication process in the clinical setting. *Journal of Nursing Education, 41*, 61–68.

Kotilainen, H. R., & Keroack, M. A. (1997). Cost analysis and clinical impact of weekly ventilator circuit changes in patients in intensive care unit. *American Journal of Infection Control, 25*, 117–120.

Kovach, C. R. (2000). Sensoristasis and imbalance in persons with dementia. *Journal of Nursing Scholarship, 32*(4), 379–384.

Kovner, C., & Gergen, P. J. (1998). Nurse staffing levels and adverse events following surgery in U.S. hospitals. *Image: Journal of Nursing Scholarship, 30*(4), 315–321.

Kovner, C., Jones, C., Zhan, C., Gergen, P. J., & Basu, J. (2002). Nurse staffing and postsurgical adverse events: An analysis of administrative data from a sample of U.S. hospitals, 1990–1996. *Health Service Research, 37*, 611–629.

Kozuki, Y., & Froelicher, E. S. (2003). Lack of awareness and nonadherence in schizophrenia. *Western Journal of Nursing Research, 25*, 57–74.

Kramer, B. J., & Lambert, J. D. (1999). Caregiving as a life course transition among older husbands. *Gerontologist, 39*, 658–667.

Kramer, B., & Thompson, E. (2002). *Men as caregivers*. New York: Springer Publishing.

Kramer, M., & Hafner, L. P. (1989). Shared values: Impact on staff nurse job satisfaction and perceived productivity. *Nursing Research, 38*, 172–177.

Kramer, M. S. (1998). Socioeconomic determinants of intrauterine growth retardation. *European Journal of Clinical Nutrition, 52*(Suppl. 1), S29–S33.

Kraus, J. B. (2000). Protecting the legacy: The nurse-patient relationship and thetherapeutic alliance. *Archives of Psychiatric Nursing, 14*, 49–50.

Krauskopf, J., Borwn, R., Tokarz, K., & Bogutz, A. (1993). *Elderlaw: Advocacy for the aging*. St. Paul: West Publishing Co.

Krebs, N. F., & Jacobson, M. S. (2003). American Academy of Pediatrics Committee on Nutrition. Prevention of pediatric overweight and obesity. *Pediatrics, 112*, 424–430.

Kressig, R. W., Wolf, S. L., Sattin, R. W., O'Grady, M., Greenspan, A., Curns, A., et al. (2001). Associations of demographic, functional, and behavioral characteristics with activity-related fear of falling among older adults transitioning to frailty. *Journal of the American Geriatrics Society, 49*, 1456–1462.

Krissovich, M. (1998). The financial side of continence promotion. *Geriatric Nursing, 19*(2), 91–98.

Krissovich, M., & Safran, R. (1997). Urinary incontinence in adults. *Lippincott's Primary Care Practice, 1*(4), 361–381.

Krueger, J. C. (1978). Utilization of nursing research: The planning process. *Journal of Nursing Administration*, 8(1), 6–9.

Kruijver, I., Kerkstra, A., Bensing, J., & van de Wiel, H. (2000). Nurse-patient communication in cancer care: A review of the literature. *Cancer Nursing, 32*(1), 20–31.

Kruijver, I., Kerkstra, A., Bensing, J., & van de Wiel, H. (2001). Communication skills of nurses during interactions with simulated cancer patients. *Journal of Advanced Nursing, 34*, 772–779.

Kuhn, T. S. (1970). *The structure of the scientific revolution* (2nd ed.). Chicago: University of Chicago Press.

Kunyk, D., & Olson, J. K. (2001). Clarification of the conceptualizations of empathy. *Journal of Advanced Nursing, 35*(3), 317–325.

Kupelian, P., Elshaikh, M., Reddy, C., Zippe, C., & Klein, E. (2002). Comparison of the efficacy of local therapies for localized prostate cancer in the prostate-specific antigen era: A large single-institution experience with radical prostectomy and external-beam radiotherapy. *Journal of Clinical Oncology, 20*(16), 3376–3385.

Kupperstein, L. (1971). Treatment and rehabilitation of delinquent youth: Some socio-cultural considerations. *Acta-Criminologica, 4*, 11–111.

Kurnat, E., & Moore, C. (1999). The impact of a chronic condition on the families of children with asthma. *Pediatric Nursing, 25*(4), 288–292.

Kurup, V. P., Alenius, H., Kelly, K. J., Castillo, L., & Fink, J. N. (1996). A two-dimensional electrophoretic analysis of latex peptides reacting with IgE and IgG antibodies from patients with latex allergy. *International Archives of Allergy & Immunology, 109*, 58–67.

Kusmer, K. (2002). *Down and out, on the road.* New York: Oxford University Press.

Kuthy, S., Grap, M. J., Penn, L., & Henderson, V. (1995). After the party's over: Evaluation of a drinking and driving prevention program. *Journal of Neuroscience Nursing, 27*, 273–277.

Labov, W. (1972). *Language in the inner city: Studies in the Black English vernacular.* Philadelphia: University of Pennsylvania Press.

Labovitz, S. (1970). The nonutility of significance tests: The significance of tests of significance reconsidered. *Pacific Sociological Review, 13*, 141–148.

Lachs, M. S., Williams, C., O'Brien, S., Hurst, L., & Horwitz, R. I. (1997). Risk factors for reported elder abuse and neglect: A nine-year observational cohort study. *Gerontologist, 37*(4), 469–474.

Lackey, M. A., & Barth, J. (2003). Gastroesophageal reflux disease: A dental concern. *General Dentistry, 1*(3), 250–254.

Ladd, R. E., Pasquarelle, L., & Smith, S. (2000). What to do when the end is near: Ethical issues in home health nursing. *Public Health Nursing, 17*(2), 103–110.

Laffrey, S. C. (1986). Development of a health conception scale. *Research in Nursing and Health, 9*, 107–113.

Laidlaw, J. K., Beeken, J. E., Whitney, F. W., & Reyes, A. A. (1999). Contracting with outpatient hemodialysis patients to improve adherence to treatment. *American Nephrology Nurses Association Journal, 26*, 37–40.

Lakatos, I. (1968). *The problem of inductive logic.* Amsterdam: North Holland.

Lakey, J. R., Singh, B., Warnock, G. L., Elliott, J. F., & Rajotte, R. V. (1995). Long-term survival of syngeneic islet grafts in BCG-treated diabetic NOD mice can be reversed by cyclophosphamide. *Transplantation, 59*, 1751–1753.

Lamaze International. (2002). Position paper—Lamaze for the 21st century. *Journal of Perinatal Education, 11*(1), x–xii.

Lambert, H. C., Gisel, E. G., Groher, M. E., & Wood-Dauphinee, S. (2003). McGill Ingestive Skills Assessment (MISA), Development and first field test of an evaluation of functional ingestive skills of elderly persons. *Dysphagia, 18*, 101–113.

Lambert, L. T. (2001). Identification and management of schizophrenia in childhood. *Journal of Child and Adolescent Psychiatric Nursing, 14*, 73–80.

La Monica, E. L., Oberst, M. T., Madea, A. R., & Wolf, R. M. (1986). Development of a patient satisfaction scale. *Research in Nursing and Health,* 9, 43–50.

Lamphear, B. P., Deitrich, K., Auinger, P., & Cox, C. (2000). Cognitive deficits associated with blood lead concentrations < 10 microg/dL in US children and adolescents. *Public Health Reports, 115*, 521–529.

Landefeld, C., Palmer, R., Kresevic, D., Fortinsky, R., & Kowal, J. (1995). A randomized trial of care in a hospital medical unit especially designed to improve the functional outcomes of acutely ill older patients. *New England Journal of Medicine, 332*(20), 1338–1344.

Landgridge, D. W. (1992). *Classification: Its kinds, elements, systems and applications.* New York: Bowker-Saur.

Landis, C. A., Frey, C. A., Lentz, M. J., Rothermel, J., Buchwald, D., & Shaver, J. L. (2003). Self-reported sleep quality and fatigue correlates with actigraphy in midlife women with fibromyalgia. *Nursing Research, 52*, 140–147.

Landrigan, P. J. (2000). Pediatric lead poisoning: Is there a threshold? *Public Health Reports, 115*, 530–531.

Lane, W. G., Rubin, D. M., Monteith, R., & Christian, C. W. (2002). Racial differences in the evaluation of pediatric fractures for physical abuse. *Journal of the American Medical Association, 288*(13), 1603–1609.

Lange, J. C. W., & Polifroni, E. C. (2000). Nurses and assistive personnel: Do patients know the difference? *Journal of Nursing Administration, 30*(11), 512–514.

Lange, L. (1996). Representation of everyday clinical nursing language in UMLS and SNOMED. In J. J. Cimino (Ed.), *Proceedings of the American Medical Informatics Association, Fall Symposium* (pp. 140–144). Philadelphia: Hanley & Belfus.

Langer, S., & Abrams, J., & Syrjala, K. (2003). Caregiver and patient marital satisfaction and affect following hematopoietic stem cell transplantation: A prospective, longitudinal investigation. *Psycho-Oncology, 12*(3), 239–253.

Langmore, S. E., Kimberly, K. A., Skarupski, K. A., Park, P. S., & Fries, B. (2002). Predictors of aspiration pneumonia in nursing home residents. *Dysphagia, 17*, 298–307.

Langmore, S. E., Terpenning, M. S., Schork, A., Chen, Y., Murray, J. T., Lopatin, D., et al. (1998). Predictors of aspiration pneumonia: How important is dysphagia? *Dysphagia, 13*(2), 69–81.

Larcombe, I., Mott, M., & Hunt, L. (2002). Lifestyle behaviours of young adult survivors of childhood cancer. *British Journal of Cancer, 87*(11), 1204–1209.

Lareau, S., Carrieri-Kohlman, V., Janson-Bjerklie, S., & Roos, P. (1994). Development and testing of the pulmonary functional status and dyspnea questionnaire (PFSDQ). *Heart & Lung: Journal of Acute & Critical Care, 23*, 242–250.

Lareau, S., Meek, P., Press, D., Anholm, J., & Roos, P. (1999). Dyspnea in patients with chronic obstructive pulmonary disease: Does dyspnea worsen longitudinally in the presence of declining lung function? *Heart & Lung: Journal of Acute & Critical Care, 28*, 65–73.

Larew, B. L. (1998). Health care provider's attitudes and practices regarding the purpose and use of advance directives in a military health care setting. *Report of Uniformed Services University of the Health Sciences, 1*.

LaRocco, J., House, J., & French, J. (1980). Social support, occupational stress, and health. *Journal of Health and Social Behavior, 21*, 202–218.

LaRosa, J. C., He, J., & Vupputuri, S. (1999). Effect of statins on risk of coronary disease: A meta-analysis of randomized controlled trials. *Journal of the American Medical Association, 282*, 2340–2346.

Larson, L. (2002, April). A new attitude: Changing organizational culture. *Trustee*, 8–14.

Laschinger, H. K. S., Finegan, J., Shamian, J., & Almost, J. (2001). Testing Karasek's demand-control model in restructured healthcare settings: Effects of job strain on staff nurses' quality of work life. *Journal of Nursing Administration, 31*, 233–243.

Lashley, F. (1998). *Clinical genetics in nursing practice* (2nd ed.). New York: Springer Publishing.

LaSorte, M. (1972). Replication as a verification technique in survey research: A paradigm. *Sociological Quarterly, 13*, 218–227.

Lasry, J. (1991). Women's sexuality following breast cancer. In D. Osoba (Ed.), *Effect of cancer on quality of life* (pp. 215–227). Boston: CRC Press.

Lassen, N. A., & Ingvar, D. H. (1972). Radioisotopic assessment of regional cerebral blood flow. *Progressive Nuclear Medicine, 1*, 376–409.

Lasser, R. A., & Sunderland, T. (1998). Newer psychotropic medication use in nursing home residents. *Journal of the American Geriatrics Society, 46*, 202–207.

Latham, N. K., Bennett, D. A., Stretton, C. M., & Anderson, C. S. (2004). Systematic review of progressive resistance strength training in older adults. *Journals of Gerontology: Biological Sciences and Medical Sciences, 59*, M48–M61.

Lau, C., Smith, E., & Schandler, R. (2003). Coordination of suck-swallow respiration in preterm infants. *Acta Paediatrica, 92*, 721–727.

Lauterbach, S. (1993). In another world: A phenomenological perspective and discovery of meaning in mothers' experience with death of a wished-for baby: Doing phenomenology. In P. L. Munhall & C. O. Boyd (Eds.), *Nursing research: A qualitative perspective* (pp. 133–179). New York: NLN Press.

Lauver, L. S. (1996). Benchmarking: Improving outcomes for the congestive heart patient population. *Journal of Nursing Care Quality, 10*(3), 7–11.

Lavie, C., & Milani, R. V. (1995). Effects of cardiac rehabilitation programs on exercise capacity, coronary risk factors, behavioral characteristics, and quality of life in a large elderly cohort. *American Journal of Cardiology, 76*, 177–179.

Lawrence, R., & Lawrence, S. (1987/88). The nurse and job related stress: Responses, Rx, and self-dependency. *Nursing Forum, 23*, 45–51.

Lawrence, R. H., & Jette, A. M. (1996). Disentangling the disablement process. *Journals of Gerontology: Psychology and Social Science, 51*, S173–S182.

Lawson, J., Fitzgerald, J., Birchall, J., Aldren, C. P., & Kenny, R. A. (1999). Diagnosis of geriatric patients with severe dizziness. *Journal of the American Geriatrics Society, 47*(1), 12–17.

Lawson, M. T. (2002). Nurse practitioner and physician communication styles. *Applied Nursing Research, 15*(2), 60–66.

Lawson, S., & Adamson, H. (1995). Informed consent readability: Subject understanding of 15 common consent form phrases. *Institutional Review Board, 17*(5–6), 16–19.

Lawton, M. P. (1991). A multidimensional view of quality of life in frail elders. In J. E. Birren, J. W. Rowe, & D. E. Deutchman (Eds.), *The concept and measurement of quality of life in the frail and elderly* (pp. 4–27). San Diego, CA: Academic Press.

Lazarus, R. (1966). *Psychological stress and the coping process*. New York: McGraw-Hill Book.

Lazarus, R. S., & Folkman, S. (1984). *Stress, appraisal, and coping*. New York: Springer.

Lea, D. (2003). How genetics changes daily practice. *Nursing Management, 34*(11), 19–25.

Lea, D. H., Jenkins, J., & Fiancomano, L. (1998). *Genetics in clinical practice: New directions for nursing and health care*. Sudbury, MA: Jones & Bartlett Publishers.

Lederman, R. P. (1995a). Part I: Relationship of anxiety, stress, and psychosocial development to reproductive health. *Behavioral Medicine, 21*, 110–112.

Lederman, R. P. (1995b). Part II: Treatment strategies for anxiety, stress, and developmental conflict during reproduction. *Behavioral Medicine, 21*, 113–122.

Lederman, R. P. (1996). *Psychosocial adaptation in pregnancy: Assessment of seven dimensions of maternal development*. New York: Springer.

Lederman, R. P., Weis, K., Brandon, J., & Mian, T. (2002, April). *Relationship of maternal prenatal adaptation and family functioning to pregnancy outcomes.* Poster presentation at the annual meeting of the Society of Behavioral Medicine, Washington, DC.

Lee, G., & Shehan, C. (1989). Retirement and marital satisfaction. *Journal of Gerontology: Social Sciences, 44,* S226–S230.

Lee, G. R., Willetts, M. C., & Seccombe, K. (1998). Widowhood and depression: Gender differences. *Research on Aging, 20,* 611–630.

Lee, K. (2003). Maternal coping skills as a moderator between depression and stressful life events: Effects on children's behavioral problems in an intervention program. *Journal of Child and Family Studies, 12,* 425–437.

Lee, K., & Carrieri, V. (2003). *Research Center for Symptom Management.* Retrieved from http://nurseweb.ucsf.edu/www/rcsm.htm

Lee, K. A. (2001). Sleep and fatigue. In *Annual review of nursing research* (Vol. 19, pp. 249–273). New York: Springer Publishing.

Lee, S. (2001). Differences among women who experience premenstrual syndrome. In J. C. Chrisler (Ed.), *A menstrual cycle: Women's reproductive health across the lifespan* (pp. 74–85). Avon, CT: Society for Menstrual Cycle Research.

Lee, S., Colditz, G. C., Berkman, L., & Kawachi, I. (2003). Caregiving to children and grandchildren and risk of coronary heart disease in women. *American Journal of Public Health, 93,* 1939–1944.

Lee, S. S., Gerberich, S. G., Waller, L. A., Anderson, A., & McGovern, P. (1999). Work related assault injuries among nurses. *Epidemiology, 10*(6), 685–691.

Lee, T., & Chu, T. (2001). The Chinese experience of male infertility. *Western Journal of Nursing Research, 23,* 714–726.

LeFort, S. M. (1993). The statistical versus clinical significance debate. *Image: Journal of Nursing Scholarship, 25,* 57–62.

LeFort, S. M., Gray-Donald, K., Rowat, K. M., & Jeans, M. E. (1998). Randomized controlled trial of a community-based psychoeducation program for the self-management of chronic pain. *Pain, 74*(2–3), 297–306.

Lehmann, L., Padilla, M., Clark, S., & Loucks, S. (1983). Training personnel in the prevention and management of violent behavior. *Hospital & Community Psychiatry, 34*(1), 40–43.

Lehna, C. (2001). A needs assessment for an end-of-life curriculum for advanced practice nursing students. *Internet Journal of Advanced Nursing Practice, 5*(2), 10.

Lehto, R. H., & Cimprich, B. (1999). Anxiety and directed attention in women awaiting breast cancer surgery. *Oncology Nursing Forum, 26,* 767–772.

Leidy, N. (1994). Functional status and the forward progress of merry-go-rounds: Toward a coherent analytical framework. *Nursing Research, 43,* 196–202.

Leigh, W. A., Lillie-Blanton, M., Martinez, R. M., & Collins, K. S. (1999). Managed care in three states: Experiences of low-income African Americans and Hispanics. *Inquiry, 36,* 318–331.

Leighton, A. H. (2000). Community mental health and information under load. *Community Mental Health Journal, 36*(1), 77–95.

Leininger, M. M. (1985a). Transcultural care diversity and universality: A theory of nursing. *Nursing and Health Care, 6,* 209–212.

Leininger, M. M. (1985b). *Qualitative research methods in nursing.* New York: Grune and Stratton.

Leininger, M. M. (1995). *Transcultural nursing: Concepts, theories, research and practices* (2nd ed.). New York: McGraw-Hill.

Leininger, M. M. (2001a). *Culture care diversity and universality: A theory of nursing.* Sudbury, MA: Jones and Bartlett.

Leininger, M. M. (2001b). A mini journey into transcultural nursing with its founder. *Nebraska Nurse, 34*(2), 16–17.

Leipzig, R., Hyer, K., Wallenstein, S., Vezina, M., Fairchild, S., Cassel, C., et al. (2002). Attitudes toward working on interdisciplinary health care teams: A comparison by disciplines. *Journal of the American Geriatrics Society, 50,* 1141–1148.

Lekan-Rutledge, D., Palmer, M., & Belyea, M. (1998). In their own words: Nursing assistants' perceptions of barriers to implementation of prompted voiding in long-term care. *Gerontologist, 38*(3), 370–378.

Lengerich, A. D. (1976). William Farr: Founder of modern concepts of surveillance. *International Journal of Epidemiology, 5,* 13–18.

Lenz, E. R., & Pugh, L. (2003). The theory of unpleasant symptoms. In M. J. Smith & P. Liehr (Eds.). *Middle range theory for nursing* (pp. 69–90). New York: Springer.

Lenz, E. R., Pugh, L. C., Milligan, R., Gift, A., & Suppe, F. (1997). The middle-range theory of unpleasant symptoms: An update. *Advances in Nursing Science, 19*(3), 14–27.

Lenz, E. R., Suppe, F., Gift, A. G., Pugh, L. C., & Milligan, R. A. (1995). Collaborative development of middle-range nursing theories: Toward a theory of unpleasant symptoms. *Advances in Nursing Science, 17*(3), 1–13.

Lesser, J., Oakes, R., & Koniak-Griffin, D. (2003). Vulnerable adolescent mothers' perceptions of maternal role and HIV risk. *Health Care for Women International, 24,* 513–528.

Letcher, D. C., & Yancey, N. R. (2004). Witnessing change with aspiring nurses: A human becoming teaching-learning process in nursing education. *Nursing Science Quarterly, 17*(1), 36–41.

Levine, C. (1998). *Rough crossings: Family caregivers' addressees through the health care system*. New York: United Hospital Fund.

Lewandowski, L., & Kositsky, A. (1983). Research priorities for critical care nursing: A study by the American Association of Critical Care Nurses. *Heart and Lung: Journal of Critical Care, 12*, 35–44.

Lewis, D. J., & Robinson, J. A. (1986). Assessment of coping strategies of ICU nurses in response to stress. *Critical Care Nurse, 6*(6), 38–43.

Lewis, E. N. (1989). *Manual of patient classification: Systems and techniques for practical application*. Rockville, MD: Aspen.

Lewis, F. M., & Hammond, M. A. (1996). The father's and mother's and adolescent's functioning with breast cancer. *Family Relations, 45*, 456–465.

Lewis, R. J., & Janda, L. H. (1988). The relationship between adult sexual adjustment and childhood experiences regarding exposure to nudity, sleeping in the parental bed, and parental attitudes toward sexuality. *Archives of Sexual Behavior, 17*, 349–362.

Lichtig, L., Knauf, R., & Milholland, K. (1999). Some impacts of nursing on acute care hospital outcomes. *Journal of Nursing Administration, 29*(2), 25–33.

Liehr, P., & Smith, M. J. (1999). Middle range theory: Spinning research and practice to create knowledge for the new millennium. *Advances in Nursing Science, 21*(4), 81–91.

Lifshitz, F. (1995). *Childhood nutrition*. Boca Raton, FL: CRC Press.

Light, D. W. (1991). Professionalism as a countervailing power. *Journal of Health Politics, Policy & Law, 16*, 499–506.

Lim, U., & Cassano, P. A. (2002). Homocysteine and blood pressure in the Third National Health and Nutrition Examination Survey, 1988–1994. *American Journal of Epidemiology, 156*(12), 1105–1113.

Lim, Y. M., & Ahn, Y. (2003). Burden of family caregivers with schizophrenic patients in Korea. *Applied Nursing Research, 16*, 110–117.

Lim, Y. W., Andersen, R., Leake, B., Cunningham, W., & Gelberg, L. (2001). How accessible is medical care for homeless women? *Medical Care, 40*(6), 510–520.

Lincoln, P. E. (2000). Comparing CNS and NP role activities: A replication. *Clinical Nurse Specialist, 14*(6), 269–277.

Lincoln, Y., & Guba, E. (1985). *Naturalistic inquiry*. Beverly Hills, CA: Sage.

Lind, C. D. (2003). Dysphagia: Evaluation and treatment. *Gastroenterology Clinics of North America, 32*(2), 553–575.

Lindeman, C. (1981). *Priorities within the health care system: A Delphi survey*. Kansas City, MO: American Academy of Nursing.

Lindgren, S., & Janzon, L. (1991). Prevalence of swallowing complaints and clinical findings among 50–70 year old men and women in an urban population. *Dysphagia, 6*, 187–192.

Lindquist, R., Banasik, J., Barnsteiner, J., Beecroft, P. C., Prevost, S., Reigel, B., et al. (1993). Determining AACN's research priorities for the 90's. *American Journal of Critical Care, 2*, 110–117.

Lindsey, A. M. (1995). Physical health of homeless adults. In *Annual review of nursing research* (Vol. 13, pp. 31–61). New York: Springer Publishing.

Linjakumpu, T., Hartikainen, S., Kalukka, T., Veijola, J., Kivela, S., & Isoaho, R. (2002). Use of medications and polypharmacy are increasing among elderly. *Journal of Clinical Epidemiology, 55*, 809–817.

Lipman, T. H., & Deatrick, J. A. (1997). Preparing advanced practice nurses for clinical decision making in specialty practice. *Nurse Educator, 22*(2), 47–50.

Lipscomb, J. A., & Love, C. C. (1992). Violence toward health care workers: An emerging occupational hazard. *American Association of Occupational Hhealth Nurses Journal, 40*(5), 219–228.

Lipson, J. (1993). Afghan refugees in California. Mental health issues. *Issues in Mental Health Nursing, 14*, 411–423.

Lipson, J. G., & Meleis, A. I. (1999). Immigrants and refugees. In A. S. Hinshaw, S. Feetham, & J. Shaver (Eds.), *Handbook of clinical nursing research* (pp. 87–106). Newbury Park, CA: Sage.

Litchfield, M. (1999). Practice wisdom. *Advances in Nursing Science, 22*, 62–73.

Littrell, K. H., Hilligoss, N. M., Kirshner, C. D., Petty, R. G., & Johnson, C. G. (2003). The effects of an educational intervention on antipsychotic-induced weight gain. *Journal of Nursing Scholarship, 35*, 237–241.

Littrell, K. H., & Littrell, S. H. (1999). Schizophrenia and comorbid substance abuse. *Journal of the American Psychiatric Nurses Association, 5*, S17–S24.

Litwin, M. (1994). Measuring health related quality of life in men with prostate cancer. *Journal of Urology, 152*(5 Pt. 2), 1882–1887.

Lloyd Jones, M., & Walters, S. (2001). The implications of contact with the mentor for preregistration: Nursing and midwifery students. *Journal of Advanced Nursing, 35*(2), 151–160.

LoBiondo-Wood, G. (2003). The theory of family stress and adaptation. In M. J. Smith & P. Liehr (Eds.), *Middle range theory for nursing* (pp. 91–109). New York: Springer.

Lobo, M. L., Barnard, K. E., & Coombs, J. B. (1992). Failure to thrive: A parent-infant interaction perspective. *Journal of Pediatric Nursing, 7*, 251–261.

Lockwood, A., & Marshall, M. (1999). Can a standardized needs assessment be used to improve the care of people with severe mental disorders? A pilot study of 'needs feedback'. *Journal of Advanced Nursing, 30*, 1408–1415.

Locsin, R. C. (1998). Technological competence as caring in critical care nursing. *Holistic Nursing Practice, 12*(4), 50–56.

Loeber, R., Farrington, D. P., & Petechuk, D. (2003, May). *Child delinquency: Early intervention and prevention. Child Delinquency Series Bulletin*. Washington, DC: U.S. Department of Justice, Office of Justice Programs, Office of Juvenile Justice and Delinquency Prevention.

Loftus, G. R. (1993). A picture is worth a thousand p values: On the irrelevance of hypothesis testing in the microcomputer age. *Behavior Research Methods, Instruments, and Computers, 25*, 250–256.

Lord, S. R., Menz, H. B., & Tiedemann, A. (2003). A physiological profile approach to falls risk assessment and prevention. *Physical Therapy, 83*, 237–252.

Lord, S. R., Sherrington, C., & Menz, H. B. (2001). *Falls in older people: Risk factors and strategies for prevention*. Cambridge, UK: Cambridge University Press.

Lorensen, M., Davis, A. J., Konishi, E., & Bunch, E. H. (2003). Ethical issues after the disclosure of a terminal illness: Danish and Norwegian hospice nurses' reflections. *Nursing Ethics: An International Journal for Health Care Professionals, 10*, 175–185.

Lorig, K. R., & Holman, H. (2003). Self-management education: History, definition, outcomes, and mechanisms. *Annals of Behavioral Medicine 26*(1), 1–7.

Lorig, K. R., Ritter, P., Stewart, A. L., Sobel, D. S., Brown, B. W., Jr., Bandura, A., et al. (2001). Chronic disease self-management programs: 2-year health status and health care utilization outcomes. *Medical Care, 39*, 1217–1223.

Love, J., Kisker, E. E., Ross, C., Schochet, P., Brooks-Gunn, J., Paulsell, D., et al. (2002). Making a difference in the lives of infants and toddlers and their families: The impact of early head start. Retrieved January 14, 2004, from http://www.acf.dhhs.gov/programs/core/ongoing_research/ehs/ehs_intro.html

Loveys, B. J., & Klaich, K. (1991). Breast cancer: Demands of illness. *Oncology Nursing Forum, 18*, 75–79.

Lu, M. C., Tache, V., Alexander, G. R., Kotelchuck, M., & Halfon, N. (2003). Preventing low birth weight: Is prenatal care the answer? *Journal of Maternal-Fetal and Neonatal Medicine, 13*, 362–380.

Ludington-Hoe, S., Ferreara, C., Swinth, J., & Ceccardi, J. J. (2003). Safe criteria and procedure for kangaroo care with intubated preterm infants. *Journal of Obstetric, Gynecologic, and Neonatal Nursing, 32*, 579–588.

Lueckenotte, A. (1996). *Gerontologic nursing*. St. Louis: Mosby.

Lundgren, I., Berg, M., & Lindmark, G. (2003). Is the childbirth experience improved by a birth plan? *Journal of Midwifery and Women's Health, 48*, 322–328.

Lunney, J. R., Lynn, J., Foley, T. J., Lipson, S., & Guaralnik, J. M. (2003). Patterns of functional decline at the end of life. *Journal of the American Medical Association, 289*(18), 2387–2392.

Lunney, M. (2003). Effects of using NANDA, NIC and NOC on health outcomes of schoolchildren: A pilot study. *International Journal of Nursing Terminology, 14*(4), Supplement: 21.

Luty, J., Kelly, C., & McCreadle, R. (2002). Smoking habits, body mass index and risk of heart disease: Prospective 2 1/2 year follow-up of first episode schizophrenic patients. *Journal of Substance Use, 7*, 15–18.

Lyder, C. H., Shannon, R., Empleo-Frazier, O., McGehee, D., & White, C. (2002). A comprehensive program to prevent pressure ulcers: Exploring cost and outcomes. *Ostomy Wound Management, 48*, 52–62.

Lyder, C., Yu, C., Emerling, J., Empleo-Frazier, O., Mangat, R., Stevenson, D., et al. (1999). Evaluating the predictive validity of the Braden scale for pressure ulcer risk in Blacks and Latino/Hispanic elders. *Applied Nursing Research, 12*, 60–68.

Lykken, D. (1968). Statistical significance in psychological research. *Psychological Bulletin, 70*, 151–159.

Lyles, J. S., Hodges, A., Collins, C., Lein, C., Given, C. W., Given, B., et al. (2003). Using nurse practitioners to implement an intervention in primary care for high-utilizing patients with medically unexplained symptoms. *General Hospital Psychiatry, 25*, 63–73.

Lynbaugh, J. E., & Fairman, J. (1992). New nurses, new spaces: A preview of the AACN history study. *American Journal of Critical Care, 1*, 19–24.

Lynch, N. A., Nicklas, B. J., Berman, D. M., Dennis, K. E., & Goldberg, A. P. (2001). Reductions in visceral fat during weight loss and walking are associated with improvements in VO_2 max. *Journal of Applied Physiology, 90*, 99–104.

Lynn, J., DeVries, K. O., Arkes, H., Stevens, M., Cohn, F., Murphy, P., et al. (2000). Ineffectiveness of the SUPPORT intervention: Review of explanations. *Journal of the American Geriatrics Society, 48*(5 Suppl.), S206–S213.

Lynn, J. (2001). Serving patients who may die soon and their families: The role of hospice and other services. *Journal of the American Medical Association, 285*(7), 925–932.

Lynn, M. R. (1986). Determination and quantification of content validity. *Nursing Resarch, 35*, 382–385.

Lyon, B. L. (1996). *Conquering stress in changing times*. Research Triangle Park, NC: Glaxo Wellcome.

Lyon, B. L. (2000). Stress, coping, and health. In V. Rice (Ed.), *Handbook of stress, coping, and health: Implications for nursing research, theory, and practice* (pp. 3–26). Thousand Oaks, CA: Sage Publications.

Lyon, B. L., & Werner, J. S. (1987). Stress. In J. J. Fitzpatrick & R. L. Tauaton (Eds.), *Annual review of nursing research* (Vol. 5, pp 3–22). New York: Springer Publishing.

Lyon, D. (2001). Human immunodeficiency virus (HIV) disease in persons with severe mental illness. *Issues in Mental Health Nursing, 22*, 109–119.

Lyotard, J. (1984). *The postmodern condition: A report on knowledge*. Manchester, England: Manchester University Press.

Maas, M., Johnson-Mekota, J. L., Buresh, K. A., Gardner, S. E., Frantz, R. A., Specht, J. K., et al. (2001). A nursing application of telecommunication: Measurements of satisfaction for patients and providers. *Journal of Gerontological Nursing, 27*(1), 28–33.

Maccines, D. L. (1998). The differences between health professionals in assessing levels of caregiver burden. *Journal of Psychiatric and Mental Health Nursing, 5*, 265–271.

Maccioli, G. A., Dorman, T., Brown, B. R., Mazuski, J. E., McLean, B. A., Kuszaj, J. M., et al. (2003). Clinical practice guidelines for the maintenance of patient physical safety in the intevensive care unit: Use of restraining therapies—American College of Critical Care Medicine Task Force 2001–2002. *Critical Care Medicine, 31*, 2665–2676.

Macdougall, M. (2000). Poor-quality studies suggest that vitamin B6 use is beneficial in premenstrual syndrome. *Western Journal of Medicine, 172*, 245.

Macduff, C. (2000). Respondent-generated quality of life measures: Useful tools for nursing or more fool's gold? *Journal of Advanced Nursing, 32*(2), 375–382. Retrieved September 29, 2003, from Ovid.

MacIntosh, J., & McCormack, D. (2000). An integrative review illuminates curricular applications of primary health care. *Journal of Nursing Education, 39*(3), 116–123.

Magavi, S. S., Leavigtt, B. R., & Macklis, J. D. (2000). Induction of neurogenesis in the neocortex of adult mice. *Nature, 405*, 951–955.

Magliano, L., Fadden, G., Economou, M., Xavier, M., Held, T., Guarneri, M., et al. (1998). Social and clinical factors influencing the choice of coping strategies in relatives of patients with schizophrenia: Results of BIOMED I study. *Social Psychiatry and Psychiatric Epidemiology, 33*, 413–419.

Magvary, D. (2002). Positive mental health: A turn of the century perspective. *Issues in Mental Health Nursing, 23*(4), 331–335.

Mahato, C. (2000). Schizophrenia patients: Duration of hospital care and returning to the self care ability. *Nursing Journal of India, 91*, 11–12.

Mahoney, D. F. (1994). Appropriateness of geriatric prescribing decisions made by nurse practitioners and physicians. *Image: Journal of Nursing Scholarship, 26*(1), 41–46.

Mahoney, E. K., Hurley, A. C., Volicer, L., Bell, M., Gianotis, P., Harsthorn, M., et al. (1999). Development and testing of the resistiveness to care scale. *Research in Nursing and Health, 22*, 27–38.

Mahoney, E. K., Volicer, L., & Hurley, A. C. (2000). Functional impairment. In E. K. Mahoney, L. Volicer, & A. C. Hurley (Eds.), *Management of challenging behaviors in dementia* (pp. 29–46). Baltimore, MD: Health Professions Press.

Mahoney, F. J., Stewart, K., Hu, H., Coleman, P., & Alter, M. J. (1997). Progress toward the elimination of hepatitis B virus transmission among health care workers in the United States. *Archives of Internal Medicine, 157*, 2601–2605.

Maison, J., Gaudet, M., Gregorie, J., & Bouchard, R. (2002). Non-compliance with drug treatment and reading difficulties with regard to prescription labelling among seniors. *Gerontology, 48*, 44–51.

Majesky, S. J., Brester, M. H., & Nishio, K. T. (1978). Development of a research tool: Patient indicators of nursing care. *Nursing Research, 27*(6), 365–371.

Mallory, J. L. (2003). The impact of a palliative care educational component on attitudes toward care of the dying in undergraduate nursing students. *Journal of Professional Nursing, 19*, 305–312.

Maloni, J. A. (1996). Bed rest and high-risk pregnancy. Differentiating the effects of diagnosis, setting, and treatment. *Nursing Clinics of North America, 31*(2), 313–325.

Maloni, J. A., Albrecht, S. A., Thomas, K. K., Halleran, J., & Jones, R. (2003). Implementing evidence-based practice: Reducing risk for low birth weight through pregnancy smoking cessation. *Journal of Obstetric, Gynecologic, and Neonatal Nursing, 32*, 676–682.

Maloni, J. A., Alexander, G. R., Schluchter, M. D., Shah, D. M., & Park, S. (2004). Antepartum bed rest: Maternal weight change and infant birth weight. *Biological Research for Nursing, 5*(3), 177–186.

Maloni, J. A., Brezinski-Tomasi, J. E., & Johnson, L. A. (2001). Antepartum bed rest: Effect upon the family. *Journal of Obstetric, Gynecologic, and Neonatal Nursing, 30*, 165–173.

Maloni, J. A., Kane, J. H., Suen, L. J., & Wang, K. K. (2002). Dysphoria among high-risk pregnant hospitalized women on bed rest: A longitudinal study. *Nursing Research, 51*, 92–99.

Maloni, J. A., & Schneider, B. S. (2002). Inactivity: Symptoms associated with gastrocnemius muscle disuse during pregnancy. *American Association of Colleges of Nursing Clinical Issues, 13*, 248–262.

Manfrin-Ledet, L., & Porche, D. J. (2003). The state of the science: Violence and HIV infection in women. *Journal of the Association of Nurses in AIDS Care, 14*(6), 56–68.

Mangram, A. J., Horan, T. C., Pearson, M. L., Silver, L. C., & Jarvis, W. R. (1999). Guideline for prevention of surgical site infection. *American Journal of Infection Control, 27*, 97–132.

Mann, H. (2003). Ethics of research involving vulnerable populations. *Lancet, 362*, 1857–1859.

Manthey, C., Ciske, K., Robertson, P., & Harris, I. (1970). Primary nursing: A return to the concept of "my nurse" and "my patient." *Nursing Forum, 9*, 64–83.

Maramba, G. G., & Hall, G. C. (2002). Meta-analyses of ethnic match as a predictor of dropout, utilization, and level of functioning. *Cultural, Diversity, Ethnicity, Minority Psychology, 8*, 290–297.

Marek, K. (1996). Nursing diagnoses and home care nursing utilization. *Public Health Nursing, 13*(3), 195–200.

Marion, L. (1996). *Nursing's vision for primary health care in the 21st century*. Washington, DC: American Nurses Association.

Marion, L., Viens, D., O'Sullivan, A. L., Crabtree, K., Fontana, S., & Price, M. M. (2003). The practice doctorate in nursing: Future or fringe? *Topics in Advanced Practice Nursing e-journal, 3*(2). Retrieved March 31, 2004, from http://www.medscape.com/viewarticle/453247_print

Mark, B. A., & Salyer, J. (1999). Methodological issues in treatment effectiveness and outcomes research. *Outcomes Management for Nursing Practice, 3*(1), 12–18.

Mark, B. A., Salyer, J., Geddes, N., & Smith, C. (1998). The Outcomes Research in Nursing Administration Project: Methodological issues in implementation. *Outcomes Management for Nursing Practice, 2*(3), 111–116.

Marks, R. M., & Sachar, E. G. (1973). Undertreatment of medical in patients with narcotic analgesics. *Annals of Internal Medicine, 78*, 173–181.

Marland, G. R. (1999). Atypical neuroleptics: Autonomy and compliance? *Journal of Advanced Nursing, 29*, 615–622.

Marland, G. R., & Cash, K. (2001). Long-term illness and patterns of medicine taking: Are people with schizophrenia a unique group? *Journal of Psychiatric and Mental Health Nursing, 8*, 197–204.

Marland, G. R., & Sharkey, V. (1999). Depot neuroleptics, schizophrenia and the role of the nurse: Is practice evidence based? A review of the literature. *Journal of Advanced Nursing, 30*, 1255–1262.

Marlatt, G. A., & Gordon, J. R. (1985). *Relapse prevention: Maintenance strategies in the treatment of addiction*. New York: Guilford Press.

Marston, M. (1970). Compliance with medical regimen: A review of the literature. *Nursing Research, 19*, 312–323.

Martens, W. (2002). Homelessness and mental disorders: A comparative review of populations in various countries. *International Journal of Mental Health, 30*(4), 79–96.

Martin, H., Slyk, M. P., Deymann, S., & Cornacchione, M. J. (2003). Safety profile assessment of risperidone and olanzapine in long-term care patients with dementia. *Journal of the American Medical Directors Association, 4*(4), 183–188.

Martin, K. S., & Scheet, N. J. (1992). *The Omaha System: Applications for community health nursing*. Philadelphia: W. B. Saunders.

Martin, K. S., & Scheet, N. J. (1995). The Omaha System: Nursing diagnoses, interventions, and client outcomes. In N. M. Lang (Ed.), *Nursing data systems: An emerging framework*. Washington, DC: American Nurses Publishing.

Martin, K. S., Scheet, N. J., & Stegman, M. R. (1993). Home health clients: Characteristics, outcomes of care, and nursing interventions. *American Journal of Public Health, 83*(12), 1730–1734.

Martin, P. (1993). Clinical settings need organizational support for research. *Applied Nursing Research, 6*, 103–104.

Maslach, C., & Pines, A. (1978). Characteristics of staff burnout in mental health settings. *Hospital Community Psychiatry, 29*, 233–237.

Massey, R., & Jedlicka, D. (2002). The Massey Bedside Swallow Screen. *Journal of Neuroscience Nursing, 34*, 252–260.

Mast, M. E. (1995). Adult uncertainty in illness: A critical review of the research. *Scholarly Inquiry for Nursing Practice, 9*, 3–24.

Master, R. J., Feltin, M., Joainchill, J., Mark, R., Kavesh, W. N., Rabkin, M. T., et al. (1987). A continuum of care for the inner city—assessment of its benefits for Boston's elderly and high-risk populations. *New England Journal of Medicine, 302*(26), 1434–1440.

Masters, W. H., & Johnson, V. E. (1966). *Human sexual response*. Boston: Little Brown.

Matney, S., Bakken, S., & Huff, S. M. (2003). Representing nursing assessments in clinical information systems using the logical observation identifiers, names, and codes database. *Journal of Biomedical Informatics, 36*(4–5), 287–293.

Matteson, M. A., Linton, A., & Barnes, S. J. (1996). Cognitive developmental approach to dementia. *Journal of Nursing Scholarship, 28*(3), 233–240.

Matteson, M. A., Linton, A., Cleary, B. L., & Lichenstein, M. J. (1993). The relationship between Piaget levels of cognitive development and cognitive impairment in persons with dementia. *Gerontologist, 33*, 207–210.

Matzo, M. L. (1996). *Registered nurses' attitudes toward and practices of assisted suicide and patient-requested euthanasia*. Master's thesis. University of Massachusetts, Boston.

Matzo, M. L., & Emanuel, E. J. (1997). Oncology nurses' practices of assisted suicide and patient requested euthanasia. *Oncology Nursing Forum, 24*, 1725–1732.

Maurin, J. T., & Boyd, C. B.. (1990). Burden of mental illness on the family: A critical review. *Archives of Psychiatric Nursing, 4*(2), 99–107.

Mausner, J. S., & Kramer, S. (1985). *Epidemiology: An introductory text*. Philadelphia: W. B. Saunders.

May, K. M., & Hu, J. (2000). Caregiving and help seeking by mothers of low birthweight infants and mothers of normal birthweight infants. *Public Health Nursing, 17*, 273–279.

Mayberry, L. J., Strange, L. B., Suplee, P. D., & Gennaro, S. (2003). Use of upright positioning with epidural analgesia: Findings from an observational study. *American Journal of Maternal Child Nursing, 28*, 152–159.

Mazure, C. M., Keita, G. P., & Blehar, M. C. (2002). *Summit on women and depression: Proceedings and recommendations*. Washington, DC: American Psychological Association. Retrieved from http://www.apa.org/pi/wpo/women&deprssion.pdf/

Mbanga, N. I., Niehaus, d. J. H., Mzamo, N. C., Wessels, C. J., Allen, A., Emsley, R. A., et al. (2002). Attitudes towards and beliefs about schizophrenia in Xhosa families with affected probands. *South African Journal of Nursing, 25*, 69–73.

McAiney, C. A. (1998). The development of the empowered aide model: An intervention for long-term care staff who care for Alzheimer's residents. *Journal of Gerontological Nursing, 24*(1), 17–22.

McAlearney, A. S. (2003). *Population health management: Strategies to improve outcomes*. Chicago, IL: Health Administration Press.

McAlister, N., Covvy, H., Tong, C., Lee, A., & Wigle, E. (1986). Randomized controlled trial of computer assisted management of hypertension in primary care. *British Medical Journal, 293*, 670–674.

McArthur, M., Brunmeier, C., Bergstrom, N., & Baun, M. (1986). The effect of a pet dog on the social interaction of mentally impaired institutionalized elderly. *People, Animals, and Environment, 4*(2), 25.

McAulay, D. (2001). Dehydration in the terminally ill patient. *Nursing Standard, 16*, 33–37.

McBride, A. B. (1993). From gynecology to GYN-ecology: Developing a practice-research agenda for women's health. *Health Care for Women International, 14*, 315–325.

McBride, A. B., & McBride, W. L. (1981). Theoretical underpinnings for women's health. *Women & Health, 6*(1–2), 37–55.

McBride, A. B., & Shore, C. P. (2001). Women as mothers and grandmothers. In J. J. Fitzpatrick, D. Taylor, & N. F. Woods (Eds.), *Annual review of nursing research* (Vol. 20, pp. 63–86). New York: Springer Publishing.

McCabe, B. W., Baun, M. M., Speich, D., & Agrawal, S. (2002). Resident dog in the Alzheimer's special care unit. *Western Journal of Nursing Research, 24*(6), 684–696.

McCabe, S. (2002). The nature of psychiatric nursing: The intersection of paradigm, evolution, and history. *Archives of Psychiatric Nursing 16*, 51–60.

McCann, E. (2000). The expression of sexuality in people with psychosis: Breaking the taboos. *Journal of Advanced Nursing, 32*, 132–138.

McCann, E. (2001). Recent developments in psychosocial interventions for people with psychosis. *Issues in Mental Health Nursing, 22*, 99–107.

McCann, T. V. (2002). Uncovering hope with clients who have psychotic illness. *Journal of Holistic Nursing, 20*, 81–99.

McCann, T. V., & Clark, E. (2003). A grounded theory study of the role that nurses play in increasing clients' willingness to access community mental health services. *International Journal of Mental Health Nursing, 12,* 279–287.

McCarthy, D., Argeriou, M., Huebner, R. B., & Lubran, B. (1991). Alcoholism, drug abuse, and the homeless. *American Psychologist, 46*(11), 1139–1148.

McCarthy, D., Murray, S., Galagan, D., Gern, J., & Hutson, P. (1998). Meperidine attenuates the secretion but not the transcription of interleukin 1 beta in human mononuclear leukocytes. *Nursing Research, 47*(1), 19–24.

McCarthy, M. C. (2003). Detecting acute confusion in older adults: Comparing clinical reasoning of nurses working in acute, long-term, and community health care environments. *Research in Nursing & Health, 26,* 203–212.

McCartney, P. R. (2000). Computer analysis of the fetal heart rate. *Journal of Obstetric, Gynecologic, and Neonatal Nursing, 29*(5), 527–536.

McCauley, J., Kern, D. E., Kolodner, K., Derogatis, L. R., & Bass, E. B. (1998). Relation of low-severity violence to women's health. *Journal of General Internal Medicine, 13*(10), 687–691.

McCay, E. A., & Seeman, M. V. (1998). A scale to measure the impact of a schizophrenic illness on an individual's self-concept. *Archives of Psychiatric Nursing, 12,* 41–49.

McCloskey, B., Grey, M., Deshefy-Longhi, T., & Grey, L. (2003). APRN practice patterns in primary care. *Nurse Practitioner, 28*(4), 39–44.

McCloskey, J. (1990). Two requirements for job contentment: Autonomy and social integration. *Journal of Nursing Scholarship, 22,* 140–143.

McCloskey, J. C., & Bulechek, G. M. (1996). *Nursing interventions classifications (NIC)* (2nd ed.). St. Louis, MO: Mosby.

McCloskey, J. C., & Bulechek, G. M. (2000). *Nursing interventions classification* (3rd ed.). St. Louis, MO: Mosby.

McCloskey, J. C., & Bulechek, G. M. (Eds.). (2004). *Nursing interventions classification (NIC)* (4th ed.). St. Louis, MO: Mosby.

McCloughen, A. (2003). The association between schizophrenia and cigarette smoking: A review of the literature and implications for mental health nursing practice. *International Journal of Mental Health Nursing, 12,* 119–129.

McClowry, S. G. (2003). *Your child's unique temperament: Insights and strategies for responsive parenting.* Champaign, IL: Research Press.

McClowry, S. G., Mayberry, L. J., Snow, D. L., & Tamis-LeMonda, C. (2004). *Conducting preventive intervention research: A focus on reducing health disparities.* Manuscript submitted for publication.

McClung, T. M. (2000). Assessing the reported financial benefits of unlicensed assistive personnel in nursing. *Journal of Nursing Administration, 30*(11), 530–534.

McCormick, K., & Jones, C. (1998). Computer based patient records require a structured vocabulary: Nursing nomenclature and needed taxonomies for health care—is one taxonomy needed for health care vocabularies and classifications? *Online Journal of Issues in Nursing.* Retrieved December, 2003, from http://www.nursingworld.org/mods/archive/mod7/cec16.htm

McCormick, K. A., Lang, N., Zielstorff, R., Milholland, D. K., Saba, V., & Jacox, A. (1994). Toward standard classification schemes for nursing language: Recommendations of the American Nurses Association Steering Committee on Databases to Support Clinical Nursing Practice. *Journal of the American Medical Informatics Association, 1*(6), 421–427.

McCormick, K. M. (2002). A concept analysis of uncertainty in illness. *Journal of Nursing Scholarship, 34*(2), 127–131.

McCreary, L., & Dancy, B. (2004). Dimensions of family functioning: Perspectives of low-income African American single-parent families. *Journal of Marriage and Therapy, 66*(3), 690–701.

McCubbin, H. I., & Patterson, J. M. (1982). Family adaptation to crisis. In H. I. McCubbin, A. Cauble, & J. Patterson (Eds.), *Family stress, coping and social support* (pp. 26–47). Springfield, IL: Charles C. Thomas.

McCubbin, H., & Patterson, J. (1983). The family stress process: The Double ABCX model of adjustment and adaptation. In H. McCubbin, M. Sussman, & J. Patterson (Eds.), *Social stress and the family: Advances and developments in family stress theory and research* (pp. 7–37). New York: Haworth Press.

McCubbin, H. I., Thompson, A. I., & McCubbin, M. A. (Eds.). *Family assessment: Resiliency, coping and adaptation (Inventories for research and practice).* Madison, WI: University of Wisconsin System.

McCubbin, M. A., & McCubbin, H. I. (1996). Resiliency and families: A conceptual model of family adjustment and adaptation in response to stress and crises. In H. I. McCubbin, A. I. Thompson, & M. A. McCubbin (Eds.), *Family assessment: Resiliency, coping and adaptation—inventories for research and practice.* Madison: University of Wisconsin System.

McDaniel, C., & Nash, J. G. (1990). Compendium of instruments measuring patient satisfaction with nursing care. *Quality Review Bulletin, May,* 182–188.

McDaniel, C., & Stumpf, L. (1993). The organizational culture: Implications for nursing service. *Journal of Nursing Administration, 23*, 54–60.

McDonald, D., & Molony, S. (in press). Postoperative pain communication skills for older adults. *Western Journal of Nursing Research.*

McDonald, J., & Badger, T. A. (2002). Social function of persons with schizophrenia. *Journal of Psychosocial Nursing and Mental Health Services, 40*, 42–50.

Mc Donnell, P., & Jacobs, M. (2003). Hospital admission resulting from preventable adverse drug reactions. *Annals of Pharmacotherapy, 36*, 1331–1336.

McDougall, G. J. (1999). Cognitive interventions among older adults. *Annual Review of Nursing Research, 17*, 219–240.

McDougall, G. J. (2001). Memory improvement program for elderly cancer survivors. *Geriatric Nursing, 22*(4), 185–190.

McDougall, G. J. (2004). Memory self-efficacy and memory performance in black and white community elders. *Nursing Research, 53*(5), 323–331.

Mc Dougall, G. J., Blixen, C., & Lee-Jen, S. (1997). The process and outcomes of life review psychotherapy with depressed homebound older adults. *Nursing Research, 46*(5), 277–283.

McDougall, G. J., Montgomery, K. S., Eddy, N., Jackson, E., Nelson, E., Stark, T., et al. (2003). Aging memory self-efficacy: Elders share their thoughts and experience. *Geriatric Nursing, 24*(3), 162–168.

McDowell, B. J., Martin, D. C., Snustad, D. G., & Flynn, W. (1986). Comparison of the clinical practice of a geriatric nurse practitioner and two internists . . . at a geriatric ambulatory care center. *Public Health Nursing, 3*(3), 140–146.

McElligott, M. (2001). Fathercraft. Antenatal information wanted by first-time fathers. *British Journal of Midwifery, 9*, 556–558.

McElmurry, B. J., & Keeney, G. B. (1999). Primary health care. In J. J. Fitzpatrick (Ed.), *Annual review of nursing research* (pp. 241–268). New York: Springer Publishing.

McElmurry, B. J., Marks, B. A., & Cianelli, R. (2002). *Primary health care in the Americas: Conceptual framework, experiences, challenges, and perspectives.* Washington, DC: PAHO/WHO.

McEwen, M. (2002). Theory development: Structuring conceptual relationships in nursing. In M. McEwen & E. M. Wills (Eds.), *Theoretical basis for nursing* (pp. 86–89, 219). Philadelphia: Lippincott Williams & Wilkins.

McFarlane, J., Malecha, A., Gist, J., Watson, K., Batten, E., Hall, I., et al. (2002). An intervention to increase safety behaviors of abused women: Results of a randomized clinical trial. *Nursing Research, 51*(6), 347–354.

McFarlane, J., Parker, B., Soeken, K., Silva, C., & Reel, S. (1998). Safety behaviors of abused women after an intervention during pregnancy. *Journal of Obstetric, Gynecologic, & Neonatal Nursing, 27*(1), 64–69.

McFarlane, J., Soeken K., Campbell, J., Parker, B., Reel, S, & Silva, C. (1998). Severity of abuse to pregnant women and associated gun access of the perpetrator. *Public Health Nursing, 15*(3), 201–206.

McGrath, J. M., & Medoff-Cooper, B. (2001). Apnea and periodic breathing during bottle feeding of premature infants . . . 34th Annual Communicating Nursing Research Conference/15th Annual WIN Assembly, "Health Care Challenges Beyond 2001: Mapping the Journey for Research and Practice," held April 19–21, 2001 in Seattle, Washington. *Community Nursing Research, 34*, 220.

McHugh, F., Lindsay, G. M., Hanlon, P., Hutton, I., Brown, M. R., Morrison, C., et al. (2001). Nurse led shared care for patients on the waiting list for coronary artery bypass surgery: A randomized controlled trial. *Heart, 86*, 317–323.

McHugh, M. (1994). Measurement of nursing intensity. Report to the American Nurses Association Database Steering Committee. *Health Care Financing Review*, suppl., 47–55.

McIntosh, J. (1974). Processes of communication, information, seeking and control aqssociated with cancer: A selective review of the literature. *Social Science & Medicine, 8*, 167–187.

McIntosh, J. (1976). Patients' awareness and desire for information about diagnosed but undisclosed malignant disease. *Lancet, 2*, 300–303.

McKenzie, N., & Erickson, R. (1996). The reliability and criterion-related validity of the infrared tympanic thermometer. *Journal of Perianesthesia Nursing, 11*(5), 300–303.

McLaughlin, C. (1999). An exploration of psychiatric nurses' and patient's opinions regarding in-patient care for suicidal patients. *Journal of Advanced Nursing, 29*(5), 1042–1051.

McLloyd, V. C., Cauce, A. M., Takeuchi, D., & Wilson, L. (2000). Marital processes and parental socialization in families of color: A decade review of research. *Journal of Marriage and the Family, 62*, 1070–1093.

McMillan, S. C. (1996). Pain and pain relief experience by hospice patients with cancer. *Cancer Nursing, 19*, 298–307.

McMillan, S. C., & Moody, L. E. (2003). Hospice patient and caregiver congruence in reporting patients' symptom intensity. *Cancer Nursing, 26*, 113–118.

McMurray, R. G., Ainsworth, B. E., Harrell, J. S., Griggs, T. R., & Williams, O. D. (1998). Is physical activity or aerobic power more influential on reducing cardiovascular disease risk factors? *Medicine & Science in Sports & Exercise*, *30*(10), 1521–1529.

McMurray-Avila, M. (1997). *Organizing health services for homeless people*. Nashville, TN: National Health Care for the Homeless Council.

McNeal, G. J. (Ed.). (2000). *AACN guide to acute care procedures in the home*. Philadelphia: Lippincott.

McQuiston, C., & Flaskerud, J. H. (2000). Sexual prevention of HIV: A model for Latinos. *Journal of the Association of Nurses in AIDS Care*, *11*(5), 70–79.

McQuiston, C., & Flaskerud, J. H. (2003). "If they don't ask about condoms, I just tell them": A descriptive case study of Latino lay health advisers' helping activities. *Health Education and Behavior*, *30*, 79–96.

McVicar, A. (2003). Workplace stress in nursing: A literature review. *Journal of Advanced Nursing*, *44*, 633–642.

McWey, R. E., Curry, N. S., Schabel, S. I., & Reines, H. D. (1988). Complications of nasoenteric feeding tubes. *American Journal of Surgery*, *155*(2), 253–257.

Meadows, A., Krejmas, N., & Belasco, J. (1980). In J. Van Eys & M. Sullivan (Eds.), *Status of the curability of childhood cancer* (pp. 263–276). New York: Raven Press.

Medical Outcomes Trust. (1993). *How to score the SF-36 health survey*. Boston: Author.

Medoff-Cooper, B. (1991). Changes in nutritive sucking patterns with increasing gestational age. *Nursing Research*, *40*(4), 245–247.

Medoff-Cooper, B. (2002). *Feeding behaviors as an index of developmental outcomes*. *International Congress of Infant Studies*. Toronto, Ontario, Canada: Lawrence Erlbaum.

Medoff-Cooper, B., Bilker, W., & Kaplan, J. (2001). Suckling behavior as a function of gestational age: A cross-sectional study. *Developmental and Behavioral Pediatrics*, *24*, 83–94.

Medoff-Cooper, B., & Gennaro, S. (1996). The correlation of sucking behaviors and Bayley Scales of Infant Development at six months of age in VLBW infants. *Nursing Research*, *45*(5), 291–296.

Medoff-Cooper, B., McGrath, J. M., & Bilker, W. (2000). Nutritive sucking and neurobehavioral development in preterm infants from 34 weeks PCA to term. *American Journal of Maternal Child Nursing*, April/May, *25*, 64–70.

Medoff-Cooper, B., McGrath, J., & Shults, J. (2002). Feeding patterns of full term and preterm infants at forty weeks post-conceptional age. *Developmental and Behavioral Pediatrics*, *23*(1), 231–236.

Meek, P. M., Nail, L. M., Barsevick, A., Schwartz, A. L., Stephen, S., Whitmer, K., et al. (2000). Psychometric testing of fatigue instruments for use with cancer patients. *Nursing Research*, *49*, 181–190.

Meiner, S. E. (2003). Polypharmacy. In M. L. Matzo & D. W. Sherman (Eds.), *Gerontologic palliative care nursing*. St. Louis, MO: Mosby.

Meleis, A. F. (1996). Culturally competent scholarship: Substance and rigor. *Advances in Nursing Science*, *19*(2), 1–16.

Meleis, A. F., & Lindgren, T. G. (2002). Man works from sun to sun, but woman's work is never done: Insights on research and policy. *Health Care for Women International*, *23*, 742–753.

Meleis, A. F., Lipson, J., Muecke, M., & Smith, G. (1998). *Immigrant women and their health: An olive paper*. Indianapolis, IN: Sigma Theta Tau International, Center for Nursing.

Meleis, A. I. (1993, June). *A passion for substance revisited: Global transitions and international commitments*. Paper presented at the 1993 National Doctoral Forum, St. Paul, MN.

Meleis, A. I. (1995). Immigrant women in borderless societies: Marginalized and empowered. *Asian Journal of Nursing Studies*, *2*(4), 39–47.

Meleis A. I. (1997). *Theoretical nursing: Development and progress* (3rd ed.). Philadelphia: J. B. Lippincott.

Meleis, A. I. (2004). *Theoretical nursing: Development and progress* (3rd ed., Rev. reprint). Philadelphia: Lippincott Williams & Wilkens.

Meleis, A. I., Omidian, P., & Lipson, J. (1993). Women's health status in the United States. An immigrant women's project.

Meleis, A. I., & Trangenstein, P. A. (1994). Facilitating transitions: Redefininition of a nursing mission. *Nursing Outlook*, *42*, 255–259.

Melia, S. (1999). Continuity in the lives of elder religious Catholic women. *International Journal of Aging and Human Development*, *48*(3), 175–189.

Melnyk, B. M., Alpert-Gillis, L., Feinstein, N. F., Fairbanks, E., Schultz-Czarniak, J., Hust, D., et al. (2001). Improving cognitive development of low-birth-weight premature infants with the COPE program: A pilot study of the benefits of early NICU intervention with mothers. *Research in Nursing and Health*, *24*, 373–389.

Melnyk, K. A. (1982). The process of theory analysis: An examination of the nursing theory of Dorothea E. Orem. *Nursing Research*, *32*(3), 170–174.

Melzack, R. (1996). Gate control theory. On the evolution of pain concepts. *Pain Forum*, *5*(2), 128–138.

Melzack, R., & Wall, P. D. (1965). Pain mechanisms: A new theory. *Science, 150*, 971–979.

Memorial Sloan-Kettering Cancer Center. (2003). *Types of cancer: Colorectal cancer*. Retrieved from http://www.mskcc.org

Mendel, B., Bergenius, J., & Langius, A. (2001). The sense of coherence: A tool for evaluating patients with peripheral vestibular disorders. *Clinical Otolaryngology & Allied Sciences, 26*(1), 19–24.

Mendes de Leon, C. F., Krumholz, H. M., Seeman, T. S., Vaccarino, V., Williams, C. S., Kasl, S. V., et al. (1998). Depression and risk of coronary heart disease in elderly men and women: New Haven EPESE, 1982–1991. Established Populations for the Epidemiologic Studies of the Elderly. *Archives of Internal Medicine, 158*, 2341–2348.

Menzies, V. (2000). Depression in schizophrenia: Nursing care as a generalized resistance resource. *Issues in Mental Health Nursing, 21*, 605–617.

Menzies, V., & Farrell, S. P. (2002). Schizophrenia, tardive dyskinesia, and the Abnormal Involuntary Movement Scale (AIMS). *Journal of the American Psychiatric Nurses Association, 8*, 51–56.

Mercadante, S., Casuccio, A., & Fulfaro, F. (2000). The course of symptom frequency and intensity in advanced cancer patients followed at home. *Journal of Pain & Symptom Management, 20*(2), 104–112.

Mercer, R. (1995). *Becoming a mother*. New York: Springer.

Mercer, R., Ferketich, S., DeJoseph, J., May, K., & Sollid, D. (1988). Effect of stress on family functioning during pregnancy. *Nursing Research, 37*, 268–275.

Mereness, D. (1983). The potential significant role of the nurse in community mental health services. *Perspectives in Psychiatric Care, 21*(4), 128–132.

Merleau-Ponty, M. (1962). *Phenomenology of perception*. London: Routledge & Kegan Paul.

Merleau-Ponty, M. (1964). *The primacy of perception* (J. Edie, Trans.). Evanston, IL: Northwestern University Press.

Merriam-Webster's Collegiate Dictionary (10th ed.). (1993). Springfield, MA: Merriam-Webster.

Merriam-Webster's Collegiate Dictionary (11th ed.). (2003). Springfield, MA: Merriam-Webster.

Merriam-Webster Online. (2004). Retrieved from http://www.m-w.com

Merton, R. K. (1968). On sociological theories of the middle range. In R. K. Merton, *Social theory and social structure* (pp. 39–72). New York: Free Press.

Merwin, E., Hinton, I., Dembling, B., & Stern, S. (2003). Shortages of rural mental health professionals. *Archives of Psychiatric Nursing, 17*, 42–51.

Merwin, E., & Mauck, A. (1995). Psychiatric nursing outcome research: The state of the science. *Archives of Psychiatric Nursing*, 9(6), 311–331.

Messert, B., Kurlanzik, A. E., & Thorning, D. R. (1976). Adult "failure to thrive" syndrome. *Journal of Nervous and Mental Disorder, 162*, 401–409.

Messler, E. C. (1974). Transforming information into nursing knowledge: A study of maternity nursing practice (Doctoral dissertation, Columbia University, 1974). *Dissertation Abstracts International, 35*, 4B.

Metheny, N. A., Eikov, R., Rountree, V., & Lengettie, E. (1999). Indicators of feeding-tube Placement in neonates. *Nutrition in Clinical Practice, 14*(5), 307–314.

Metheny, N., McSweeney, M., Wehrle, M. A., & Wiersema, L. (1990). Effectiveness of the auscultatory method in predicting feeding tube location. *Nursing Research, 39*(5), 262–267.

Metheny, N., Reed, L., Berglund, B., & Wehrle, M. A. (1994). Visaual characteristics of aspirates from feeding tubes as a method for predicting tube location. *Nursing Research, 43*(5), 282–287.

Metheny, N., Reed, L., Wiersema, L., McSweeney, M., Wehrle, M. A., & Clark, J. (1993). Effectiveness of pH measurements in predicting feeding tube placement: An update. *Nursing Research, 42*(6), 324–331.

Metheny, N. A., Smith, L., & Stewart, B. J. (2000). Development of a reliable and valid bedside test for bilirubin and its utility for improving prediction of feeding tube location. *Nursing Research, 49*(6), 302–309.

Metheny, N. A., Spies, M., & Eisenberg, P. (1986). Frequency of nasoenteral tube displacement and associated risk factors. *Research in Nursing and Health*, 9(3), 241–247.

Metheny, N. A., & Stewart, B. J. (2002). Testing feeding tube placement during continuous tube feedings. *Applied Nursing Research, 15*(4), 254–258.

Metheny, N. A., Stewart, B. J., Smith, L., Yan, H., Diebold, M., & Clouse, R. E. (1999). pH and concentration of bilirubin in feeding tube aspirates as predictors of tube placement. *Nursing Research, 48*(4), 189–197.

Meyer, E. C., Garcia Coll, C. T., Seifer, R., Ramos, A., Kilis, E., & Oh, W. (1995). Psychological distress in mothers of preterm infants. *Journal of Developmental and Behavioral Pediatrics, 16*, 412–417.

Meyer, L. (1956). *Emotion and meaning in music*. Chicago: University of Chicago Press.

Mezey, M., Dubler, N. N., Mitty, E., & Brody, A. A. (2002). What impact do setting and transitions have on the quality of life at the end of life and the quality of the dying process? *Gerontologist, 42*(Special Issue iii), 54–67.

Mezey, M., & Fulmer, T. (1998). Quality care for the frail elderly. *Nursing Outlook, 46*(6), 291–292.

Mezey, M., Kluger, M., Maislin, G., & Mittelman, M. (1996). Life-sustaining treatment decisions by spouses of patients with Alzheimer's disease. *Journal of the American Geriatrics Society, 44*(2), 144–150.

Mezey, M., Teresi, J., Ramsey, G., Mitty, E., & Bobrowitz, T. (2000). Decision-making capacity to execute a Health Care Proxy: Development and testing of guidelines. *Journal of the American Geriatrics Society, 48*(2), 179–187.

Mezey, M. D., Leitman, R., Mitty, E. L., Bottrell, M. M., & Ramsey, G. C. (2000). Why hospital patients do and do not execute an advance directive. *Nursing Outlook, 48*(4), 165–171.

Mickley, J. R., Soeken, K., & Belcher, A. (1992). Spiritual well-being, religiousness and hope among women with breast cancer. *Image: Journal of Nursing Scholarship, 24*(4), 267–272.

Midanik, L., Soghikian, K., Ransom, L., & Tekawa, S. (1995). The effect of retirement on mental health and health behaviors: The Kaiser Permanente Retirement Study. *Journals of Gerontology: Social Sciences, 50*, S59–S61.

Miles, M. S. (2003). Parents of children with chronic health problems: Programs of nursing research and their relationship to developmental science. In J. J. Fitzpatrick, M. S. Miles, & D. Holditch-Davis (Eds.), *Annual review of nursing research* (Vol. 21, pp. 247–277). New York: Springer Publishing.

Miles, M. S., Funk, S. G., & Carlson, J. (1993). Parental Stressor Scale: Neonatal Intensive Care Unit. *Nursing Research, 42*, 148–152.

Miles, M. S., Funk, S., & Kasper, M. A. (1992). The stress response of mothers and fathers of preterm infants. *Research in Nursing and Health, 15*, 261–269.

Miles, M. S., & Holditch-Davis, D. (1997). Parenting the prematurely-born child: Pathways of influence. *Seminars in Perinatology, 213*, 254–266.

Miles, M. S., & Holditch-Davis, D. (2003). Enhancing nursing research with children and families using a developmental science perspective. In J. J. Fitzpatrick, M. S. Miles, & D. Holditch-Davis (Eds.), *Annual review of nursing research* (Vol. 21, pp. 1–20). New York: Springer Publishing.

Miles, M. S., Holditch-Davis, D., Burchinal, P., & Nelson, D. (1999). Distress and growth outcomes in mothers of medically fragile infants. *Nursing Research, 48*, 129–140.

Miles, S., Koepp, R., & Weber, E. (1996). Advanced end of life treatment planning: A research review. *Archives of Internal Medicine, 156*(10), 1062–1068.

Miles, S. H., & Irvine, P. (1992). Deaths caused by physical restraints. *Gerontologist, 32*, 762–766.

Millar, K., Asbury, A. J., & Murray, G. D. (2001). Pre-existing cognitive impairment as a factor influencing outcome after cardiac surgery. *British Journal of Anaesthesia, 86*(1), 63–67.

Miller, E. T., & Spilker, J. (2003). Readiness to change and brief educational interventions: Successful strategies to reduce stroke risk. *Journal of Neuroscience Nursing, 35*, 215–222.

Miller, I. W., Keitner, G. I., Whisman, M. A., Ryan, C. E., Epstein, N. B., & Bishop, D. S. (1992). Depressed patients with dysfunctional families: Description and course of illness. *Journal of Abnormal Psychology, 101*, 637–646.

Miller, J. C. (1981). Theoretical basis for the practice of community mental health nursing. *Issues in Mental Health Nursing, 3*, 319–339.

Miller, J. M. (2002). Criteria for therapeutic use of pelvic floor muscle training in women. *Journal of Wound, Ostomy, and Continence Nurses, 29*, 301–311.

Miller, N. H., Smith, P. M., DeBusk, R. F., Sobel, D. S., & Taylor, C. B. (1997). Smoking cessation and hospitalized patients: Results of a randomized trial. *Archives of Internal Medicine, 157*, 409–415.

Miller, S. K. (1997). Impact of a gerontological nurse practitioner on the nursing home elderly in the acute care setting. *AACN Clinical Issues: Advanced Practice in Acute & Critical Care, 8*(4), 609–615.

Miller, S. K. (2002). Acute care of the elderly units: A positive outcomes case study. *Advanced Practice in Acute and Critical Care, 13*(1), 34–42.

Millette, B. E. (1994). Using Gilligan's framework to analyze nurses' stories of moral choices. *Western Journal of Nursing Research, 16*(6), 660–674.

Milligan, R. A., & Pugh, L. C. (1994). Fatigue during the childbearing period. In J. J. Fitzpatrick & J. S. Stevenson (Eds.), *Annual review of nursing research* (Vol. 12, pp. 33–49). New York: Springer Publishing.

Milliken, P. J. (2001). Disenfranchised mothers: Caring for an adult child with schizophrenia. *Health Care of Women International, 22*, 149–166.

Milliken, P. J., & Northcott, H. C. (2003). Redefining parental identity: Caregiving and schizophrenia. *Qualitative Health Research, 13*, 100–113.

Milliken, P. J., & Rodney, P. A. (2003). Parents as caregivers for children with schizophrenia: Moral dilemmas and moral agency. *Issues in Mental Health Nursing, 24*, 757–773.

Miltner, R. S. (2002). More than support: Nursing interventions provided to women in labor. *Journal of Obstetric, Gynecologic, and Neonatal Nursing, 31*(6), 753–761.

Mimura, C., & Griffiths, P. (2003). The effectiveness of current approaches to workplace stress management in the nursing profession: An evidence based literature review. *Occupational and Environmental Medicine*, 60(1), 10–15.

Minino, A. M., Arias, E., Kochanek, K. D., Murphy, S. L., & Smith, B. L. (2002). Deaths: Final data for 2000. *National vital statistics reports, (50)*, 15. Hyattsville, MD: National Center for Health Statistics. Retrieved from http://www.cdc.gov/nchs/data/nvsr/nvsr50/nvsr50_15.pdf

Minkler, M., & Fuller-Thomson, E. (2001). Physical and mental health status of American grandparents providing extensive child care to the grandchildren. *Journal of the American Medical Women's Association*, 56, 199–205.

Minkler, M., & Roe, K. M. (1993). *Grandmothers as caregivers: Raising children of the crack cocaine epidemic*. Newbury Park, CA: Sage Publications.

Minnick, A. F., Mion, L. C., Leipzig, R., Lamb, K., & Palmer, R. M. (1998). Prevalence and patterns of physical restraint use in the acute care setting. *Journal of Nursing Administration, 28*(11), 19–24.

Miota, P., Yahle, M., & Bartz, C. (1991). Premenstrual syndrome: A biopsychosocial approach to treatment. In D. Taylor & N. F. Woods (Eds.), *Menstruation, health and illness* (pp. 143–152). Washington, DC: Hemisphere.

Miota, P., Yahle, M., & Bartz, C. (1991). Premenstrual syndrome: A biopsychosocial approach to treatment. In D. Taylor & N. F. Woods (Eds.), *Menstruation, health and illness* (pp. 143–152). New York: Hemisphere.

Miranda, J., Azocar, F., Komaromy, M., & Golding, J. M. (1998). Unmet mental health needs of women in public-sector gynecologic clinics. *American Journal of Obstetrics and Gynecology, 178*(2), 212–217.

Miranda, J., Chung, J. Y., Green, B. L., Krupnick, J., Siddique, J., Revicki, D. A., et al., (2003). Treating depression in predominantly low-income young minority women. *Journal of the American Medical Association, 290*(1), 57–65.

Miranda, J., Hohmann, A. A., Attkisson, C. C., & Larson, D. B. (Eds.). (1994). *Mental disorders in primary care*. San Francisco, CA: Jossey-Bass.

Miranda, J., Lawson, W., & Escobar, J. (2002). Ethnic minorities. *Mental Health Services Research, 4*, 231–237.

Miranda, J., Nakamura, R., & Bernal, G. (2003). Including ethnic minorities in mental health intervention research: A practical approach to a long-standing problem. *Culture, Medicine, and Psychiatry, 27*, 467–486.

Mishel, M. H. (1981). The measurement of uncertainty in illness. *Nursing Research, 30*, 258–263.

Mishel, M. H. (1983a). Adjusting the fit: Development of uncertainty scales for specific clinical populations. *Western Journal of Nursing Research, 5*, 355–370.

Mishel, M. H. (1983b). Parents' perception of uncertainty concerning their hospitalized child. *Nursing Research, 32*, 324–330.

Mishel, M. H. (1988). Uncertainty in illness. *Image: Journal of Nursing Scholarship, 20*, 225–231.

Mishel, M. H. (1990). Reconceptualization of the uncertainty in illness theory. *Image: Journal of Nursing Scholarship, 22*, 256–262.

Mishel, M. H. (1990). Reconceptualization of the uncertainty in illness theory. *Image, 22*(4), 256–262.

Mishel, M. H. (1997). Uncertainty in acute illness. In J. J. Fitzpatrick & J. S. Norbeck (Eds.), *Annual review of nursing research* (Vol. 15, pp. 57–80). New York: Springer Publishing.

Mishel, M. H. (1999). Uncertainty in chronic illness. In J. J. Fitzpatrick & J. J. Norbeck (Eds), *Annual review of nursing research* (Vol. 17, pp. 269–294). New York: Springer Publishing.

Mishel, M., Belyea, M., Germino, B. B., Stewart, J. L., Bailey, D. E., Robertson, C., et al. (2002). Helping patients with localized prostate cancer manage uncertainty and treatment side effects: Nurse delivered psycho-educational intervention via telephone. *Cancer, 94*(6), 1854–1866.

Mishel, M. H., & Clayton, M. F. (2003). Theories of uncertainty in illness. In M. J. Smith & P. L. Liehr (Eds.), *Middle range theory for nursing* (pp. 25–48). New York: Springer Publishing.

Mishler, E. G. (1995). Models of narrative analysis: A typology. *Journal of Narrative and Life History*, 5, 87–123.

Miskella, C., & Avis, M. (1998). Care of the dying person in the nursing home: Exploring the care assistants' contribution. *European Journal of Oncology Nursing, 2*(2), 80–88.

Mistry, R. S., Vandewater, E. A., Huston, A. C., & McLloyd, V. C. (2002). Economic well-being and children's social adjustment: The role of family process in an ethnically diverse low-income sample. *Child Development, 73*, 935–951.

Mitby, P., Robison, L., Whitton, J., Zevon, M., Gibbs, I., Tersak, J., et al. (2003). Utilization of special education services and educational attainment among long-term survivors of childhood cancer:

A report from the Childhood Cancer Survivor Study. *Cancer, 97*(4), 1115–1126.

Mitchell, E. S. (1986). Multiple triangulation: A methodology for nursing science. *Advances in Nursing Science, 8*(3), 18–26.

Mitchell, E. S. (1999). Tips, tricks and trials of longitudinal research on the menstrual cycle [Abstract]. *Abstracts of the 13th Conference of the Society for Menstrual Research, 4*.

Mitchell, E. S., & Woods, N. F. (2001). Midlife women's attributions about perceived memory changes: Observations from the Seattle Midlife Women's Health Study. *Journal of Women's Health and Gender Based Medicine, 10*(4), 351–362.

Mitchell, E. S., Woods, N. F., & Lentz, M. J. (1987). Distinguishing among menstrual cycle symptom severity patterns [Abstract]. *Abstracts of the 7th Conference of the Society for Menstrual Cycle Research, 44*.

Mitchell, E. S., Woods, N. F., & Lentz, M. J. (1993). Stressors, coping and psychological distress: Experiences of women with three perimenstrual symptom patterns [Abstract]. *Abstracts of the 10th Conference of the Society for Menstrual Cycle Research, 6*.

Mitchell, E., Woods, N., Lentz, M., & Taylor, D. (1991). Recognizing PMS when you see it: Criteria for PMS sample selection. In D. L. Taylor & N. F. Woods (Eds.), *Menstruation, health and illness* (pp. 89–102). New York: Hemisphere.

Mitchell, E. S., Woods, N. F., Lentz, M. J., Taylor, D., & Lee, K. (1992). Methodological issues in the definition of perimenstrual symptoms. In A. Dan & L. Lewis (Eds.), *Menstrual health in women's lives* (pp. 7–14). Urbana: University of Illinois Press.

Mitchell, E. S., Woods, N. F., & Mariella, A. (2002). Three stages of the menopausal transition from the Seattle Study: Toward a more precise definition. *Menopause, 7*, 334–349.

Mitchell, E. S., Woods, N. F., & Mariella, A. (2003). FSH and estrogen patterns during the menopausal transition [Abstract]. *Abstracts of the 15th Conference of the Society for Menstrual Cycle Research.*

Mitchell, S. L., Teno, J. M., Roy, J., Kabumoto, G., & Mor, V. (2003). Clinical and organizational factors associated with feeding tube use among nursing home residents with advanced cognitive impairment. *Journal of the American Medical Association, 290*, 73–80.

Mittelmark, M. B., Psaty, B. M., Rautaharju, P. M., Fried, L. P., Borhani, N. O., Tracy, R. P., et al. (1993). Prevalence of cardiovascular diseases among older adults. *American Journal of Epidemiology, 137*, 311–317.

Mittelstadt, P. (1991). *PPRC recommends payment levels for non-physician providers. Capitol Update* (pp. 7–8). Washington, DC: American Nurses Association. Retrieved from http://www.ama.assn.org/ama/pub/category/3883.html

Mitty, E. (2001). Ethnicity and end-of-life decision making. *Reflections on Nursing Leadership, 27*(1), 28–31.

Mitty, E. (2003). *Assisted living: Aging-in-place and end-of-life care*. Manuscript submitted for publication.

Mobily, K., Lemke, J., & Gisin, G. (1991). The idea of leisure repertoire. *Journal of Applied Gerontology, 10*, 208–223.

Moen, P., Robison, J., & Dempster-McClain, D. (1995). Caregiving and women's well-being: A life course approach. *Journal of Health and Social Behavior, 36*(6), 752–761.

Mohr, W. K., Lutz, M. J. N., Fantuzzo, J. W., & Perry, M. A. (2000). Children exposed to family violence: A review of empirical research from a developmental ecological perspective. *Trauma, Violence, & Abuse, 1*(3), 263–283.

Mok, E., Chan, F., Chan, V., & Yeung, E. (2002). Perception of empowerment by family caregivers of patients with a terminal illness in Hong Kong. *International Journal of Palliative Nursing, 8*, 137–145.

Mokhlesi, B. (2003). Clinical implications of gastroesophageal reflux disease and swallowing dysfunction in COPD. *American Journal of Respiratory Medicine, 2*(2), 117–121.

Molloy, D. W., Silberfeld, M., Darzins, P., Guyatt, G. H., Singer, P. A., Rush, B., et al. (1996). Measuring capacity to complete an advance directive. *Journal of the American Geriatrics Society, 44*(6), 660–664.

Money, J. (1955). Linguistic resources and psychodynamic theory. *British Journal of Medical Psychology, 28*, 264–266.

Money, J., & Ehrhardt, A. A. (1972). *Man & woman, boy & girl.* Baltimore: Johns Hopkins University Press.

Monninkhof, E., van der Valk, P., van der Palen, J., van Herwaarden, C., Partridge, M. R., & Zielhuis, G. (2003). Self-management education for patients with chronic obstructive pulmonary disease: A systematic review. *Thorax, 58*, 394–398.

Montag, M. (1959). *Community college education for nursing.* New York: McGraw-Hill.

Montgomery, K. S. (2000). Creating consistency and control out of chaos: A qualitative view of planned pregnancy during adolescence. *Journal of Perinatal Education, 9*(4), 7–14.

Montgomery, K. S. (2001). Planned adolescent pregnancy: What they needed. *Issues in Comprehensive Pediatric Nursing, 24*(3), 19–29.

Montgomery, K. S. (2002). Planned adolescent pregnancy: What they wanted. *Journal of Pediatric Health Care, 16*, 282–289.

Moore, G., & Showstack, J. (2003). Primary care medicine in crisis: Toward reconstruction and renewal. *Annals of Internal Medicine, 138*, 244–247.

Moore, J. (1998). CCRCs shine in the shadows. *Contemporary Long Term Care, 21*, 39–40.

Moore, L. W., & Miller, M. (1999). Initiating research with doubly vulnerable populations. *Journal of Advanced Nursing, 30*(5), 1034–1040.

Moore, S. L. (1997). A phenomenological study of meaning in life in suicidal older adults. *Archives of Psychiatric Nursing, 11*, 29–36.

Moore, S. M. (2004). Critical analysis exercises. Chapter 3 analysis exercise: Pain: A balance between analgesia and side effects. In S. J. Peterson & T. S. Bredow (Eds.), *Middle range theories: Application to nursing research* (pp. 369–371). Philadelphia: Lippincott Williams & Wilkins.

Moore, S. M., Dolansky, M. A., Ruland, C. M., Pashkow, F. J., & Blackburn, G. G. (2003). Predictors of women's exercise maintenance after cardiac rehabilitation. *Journal of Cardiopulmonary Rehabilitation, 23*(1), 40–49.

Moorhead, S., Head, B., Johnson, M., & Maas, M. (1998). The nursing outcomes taxonomy: Development and coding. *Journal of Nursing Care Quality, 12*(6), 56–63.

Moorhead, S., Johnson, M., & Maas, M. (2004). *Nursing outcomes classification (NOC)* (3rd ed.). St. Louis, MO: Mosby.

Morgan, B. S., & Littell, D. H. (1988). A closer look at teaching and contingency contracting with type II diabetes. *Patient Education and Counseling, 12*, 145–158.

Morgan, S. (1990). A comparison of three methods of managing fever in the neurologic patient. *Journal of Neuroscience Nursing, 22*(1), 19–24.

Morley, J. (2003). Anorexia and weight loss in older persons. *Journal of Gerontology, 58A*, 131–137.

Morrell-Bellai, T., Goering, P. N., & Boydell, K. M. (2000). Becoming and remaining homeless: A qualitative investigation. *Issues in Mental Health Nursing, 21*(6), 581–604.

Morris, A. (2001). Rational use of computerized protocols in the intensive care unit. *Critical Care, 5*, 249–254.

Morris, J., & Ingham, R. (1988). Choice of surgery for early breast cancer psychosocial considerations. *Social Science and Medicine, 27*, 583–585.

Morris, J. N. (1964). *Uses of epidemiology*. Baltimore: Williams and Wilkins.

Morrison, E. F. (1992). A coercive interactive style as an antecedent to aggression and violence in psychiatric inpatients. *Research in Nursing and Health, 15*, 421–431.

Morrison-Beedy, D. (2001). Mentoring students and junior faculty in faculty research: A win-win scenario. *Journal of Professional Nursing, 17*(6), 291–296.

Morse, C., Bernard, M., et al. (1989). The effects of rational-emotive therapy and relaxation training on premenstrual syndrome: A preliminary study. *Journal of Rational-Emotive & Cognitive-Behavioral Therapy, 7*, 98–110.

Morse, C., Dennerstein, L., Farrell, E., & Varnavides, K. (1991). A comparison of hormone therapy, coping skills training, and relaxation for the relief of premenstrual syndrome. *Journal of Behavioral Medicine, 14*, 469–489.

Morse, G. (1999). Positively reframing perceptions of the menstrual cycle among women with premenstrual syndrome. *Journal of Obstetric, Gynecological, and Neonatal Nursing, 28*, 165–174.

Morse, J. E. (2001). The cultural sensitivity of grounded theory. *Qualitative Health Research, 11*, 721–722.

Morse, J. M., Bottoroff, J., Neander, W., & Solberg, S. (1991). Comparative analysis of conceptualizations and theories of caring. *Image: Journal of Nursing Scholarship, 23*, 119–127.

Morse, J. M., & Field, D. A. (1995). *Qualitative research methods for health professionals*. Newbury Park, CA: Sage.

Moss, J., Coenen, A., & Mills, M. (2003). Evaluation of the draft international standard for a reference terminology model for nursing actions. *Journal of Biomedical Informatics, 36*(4–5), 271–278.

Mostaghel, E., & Waters, D. (2003). Women benefit from lipid-lowering: Latest clinical trial data. *Cardiology in Review, 11*, 4–12.

Motzer, S. A., Hertig, V., Jarrett, M., & Heitkemper, M. M. (2003). Sense of coherence and quality of life in women with and without irritable bowel syndrome. *Nursing Research, 52*(5), 329–337.

Moyer, B. (1996). *The effects of interactive video on the problem-solving ability of senior level nursing students in group settings*. Unpublished doctoral dissertation, Lehigh University, Bethlehem, PA.

Mueller, C., & McCloskey, J. C. (1990). Nurses' job satisfaction: A proposed measure. *Nursing Research, 39*, 113–117.

Muender, M. M., Moore, M., Chen, G. J., & Sevick, M. (2000). Cost-benefit of a nursing telephone intervention to reduce preterm and low-birthweight births in an African American clinic population. *Prevention Medicine, 30*, 271–276.

Muir-Cochrane, E. C. (1998). The role of the community mental health nurse in the administration of depot neuroleptic medication: "Not just the needle nurse!" *International Journal of Nursing Practice, 4*, 254–260.

Mujic, V. R., & Rao, S. S. (1999). Recognizing atypical manifestations of GERD. Asthma, chest pain, and otolaryngologic disorders may be due to reflux. *Postgraduate Medicine, 105*, 53.

Mulley, G. (1995). Preparing for the late years. *Lancet, 345*, 1409–1413.

Mumford, E., Schlesinger, H. J., & Glass, G. V. (1982). The effects of psychological intervention on recovery from surgery and heart attacks: An analysis of the literature. *American Journal of Public Health, 72*(2), 141–151.

Mundinger, M. O., Kane, R. L., Lenz, E. R., Totten, A. M., Tsai, W., Cleary, P. D., et al. (2000). Primary care outcomes of patients treated by nurse practitioners or physicians: A randomized trial. *Journal of the American Medical Association, 283*(1), 59–68.

Munet-Vilaro, F. (1998). Forum focus: Grieving and death rituals of Latinos. *Oncology Nurses Forum, 25*(10), 1761–1763.

Munro, B., Jacobsen, D., & Brooten, D. (1994). Reexamination of the psychometric characteristics of the La Monica–Oberst Patient Satisfaction Scale. *Research in Nursing and Health, 17*, 119–125.

Murkies, A. L., Wilcox, G., & Davis, S. R. (1998). Clinical review 92: Phytoestrogens. *Journal of Clinical Endocrinology and Metabolism, 83*(2), 297–303.

Murphy, L. (1978). *Methods for studying nurse staffing on a patient unit* (Publication No. HRA 78-3). Washington, DC: DHEW.

Murphy, S., Johnson, C., Wu, L., Fan, J., & Lohan, J. (2003). Bereaved parents' outcomes 4 to 60 months after their children's deaths by accident, suicide, or homicide: A comparative study demonstrating differences. *Death Studies, 27*, 39–61.

Murphy, S. A. (2001). Traumatic events: Individual and collective responses. In J. J. Fitzpatrick & P. A. Wilke (Eds.), *Psychiatric mental health nursing research digest* (pp. 230–233). New York: Springer Publishing.

Murray, L., Sinclair, D., Cooper, P., Ducournau, P., & Turner, P. (1999). The socioemotional development of 5-year-old children of postnatally depressed mothers. *Journal of Child Psychology and Psychiatry, 40*, 1259–1271.

Musil, C. M. (1998). Health, stress, coping, and social support in grandmother caregivers. *Health Care for Women International, 19*, 441–445.

Musil, C., Morris, D., Warner, C., & Saied, H. (2003). Issues in caregivers' stress and providers' support. *Research on Aging, 25*(5), 505–526.

Mwaba, K., & Molamu, R. B. (1998). Perceived causes of relapse among a sample of recovering psychiatric patients at a Mafikeng hospital. *South African Journal of Nursing, 221*, 55–57.

Myhrman, A. (1988). The Northern Finland cohort, 1966–82: A follow-up study of children unwanted at birth. In H. P. David, Z. Dytrych, Z. Matejcek, & V. Schuller (Eds.), *Born unwanted* (pp. 103–110). New York: Springer.

Nadler, A. (1990). Help-seeking behavior as a coping resource. In M. Rosenbaum (Ed.), *Learned resourcefulness: On coping skills, self-control, and adaptive behavior* (pp. 127–162). New York: Springer Publishing.

Nagengast, S. L., Baun, M. M., Megel, M., & Leibowitz, M. J. (1997). The effects of the presence of a companion animal on physiological and behavioral distress in children during a physical examination. *Journal of Pediatric Nursing, 12*(6), 323–330.

Nagi, S. (1991). Disability concepts revisited: Implications for prevention. In Institute of Medicine *Disability in America: Toward a national agenda for prevention* (pp. 304–327). Washington, DC: National Academy Press.

Nail, L. M. (2002). Fatigue in patients with cancer. *Center for Leadership, Information & Research, 29*, 537–546.

Nathaniel, A. K. (2004). A grounded theory of moral reckoning in nursing. *Grounded Theory Review, 4*(1), 43–58.

National Cancer Institute. (2003). *Annual report*. Washington, DC: Author.

National Center for Health Statistics. (n.d.). *Highlights from trend tables and chartbook. Health, United States, 2003*. Retrieved January 9, 2004, from http://www.cdc.gov/nchs/products/pubs/pubd/hus/highlits.pdf

National Center for Nursing Quality. (2003). *National Database for Nursing Quality Indicators (NDNQI)*. Retrieved January 10, 2004, from http://www.nursingquality.org/ndnqi/

National Center for Nursing Research. (1993). *Nursing informatics: Enhancing patient care* (NIH Publication No. 93-2419). Bethesda, MD: National Institutes of Health.

National Center on Addiction and Substance Abuse at Columbia University. (2002). *Teen tipplers: America's underage drinking epidemic*. New York: Columbia University.

National Center on Elder Abuse. (n.d.). *Types of elder abuse in domestic settings*. Retrieved from http://www.elderabusecenter.org

National Coalition for Cancer Survivors. (2003). *Annual report*. Silver Springs, MD: Author.

National Coalition for Health Professional Education in Genetics. (2001). *Core competencies in genetics essentials for health care professionals*. Lutherville, MD: Author.

National Coalition for the Homeless. (1999). Retrieved from http://nch.ari.net

National Coalition for the Homeless. (1999, March). *Rural homelessness* (Fact Sheet #13). Retrieved from http://www.nationalhomeless.org/rural.html

National Coalition for the Homeless. (2002). Retrieved December 15, 2003, from http://www.nationalhomeless.org.

National Coalition for the Homeless. (2002, September). *How many people experience homelessness?* (Fact Sheet #2). Washington, DC.

National Commission for the Protection of Human Subjects of Biomedical and Behavioral Research. (1979). *The Belmont report* (GPO No. 887–809). Washington, DC: U.S. Government Printing Office.

National Committee for Quality Assurance. (2003, June). *NCQA overview: Measuring the quality of America's health care*. Washington, DC.

National Family Caregivers Association. (2002). *NFCA caregiver survey*. Retrieved from http://www.nfcacares.org/survrpt2002.html

National Guideline Clearinghouse. *Guidelines for Alzheimer's disease management*. Issued January 8, 1999. Revised January 1, 2002. Retrieved from http://www.guidelines.gov/summary/summary.aspx?doc_id=3157

National Heart Lung and Blood Institute, National Institutes of Health. (1998). *Clinical guidelines on the identification, evaluation, and treatment of overweight and obesity in adults: The evidence report*. U.S. Department of Health and Human Services, Public Health Service.

National Highway Traffic Safety Administration. (2002). *Traffic safety facts—alcohol*. Washington, DC: U.S. Department of Transportation.

National Institute for Nursing Research. (1993). *Nursing informatics: Enhancing patient care* (NIH Publication No. 93-2419). Bethesda, MD: U.S. Department of Health and Human Services.

National Institute of Diabetes and Digestive and Kidney Diseases. (2003). *Conquering diabetes: A strategic plan for the 21st century* (NIH Publication No. 99–4398). Retrieved November 25, 2003, from http://www.niddk.nih.gov/federal/dwgsummary.htm

National Institute of Mental Health (NIMH). (1994). *Epidemiological Catchment Area Project* (ECA). Washington, DC: Author.

National Institute of Mental Health. (1998a). *Priorities for prevention research at NIMH* (NIH Publication No. 98–4321). Retrieved April 21, 2003, from http://www.nimh.nih.gov/publist/984321.html

National Institute of Mental Health. (1998b). *Bridging science and service*. [National Advisory Mental Health Council Clinical Treatment and Services Research Workgroup.] Bethesda, MD: Author.

National Institute of Mental Health. *Research on women's mental health, FY2001–FY2002*. Retrieved from http://www.nimh.nih.gov/wmhc/0102highlights.pdf

National Institute of Mental Health. (2003). *Mental health services research fact sheet* (NIH Publication. No. 03-5409). Bethesda, MD: Author.

National Institute of Mental Health Depression Awareness, Recognition, and Treatment Program. (2003). Rockville, MD: National Institute of Mental Health. Available at http://www.nimh.nih.gov/DART/

National Institute of Nursing Research. (1993). Report on Nursing Information, US PHS.

National Institute of Nursing Research. (2000). *Minority health research development for nurse investigators. Executive Summary*. Retrieved from http://www.nih.gov/ninr/research/diversity/exec_sum_mhrdni.pdf

National Institute of Nursing Research Priority Expert Panel on Nursing Informatics. (1993). *Nursing informatics: Enhancing patient care*. Bethesda, MD: U.S. Department of Health and Human Services, U.S. Public Health Service, National Institutes of Health.

National Institute of Nursing Research Priority Expert Panel. (1995). *Community-based health care: Nursing strategies* (NIH Publication No. 95-3917). Bethesda, MD: U.S. Department of Health and Human Services.

National Institute of Occupational Safety and Health. (1996). *Violence in the workplace: Risk factors and prevention strategies*. Department of Health and Human Services CIB 57.

National Institute of Occupational Safety and Health (NIOSH). (1997). *Reducing healthcare worker risk of sharp object injury through safer sharps disposal*. Retrieved from www.cdc.gov/niosh/homepage

National Institute of Occupational Safety and Health. (1999). Control of smoke from laser/electric surgical procedures. *Journal of Applied Occupational and Environmental Hygiene, 14*, 71.

National Institute of Occupational Safety and Health. (2002). *Violence: Occupational hazards in hospitals*. Department of Health and Human Services 2002-101.

National Institute on Aging. (1995). *Progress report on Alzheimer's disease 1995*. (NIH Publication No.

95-3994). Washington, DC: U.S. Government. Printing Office.

National Institutes of Health. (1997, February 11–13). *Interventions to prevent HIV risk behaviors.* (Consensus Development Statement). Bethesda, MD: Author.

National Institutes of Health. (1999). *Agenda for research on women's health for the 21st century. A report of the task force on the NIH Women's Health Research Agenda for the 21st century*, Volume 1. Executive Summary (NIH Publication No. 99-4385, pp. 49–50). Bethesda, MD: Author.

National Institutes of Health. (2000). *Consensus development conference statement: Osteoporosis: Prevention, diagnosis, and therapy.* Retrieved November 16, 2003, from http://consensus.nih.gov/cons/111/111_statement.htm

National Institutes of Health. (2003). *CRISP: Computer Retrieval of Information on Scientific Projects.* Retrieved October 9, 2003, from http://crisp.cit.nih.gov/crisp/crisp_lib.query

National Institutes of Health. (n.d.). *NIH roadmap.* Retrieved March 31, 2004, from http://nihroadmap.nih.gov/

National Institutes of Health Consensus and State-of-the-Science Statements. (2002). Symptoms management in cancer: Pain, depression, and fatigue. *National Institutes of Health, 19*(4), 1–29.

National Institutes of Health Guide. (1997). Opportunities in genetics and nursing research. *Nursing Research NIH Guide, 26*(9), (PA number: PA-97-047 PT 34).

National Institutes of Health Guide: *Opportunities in genetics and nursing research.* Retrieved from http://grants.nih.gov/grants/guide/pa-files/PA-97-047.html/

National Institutes of Health, Office of the Director. (1996). *NIH almanac 1995–1996* (NIH Publication No. 96-50). Washington, DC: Author.

National Library of Medicine. (1960). *Medical subject headings.* Washington, DC: Author.

National Mental Health Association. (2003). Retrieved from http://nmha.org

National Organization of Nurse Practitioner Faculties. (2002). *Nurse practitioner primary care competencies in specialty areas: Adult, family, gerontological, pediatric, and women's health.* Retrieved March 31, 2004, from http://www.nonpf.com

National Osteoporosis Foundation. (2002, February). *America's bone health: The state of osteoporosis and low bone mass in our nation.* Washington, DC.

National Osteoporosis Foundation. (2003). *Physician's guide to prevention and treatment of osteoporosis.* Washington DC.

National Research Council. (1989). *Recommended dietary allowances.* Washington, DC: National Academy Press.

National Research Council Institute of Medicine. (2000). *From neurons to neighborhoods.* Washington, DC: National Academy Press.

National Women's Health Information Center. (2003). *Osteoporosis.* 4woman.gov, a project of the U.S. Department of Health and Human Services, Office on Women's Health, Washington, DC. Retrieved October 13, 2003, from http://www.4woman.gov/faq/osteopor.htm

Navon, L., & Ozer, N. (2003). Ordinary logic in unordinary lay theories: A key to understanding proneness to medication nonadherence in schizophrenia. *Archives of Psychiatric Nursing, 17*, 108–116.

Naylor, M. D. (2003). Nursing intervention research and quality of care: Influencing the future of healthcare. *Nursing Research, 52*(60), 380–385.

Naylor, M., Bowles, K., & Brooten, D. (2000). Patient problems and advanced practice nurse interventions during transitional care. *Public Health Nursing, 72*(2), 94–102.

Naylor, M. D., Brooten, D., Campbell, R., Jacobsen, B. S., Mezey, M., Pauly, M. V., et al. (1999). Comprehensive discharge planning and home follow-up of hospitalized elders—a randomized clinical trial. *Journal of the American Medical Association, 281*(7), 613–620.

Naylor, M. D., Brooten, D. A., Campbell, R. L., Maislin, G., McCauley, K. M., & Schwartz, J. S. (2004). Transitional care of older adults hospitalized with heart failure: A randomized, controlled trial. *Journal of the American Geriatric Society, 52*, 675–684.

Naylor, M., Brooten, D., Jones, R., Lavizzo, O., Mourey, R., Mezey, M., et al. (1994). Comprehensive discharge planning for hospitalized elderly. *Annals of Internal Medicine, 120*, 999–1006.

Naylor, M. D., Munro, B. H., & Brooten, D. A. (1991). Measuring the effectiveness of nursing practice. *Clinical Nurse Specialist, 5*(4), 210–215.

Needleman, H. L., Gunnoe, C., Leviton, A., Reed, R., Peresie, H., Maher, C., et al. (1979). Deficits in psychologic and classroom performance of children with elevated dentine lead levels. *New England Journal of Medicine, 300*(13), 689–695.

Needleman, H. L., & Landrigan, P. J. (2004). What level of lead in blood is toxic for a child? *American Journal of Public Health, 94*, 8.

Needleman, H. L, Riess, J. A., Tobin, M. J., Biesecker, G. E., & Greenhouse, J. B. (1996). Bone lead levels and delinquent behavior. *Journal of the American Medical Association, 275*, 363–369.

Needleman, J., Buerhaus, P. I., Mattke, S., Stewart, M., & Zelevinsky, K. (2001). *Nurse staffing and patient outcomes in hospitals* (Report 230-99-0021). Health Resources Services Administration.

Needleman, J., Buerhaus, P., Mattke, S., Stewart, M., & Zelevinsky, K. (2002). Nurse-staffing levels and the quality of care in hospitals. *New England Journal of Medicine, 346*, 1715–1722.

Neglia, J., Friedman, D., Yasui, Y., Mertens, A., Hammond, S., Stovall, M., et al. (2001). Second malignant neoplasms in five-year survivors of childhood cancer: Childhood cancer survivor study. *Journal of the National Cancer Institute*, 93(8), 618–629.

Negri, E., Franceschi, S., Parpinel, M., & LaVecchia, C. (1998). Fiber intake and risk of colorectal cancer. *Cancer Epidemiological Biomarkers Prevention, 7*(8), 667–771.

Neidig, J. L., Smith B. A., & Brashers, D. E. (2003). Aerobic exercise training for depressive symptom management in adults living with HIV infection. *Journal of the Association of Nurses in AIDS Care, 14*(2), 30–40.

Neinstein, L. S., Radzik, M., & Sherer, S. (2002). Common concerns of adolescents and their parents. In L. S. Neinstein (Ed.), *Adolescent health care* (pp. 1397–1401). Philadelphia: Lippincott, Williams and Wilkins.

Nelson, A., Fragala, G., & Menzel, N. (2003). Myths and facts about back injuries in nursing. *American Journal of Nursing, 103*(2), 32–41.

Nelson, H. D., Humphrey, L. L., Nygren, P., Teutsch, S. M., & Allan, J. A. (2002). Postmenopausal hormone replacement therapy. *Journal of the American Medical Association, 288*(7), 872–884.

Nesse, R. E. (2002). The demographics and economics of chronic disease: The future of medicare depends on how well we learn to manage chronic disease. *Health Affairs*, W125–W126.

Neugarten, B. (1968). *Middle age and aging*. Chicago: University of Chicago Press.

Neuman, B. (Ed.). (1982). *The NSM: Applications to nursing education and practice*. New York: Appleton-Century-Crofts.

Neuman, B. (Ed.). (1989). *The NSM* (2nd ed.). Norwalk, CT: Appleton & Lange.

Neuman, B. (Ed.). (1995). The NSM. In B. Neuman (Ed.), *The NSM* (3rd ed., pp. 3–62). Norwalk, CT: Appleton & Lange.

Neuman, B. (Ed.). (2001). The Neuman Systems Model. In B. Neuman & J. Fawcett (Eds.), *The NSM* (4th ed.). Upper Saddle River, NJ: Prentice Hall.

Neuman, B., & Fawcett, J. (Eds.). (2001). *The Neuman Systems Model* (4th ed.). Upper Saddle River, NJ: Prentice Hall.

Neville, K. L. (2003). Uncertainty in illness. *Orthopaedic Nursing, 22*(3), 206–214.

New, P., Nite, G., & Callahan, J. (1959). Too many nurses may be worse than too few. *Modern Hospital*, 93, 104–108.

Newacheck, P. W., & Taylor, W. R. (1992). Childhood chronic illness: Prevalence, severity, and impact. *American Journal of Public Health, 82*, 364–371.

Newbern, V. B. (1992). Failure to thrive: A growing concern in the elderly. *Journal of Gerontological Nursing, 18*(8), 21–25.

Newbrander, W., & Eichler, R. (2001). Managed care in the United States: Its history, forms, and future. In R. Aviva & X. Scheil-Adbury (Eds.), *Recent health policy in social security*. Somerset, NJ: Transaction Publishers.

Newcomer, S. F., & Udry, J. R. (1985). Oral sex in an adolescent population. *Archives of Sex Research, 14*, 41–46.

Newell, A., & Simon, H. (1972). *Human problem solving*. Englewood Cliffs, NJ: Prentice-Hall.

Newell, K. W. (Ed.). (1975). *Health by the people*. Geneva, Switerzerland: World Health Organization.

Newman, M. A. (1979). *Theory development in nursing*. Philadelphia: F A. Davis.

Newman, M. A. (1986). *Health as expanding consciousness*. St. Louis, MO: C. V. Mosby.

Newman, M. A. (1990a). Newman's theory of health as praxis. *Nursing Science Quarterly*, 3, 37–41.

Newman, M. A. (1990b). Shifting to a higher consciousness. In M. E. Parker (Ed.), *Nursing theories in practice*. New York: National League for Nursing Press.

Newman, M. A. (1994). *Health as expanding consciousness* (2nd ed.). New York: National League for Nursing Press.

Newman, M. A. (2002). The pattern that connects. *Advances in Nursing Science, 24*(3), 1–7.

Newman, M. A., Sime, A. M., & Corcoran-Perry, S. A. (1991). The focus of the discipline of nursing. *Advances in Nursing Science, 14*(1), 1–6.

Newschaffer, C. (1997). The impact of co-morbidity on life expectancy among men with localized prostate cancer. *Journal of Urology, 157*(3), 964–965.

Newton, R. (2000). Osteoporosis and fall prevention. In S. H. Gueldner, M. S. Burke, & H. Smiciklas-Wright (Eds.), *Preventing and managing osteoporosis* (pp. 117–130). New York: Springer Publishing.

Ng, D. T., Chan, S. W., & MacKenzie, A. (2000). Case management in the community psychiatric nursing service in Hong Kong: Describing the process. *Perspectives in Psychiatric Care*, 36, 59–66.

Nguyen, J. D., Carson, M. L., Parris, K. M., & Place, P. (2003). A comparison pilot study of public health field nursing home visitation program interventions for pregnant Hispanic adolescents. *Public Health Nursing, 20*, 412–418.

Nicholas, P. K., Kemppainen, J. K., Holzemer, W. L., Nokes, K. M., Eller, L. S., Corless, I. B., et al. (2002). Self-care management for neuropathy in HIV disease. *AIDS Care, 14*(6), 763–771.

Nicklas, B. J., Berman, D. M., Davis, D. C., Dobrovolny, C. L., & Dennis, K. E. (1999). Racial differences in metabolic predictors of obesity among postmenopausal women. *Obesity Research, 7*(5), 463–468.

Nicklas, B. J., Dennis, K. E., Berman, D. M., Sorkin, J., Ryan, A. S., & Goldberg, A. P. (2003). Lifestyle intervention of hypocaloric dieting and walking reduces abdominal obesity and improves coronary heart disease risk factors in obese, postmenopausal, African-American and Caucasian women. *Journal of Gerontology, 58*(2), M181–M189.

Nicklas, B. J., Katzel, L. I., Bunyard, L. B., Dennis, K. E., & Goldberg, A. P. (1997). Effects of an American Heart Association diet and weight loss on lipoprotein lipids in obese, postmenopausal women. *American Journal of Clinical Nutrition*, 66, 853–859.

Nicklas, B. J., Penninx, B. W., Ryan, A., Berman, D. M., Lynch, N. A., & Dennis, K. (2003). Visceral adiose tissue cutoffs associated with metabolic risk factors for coronary heart disease in women. *Diabetes Care, 26*(5), 1413–1420.

Nies, M. A., Chrusical, H., & Hepworth, J. (in press). An intervention to promote walking in sedentary women in the community. *American Journal of Health Behavior*.

Nightingale, F. (1858). *Notes on matters affecting the health, efficiency, and hospital administration of the British army, founded chiefly on the experience of the late war*. London: Harrison and Sons.

Nightingale, F. (1863a). *How people may live and not die in India*. London: Emil Faithfull.

Nightingale, F. (1863b). *Notes on hospitals* (3rd ed.). London: Longman, Green, Longman, Roberts, and Green.

Nightingale, F. (1885). Nursing the sick. In R. Quain (Ed.), *A dictionary of medicine* (9th ed., pp. 1043–1056). New York: Appleton.

Nightingale, F. (1892). Introduction. In D. Gidumal (Ed.), *Behramji M. Malabari: A biographical sketch*. London: T. Fisher Unwin.

Nightingale, F. (1949). Sick nursing and health nursing. In I. A. Hampton (Ed.), *Nursing of the sick*. New York: McGraw Hill. (Original work published 1893)

Nightingale, F. (1956). *The institution of Kaiserwerth on the Rhine for the practical training of deaconesses under the direction of the Rev. Pastor Fliedner embracing the support and care of a hospital, infant and industrial schools, and a female penitentiary*. Duesseldorf-Kaiserwerth, Germany: Diakonissenanstalt. (Original work published 1851)

Nightingale, F. (1969). *Notes on nursing: What it is and what it is not*. New York: Dover. (Original work published 1859)

NIH Technology Assessment Panel. (1996). Integration of behavioral and relaxation approaches into the treatment of chronic pain and insomnia. *Journal of the American Medical Association, 276*, 313–318.

Nissen, S. E., Tuzcu, E. M., Schoenhagen, P., Brown, B. G., Ganz, P., Vogel, R. A., et al (2004). Effect of intensive compared with moderate lipid-lowering therapy on progression of coronary atherosclerosis: A randomized controlled trial. *Journal of the American Medical Association, 291*, 1071–1080.

Nite, G., & Willis, F. (1964) *The coronary patient: Hospital care and rehabilitation*. New York: Macmillan.

Niv, Y., & Abu-Avid, S. (1988). On the positioning of a nasogastric tube. *American Journal of Medicine, 84*(3 Pt. 1), 563–564.

Noble, M. A. (1982). *The ICU environment: Directions for nursing*. Reston, VA: Reston Publishing.

Noddings, N. (1994). Moral obligation or moral support for high-tech home care? *Hastings Center Report, 24*(5), S6–S10.

Noe, R., Greenberer, B., & Wang, S (2002). Mentoring: What we know and where we might go. *Research in Personnel and Human Resource Management, 21*, 129–173.

Nokes, K. M., Chew, L., & Altman C. (2003). Using a telephone support group for HIV-positive persons aged 50+ to increase social support and health-related knowledge. *AIDS Patient Care and STDs, 17*(7), 345–351.

Nolan, J. R., & Nolan-Haley, J. M. (Eds.). (1990). *Black's law dictionary* (16th ed.). St. Paul, MN: West.

Nomura, Y., Wickramaratne, P. J., Warner, V., Mufson, L., & Weissman, M. M. (2002). Family discord, parental depression, and psychopathology in offspring: Ten year follow-up. *Journal of the American Academy of Child and Adolescent Psychiatry, 41*, 402–409.

Norbeck, J. S., DeJoseph, J. F., & Smith, R. T. (1996). A randomized trial of an empirically-derived social support intervention to prevent low birthweight among African-American women. *Social Science and Medicine, 43*(6), 947–954.

Nordentoft, M., Lou, H., Hansen, D., Nim, J., Pryds, O., Rubin, P., et al. (1996). Intrauterine growth retardation and premature delivery: The influence of maternal smoking and psychosocial factors. *American Journal of Public Health, 86*(3), 347–354.

Norman, D. A. (2002). *The design of everyday things.* New York. Basic Books.

Normand, S. T., Glickman, M. E., Sharma, R. G. V. R. K., & McNeil, B. J. (1996). Using admission characteristics to predict short-term mortality from myocardial infarction in elderly patients. *Journal of the American Medical Association, 275,* 1322–1328.

Norris, F. (1992). Epidemiology of trauma: Frequency and impact of different potentially traumatic events on different demographic groups. *Journal of Consulting and Clinical Psychology, 60,* 409–418.

Norris, F. H., Friedman, M. J., Watson, P. J., Byrne, C. M., Diaz, E., & Kaniasty, K. (2002). 60,000 disaster victims speak: Part I. An empirical review of the empirical literature, 1981–2001. *Psychiatry, 65*(3), 207–260.

Norris, J. R. (2002). One-to-one teleapprenticeship as a means for nurses teaching and learning Parse's theory of human becoming. *Nursing Science Quarterly, 15*(2), 143–149.

North American Nursing Diagnosis Association. (2003). *Nursing diagnoses: Definitions & classifications 2003–2004.* Philadelphia: Author.

Northouse, L. L. (1990). A longitudinal study of the adjustment of patients and husbands to breast cancer. *Oncology Nursing Forum, 17,* 39–45.

Northouse, L. L., Dorris, G., & Charron-Moore, C. (1995). Factors affecting couples' adjustment to recurrent breast cancer. *Social Science Medicine, 41,* 69–76.

Northouse, L. L., Laten, D., & Reddy, P. (1995). Adjustment of women and their husbands to recurrent breast cancer. *Research in Nursing and Health, 18,* 515–524.

Northouse, L. L., & Swain, M. A. (1987). Adjustment of patients and their husbands to the initial impact of breast cancer. *Nursing Research, 36,* 221–225.

Northrup, C. (1997). Shedding light on sunlight. *Health Wisdom for Women, 4*(6), 6.

Norton, D., McLaren, R., & Exton-Smith, A. (Eds.). (1975). *An investigation of geriatric nurse problems in hospitals.* Edinburgh, United Kingdom: Churchill Livingston.

Norton, S. A., & Talerico, K. A. (2000). Facilitating end-of-life decision making: Strategies for communicating and assessing. *Journal of Gerontological Nursing, 26*(9), 6–13.

Norusis, M. J. (1994). *SPSS for Windows 6.1. advanced statistics.* Chicago: SPSS.

Nunnally, J. C. (1978). *Psychometric theory* (2nd ed.). New York: McGraw-Hill.

Nunnally, J. C., & Bernstein, I. H. (1994). *Psychometric theory* (3rd ed.). New York: McGraw-Hill.

Nutrition Screening Initiatives. (1991). *Nutrition screening manual for professionals caring for older Americans.* Washington, DC: Greer, Margolis, Mitchell, Grunwald, and Associates.

Oakley, A., Hickey, D., Rajan, L., & Rigby, A. S. (1996). Social support in pregnancy: Does it have long-term effects? *Journal of Reproductive and Infant Psychology, 14,* 7–22.

O'Brien, B., Evans, M., & White-McDonald, E. (2002). Isolation from "being alive": Coping with severe nausea and vomiting of pregnancy. *Nursing Research, 51,* 302–308.

O'Brien-Pallas, L. L., Cockerill, R., & Leatt, P. (1991). *A comparison of the workload estimated by five patient classification systems in nursing* (Final report No. 6606-3706-57). Ottawa, Ontario: Health and Welfare Canada.

O'Brien-Pallas, L. L., Irvine, D., Peereboom, E., & Murray, M. (1997). Measuring nursing workload: Understanding the variability. *Nursing Economic$, 15*(4), 171–182.

O'Brien-Pallas, L., Irvine Doran, D., Murray, M., Cockerill, R., Sidani, S., Laurie-Shaw, B., et al. (2001). Evaluation of a client care delivery model part 1: Variability in nursing utilization in community home nursing. *Nursing Economic$, 19*(6), 267–276.

O'Brien-Pallas, L., Irvine Doran, D., Murray, M., Cockerill, R., Sidani, S., Laurie-Shaw, B., et al. (2002). Evaluation of a client care delivery model part 2: Variability in client outcomes in community home nursing. *Nursing Economic$, 20*(1), 13–21.

Obrist, W. D. (2001). History of cerebral blood flow assessment. *Intensive Care and Emergency Medicine, 37,* 3–6.

Ockene, I. S., Hayman, L. L., Pasternak, R. C., Schron, E., & Dunbar-Jacob, J. (2002). Task Force #4: Adherence issues and behavior change: Achieving a long term solution. *Journal of the American College of Cardiology, 40*(4), 630–640.

O'Connor, A., Drake, E., Fiset, V., Page, J., Curtin, D., & Llewellyn-Thomas, H. (1997). Annotated bibliography: Studies evaluating decision-support interventions for patients. *Canadian Journal of Nursing Research, 29*(3), 113–120.

O'Connor, A. M., Stacey, D., Rovner, D., Homes-Rovner, M., Tetroe, J., Llewellyn-Thomas, H., et al. (2002). *Decision aids for people facing health treatment or screening decisions (Cochrane Review) in the*

Cochrane Library. Oxford, England: Update Software.

Odegard, S., & Andersson, D. K. G. (2001). Knowledge of diabetes among personnel in home-based care: How does it relate to medical mishaps? *Journal of Nursing Management, 9*, 107–114.

Oetting, K., Baun, M., Bergstrom, N., & Langston, N. (1985). Petting a companion dog and autogenic relaxation effects on systolic and diastolic blood pressure, heart rate, and peripheral skin temperature. *Journal of the Delta Society, 2*(1), 72.

Office of Communications, Office of the Director. (1996). *National Institutes of Health*. Washington, DC: National Institutes of Health.

Office of Disease Prevention and Health Promotion. (2002). Retrieved from http://odphp.osophs.dhhs.gov/pubs/LeadingIndicators/ldgsec1.html

Office of Juvenile Justice and Delinquency Prevention. (1995). *Delinquency prevention works. Summary*. Washington, DC: U.S. Department of Justice, Office of Justice Programs, Office of Juvenile Justice and Delinquency Prevention.

Office of the U.S. Surgeon General. (1999). *Mental health: A report of the Surgeon General*. Washington, DC: Author.

O'Grady, N. P., Alexander, M., Dellinger, E. P., Gerberding, J. L., Heard, S. L., Maki, D. G., et al. (2002). Guidelines for the prevention of intravascular catheter-related infections. *Morbidity and Mortality Weekly Report, 51*(RR-10), 1–26.

Ohr, W. K., Fantuzzo, J. W., & Abdul-Kabir, S. (2001). Safeguarding themselves and their children: Mothers share their strategies. *Journal of Family Violence, 16*(1), 75–92.

Okami, P., Olmstead, R., Abramson, P. R., & Pendleton, L. (1998). Early childhood exposure to parental nudity and scenes of parental sexuality. *Archives of Sexual Behavior, 27*, 361–384.

Olds, D., Eckenrode, J., Henderson, C., Kitzman, H., Powers, J., Cole, R., et al. (1997). Long term effects of home visitation on maternal life course and child abuse and neglect. *Journal of the American Medical Association, 278*, 637–643.

Olds, D., Henderson, C., Jr., Kitzman, H., Eckenrode, J., Cole, R., & Tatelbaum, R. (1998). The promise of home visitation: Results of two randomized trials. *Journal of Community Psychology, 26*(1), 5–21.

Olds, D., Robinson, J., O'Brian, R., Luckey, D., Pettitt, L., Henderson, C., et al. (2002). Home visiting by paraprofessionals and by nurses: A randomized, controlled trial. *Pediatrics, 110*(3), 486–496.

Oleske, J. M., Rothpletz-Puglia, P. M., & Winter, H. (1996). Historical perspectives on the evolution in understanding the importance of nutritional care in pediatric HIV infection. *Journal of Nutrition, 126*(10 suppl.), 2616S–2619S.

Oleson, V., & Woods, N. F. (1986). *Culture, society, and menstruation*. New York: Hemisphere, Harper & Row.

Oliver, D., Britton, M., Seed, P., Martin, F. C., & Hopper, A. H. (1997). Development and evaluation of evidence based risk assessment tool (STRATIFY) to predict which elderly inpatients will fall: Case-control and cohort studies. *British Medical Journal, 315*, 1049–1053.

Oliver, S., & Redfern, S. (1991). Interpersonal communication between nurses and elderly patients: Refinement of an observation schedule. *Journal of Advanced Nursing, 16*, 30–38.

Olsen, D. (2003). Ethical considerations in international nursing research: A report from the International Centre for Nursing Ethics. *Nursing Ethics, 10*(2), 122–137.

Olson, R. (1995). Mentoring through predoctoral fellowships to enhance research productivity. *Journal of Professional Nursing, 11*(5), 270–275.

O'Malley, M., & Orem, D. E. (1952). Diagnosis of hospital nursing problems. *Hospitals, 26*(8), 63–65.

Ondeck, M. (2000). Historical development. In F. H. Nichols & S. S. Humenick, *Childbirth education: Practice, research, and theory* (pp. 18–31). Philadelphia: Saunders.

Oppenheim, R. W. (1981). Ontogenetic adaptations and retrogressive processes in the development of the nervous system and behavior. In K. Connolly & H. Prechtl (Eds.), *Maturation and behavior development* (pp. 73–109). London: Spastic Society.

Orem, D. E. (1956). Hospital nursing service: An analysis. *Division of Hospital and Institutional Services, Indiana State Board of Health, Indianapolis*, 85.

Orem, D. E. (1991). *Nursing: Concepts of practice* (4th ed.). St. Louis, MO: Mosby Year-Book.

Orem, D. E. (2001). *Nursing: Concepts of practice* (6th ed.). St. Louis, MO: Mosby.

Orlando, I. J. (1961). *The dynamic nurse-patient relationship*. New York: Putnam.

Orlando, I. J. (1990). *The dynamic nurse-patient relationship* (2nd ed.). New York: National League for Nursing.

Orr, S. T., James, S. A., Miller, C. A., Barakat, B., Daikoku, N., Pupkin, M., et al. (1996). Psychosocial stressors and low birth weight in an urban population. *American Journal of Preventive Medicine, 12*(6), 459–466.

Orrell, M. W., & Blazer, D. G. (Eds.). (2004). Behavioral symptoms of dementia: Their measurement and intervention (special issue). *Aging and Mental Health, 8*(2), 106–108.

Ortiz, E., & Clancy, C. (2003). Use of information technology to improve the quality of health care in the United States (AHRQ Update). *Health Services Research, April*, 1–8.

Orwell, E. S., & Klein, R. F. (1996). Osteoporosis in men: Epidemiology, pathophysiology, and clinical characterization. In R. Marcus, D. Feldman, & J. Kelsey (Eds.), *Osteoporosis* (pp. 86–101). San Diego, CA: Academic Press.

Ory, M. G., Hoffman, R. R., Yee, J. L., Tennstedt, S., & Schultz, R. (1999). Prevalence and impact of caregiving: A detailed comparison between dementia and nondementia caregivers. *Gerontologist, 39*(2), 177–185.

Ory, M. G., Williams, T. F., Emr, M., Lebowitz, B., Rabins, P., Salloway, J., et al. (1985). Families, informal supports, and Alzheimer's disease. *Research on Aging, 7*, 623–644.

Osato, E. E., Stone, J. T., Phillips, S. L., & Winne, D. M. (1993). Clinical manifestations. Failure to thrive in the elderly. *Journal of Gerontological Nursing, 19*, 28–34.

Ossip-Klein, D. J., Bigelow, G., Parker, S. R., Curry, S., Hall, S., & Kirkland, S. (1986). Classifcation and assessment of smoking behavior. *Health Psychology, 5*(Suppl.), 3–11.

O'Sullivan, A. L., & Schwarz, D. F. (2000). Preventing injuries to infants of adolescent mothers. *Nurse Practitioner Forum, 11*, 124–131.

O'Sullivan, J. (2003). *My family is the pits: An ethnographic study of homeless adolescents.* Unpublished doctoral dissertation, Boston College, Chestnut Hill, MA.

O'Toole, A., & Welt, S. (Eds.). (1989). *Interpersonal theory in nursing practice: Selected works of Hildegard E. Peplau.* New York: Springer Publishing.

Ouslander, J. G., Blaustein, J., Connor, A., & Pitt, A. (1988). Habit training and oxybutin for incontinence in nursing homepatients: A placebo control trial. *Journal of the American Geriatrics Society, 36*, 40–46.

Ouslander, J. G., & Schnelle, J. F. (1995). Incontinence in the nursing home. *Annals of Internal Medicine, 122*(6), 438–449.

Overhage, J. M., Tierney, W. M., Zhou, X. H., & McDonald, C. J. (1997). A randomized trial of "corollary orders" to prevent errors of omission. *Journal of the American Medical Informatics Association, 4*, 364–375.

Overpeck, M. D., Brenner, R. A., Trumble, A. C., Trifiletti, L. B., & Berendes, H. W. (1998). Risk factors for infant homicide in the United States. *New England Journal of Medicine, 339*, 1211–1216.

Owens, J. E., Taylor, A. G., & DeGood, D. (1999). Complementary and alternative medicine and psychologic factors: Toward an individual differences model of complementary and alternative medicine use and outcomes. *Journal of Alternative & Complementary Medicine, 5*(6), 529–542.

Owens, J. L., France, K. G., & Wiggs, L. (1999). Behavioural and cognitive-behavioural interventions for sleep disorders in infants and children: A review. *Sleep Medicine Review, 3*(4), 281–302.

Oyserman, D., Bybee, D., & Mowbray, C. (2002). Influences of maternal mental illness on psychological outcomes for adolescent children. *Journal of Adolescence, 25*, 587–602.

Oz, F. (2001). Impact of training on empathetic communication skills and tendency of nurses. *Clinical Excellence for Nurse Practitioners, 5*(1), 44–51.

Ozbolt, J. G. (1996). From minimum data to maximum impact: Using clinical data to strengthen patient care. *Advanced Practice Nursing Quarterly, 1*(4), 62–69.

Ozbolt, J. G. (2000). Terminology standards for nursing: Collaboration at the summit. *Journal of the American Medical Informatics Association, 7*(6), 517–522.

Ozbolt, J. G., Fruchtnicht, J. N., & Hayden, J. R. (1994). Toward data standards for clinical nursing information. *Journal of the American Medical Informatics Association, 1*, 175–185.

Paarlberg, K. M., Vingerhoets, A. J., Passchier, J., Dekker, G. A., Heinen, A. G., & van Geijn, H. P. (1999). Psychosocial predictors of low birthweight: A prospective study. *British Journal of Obstetrics and Gynaecology, 106*, 834–841.

Paarlberg, K. M., Vingerhoets, A. J., Passchier, J., Dekker, G. A., & van Geijn, H. P. (1995). Psychosocial factors and pregnancy outcome: A review with emphasis on methodological issues. *Journal of Psychosomatic Research, 39*(5), 563–595.

Page, A. (Ed.). (2003). *Keeping patients safe. Transforming the work environment of nurses.* Washington, DC: National Acadamies Press.

Pajares, F. (2003). *Information on self-efficacy.* Atlanta, GA: Emory University. Retrieved from http://www.emory.edu/EDUCATION/mfp/effpage.html - info

Paley, G., & Shapiro, D. (2001). Transactional analysis functional ego states in people with schizophrenia and their immediate relatives. *International Journal of Psychiatric Nursing Research, 6*, 737–745.

Palmer, J. B. (2002). Dysphagia. In W. R. Frontera & J. K. Silver (Eds.), *Essentials of physical medicine and rehabilitation* (pp. 547–551). Philadelphia: Hanley & Belfus.

Palmer, R. (1969). *Hermeneutics: Interpretation theory in Schleiermacher, Dilthey, Heidegger, and Gadamer.* Evanston, IL: Northwestern University Press.

Palmer, R. M., Landefeld, C. S., Kresevic, D. M., & Kowal, J. (1994). A medical unit for the acute care of the elderly. *Journal of the American Geriatrics Society, 42*(5), 545–552.

Palmer, S., & Glass, T. (2003). Family function and stroke recovery: A review. *Rehabilitation Psychology, 48*(4), 255–265.

Pan American Health Organization. (2004, September 27). *A renewed commitment to Health for All in the 21st century* (News Release). Washington, DC: Author. Retrieved October 1, 2004, from http://www.paho.org/English/DD/PIN/pr040824.htm

Pang, S. M., & Wong, T. K. (1998). Predicting pressure sore risk with the Norton, Braden, and Waterlow Scales in a Hong Kong rehabilitation hospital. *Nursing Research, 47*, 147–153.

Paolella, L. P., Dorfman, G. S., Gronan, J. J., & Hasa, F. M. (1988). Topographic location of the left atrium by computed tomography: Reducing pulmonary artery calibration error. *Critical Care Medicine, 16*, 1154–1156.

Papia, G., Louie, M., Tralla, A., Johnson, C., Collins, V., & Simor, A. E. (1999). Screening high-risk patients for methicillin-resistant *Staphylococcus aureus* on admission to the hospital: Is it cost effective? *Infection Control and Hospital Epidemiology, 20*, 473–477.

Park, D. C., Hertzog, C., Leventhal, H., Morrell, R. W., Leventhal, E., Birchmore, D., et al. (1999). Medication adherence in rheumatoid arthritis patients: Older is wiser. *Journal of the American Geriatrics Society, 47*, 172–183.

Parker, C., Power, M., Hamdy, S., Bowen, A., Tyrell, P., & Thompson, D. G. (2004). Awareness of dysphagia by patients following stroke predicts swallowing performance. *Dysphagia, 19*, 28–35.

Parker, K. P. (2003). Sleep disturbances in dialysis patients. *Sleep Medicine Reviews, 7*, 131–143.

Parker, L. D., Cantrell, C., & Demi, A. (1997). Older adults attitudes toward suicide: Are there race and gender differences? *Death Studies, 21*, 289–298.

Parkin, D., Pisani, P., & Ferlay, J. (1999). Global cancer statistics. *CA Cancer Journal for Clinicians, 49*(1), 33–64.

Parlee, M. B. (1973). The premenstrual syndrome. *Psychology Bulletin, 80*(6), 454–465.

Parlocha, P. K., & Henry, S. B. (1998). The usefulness of the Georgetown Home Health Care Classification system for coding patient problems and nursing interventions in psychiatric home care. *Computers in Nursing, 16*(1), 45–52.

Parse, R. R. (1981). *Man-living-health: A theory of nursing*. New York: Wiley.

Parse, R. R. (1992). Human becoming: Parse's theory of nursing. *Nursing Science Quarterly, 5*, 35–42.

Parse, R. R. (1995). The theory of human becoming. In R. R. Parse (Ed.), *Illuminations: The human becoming theory in practice and research*. New York: National League for Nursing Press.

Parse, R. R. (1998). *The human becoming school of thought: A perspective for nurses and other health professionals*. Thousand Oaks, CA: Sage.

Parse, R. R. (2004). A human becoming teaching-learning model. *Nursing Science Quarterly, 17*(1), 33–35.

Parshall, M. (1999). Adult emergency visits for chronic cardiorespiratory disease: Does dyspnea matter? *Nursing Research, 48*(2), 62–70.

Parson, C. (1999). Managed care: The effect of case management on state psychiatric clients. *Journal of Psychiatric Nursing, 37*(10), 16–21.

Parsons, S. K., Simmons, W. P., Penn, K., & Furlough, M. (2003). Determinants of satisfaction and turnover among nursing assistants: The results of a statewide survey. *Journal of Gerontological Nursing, 29*(3), 51–58.

Pascreta, J. V. (1997). Depressive phenomena, physical symptom distress, and functional status among women with breast cancer. *Nursing Research, 46*, 214–221.

Pasquali, E. A. (1999). The impact of premature menopause on women's experience of self [Abstract]. *Journal of Holistic Nursing, 17*, 346–364.

Pasquali, S., Alexander, K., & Peterson, E. (2001). Cardiac rehabilitation in the elderly. *American Heart Journal, 142*, 748–754.

Paterson, J., & Zderad, L. (1976). *Humanistic nursing*. New York: John Wiley and Sons.

Patton, M. Q. (1990). *Qualitative evaluation and research methods*. Newbury Park, CA: Sage Publications.

Paul-Allen, J., & Ostrow, L. (2000). Survey of nursing practices with closed system suctioning. *American Journal of Critical Care, 9*, 9–17.

Payne, S. A., Dean, S. J., & Kalus, C. (1998). A comparative study of death in hospice and emergency nurses. *Journal of Advanced Nursing, 28*, 700–706.

Peacock, J. L., Bland, J. M., & Anderson, H. R. (1995). Preterm delivery: Effects of socioeconomic factors, psychological stress, smoking, alcohol, and caffeine. *British Medical Journal, 311*, 531–535.

Pearls, F. (1973). *The Gestalt approach: Eyewitness to therapy*. Palo Alto, CA: Science and Behavior Books.

Pearson, T. A., Blair, S. N., Daniels, S. R., Eckel, R. H., Fair, J. M., & Fortman, S. P. (2002). AHA Guidelines for primary prevention of cardiovascular disease and stroke: 2002 update. *Circulation, 106*, 388–391.

Peck, M. L. (1992). The future of nursing in a technological age: Computers, robots, and TLC. *Journal of Holistic Nursing 10*(2), 183–191.

Peckover, S. (2002). Supporting and policing mothers: An analysis of the disciplinary practices of health visiting. *Journal of Advanced Nursing, 38*(4), 369–377.

Peden, A. R. (1998). The evolution of an intervention—the use of Peplau's process of practice-based theory development. *Journal of Psychiatric and Mental Heath Nursing, 5*, 173–178.

Peden, A. R., Hall, L. A., Rayens, M. K., & Beebe, L. (2000). Negative thinking mediates the effect of self-esteem on depressive symptoms in college women. *Nursing Research, 49*(4), 201–207.

Pedhazur, E. J. (1982). *Multiple regression in behavioral research* (2nd ed.). New York: Holt, Rinehart, and Winston.

Pejlert, A., Asplund, K., & Norberg, A. (1999). Towards recovery: Living in a home-like setting after the move from a hospital ward. *Journal of Clinical Nursing, 8*, 663–73.

Pelton, J. (2001). Insight into schizophrenia: Planning mental health service provision for schizophrenia using a brief psychological intervention. *International Journal of Clinical Practice, 55*, 135–137.

Peluchette, J. V., & Jenaquart, S. (2000). Professionals' use of different mentor sources at various career stages: Implications for career success. *Journal of Social Psychology, 140*(5), 549–564.

Pender, N. (1985). Effects of progressive muscle relaxation training on anxiety and health locus of control among hypertensive adults. *Research in Nursing and Health, 8*, 67–72.

Pender, N. J. (1982). *Health promotion in nursing practice* (1st ed.). Norwalk, CT: Appleton Century-Crofts.

Pender, N. J. (1987). *Health promotion in nursing practice* (2nd ed.). Norwalk, CT: Appleton & Lange.

Pender, N. J. (1996). *Health promotion in nursing practice* (3rd ed.). Norwalk, CT: Appleton & Lange.

Pender, N. J. (2001a). *Biographical sketch*. Retrieved September 2, 2004, from http://www.nursing.umich.edu/faculty/pender/pender_bio.html

Pender, N. J. (2001b). *Most frequently asked questions about the Health Promotion Model and my professional work and career*. Retrieved September 2, 2004, from http://www.nursing.umich.edu/faculty/pender/pender_questions.html

Pender, N. J., Barkauskas, V. H., Hayman, L., Rice, V. H., & Anderson, E. T. (1992). Health promotion and disease prevention: Toward excellence in nursing practice and education. *Nursing Outlook, 40*, 106–112.

Pender, N. J., Murdaugh, C. L., & Parsons, M. A. (2002). *Health promotion in nursing practice* (4th ed.). Upper Saddle River, NJ: Prentice Hall.

Pengelly, A. W., & Booth, C. M. (1980). A prospective trial of bladder training as treatment for detrusor instability. *British Journal of Urology, 52*, 463–466.

Penner, L. A., Ludenia, K., & Mead, G. (1984). Staff attitudes: Image or reality. *Journal of Gerontological Nursing, 10*, 110–117.

Penninx, B. W., Beekman, A. T., Honig, A., Deeg, D. J., Schoevers, R. A., van Eijk, J. T., et al. (2001). Depression and cardiac mortality: Results from a community-based longitudinal study. *Archives of General Psychiatry, 58*, 221–227.

Peplau, H. E. (1952). *Interpersonal relations in nursing*. New York: G. P. Putnam & Sons.

Peplau, H. E. (1988). The art and science of nursing: Similarities, differences, and relations. *Nursing Science Quarterly, 1*, 8–15.

Peplau, H. E. (1992). Interpersonal relations: A theoretical framework for application in nursing practice. *Nursing Science Quarterly, 5*, 13–18.

Peplau, H. E. (1997). Peplau's theory of interpersonal relations. *Nursing Science Quarterly, 10*, 162–167.

Peplau, L. A., & Garnets, L. D. (2000). A new paradigm for understanding women's sexuality and sexual orientation. *Journal of Social Issues, 56*, 329–350.

Peplau, L. A., Spalding, L. R., Conley, T. D., & Veniegas, R. C. (1999). The development of sexual orientation in women. *Annual Review of Sex Research, 10*, 70–99.

Perell, K. L., Nelson, A., Goldman, R. L., Luther, S. L., Prieto-Lewis, N., & Rubenstein, L. Z. (2001). Fall risk assessment measures: An analytic review. *Journals of Gerontology Series A: Biological and Medical Sciences, 56*, M761–M766.

Perkins, D. O., Leserman, J., Stern, R. A., Baum, S. F., Liao, D., Golden, R. N., et al. (1995). Somatic symptoms and HIV infection: Relationship to depressive symptoms and indicators of HIV disease. *American Journal of Psychiatry, 152*, 1776–1781.

Perkins, H. S. (2000). Time to move advance care planning beyond advance directives. *Chest, 117*, 1228–1231.

Perkins, K. (1992). Psychosocial implications of women and retirement. *Social Work, 37*, 526–532.

Perla, L. (2002). The future role of nurses. *Journal of Nursing Staff Development, 18*(4), 194–197.

Perrin, E. C., Newacheck, P., Pless, I. B., Drotar, D., Gortmaker, S. L., Leventhal, J., et al. (1993). Issues involved in the definition and classification of chronic health conditions. *Pediatrics, 91*, 787–793.

Perry, L., & McLaren, S. (2003). Eating difficulties after stroke. *Journal of Advanced Nursing, 43*, 360–369.

Perseius, A., Ojehagen, A., Ekdahl, S., Asberg, M. Y., & Samuelsson, M. (2003). Treatment of suicidal and deliberate self-harming patients with borderline personality disorder using dialectical behavior therapy: The patient's and the therapist's perceptions. *Archives of Psychiatric Nursing, 17*(5), 218–227.

Persily, C. A., & Hildebrandt, E. (2003). The theory of community empowerment. In M. J. Smith & P. L. Liehr (Eds.), *Middle range theory for nursing* (pp. 111–123). New York: Springer Publishing.

Perski, A., Feleke, E., Anderson, G., Samad, B. A., Westerlund, H., Ericsson, C. G., et al. (1998). Emotional distress before coronary bypass grafting limits the benefits of surgery. *American Heart Journal, 136*(3), 510–517.

Perski, A., Osuchowski, K., Andersson, L., Sanden, A., Feleke, E., & Anderson, G. (1999). Intensive rehabilitation of emotionally distressed patients after coronary by-pass grafting. *Journal of Internal Medicine, 246*, 253–263.

Peterman, B. A., Springer, P., & Farnsworth, J. (1995). Analyzing job demands and coping techniques. *Nursing Management, 26*(2), 51–53.

Peters, M. (1996). Decision support systems in diagnostic pathology [Editorial]. *British Journal of Hospital Medicine, 10*, 502–503.

Peterson, A., Takiya, L., & Finley, R. (2003). Meta-analysis of trials of interventions to improve medication adherence. *American Journal of Health-System Pharmacy, 60*, 657–665.

Peterson, L., & Brown, D. (1994). Integrating child injury and abuse-neglect research: Common histories, etiologies and solutions. *Psychological Bulletin, 116*, 293–315.

Peterson, T. J., Alpert, J. E, Papakostas, G. I., Bernstein, E. M., Freed, R., Smith, M. M., et al. (2003). Early-onset depression and the emotional and behavioral characteristics of offspring. *Depression and Anxiety, 18*, 104–108.

Petit, J. (1994). Continuing care retirement communities and the role of the wellness nurse. *Geriatric Nursing, 15*, 28–31.

Petrucci, K., Petrucci, P., Canfield, K., McCormick, K., Kjerulff, K., & Parks, P. (1992). Evaluation of UNIS: Urological Nursing Information Systems. In P. D. Clayton (Ed.), *Proceedings of the Fifteenth Annual Symposium on Computer Applications in Medical Care* (pp. 43–47). New York: McGraw-Hill.

Petterson, S. M., & Albers, A. B. (2002). Effects of poverty and maternal depression on early child development. *Child Development, 72*(6), 1794–1813.

Pfeiffer, E. (1998). Why teams? In E. L. Siegler, K. Hyer, T. Fulmer, & M. Mezey (Eds.), *Geriatric interdisciplinary team training* (pp. 13–21). New York: Springer.

Phillips, C. D., Hawes, C., & Fries, B. E. (1993). Reducing the use of physical restraints in nursing homes: Will it increase costs? *American Journal of Public Health, 83*, 342–348.

Phillips, C. Y., Castorr, A., Prescott, P. A., & Soeken, K. (1992). Nursing intensity: Going beyond patient classification. *Journal of Nursing Administration, 22*(4), 46–52.

Phillips, E. L. (1999). *A guide for therapists and patients to short-term psychotherapy*. Springfield, IL: Charles C. Thomas Publisher.

Phillips, J., Cohen, M., & Moses, G. (1999). Breast cancer screening and African American women: Fear, fatalism, and silence. *Oncology Nursing Forum, 26*(3), 561–571.

Phillips, J., & Weekes, D. (2002). Incorporating multiculturalism into oncology nursing research: The last decade. *Oncology Nursing Forum, 29*(5), 807–816.

Phillips, L. R., & Rempusheski, V. F. (1985). A decision-making model for diagnosing and intervening in elder abuse and neglect. *Nursing Research, 34*, 134–139.

Phillips, P. A., Rolls, B. J., Ledingham, J. G., Forsling, M. L., Morton, J. J., Crowe, M. J., et al. (1984). Reduced thirst after water deprivation in healthy elderly men. *New England Journal of Medicine, 311*, 753–759.

Phillips, R. (1997). Alterations in cardiac effort and oxygenation during shivering after cardiac surgery. *Seminars in Perioperative Nursing, 6*(3), 176–184.

Phillips, R. A. (1999). *Thermoregulatory and inflammatory mechanisms of shivering after cardiopulmonary bypass in cardiac surgery patients*. Unpublished dissertation, University of Texas Health Science Center at San Antonio, Texas.

Phillips, R. M., & Baldwin, B. A. (1997). Teaching psychosocial care to long-term care nursing assistants. *Journal of Continuing Education in Nursing, 28*(3), 130–134.

Picker Institute. (1998). *Improving healthcare through the patient's eyes report*. Boston, MA.

Picker Institute. (2005). *Improving continuity of healthcare through the patient's eyes report*. Boston, MA.

Picot, S. J. (1995). Rewards, costs, and coping of African American caregivers. *Nursing Research, 44*, 147–152.

Pienta, K., & Esper, P. (1993). Is dietary fat a risk factor for prostate cancer? *Journal of the National Cancer Institute, 85*(19), 1538–1540.

Pienta, K., Goodson, J., & Esper, P. (1996). Epidemiology of prostate cancer: Molecular and environmental clues. *Urology, 48*(5), 676–683.

Pierce, J. P., & Gilpin, E. A. (2002). Impact of over-the-counter sales on effectiveness of pharmaceuticals for smoking cessation. *Journal of the American Medical Association, 288*(10), 1260–1264.

Pignay-Demaria, V., Lespèrance, D., Roland G., Frasure-Smith, N., & Perrault, L. P. (2003). Depression and anxiety and outcomes of coronary artery bypass surgery. *Annals of Thoracic Surgery, 75*, 314–321.

Pilkington, F. B., & Mitchell, G. J. (2003). Mistakes across paradigms. *Nursing Science Quarterly, 16*(2), 102–108.

Pillemer, K. A., & Finkelhor, D. (1988). The prevalence of elder abuse: A random sample survey. *Gerontologist, 28*(1), 51–57.

Pincharoen, S., & Congdon, J. G. (2003). Spirituality and health in older Thai persons in the United States. *Western Journal of Nursing Research, 25*(1), 93–108.

Pinikahana, J., Happell, B., Hope, J., & Keks, N. A. (2002). Quality of life in schizophrenia: A review of the literature from 1995 to 2000. *International Journal of Mental Health Nursing, 11*, 103–111.

Pinikahana, J., Happell, B., & Keks, N. A. (2003). Suicide and schizophrenia: A review of literature for the decade (1990–1999) and implications for mental health nursing. *Issues in Mental Health Nursing, 24*, 27–43.

Pinikahana, J., Happell, B., Taylor, M., & Keks, N. A. (2002). Exploring the complexity of compliance in schizophrenia. *Issues in Mental Health Nursing, 23*, 513–528.

Pinn, W. W. (2001). Science and advocacy as partners: The office of Research on Women's Health in the 1990s. *Journal of the American Medical Women's Association, 56*(2), 77–78.

Piper, B. F. (1989). Fatigue: Current bases for practice. In S. G. Funk, E. M. Tornquist, M. T. Champagne, L. A. Copp, & R. Wiese (Eds.), *Key aspects of comfort* (pp. 187–240). New York: Springer Publishing.

Piper, B. F., Lindsey, A. M., & Dodd, M. J. (1987). Fatigue mechanisms in cancer patients: Developing a nursing theory. *Oncology Nursing Forum, 14*(6), 17–23.

Pirkle, J. L., Brody, D. J., Gunter, E. W., Kramer, R. A., Paschal, D. C., Flegal, K. M., et al. (1994). The decline in blood lead levels in the United Stest: The national health and nutrition examination surveys (NHANES). *Journal of the American Medical Association, 272*, 284–291.

Pirl, W., & Mello, J. (2002). Psychological complications of prostate cancer. *Oncology, 16*(11), 1448–1453.

Pirraglia, P. A., Petreson, J. C., Williams-Russo, P., Gorkin, L., & Charlson, M. E. (1999). Depressive symptomatology in coronary artery bypass graft surgery patients. *International Journal of Geriatric Psychiatry, 14*, 668–680.

Pittet, D. (2001). Improving adherence to hand hygiene practice: A multidisciplinary approach. *Emerging Infectious Diseases, 7*, 234–240.

Plotnikoff, G. A., & Quigley, J. M. (2003). Prevalence of severe hypovitaminosis D in patients with persistent, nonspecific musculoskeletal pain. *Mayo Clinic Proceedings, 78*(12), 1463–1470.

Podsiadlo, D., & Richardson, S. (1991). The timed "Up & Go": A test of basic functional mobility for frail elderly persons. *Journal of the American Geriatrics Society, 39*, 142–148.

Pohl, J. M., Vonderheid, S. C., Barkauskas, V. H., & Nagelkerk, J. (2004). The safety net: Academic nurse managed centers' role. *Policy, Politics, & Nursing Practice, 5*(2), 84–94.

Polit, D. F., & Beck, C. T. (2004). *Nursing research: Principles and methods* (7th ed.). Philadelphia: Lippincott, Williams, & Wilkins.

Polit, D., & Hungler, B. (1995). *Nursing research: Principles and methods* (5th ed.). Philadelphia: J. B. Lippincott.

Polit, D. F., & Hungler, B. P. (1999). *Nursing research: Principles and methods* (6th ed.). Philadelphia: Lippincott.

Pollock, S. E. (1987). Adaptation to chronic illness: Analysis of nursing research. *Nursing Clinics of North America, 22*(3), 631–644.

Pollack, S. E. (1993). Adaptation to chronic illness: A program of research for testing nursing theory. *Nursing Science Quarterly, 6*, 86–92.

Pompili, M., Mancinelli, I., Girardi, P., & Tatarelli, R. (2003). Nursing schizophrenic patients who are at risk of suicide. *Journal of Psychiatric Mental Health Nursing, 10*, 622–624.

Pope, A., & Tarlov, A. (1991). *Disability in America: Toward a national agenda for prevention*. Washington, DC: National Academy Press.

Pope, J. H., Aufderheide, T. P., Ruthazer, R., Woolard, R. H., Feldman, J. A., Beshansky, J. R., et al. (2000). Missed diagnoses of acute cardiac ischemia in the emergency department. *New England Journal of Medicine, 342*(16), 1163–1170.

Popkess-Vawter, S., Brandau, C., & Straub, J. (1998). Triggers of overeating and related intervention strategies for women who weight cycle. *Applied Nursing Research, 11*, 69–76.

Popper, K. (1969). *Conjectures and refutations*. London: Rutledge & Kegan Paul.

Porter, C. P., & Villarruel, A. M. (1993). Nursing research with African American and Hispanic people: Guidelines for action. *Nursing Outlook, 41*, 59–67.

Porter, E. J. (1998a). Older widows' intention to keep the generations separate. *Health Care of Women International, 19*, 395–410.

Porter, E. J. (1998b). 'Staying close to shore': A context for older rural widows' use of health care. *Journal of Women & Aging, 10*(4), 25–39.

Porter, E. J. (2000). Widows and widowers. In J. J. Fitzpatrick & T. J. Fulmer (Eds.), *Geriatric nursing research digest* (pp. 93–98). New York: Springer Publishing.

Porter, E. J. (2001). An older rural widow's transition from home care to assisted living. *Care Management Journals, 3*(1), 25–32.

Porter, M. L. (2000). Fetal pulse oximetry: An adjunct to electronic fetal heart rate monitoring. *Journal of Obstetric, Gynecologic, and Neonatal Nursing, 29*(5), 537–548.

Posch, A., Chen, Z., Wheeler, C., Dunn, M. J., Raulf-Heimsoth, M., & Baur, X. (1997). Characterization and identification of latex allergens by two-dimensional electrophoresis and protein microsequencing. *Journal of Allergy and Clinical Immunology, 99*, 385–394.

Posmontier, B., & Horowitz, J. A. (2004). Postpartum practices and depression prevalences: Technocentric and ethnocentric cultural perspectives. *Journal of Transcultural Nursing, 15*, 34–43.

Poster, E. C., Dee, V., & Randell, B. P. (1997). The Johnson Behavioral System Model as a framework for patient outcome evaluation. *Journal of the American Psychiatric Nurses Association, 3*(3), 73–80.

Poston, W. S., Haddock, C. K., Conard, M. W., Jones, P., & Spertus, J. (2003). Assessing depression in the cardiac patient. *Behavior Modification, 27*(1), 26–36.

Poston, W. S. C., Haddock, C. K., Dill, P. l. L., Thayer, B., & Foreyt, J. P. (2001). Lifestyle treatments in randomized clinical trials of pharmacotherapies for obesity. *Obesity Research*, 9, 552–563.

Potempa, K. M. (1993). Chronic fatigue. In J. J. Fitzpatrick & J. S. Stevenson (Eds.), *Annual review of nursing research* (Vol. 11, pp. 57–76). New York: Springer Publishing.

Pound, C., Partin, A, Eisenberger, M., Chan, D., Pearson, J., & Walsh, P. (1999). Natural history of progression after PSA elevation following radical prostatectomy. *Journal of the American Medical Association, 281*(17), 1591–1597.

Powel, L. (2002). *Incontinence morbidity, psychosocial adjustment, and quality of life after prostatectomy.* Unpublished dissertation, University of Maryland, Baltimore.

President's Commission for the Study of Ethical Problems in Medicine and Biomedical and Behavioral Research. (1981). *Defining death: Medical, legal and ethical issues in the determination of death.* Washington, DC: U.S. Government Printing Office.

President's New Freedom Commission on Mental Health. (2003). Retrieved from www.mentalheathcommission.gov/reports/FinalReports/fullre, 1–17.

President's New Freedom Commission on Mental Health. (2003). *Achieving the promise: Transforming mental health care in America*. Final report (DHHS Publication No. SMA-03-3832). Rockville, MD: Author. Retrieved from http://mentalhealthcommission.gov/reports/finalreport/

Pressler, J. L., & Montgomery, K. S. (2005). Fitzpatrick's life perspective rhythm model. In J. J. Fitzpatrick & A. L. Whall (Eds.), *Conceptual models of nursing: Analysis and application* (4th ed., pp. 325–347). Upper Saddle River, NJ: Pearson, Prentice Hall.

Price, C. R., & Balough, J. (2001). Using alumni to mentor students at risk. *Nurse Educator, 26*(5), 209–211.

Price, J. D., Hermans, D. G., & Grimley, E. J. (2000). *Subjective barriers to prevent wandering of cognitive impaired people*. Cochrane Database of Systematic Reviews (4). CD001932.

Pritchard, A. (1969). Statistical bibliography or bibliometrics? *Journal of Documentation, 25*, 348–349.

Prochaska, J. O., & DiClemente, C. C. (1983). Stages and process of self-change of smoking: Toward an integrative model of change. *Journal of Consulting and Clinical Psychology, 51*, 390–395.

Prochaska, J. O., Velicer, W. F., Rossi, J. S., Goldstein, M. G., Marcus, B. H., Rakowski, W., et al. (1994). Stages of change and decisional balance for 12 problem behaviors. *Health Psychology, 13*, 39–46.

Project Achieve. (2003). Retrieved from http://homelessness.net/

Propp, V. (1968). *Morphology of the Russian folktale*. Austin: University of Texas Press.

Pruchno, R. A., & McKenney, D. (2002). Psychological well-being of black and white grandmothers raising grandchildren: Examination of a two-factor model. *Journal of Gerontology, 57B*, 444–452.

Public Health Foundation. (1997). *Measuring health objectives and indicators: 1997 state and local capacity survey*. Washington, DC: Author.

Puddey, I. (2000). Large multicentre hypertension trials. *Current Opinion in Nephrology & Hypertension*, 9, 285–292.

Pullen, L., Tuck, I., & Wallace, D. C. (1999). Research priorities in mental health nursing. *Issues in Mental Health Nursing, 20*, 217–227.

Puntillo, K. (2003). Pain assessment and management in the critically ill: Wizardry or science? *American Journal of Critical Care, 12*(4), 310–316.

Punyahotra, S., & Street, A. (1998). Exploring the discursive construction of menopause for Thai women. *Nursing Inquiry, 5*, 96–103.

Putnam, F. W. (2003). Ten-year research update review: Child sexual abuse *Journal of the American Academy of Child and Adolescent Psychiatry, 42*(3), 269–278.

Putnam, R. (1992, October). *Theory of action from the action science perspective*. Paper presented at the Third Knowledge Development Symposium, University of Rhode Island College of Nursing, Newport.

Putnam, R. (1996). The reflective mode: Interpersonal reflections regarding espoused theories and theories in use. In *Building a cumulative knowledge base for nursing: From fragmentation to congruence of philosophy, theory, methods of inquiry and practice* (Invited papers of the 4th and 5th symposia of the Knowledge of Development Series, pp. 45–52). Kingston: University of Rhode Island, College of Nursing.

Pyne, J. M., Smith, J., Fortney, J., Zhang, M., Williams, D. K., & Rost, K. (2003). Cost-effectiveness of a primary care intervention for depressed females. [Clinical Trial. Journal Article. Randomized Controlled Trial] *Journal of Affective Disorders, 74*(1), 23–32.

Quinn, J. A., Smith, M. C., Ritenbaugh, C., Swanson, K., & Watson, M. J. (2003). Research guidelines for assessing the impact of the healing relationship in clinical nursing. *Alternative Therapies*, 9(3), A65–A79.

Rabins, P. V., Black, B. S., Roca, R., German, P., McGuire, M., Robbins, B., et al. (2000). Effectiveness of a nurse-based outreach program for identifying and treating psychiatric illness in the elderly. *Journal of the American Medical Association, 283*, 2802–2809.

Ragucci, A. T. (1990). The ethnographic approach and nursing research. In P. J. Brink (Ed.), *Transcultural nursing* (pp. 163–174). Prospect Heights, IL: Waveland Press. (Original work published 1972)

Rahimtola, S. H. (1982). Coronary artery bypass surgery for chronic angina—1981. *Circulation, 65*, 225–241.

Raik, B. (2001). Polypharmacy: Drug-drug interactions. In M. Mezey (Ed.), *The encyclopedia of elder care* (pp. 514–517). New York: Springer Publishing.

Raingruber, B. (2003). Nurture: The fundamental significance of relationship as a paradigm for mental health. *Perspectives in Psychiatric Care, 39*(3), 104–112, 132–135.

Raisig, M. (1964). The index to current nursing periodical literature in the United States. *Nursing Forum, 3*, 97–109.

Rakowski, W., Dube, C., Marcus, B. H., Prochaska, J. O., Velicer, W., & Abrams, D. (1992). Assessing elements of women's decisions about mammography. *Healthy Psychology, 11*, 111–118.

Ramirez, F. C. (2000). Diagnosis and treatment of gastroesophageal reflux disease in the elderly. *Cleveland Clinics Journal of Medicine, 67*(10), 755–766.

Ramirez, M., Teresi, J., Holmes, D., & Fairchild, S. (1998). Ethnic and racial conflict in relation to staff burnout, demoralization, and job dissatisfaction in SCUs and non-SCUs. *Journal of Mental Health & Aging, 4*(4), 459–479.

Ramsay, J. A., McKenzie, J. K., & Fish, D. G. (1982). Physicians and nurse practitioners: Do they provide equivalent care? *American Journal of Public Health, 72*(1), 55–57.

Rando, T. (1993). *Treatment of complicated mourning*. Champaign, IL: Research Press.

Rantanen, T., Guralnik, J. M., Ferrucci, L., Penninx, B. W., Leveille, S., Sipila, S., et al. (2001). Coimpairments as predictors of severe walking disability in older women. *Journal of the American Geriatrics Society, 49*, 21–27.

Rantanen, T., Guralnik, J. M., Sakari-Rantala, R., Leveille, S., Simonsick, E. M., Ling, S., et al. (1999). Disability, physical activity, and muscle strength in older women: The Women's Health and Aging Study. *Archives of Physical Medicine and Rehabilitation, 80*, 130–135.

Rapp, C. G. & Iowa Veterans Affairs Nursing Research Consortium. (1998). *Acute confusion/delirium: A research-based protocol*. Retrieved from http://www.nursing.uiowa.edu/centers/gnirc/protocols.htm

Rapp, C. G., Wakefield, B., Kundrat, M., Mentes, J., Tripp-Reimer, T., Culp, K., et al. (2000). Acute confusion assessment instruments: Clinical versus research usability. *Applied Nursing Research, 13*(1), 37–45.

Rapp, S. R., Shumaker, S., Schmidt, S., Naughton, M., & Anderson, R. (1998). Social resourcefulness: Its relationship to social support and well-being among caregivers of dementia victims. *Aging and Mental Health, 2*(1), 40–48.

Rasmussen, B. H., & Sandman, P. O. (1998). How nurses spend their time in a hospice and in an oncological unit. *Journal of Advanced Nursing, 28,* 818–828.

Raudonis, B. M., & Acton, G. J. (1997). Theory-based nursing practice. *Journal of Advanced Nursing, 26*(1), 138–145.

Ravert, P. (2002). An integrative review of computer-based simulation in the education process. *CIN: Computers, Informatics, Nursing, 20*(5), 203–208.

Ray, C. (1991). Chronic fatigue syndrome and depression: Conceptual and methodological ambiguities. *Psychological Medicine, 21,* 1–9.

Raymond, S. J. (1995). Normal saline instillation before suctioning: Helpful or harmful? A review of the literature. *American Journal of Critical Care, 4,* 267–271.

Reame, N. E. (2001). Female troubles: An analysis of menstrual cycle research in the NINR portfolio as a model for science development in women's health. In J. J. Fitzpatrick, D. Taylor, & N. Woods (Eds.), *Annual review of nursing* (Vol. 19, pp. 325–338). New York: Springer Publishing.

Reame, N. E., Kelch, R. P., Beitins, I. Z., Yu, M. Y., Zawacki, C., & Padmanabhan, V. (1996). Age effects of FSH and pulsatile LH secretion across the menstrual cycle of premenopausal women. *Journal of Clinical Endocrinology and Metabolism, 81,* 1512–1518.

Reckling, J. B. (1997). Who plays what role in decisions about withholding and withdrawing life-sustaining treatment. *Journal of Clinical Ethics, 8*(1), 39–45.

Reason, J. (1990). *Human error.* Cambridge, MA: Cambridge University Press.

Records, K. (2003). Mentoring for research skill development. *Journal of Nursing Education, 42*(12), 553–557.

Redeker, N. S. (2000). Sleep in acute care settings: An integrative review. *Journal of Nursing Scholarship, 32*(1), 31–38.

Reed, P. G. (1987). Spirituality and well-being in terminally ill hospitalized adults. *Research in Nursing & Health, 10,* 335–344.

Reed, P. G. (1991). Toward a theory of self-transcendence: Deductive reformulation using developmental theories. *Advances in Nursing Science, 13*(4), 64–77.

Reed, P. G. (1992). An emerging paradigm for the investigation of spirituality in nursing. *Research in Nursing & Health, 15,* 349–357.

Reed, P. G. (1996a). Transcendence: Formulating nursing perspectives. *Nursing Science Quarterly, 9*(1), 2–4.

Reed, P. G. (1996b). Transforming Peplau's interpersonal relations model: A revisionist analysis of Peplau. *Journal of Nursing Scholarship, 29,* 29–33.

Reed, P. G. (2003). The theory of self-transcendence. In M. J. Smith & P. L. Liehr (Eds.), *Middle range theory for nursing* (pp. 145–165). New York: Springer Publishing.

Reed, P. G. (2005). Peplau's theory of interpersonal relations. In J. J. Fitzpatrick & A. L. Whall (Eds.), *Conceptual models of nursing: Analysis and application* (4th ed, pp. 46–67). Upper Saddle River, NJ: Pearson/Prentice Hall.

Reeves, W. C., Lloyd, A., Vernon, S. D., Klimas, N., Jason, L. A., Blijenberg, G., et al. (2003). Identification of ambiguities in the 1994 chronic fatigue syndrome research case definition and recommendations for resolution. *BMC Health Services Research.* Retrieved from http://www.biomedcentral.com/1472-6963/3/25

Regenstein, M., Meyer, J., & Bagby, N. (1998). *Geriatric teams in managed care: A promising strategy for costs and outcomes.* Washington, DC: Economic and Social Research Institute.

Reichers, A., & Schneider, B. (1990). Climate and culture: An evolution of constructs. In B. Schneider (Ed.), *Organizational climate and culture* (pp. 5–39). San Francisco: Jossey-Bass.

Reif-Lehrer, L. (1995). *Grant application writer's handbook.* Boston: Jones and Bartlett.

Reilly, A., Dracup, K., & Dattolo, J. (1994). Factors influencing prehospital delay in patients experiencing chest pain. *American Journal of Critical Care, 3,* 300–306.

Reiss, B. S., & Evans, M. E. (2002). *Pharmacological aspects of nursing care* (6th ed.). Albany, NY: Delmar Publishers.

Reiss, D., & Price, R. H. (1996). National research agenda for prevention research: The National Institute of Mental Health report. *American Psychologist, 51,* 1109–1115.

Reizian, A., & Meleis, A. I. (1987). Symptoms reported by Arab American patients on the Cornell Medical Index. *Western Journal of Nursing Research, 9,* 368–384.

Relf, M. V. (1997). Illuminating meaning and transforming issues of spirituality in HIV disease and AIDS: An application of Parse's theory of human becoming. *Holistic Nursing Practice, 12,* 1–8.

Rempfer, M. V., Hamera, E. K., Brown, C. E., & Cromwell, R. L. (2003). The relations between cognition and the independent living skill of shopping in people with schizophrenia. *Psychiatry Research, 117*, 103–112.

Rescher, N. (2001). *Philosophical reasoning: A study in the methodology of philosophizing*. Maldon, MA: Blackwell.

Resnick, B. (in press). Falls in a comminuty of older adults: Putting research into practice. *Clinical Nursing Research*.

Resnick, B. (1989). Care of life. *Geriatric Nursing, 10*, 130–132.

Resnick, B. (1998a). Health care practices of the old-old. *American Academy Journal Nurse Practitioners, 10*, 147–155.

Resnick, B. (1998b). Functional performance of older adults in a long term care setting. *Clinical Nursing Research, 7*, 230–246.

Resnick, B. (1999). Motivation in the older adult: Can a leopard change its spots? *Journal of Advanced Nursing, 29*, 792–799.

Resnick, B. (2003). The theory of self-efficacy. In M. J. Smith & P. Liehr (Eds.), *Middle range theory for nursing* (pp. 49–68). New York: Springer Publishing.

Resnick, B., & Andrews, C. (2002). End-of-life treatment preferences among older adults: A nurse practitioner initiated intervention. *Journal of the American Academy of Nurse Practitioners, 14*(11), 517–522.

Resnick, B., Palmer, M. H., Jenkins, L., & Spellbring, A. M. (in press). Efficacy expectations and exercise behavior in older adults: A path analysis. *Journal of Advanced Nursing*.

Resnick, B., & Spellbring, A. M. (in press). Understanding what motivates older adults to exercise. *Journal of Gerontologic Nursing*.

Rew, L. (1988). Intuition in decision making. *Image: Journal of Nursing Scholarship, 20*, 150–154.

Rew, L., & Horner, S. D. (2003). Personal strengths of homeless adolescents living in a high risk environment. *Advances in Nursing Science, 26*(2), 90–101.

Rew, L., Taylor-Seehafer, M., & Fitzgerald, M. L. (2001). Sexual abuse, alcohol and other drug use, and suicidal behaviors in homeless adolescents. *Issues in Comprehensive Pediatric Nursing, 24*, 225–240.

Rew, L., Taylor-Seehafter, M., Thomas, N., & Yockey, R. (2001). Correlates of resilience in homeless adolescents. *Journal of Nursing Scholarship, 33*(1), 33–40.

Rew, L., Thomas, N., Horner, S. D., Resnick, M. D., & Beuhring, T. (2001). Correlates of recent suicide attempts in a triethnic group of adolescents. *Journal of Nursing Scholarship, 33*, 361–367.

Reynolds, N. R., Timmerman, G., Anderson, J., & Stevenson, J. S. (1992). Meta-analysis for descriptive research. *Research in Nursing and Health, 15*, 467–475.

Reynolds, W., & Cormack, D. (1991). An evaluation of the Johnson Behavioral System Model of nursing. *Journal of Advanced Nursing, 16*, 1122–1130.

Rhodes, V. A., McDaniel, R. W., & Matthews, C. A. (1998). Hospice patients' and nurses' perceptions of self-care deficits based on symptom experience. *Cancer Nursing, 21*, 312–319.

Rice, V. H. (2000). *Handbook of stress, coping and health: Implications for nursing research, theory, and practice*. Thousand Oaks, CA: Sage Publications.

Rice, V. H., Beck, C., & Stevenson, J. S. (1997). Ethical issues relative to autonomy and personal control in independent and cognitively impaired elders. *Nursing Outlook, 45*(1), 27–34.

Rich, M. W., Beckham, V., Wittenburg, C., Leven, C., Freddland, K., & Carney, R. (1995). A multidisciplinary intervention to prevent readmission of elderly patients with congestive heart failure. *New England Journal of Medicine, 333*, 1190–1195.

Richards, K. C. (1998). Effect of a back massage and relaxation intervention on sleep in critically ill patients. *American Journal of Critical Care, 7*, 288–299.

Richards, S. M. (1995). Meta-analyses and overview of randomized trials [Review]. *Blood Reviews, 9*, 85–91.

Richardson, V. (1993). *Retirement counseling: A handbook for gerontology practitioners*. New York: Springer Publishing.

Richie, M. F. (1996). Meeting the challenge of disruptive behaviors in the nursing home. *Journal of Gerontological Nursing, 22*(11), 3.

Richmond, C. (2002). Effects of hydration on febrile temperature patterns in rabbits. *Biological Research for Nursing, 2*(3), 277–291.

Ricoeur, P. (1984). *Time and narrative*. Chicago: University of Chicago Press.

Ridling, D. A., Martin, L. D., & Bratton, S. L. (2004). Endotracheal suctioning with or without instillation of isotonic sodium chloride solution in critically ill children. *American Journal of Critical Care, 12*(3), 212–219.

Riemsma, R. P., Kirwan, J. R., Taal, E., & Rasker, J. J. (2003). Patient education for adults with rheumatoid arthritis. *Cochrane Database of Systematic Reviews*. CD 003688.

Riessman, C. K. (1993). *Qualitative research methods series. Vol. 30. Narrative analysis*. Newbury Park, CA: Sage Publications.

Righter, B. M. (1995). Uncertainty and the role of the credible authority during an ostomy experience.

Wound, Ostomy, and Continence Nurses Society, 22, 100–104.

Rimmer, J., Silverman, K., Braunschweig, C., Quinn, L., & Liu, Y. (2002). Feasibility of a health promotion intervention for a group of predominantly African American women with type 2 diabetes. *Diabetes Educator, 28*, 571–580.

Rind, B., Tromovitch, P., & Bauserman, P. (1998). A meta-analytic examination of assumed properties of child sexual abuse using college samples. *Psychological Bulletin, 124*, 22–53.

Ringel, Y., Sperber, A. D., & Drossman, D. A. (2001). Irritable bowel syndrome. *Annual Review of Medicine, 52*, 319–338.

Ringwalt, C. L., Greene, J. M., Robertson, M., & McPheetes, M. (1998). The prevalence of homelessness among adolescents in the United States. *American Journal of Public Health, 88*(9), 1325–1329.

Riordan, J., Bibb, D., Miller, M., & Rawlins, T. (2001). Predicting breastfeeding duration using the LATCH breastfeeding assessment tool. *Journal of Human Lactation, 17*(1) 20–23.

Ripich, S., Moore, S. M., & Brennan, P. F. (1992). A new nursing medium: Computer networks for group intervention. *Journal of Psychosocial Nursing and Mental Health Services, 30*(7), 15–20.

Risser, N. L. (1975). Development of an instrument to measure patient satisfaction with nurses and nursing in primary care settings. *Nursing Research, 24*, 45–52.

Ritchie, B. (1996). *Compelled to crime: The gender entrapment of battered black women*. New York: Routledge.

Rizzolo, M. A. (Ed.). (1994). *Interactive video: Expanding horizons in nursing*. New York: American Journal of Nursing.

Rizzuto, C., & Mitchell, M. (1988a). Research in service settings: Part I. Consortium project outcomes. *Journal of Nursing Administration, 18*(2), 32–37.

Rizzuto, C., & Mitchell, M. (1988b). Research in service settings: Part 2. Consortium project outcomes. *Journal of Nursing Administration, 18*(3), 19–24.

Rizzuto, C., & Mitchell, M. (1990). Outcomes of research consortium project. *Journal of Nursing Administration, 20*(4), 13–17.

Robb, S. S., Boyd, M., & Pristash, C. L. (1980). A wine bottle, plant, and puppy. Catalysts for social behavior. *Journal of Gerontological Nursing, 6*(12), 721–728.

Roberto, K. A., Wacker, R. R., Jewell, E. M., & Rickard, M. (1997). Resident rights: Knowledge of and implementation by nursing staff in long-term care facilities. *Journal of Gerontological Nursing, 23*(12), 32–40.

Roberts, B. L. (1999). Activities of daily living: Factors related to independence. In A. Hinshaw, S. Feetham, & J. Shaver (Eds.), *Handbook of clinical nursing research* (pp. 561–577). New York: Sage.

Roberts, B. L., Anthony, M. K., Matejczyk, M. B., & Moore, D. (1994). The relationship of social support to functional limitations, pain, and well being among men and women. *Journal of Women and Aging, 6*, 3–19.

Roberts, D. C., & Cleveland, L. A. (2001). Surrounded by ocean, a world apart . . . The experience of elder women living alone. *Holistic Nursing Practice, 15*(3), 45–55.

Roberts, J., Brown, G. B., Streiner, D., Gafni, A., Pallister, R., Hoxby, H., et al. (1995). Problem solving counseling or phone-call support for outpatients with chronic illness: Effective for whom? *Canadian Journal of Nursing Research, 27*, 111–137.

Roberts, K. (1997). Nurse academics' scholarly productivity: Framed by the system, facilitated by mentoring. *Australian Journal of Advanced Nursing, 14*, 5–14.

Roberts, S. J., & Garling, J. (1980). An investigation of cyclic distress among staff nurses. In A. Dan, E. Graham, & C. Beecher (Eds.), *The menstrual cycle: A synthesis of interdisciplinary research*. (Vol. 1, pp. 305–311). New York: Springer Publishing.

Robinson, J. C. (1995). Healthcare purchasing and market changes in California. *Health Affairs, 14*(4), 117–130.

Robinson, K. (1997). Systems and cycles: Mother-daughter perceptions of interaction across the menstrual cycle [Abstract]. *Abstracts of the 12th Conference of the Society for Menstrual Cycle Research*, 4.

Robinson, K. R. (1988). Denial and anxiety in second day myocardial infarction patients. In C. F. Waltz, & O. L. Strickland (Eds.), *Measurement of nursing outcomes*. (Vol. 1, pp. 47–60). New York: Springer Publishing.

Robinson, K. R. (1993). Denial: An adaptive response. *Dimensions of Critical Care Nursing, 12*(2), 102–106.

Robinson, K. R. (1994). Developing a scale to measure denial levels of clients with actual or potential myocardial infarctions. *Heart & Lung: Journal of Critical Care, 23*(1), 36–44.

Robinson, K. R. (2003). A measure of denial in coronary clients: The Robinson Self-Appraisal Inventory. In O. L. Strickland & C. DiIorio (Eds.), *Measurement of nursing outcomes. Vol. 2: Client outcomes and quality of care* (2nd ed.). New York: Springer Publishing.

Robinson, K. R., & Griffith, H. M. (1997). Identification of current procedural terminology-coded services provided by family nurse practitioners. *Clinical Excellence for Nurse Practitioners, 1*, 397–404.

Robinson, K. R., Griffith, H. M., & Sullivan-Marx, E. M. (2001). Nursing practice reimbursement issues in the 21st century. In N. L. Chaska (Ed.), *The nursing profession: Tomorrow and beyond* (pp. 501–513). Thousand Oaks, CA: Sage Publications.

Robinson, S. B., & Rosher, R. B. (2002). Can a beverage cart help improve hydration? *Geriatric Nursing, 23*, 208–211.

Rockefeller University Hospital. Retrieved from http://www.ceneewatch.com/professional/pro

Rockwell, J. M., & Riegel, B. (2001). Predictors of self-care in persons with heart failure. *Heart and Lung, 30*, 18–25.

Rodgers, J., Black, G., Stobbart, A., & Foster, J. (2003). Audit of primary care of people with schizophrenia. *Quality in Primary Care, 11*, 133–140.

Rodgers, S. (1994). An exploratory study of research utilization by nurses in general medical and surgical wards. *Journal of Advanced Nursing, 20*, 904–911.

Rodney, P. (1988). Moral distress in critical care nursing. *Canadian Critical Nursing Journal, 5*(2), 9–11.

Roffwarg, H. P., Muzio, J. N., & Dement, W. C. (1966). Ontogenetic development of the human sleep-dream cycle. *Science, 152*, 604–619.

Rogers, A. E., & Dreher, H. M. (2002). Narcolepsy. *Nursing Clinics of North America, 37*, 675–692.

Rogers, B. (1997). Health hazards in nursing and health care: An overview. *American Journal of Infection Control, 25*(3), 248–261.

Rogers, B., & Emmett, E. A. (1987). Handling antineoplastic agents: Urine mutagenicity in nursing personnel. *Image: Journal of Nursing Scholarship, 19*, 108–113.

Rogers, C. (1961). *On becoming a person*. Boston: Houghton Miffin.

Rogers, E. (1995). *Diffusion of innovations* (4th ed.). New York: Free Press.

Rogers, M. E. (1970). *An introduction to the theoretical basis of nursing*. Philadelphia: F. A. Davis.

Rogers, M. E. (1990). *Nursing: Science of unitary, irreducible, human beings*: Update 1990. NLN Publications (15-2285), 5–11.

Rogers, M. E. (1992). Nursing science and the space age. *Nursing Science Quarterly, 5*, 27–34.

Rogers, M. E. (1994). The science of unitary human beings: Current perspectives. *Nursing Science Quarterly, 7*, 33–35.

Rogers, M. E. (1998). Nursing science and art: A perspective. *Nursing Science Quarterly, 1*, 99–102.

Rolka, D. B., Fagot-Campagna, A., & Narayan, K. M. V. (2001). Aspirin use among adults with diabetes. *Diabetes Care, 24*, 197–201.

Rolland, J. S. (1999). Families and genetic fate: A millennial challenge. *Families, Systems & Health, 17*(1), 123–133.

Rolland, J. S., & Williams, J. K. (in press). Toward a psychosocial typology of 21st century genetics. In S. Miller, S. L. Feetham, J. S. Rolland, & S. H. McDaniels (Eds.), *Individuals, families, and the new era of genetics: Biopsychosocial perspectives*. New York: Norton.

Romer, D. (2003). *Reducing adolescent risk: Toward an integrated approach*. Thousand Oaks, CA: Sage.

Rose, K. E. (1998). Perceptions related to time in a qualitative study of informal carers of terminally ill patients. *Journal of Clinical Nursing, 7*, 343–350.

Rose, L. (1998). Benefits and limitations of professional-family interactions: The family perspective. *Archives of Psychiatric Nursing, 12*(3), 140–147.

Rosenbaum, M. (1990). The role of learned resourcefulness in the self-control of health behavior. In M. Rosenbaum (Ed.), *Learned resourcefulness: On coping skills, self-control, and adaptive behavior* (pp. 3–30). New York: Springer Publishing.

Rosenkoetter, M., & Garris, J. (1998). Psychosocial changes following retirement. *Journal of Advanced Nursing, 27*, 966–976.

Rosenkoetter, M., Garris, J., & Engdahl, R. (2001). Postretirement use of time: Implications for preretirement planning and postretirement management. *Activities, Adaptation, and Aging, 25*, 1–18.

Rosenkoetter, M., Garris, J., & Hendricksen, S. (1997). Perceptions of retirees: Depression in retirement. *Journal of Nursing Science, 2*, 142–152.

Rosenstock, I. M. (1966). Why people use health services. *Milbank Memorial Fund Quarterly, 44*, 94–121.

Rosenstock, I. M. (1974). The health belief model and preventive health behavior. *Health Education Monographs, 2*, 354–385.

Rosenthal, G., Halloran, E., Kiley, M., & Landefeld, S. (1995). Validation of the nursing severity index in the assessment of hospital outcomes in patients with musculoskeletal disease. *Journal of Clinical Epidemiology, 48*(2), 179–188.

Rosenthal, G., Halloran, E., Kiley, M. L., Pinkley, C., & Landefeld, S. (1992). Development and validation of the nursing severity index: A new method for measuring severity of illness using nursing diagnosis. *Medical Care, 30*(12), 1127–1141.

Rosenthal, R. (1979). The file drawer problem and tolerance for null results. *Psychological Bulletin, 86*, 638–641.

Ross, L. A. (1996). Teaching spiritual care to nurses [Abstract]. *Nurse Education Today, 16*, 38–43.

Rossi, P. H., & Freeman, H. E. (1985). *Evaluation: A systematic approach* (3rd ed.). Beverly Hills, CA: Sage.

Rössler, W., & Haker, H. (2003). Conceptualizing psychosocial interventions. *Current Opinion in Psychiatry, 16*(6), 709–712.

Roter, D., Hall, J., Merisca, R., Nordstrom, B., Cretin, D., & Svarstad, B. (1998). Effectiveness of interventions to improve patient compliance: A meta-analysis. *Medical Care, 36*, 1138–1161.

Roter, D. L. (2003). Observations on methodological and measurement challenges in the assessment of communication during medical exchanges. *Patient Education and Counseling, 50*, 17–21.

Rothert, M., & O'Connor, A. (2001). Health decisions and decision support for women. In J. J. Fitzpatrick, D. Taylor, & N. Woods (Eds.), *Annual review of nursing* (Vol. 19, pp. 307–324). New York: Springer Publishing.

Roubenoff, R. (2003). Catabolism of aging: Is it an inflammatory process? *Current Opinion Clinical Nutrition and Metabolism Care, 6*, 295–299.

Rowland, J., Aziz, N., Tesauro, G., & Feuer, E. (2001). The changing face of cancer survivorship. *Seminars in Oncology Nursing, 17*(4), 236–240.

Rowles, G. D., & Dallas, M. (1996). Individualizing care: Family roles in nursing home decision making. *Journal of Gerontological Nursing, 22*(3), 20–25.

Rowsey, P., & Gordon, C. (2000). A peripheral mechanism of fever: Differential sensitivity to the antipyretic action of methyl scopolamine. *Autonomic Neuroscience, 85*(1–3), 148–155.

Rowsey, P., Metzger, B., & Gordon, C. (2001). Effects of exercise conditioning on thermoregulatory response to anticholinesterase insecticide toxicity. *Biological Research for Nursing, 2*(4), 267–276.

Roy, C., & Andrews, H. A. (1999). *The Roy Adaptation Model* (2nd ed.). Stanford, CT: Appleton & Lange.

Roy, C. S., & Sherrington, C. S. (1890). On the regulation of the blood supply of the brain. *Journal of Physiology, 11*, 85–108.

Roykulcharoen, V., & Good, M. (in press). Systematic relaxation relieves postoperative pain in Thailand. *Journal of Advanced Nursing.*

Rozeboom, W. W. (1960). The fallacy of the null hypothesis significance test. *Psychological Bulletin, 57*, 416–428.

Rubenstein, L., Friedrich, R. M., Liveley, S., & Buckwalter, K. (2002). The Friedrich-Lively Instrument to assess the Impact of Schizophrenia on Siblings (FLIISS): Part II—reliability and validity assessment. *Journal of Nursing Measures, 10*, 231–248.

Rubin, E. (1997). Rehabilitation problems of women who are blind. *Sexuality and Disability, 15*, 41–45.

Rubin, R. (1975). Maternal tasks in pregnancy. *Maternal-Child Nursing Journal, 4*(3), 143–153.

Rubinow, D. R., Hoban, M., et al. (1988). *Medical and psychiatric perspectives*. Philadelphia: W. B. Saunders.

Rubinow, D. R., & Schmidt, P. J. (1995). The neuroendocrinology of menstrual cycle mood disorders. *Annals of the New York Academy of Sciences, 771*, 648–659.

Ruchlin, H., Morris, S., & Morris, J. (1993). Resident medical care utilization patterns in continuing care retirement communities. *Health Care Financing Review, 14*, 151–161.

Rudy, E. B., Turner, B. S., Baun, M., Stone, K. S., & Brucia, J. (1991). Endotracheal suctioning in adults with head injury. *Heart & Lung, 20*, 667–674.

Ruiz, B. A., Tabloski, P. A., & Frazier, S. M. (1995). The role of gerontological advanced practice nurses in geriatric care. *Journal of the American Geriatrics Society, 44*(5), 6–11.

Ruland, C. M., & Moore, S. M. (1998). Theory construction based on standards of care: A proposed theory of the peaceful end of life. *Nursing Outlook, 46*(4), 169–175.

Rungreangkulkij, S., & Chesla, C. (2001). Smooth a heart with water: Thai mothers care for a child with schizophrenia. *Archives of Psychiatric Nursing, 15*, 120–127.

Rungreangkulkij, S., Chafetz, L., Chesla, C., & Gilliss, C. (2002). Psychological morbidity of Thai families of a person with schizophrenia. *International Journal of Nursing Studies, 39*, 35–50.

Runyan, C. W., Zakocs, R. C., & Zwerling, C. (2000). Administrative and behavioral interventions for workplace violence prevention. *American Journal of Preventive Medicine, 18*(4 Suppl.), 116–127.

Russell, C. (1994). Elder care recipients' care-seeking process. *Western Journal of Nursing Research, 18*, 43–62.

Russo, J. M., & Lancaster, D. R. (1995). Evaluating unlicensed assistive personnel models: Asking the right questions, collecting the right data. *Journal of Nursing Administration, 25*(9), 51–57.

Ryan, C. (1997). Long term care employees: Attitudes regarding feeding the older adult: A pilot study. *Journal of Nutrition for the Elderly, 16*(4), 17–25.

Ryden, M., Bossenmaier, M., & McLachlan, C. (1991). Aggressive behavior in cognitively impaired nursing home residents. *Research in Nursing and Health, 14*(2), 87–95.

Saba, V., & McCormick, K. (2001). *Essentials of computers for nurses: Informatics for the new millennium* (3rd ed.). New York: McGraw-Hill Companies.

Saba, V. K. (1992). The classification of home health care nursing: Diagnoses and interventions. *Caring Magazine, 11*, 50–57.

Sable, J. A., Dunn, L. B., & Zisook, S. (2002). Late-life depression: How to identify its symptoms and provide effective treatment. *Geriatrics, 57*(2), 18–19, 22–23, 26.

Sabourin, C. B., & Funk, M. (1999). Readmission of patients after coronary artery bypass graft surgery. *Heart & Lung, 28*, 243–250.

Sackett, D. L., & Cook, D. J. (1993). Can we learn anything from small trials? [Review]. *Annals of the New York Academy of Sciences, 703*, 25–32.

Sackett, D. L., Rosenberg, W., Muir Gray, J. A., Haynes, R., & Richardson, W. (1996). Evidence-based medicine: What it is and what it isn't. *British Medical Journal, 312*, 71–72.

Sacks, H. (1967). The search for help: No one to turn to. In E. S. Schneidman (Ed.), *Essays in self destruction* (pp. 203–223). New York: Science House.

Saks, E. R., Jeete, D. V., Granholm, E., Palmer, B. W., & Schneiderman, L. (2002). Ethical issues in psychosocial interventions research involving controls. *Ethical Behavior, 12*, 87–101.

Salantera, S., Eriksson, E., Junnola, T., Salminen, E. K., & Lauri, S. (2003). Clinical judgement and information seeking by nurses and physicians working with cancer patients. *Psychooncology, 12*(3), 280–290.

Salerno, E. S. (2002). Hope, power, and perception of self in individuals recovering from schizophrenia: A Rogerian perspective. *Visions: The Journal of Rogerian Nursing Science, 10*, 23–36.

Samms, M. C. (1999). The husband's untold account of his wife's breast cancer: A chronologic analysis. *Oncology Nursing Forum, 26*, 1351–1358.

Sampselle, C. M., Burns, P. A., Dougherty, M. C., Newman, D. K., Thomas, K. K., & Wyman, J. F. (1997). Continence for women: Evidence-based practice. *Journal of Obstetric, Gynecologic, & Neonatal Nursing, 26*(4), 375–385.

Sarna, L., & Lillington, L. (2002). Tobacco: An emerging topic in nursing research. *Nursing Research, 51*, 245–253.

Sasaki, C. T., & Leder, S. B. (2003). Comments on selected recent dysphagia literature. *Dysphagia, 18*, 223–226.

Saunders, J. C. (1999). Family functioning in families providing care for a family member with schizophrenia. *Issues in Mental Health Nursing, 20*, 95–113.

Saunders, J. (2003). Families living with severe mental illness: A literature review. *Issues in Mental Health Nursing, 24*, 175–198.

Saunders, J. C., & Byrne, M. M. (2002). A thematic analysis of families living with schizophrenia. *Archives of Psychiatric Nursing, 16*, 217–223.

Saur, C. D., Granger, B. B., Muhlbaier, L. H., Forman, L. M., McKenzie, R. J., Taylor, M. C., et al. (2001). Depressive symptoms and outcome of coronary artery bypass grafting. *American Journal of Critical Care, 10*(1), 4–10.

Sayer, J., Ritter, S., & Gournay, K. (2000). Beliefs about voices and their effects on coping strategies. *Journal of Advanced Nursing, 31*, 1199–2005.

Schaefer, K. M., Swavely, D., Rothenberger, C., Hess, S., & Williston, D. (1996). Sleep disturbances post coronary artery bypass surgery. *Progress in Cardiovascular Nursing, 11*(1), 5–14.

Scheff, T., & Retzinger, S. (1991). *Emotions and violence: Shame and rage in destructive conflicts*. Lexington, MA: Lexington Books.

Scheier, M. F., Matthews, K. A., Owens, J. F., Schulz, R., Bridges, M. W., Magovern, G. J., et al. (1999). Optimism and rehospitalization after coronary artery bypass graft surgery. *Archives of Internal Medicine, 159*, 829–835.

Schein, L. A., Bernard, H. S., Spitz, H. I., & Muskin, P. R. (Eds.). (2003). *Psychosocial treatment of medical conditions*. New York: Brunner-Routledge.

Schepp, K. G., O'Connor, F. W., Kennedy, M., Tsi, J. H. C., Davidson, B., Sekijima, M., et al. (1999). Family centered program for adolescents with mental illness. *Communicating Nursing Research*, 32.

Scherb, C. A., Rapp, C. G., Johnson, M., & Maas, M. (1998). The nursing outcomes classification: Validation by rehabilitation nurses [In Process Citation]. *Rehabilitation Nursing, 23*(4), 174–178, 191.

Schim, S. M., Jackson, F., Seely, S., Gruinow, K., & Baker, J. (2000). Knowledge and attitudes of home care nurses toward hospice referral. *Journal of Nursing Administration, 30*, 273–277.

Schindul-Rothschild, J., Berry, D., & Long-Middleton, E. (1996). Where have all the nurses gone? Final results of the AJN patient care survey. *American Journal of Nursing, 96*(11), 26–31.

Schirm, V., & Stachel, L. (1996). The values history as a nursing intervention to encourage use of advance directives among older adults. *Applied Nursing Research, 9*(2), 93–96.

Schlegel, K. L., & Shannon, S. E. (2000). Legal guidelines related to end-of-life decisions: Are nurse practitioners knowledgeable? *Journal of Gerontological Nursing, 26*(9), 14–24.

Schlotfeldt, R. (1975). The need for a conceptual framework. In P. Verhonic (Ed.), *Nursing research* (pp. 3–25). Boston: Little & Brown.

Schmidt, J. V., & McCartney, P. R. (2000). History and development of fetal heart assessment: A composite. *Journal of Obstetric, Gynecologic, and Neonatal Nursing, 29*(5), 295–305.

Schmied, V., Myors, K., Wills, J., & Cooke, M. (2002). Preparing expectant couples for new-parent experiences: A comparison of two models of antenatal education. *Journal of Perinatal Education, 11*(3), 20–27.

Schoenhofer, S. O., Bingham, V., & Hutchins, G. C. (1998). Giving of oneself on another's behalf: The phenomenology of everyday caring. *International Journal for Human Caring, 2*(2), 23–29.

Scholle, S. H., Rost, K. M., & Golding, J. M. (1998). Physical abuse among depressed women. *Journal of General Internal Medicine, 13*(9), 607–613.

Schön, D. (1983). *The reflective practitioner: How professionals think in action*. New York: Basic Books.

Schramm, C. J. (1996). Capitation in managed care. *Endocrine Practice, 2*(6), 429–431.

Schroder, K. E. E., Carey, M. P., & Vanable, P. A. (2003). Methodological challenges in research on sexual risk behavior: II. Accuracy of self-reports. *Annals of Behavioral Medicine, 26*(2), 104–123.

Schroeder, S. A. (2004). Tobacco control in the wake of the 1998 master agreement settlement. *New England Journal of Medicine, 350*, 293–301.

Schuelke, S. T., Trask, B., Wallace, C., Baun, M. M., Bergstrom, N., & McCabe, B. (1991/92, Winter). Physiological effects of the use of a companion dog as a cue to relaxation in diagnosed hypertensives. *The Latham Letter*, 14–17.

Schultz, R. (2000). *Handbook of dementia caregiving: Evidence-based interventions for family caregivers*. New York: Springer Publishing.

Schultz, R., & Beach, S. (1999). Caregiving is a risk factor for mortality: The caregiver health effects study. *Journal of the American Medical Association, 282*, 2215–2219.

Schultz, R., Beach, S. R., Ives, D. G., Martire, L. M., Ariyo, A. A., & Kop, W. J. (2000). Association between depression and mortality in older adults: The Cardiovascular Health Study. *Archives of Internal Medicine, 160*, 1761–1768.

Schultz, R., Lustig, A., Handler, S., & Martire, L. M. (2002). Technology based caregiver intervention research: Current status and future directions. *Gerontechnology, 2*(1), 15–47.

Schumacher, K., Stewart, B., Archbold, P., Dodd, M., & Dibble, S. (2000). Family caregiving skill: Development of the concept. *Research in Nursing & Health, 23*, 191–203.

Schupak-Neuberg, E., & Nemeroff, C. (1993). Disturbances in identity and self-regulation in bulimia nervosa: Implications for a metaphorical perspective of "body as self." *International Journal of Eating Disorders, 13*, 335–347.

Schuster, M. A., Stein, B. D., Jaycox, L. H., Collins, R. L., Marshall, G. N., Elliott, M. N., et al. (2001). A national survey of stress reactions after the September 11, 2001, terrorist attacks. *New England Journal of Medicine, 345*(20), 1507–1512.

Schutz, A. (1973). *Collected papers I: The problem of social reality*. The Hague, Netherlands: Martinus Nijhoff.

Schutzenofer, K. K., & Potter, P. (1989). Collaboration by consortium. *Nursing Connections, 2*(2), 39–47.

Schwab, J. J., Stephenson, J. J., & Ice, J. F. (1993). Family research. In J. J. Schwab, J. J. Stephenson, & J. F. Ice, *Evaluating family mental health: History, epidemiology and treatment issues* (pp. 157–226). New York: Plenum.

Schwab-Stone, M., Chen, C., Greenberger, E., Silver, D, Lichtman, J., & Voyce, C. (1999). No safe haven II: The effects of violence exposure on urban youth. *Journal of the American Academy of Child and Adolescent Psychiatry, 38*, 359–367.

Schwartz, C. E., & Fox, B. H. (1995). Who says yes? Identifying selection biases in a psychosocial intervention study of multiple sclerosis. *Social Science and Medicine, 40*, 359–370.

Schwartz, C. E., Wheeler, H. B., Hammes, B., Basque, N., Edmunds, J., Reed, G., et al. (2002). Early intervention in planning end-of-life care with ambulatory geriatric patients: Results of a pilot trial. *Archives of Internal Medicine, 162*(14), 1611–1618.

Schwartz, I. D. (2002). Failure to thrive: An old nemesis in the new millennium. *Pediatrics in Review, 21*, 257–264.

Schwartz, J. K. (1999). Assisted dying and nursing practice. *Image: The Journal of Nursing Scholarship, 31*(4), 367–373.

Schwartz, W. B., Gorry, G. A., Kassirer, J. P., & Essig, A. (1973). Decision analysis and clinical judgment. *American Journal of Medicine, 55*(3), 459–472.

Schwarz, D. F., Grisso, J. A., Holmes, J. H., Miles, C. G., Wishner, A. R., & Sutton, R. L. (1994). Injuries in an urban African American population. *Journal of the American Medical Association, 271*, 755–760.

Scientific Advisory Committee of the Medical Outcomes Trust. (2002). Assessing health status and quality of life instruments. *Quality of Life Research, 11*, 193–205.

Scott, J., Sochalski, J., & Aiken, L. (1999). Review of Magnet Hospital research: Findings and implications for professional nursing practice. *Journal of Nursing Administration, 29*(1), 9–19.

Scott, J. D. (1996). *Hypothesis generation research: The role of medical treatment effectiveness research in hypothesis generation*. Center for Medical Effectiveness Research, Agency for Health Care Policy and Research. Rockville, MD: U.S. Public Health Services.

Scott, J. G., Sochalski, J., & Aiken, L. (1999). Review of magnet hospital research: Findings and implications for professional nursing practice. *Journal of Nursing Administration, 29*, 9–19.

Scott, L. D. (2001). Technological caregiving: A qualitative perspective. *Home Health Care Management & Practice, 13*(3), 227–235.

Screeche-Powell, C., & Owen, S. (2003). Early experiences of patients waiting to be accepted for CABG. *British Journal of Nursing, 12*(10), 613–619.

Seago, J. A. (2000). Registered Nurses, Unlicensed Assistive Personnel, and organizational culture in hospitals. *Journal of Nursing Administration, 30*(5), 278–286.

Searle, J. R., Kiefer, F., & Bierwisch, M. (Eds.). (1980). *Speech act theory and pragmatics*. Dordrecht, Netherlands: Reidel.

Sebastian, J., Barkauskas, V. H., Stanhope, M., Pohl, J. M., & Vonderheid, S. (2004, October 15–17). *Organizational and business processes of academic nurse managed centers: A report from a national survey*. Paper presented at the National Nursing Centers Consortium Third Annual Conference, Nashville, TN.

Sechrist, K., & Pravikoff, D. (2002). *Physiological studies*. Glendale, CA: Cinhal Information Systems.

Seeman, T. E., Bruce, M. L., & McAvay, G. J. (1996). Social network characteristics and onset of ADL disability: MacArthur studies of successful aging. *Journals of Gerontology: Psychology and Social Science, 51*, S191–S200.

SEER. (2004). *Surveillance, Epidemiology, & End Results*. Retrieved from http://seer.cancer.gov/

Segar, J. L., Merrill, D. C., Chapleau, M. W., & Robillard, J. E. (1993). Hemodynamic changes during endotracheal suctioning are mediated by increased autonomic activity. *Pediatric Research, 33*(6), 649–652.

Selye, H. (1976). *The stress of life* (2nd ed.). New York: McGraw-Hill.

Serdula, M. K, Khan, L. K., & Dietz, W. H. (2003). Weight loss counseling revisited. *Journal of the American Medical Association, 289*, 1747–1750.

Sermon, F., Vanden Brande, S., Roosens, B., Mana, F., Deron, P., & Urbain, D. (2004). Is ambulatory 24-h dual-probe pH monitoring useful in suspected ENT manifestations of GERD? *Digest of Liver Diseases, 36*(2), 105–110.

Seventh Day Adventist Hospital Association. (1961–1967). *Cumulative index to nursing literature*. Glendale, CA: Author.

Seyle, H. (1950). *The physiology and pathology of exposure to stress*. Montreal, Quebec, Canada: ACTA.

Shamian, J. (1991). Effect of teaching decision analysis on student nurses' clinical intervention decision making. *Research in Nursing & Health, 14*(1), 59–66.

Sharber, J. (1997). The efficacy of tepid sponge bathing to reduce fever in young children. *American Journal of Emergency Medicine, 15*(2), 188–192.

Shariat, S., Mallonee, S., Kruger, E., Farmer, K., & North, C. (1999). A prospective study of long-term health outcomes among Oklahoma City bombing survivors. *Journal of Oklahoma State Medical Association, 92*(4), 178–186.

Shaver, J. L. (2002). Women and sleep. *Nursing Clinics of North America, 37*, 707–718.

Shaver, J. L. F., Giblin, E., Lentz, M., & Lee, K. (1988). Sleep patterns and stability in perimenopausal women. *Sleep, 11*, 556–561.

Shaver, J. F., & Woods, N. F. (1985). Concordance of perimenstrual symptoms across two cycles. *Research in Nursing & Health, 8*, 313–319.

Shavers, V., & Brown, M. (2002). Racial and ethnic disparities in the receipt of cancer treatment. *Journal of the National Cancer Institute, 94*(5), 334–357.

Shaw, B. R., McTavish, F., Hawkins, R., Gustafson, D. H., & Pingree, S. (2000). Experiences of women with breast cancer: Exchanging social support over the CHESS computer network. *Journal of Health Communication, 5*(2), 135–159.

Shea, B., Wells, G., Cranney, A., Zytaruk, N., Robinson, V., Griffith, L., et al. (2002). VII. Meta-analysis of calcium supplementation for the prevention of postmenopausal of osteoporosis. *Endocrine Review, 23*(4), 552–559.

Sheers, N. J., Rutherford, G. W., & Kemp, J. S. (2003). Where should infants sleep? A comparison of risk for suffocation of infants sleeping in cribs, adult beds, and other sleeping locations. *Pediatrics, 112*, 883–889.

Shelley, P. (2002). Serious and enduring mental illness—schizophrenia. *International Journal of Psychiatric Nursing Research, 7*, 856–870.

Shepard, J., & Faust, S. (1994). Refugee health care and the problem of suffering. *Bioethics Forum, 9*, 3–7.

Sherrell, K., Anderson, R., & Buckwalter, K. (1998). Invisible residents: The chronically mentally ill elderly in nursing homes. *Archives of Psychiatric Nursing, 12*(3), 131–139.

Sherrell, K., & Buckwalter, K. C. (1997). Geropsychiatry. Barriers to follow-up studies with the chronically mentally ill elderly in long-term care settings. *Journal of Gerontological Nursing, 23*(8), 37–40.

Sherrell, K., Buckwalter, K. C., Bode, R., & Strozdas, L. (1999). Use of the cognitive abilities screening instrument to assess elderly persons with schizophrenia in long-term care settings. *Issues in Mental Health Nursing, 20,* 541–558.

Sherwood, G. (1997). Meta-synthesis of qualitative analyses of caring: Defining atherapeutic model of nursing. *Advanced Practice Nursing Quarterly, 3*(1), 32–42.

Sherwood, P., Given, B., Given, C., Schiffman, R., Murman, D., & Lovely, M. (2004). Caregivers of persons with a brain tumor: A conceptual model. *Nursing Inquiry, 11*(1), 43–53.

Shiao, S-Y. (1993). *Nasal gastric tube placement: Effect on sucking and breathing in very low birth weight infants.* Unpublished doctoral dissertation, Case Western Reserve University, Cleveland, OH.

Shiao, S-Y. (2002). Desaturation events in neonates during mechanical ventilation. *Critical Care Nursing Quarterly, 24*(4), 14–29.

Shiao, S-Y., & DiFiore, T. E. (1996). A survey of gastric tube practices in level II and level III nurseries. *Issues in Comprehensive Pediatric Nursing, 19*(3), 209–220.

Shields-Poe, D., & Pinelli, J. (1997). Variables associated with parental stress in neonatal intensive care units. *Neonatal Network, 16*(1), 29–37.

Shinn, M., & Wietzman, B. (1996). Homeless families are different. In J. Baumohl (Ed.), *Homelessness in America* (pp. 109–122). Washington, DC: National Coalition for the Homeless.

Shires, B., & Tappan, T. (1992). The clinical nurse specialist as brief psychotherapist. *Perspectives in Psychiatric Care, 28*(4), 15–18.

Shore, E. R., & Compton, K. L. (1998). Wadda ya mean, I can't drive? *Journal of Prevention and Intervention in the Community, 17,* 45–52.

Shore, E. R., & Compton, K. L. (2000). Individual interventions to prevent drunk driving: Types, efficacy, and a theoretical perspective. *Journal of Drug Education, 30,* 281–289.

Shors, T. J., & Leuner, B. (2003). Estrogen-mediated effects on depression and memory formation in females. *Journal of Affective Disorders, 74,* 85–96.

Showers, C., & Larson, B. (1999). Looking at body image: The organization of self-knowledge about physical appearance and its relation to disordered eating. *Journal of Personality, 67,* 659–700.

Shreve, W. S. (1998). Trauma prevention: An evaluation tool for youth and alcohol trauma-prevention programs. *Journal of Trauma Nursing, 5,* 12–16.

Shumway-Cook, A., Brauer, S., & Woollacott, M. (2000). Predicting the probability for falls in community-dwelling older adults using the Timed Up & Go Test. *Physical Therapy, 80,* 896–903.

Shyu, Y. L. (2000). Role tuning between caregiver and care receiver during discharge transition: An illustration of role function mode in Roy's adaptation model. *Nursing Science Quarterly, 13*(4), 323–331.

Sichel, D., & Driscoll, J. W. (1999). *Women's moods.* New York: Harper Collins.

Siddle, R., & Kingdon, D. (2000). The management of schizophrenia: Cognitive behavioural therapy. *British Journal of Community Nursing, 5,* 20–25.

Siegel, C. D., Graves, P., Maloney, K., Norris, J. M., Colonge, B. N., & Lezotte, D. (1996). Mortality from intentional and unintentional injury among infants of young mothers in Colorado, 1986 to 1992. *Archives of Pediatric and Adolescent Medicine, 150,* 1077–1083.

Siegel, S., & Rees, B. (1992). Preparing the public employee for retirement. *Public Personnel Management, 21,* 89–100.

Siegler, E. L., Capezuti, E., Maislin, G., Baumgarten, M., Evans, L., & Strumpf, N. (1997). Effects of a restraint reduction intervention and OBRA '87 regulations on psychoactive drug use in nursing homes. *Journal of the American Geriatrics Society, 45,* 791–796.

Siegler, E. L., Glick, D., & Lee, J. (2002). Optimal staffing for Acute Care of the Elderly (ACE) units. *Geriatric Nursing, 23*(3), 152–155.

Siehoff, A. M. (1998). Impact of unlicensed assistive personnel on patient satisfaction: An integrative review of the literature. *Journal of Nursing Care Quality, 13*(2), 1–10.

Sieloff, C. L. (2003). Measuring nursing power within organizations. *Journal of Nursing Scholarship, 35*(2), 183–187.

Sieloff, C. L., Frey, M. A., & Killeen, M. B. (in press). Application of King's work to practice. In M. Parker (Ed.), *Nursing theories and nursing practice* (2nd ed.). Philadelphia: F. A. Davis.

Siesjo, B. K. (1992). Pathophysiology and treatment of focal cerebral ischemia. Part I: Pathophysiology. *Journal of Neurosurgery, 77*(2), 169–184.

Sigma Theta Tau International. (2003). Evidence-based nursing. Retrieved from http://www.nursingsociety.org/research/main.html

Silber, J. H., Rosenbaum, P. R., & Ross, R. N. (1995). Comparing the contributions of groups of predictors: Which outcomes vary with hospital rather than patient characteristics. *Journal of the American Statistical Association*, 90(429), 7–18.

Silbert, B. S., Santamaria, J. D., Kelly, W. J., O'Brien, J. L., Blyth, C. M., Wong, M. Y., et al. (2001). Early extubation after cardiac surgery: Emotional status in the early postoperative period. *Journal of Cardiothoracic and Vascular Anesthesia*, *15*(4), 439–444.

Sills, G. M. (1998). Peplau and professionalism: The emergence of the paradigm of professionalization. *Journal of Psychiatric and Mental Health Nursing*, 5, 167–171.

Silva, M. C. (1997). Philosophy, theory, and research in nursing: A linguistic journey to nursing practice. In I. M. King & J. Fawcett (Eds.), *The language of nursing theory and metatheory* (pp. 51–59). Indianapolis, IN: Sigma Theta Tau's International Center Nursing Press.

Silver, H. J., & Wellman, N. S. (2002). Nutrition education may reduce burden in family caregivers of older adults. *Journal of Nutrition Education & Behavior*, *34*, S53–S58.

Simmons, B., Lanuza, D., Fonteyn, Hicks, F., & Holm, K. (2003). Clinical reasoning in experienced nurses. *Western Journal of Nursing Research*, *25*(6), 701–719.

Simmons, L., & Henderson, V. (1964). *Nursing research: A review and assessment*. New York: Macmillan.

Simmons, S. F., Alessi, C., & Schnelle, J. F. (2001). An intervention to increase fluid intake in nursing home residents: Prompting and preference compliance. *Journal of the American Geriatrics Society*, *49*, 926–933.

Simon, J. (1993). *Poor discipline: Parole and the social control of the underclass, 1890–1990*. Chicago: University of Chicago Press.

Simpson, H. (1991). *Peplau's model in action*. London: Macmillan.

Simpson, K. R. (2000). A critical evaluation of the past 25 years of perinatal nursing practice: Opportunities for improvement. *Maternal Child Nursing*, *25*(6), 300–304.

Sin, J., & Gamble, C. (2003). Managing side-effects to the optimum: Valuing a client's experience. *Journal of Psychiatric Mental Health Nursing*, *10*, 147–153.

Singh, U., & Saxena, M. S. (1991). Anxiety during pregnancy and after childbirth. *Psychological Studies*, *36*(2), 108–111.

Siris, E. S., Miller, P. D., Barrett-Connor, E., Faulkner, K. G., Wehren, L. E., Abbott, T. A., et al. (2001). Identification and fracture outcomes of undiagnosed low bone mineral density in postmenopausal women: Results from the National Osteoporosis Risk Assessment. *Journal of the American Medical Association*, *286*(22), 2815–2822.

Sisk, J. E. (1998). How are health care organizations using clinical guidelines? *Health Affairs*, *17*(5), 91–109.

Sjostrom, A. C., Holmberg, B., & Strang, P. (2002). Parkinsons-plus patients: An unknown group with severe symptoms. *Journal of Neuroscience Nursing*, *34*, 314–319.

Skov, L., Ryding, J., Pryds, O., & Greisen, G. (1992). Changes in cerebral oxygenation and cerebral blood volume during endotracheal suctioning in ventilated neonates. *Acta Paediatrica*, *81*(5), 389–393.

Skybo, T., & Ryan-Wenger, N. (2002). A school-based intervention to teach third grade children about the prevention of heart disease. *Pediatric Nursing*, *22*(3), 223–229.

Slavinsky, A. T., & Krauss, J. B. (1982). Two approaches to the management of long-term psychiatric outpatients in the community. *Nursing Research*, *31*, 284–289.

Sleutel, M. (2000). Climate, culture, context, or work environment? Organizational factors that influence nursing practice. *Journal of Nursing Administration*, *30*, 53–58.

Sleutel, M. R. (2002). Development and testing of the Labor Support Scale. *Journal of Nursing Measurement*, *10*, 249–262.

Slevin, K., & Wingrove, C. (1995). Women in retirement: A review and critique of empirical research since 1976. *Sociological Inquiry*, *65*, 1–21.

Sloane, P. D., Coeytaux, R. R., Beck, R. S., & Dallara, J. (2001). Dizziness: State of the science. *Annals of Internal Medicine*, *134*(2 Suppl.), 823–832.

Smart, R. G., & Stoduto, G. (1997). Interventions by students in friends' alcohol, tobacco, and drug use. *Journal of Drug Education*, *27*, 213–222.

Smeltzer, C. H., Leighty, S., & Williams-Brinkley, R. (1997). In J. C. McCloskey & H. K. Grace (Eds.), *Current issues in nursing* (5th ed., pp. 93–98). St. Louis, MO: C. V. Mosby.

Smets, E. M., Garssen, B., Schuster-Uitterhoeve, A. L., & de Haes, J. C. (1993). Fatigue in cancer patients. *British Journal of Cancer*, *68*, 220–224.

Smith, C. E. (1994). A model of caregiving effectiveness for technologically dependent adults. *Advances in Nursing Science*, *17*(2), 27–40.

Smith, C. E. (1995). Technology home care: Part I. In J. Fitzpatrick & A. Jacox (Eds.), *Annual review of nursing research* (Vol. 13, pp. 137–167). New York: Springer Publishing.

Smith, C. E. (1996). Quality of life and caregiving in technological home care. In J. Fitzpatrick & A. Jacox (Eds.), *Annual review of nursing research* (Vol. 14, pp. 95–118). New York: Springer Publishing.

Smith, C. E., Curtas, S., Kleinbeck, S., Werkowitch, M., Mosier, M., Seidner, D., et al. (2003). Clinical trial of interactive and videotaped educational interventions reduce infection, reactive depression and rehospitalizations for sepsis in patients on home parenteral nutrition. *Journal of Parenteral & Enteral Nutrition, 27*(2), 137–145.

Smith, C. E., Kleinbeck, S. V. M., Boyle, D., Kochinda, C., & Parker, S. (2002). Family caregivers' motives for helping scale derived from motivation-to-help theory. *Nursing Measurement*, 9(3), 239–257.

Smith, C. E., Pace, K., Kochinda, C., Kleinbeck, S. V. M., Koehler, J., & Popkess-Vawter, S. (2002). Caregiving effectiveness: Evolution of a nursing model for home care. *Advances in Nursing Science, 25*(1), 51–65.

Smith, D., & Clark, M. S. (1995). Competence and performance in activities of daily living of patients following rehabilitation from stroke. *Disability and Rehabilitation, 17*, 15–33.

Smith, D., Zhou, X., Weinberger, M., Smith, F., & McDonald, R. (1999). Mailed reminders for area-wide influenza immunization: A randomized controlled trial. *Journal of the American Geriatrics Society, 47*, 1–5.

Smith, E. (1979). Nonclinical practice: CE meeting the needs of the demanding nursing profession. *CE Focus, 2*, 8–10.

Smith, J. A. (1981). The idea of health: A philosophical inquiry. *Advances in Nursing Science, 3*, 43–50.

Smith, J. A. (1983). *The idea of health implications for the nursing professional.* New York: Columbia University.

Smith, M., & Hare, M. (2004). An overview of progress in childhood cancer survival. *Journal of Pediatric Oncology Nursing, 21*(3), 160–164.

Smith, M. A., & Gloeckler Ries, L. A. (2002). Childhood cancer incidence survival, and mortality. In P. A. Pizzo & D. G. Poplack (Eds.), *Principles and practice of pediatric oncology* (4th ed.). Philadelphia: J. B. Lippincott.

Smith, M. A., Ruffin, M. T., & Green, L. A. (1993). The rational management of labor. *American Family Physician, 47*, 1471–1481.

Smith, M. C. (2004). Review of research related to Watson's theory of caring. *Nursing Science Quarterly, 17*(1), 13–25.

Smith, M. J., Kennison, M., Gamble, S., & Loudin, B. (in press). Intervening as a passenger in drinking/driving situations. *Applied Nursing Research.*

Smith, M. J., & Liehr, P. (1999). Attentively embracing story: A middle range theory with practice and research implications. *Scholarly Inquiry for Nursing Practice: An International Journal, 13*, 187–204.

Smith, M. J., & Liehr, P. L. (2003a). *Middle range theory for nursing.* New York: Springer Publishing.

Smith, M. J., & Liehr, P. (2003b). The theory of attentively embracing story. In M. J. Smith & P. Liehr (Eds.), *Middle range theory for nursing* (pp. 167–188). New York: Springer Publishing.

Smith, N. (1999). Antenatal classes and the transition to fatherhood: A study of some fathers' views. *Midwifery Digest, 9*, 463–468.

Smith, P. M., Reilly, K. R., Miller, N. H., DeBusk, R. F., & Taylor, C. B. (2002). Application of a nurse-managed inpatient smoking cessation program. *Nicotine & Tobacco Research, 4*, 211–222.

Smith, S. S., Blair, S. N., Bonow, R. O., Brass, L. M., Cerqueira, M. D., & Dracup, K. (2001). AHA/ACC guidelines for preventing heart attack and death in patients with atherosclerotic cardiovascular disease: 2001 update. *Circulation, 104*, 1577–1579.

Snyder, H. N. (2001). Epidemiology of official offending. In R. Loeber & D. P. Farrington (Eds.), *Child delinquents: Development, intervention, and service needs* (pp. 25–46). Thousand Oaks, CA: Sage Publications.

Snyder, L. H., Rupprecht, P., Pyrek, J., Brekhus, S., & Moss, T. (1978). Wandering. *Gerontologist, 29*(3), 272–280.

Snyder, M. (1993). The influence of interventions on the stress-health outcome linkage. In J. S. Barnfather & B. L. Lyon (Eds.), *Stress and coping: State of the science and implications for nursing theory, research and practice* (pp. 159–170). Indianapolis, IN: Sigma Theta Tau International.

Snyder, M. (2000). The influence of interventions on the stress-health outcome linkage. In J. S. Werner & M. H. Forst (Eds.), *Stress and coping: State of the science and implications for nursing theory, research, and practice, 1991–1995.* Glenview, IL: Midwest Nursing Research Society.

Snyder, M., & Chlan, L. (1999). Music therapy. *Annual Review of Nursing Research, 17*, 3–25.

Sochalski, J. (2004). Is more better? The relationship between nurse staffing and the quality of nursing care in hospitals. *Medical Care, 42*(2 suppl.), 67–73.

Social Security Administration. (2003). *Social Security basic fact.* Retrieved October 3, 2003, from http://www.ssa.gov/pressoffice/basicfact.htm

Society for Research on Nicotine and Tobacco Subcommittee on Biochemical Verification. (2002).

Biochemical verification of tobacco use and cessation. *Nicotine & Tobacco Research, 4*, 149–159.

Soehren, P. M., & Schumann, L. L. (1994). Enhanced role opportunities available to the CNS/Nurse Practitioner. *Clinical Nurse Specialist, 8*(3) 123–127.

Sokal, R. R. (1974). Classification: Purposes, principles, progress, prospects. *Science, 185*, 1115–1123.

Sole, M. L., Byers, J. F., Ludy, J. E., Zhang, Y., Banta, C. M., & Brummel, K. (2004). A multi-site survey of suctioning techniques and airway management practices. *American Journal of Critical Care, 12*(3), 220–230.

Sommers, L., Marton, K., Barbaccia, J., & Randolph, J. (2000). Physician, nurse and social worker collaboration in primary care for chronically ill seniors. *Archives of Internal Medicine, 160*, 1825–1833.

Son, G., Therrien, B., & Whall, A. (2002). Implicit memory and familiarity among elders with dementia. *Journal of Nursing Scholarship, 34*(3), 263–267.

Sousa, K. H., Holzemer, W. L., Henry, S. B., & Slaughter, R. (1999). Dimensions of health-related quality of life in persons living with HIV disease. *Journal of Advanced Nursing, 29*(1), 178–187.

Sovie, M. D., & Jawad, A. F. (2001). Hospital restructuring and its impact on outcomes: Nursing staff regulations are premature. *Journal of Nursing Administration, 31*, 588–600.

Sowan, N., & Stember, M. (2000). Parental risk factors for infant obesity. *Maternal Child Nursing, 25*(5), 234–241.

Sowell, R. L., & Misener, T. R. (1997). Decisions to have a baby by HIV-infected women. *Western Journal of Nursing Research, 19*, 56–70.

Sox, H. C. (1979). Quality of patient care by nurse practitioners and physician assistants: A 10 year perspective. *Annals of Internal Medicine, 91*, 459–468.

Sparks, S. M. (1993). Electronic networking for nurses. *Image: Journal of Nursing Scholarship, 25*, 245–248.

Sparks, S. M. (1995). Integrating nursing diagnosis in nursing education. In M. J. Rantz (Eds.), *Classification of nursing diagnoses: Proceedings of the eleventh conference of the North American Nursing Diagnosis Association*, 3–11.

Sparks, S. M., & Lien-Gieschen, T. (1994). Modification of the diagnostic content validity model. *Nursing Diagnosis, 5*, 31–35.

Spector, W. D., Katz, S., Murphy, J. B., & Fulton, J. P. (1987). The hierarchical relationship between activities of daily living and instrumental activities of daily living. *Journal of Chronic Disease, 40*, 481–489.

Spellbring, A. M., & Ryan, J. W. (2003). Medication administration by unlicensed caregivers. A model program. *Journal of Gerontological Nursing, 29*(6), 48–54.

Spence, J. T., & Helmreich, R. L. (1974). *Masculinity and femininity*. Austin: University of Texas Press.

Speroff, L. (1988). Letter from Erle Henriksen, MD on the "melancholies of menstruation."

Speroff, L., Glass, R., & Kase, N. (1999). *Clinical gynecology, endocrinology and infertility* (6th ed.). New York: Lippincott, Williams & Wilkins.

Spielmeyer, W. (1922). *Histopathologic des Nervensystems*. Berlin: Springer-Verlag.

Spilker, J., Kongable, G., Barch, C., Braimab, J., Brattina, P., Daley, S., et al. (1997). Using the NIH Stroke Scale to assess stroke patients. *Journal of Neuroscience Nursing, 29*, 384–392.

Spitz, R. (1945). Hospitalism: An inquiry into the genesis of psychiatric conditions in early childhood. *Psychoanalytic Study of the Child, 1*, 52–74.

Spitzer, W. O., Sackett, D. L., Sibley, J. C., Roberts, R. S., Gent, M., Kergin D. J., et al. (1974). The Burlington randomized trial of the nurse practitioner. *New England Journal of Medicine, 290*(5), 251–256.

St. Lawrence, J. S., Brasfield, T. L., Jefferson, K. W., Alleyne, E., O'Bannon, R. E., & Shirley, A. (1995). Cognitive-behavioral intervention to reduce African American adolescents' risk for HIV infection. *Journal of Consulting and Clinical Psychology, 63*(2), 221–237.

Staggers, N., Gassert, C., Kwai, J, Hunter, D., Nelson, R., Sensmeier, J., et al. (2001). *Scope and standards of nursing informatics practice*. Washington, DC: American Nurses Publishing.

Stake, R. (1994). Case studies. In N. Denzin & Y. Lincoln (Eds.), *Handbook of qualitative research* (pp. 435–454). Thousand Oaks, CA: Sage.

Stamps, P. L. (1997). *Nurses and work satisfaction: An index for measurement* (2nd ed.). Chicago: Health Administration Press.

Standing, T., Anthony, M. K., & Hertz, J. E. (2001). Nurses' narratives of outcomes after delegation to unlicensed assistive personnel. *Journal of Nursing Administration, 5*(1), 18–23.

Standley, J. M., & Hanser, S. B. (1995). Music therapy research and applications in pediatric oncology treatment. *Journal of Pediatric Oncology Nursing, 12*(1), 3–8; discussion 9–10.

Stanley, M., & Beare, P. (1999). *Gerontological nursing*. Philadelphia: F. A. Davis.

Stanley, M., & Prasun, M. (2002). Heart failure in older adults: Keys to successful management. *AACN Clinical Issues, 13*, 94–102.

Starck, P. L. (2003). The theory of meaning. In M. J. Smith & P. L. Liehr (Eds.), *Middle range theory for nursing* (pp. 125–144). New York: Springer Publishing.

Starfield, B. (1998). *Balancing health needs, services, and technology*. New York: Oxford University Press.

Stechmiller, J. K., Childress, B., & Porter, T. (2004). Arginine immunonutrition in critically ill patients: A clinical dilemma. *American Journal of Critical Care, 13*, 17–23.

Steckel, S. B. (1974). The use of positive reinforcement in order to increase patient compliance. *American Association of Nephrology Nurses and Technicians Journal, 1*, 39–41.

Steckel, S. B. (1982). *Patient contracting*. Norwalk, CT: Appleton-Century-Crofts.

Steckel, S. B., & Funnell, M. M. (1981). *Increasing adherence of outpatients to therapeutic regimens*. Final report on Veterans Administration Health Service Research and Development Project, #343. Ann Arbor, MI.

Steckel, S. B., & Swain, M. A. (1977). Contracting with patients to improve compliance. *Hospitals, 51*, 81–84.

Steele, N. M., French, J., Gatherer-Boyles, J., Newman, S., & Leclaire, S. (2001). Effect of acupressure by Sea-Bands on nausea and vomiting of pregnancy. *Journal of Obstetric, Gynecologic, and Neonatal Nursing, 30*, 61–70.

Steele, R. G. (2002). Experiences of families in which a child has a prolonged terminal illness: Modifying factors. *International Journal of Palliative Nursing, 418*(8), 420–434.

Steeman, E., Abraham, I., & Godderis, J. (in press). Risk profiles for institutionalization in a cohort of elderly people with dementia or depression. *Archives of Psychiatric Nursing*.

Steeves, R., Cohen, M. Z., & Wise, C. (1994). An analysis of critical incidents describing the essence of oncology nursing. *Oncology Nursing Forum, 21*(Suppl. 8), 19–25.

Steeves, R. H. (2002). The rhythms of bereavement. *Family and Community Health, 25*(1), 1–10.

Steiger, E., & Ireton-Jones, C. (2001). The evolution of home parenteral nutrition in the United States. *Nutrition Clinical Practice, 16*, 236–239.

Stein, B. D., Jaycox, L. H., Kataoka, S. H., Wong, M., Tu, W., Elliott, M. N., & et al. (2003). A mental health intervention for students exposed to violence: A randomized controlled trial. *Journal of the American Medical Association, 290*(5), 603–611.

Stein, K. F., Corte, C. M., & Nyquist, L. (2004). *The impoverished self and valenced self-schemas: Is it only the absence of positive selves?* Revision of manuscript in preparation.

Stein, R. E. K. (1996). To be or not to be . . . noncategorical. *Developmental and Behavioral Pediatrics, 17*, 36–37.

Steiner, M., Dunn, E., & Born, L. (2003). Hormones and mood: From menarche to menopause and beyond. *Journal of Affective Disorders, 74*, 67–83.

Steinhauser, K. E., Clipp, E. C., McNeilly, M., Christakis, N. A., McIntyre, L. M., & Tulsky, J. A. (2000). In search of a good death: Observations of patients, families, and providers. *Annals of Internal Medicine, 132*(10), 825–832.

Steinman, M., Sands, L., & Covinsky, K. (2001). Self-restriction of medications due to cost in seniors without prescription coverage. *Journal of General Internal Medicine, 16*, 793–799.

Stetler, C. B. (1994). Refinement of the Stetler/Marram model for application of research findings to practice. *Nursing Outlook, 42*, 15–25.

Stetler, C. B., Morsi, D., Rucki, S., Broughton, S., Corigan, B., Fitzgerald, J., et al. (1998). Utilization-focused integrative reviews in a nursing service. *Applied Nursing Research, 11*, 195–206.

Stevenson, J. S. (1990). Quantitative care research: Review of content, process, and product. In J. S. Stevenson & T. Tripp-Reimer (Eds.), *Knowledge about care and caring: State of the art and future developments* (pp. 97–118). Kansas City, MO: American Academy of Nursing.

Stevenson, J. S. (1993). Adult development is NOT (JUST) a demographic variable: A call for contextual content in doctoral programs. In M. Snyder & M. Newman (Eds.), *Annual Forum on Doctoral Nursing Education: 1993 Proceedings* (pp. 23–31). Minneapolis: University of Minnesota.

Steward, D. K. (2001). Behavioral characteristics of infants with nonorganic failure to thrive during a play interaction. *American Journal of Maternal/Child Nursing, 26*, 79–85.

Steward, D. K., Ryan-Wenger, N. A., & Boyne, L. J. (2003). Selection of growth parameters to define failure to thrive. *Journal of Pediatric Nursing, 18*, 52–59.

Stewart, D. W., & Kamins, M. A. (1993). *Secondary research: Information sources and methods*. Newbury Park, CA: Sage.

Stewart, J. L. (2003). Children living with chronic illness: An examination of their stressors, coping responses, and health outcomes. In *Annual review of nursing research* (Vol. 21, pp. 203–243), New York: Springer Publishing.

Stewart, J. L., & Mishel, M. H. (2000). Uncertainty in childhood illness: A synthesis of the parent child

literature. *Scholarly Inquiry for Nursing Practice: An International Journal, 14*(4), 299–319.
Stewart, M., Craig, D., MacPherson, K., & Alexander, S. (2001). Promoting positive affect and diminishing loneliness of widowed seniors through a support intervention. *Public Health Nursing, 18*(1), 54–63.
Stewart, W., & Barling, J. (1996). Daily work stress, mood and interpersonal job performance: A mediational model. *Work and Stress, 10*, 336–351.
Stiller, A., Molloy, D. W., Russo, R., Dubois, S., Kavsak, H., & Bedard, M. (2001). Development and evaluation of a new instrument that measures barriers to implementing advance directives. *Journal of Clinical Outcomes Management*, 8(4), 26–31.
Stillman, M. J. (1977). Women's health beliefs about breast cancer and breast self-examination. *Nursing Research, 26*, 121–127.
Stinson, N. (2003). Closing the gap working toward our goal. *Office of Minority Health Newsletter*, 1–20. Washington, DC: Department of Health & Human Services, Office of Minority Health.
Stone, K. L., Seeley, D. G., Cauley, J. A., Ensrud, J. A., Browner, W. S., Nevitt, M. C., et al. (2003). BMD at multiple sites and risk of fracture of multiple types: Long term results from the Study of Osteoporotic Fractures [Abstract]. *Journal of Bone Mineral Research, 18*(11), 1947–1954.
Stone, K. S. (1990). Ventilator versus manual resuscitation bag as the method for delivering hyperoxygenation before endotracheal suctioning. *AACN's Clinical Issues in Critical Care Nursing, 1*, 289–299.
Stone, K. S., Bell, S. D., & Preusser, B. A. (1991). The effect of repeated endotracheal suctioning on arterial blood pressure. *Applied Nursing Research, 4*, 150–158.
Stone, K. S., & Turner, B. (1989). Endotracheal suctioning. In *Annual review of nursing research* (Vol. 7, pp. 27–49). New York: Springer Publishing.
Stone, P. W., Larson, E., & Kawar, L. N. (2002). A systematic audit of economic evidence linking nosocomial infections and infection control interventions: 1990–2000. *American Journal of Infection Control, 30*, 145–152.
Stone, T. H. (2003). The invisible vulnerable: The economically and educationally disadvantaged subjects of clinical research. *Currents in Contemporary Ethics, 31*(1), 149–153.
Storch, J. L., & Dossetor, J. (1994). Public attitudes toward end-of-life treatment decisions: Implications for nurse clinicians and nursing administrators. *Canadian Journal of Nursing Administration, 7*(3), 65–89.
Storr, M., Meining, A., & Allescher, H. D. (2000). Pathophysiology and pharmacological treatment of gastroesophageal reflux disease. *Digestive Diseases, 18*(2), 93–102.
Stoudemire, A., & Smith, D. A. (1996). OBRA regulations and the use of psychotropic drugs in long-term care facilities: Impact and implications for geropsychiatric care. *General Hospital Psychiatry, 18*, 77–94.
Strauman, T. J., Vookles, J., Berenstein, V., Chaiken, S., & Higgins, E. T. (1991). Self-discrepancies and vulnerability to body dissatisfaction and disordered eating. *Journal of Personality and Social Psychology, 61*, 946–956.
Street, E., & Soldan, J. (1998). A conceptual framework for the psychosocial issues faced by families with genetic conditions. *Families, Systems & Health, 16*(3), 217–233.
Street, K., Ashcroft, R., Henderson, J., & Campbell, A. V. (2000). The decision-making process regarding the withdrawal or withholding of potential life-saving treatments in a children's hospital. *Journal of Medical Ethics, 26*(5), 346–352.
Street, L. L., & Luoma, J. B. (2002). Control groups in psychosocial intervention research: Ethical and methodological issues. *Ethics Behavior, 12*, 1–30.
Strehlow, A. J., & Amos-Jones, T. (1999). The homeless as a vulnerable population. *Nursing Clinics of North America, 34*(2), 261–274.
Strickland, O., & Waltz, C. (1986). Measurement of research variables in nursing. In P. Chinn (Ed.), *Nursing research methodology: Issues and implementation* (pp. 79–90). Rockville, MD: Aspen Publishers.
Strickland, O. L. (1995). Assessment of perinatal indicators for the measurement of programmatic effectiveness. *Journal of Perinatal and Neonatal Nursing*, 9(1), 52–67.
Strober, M. (1991). Disorders of the self in anorexia nervosa: An organismic-developmental paradigm. In C. Johnson (Ed.), *Psychodynamic treatment of anorexia nervosa and bulimia* (pp. 354–373). New York: Guilford Press.
Stroebe, M., & Schut, H. (1999). The dual process model of coping with bereavement: Rationale and description. *Death Studies, 23*, 197–224.
Stroebe, W., & Stroebe, M. S. (1995). *Social psychology and health*. Buckingham, England: Open University Press.
Stroud, S. D., Smith, C. A., Edlund, B. J., & Erkel, E. A. (1999). Evaluating clinical decision-making skills of nurse practitioner students. *Clinical Excellence for Nurse Practitioners*, 3(4), 230–237.
Strube, M., & Hartman, D. (1983). Meta-analysis: Techniques, applications, and functions. *Journal of Consulting and Clinical Psychology, 51*, 14–27.
Strumpf, N. E., & Evans, L. K. (1988). Physical restraint of the hospitalized elderly: Perceptions of patients and nurses. *Nursing Research, 37*, 132–137.

Strumpf, N. E., Robinson, J. P., Wagner, J. S., & Evans, L. K. (1998). *Restraint-free care: Individualized approaches for frail elders*. New York: Springer Publishing.

Stryer, D., Tunis, S., Hubbard, H., & Clancy, C. (2000). The outcomes of outcomes and effectiveness research: Impacts and lessons from the first decade. *Health Services, Research, 35*(5), 977–993.

Stuart, A. (1968). Sample surveys: Non-probability sampling. In D. L. Sills (Ed.), *International encyclopedia of the social sciences* (Vol. 13, pp. 612–616). New York: MacMillan.

Stuart-Shor, E., Buselli, E., Carroll, D., & Forman, D. (2003). Are psychosocial factors associated with the pathogenesis and consequences of cardiovascular disease in the elderly? *Journal of Cardiovascular Nursing, 18*, 169–183.

Stuifbergen, A. K., Becker, H., Blozis, S., Timmerman, G., & Kullberg, V. (2003). A randomized clinical trial of a wellness intervention for women with multiple sclerosis. *Archives of Physical Medicine and Rehabilitation, 84*(4), 467–476.

Stuifbergen, A., Becker, H., Rogers, S., Timmerman, G., & Kullberg, V. (1999). Promoting wellness for women with multiple sclerosis. *Journal of Neuroscience Nursing, 31*(2), 73–79.

Styron, W. (1990). *Darkness visible*. New York: Random House.

Sue, S. (2003). In defense of cultural competency in psychotherapy and treatment. *American Psychologist, 58*, 964–970.

Suen, L. K., & Chow, F. L. (2001). Student perceptions of effectiveness of mentors in an undergraduate nursing program. *Journal of Advanced Nursing, 36*(4), 505–511.

Sullivan, E. (1987). Comparison of chemically dependent and nondependent nurses on familial, personal and professional characteristics. *Journal of Studies on Alcohol, 48*, 563–568.

Sullivan, E., Bissell, I., & Leffler, D. L. (1990). Drug use and disciplinary actions among 300 nurses. *International Journal of Addictions, 25*(4), 375–391.

Sullivan, J. A. (1982). Research on nurse practitioners: Process behind the outcome. *American Journal of Public Health, 72*(1), 8–9.

Sullivan, M. D., LaCroix, A. Z., Spertus, J. A., & Hecht, J. (2000). Five-year prospective study of the effects of anxiety and depression in patients with coronary artery disease. *American Journal of Cardiology, 86*, 1135–1138.

Sullivan-Bolyai, S., Knafl, K., Sadler, L., & Gilliss, C. (2004). Great expectations: A position description for parents as caregivers: Part II. *Pediatric Nursing, 30*(1), 52–56.

Sullivan-Bolyai, S., Sadler, L., Knafl, K., & Gilliss, C. (2003). Great expectations: A position description for parents as caregivers: Part I. *Pediatric Nursing, 29*(6), 457–461.

Sullivan-Marx, E. M., & Mullinix, C. (1999). Payment for advanced practice nurses: Economic structures and systems. In M. D. Mezey & D. O. McGivern (Eds.), *Nurses, nurse practitioners* (3rd ed., pp. 345–368). New York: Springer Publishing.

Sullivan-Marx, E. M., Strumpf, N. E., Evans, L. K., Capezuti, E. A., & Maislin, G. (under review). An advanced practice nurse implemented restraint reduction for hospitalized nursing home residents. *Journal of the American Geriatrics Society*.

Sund-Levander, M., & Wahren, L. K. (2000). Assessment and prevention of shivering in patients with severe cerebral injury. A pilot study. *Journal of Clinical Nursing, 9*(1), 55–61.

Sundström, I. M. E., Bixo, M., Björn, I., & Aström, M. (2001). Prevalence of psychiatric disorders in gynecologic outpatients. *American Journal of Obstetrics & Gynecology, 184*, 8–13.

Sundt, T. M., Jr., Sharbrough, F. W., Anderson, R. E., & Michenfelder, J. D. (1974). Cerebral blood flow measurements and electroencephalograms during carotid endarterectomy. *Journal of Neurosurgery, 41*(3), 310–320.

Suppe, F. (1996). *Middle range theories: Historical and contemporary perspectives*. Keynote presentation at the Eleventh Annual Summer Research Conference: Advancing Nursing Science through Middle Range Theory, Wayne State University College of Nursing, Detroit MI.

Suppes, T., & Rush, J. (1996). Evolving clinical characteristics or distinct disorders? In K. I. Shulman, M. Tohen, & S. P. Kutcher (Eds.), *Mood disorders across the lifespan* (pp. 3–16). New York: Wiley-Liss.

SUPPORT Principal Investigators. (1995). A controlled trial to improve care for seriously ill hospitalized patients. *Journal of the American Medical Association, 274*(20), 1591–1598.

Susman, E., Dorn, L., & Fletcher, J. (1992). Participation in biomedical research: The consent process as viewed by children, adolescents, young adults, and physicians. *Journal of Pediatrics, 121*, 547–552.

Suwanwalaikorn, S., & Baran, D. (1996). Thyroid hormone and the skeleton. In R. Marcus, D. Feldman, & J. Kelsey (Eds.), *Osteoporosis*. San Diego, CA: Academic Press.

Svedberg, B., Hallstrom, T., & Lutzen, K. (2000). The morality of treating patients with depot neuroleptics: The experience of community psychiatric nurses. *Nursing Ethics: An International Journal for Health Care Professionals, 7*, 35–46.

Swafford, S. (1997). Older people take too many drugs. *British Medical Journal, 314*, 1369.
Swain, M. A., & Steckel, S. B. (1981). Influencing adherence among hypertensives. *Research in Nursing and Health, 4*, 213–233.
Swan, J. H. C., Ganz, W., Forrester, J., Marcus, H., Diamond, G., & Chonette, D. (1970). Catheterization of heart in man with use of flow-directed balloon tipped catheter. *New England Journal of Medicine, 283*, 447–451.
Swanson, K. M. (1991). Empirical development of a middle range theory of caring. *Nursing Research, 40*(3), 161–165.
Swanson, K. M. (1999). What is known about caring in nursing science. In A. S. Hinshaw, S. Feetham, & J. Shaver (Eds.), *Handbook of clinical nursing research* (pp. 31–60). Thousand Oaks, CA: Sage.
Swartz, C. (1999). Long-term survivors of childhood cancer: The late effects of therapy. *Oncologist, 4*, 45–54.
Swenson, M. M. (1998). The meaning of home to five elderly women. *Healthcare for Women International, 19*, 381–393.
Symon, A. G., & Wrieden, W. L. (2003). A qualitative study of pregnant teenagers' perceptions of the acceptability of a nutritional education intervention. *Midwifery, 19*, 140–147.
Szarka, L. A., DeVault, K. R., & Murray, J. A. (2001). Diagnosing gastroesophageal reflux disease. *Mayo Clinic Proceedings, 76*(1), 91–101.
Szinovacz, M., & Harpster, P. (1994). Couples' employment/retirement status and the division of household tasks. *Journals of Gerontology: Social Sciences, 49*, S125–S136.
Szinovacz, M., & Washo, C. (1992). Gender differences in exposure to life events and adaptation to retirement. *Journals of Gerontology: Social Sciences, 47*, S191–S196.
Szinovacz, M. E., DeViney, S., & Atkinson, M. P. (1999). Effects of surrogate parenting on grandparents' well being. *Journal of Gerontology, 54B*, S376–S388.
Szreter, S. (2003). The population health approach in historical perspective [Electronic Version]. *American Journal of Public Health, 93*(3), 421–431.
Taber's Cyclopedic Medical Dictionary. (1997). (18th ed.). Philadelphia: F. A. Davis.
Tablan, O. C., Anderson, L. J., Arden, N. H., Breiman, R. F., Butler, J. C., & McNeil, M. M. (1994). *Guideline for prevention of nosocomial pneumonia.* Retrieved from http://www.cdc.gov/ncidod/hip/pneumonia/pneu_mmw.htm
Tahan, H. (1998). Case management: A heritage more than a century old. *Nursing Case Management, 3*(2), 55–60.
Tahan, H. (2003). *A substantive theory in acute care case management delivery: Provision of integrated care using a collaborative core team.* Doctoral dissertation. (UMI # 3088430)
Talcott, J., Rieker, P., Clark, J., Propert, K., Weeks, J., Beard, C., et al. (1998). Patient-reported symptoms after primary therapy for early prostate cancer: Results of a prospective cohort study. *Journal of Clinical Oncology, 16*, 275–283.
Talley, N. J., Young, L., Bytzer, P., Hammer, J., Leemon, M., & Jones, M. (2001). Impact of chronic gastrointestinal symptoms in diabetes mellitus on health-related quality of life. *American Journal of Gastroenterology*, 96(1), 71–76.
Talley, S., & Richens, S. (2001). Prescribing practices of advanced practice psychiatric nurses: Part I—demographic, educational, and practice characteristics. *Archives of Psychiatric Nursing, 15*, 205–213.
Tang, W. R., Aaronson, L. S., & Forbes, S. A. (2004). Quality of life in hospice patients with terminal illness. *Western Journal of Nursing Research, 26*, 113–128.
Tanner, C., Pohl, J., Ward, S., & Dontje, K. (2003). Education of nurse practitioners in academic nurse managed centers: Student perspectives. *Journal of Professional Nursing, 19*(6), 354–363.
Tanner, C. A., Padrick, K. P., Westfall, U. E., & Putzier, D. J. (1987). Diagnostic reasoning strategies of nurses and nursing students. *Nursing Research, 36*(6), 358–363.
Tappen, R., & Barry, C. (1995). Assessment of affect in advanced Alzheimer's disease: The dementia mood picture test. *Journal of Gerontological Nursing, 21*(3), 44–46.
Tarrier, N., Barrowclough, C., Haddock, G., & McGovern, J. (1999). The dissemination of innovative cognitive-behavioral psychosocial treatments for schizophrenia. *Journal of Mental Health*, 8(6), 569–582.
Tatara, T. (1993). Understanding the nature and scope of domestic elder abuse with the use of state aggregate data: Summaries of key findings of a national survey of state APS and aging agencies. *Journal of Elder Abuse and Neglect, 5*, 35–57.
Tate, D. F., Wing, R. R., & Winett, R. A. (2001). Using Internet technology to deliver a behavioral weight loss program. *Journal of the American Medical Association, 285*, 1172–1177.
Taunton, R. L., Bott, M. J., Koehn, M. L., Miller, P., Rindner, E., Pace, K., et al. (in press). The NDNQI-Adapted Index of Work Satisfaction. *Journal of Nursing Measurement.*
Taylor, A. G. (1998). A nurse-directed interdisciplinary center for the study of complementary therapies. *Journal of Emergency Nursing, 24*(6), 486–487.

Taylor, C. B., Houston-Miller, N. H., Killen, J. D., & DeBusk, R. F. (1990). Smoking cessation after acute myocardial infarction: Effects of a nurse-managed intervention. *Annals of Internal Medicine, 13*, 118–123.

Taylor, D. (1990). Time-series analysis: Use of autocorrelation as an analytic strategy for describing pattern and change. *Western Journal of Nursing Research, 12*(2), 254–261.

Taylor, D. (1996). The perimenstrual symptom management program: Elements of effective treatment. *Capsules & Comments in Perinatal/Women's Health Nursing, 2*, 140–151.

Taylor, D. (1999). Effectiveness of professional-peer group treatment: Symptom management for women with PMS. *Research in Nursing & Health, 22*(6), 496–511.

Taylor, D. (1996a). The perimenstrual symptom management program: Elements of effective treatment. *Capsules & Comments in Perinatal/Women's Health Nursing, 2*, 140–151.

Taylor, D. (1999b). Effectiveness of professional-peer group treatment: Symptom management for women with PMS. *Research in Nursing & Health, 22*(6), 496–511.

Taylor, D. (2000). More than personal change: Effective elements of symptom management. *Nurse Practitioner Forum, 11*(2), 79–86.

Taylor, D., & Bledsoe, L. (1986). PMS, stress and social support: Results from a pilot study. In V. Oleson & N. F. Woods (Eds.), *Culture, society, and menstruation* (pp. 158–171). New York: Hemisphere, Harper & Row.

Taylor, D., & Colino, S. (2002). *Taking back the month: A personalized solution to managing PMS and enhancing your health*. New York: Perigee/Putnam-Penguin.

Taylor, D., & Woods, N. (Eds.). (1991). *Menstruation, health and illness*. New York: Hemisphere.

Taylor, D., Woods, N., Lentz, M. J., Mitchell, E. S., & Lee, K. A. (1991). Perimenstrual negative affect: Development and testing of an explanatory model. In D. Taylor & N. Woods (Eds.), *Menstruation, health and illness* (pp. 103–118). New York: Hemisphere.

Taylor, D., Woods, N. F., Mitchell, E. S., & Lentz, M. J. (1987). Perimenstrual symptoms: Towards a therapeutic model [Abstract]. *Abstracts of the 7th Conference of the Society for Menstrual Cycle Research*, 46.

Taylor, F. W. (1911). *The principles of scientific management*. New York: Harper.

Technical Committee ISO/TC 215 *Health Informatics*, Working Group 3 *Health Concept Representation*. (2003). Health Informatics—Integration of a reference terminology model for nursing. (Draft for International Standard ISO 18104.) International Organization of Standardization.

Tegtmeyer, K., Ibsen, L., & Goldstein, B. (2001). Computer-assisted learning in critical care: From ENIAC to HAL. *Critical Care Medicine, 29*(8), 177–182.

Tejada de Rivero, D. A. (2003). Alma-Ata revisited. *Perspectives in Health Magazine, 8*(2). Retrieved from http://www.paho.org/English/DD/PIN/Number17_article1_4.htm

Teno, J. M., Clurridge, B. R., Casey, V., Welch, L. C., Wetle, T., Shield, R., et al. (2004). Family perspectives on end of life care at the last place of care. *Journal of the American Medical Association, 291*(1), 88–93.

Teo, K. K., Spoor, M., Pressey, T., Williamson, H., Calder, P., Gelfand, E. T., et al. (1998). Impact of managed waiting for coronary artery bypass graft surgery on patients' perceived quality of life. *Circulation*, 98, II-29–II-34.

Teresi, J., Homes, D., Benenson, E., Monaco, C., Barrett, V., Ramirez, M., et al. (1993). A primary care nursing model in long-term care facilities: Evaluation of impact on affect, behavior and socialization. *Gerontoloigst, 33*(5), 667–674.

Teresi, J. A., Grant, L. A., Holmes, D., & Ory, M. G. (1998). Staffing in traditional and special dementia care units: Preliminary findings from the National Institute on Aging Collaborative Studies. *Journal of Gerontological Nursing, 24*(1), 49–53.

Teri, L., Logsdon, R. G., Peskind, E., Raskind, M., Weiner, M. F., Tractenberg, R. E., et al. (2000). Treatment of agitation in AD. A randomized, placebo-controlled clinical trial. *Neurology, 55*, 1271–1278.

Teschinsky, U. (2000). Living with schizophrenia: The family illness experience. *Issues in Mental Health Nursing, 21*, 387–396.

Tesio, L., Alpini, D., Cesarani, A., & Perucca, L. (1999). Short form of the Dizziness Handicap Inventory: Construction and validation through Rasch analysis. *American Journal of Physical Medicine and Rehabilitation, 78*, 233–241.

Thibaut, J., & Kelley, H. (1959). *The social psychology of groups*. New York: Wiley.

Thiele, J. R. (1989). Guidelines for collaborative research. *Applied Nursing Research, 2*, 150–153.

Thielemann, P. (2000). Educational needs of home caregivers of terminally ill patients: A literature review. *American Journal of Hospice & Palliative Care, 17*(4), 253–257.

Thoman, E. B. (1982). A biological perspective and a behavioral model for assessment of premature infants. In L. A. Bond & J. M. Joffee (Eds.), *Primary prevention of psychopathology: Facilitating infant and early childhood development* (Vol. 6, pp. 159–179). Hanover, NH: University Press of New England.

Thomas, B. W., & Falcone, R. E. (1998). Confirmation of nasogastric tube placement by colorimetric indicator detection of carbon dioxide: A preliminary report. *Journal of the American College of Nutrition, 17*(2), 195–197.

Thomas, K. A., & Burr, R. (2002). Preterm infant temperature circadian rhythm: Possible effect of parental cosleeping. *Biological Research for Nursing, 3*(3), 150–159.

Thomas, S. A., Barter, M., & McLaughlin, F. E. (2000). State and territorial boards of nursing approaches to the use of unlicensed assistive personnel. *JONAs Healthcare Law, Ethics & Regulation, 2*(1), 13–21.

Thomas, V. S., & Hageman, P. A. (2003). Can neuromuscular strength and function in people with dementia be rehabilitated using resistance-exercise training? Results from a preliminary intervention study. *Journals of Gerontology: Biological and Medical Sciences, 58*, M746–M751.

Thompson, F. E., & Dennison, B. A. (1995). Dietary sources of fats and cholesterol in US children aged 2 through 5 years. *American Journal of Public Health, 84*, 799–806.

Thompson, J. (1991). Exploring gender and culture with Khmer refugee women. Reflections on participatory feminist research. *Advances in Nursing Science, 13*(3), 30–48.

Thompson, T. G., & Brailer, D. J. (2004). *The decade of health information technology: Delivering consumer-centric and information-rich health care. Framework for strategic action*. Washington, DC: U.S. Department of Health and Human Services, Office of the National Coordinator for Health Information Technology.

Thompson, W. G., Longstreth, G. F., Drossman, D. A., Heaton, K. W., Irvine, E. J., & Mueller-Lissner, S. A. (2000). Functional bowel disorders and functional abdominal pain. In D. A. Drossman, N. J. Talley, W. G. Thompson, W. E. Whitehead, & E. Corazziari (Eds.), *Rome II: Functional gastrointestinal disorders: Diagnosis, pathophysiology, and treatment* (2nd ed., pp. 351–432). McLean, VA: Degnon Associates.

Thomson, M., & Burke, K. (1998). A nursing assistant training program in a long term care setting. *Gerontology and Geriatrics Education, 19*(1), 23–35.

Thoresen, C. J., Kaplan, S. A., Barsky, A. P., Warren, C. R., & de Chermont, K. (2003). The affective underpinnings of job perceptions and attitudes: A meta-analytic review and integration. *Psychological Bulletin, 129*, 914–945.

Thorne, S. E., & Paterson, B. L. (2000). Two decades of insider research: What we know and don't know about chronic illness experience. In *Annual review of nursing research* (Vol. 18, pp. 3–25). New York: Springer Publishing.

Thorne, S. E., & Paterson, B. L. (2000). Two decades of insider research: What we know and don't know about chronic illness experiences. In J. Fitzpatrick & J. Goeppinger (Eds.), *Annual review of nursing research* (pp. 3–25). New York: Springer Publishing.

Tideiksaar, R. (2002). *Falls in older people: Prevention and management* (3rd ed.). Baltimore: Health Professions Press.

Tierney, W. M., Dexter, P. R., Gramelspacher, G. P., Perkins, A. J., Zhou, X. H. & Wolinksy, F. D. (2001). The effect of discussions about advance directives on patients' satisfaction with primary care. *Journal of General Internal Medicine, 16*, 32–40.

Tilden, V. P., Tolle, S. W., Garland, M. J., & Nelson, C. A. (1995). Decisions about life-sustaining treatment. Impact of physician's behaviors on the family. *Archives of Internal Medicine, 155*(6), 633–638.

Tillett, L. A. (1994). Nola J. Pender: The Health Promotion Model. In A. Marriner-Tomey (Ed.), *Nursing theorists and their work* (3rd ed., pp. 507–513). Boston: Mosby.

Timm, S. E. (2003). Effectively delegating nursing activities in home care. *Home Healthcare Nurse, 21*(4), 260–265.

Timmerman, G. M., & Gregg, E. K. (2003). Dieting, perceived deprivation, and preoccupation with food. *Western Journal of Nursing Research, 25*, 405–418.

Tinetti, M. E., Williams, N. A., & Gill, T. M. (2000). Dizziness among older adults: A possible geriatric syndrome. *Annals of Internal Medicine, 132*(5), 337–344.

Titler, M., & Mentes, J. (1999). Research utilization in gerontological nursing practice. *Journal of Gerontological Nursing, 25*, 6–9.

Titler, M. G., Kleiber, C., Steelman, V., Goode, C., Rakel, B., Barry-Walker, J., Small, S., & Buckwalter, K. (1994). Infusing research into practice to promote quality care. *Nursing Research, 43*, 307–313.

Tonelli, M. R. (1996). Pulling the plug on living wills: A critical analysis of advance directives. *Chest, 110*, 816–922.

Topol, E. J. (2004). Intensive statin therapy—a sea change in cardiovascular prevention. *New England Journal of Medicine, 350*, 1562–1564.

Tornstam, L. (1999). Gerotranscendence and the functions of reminiscence. *Journal of Aging and Identity, 4*, 155–166.

Torres, S., & Han, H. (2000). Psychological distress in non-Hispanic white and Hispanic abused women. *Archives of Psychiatric Nursing, 14*(1), 19–29.

Torrisi, D., & McDanel, H. (2003). Better outcomes for depressed patients. *Nurse Practitioner: American Journal of Primary Health Care, 28*(8), 32–38.

Travelbee, J. (1971). *Interpersonal aspects of nursing*. Philadelphia: F. A. Davis.

Travelbee, J. (1972). *Interpersonal aspects of nursing* (2nd ed.). Philadelphia: F. A. Davis.

Treolar, A. E., Boynton, R. E., Borghild, B. G., & Brown, B. W. (1967). Variation of the human menstrual cycle through reproductive life. *International Journal of Fertility, 12*(1), 77–126.

Tresch, D. D., & Alla, H. (2001). Diagnosis and management of myocardial ischemia(angina) in the elderly patient. *American Journal of Geriatric Cardiology, 10*, 337–344.

Trinkoff, A. M., Eaton, W. W., & Anthony, J. C. (1991). The prevalence of substance abuse among registered nurses. *Nursing Research, 40*(30), 172–175.

Trinkoff, A. M., & Storr, C. L. (1998a). Substance use among nurses: Differences between specialities. *American Journal of Public Health, 88*, 581–584.

Trinkoff, A. M., & Storr, C. L. (1998b). Work schedule characteristics and substances use among nurses. *American Journal of Industrial Medicine, 34*, 266–271.

Tronick, E. Z., & Weinberg, M. K. (1997). Depressed mothers and infants: Failure to form dyadic states of consciousness. In L. Murray & P. J. Cooper (Eds.), *Postpartum depression and child development* (pp. 54–81). New York: Guilford Press.

Truman, B., & Ely, E. W. (2003). Monitoring delirium in critically ill patients: Using the confusion assessment method for the intensive care unit. *Critical Care Nurse, 23*(2), 25–36.

Trygstad, L., Buccheri, R., Dowling, G., Zind, R., White, K., & Griffin, J. J. (2002). Behavioral management of persistent auditory hallucinations in schizophrenia: Outcomes from a 10-week course. *Journal of the American Psychiatric Nurses Association, 8*, 1–8.

Trzcieniecka-Green, A., & Steptoe, A. (1996). The effects of stress management on the quality of life of patients following acute myocardial infarction or coronary artery bypass surgery. *European Heart, 17*, 1663–1670.

Trzepacz, P. (1999). Update on the neuropathogenesis of delirium. *Dementia and Geriatric Cognitive Disorders, 10*, 330–334.

Tulman, L., & Fawcett, J. (1990). A framework for studying functional status after diagnosis of breast cancer. *Cancer Nursing, 13*, 95–99.

Tuomilehto, J., Lindstrom, J., Eriksson, J. G., Valle, T. T., Hamalainen, H., Ilanne-Parikka, P., et al. (2001). Prevention of type 2 diabetes mellitus by changes in lifestyle among subjects with impaired glucose tolerance. *New England Journal of Medicine, 344*, 1343–1350.

Turner, B. S., & Loan, L. A. (2000). Tracheobronchial trauma associated with airway management in neonates. *AACN Clinical Issues, 11*(2), 283–299.

Twitchell, K. T. (2003a). Bloodborne pathogens: What you need to know—part I. *Journal of the American Association of Occupational Health Nursing, 51*(1), 38–47.

Twitchell, K. T. (2003b). Bloodborne pathogens: What you need to know—part II. *Journal of the American Association of Occupational Health Nursing, 51*(2), 89–99.

UNAIDS. (2004a). *Understanding the latest estimates of the global AIDS epidemic—July 2004*. Retrieved September 27, 2004, from http://www.unaids.org/bangkok2004/docs/QA_Epi_en.doc

UNAIDS. (2004b). *UNAIDS 2004 Report on the global AIDS epidemic*. Retrieved September 27, 2004, from http://www.unaids.org/bangkok2004/report.html

Underwood, P. W. (2000). Social support: The promise and the reality. In V. H. Rice (Ed.), *Handbook of stress, coping, and health: Implications for nursing research, theory, and practice*. Thousand Oaks, CA: Sage.

University of California, San Francisco School of Nursing Symptom Management Faculty Group. (1994). A model for symptom management. *Image, 26*, 272–276.

United Kingdom Central Council. (1999). *Nursing in secure environments*. London: United Kingdom Central Council for Nursing, Midwifery and Health Visiting.

United Kingdom Prospective Diabetes Group Study. (1998). Effects of intensive blood glucose control with Metformin on complications in overweight patients with type 2 diabetes. *Lancet, 352*, 854–865.

United Nations Scientific Committee on the Effects of Atomic Radiation. (1993). *Sources and effects of ionizing radiation*. New York: United Nations.

Urban Institute. (2000). *A new look at homelessness in America*. Washington, DC: Urban Institute.

Urden, L. D., & Walston, S. L. (2001). Outcomes of hospital restructing and reengineering: How is

success or failure being measured? *Journal of Nursing Administration, 31*(4), 203–209.
U.S. Agency for Healthcare Research and Quality. (1996). Medical Expenditure Panel Survey.
U.S. Bureau of the Census. (2001). *Census 2000 Supplemental Survey: Profile of selected social characteristics*. Retrieved from www.factfinder.census.gov
U.S. Bureau of the Census. (2002). *American community survey profile 2002—United States general demographic characteristics*. Retrieved January 14, 2004, from http://www.census.gov/acs/www/products/profiles/single/2002/ACS/tabular/010/01000US1.htm
U.S. Cancer Statistics Working Group. (2003). *United States Cancer Statistics: 2000 Incidence*. Atlanta, GA:, Department of Health and Human Services, Centers for Disease Control and Prevention and National Cancer Institute.
U.S. Centers for Disease Control. (1991). *Preventing lead poisoning in young children*. Atlanta, GA: Department of Health and Human Services.
U.S. Conference of Mayors. (1998). *A status report on hunger and homelessness in America's cities*. Washington, DC: Author.
U.S. Department of Agriculture. (1992). *The food pyramid guide*. Washington, DC: Government Printing Office.
U.S. Department of Health and Human Services. (1983). *Protection of human subjects*. Code of Federal Regulation, title 45, part 46.
U.S. Department of Health and Human Services. (1985). *Report of the Secretary's Task Force on Black and Minority Health*. Washington, DC: Government Printing Office.
U.S. Department of Health and Human Services. (1998a). *Leading indicators for Healthy People 2010*. Retrieved from http://odphp.osophs.dhhs.gov/pubs/LeadingIndicators/ldgindtoc.html
U.S. Department of Health and Human Services. (1998b). *The initiative to eliminate racial and ethnic disparities in health*. Retrieved August 16, 1999, from http://raceandhealth.hhs.gov
U.S. Department of Health and Human Services, Children's Bureau. (1999). *Child maltreatment 1997: Reports from the states to the national child abuse and neglect data system*. Washington, DC: U.S. Government Printing Office.
U.S. Department of Health and Human Services. (1999a). *Healthy People 2000*. Retrieved February 22, 2004, from http://odphp.osophs.dhhs.gov/pubs/hp2000/
U.S. Department of Health and Human Services. (2000). *Healthy People 2010*. Washington, DC: Office of Disease Prevention and Health Promotion.
U.S. Department of Health and Human Services. (2000). *Healthy People 2010: National health promotion and disease prevention objectives*. Washington, DC: U.S. Government Printing Office. Retrieved from http://www.health.gov/healthypeople
U.S. Department of Health and Human Services. Health Resources and Services Administration. (2001). *Cultural competence works*. Merrifield, VA: HRSA Information Center. Retrieved from http://www.hrsa.gov/cmc
U.S. Department of Health and Human Services. (2001a). *Youth violence: A report of the Surgeon General*. Rockville, MD: Author.
U.S. Department of Health and Human Services. (2001b). *Mental health: Culture, race, and ethnicity—a supplement to Mental Health: A report of the Surgeon General*. Rockville, MD: U.S. Department of Health and Human Services, Substance Abuse and Mental Health Services Administration, Center for Mental Health Services.
U.S. Department of Health and Human Services. (2003a). *Child Maltreatment 2001*. Administration on Children, Youth and Families. Washington, DC: U.S. Government Printing Office.
U.S. Department of Health and Human Services. National Center for Health Statistics. (1996). *Healthy People 2000 review, 1995–1996*. Hyattsville, MD: Public Health Service.
U.S. Department of Justice, Office of Justice Programs. (2003). *Violent crime and property crime levels all to the lowest level since 1973*. Retrieved January 5, 2004, from http://www.ojp.usdoj.gov/bjs/pub/press/cv02pr.htm
U.S. Department of Labor. (1991). *Occupation exposure to bloodborne pathogens* (Federal Register, 29 CFR 1910.1030). Washington, DC: Government Printing Office.
U.S. Nuclear Regulatory Commission. (1997). *Release of patients administered radioactive materials* (USNRC Regulatory Guide 8.39). Washington, DC: Author.
U.S. Preventive Services Task Force. (1996). *Guide to clinical preventive services* (2nd ed.). Washington, DC: U.S. Department of Health and Human Services, Office of Disease Prevention and Health Promotion.
U.S. Preventive Services Task Force. (2000). *Guide to clinical preventive services* (3rd ed.). Washington, DC: Office of Disease Prevention and Health Promotion, Government Printing Office.
U.S. Preventive Services Task Force. (2002). *Screening for osteoposis in postmenopausal women*. Retrieved October, 14, 2003, from http://www.ahrq.gov/clin/3rduspstf/osteoporosis/osteorr.htm

U.S. Public Health Service. (1985). *Women's health: Report of the Public Health Service Task Force on Women's Health Issues*, Vol. 1. Bethesda, MD: National Institutes of Health.

U.S. Public Health Service. (1994). Put prevention into practice: Implementing primary care. *Journal of the American Academy of Nursing Practice, 6*, 257–266.

U.S. Public Health Service. (1999). *Agenda for research on women's health research for the 21st century. A report of the Task Force on the NIH Women's Health Research Agenda for the 21st century*, Vol. 2. Bethesda, MD: National Institutes of Health.

U.S. Public Health Service. Office of the Surgeon General. (1999). *Mental health: A report of the Surgeon General.* Rockville, MD: Department of Health and Human Services, U.S. Public Health Service.

Vaccarino, V., Abramson, J., Veledar, E., & Weintraub, W. S. (2002). Sex differences in hospital mortality after coronary artery bypass surgery. *Circulation, 105*, 1176–1181.

Vaccarino, V., Lin, Z. Q., Kasl, S. V., Mattera, J. A., Roumanis, S. A., Abramson, J. L., et al. (2003). Gender differences in recovery after coronary artery bypass surgery. *Journal of the American College of Cardiology, 41*(2), 307–314.

Vaezi, M. F., Hicks, D. M., Abelson, T. I., & Richter, J. E. (2003). Laryngeal signs and symptoms and gastroesophageal reflux disease: A critical assessment of cause and effect association. *Clinical Gastroenterology & Hepatology, 1*(5), 333–344.

Vahey, D. C., Aiken, L. H., Sloane, D. M., Clarke, S. P., & Vargas, D. (2004). Nurse burnout and patient satisfaction. *Medical Care, 42*(2 Suppl.), II 57–66.

Valanis, B., Vollmer, W. M., & Steele, P. (1999). Occupational exposure to antineoplastic agents: Self-reported miscarriages and stillbirths among nurses and pharmacists. *Journal of Occupational and Environmental Medicine, 41*, 632–638.

Valente, S. M. (1994). Messages of psychiatric patients who attempted or committed suicide. *Clinical Nursing Research, 3*, 316–333.

Van, P., & Meleis, A. (2003). Coping with grief after involuntary pregnancy loss: Perspectives of African American women. *Journal of Obstetric, Gynecologic, and Neonatal Nursing, 32*, 28–39.

Van Cott, M. L., Tittle, M. B., Moody, L. E., & Wilson, M. E. (1991). Analysis of a decade of critical care nursing practice: 1979–1988. *Heart & Lung, 20*, 394–397.

Van Dijk, D., Jansen., E. W., Hijman, R., Nierich, A. P., Moons, K. G., Lahpor, J. R., et al. (2002). Cognitive outcome after off-pump and on-pump coronary artery bypass graft surgery. *Journal of the American Medical Association, 287*(11), 1405–1412.

Van Dijk, T. A. (Ed.). (1985). *Handbook of discourse analysis: Vol. 1. Disciplines of discourse.* London: Academic Press.

Van Dover, L. (1986). Influence of nurse-client contracting on family planning knowledge and behaviors in a university student population. University of Michigan, Dearborn. *Dissertation Abstracts International, 46*, 3787B.

Van Eijken, M., Tsang, S., Wensing, M., de Smet, P., & Grol, R. (2003). Internvetions to improve medication compliance in older patients living in the community: A systematic review of the literature. *Drugs Aging, 20*, 229–240.

van Elderen, T., Maes, S., & Dusseldorp, E. (1999). Coping with coronary heart disease: A longitudinal study. *Journal of Psychosomatic Research, 47*, 175–183.

Van Kaam, A. (1966). *Existential foundations of psychology.* Pittsburgh, PA: Duquesne University Press.

Van Manen, M. (1990). *Researching lived experiences.* New York: State University of New York Press.

van Meijel, B., van der Gaag, M., Kahn, R. S., & Grypdonck, M. (2002a). The practice of early recognition and early intervention to prevent psychotic relapse in patients with schizophrenia: An exploratory study. Part 1. *Journal of Psychiatric and Mental Health Nursing, 9*, 347–355.

van Meijel, B., van der Gaag, M., Kahn, R. S., & Grypdonck, M. H. (2002b). The practice of early recognition and early intervention to prevent psychotic relapse in patients with schizophrenia: An exploratory study. Part 2. *Journal of Psychiatric and Mental Health Nursing, 9*, 357–363.

van Meijel, B., van der Gaag, M., Kahn, R. S., & Grypdonck, M. H. (2003a). Relapse prevention in patients with schizophrenia. *Archives of Psychiatric Nursing, 17*, 117–125.

van Meijel, B., van der Gaag, M., Kahn, R. S., & Grypdonck, M. H. (2003b). Relapse prevention in patients with schizophrenia: The application of an intervention protocol in nursing practice. *Archives of Psychiatric Nursing, 17*, 165–172.

Van Roekel, N. B. (2003). Gastroesophageal reflux disease, tooth erosion, and prosthodontic rehabilitation: A clinical report. *Journal of Prosthodontology, 12*(4), 255–259.

van Tilburg, T. (1992). Support networks before and after retirement. *Journal of Social and Personal Relationships, 9*, 433–445.

Vance, C., & Olson, R. (1998). *The mentor connection in nursing*. New York: Springer Publishing.

Varcoe, C. (2001). Abuse obscured: An ethnographic account of emergency nursing in relation to violence against women. *Canadian Journal of Nursing Research, 32*(4), 95–115.

Vaughn, K., Webster, D. C., Orahood, S., & Young, B. C. (1995). Brief inpatient psychiatric treatment: Finding solutions. *Issues in Mental Health Nursing, 16*, 519–531.

Veena, J. (2001). A computer expert system prototype for mechanically ventilated neonates: Development and impact on clinical judgment and information access capability of nurses. *Computers in Nursing, 19*(5), 194–202.

Venner, G., & Solitro-Seelbinder, J. (1996). Team management of congestive heart failure across the continuum. *Journal of Cardiovascular Nursing, 10*(2), 71–84.

Ventura, M. J. (1999). Staffing issues. *RN, 62*(2), 26–30.

Ventura, S. J., Abma, J. C., Mosher, W. D., & Henshaw, S. (2003). Revised pregnancy rates, 1990–97 and new rates for 1998–1999: United States. *National Vital Statistics Reports, 52*(7). Retrieved from http://www.cdc.gov/nchs/data/nvsr/nvsr52/nvsr52_07.pdf

Verbrugge, L. M., & Jette, A. M. (1994). The disablement process. *Social Science and Medicine, 38*, 1–14.

Verdery, R. B. (1996). Failure to thrive in older people. *Journal of American Gerontological Association, 44*, 465–466.

Verdery, R. B. (1997). Clinical evaluation of failure to thrive in older people. *Clinics in Geriatric Medicine, 13*, 769–778.

Vessey, J. A., Duffy, M., O'Sullivan, P., & Swanson, M. (2003). Assessing teasing in school-age youth. *Issues in Comprehensive Pediatric Nursing, 26*(1), 1–11.

Viguera, A. C., & Rothschild, A. J. (1996). Depression: Clinical features and pathogenesis. In K. I. Shulman, M. Tohen, & S. P. Kutcher (Eds.), *Mood disorders across the lifespan* (pp. 189–215). New York: Wiley-Liss.

Villareal, E. (2003). Using Roy's adaptation model when caring for a group of young women contemplating quitting smoking. *Public Health Nursing, 20*(5), 377–384.

Villarruel, A. M. (1996). Culturally competent nursing: Are we there yet? *Capsules and Comments in Pediatric Nursing, 1*, 18–26.

Vincent, D., Mackey, T., Pohl, J. M., Oakley, D., & Hirth, R. (1999). A tale of two nursing centers: A cautionary study of profitability. *Nursing Economics, 17*(5), 257–262.

Vingerhoets, G., De Soete, G., & Jannes, C. (1995). Subjective complaints versus neuropsychological test performance after cardiopulmonary bypass. *Journal of Psychosomatic Research, 39*(7), 843–853.

Viseoli, C., Bruzzi, P., & Glauser, M. (1995). An approach to the design and implementation of clinical trials of empirical antibiotic therapy in febrile and neutropenic cancer patients [Review]. *European Journal of Cancer, 31A*, 2013–2022.

Vitousek, K. B., & Ewald, L. S. (1993). Self-representation in the eating disorders: A cognitive perspective. In Z. Segal & S. Blatt (Eds.), *The self in emotional disorders: Cognitive and psychodynamic perspectives* (pp. 221–257). New York: Guilford Press.

Vivian, B., & Wilcox, J. (2000). Compliance communication in home health care: A mutually reciprocal process. *Qualitative Health Research, 10*, 103–116.

Vlieland, T. P. M. V. (2003). Managing chronic disease: Evidence-based medicine or patient centered medicine? *Health Care Analysis, 10*, 289–298.

Voda, A. M. (1991). The Tremin Trust: An intergenerational research program on events associated with women's menstrual and reproductive lives. In D. Taylor & N. F. Woods (Eds.), *Menstruation, health and illness* (pp. 5–18). Washington, DC: Hemisphere.

Voda, A. M., & Mansfield, P. K. (1993). Changes in the pattern of menstrual bleeding. In D. Golgert (Ed.), *Proceedings of the 9th Conference, Society for Menstrual Cycle Research*. Seattle, WA: Hamilton and Cross.

Vogelzang, J. L. (1999). Elusive hunger. *Home Healthcare Nurse, 17*(4), 261–262.

Volicer, L., & Hurley, A. C. (2003). Management of behavioral symptoms in progressive degenerative dementias. *Journal of Gerontology: Medical Sciences, 58A*(9), 837–845.

Volicer, L., Hurley, A. C., & Camberg, L. (1999). A model of psychological well-being in advanced dementia. *Journal of Mental Health and Aging, 5*(1), 83–94.

Volicer, L., Hurley, A. C., Lathi, D. C., & Kowall, N. W. (1994). Measurement of severity in advanced Alzheimer's disease. *Journal of Gerontology, 49*, M223–M226.

Volker, D. L. (2001). Oncology nurses' experiences with requests for assisted dying from terminally ill patients with cancer. *Oncology Nurses Forum, 28*(1), 39–49.

Von Bertalanffy, L. (1968). *General systems theory*. New York: George Braziller.

Vonderheid, S., Pohl, J., Barkauskas, V., Gift, D., & Hughes-Cromwick, P. (2003). Financial performance of academic nurse-managed primary care centers. *Nursing Economics, 21*(4), 167–175.

Vonderheid, S., Pohl, J., Schafer, P., Forrest, K., Poole, M., Barkauskas, V., et al. (2004). Using FTE and RVU performance measures to assess the financial viability of academic nurse-managed primary care centers. *Nursing Economics, 22*(3), 124–134.

Wadden, T. A., Anderson, D. A., Foster, G. D., Bennett, A., Steinberg, C., & Sarwer, D. B. (2000). Obese women's perceptions of their physicians' weight management attitudes and practices. *Archives of Family Medicine*, 9, 854–860.

Wade, T. D., & Kendler, K. S. (2000). The relationship between social support and major depression: Cross-sectional, longitudinal, and genetic perspectives. *Journal of Nervous and Mental Disease, 188*(5), 251–258.

Wade, T. J., & Cairney, J. (2000). Major depressive disorder and marital transition among mothers: Results from a national panel study. *Journal of Nervous and Mental Disease, 188*(11), 741–750.

Wadwha, P. D., Sandman, C. A., Porto, M., Dunkel-Schetter, C., & Garite, T. J. (1993). The association between prenatal stress and infant birth weight and gestational age at birth: A prospective investigation. *American Journal of Obstetrics and Gynecology, 169*(4), 858–865.

Wagner, E. H., Davis, C., Schaefer, J., Von Korff, M., & Austin, B. (2002). A survey of leading chronic disease management programs: Are they consistent with the literature? *Journal of Nursing Care Quality, 16*, 67–80.

Wagner, L. K., Lester, R. G., & Saldana, L. R. (1997). *Exposure of the pregnant patient to diagnostic radiations: A guide to medical management* (2nd ed.). Madison, WI: Medical Physics Publishing.

Wahbeh, G., Wyllie R., & Kay, M. (2002). Foreign body ingestion in infants and children: Location, location, location. *Clinical Pediatrics, 41*, 633–641.

Wakefield, B., Flanagan, J., & Specht, J. K. P. (2001). Telehealth: An opportunity for gerontological practice. *Journal of Gerontological Nursing, 27*(1), 10–14.

Wakefield, B., Mentes, J., Diggelmann, L., & Culp, K. (2002). Monitoring hydration status in elderly veterans. *Western Journal of Nursing Research, 24*(2), 132–142.

Waldrop, J., & Stern, S. M. (2003). *Disability status: 2000 Census brief*. Washington, DC: U.S. Department of Commerce.

Walker, A. M. (1986). Reporting the results of epidemiologic studies. *American Journal of Public Health, 76*, 556–558.

Walker, B. L., Nail, L. M., & Croyle, R. T. (1999). Does emotional expression make a difference in reactions to breast cancer? *Oncology Nursing Forum, 26*, 1025–1032.

Walker, B. L., Nail, L. M., Larsen, L., Magill, J., & Schwartz, A. (1996). Concerns, affect, and cognitive disruption following completion of radiation treatment for localized breast or prostate cancer. *Oncology Nursing Forum, 23*, 1181–1187.

Walker, K., McGowan, A., Jantos, M., & Anson, J. (1997). Fatigue, depression, and quality of life in HIV-positive men. *Journal of Psychosocial Nursing and Mental Health Services, 35*(9), 32–40.

Walker, L. O. (1996). Predictors of weight gain at 6 and 18 months after childbirth: A pilot study. *Journal of Obstetric, Gynecologic, and Neonatal Nursing, 25*, 39–48.

Walker, P. H. (2004). In J. Fitzpatrick & A. L. Whall (Eds.), *Conceptual models in nursing* (4th ed.). Upper Saddle River, NJ: Prentice Hall.

Walker, P. H., & Redman, R. (1999). Theory-guided, evidence-based reflective practice. *Nursing Science Quarterly, 12*, 298–303.

Walker, S. N., Sechrist, K. R., & Pender, N. (1987). The Health Promoting Lifestyle Profile: Development and psychometric characteristics. *Nursing Research, 36*, 76–81.

Walker, T., Porter, M., Gruman, C., & Michalski, M. (1999). Developing individualized care in nursing homes: Integrating the views of nurses and certified nurse aides. *Journal of Gerontological Nursing, 25*(3), 30–35.

Wallace, D. C., Molavi, G., Hemphill, J. C., & Fields, B. (1999). The relation of widowhood and living arrangements to function and health service use among elderly African-American men and women. *Journal of Multicultural Nursing & Health, 5*(2), 19–27.

Walton, J. (2000). Schizophrenia and life in the world of others. *Canadian Journal of Nursing Research, 32*, 69–84.

Wandelt, M. (1970). *Guide for the beginning researcher*. New York: Appleton-Century Crofts.

Wang, P. S., Berglund, P., & Kessler, R. C. (2000). Recent care of common mental disorders in the United States: Prevalence and conformance with evidence-based recommendations. *Journal of General Internal Medicine, 15*(5), 284–292.

Warchol, G. (1998). *Workplace violence 1992–1996: Report from the Bureau of Justice Statistics National Crime Victimization Survey* (NCJ 168634). Retrieved from www.ojp.usdoj.gov

Ward, A. J. (1991). Prenatal stress and childhood psychopathology. *Child Psychiatry and Human Development, 22*(2), 97–110.

Ware, J. E., & Berwick, D. M. (1990). Patient judgments of hospital quality: Report of a pilot study. Conclusions and recommendations. *Medical Care, 28*(Suppl.), S39–S42.

Ware, J. E., Davies-Avery, A., & Stewart, A. L. (1978). The measurement and meaning of patient satisfaction: A review of the literature. *Health and Medical Services Review, 1*, 1–15.

Watchirs, H. (2002). Review of methodologies measuring human rights implementation. *Journal of Law and Ethics, 30*, 716–733.

Waterreus, A., Blanchard, M., & Mann, A. (1994). Community psychiatric nurses for the elderly: Well tolerated, few side-effects and effective in the treatment of depression. *Journal of Clinical Nursing, 3*, 299–306.

Waters, B. L., & Raisler, J. (2003). Ice massage for reduction of labor pain. *Journal of Midwifery & Women's Health, 48*(5), 317–321.

Watson, J. (1979). *Nursing: The philosophy and science of caring*. Boston: Little, Brown.

Watson, J. (1985a). *Nursing: Human science and human care: A theory of nursing*. Norwalk, CT: Appleton-Century-Crofts.

Watson, J. (1985b). *Nursing: The philosophy and science of caring*. Boulder, CO: Colorado Associated University Press.

Watson, J. (1988). *Nursing: Human science and human care: A theory of nursing*. New York: National League for Nursing.

Watson, J. (1996). Watson's theory of transpersonal caring. In P. Hinton Walker & B. Neuman (Eds.), *Blueprint for use of nursing models*. Sudbury: Jones & Bartlett.

Watson, J. (1997). The theory of human caring: Retrospective and prospective. *Nursing Science Quarterly, 10*, 49–52.

Watson, J. (1999). *Postmodern nursing and beyond*. Edinburgh, Scotland: Churchill-Livingstone.

Watson, J. (2001). Jean Watson, theory of human caring. In M. Parker (Ed.), *Nursing theories and nursing practice* (pp. 343–354). Philadelphia: F. A. Davis.

Watson, J. (2001). *Assessing and measuring caring in nursing and health science*. New York: Springer Publishing.

Watson, J., & Smith, M. C. (2002). Caring science and the science of unitary human beings: A transtheoretical discourse for nursing knowledge development. *Journal of Advanced Nursing, 37*(5), 452–461.

Watts, A. (1987). Stress in retirement and its management. *Stress Medicine, 3*, 205–210.

Webster, J. D. (2003). The reminiscence circumplex and autobiographical memory functions. *Memory, 11*(2), 203–215.

Webster, J. D., & Haight, B. K. (Eds.). (2002). *Critical advances in reminiscence work: From theory to application*. New York: Springer Publishing.

Webster, J., & McCall, M. (1999). Reminiscence functions across adulthood: A replication and extension. *Journal of Adult Development, 6*(1), 73–85.

Webster's New World College Dictionary. (2001). (5th ed., p. 1451). Foster City, CA: IDG Books Worldwide.

Weibley, T. T., Adamson, M., Clinkscales, N., Curran, J., & Bramson, R. (1987). Gavage tube insertion in the premature infant. *Maternal Child Nursing, 12*(1), 24–27.

Weinberg, A. D., & Minaker, K. L. (1995). Dehydration: Evaluation and management in older adults. *Journal of the American Medical Association, 274*(19), 1552–1556.

Weinberg, B. H. (1987). Why indexing fails the researcher. *Proceedings of the 50th Annual Meeting of the American Society for Information Science, 24*, 241–244.

Weiner, J. M., Stowe, S. M., Shirley, S., & Gilman, N. J. (1981). Information processing using document data management techniques. *Proceedings of the 44th Annual Meeting of the American Society for Information Science, 18*, 291–294.

Weiner, M., & Pifer, E. (2000). Computerized decision support and the quality of care. *Managed Care, 9*(5), 48–51.

Weinert, C. (2002). Rural nursing research: Riddle, rhyme, reality. *Communicating Nursing Research, 35*, 37–49.

Weinert, C., & Catanzaro, M. (1994). [Family health study]. Unpublished raw data.

Weingourt, R., Maruyama, T., Sawada, I., & Yoshino, J. (2001). Domestic violence and women's mental health in Japan. *International Nursing Review, 48*(2), 102–108.

Weinrich, S. P., Boyd, M. D., & Herman, J. (2004). Tool adaptation to reduce health disparities. In M. Frank-Stromberg & S. J. Olsen (Eds.), *Instruments for clinical healthcare research* (3rd ed., pp 20–32). Sudbury, MA: Jones and Bartlett.

Weinsier, R. L., & Krumdieck, C. L. (2000). Dairy foods and bone health: Examination of the evidence. *American Journal of Clinical Nutrition, 72*(3), 681–689.

Weis, P. A., & Guyton-Simmons, J. (1998). A computer simulation for teaching critical thinking skills. *Nurse Educator, 23*(2), 30–33.

Weiss, C. (1980). Knowledge creep and decision accretion. *Image: Journal of Nursing Scholarship, 1*, 381–404.

Weiss, E. L., Longhurst, J. G., & Mazure, C. M. (1999). Childhood sexual abuse as a risk factor for depression in women: Psychosocial and neurobiological correlates. *American Journal of Psychiatry, 156*, 816–818.

Welch, M. (1986). Nineteenth century philosophic influences on Nightingale's concept of the person. *Journal of Nursing History, 1*(2), 3–11.

Welch, T. (1998). Liquid assets: Hydration in the older adult. *Consultant Dietician, 22*(3), 3–7.

Wells, G., Tugwell, P., Shea, B., Guyatt, G., Peterson, J., Zytaruk, N., et al. (2002). V. Meta-analysis of the efficacy of hormone replacement therapy in treating and preventing osteoporosis in postmenopausal women. *Endocrine Review, 23*(4), 529–539.

Wells, R., & Gionnetti, V. (1990). *Handbook of brief psychotherapies*. New York: Plenum Press.

Wells-Federman, C., Arnstein, P., & Caudill, M. (2002). Nurse-led pain management program: Effect on self-efficacy, pain intensity, pain-related disability, and depressive symptoms in chronic pain patients. *Pain Management Nursing, 3*(4), 131–140.

Wennberg, J., & Cooper, M. (Eds.). (1999). *The quality of medical care in the United States: A report on the Medicare program*. Chicago: Dartmouth Atlas of Health Care, AHA Press.

Wenzel, R. P., & Edmond, M. B. (2001). The impact of hospital-acquired bloodstream infections. *Emerging Infectious Diseases, 7*, 174–177.

Werley, H. H., Devine, E. C., & Zorn, C. R. (1988). *Nursing Minimum Data Set data collection manual*. Milwaukee: School of Nursing, University of Wisconsin.

Werley, H., Devine, E., Zorn, C., Ryan, P., & Westra, B. L. (1991). The nursing minimum data set: Abstraction tool for standardized, comparable, essential data. *American Journal of Public Health, 81*(4), 421–426.

Werley, H. H., & Lang, N. M. (Eds.). (1988). *Identification of the nursing minimum data set*. New York: Springer Publishing.

Werner, J. S. (1993). Stressors and health outcomes: Synthesis of nursing research, 1980–1990. In J. S. Barnfather & B. L. Lyon (Eds.), *Stress and coping: State of the science and implications for nursing theory, research and practice* (pp. 11–41). Indianapolis, IN: Sigma Theta Tau International.

Werner, J. S., & Frost, M. H. (2000). *Stress & coping: State of the science and implications for nursing theory, research, and practice 1991–1995*. Glenview, IL: Midwest Nursing Research Society.

Werner, J. S., Frost, M., & Orth, K. S. (2000). Stressors and health outcomes: Synthesis of nursing research, 1991–1995. In J. S. Werner & M. H. Frost (Eds.), *Stress and coping: State of the science and implications for nursing theory, research, and practice 1991–1995*. Glenview, IL: Midwest Nursing Research Society.

Westergren, A., Ohlsson, O., & Rahm Hallberg, I. (2001). Eating difficulties, complications and nursing interventions during a period of three months after a stroke. *Journal of Advanced Nursing, 35*, 416–426.

Wetherill, J., Kelly, T., & Hore, B. (1987). The role of the community psychiatric nurse in improving treatment compliance in alcoholics. *Journal of Advanced Nursing, 12*, 707–711.

Whaley, A. L. (2000). Sociocultural differences in the developmental consequences of the use of physical discipline during childhood for African Americans. *Cultural Diversity and Ethnic Minority Psychology, 6*, 5–12.

Whall, A. L. (2002). Deriving interventions from the NDG model: Using natural environment and implicit memory theories. *Journal of Gerontological Nursing, 28*(10), 21–23.

Wheeler, S. Q. (1993). *Telephone triage: Theory, practice, and protocol development*. Albany, NY: Delmar Publishers.

White, J. E., Nativio, D. G., Kobert, S. N., & Engberg, S. J. (1992). Content and process in clinical decision-making by nurse practitioners. *Image: Journal of Nursing Scholarship, 24*(2), 153–158.

White, J. H. (2000). Developing a CNS role to meet the mental health needs of the underserved. *Clinical Nurse Specialist, 14*, 141–149.

Whitley, D. M., White, K. R., Kelley, S. J., & Yorker, B. C. (1999). Strengths-based case management: The application to grandparents raising grandchildren. *Families in Society, 80*, 110–119.

Whitman, G. R., Davidson, L. J., Sereika, S. M., & Rudy, E. B. (2001). Staffing and pattern of mechanical restraint use across a multiple hospital system. *Nursing Research, 50*(6), 356–362.

Whitney, S. L., Wrisley, D. M., Marchetti, G. F., & Furman, J. M. (2002). The effect of age on vestibular rehabilitation outcomes. *Laryngoscope, 112*(10), 1785–1790.

Whitten, P., Cook, D. J., & Doolittle, G. (1998). An analysis of provider perceptions for telehospice. *American Journal of Hospice & Palliative Care, 15*(5), 267–274.

Whitten, P., Mair, F., & Collins, B. (1997). Home telenursing in Kansas: Patients' perceptions of uses and benefits. *Journal of Telemedicine & Telecare 3*(Suppl. 1), 67–69.

Wicks, M. N. (1995). Family health as derived from King's framework. In M. A. Frey & C. L. Sieloff (Eds.), *Advancing King's systems framework and the-*

ory of nursing (pp. 97–108). Thousand Oaks, CA: Sage.

Widiger, T. A., & Anderson, K. G. (2003). Personality and depression in women. *Journal of Affective Disorders, 74*, 59–66.

Wikstrom, B. (2001). Work of art: An educational technique by which students discover personal knowledge of empathy. *International Journal of Nursing Practice, 7*(1), 24–29.

Wiles, R. (1998). The views of women of above average weight about appropriate weight gain in pregnancy. *Midwifery, 14*, 254–260.

Wilford, S. L. (1989). Knowledge development in nursing: Emergence of a paradigm (Doctoral dissertation: University of Minnesota, 1989). *Dissertation Abstracts International, 50*, 8B.

Wilhite, M. J., & Johnson, D. M. (1976). Changes in nursing student's stereotypic attitudes toward old people. *Nursing Research, 25*, 430–432.

Wilk, J. (1999). Health care for the homeless: A model for nursing education. *International Nursing Review, 46*(6), 171–175.

Wilkinson, C. L. (1999). An evaluation of an educational program on the management of assaultive behaviors. *Journal of Gerontological Nursing, 25*(4), 6–11.

Wilkinson, J. M. (1987–88). Moral distress in nursing practice: Experience and effect. *Nursing Forum, 23*(1), 16–29.

Wilkinson, P., & Mynors-Wallis, L. (1994). Problem-solving therapy in the treatment of unexplained physical symptoms in primary care: A preliminary study. *Journal of Psychosomatic Research, 38*, 591–598.

Wilkinson, S., Roberts, A., & Aldridge, J. (1998). Nurse-patient communication in palliative care: An evaluation of a communication skills program. *Palliative Medicine, 12*, 13–22.

Williams, A. B. (2003). Gynecologic care for women with HIV infection. *Journal of Obstetric, Gynecologic, and Neonatal Nursing, 32*(1), 87–93.

Williams, B. (1994). Patient satisfaction: A valid concept? *Social Science & Medicine, 38*, 509–516.

Williams, C. A. (1977). Community health nursing—what is it? *Nursing Outlook, 25*, 250–254.

Williams, C. A., Pesut, D. J., Boyd, M., Russell, S. S., Morrow, J., & Head, K. (1998). Toward an integration of competencies for advanced practice mental health nursing. *Journal of the American Psychiatric Nurses Association, 4*, 48–56.

Williams, C. C., & Collins, A. A. (2002). The social construction of disability in schizophrenia. *Qualitative Health Research, 12*, 297–309.

Williams, J. L. (2003). Gastroesophageal reflux disease: Clinical manifestations. *Gastroenterology Nursing, 26*(5), 195–200.

Williams, L. S., Weinberger, M., Harris, L. E., Clark, D. O., & Biller, J. (1999). Development of a stroke-specific quality of life scale. *Stroke, 30*, 1362–1369.

Williams, M. A., Fleg, J. L., Ades, P. A., Chaitman, B. R., Miller, N. H., Mohuiddin, S. M., et al. (2002). Secondary prevention of coronary heart disease in the elderly (with emphasis on patients > 75 years of age). *Circulation, 105*, 1735–1743.

Williams, S. A., Kasl, S. V., Heiat, A., Abramson, J. L., Krumholz, H. M., & Vaccarino, V. (2002). Depression and risk of heart failure among the elderly: A prospective community-based study. *Psychosomatic Medicine, 64*, 6–12.

Wilson, H. (1993). *Introducing nursing research*. Redwood City, CA: Addison-Wesley.

Wilson, H. S., & Hutchinson, S. A. (1996). *The consumer's guide to nursing research: Exercises, learning activities, tools and resources*. Albany, NY: Delmar.

Wilson, I. B., & Cleary, P. D. (1995). Linking clinical variables with health-related quality of life: A conceptual model of patient outcomes. *Journal of the American Medical Association, 273*, 59–65.

Wilson, S., Andersen, M., & Meischke, H. (2000). Meeting the needs of rural breast cancer survivors: What still needs to be done? *Journal of Women's Health & Gender-Based Medicine, 9*(6), 667–677.

Wilson, S., & Morse, J. (1991). Living with a wife undergoing chemotherapy. *Image: Journal of Nursing Scholarship, 23*, 1181–1187.

Wilson, S. A., & Daley, B. J. (1999). Family perspectives on dying in long-term care settings. *Journal of Gerontological Nursing, 25*(11), 19–25.

Winland-Brown, J. E. (1998). Death, denial and defeat: Older patients and advance directives. *Advanced Practice Nursing Quarterly, 4*(2), 36–40.

Winningham, M. L., Nail, L. M., Burke, M. B., Brophy, L., Cimprich, B., Jones, L. S., et al. (1994). Fatigue and the cancer experience: The state of the knowledge. *Oncology Nursing Forum, 21*(1), 23–36.

Wolf, R. (2003). *Risk assessment instruments*. Retrieved January 5, 2004, from http://www.elderabusecenter.org/default.cfm?p=riskassessment.cfm

Wolfe, R. L., Penrold, J., & Cauley, J. A. (2000). Epidemiology: The magnitude of concern. In S. H. Gueldner, M. S. Burke, & H. Smiciklas-Wright (Eds.), *Preventing and managing osteoporosis* (pp. 5–16). New York: Springer Publishing.

Wolff, P. (1968). The serial organization of sucking in the young infant. *Pediatrics, 42*(6), 943–956.

Wong, J., & Wong, S. (2002). Trends in lifestyle cardiovascular risk factors in women: Analysis from the Canadian National Population Health Survey. *International Journal of Nursing Studies, 39*, 229–242.

Wood, P., Hurburt, M., Hough, R., & Hofstetter, C. (1998). Longitudinal assessment of family support among homeless mentally ill participants in a housing program. *Journal of Community Psychology, 26*(4), 327–344.

Wood, W. (2000). Attitude change: Persuasion and social influence. *Annual Review of Psychology, 51*, 539–570.

Woodgate, R. L., & Degner, L. F. (2003). Expectations and beliefs about children's cancer symptoms: Perspective of children and their families. *Oncology Nursing Forum, 30*(3), 479–491.

Woodham-Smith, C. (1951). *Florence Nightingale*. New York: McGraw-Hill.

Woods, N. (1985). Relationship of socialization and stress to perimenstrual symptoms, disability, and menstrual attitudes. *Nursing Research, 34*, 145–149.

Woods, N. (1988). Women's health. In J. J. Fitzpatrick, R. L. Taunton, & J. Q. Benoliel (Eds.), *Annual review of nursing* (Vol. 6). New York: Springer Publishing.

Woods, N., & Catanzaro, M. (1988). *Nursing research: Theory and practice*. St. Louis, MO: C. V. Mosby.

Woods, N., Mitchell, E., & Taylor, D. (1999). From menarche to menopause: Contributions from nursing research and recommendations for practice. In A. Hinshaw, S. Feetham, & J. Shaver (Eds.), *Handbook of clinical nursing research* (pp. 459–484). Thousand Oaks, CA: Sage.

Woods, N., Most, A., & Dery, G. (1982). Estimating the prevalence of perimenstrual symptoms. *American Journal of Public Health, 72*, 1257–1264.

Woods, N. F. (2002). *Hormones and women's health: Update 10/2002*. Retrieved from http://www.uwcwhr.org/health-topics2.asp

Woods, N. F., & Hulka, B. S. (1979). Symptom reports and illness behavior among employed women and homemakers. *Journal of Community Health, 5*(1), 36–45.

Woods, N. F., Lentz, M., Mitchell, E. S., & Kogan, H. (1994). Arousal and stress response across the menstrual cycle in women with three perimenstrual symptom patterns. *Research in Nursing & Health, 17*, 99–110.

Woods, N. F., Mariella, A., & Mitchell, E. S. (2002). Patterns of depressed mood across the menopausal transition: Approaches to studying patterns in longitudinal data. *Acta Obstetrica Et Gynecologica Scandinavica, 81*(7), 623–632.

Woods, N. F., Mitchell, E. S., & Lentz, M. (1999). Premenstrual symptoms: Delineating symptom clusters. *Journal of Women's Health and Gender-Based Medicine, 8*, 1053–1062.

Woods, N. F., Mitchell, E. S., Lentz, M. J., Taylor, D., & Lee, K. (1987). Premenstrual symptoms: Another look. *Public Health Reports, July-August*(Suppl.), 106–112.

Woods, N., Most, A., & Dery, G. (1982). Estimating the prevalence of perimenstrual symptoms. *American Journal of Public Health, 72*, 1257–1264.

Woods, N. F., Most, A., & Longenecker, G. D. (1985). Major life events, daily stressors, and perimenstrual symptoms. *Nursing Research, 34*, 263–267.

Woolery, L., Grzymala-Busse, J., Summers, S., & Budihardjo, A. (1991). The use of machine learning program LERS LB 2. 5 in knowledge acquisition for expert system development in nursing. *Computers in Nursing, 9*, 227–234.

Woolf, L., & Jackson, B. (1996). 'Coffee & condoms': The implementation of a sexual health programme in acute psychiatry in an inner city area. *Journal of Advanced Nursing, 23*, 299–304.

Wootton, R., Loane, M., Mair, F., Allen, A., Doolittle, G., & Begley, M. (1998). A joint US-UK study of home telenursing. *Journal of Telemedicine & Telecare, 4*(Suppl. 1), 83–85.

Worden, J. W. (1991). *Grief counseling and grief therapy: A handbook for the mental health practitioner*. New York: Springer Publishing.

World Congress of Self-Care Deficit Nursing Theory. (2004). Retrieved September 15, 2004, from http://www.worldcongress-scdnt.com/

World Health Organization. (1977). *Development of designs in, and the documentation of the nursing process* (Report on a Technical Advisory Group, Regional Office for Europe, Copenhagen). Geneva, Switzerland: Author.

World Health Organization. (1978). *Primary health care: Report of the International Conference on Primary Health Care, Alma Ata, USSR* (Serican No. 1). Geneva: Author.

World Health Organization. (1978a). *Primary health care:* Report of the international conference on primary health care. Geneva, Switzerland: Author.

World Health Organization. (1978b). *Declaration of Alma-Ata*: International conference on Primary Health Care, Alma-Ata, USSR, 6-12 September 1978. Geneva, Switzerland: Author. Retrieved October 5, 2004, from http://www.who.int/hpr/NPH/docs/declaration_almaata.pdf

World Health Organization. (1980). *International classification of impairment, disabilities and handicaps*. Geneva, Switzerland: Author.

World Health Organization. (1985). *Evolution of primary health care* (HFA Leadership/IM.1). Geneva, Switzerland: Author.

World Health Organization. (1986). *Regulatory mechanisms for nursing training and practice: Meeting primary health care needs* (Technical Report Series #738). Geneva, Switzerland: Author.

World Health Organization. (1989). *World Health Organization: Cancer pain and relief*. Geneva, Switzerland: Author.

World Health Organization. (2001). *The world health report 2001—Mental health: New understanding, new hope*. Geneva, Switzerland: Author.

World Health Organization. Department of Reproductive Health and Research. (2003a). *Kangaroo mother care: A practical guide* (No. 1150508). Geneva, Switzerland: Author. Retrieved from http://www.who.int.bookorders

World Health Organization. (2003b). *The burden of musculoskeletal conditions at the start of the new millennium: Report of the WHO Scientific Group* (WHO technical report series: 919). Geneva, Switzerland: Author.

Wright, D. (2001). Hospice nursing: The specialty. *Cancer Nursing, 24*, 20–27.

Wright, T. F., Blache, C. F., Ralph, J., & Luterman, A. (1993). Hardiness, stress, and burnout among intensive care nurses. *Journal of Burn Care & Rehabilitation, 14*(3), 376–381.

Wrightson, D. D. (1999). Suctioning smarter: Answers to eight common questions about endotracheal suctioning in neonates. *Neonatal Network, 18*(1), 51–55.

Writing Group for the Women's Health Initiative Investigators. (2002). Risks and benefits of estrogen plus progestin in healthy postmenopausal women: Principal results from the Women's Health Initiative randomized controlled trial. *Journal of the American Medical Association, 288*(3), 321–333.

Wuerker, A. K. (2000). The family and schizophrenia. *Issues in Mental Health Nursing, 21*, 127–141.

Wunderlich, G., Sloan, F., & Davis, C. (1996). *Nursing staff in hospitals and nursing homes: Is it adequate?* Washington, DC: National Academy Press.

Wurzbach, M. E. (1992). Assessment and intervention for certainty and uncertainty. *Nursing Forum, 27*(2), 29–35.

Wurzbach, M. E. (1995). Long-term care nurses' moral convictions. *Journal of Advanced Nursing, 21*(6), 1059–1064.

Wyatt, G. K., & Friedman, L. L. (1998). Physical and psychosocial outcomes of midlife and older women following surgery and adjuvant therapy for breast cancer. *Oncology Nursing Forum, 25*, 761–768.

Wyatt, J., & Spiegelhalter, D. (1990). Evaluating medical expert systems: What to test and how? *Medical Informatics, 15*, 205–217.

Wykes, T., Parr, A. M., & Landau, S. (1999). Group treatment of auditory hallucinations: Exploratory study of effectiveness. *British Journal of Psychiatry, 175*, 180–185.

Xakellis, G. C., Frantz, R. A., Lewis, A., & Harvey, P. (1998). Cost-effectiveness of an intensive pressure ulcer prevention protocol in long term care. *Advances in Wound Care, 11*, 22–29.

Yamada, Y. (2002). Profile of home care aides, nursing home aides, and hospital aides: Historical changes and data recommendations. *Gerontologist, 42*(2), 199–206.

Yamashita, M. (1999). Newman's theory of health applied in family caregiving in Canada. *Nursing Science Quarterly, 12*, 73–79.

Yanovski, J. A., & Yanovski, S. Z. (2002). Recent advances in basic obesity research. *Journal of the American Medical Association, 282*, 1504–1506.

Yarcheski, A., & Mahon, N. E. (1995). Rogers' pattern manifestations and health in adolescents. *Western Journal of Nursing Research, 17*(4), 383–397.

Yardley, L., Masson, E., Verschuur, C., Haacke, N., & Luxon, L. (1995). Symptoms, anxiety and handicap in dizzy patients: Development of the vertigo symptom scale. *Journal of Psychosomatic Research, 36*, 731–741.

Yardley, L. (2000). Overview of the psychological effects of chronic dizziness and balance disorders. *Otolaryngologic Clinics of North America, 33*(3), 603–616.

Yardley, L., & Beech, S. (1999). Nurse-delivered exercise therapy for dizziness. *Nursing Times, 95*, 50–51.

Yardley, L., Beech, S., Zander, L., Evans, T., & Weinman, J. (1998). A randomized controlled trial of exercise therapy for dizziness and vertigo in primary care. *British Journal of General Practice, 48*, 1136–1140.

Yates, T. M., Dodds, M. F., Sroufe, L. A., & Egeland, B. (2003). Exposure to partner violence and child behavior problems: A prospective study controlling for child physical abuse and neglect, child cognitive ability, socioeconomic status and life stress. *Development and Psychopathology, 15*(1), 199–218.

Yeh, C. (2001). Adaptation in children with cancer: Research with Roy's model. *Nursing Science Quarterly, 14*(2), 141–148.

Yeh, C. (2003). Psychological distress: Testing hypotheses based on Roy's adaptation model. *Nursing Science Quarterly, 16*(3), 255–263.

Yeung, E. W. F., French, P., & Leung, A. O. S. (1999). The impact of hospice inpatient care on the quality of life of patients terminally ill with cancer. *Cancer Nursing, 22*, 350–357.

Yin, R. (1989). *Case study research: Design and methods* (Rev. ed.). Newbury Park, CA: Sage.

Yin, T., Zhou, Q., & Bashford, C. (2002). Burden on family members: Caring for frail elderly: A meta-analysis of interventions. *Nursing Research, 51*(3), 199–208.

Yoder, M. E. (1994). Preferred learning style and education technology: Linear vs. interactive video. *Nursing and Health Care, 15*(3), 128–132.

Yonas, H., Sekhar, L., Johnson, D. W., & Gur, D. (1989). Determination of irreversible ischemia by xenon-enhanced computed tomographic monitoring of cerebral blood flow in patients with symptomatic vasospasm. *Neurosurgery, 24*(3), 368–372.

Yorker, B., Kelley, S., Whitley, D., Lewis, A., Magis, J., Bergeron, A., et al. (1998). Custodial relationships of grandparents raising grandchildren: Results of a home-based intervention study. *Juvenile and Family Court Journal, 49*(2), 15–25.

Young, A. S., Klap, R., Sherbourne, C. D., & Wells, K. B. (2001). The quality of care for depressive and anxiety disorders in the United States. *Archives of General Psychiatry, 58*, 55–61.

Young, J., Giovanetti, P., Lewison, D., & Thoms, M. (1981). *Factors affecting nurse staffing in acute care hospitals: A review and critique of the literature* (DHEW Publication No. HRA 81-10). Washington, DC: U.S. Department of Health and Human Services.

Young, L. J., & George, J. (2003). Do guidelines improve the process and outcomes of care in delirium? *Age and Ageing, 32*, 525–528.

Youngblut, J. M. (1998). Integrative review of assessment models for examining children's and families' responses to acute illness. In M. E. Broome, K. Knafl, K. Pridham, & S. Feethan (Eds.), *Children and families in health and illness* (pp. 115–141). Thousand Oaks, CA: Sage Publications.

Yu, L. C. (1987). Incontinence Stress Index: Measuring psychological impact. *Journal of Gerontological Nursing, 13*(7), 18–25.

Zabalegui, A. (1999). Coping strategies and psychological distress in patients with advanced cancer. *Oncology Nursing Forum, 26*, 1511–1518.

Zahlis, E. H., & Shands, M. E. (1993) The impact of breast cancer on the partner 18 months after diagnosis. *Seminars in Oncology Nursing, 9*, 83–87.

Zalar, M. K., Welches, L. J., & Walker, D. D. (1985). Nursing consortium approach to increase research in service settings. *Journal of Nursing Administration, 15*(7–8), 36–41.

Zambrana, R. E. (2001). Improving access and quality for ethnic minority women—panel discussion. *Women's Health Issues, 11*(4), 354–358.

Zambroski, C. (2004). Faculty role transition from a community college to a research-intensive university. *Journal of Nursing Education, 43*(3), 104–106.

Zauszniewski, J. A. (1995). Health-seeking resources in depressed outpatients. *Archives of Psychiatric Nursing, 9*(4), 179–187.

Zauszniewski, J. A. (1996). Self-help and help-seeking behavior patterns in healthy elders. *Journal of Holistic Nursing, 14*(3), 223–236.

Zauszniewski, J. A., & Chung, C. (2001). Resourcefulness and health practices of diabetic women. *Research in Nursing and Health, 24*(2), 113–121.

Zauszniewski, J. A., Chung, C., & Krafcik, K. (2001). Social cognitive factors predicting the health of elders. *Western Journal of Nursing Research, 23*(5), 490–503.

Zebrack, B., Zeltzer, L., Whitton, J., Mertens, A., Odom, L., Berkow, R., et al. (2002). Psychological outcomes in long-term survivors of childhood leukemia, Hodgkin's disease, and non-Hodgkin's lymphoma: A report from the Childhood Cancer Survivor Study. *Pediatrics, 110*(1 Pt. 1), 42–52.

Zembrzuski, C. D. (1997). A three-dimensional approach to hydration of elders: Administration, clinical staff, and inservice education. *Geriatric Nursing, 18*, 20–26.

Zhan, L. (2000). Cognitive adaptation and self-consistency in hearing-impaired older persons: Testing Roy's adaptation model. *Nursing Science Quarterly, 13*(2), 158–165.

Zhou, Q., O'Brien, B., & Soeken, K. (2001). Rhodes Index of Nausea and Vomiting—Form 2 in pregnant women. A confirmatory factor analysis. *Nursing Research, 50*, 251–257.

Zielstorff, R., Delaney, C., Marek, K., Kneedler, J., Marr, P., Averil, C., et al. (1997). *NIDSEC standards and scoring guidelines*. Washington, DC: American Nurses Publishing.

Zielsdorff, R., Hudgings, C., & Grobe, S. (1993). *Next-Generation Information Systems: Essential characteristics for professional practice*. Washington, DC: American Nurses Publishing.

Ziemer, M., & Carroll, J. S. (1978). Infant gavage reconsidered. *American Journal of Nursing, 78*(9), 1543–1544.

Zimmerman, P. G. (2000). The use of unlicensed yassistive personnel: An update and skeptical look at a role that may present more problems than solutions. *Journal of Emergency Nursing, 26*(4), 312–317.

Zonnebelt-Smeenge, S., & DeVries, R. (2003). The effects of gender and age on grief work associated with grief support groups. *Illness, Crisis & Loss, 11*, 226–241.

Appendix: Contributors to First Edition

Lauren S. Aaronson, PhD, RN, FAAN
Associate Dean for Research and Professor
University of Kansas
School of Nursing
Kansas City, KS

Faye G. Abdellah, EdD, ScD, FAAN
Dean and Professor
Uniformed Services University of the Health Sciences
Bethesda, MD

Ivo L. Abraham, PhD, RN, CS, FAAN
Chief Executive Officer and Principal
Epsilon Group, LLC
Charlottesville, VA

Dyanne D. Affonso, PhD, RN, FAAN
Dean and Professor
Emory University
Nell Hodgson Woodruff School of Nursing
Atlanta, GA

Jerilyn K. Allen, ScD, RN
Associate Professor
The Johns Hopkins University
School of Nursing
Baltimore, MD

Carole A. Anderson, PhD, RN, FAAN
Dean and Professor
The Ohio State University
College of Nursing
Columbus, OH

Gene Cranston Anderson, PhD, RN, FAAN
Mellen Professor
Case Western Reserve University
Frances Payne Bolton School of Nursing
Cleveland, OH

Patricia G. Archbold, PhD, RN, FAAN
Professor
Oregon Health Sciences University
School of Nursing
Portland, OR

Carol A. Ashton, PhD, RN
Director of Nursing Research
LDS, Cottonwood, and Alta View Hospitals
Salt Lake City, UT

Regina C. Aune, PhD, RN
Associate Professor; Lieutenant Colonel, USAF
Uniformed Services University of the Health Sciences
Bethesda, MD

Joan Kessner Austin, DNS, RN, FAAN
Professor
Indiana University School of Nursing
Indianapolis, IN

Susan Auvil-Novak, PhD, RN
Assistant Professor
Case Western Reserve University
School of Nursing
Cleveland, OH

Kay C. Avant, PhD, RN, FAAN
Associate Professor
University of Texas
School of Nursing
Austin, TX

Judith A. Baigis, PhD, RN, FAAN
Associate Dean for Research and Scholarship
Georgetown University
School of Nursing
Washington, DC

Jane H. Barnsteiner, PhD, RN, FAAN
Professor and Director
University of Pennsylvania
School of Nursing
Philadelphia, PA

Cheryl Tatano Beck, DNSc, CNM, FAAN
University of Connecticut
Storrs, CT

Barbara E. Berger, PhD, RN
Clinical Assistant Professor and Clinical Scientist
University of Illinois at Chicago and University of Illinois at Chicago Medical Center
Chicago, IL

Nancy Bergstrom, PhD, RN, FAAN
Professor
University of Nebraska Medical Center
College of Nursing
Omaha, NE

Barbara Bishop, MN, RN, FAAN
Editor
The American Journal of Maternal/Child Nursing
New York, NY

Suzanne Blancett, EdD, RN, FAAN
Editor-in-Chief
The Journal of Nursing Administration
Bradenton, FL

Carol E. Blixen, PhD, RN
Senior Nurse Researcher
Cleveland Clinic Foundation
Department of Nursing Education and Research
Cleveland, OH

Eleanor J. Bond, PhD, RN
Associate Professor
University of Washington
Department of Biobehavioral Nursing and Health Systems
Seattle, WA

Joan L. Bottorff, PhD, RN
Associate Professor and NHRDP Health Researcher
University of British Columbia
School of Nursing
Vancouver, British Colombia, Canada

Barbara J. Braden, PhD, RN, FAAN
Professor and Dean
Creighton University
Graduate School
Omaha, NE

Patricia Flatley Brennan, PhD, RN, FAAN
Professor
University of Wisconsin
School of Nursing
Madison, WI

Pamela J. Brink, PhD, RN, FAAN
Executive Editor
University of Alberta
Faculty of Nursing
Edmonton, Alberta

Dorothy Brooten, PhD, FAAN
Burry Professor and Dean
Case Western Reserve University
Frances Payne Bolton School of Nursing
Cleveland, OH

Emma J. Brown, PhD, RN
University of Pennsylvania
School of Nursing
Philadelphia, PA

Kathleen C. Buckwalter, PhD, RN, FAAN
Professor
University of Iowa
College of Nursing
Iowa City, IA

Helen Kogan Budzynski, RN, PhD, FAAN
Professor
University of Washington School of Nursing
Psychosocial and Community Health
Seattle, WA

Vern L. Bullough, PhD, RN, FAAN
Visiting Professor
University of Southern California
Department of Nursing
Northridge, CA

Cynthia F. Cameron, PhD, RN
Associate Professor and Associate Dean
The University of Manitoba
Faculty of Nursing
Winnipeg, Manitoba

Jacquelyn C. Campbell, PhD, RN, FAAN
Professor
Johns Hopkins University
School of Nursing
Baltimore, MD

Sara Campbell, MS, RN
Coordinator for Student Development and
Mennonite College of Nursing
Bloomington, IL

Victoria Champion, DNS, RN, FAAN
Associate Dean of Research
Indiana University
School of Nursing
Indianapolis, IN

Peggy L. Chinn, PhD, RN, FAAN
Editor
Advances in Nursing Science
University of Connecticut
Storrs, CT

Marlene Zichi Cohen, PhD, RN
Associate Professor
University of Maryland
School of Nursing
Baltimore, MD

Kathleen Byrne Coiling, PhD, RN
University of Michigan
School of Nursing
Ann Arbor, MI

Inge B. Corless, PhD, RN, FAAN
Associate Professor and Director
Massachusetts General Hospital
Institute of Health Professions
Boston, MA

Cynthia L. Corritore, PhD
Assistant Professor
Creighton University
College of Business Administration
Omaha, NE

Marie J. Cowan, PhD, RN, FAAN
Professor and Dean
University of California, Los Angeles
School of Nursing
Los Angeles, CA

Diane Cronin-Stubbs, PhD, RN, FAAN
Professor
Rush University College of Nursing
Riverside, IL

Leah Curtin, ScD, RN, FAAN
Consultant
Cincinnati, OH

Jennifer P. D'Auria, PhD, RN
Assistant Professor
University of North Carolina
School of Nursing
Chapel Hill, NC

Barbara Daly, PhD, RN, FAAN
Associate Professor
Case Western Reserve University
School of Nursing
Cleveland, OH

Sabina De Geest, PhD, RN
Assistant Professor
Katholieke Universitieit Leuven
Leuven, Belgium

Alice S. Demi, DNS, RN, FAAN
Professor
Georgia State University
School of Nursing
Atlanta, GA

Karen E. Dennis, PhD, RN, FAAN
Associate Professor
University of Maryland
School of Nursing
Baltimore, MD

Elizabeth C. Devine, PhD, FAAN
Professor
University of Wisconsin
School of Nursing
Milwaukee, WI

Nancy Diekelmann, PhD, RN, FAAN
Helen Denne Shulte Professor
University of Wisconsin
School of Nursing
Madison, WI

Sue K. Donaldson, PhD, RN, FAAN
Dean and Professor
Johns Hopkins University
School of Nursing
Baltimore, MD

Rosemary Donley, PhD, RN, FAAN
Executive Vice President
Catholic University of America
School of Nursing
Washington, DC

Molly C. Dougherty, PhD, RN, FAAN
Editor
School of Nursing
University of North Carolina
Chapel Hill, NC

Karen Hassey Dow, PhD, RN
Associate Professor
University of Central Florida
School of Nursing
Orlando, FL

Jacqueline Dunbar-Jacob, PhD, RN, FAAN
Professor
University of Pittsburgh
School of Nursing
Pittsburgh, PA

Marsha L. Ellett, DNS, RN
Assistant Professor
Indiana University
School of Nursing
Indianapolis, IN

Veronica F. Engle, PhD, RN, FAAN
Professor
University of Tennessee
College of Nursing
Memphis, TN

Janet Enslein, RN, MA
University of Iowa
College of Nursing
Iowa City, IA

W. Scott Erdley, RN, MS
State University of New York
School of Nursing
Buffalo, NY

Lois K. Evans, DNSc, RN, FAAN
Associate Professor
University of Pennsylvania
School of Nursing
Philadelphia, PA

Sarah P. Farrell, PhD, RN, CS
Assistant Professor
University of Virginia
Charlottesville, VA

Jacqueline Fawcett, PhD, RN, FAAN
Professor
University of Pennsylvania
School of Nursing
Philadelphia, PA

Suzanne Lee Feetham, PhD, RN, FAAN
Professor, Harriet L. Werley Research Chair
University of Illinois at Chicago
College of Nursing
Chicago, IL

Harriet R. Feldman, PhD, RN, FAAN
Editor
Pace University
Lienhard School of Nursing
Pleasantville, NY

Mary L. Fisher, PhD, RN
Associate Professor
Indiana University
School of Nursing
Indianapolis, IN

Joyce J. Fitzpatrick, RN, PhD, FAAN
Elizabeth Brooks Ford Professor
Case Western Reserve University
Frances Payne Bolton School of Nursing
Cleveland, OH

Jacquelyn H. Flaskerud, PhD, RN, FAAN
Professor
University of California
School of Nursing
Los Angeles, CA

Juanita W. Fleming, PhD, RN, FAAN
Professor and Special Assistant to the President
University of Kentucky
Lexington, KY

Beverly C. Flynn, PhD, RN, FAAN
Professor and Director
Indiana University School of Nursing
Institute of Action Research and Community
Indianapolis, IN

Marquis D. Foreman, PhD, RN
Associate Professor
University of Illinois at Chicago
College of Nursing
Chicago, IL

Jeanne C. Fox, PhD, RN, FAAN
Director, SRMHRC
University of Virginia
SE Rural Research Center
Charlottesville, VA

Marilyn Frank-Stromborg, EdD, JD, RN, FAAN
Professor
Northern Illinois University
Dekalb, IL

Maureen Frey, PhD, RN
Director of Research and Advanced Practice
Children's Hospital of Michigan
School of Nursing
Detroit, MI

Sara T. Fry, PhD, RN, FAAN
Professor of Nursing Ethics
Boston College
School of Nursing
Chestnut Hill, MA

Teresa T. Fulmer, PhD, RN, FAAN
Professor
New York University
School of Nursing
New York, NY

John F. Garde, CRNA, MS, FAAN
Executive Director
American Association of Nurse Anesthetists
School of Nursing
Park Ridge, IL

Susan Gardner, MSN, RN
University of Iowa
College of Nursing
Iowa City, IA

Carol Gaskamp, MA, RN
Associate Professor
Kansas Newman College
Division of Nursing
Wichita, KS

Carole Gassert, PhD, RN
Officer
American Medical Informatics Association
Rockville, MD

Denise H. Geolot, PhD, RN, FAAN
Deputy Director
Division of Nursing
Rockville, MD

Carol P. Germain, EdD, FAAN
Associate Professor and Chairperson
University of Pennsylvania
School of Nursing
Philadelphia, PA

Phyllis B. Giovannetti, ScD, RN
Professor and Associate Dean (Graduate)
University of Alberta
Faculty of Nursing
Edmonton, Alberta, Canada

Greer Glazer, RNC, PhD, FAAN
Professor
Kent State University
School of Nursing
Solon, OH

Jody E. Glittenberg, PhD, RN, FAAN
Professor
University of Arizona
College of Nursing
Tucson, AZ

Marion Good, PhD, RN
Assistant Professor
Case Western Reserve University
Frances Payne Bolton School of Nursing
Cleveland, OH

Patricia A. Grady, PhD, RN, FAAN
Director
National Institute of Health
National Institute of Nursing Research
Bethesda, MD

Judith R. Graves, PhD, RN, FAAN
Director
Virginia Henderson Nursing Library
Sigma Theta Tau, Inc.
Indianapolis, IN

Margaret Grey, DrPH, RN, FAAN
Associate Dean for Research and Doctoral Studies
Yale University
School of Nursing
New Haven, CT

Hurdis M. Griffith, PhD, RN, FAAN
Dean and Professor
Rutgers College of Nursing
Newark, NJ

Deborah Gross, DNSc, RN, FAAN
Professor
Rush University
College of Nursing
Chicago, IL

Ira P. Gunn, CRNA, MLN
Consultant
El Paso, TX

Linda C. Haber, DNS, RN, CS
Clinical Specialist
Veterans Affairs
Northern Indiana Health Care System
Fort Wayne, IN

Edward J. Halloran, PhD, RN, FAAN
Associate Professor
University of North Carolina at Chapel Hill
Chapel Hill, NC

Charlene M. Hanson, EdD, RN, CS, FAAN
Professor
Georgia Southern University
Center for Rural Health & Research
Statesboro, GA

Gail A. Harkness, DrPH, RN, FAAN
Professor
University of Connecticut
School of Nursing
Storrs, CT

Roseanne Harrigan, EdD, CPNP, RN, FAAN
Dean and Professor
University of Hawaii
School of Nursing
Honolulu, HI

Emily J. Hauenstein, PhD, RN, CS
Associate Professor
University of Virginia
School of Nursing
Charlottesville, VA

Patricia Hayes, RN, MHSA
Co-Editor
Clinical Nursing Research
Edmonton, Alberta
Canada

Laura L. Hayman, PhD, RN, FAAN
Walter Professor
Case Western Reserve University
Frances Payne Bolton School of Nursing
Cleveland, OH

Janet Heinrich, DrPH, RN, FAAN
Executive Director
American Academy of Nursing
Washington, DC

Margaret Heitkemper, PhD, RN, FAAN
Professor
University of Washington
Department of Biobehavioral Nursing and Health
Seattle, WA

Marion M. Hemstrom, DNSc, RN
Assistant Professor
Case Western Reserve University
Frances Payne Bolton School of Nursing
Cleveland, OH

Beverly Henry, RN, PhD, FAAN
Editor
University of Illinois
College of Nursing
Chicago, IL

Suzanne Bakken Henry, DNSc, RN, FAAN
Associate Professor
University of California
School of Nursing
San Francisco, CA

Nancy Olson Hester, PhD, RN, FAAN
Professor
University of Colorado
School of Nursing
Denver, CO

Martha N. Hill, PhD, RN, FAAN
Professor
Johns Hopkins University
School of Nursing
Baltimore, MD

Ada Sue Hinshaw, PhD, RN, FAAN
Dean and Professor
University of Michigan
School of Nursing
Ann Arbor, MI

Diane Holditch-Davis, RN, PhD, FAAN
Professor
University of North Carolina
School of Nursing
Chapel Hill, NC

Barbara J. Holtzclaw, PhD, RN, FAAN
Director of Research
University of Texas
Health Science Center
San Antonio, TX

William L. Holzemer, PhD, RN, FAAN
Professor and Chair
University of California
School of Nursing
San Francisco, CA

Lois M. Hoskins, PhD, RN, FAAN
Professor
The Catholic University of America
School of Nursing
Washington, DC

Sally A. Hutchinson, PhD, RN, FAAN
Professor
University of Florida
College of Nursing
Jacksonville, FL

Kathleen Huttlinger, PhD, RN
Professor
Samuel Merritt College of Nursing
Oakland, CA

Gail L. Ingersoll, EdD, RN, FAAN
Professor and Associate Dean of Research
Vanderbilt University
School of Nursing
Nashville, TN

Pamela Magnussen Ironside, PhD, RN
Assistant Professor
Clarke College
Dubuque, IA

Sharol F. Jacobson, PhD, RN, FAAN
Professor and Director of Nursing Research
University of Oklahoma
Health Sciences College of Nursing
Oklahoma City, OK

Ada Jacox, PhD, RN, FAAN
Professor and Associate Dean for Research
Wayne State University
College of Nursing
Detroit, MI

Monica E. Jarrett, PhD, RN
Research Associate Professor
University of Washington
Department of Biobehavioral Nursing and Health
Seattle, WA

Loretta Sweet Jemmott, PhD, RN, FAAN
Associate Professor and Director
University of Pennsylvania
School of Nursing
Philadelphia, PA

John B. Jemmott, III, PhD
Professor
Princeton University
Department of Psychology
Princeton, NJ

Jean E. Johnson, PhD, RN, FAAN
Professor Emerita
University of Rochester
School of Nursing
Rochester, NY

Marion Johnson, PhD, RN
Associate Professor
University of Iowa
College of Nursing
Iowa City, IA

Dorothy A. Jones, EdD, RNC, FAAN
Associate Professor
Boston College
School of Nursing
Chestnut Hill, MA

Catherine F. Kane, PhD, RN, FAAN
Associate Professor
University of Virginia
School of Nursing
Charlottesville, VA

Gwen Brumbaugh Keeney, MS, RN
University of Illinois
College of Nursing
Chicago, IL

Maureen Keickeisen
Clinical Nurse Specialist
UCLA Medical Center
Department of Nursing
Los Angeles, CA

Lisa Skemp Kelly, RN, MA
University of Iowa
College of Nursing
Iowa City, IA

Mary E. Kerr, RN, PhD
Associate Professor
University of Pittsburgh
School of Nursing
Pittsburgh, PA

Shaké Ketefian, EdD, RN
Professor
University of Michigan
School of Nursing
Ann Arbor, MI

Hesook Suzie Kim, PhD, RN
Professor
University of Rhode Island
College of Nursing
Kingston, RI

Karin T. Kirchhoff, PhD, RN, FAAN
Professor
University of Utah
College of Nursing
Salt Lake City, UT

Katharine Y. Kolcaba, PhD, RN
Assistant Professor
University of Akron
College of Nursing
Akron, OH

Christine T. Kovner, PhD, RN, FAAN
Associate Professor
New York University
Division of Nursing
New York, NY

Heidi vonKoss Krowchuck, PhD, RN
Associate Professor
The University of North Carolina at Greensboro
School of Nursing
Greensboro, NC

Joan Kub, PhD, RN
Assistant Professor
Johns Hopkins University
School of Nursing
Baltimore, MD

Alice M. Kuramoto, PhD, RNC, FAAN
Professor
University of Wisconsin
School of Nursing
Milwaukee, WI

Hae-OK Lee, DNSc, RN
Assistant Professor
Case Western Reserve University
School of Nursing
Cleveland, OH

Elizabeth R. Lenz, PhD, FAAN
Professor and Associate Dean
Columbia University
School of Nursing
New York, NY

Eugene Levine, PhD
Professor
Uniformed Services University of the Health Sciences
Bethesda, MD

Linda Lewandowski, PhD, RN
Assistant Professor
Johns Hopkins University
School of Nursing
Baltimore, MD

Ada M. Lindsey, PhD, RN, FAAN
Dean and Professor
University of Nebraska Center
College of Nursing
Omaha, NE

Terri H. Lipman, PhD, CRNP
Assistant Professor/Clinical Nurse Specialist
University of Pennsylvania
Diabetes/Endocrinology
Philadelphia, PA

Juliene G. Lipson, PhD, RN
Assistant Professor/Clinical Nurse
University of California
Department of Community Health Systems
San Francisco, CA

Carol Loveland-Cherry, PhD, RN, FAAN
Associate Professor
The University of Michigan
School of Nursing
Ann Arbor, MI

Brenda L. Lyon, DNS, RN, FAAN
Associate Professor
Indiana University School of Nursing
Adult Health Nursing
Indianapolis, IN

Meridean Maas, PhD, RN, FAAN
Professor
University of Iowa
College of Nursing
Iowa City, IA

Susan L. MacLean, PhD, RN
Director
Research Science
Park Ridge, IL

Beverly Malone, PhD, RN
President
American Nurses Association
Washington, DC

Lucy N. Marion, PhD, RN, FAAN
Associate Professor
University of Illinois
College of Nursing
Chicago, IL

Karen S. Martin, RN, MSN, FAAN
Health Care Consultant
Martin Associates
Omaha, NE

Patricia A. Martin, PhD, RN
Director for Nursing Research
Wright State-Miami Valley College of Nursing and Health
Dayton, OH

Margaret Fisk Mastal, PhD, MSN
Clinical Coordinator
Kaiser Permanente
Springfield, VA

Linda J. Mayberry, PhD, RN
Adjunct Professor
Emory University
Nell Hodgson Woodruff School of Nursing
Atlanta, GA

Angela Barron McBride, PhD, RN, FAAN
Distinguished Professor and University Dean
Indiana University
School of Nursing
Indianapolis, IN

Maureen P. McCausland, DNSc, RN, FAAN
Associate Dean for Nursing & Chief Nursing
University of Pennsylvania
School of Nursing
Philadelphia, PA

Joanne Comi McCloskey, PhD, RN, FAAN
Distinguished Professor
University of Iowa
College of Nursing
Iowa City, IA

Kathleen A. McCormick, PhD, RN, FAAN
Agency for Health Care Policy and Research
Rockville, MD

Charlotte McDaniel, PhD, RN
Director and Clinical Professor
The University of Pittsburgh Medical Center
Pittsburgh, PA

Patricia McDonald, PhD, RN
Assistant Professor
Case Western Reserve University
School of Nursing
Cleveland, OH

Graham McDougall, PhD, RN
Associate Professor
Case Western Reserve University
School of Nursing
Cleveland, OH

Beverly J. McElmurry, EdD, FAAN
Professor and Associate Dean
University of Illinois at Chicago
College of Nursing
Chicago, IL

Mary L. McHugh, PhD, RN
Associate Professor
Wichita State University
School of Nursing
Wichita, KS

Mary J. McNamee, PhD, RN
Assistant Dean and Assistant Professor
University of Nebraska Medical Center
College of Nursing
Omaha, NE

Barbara Medoff-Cooper, PhD, RN, FAAN
Associate Professor
University of Pennsylvania
School of Nursing
Philadelphia, PA

Paula M. Meek, PhD, RN
Assistant Professor
University of Arizona
College of Nursing
Tucson, AZ

Janet C. Meininger, PhD, RN
Professor
University of Texas at Houston
School of Nursing
Houston, TX

Afaf Ibrahim Meleis, PhD, RN, FAAN
Professor
University of California
Department of Community Health Systems
San Francisco, CA

Bonnie L. Metzger, PhD, RN, FAAN
Associate Professor
University of Michigan
School of Nursing
Ann Arbor, MI

Mathy Mezey, EdD, RN, FAAN
Professor
New York University
Division of Nursing
New York, NY

Margaret Shandor Miles, PhD, RN, FAAN
Professor
University of North Carolina
School of Nursing
Chapel Hill, NC

D. Kathleen Milholland, PhD, RN
Research Associate Professor
University of South Florida
Tampa, FL

Nancy Milio, PhD, RN, FAAN
Professor
University of North Carolina
School of Nursing
Chapel Hill, NC

Nancy Houston Miller, RN, BSN
Associate Director
Stanford University School of Medicine
Division of Cardiovascular Medicine
Palo Alto, CA

Susan M. Miovech, PhD, RNC
Clinical Instructor
University of Pennsylvania
School of Nursing
Philadelphia, PA

Pamela H. Mitchell, PhD, RN, FAAN
Professor
School of Nursing
University of Washington
Seattle, WA

Ethel L. Mitty, EdD, RN
Adjunct Assistant Professor
Associate Research Scientist
New York University
Division of Nursing
New York, NY

Doris M. Modly, PhD, RN, FAAN
Professor
Case Western Reserve University
School of Nursing
Cleveland, OH

Rita Black Monsen, DSN, MPH, RN
Professor and Chairperson
Henderson State University
Department of Nursing
Arkadelphia, AR

Ida M. Moore, DNSc, RN, FAAN
Associate Professor
The University of Arizona
College of Nursing
Tucson, AZ

Mary Lou Moore, PhD, RNC
Research Assistant Professor
Bowman Gray School of Medicine of Wake Forest University
Winston-Salem, NC

Shirley M. Moore, PhD, RN
Associate Professor
Case Western Reserve University
Frances Payne Bolton School of Nursing
Cleveland, OH

Patricia Moritz, PhD, FAAN
Associate Professor
University of Colorado Health Sciences Center
School of Nursing
Denver, CO

Diana Lynn Morris, PhD, RN, FAAN
Case Western Reserve University
School of Nursing
Cleveland, OH

Evelyn Moses
Chief, Nursing Data and Analysis Staff
Division of Nursing
Rockville, MD

Barbara Munro, PhD, RN, FAAN
Dean and Professor
Boston College
School of Nursing
Chestnut Hill, MA

Carol M. Musil, PhD, RN
Assistant Professor
Case Western Reserve University
Frances Payne Bolton School of Nursing
Cleveland, OH

Mary Duffin Naylor, PhD, RN, FAAN
Associate Dean
University of Pennsylvania
School of Nursing
Philadelphia, PA

Leslie H. Nicoll, PhD, MBA
Editor-in-Chief
Muskie Institute of Public Affairs
University of Southern Maine
Portland, ME

Kathleen M. Nokes, PhD, RN, FAAN
Professor
CUNY, Hunter College
Hunter-Bellevue
New York, NY

Jane S. Norbeck, RN, DNSc, FAAN
Dean and Professor
University of California
School of Nursing
San Francisco, CA

Kathleen A. O'Connell, PhD, RN, FAAN
Professor
University of Kansas Medical Center
School of Nursing
Kansas City, KS

Ann L. O'Sullivan, PhD, CPNP, FAAN
Professor
University of Virginia
School of Nursing
Charlottesville, VA

Lisa Onega, PhD, RN
Assistant Professor
Oregon Health Sciences University
School of Nursing
Portland, OR

Judy G. Ozbolt, PhD, RN, FAAN
Professor
Vanderbilt University
School of Nursing
Nashville, TN

John R. Phillips, PhD, RN
Professor
New York University
School of Education
New York, NY

Linda R. Phillips, PhD, RN, FAAN
Professor
University of Arizona
College of Nursing
Tucson, AZ

Sally Phillips, PhD, RN
Director, Nursing Doctorate Program
University of Colorado
Health Sciences Center
Denver, CO

Bonita Ann Pilon, DSN, RN
Associate Professor for the Practice Nursing
Vanderbilt University
School of Nursing
Nashville, TN

Denise F. Polit, PhD
President
Humanalysis, Inc.
Saratoga Springs, NY

Sue Popkess-Vawter, PhD, RN
Professor
University of Kansas Medical Center
School of Nursing
Kansas City, KS

Diane Shea Pravikoff, PhD, RN
Director of Research/ Professional Liaison
CINAHL Information Systems
Glendale, CA

Jana L. Pressler, PhD, RN
Assistant Professor
Pennsylvania State University
School of Nursing
University Park, PA

Linda C. Pugh, PhD, RNC
Director, Center for Nursing Research and
Pennsylvania State University
Center for Nursing Research
Hershey, PA

Joanne W. Rains, DNS, RN
Dean and Associate Professor
Indiana University East
Division of Nursing
Richmond, IN

Barbara Rakel, RN, MA
Advanced Practice Nurse
University of Iowa
Hospitals and Clinics
Iowa City, IA

Gloria C. Ramsey, RN, BSN, JD
Project Director
New York University
Division of Nursing
New York, NY

Nancy E. Reame, PhD, MSN, FAAN
Professor
University of Michigan
Center for Nursing Research
Ann Arbor, MI

Richard W. Redman, PhD, RN, FAAN
Interim Associate Dean for Community
University of Michigan
School of Nursing
Ann Arbor, MI

Pamela G. Reed, PhD, RN, FAAN
Professor and Associate Dean for Academic
University of Arizona
College of Nursing
Tucson, AZ

Susan K. Riesch, DNSc, RN, FAAN
Professor and Associate Dean, Graduate Studies
University of Wisconsin, Madison
School of Nursing
Madison, WI

Mary Anne Rizzolo, EdD, RN, FAAN
Director
Interactive Technologies
Lippincott-Raven Publishers
New York, NY

Beverly L. Roberts, PhD, RN, FAAN
Associate Professor
Case Western Reserve University
Frances Payne Bolton School of Nursing
Cleveland, OH

Joyce Roberts, PhD, CNM, FAAN
Professor and Head
University of Illinois at Chicago
Department of Maternal–Child Nursing
Chicago, IL

Bonnie Rogers, DrPH, RN, FAAN
Associate Professor
University of North Carolina at Chapel Hill
School of Public Health
Chapel Hill, NC

Carol A. Romano, PhD, RN, FAAN
Director
National Institutes of Health Clinical Informatics Services
Bethesda, MD

Sheila Ryan, PhD, RN, FAAN
Dean and Professor
University of Rochester
School of Nursing
Rochester, NY

Virginia K. Saba, EdD, RN, FAAN
Clinical Associate Professor
Georgetown University
School of Nursing
Washington, DC

Marla E. Salmon, ScD, RN, FAAN
Professor
University of Pennsylvania
School of Nursing
Philadelphia, PA

Pamela J. Salsberry, PhD, RN
Associate Professor
The Ohio State University
College of Nursing
Columbus, OH

Loretta M. Schlachta, RN, MSHP
Clinical Director of Telemedicine
Strategic Monitored Services
New York, NY

Elizabeth A. Schlenk, PhD, RN
Assistant Professor
University of Pittsburgh
School of Nursing
Pittsburgh, PA

Madeline H. Schmitt, PhD, RN, FAAN
Professor
University of Rochester
School of Nursing
Rochester, NY

Susan M. Schneider, RN
Case Western Reserve University
Frances Payne Bolton School of Nursing
Richmond Heights, OH

Karen L. Schumaker, PhD, RN
Assistant Professor
University of California at San Francisco
School of Nursing
San Francisco, CA

Donald F. Schwarz, MD, MPH
Associate Professor of Pediatrics
University of Pennsylvania
School of Nursing and Medicine
Philadelphia, PA

Joan L. Shaver, PhD, RN, FAAN
Professor and Dean
University of Illinois at Chicago
College of Nursing
Chicago, IL

Nelma B. Shearer, MEd, MS
University of Arizona
College of Nursing
Tucson, AZ

Grayce M. Sills, PhD, RN, FAAN
Visiting Professor
Case Western Reserve University
Frances Payne Bolton School of Nursing
Cleveland, OH

Mary Cipriano Silva, PhD, RN, FAAN
Professor
George Mason University
College of Nursing and Health
Fairfax, VA

Carol E. Smith, RN, PhD
Professor
University of Kansas
School of Nursing
Kansas City, KS

Mariah Snyder, PhD, RN, FAAN
Professor
University of Minnesota
School of Nursing
Minneapolis, MN

Julie Sochalski, PhD, RN
Research Associate Professor
University of Pennsylvania
School of Nursing
Philadelphia, PA

Gwi-Ryung Son, RN, MN
Case Western Reserve University
School of Nursing
Cleveland, OH

Bernard Sorofman, PhD
Associate Professor
University of Iowa
College of Pharmacy
Iowa City, IA

Susan M. Sparks, PhD, RN, FAAN
Senior Education Specialist
National Library of Medicine
Bethesda, MD

Janet Specht, PhD, RN
Research Scientist
University of Iowa
College of Nursing
Iowa City, IA

Theresa Standing, PhD, RN
Assistant Professor
Case Western Reserve University
Frances Payne Bolton School of Nursing
Cleveland, OH

Joanne Sabol Stevenson, PhD, RN, FAAN
Professor and Associate Dean
Rutgers University
College of Nursing
Newark, NJ

Barbara J. Stewart, PhD, RN
Professor
Oregon Health Sciences University
School of Nursing
Portland, OR

Kathleen S. Stone, PhD, RN, FAAN
Professor
The Ohio State University
College of Nursing
Columbus, OH

Ora L. Strickland, PhD, RN, FAAN
Professor
Emory University
Nell Hodgson School of Nursing
Atlanta, GA

Neville E. Strumpf, PhD, RN, FAAN
Associate Professor
University of Pennsylvania
School of Nursing
Philadelphia, PA

Eleanor J. Sullivan, PhD, RN, FAAN
Professor
University of Kansas
School of Nursing
St. Louis, MO

Susan Dale Tannenbaum, RN, BSN
Staff Nurse—Cardiac Unit
Johns Hopkins University
School of Nursing
Baltimore, MD

Anita J. Tarzian, MS, RN
Department of Acute Long-Term Care
University of Maryland
Baltimore, MD

Roma Lee Taunton, PhD, RN, FAAN
Professor
University of Kansas Medical Center
School of Nursing
Kansas City, KS

Ann Gill Taylor, RN, EdD, FAAN
Professor of Nursing
University of Virginia
Center for the Study of Complementary and Alternative Therapies
Charlottesville, VA

Debera Jane Thomas, DNS, RN, CS
Associate Professor
Florida Atlantic University
Boca Raton, FL

Carol Lynn Thompson, PhD, RN
Associate Professor and Chair
University of Tennessee
College of Nursing
Memphis, TN

Mary E. Tiedeman, PhD, RN
Visiting Assistant Professor
Brigham Young University
College of Nursing
Provo, UT

Virginia P. Tilden, RN, DNSc, FAAN
Professor
Oregon Health Sciences University
School of Nursing
Portland, OR

Toni Tripp-Reimer, PhD, RN, FAAN
Professor and Associate Dean
University of Iowa
College of Nursing
Iowa City, IA

Barbara S. Turner, RN, DNSc, FAAN
Associate Dean
Duke University
School of Nursing
Durham, NC

Sharon Williams Utz, PhD, RN
Associate Professor and Chair
University of Virginia
School of Nursing
Charlottesville, VA

Barbara Valanis, PhD, FAAN
Director of Nursing Research
Kaiser-Permanente Center for Health Research
Portland, OR

Connie Vance, EdD, RN, FAAN
Dean and Professor
College of New Rochelle
New Rochelle, NY

Joyce A. Verran, PhD, RN, FAAN
Professor
University of Arizona
College of Nursing
Tucson, AZ

Antonia M. Villarruel, PhD, RN, FAAN
University of Pennsylvania
School of Nursing
Philadelphia, PA

Madeline Musante Wake, PhD, RN, FAAN
Dean
Marquette University
College of Nursing
Milwaukee, WI

Patricia Hinton Walker, PhD, FAAN
Dean and Professor
University of Colorado Health Sciences Center
School of Nursing
Denver, CO

Lynn I. Wasserbauer, PhD, RN
Assistant Professor
University of Akron
College of Nursing
Akron, OH

Clarann Weinert, SC, PhD, RN, FAAN
Associate Professor
Montana State University
College of Nursing
Bozeman, MT

Joan Stehle Werner, RN, DNS
Professor
University of Wisconsin-Eau Claire
School of Nursing
Eau Claire, WI

Ann L. Whall, PhD, RN, FAAN
Professor
University of Michigan
School of Nursing
Ann Arbor, MI

Carolyn A. Williams, PhD, RN, FAAN
Dean and Professor
University of Kentucky
Chandler Medical Center
Lexington, KY

Reg Williams, PhD, RN, FAAN
Associate Professor
University of Michigan
School of Nursing
Ann Arbor, MI

Holly Skodol Wilson, PhD, RN, FAAN
Professor
University of California
School of Nursing
San Francisco, CA

Chris Winkleman
Case Western Reserve University
Frances Payne Bolton School of Nursing
Cleveland, OH

Mary A. Woo, DNSc, RN
Assistant Professor
UCLA
School of Nursing
Los Angeles, CA

Marilynn J. Wood, RN, DrPH
Co-Editor
Clinical Nursing Research
Edmonton, Alberta
Canada

May L. Wykle, PhD, RN, FAAN
Professor and Associate Dean for Community
Case Western Reserve University
Frances Payne Bolton School of Nursing
Cleveland, OH

JoAnne M. Youngblut, PhD, RN, FAAN
Associate Professor
Case Western Reserve University
Frances Payne Bolton School of Nursing
Cleveland, OH

Renzo Zanotti, PhD
Professor
University of Padova
Padova, Italy

Jaclene A. Zauszniewski, PhD, RN
Associate Professor
Case Western Reserve University
Frances Payne Bolton School of Nursing
Cleveland, OH

Index